An Introduction to the Neurosciences

BRIAN A. CURTIS, Ph.D.

Assistant Dean, Tufts University School of Medicine and Associate Professor of Physiology, Tufts University Schools of Medicine and Dental Medicine

STANLEY JACOBSON, Ph.D.

Associate Professor of Anatomy, Tufts University Schools of Medicine and Dental Medicine

ELLIOTT M. MARCUS, M.D.

Associate Professor of Neurology and Subject Matter Chairman for Neurosciences, Tufts University School of Medicine; Neurologist, New England Medical Center Hospitals.

illustrated by marc bard
Tufts University School of Medicine

W. B. SAUNDERS COMPANY · PHILADELPHIA · LONDON · TORONTO

W. B. Saunders Company: West Washington Square
Philadelphia, Pa. 19105

12 Dyott Street
London, WC1A   1DB

833 Oxford Street
Toronto, Ontario M8Z 5T9, Canada

An Introduction to the Neurosciences   ISBN 0-7216-2810-9

Print No.:   9   8   7   6   5   4

*To our wives
and
children*

Preface

In order to make intelligent diagnoses and provide rational treatment in disorders of the nervous system, it is necessary to develop a capacity to answer the basic questions of clinical neurology: *Where is the disease process located? What is the nature of the disease process?* It is perhaps more true in neurology than in any other system of medicine that a firm knowledge of basic subject matter — the anatomy, physiology, and pathology of the nervous system — can enable one to readily arrive at a diagnosis of where the disease process is located. We have found that a well-trained first year student in neurosciences is often better able to make a correct diagnosis than a poorly prepared resident in medicine or neurology. It is the joy of the neurosciences that the student can directly and immediately apply his knowledge to solving problems in a clinical situation. This immediate application of basic knowledge to the clinical situation reinforces the subject matter learned by markedly increasing the interest of the student in the basic science material.

This book is designed to provide a single integrated text for medical school courses in the neurosciences. An integrated presentation of neuroanatomy, neurophysiology, neuropathology, and clinical neurology is provided. The book is an outgrowth of a course in neurosciences evolved by the authors over the last six years at Tufts University School of Medicine. It is the result of the collaboration of a cell physiologist (Dr. B. Curtis), a neuroanatomist (Dr. S. Jacobson), and a clinical neurologist with a background in neurological sciences (Dr. E. Marcus).

This book is designed to meet the needs of those medical schools with an evolving curriculum where integrated system teaching is in progress and where greater relevant clinical material is presented during basic science courses. The main approach of the textbook is to have the student immediately apply neurological basic science material in a problem-solving situation. While the textbook is designed primarily for first and second year medical students who are enrolled in an integrated neuroscience course, it is expected that the text may be of considerable value as a companion in neurology or an introduction to neurological diagnosis for a second, third, or fourth year student.

The authors' course is designed so that the problem-solving exercises at the end of Chapters 8, 15, 22, and 28 are used in weekly discussion groups, which include six to eight medical students who meet with a discussion leader, usually a neurologist, neurosurgeon, senior neurology resident, senior neurosurgical resident, or one of the three authors. Two conferences are spent on the Appendix to Chapter 8 (spinal cord), two periods on the Appendix to Chapter 15 (brain stem), and two periods on the Appendix to Chapter 22 (cerebral hemispheres). A single period is then spent on the details and practice of the neurological history and examination, with the students then divided into even smaller groups for a series of hospital trips for the evaluation of patients with neurological disease. During the last two weeks of the course, the final problem-solving exercises of Chapter 28 are considered in a series of three conferences; the first conference deals with case histories 2, 8, 11, 12, 13, 16, 18; the second with 1, 3, 4, 5, 6, 7, 9, and 10; and the final conference with case histories 14, 15, 17, 19, 20, 21, and 22.

The case histories which have been used to illustrate specific points of functional localization or neurological diagnosis and those which have been used for the problem-solving exercises are drawn primarily from Dr. Marcus's files. In many instances, however, his associates in the Neurology and Neurosurgical Departments of the New England Medical Center Hospital have made freely available the information in their own files. Particular thanks are due to Dr. John Sullivan, Dr. John Hills, Dr. Huntington Porter and Dr. C. Wesley Watson, Dr. Daniel Drachman, Dr. Bertram Selverstone, Dr. Samuel Brendler, Dr. Peter Carney, and Dr. Robert Yuan. The case histories in all instances present actual patients. It is our impression that such cases are more instructive and more interesting to students than manufactured, stereotype case histories. Because these are cases based upon clinical reality, at times there are minor deviations from the classic picture of disease. In the problem-solving exercises, in general, the cases have been arranged in the order of degree of difficulty—the more difficult case histories are found toward the conclusion of the section. An answer sheet is available for instructors and other senior students on request from Dr. Marcus.

An optional series of exercises is provided with Chapters 4 and 5 for those instructors and courses utilizing problems in cell and nerve physiology. An answer sheet is available for instructors and senior students on request from Dr. Curtis.

We wish to extend our appreciation to Dr. John Hills, Dr. Jose Segarra, Dr. Emanual Ross, and Dr. David Cowen for allowing us to photograph material from their neuropathological files and to Dr. Samuel Wolpert for allowing us to use neuroradiological material from his files. The brain scans were provided by Dr. Selverstone. Miss Renette Bowker provided assistance in the preparation of illustrations for the EEG chapter. Critical review of particular chapters was provided by Dr. Robert DeVoe, Dr. John Sullivan, Dr. Thomas Twitchell, and Dr. C. Wesley Watson. We would like to thank Dr. Herbert Schaumburg for use of slides of the spinal cord.

For secretarial assistance we must commend Miss Evelyn Losh, Miss Sherry Johnson, Mrs. Kathy Begley Hayes, and Mrs. Denise Solso, and for assistance with the photography we thank Mrs. Marcene Li Heung.

Finally, it is with great pleasure that we extend our thanks to our publishers, the W. B. Saunders Company. Without their cooperation and assistance we would never have been able to move from conception to finished product. We must single out for particular mention Mr. John Dusseau, Miss Diana Intenzo, and Mr. Al Beringer.

Any faults or errors are those of the authors. We would therefore appreciate any suggestions and comments from our colleagues.

BRIAN A. CURTIS

STANLEY JACOBSON

ELLIOTT M. MARCUS

Contents

4

5

6

7

8

CLINICAL CONSIDERATIONS OF THE SPINAL CORD

9

BRAIN STEM: GROSS ANATOMY

10

CRANIAL NERVES

11

MICROSCOPIC ANATOMY OF THE BRAIN STEM

12

DIENCEPHALON

21

22

23

24

25

THE CEREBELLUM AND MOVEMENT 696

Elliott M. Marcus

26

THE ELECTROENCEPHALOGRAM: SEIZURES, SLEEP, COMA, AND CONSCIOUSNESS 710

Elliott M. Marcus

27

LEARNING, MEMORY, AND INSTINCTIVE BEHAVIOR.............. 753

Elliott M. Marcus

28

GENERAL CASE HISTORY PROBLEM SOLVING........................ 778

Elliott M. Marcus

29

DESCRIPTIVE ATLAS OF THE SPINAL CORD, BRAIN STEM, AND CEREBRUM.................................. 797

Stanley Jacobson

1

An Overview

BRIAN CURTIS

Man has always wondered and speculated about the function of the brain. It was clear to the ancients that the brain was the seat of thought and behavior, and to satisfy their curiosity they began dissecting brains and speculating on the functions of its various parts. Scientific inquiry over the last 300 years has revealed a great deal about the functions of the human nervous system and the localization of that function within the various structures of the nervous system. Careful, systematic investigation has revealed the rich interconnections between these structures.

The major concern of this book is the localization of function to specific structures of the nervous system. This knowledge is of great importance to the physician since correct diagnosis of diseases of the nervous system is based on a firm understanding of the correlations of structure and function and on a detailed knowledge of the major connections of the nervous system. Correct diagnosis must, of course, precede rational therapy.

The student as he begins his study of the nervous system usually has a fair understanding of the gross functions of the nervous system—functions such as sensory perception, movement, and speech. However, he usually has very little knowledge of its component parts. Therefore, an introduction to the major structures of the nervous system

and a few examples of functional localization should prove useful to the student. Thus we will begin with an overview of the nervous system and of how its complex parts function in relation to each other and to the whole.

The building blocks of the nervous system are called *nerve cells* each having a *cell body* and one long process, the *axon*, and many short processes, the *dendrites*. The cell is capable of propagating an electrical disturbance received by the dendrites through the cell body and down the axon. The axon forms many connections or *synapses* with dendrites.

The nervous system can be divided into manageable parts, with each part being considered at several levels of complexity. However, the student should never forget that these parts work together in the integrated, purposeful action of the complete nervous system.

There are two basic divisions of the nervous system: the peripheral nervous system and the central nervous system. The peripheral nervous system (PNS) connects the central nervous system to the rest of the body. Consequently, it lies primarily outside the bony structures of the skull and vertebral column.

The central nervous system (CNS) is completely encased in these bony structures (Fig. 1–1). It forms the integrative and thinking portions of the nervous system. Our

1

Central Nervous System

Brain

Spinal cord

Peripheral
nerve

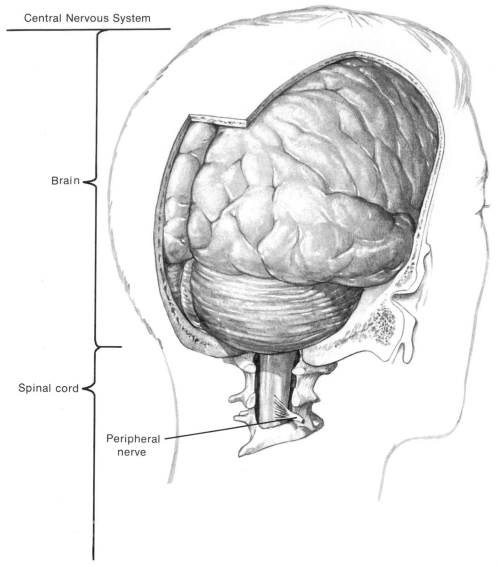

Figure 1-1 The major components of the central nervous system in relationship to the head and neck.

See Filmstrip, Frame 2.

actions and our dreams originate there, so we will begin our discussion with it.

THE CENTRAL NERVOUS SYSTEM

The central nervous system consists of the *spinal cord,* lying within the vertebral column, and the *brain,* lying within the skull (Fig. 1–1).

The spinal cord serves both as a connecting link between the brain and the body and as a lower level center for the integration of motor activity. For example, the classic knee-jerk reflex is completed within the spinal cord.

The *brain* consists of three major parts: the cerebrum, the brain stem, and the cerebellum. The cerebrum is by far the largest part and occupies the upper portion of the skull (Fig. 1–1). Inferior to (beneath) the cerebrum lie the brain stem and the cerebellum. In Figure 1–1 the brain stem is largely hidden.

The *brain stem* is phylogenetically the most ancient part of the brain. Its size and functions have changed very little with the evolution of the vertebrates. The brain stem serves three major functions: (1) it is a connecting link between the cerebral cortex, the spinal cord, and the cerebellum; (2) it is a center of integration for several visceral functions, such as control of heart and respiratory rates; and (3) it is a center of integration for various motor reflexes.

The *cerebellum* is a coordinator in the efferent, voluntary muscle system. It acts in conjunction with the brain stem and cerebral cortex to maintain balance and to provide harmonious muscle movements. The staggering gait which results from an excessive intake of alcohol is due primarily to the selective alteration of cerebellar function.

The *cerebrum* occupies a special dominant position in the central nervous system; here are localized the conscious functions of the nervous system.

LOCALIZATION OF SOME GROSS CONSCIOUS FUNCTIONS IN THE CEREBRUM

Most of those functions of the nervous system with which you are familiar are conscious functions which are located in the cerebrum; that is, the final integrative or "conscious" action occurs in the cerebrum. Thus we will concentrate first on the cerebrum, for in man the cerebrum dominates all the other parts of the nervous system; it is impossible to discuss the functions of these parts without referring to the cerebrum. Once we have established some understanding of cerebral function we can discuss the spinal cord and other parts of the brain in more detail.

The *cerebrum* is a paired structure, with right and left cerebral hemispheres, each relating to the opposite side of the body. Voluntary movements of the right hand are "willed" in the left cerebral hemisphere. The surface of the hemisphere called the cortex receives sensory information from skin, eyes, ears, and other sensory receptors on the opposite side of the body. This information is compared to previous experience and produces movements in response to these stimuli.

Each hemisphere consists of several layers. The outer layer consists of a dense collection of nerve cells which look gray when examined in a fresh state and are thus called *gray matter*. This outer layer, about 3 mm. in thickness, is called the *cerebral cortex* and is molded into gyri (ridges) and sulci (valleys), the deepest sulci being termed fissures. The deeper layers of the hemisphere consist of axons, or *white matter*, and collections of cell bodies (nuclei).

Some of the integrative functions of the cerebrum can be localized within specific regions of the cortex, whereas others are more diffusely distributed.

THE LATERAL SURFACE OF THE CEREBRUM

The major dividing landmark of the cerebral cortex is the *lateral fissure* (Fig. 1–2), which runs on the lateral surface of the brain from the open end in front, posteriorly and dorsally (backwards and up). The lateral fissure defines a tongue of cortex ventral to it, the *temporal lobe* (Fig. 1–3). This lobe contains the primary auditory cortex, which is that part of the cortex receiving auditory impulses via pathways leading from the auditory receptors in the inner ear.

The *primary auditory cortex* is localized on the *transverse temporal gyrus* which is located at the posterior and dorsal margin of the temporal lobe (Fig. 1–4), buried on the inner slope of the lateral fissure. To see it, we must reflect (pull) the temporal lobe out and down. When a recording electrode is placed on this gyrus at the time of neurosurgery, a large and characteristic electrical response follows when noise is played into the patient's ear (Fig. 1–5). If a weak current is passed into a stimulating electrode in this same location, the conscious patient will report "hearing" tones or noise. The primary auditory cortex, then, is an excellent example of a function which can be precisely located on the cortex.

In right-handed individuals, the left temporal lobe surrounding the transverse temporal gyrus is involved in the more complex interpretation of auditory signals. If the cells of this area die the patient will not be able to interpret sounds as words. The function of the cells on the homologous surface of the right hemisphere is unknown. They can be removed without causing any overt clinical problems. Consequently, the neurosurgeon will not hesitate to cut through the right temporal lobe of a right-handed person to reach a tumor, but he will try some other approach on the left side. The functions of the rest of the temporal lobe, particularly the anterior tip, are more difficult to specify, but storage of long-term memory is one of them.

Another major landmark of the cerebral cortex is the *central sulcus* (Fig. 1–6). It is not

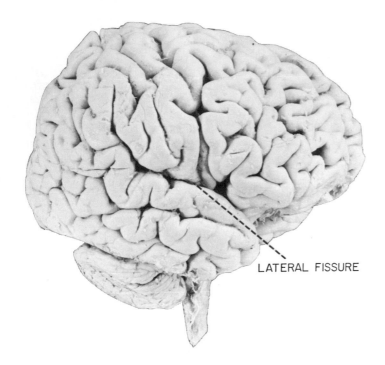

LATERAL FISSURE

Figure 1–2 The lateral fissure is shown on a lateral view of the right side of the brain.

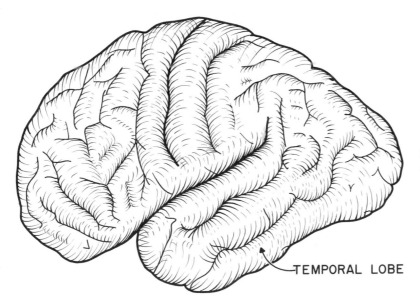

TEMPORAL LOBE

Figure 1–3 The temporal lobe shown on a lateral view of the left cerebrum.

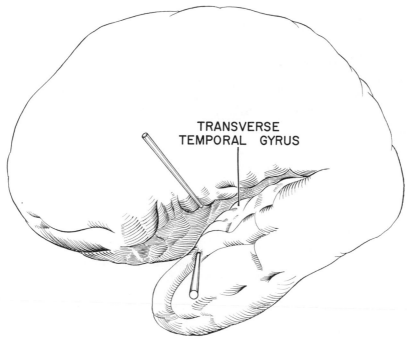

Figure 1-4 A view of the transverse temporal gyrus. The temporal lobe has been retracted to open the lateral fissure.

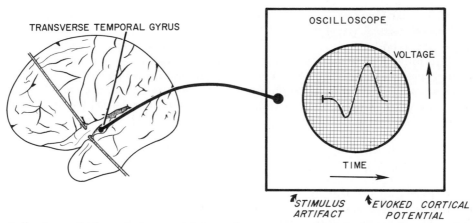

Figure 1-5 An evoked cortical potential from the transverse temporal gyrus in response to a brief noise in the ears.

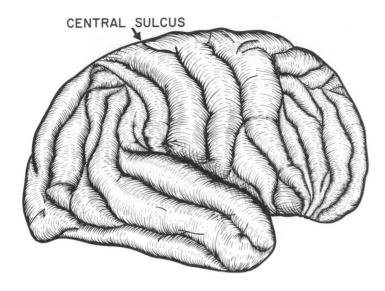

CENTRAL SULCUS

Figure 1–6 The central sulcus shown on the right cerebrum.

as prominent and unvarying a landmark as is the lateral fissure. The central sulcus runs from the medial surface over the convexity of the hemisphere to the lateral fissure. There are usually two well-formed and continuous gyri on either side of this sulcus. It will take some experience to pick it out.

This sulcus delimits the posterior border of the *frontal lobe* (Fig. 1–7). The gyrus immediately anterior to the central sulcus is the *precentral gyrus* (Fig. 1–8) which functions as the primary motor cortex. From this gyrus, signals run down through the brain stem to the spinal cord and out via the peripheral nervous system to control the skeletal muscles. Lesions (destruction) of part of the precentral gyrus will cause partial paralysis on the opposite side of the body.

Further anterior in the frontal lobe there is an area of *premotor cortex* (Fig. 1–9). Here more complex motor movements, such as speech, are organized. This is a larger area and is not readily definable in terms of gyri. Its anterior border is somewhat vague.

The anterior and inferior portions of the frontal lobe are involved in control of emotional behavior. These areas, referred to as *prefrontal* (Fig. 1–9), appear to have an inhibitory function predicated on the future consequences of present actions. Patients who have had prefrontal lobectomies (removal of the lobe) seem to have little awareness of the social consequences of their actions, i.e., they don't see anything wrong with urinating on the floor at a cocktail party.

Immediately behind the central sulcus lies the *parietal lobe* (Fig. 1–10). Its anterior

boundary is the central sulcus. The ventral boundary is the lateral sulcus or a line continuing in the same direction. Its posterior boundary is poorly defined on the lateral surface.

Several component areas of the parietal lobe may be distinguished. Immediately posterior to the central sulcus is the *postcentral gyrus* (Fig. 1–10). This is the primary sensory cortex which receives impulses from all of the sensory receptors in the skin. Each little area along the gyrus is related to a particular part of the body; for example, the legs on the medial end, the hand in the center, and the face on the end next to the lateral fissure. We can "feel" pain, touch, and pressure at lower levels of the nervous system, particularly the brain stem, but we cannot determine where the stimulus was applied. The following example is useful. A patient loses a small portion of the hand-area in the left postcentral gyrus. When a pin is stuck into his right hand, the patient will still know that a pin has been stuck into him, but he cannot tell the examiner where the pin was placed.

If a recording electrode (Fig. 1–11) is appropriately placed during a neurosurgical procedure, cortical response can be elicited by tactile stimuli to the contralateral (opposite side of the body) hand. Likewise, if a stimulus is applied through the same electrode, the patient will report a tingling sensation in his contralateral hand. Higher order sensory discrimination, such as recognizing a number drawn on the palm of the hand, is organized solely in the parietal lobe. Destruction of the

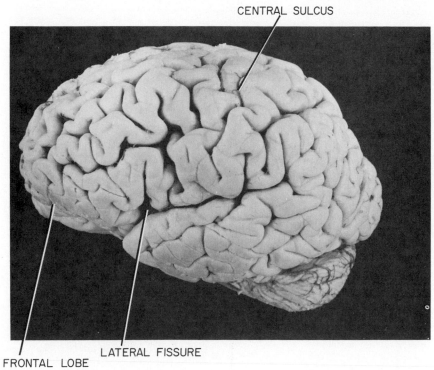

CENTRAL SULCUS

FRONTAL LOBE

LATERAL FISSURE

Figure 1–7 The frontal lobe shown on a photograph of a markedly atrophied human brain. The sulci are much wider than normal.

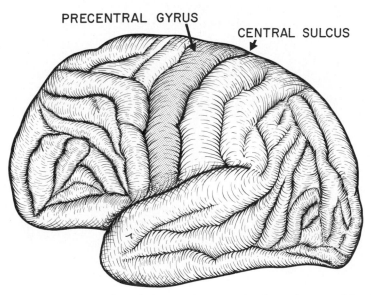

PRECENTRAL GYRUS

CENTRAL SULCUS

Figure 1–8 The precentral gyrus in relation to the central sulcus. Can you identify the precentral gyrus on the brain in Figure 1–7?

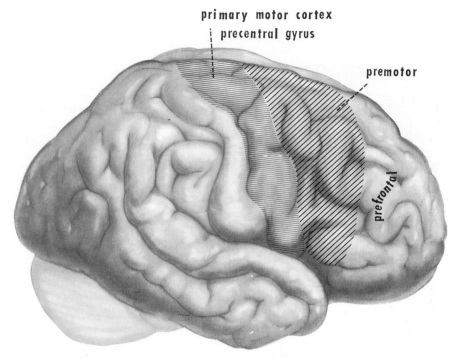

Figure 1–9   The premotor and prefrontal areas.

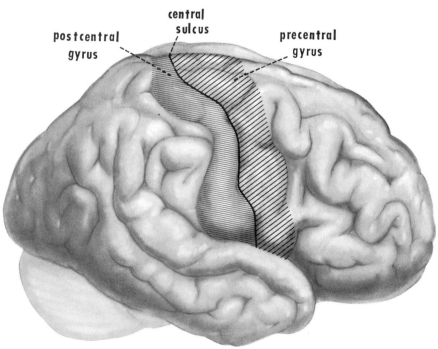

Figure 1–10   The postcentral gyrus and the boundaries of the parietal lobe. Can you identify the postcentral gyrus on the brain in Figure 1–7?

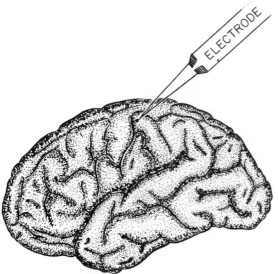

Figure 1–11 This electrode, on the postcentral gyrus, will record evoked cortical potentials in response to stimuli on the opposite (right) hand.

parietal lobe will lead to a loss of this ability, although the patient will still know he is being touched but cannot tell where or what is being drawn. The awareness of body is also organized in the parietal lobe. A patient with a lesion in the posterior parietal lobe will often forget to put the contralateral arm into his shirt.

The *occipital lobe* (Fig. 1–12) is the last and most posterior lobe. Only a small portion is present on the lateral surface of the cerebrum.

THE MEDIAL SURFACE OF THE CEREBRUM

When the cerebral hemispheres are cut apart at the midline and the hemispheres are separated, the medial surface is seen. All four lobes extend onto the medial surface, as shown in Figure 1–13. The tissue on either side of the *calcarine fissure* in the occipital lobe is the primary visual cortex. Light flashed into the eye evokes large electrical potentials from electrodes placed over this area of the cortex. The remainder of the occipital lobe is involved in interpreting and categorizing visual sensations.

A prominent structure on the medial surface is the *corpus callosum*. This wide band of nerve fibers interconnects the two cerebral hemispheres and serves to transfer information between the two cerebral hemispheres.

Immediately surrounding the corpus callosum is the *cingulate gyrus*. This area is involved in emotional responses. It functions in conjunction with other areas of the brain, such as the phylogenetically newer frontal lobe and other phylogenetically older areas

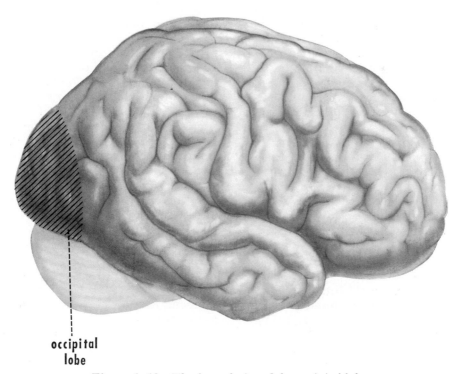

occipital
lobe

Figure 1–12 The boundaries of the occipital lobe.

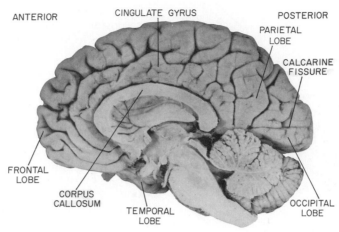

ANTERIOR   CINGULATE GYRUS   POSTERIOR

PARIETAL LOBE

CALCARINE FISSURE

FRONTAL LOBE

CORPUS CALLOSUM

TEMPORAL LOBE

OCCIPITAL LOBE

Figure 1–13 The four lobes of the cerebrum shown on a photograph of the medial surface of a hemisection of the same atrophied brain shown in Figure 1–7.

See Filmstrip, Frame 3.

of the brain stem. This illustrates one of the difficulties in studying the nervous system; the system evolved slowly with phylogenetically newer structures being added on top of older structures. The older structures did not, however, have the good grace to disappear.

THE SPINAL CORD

The segmental nature of the spinal cord is quite evident upon gross inspection. The nerves which enter and leave the cord do so at regular intervals, as seen in Figure 1–14.

There are two pairs of nerve roots for each segment. While the segmental nature of the spinal cord is evident, the segmental nature of the body regions which it innervates is not. In an earthworm the segment is simply a cylinder of body wall, and each segment of the worm's spinal cord supplies both sensory and motor innervation to "its" segment. In the human the segments are of variable size and shape, yet the principle still holds; each segment of the spinal cord provides both sensory and motor innervation to "its" segment.

In cross section (Fig. 1–15), the spinal cord is composed of two distinct areas: the gray matter and the white matter. The *gray matter* is the central, butterfly-shaped area, which appears gray on gross examination and is composed largely of cell bodies. The cell bodies of the axons which run out to control the muscles are located in the large anterior horn of the gray matter and are

known as *anterior horn cells* (Fig. 1–15). Their axons leave the cord by the anterior root. The only way that the muscle at the end of the axon can contract is through the stimulation of this anterior horn cell. Therefore, all motor commands from higher centers, such as the precentral gyrus, are conducted via the anterior horn cells of the appropriate spinal cord segments. The sensory fibers enter via the posterior root and then branch and synapse many times in the gray matter. In some instances a sensory fiber may synapse directly on an anterior horn cell.

The neurons of each segment are organized to give a few stereotype responses to specific stimuli. The jerking of the knee in response to tapping the patellar tendon is an example of such a stereotyped response.

In addition to its role in segmental responses, the spinal cord also conducts signals to and from the higher centers (brain stem, cerebellum, and cerebral cortex). These *ascending* and *descending* tracts lie in the lateral spaces surrounding the gray matter. The myelin sheaths of the axons in these areas account for the appearance of the *white matter* (Fig. 1–16). In addition to receiving motor commands from the descending tracts, each segment adds sensory information to the ascending tracts. Most of the axons in the white matter of a segment bypass that segment; they are connecting other segments to the brain.

Each segment of the spinal cord has, then, several functions. It provides a locus for sensory input, a modest integration of information, and motor control of "its" seg-

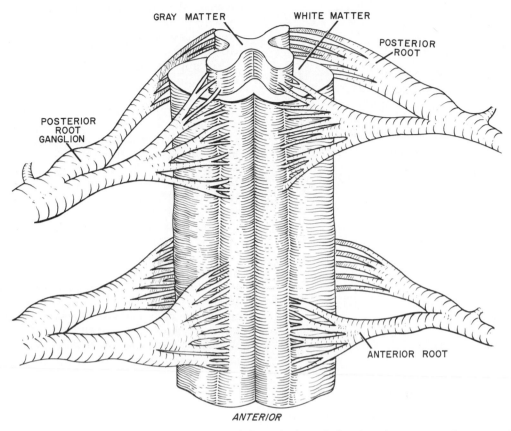

Figure 1–14 A view of the anterior aspect of the spinal cord showing the segmental nature of the spinal cord roots.

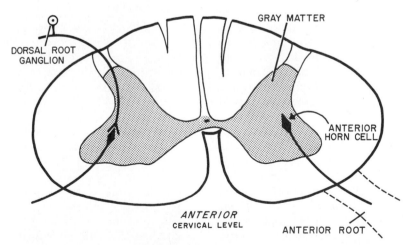

Figure 1–15 A cross section of the spinal cord showing the synaptic connection between a sensory fiber, entering the spinal cord through the posterior root, and a motor fiber, leaving via the anterior root. This particular section is from the neck region.

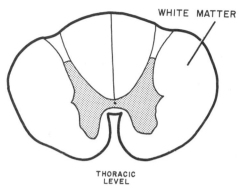

WHITE MATTER

THORACIC LEVEL

Figure 1–16 A cross section of the spinal cord taken at the middle back region. Note the different ratio of white and grey matter than seen in Figure 1–15.

ment. In addition, it serves as a conduction pathway for ascending and descending tracts.

THE BRAIN

THE BRAIN STEM

The brain stem is composed of four regions: medulla oblongata, pons, midbrain, and diencephalon (Fig. 1–17). These regions have discrete functions, and each of them contains groupings of cell bodies (nuclei) and bundles of axons (tracts). In contrast to the spinal cord, the tracts and nuclei are intermingled. The *medulla oblongata* is a direct continuation of the spinal cord. At the upper limit of the medulla is a very distinctive bulge, the pons.

The medulla contains fiber tracts just as does the spinal cord. It also contains groups of motor and sensory nuclei for "its" segments, mainly the throat, neck, and mouth. In addition, the medulla exhibits integrative functions as regards reflex activities involved in the control of respiratory and cardiovascular systems.

The nerves that connect directly to the brain are known as *cranial nerves*. There are 12 pairs of cranial nerves, 11 of which enter the brain stem. The olfactory nerve (from the nose) enters the cerebrum. The cell bodies of each cranial nerve, both sensory and motor, are grouped and are very distinct within the brain stem, in contrast to the continuous nature of the gray matter of the spinal cord. A detailed consideration of each cranial nerve will be found in the chapters on the brain stem.

The *pons* contains cranial nerve nuclei associated with sensory input and motor outflow to the face. The large bulge of the brain stem which is so typical of the pons is made up of fibers coursing down from the cerebrum and turning and running up into the cerebrum.

The *midbrain* contains the major motor nuclei controlling eye movement. It contains a huge pair of tracts carrying signals down from the cerebral hemispheres. It also contains the sensory tracts which arise in the spinal cord and continue, with additional fibers added, through the brain stem. The midbrain exerts control over the state of wakefulness of the entire brain.

The most superior portion of the brain stem is the *diencephalon* (Fig. 1–18) which is almost completely covered by the cerebrum. For the diencephalon to be visible, the cerebral hemisphere on the same side must be dissected away (Fig. 1–18). In this figure the brain stem has not been dissected. The diencephalon is a paired structure with a thin fluid space between the two parts. The largest structure within the diencephalon

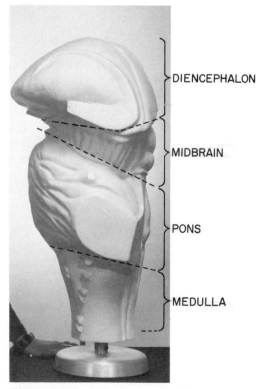

DIENCEPHALON

MIDBRAIN

PONS

MEDULLA

Figure 1–17 The brain stem. This photograph of the oversized Tuft's Brain Stem Model shows the major subdivisions.

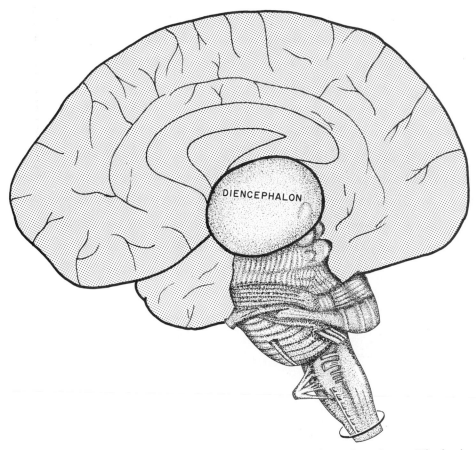

Figure 1-18   The diencephalon shown in relationship to a hemisected cerebrum. The brain stem has not been dissected.

is the *thalamus.* It is the major relay and integration center for all of the sensory systems, except smell. We can "feel" pain and crude touch at the level of the thalamus.

THE CEREBELLUM

The cerebellum (Fig. 1-19) has three major connections with the rest of the nervous system. (Be sure you can identify the cerebellum in Figures 1-7 and 1-13.) Fibers from the spinal cord carrying information concerning the position of the trunk and limbs enter via the *inferior cerebellar peduncles* (Fig. 1-20). The *middle cerebellar peduncle* conveys information which has originated in the cerebral cortex. From the cerebral cortex, fibers descend to the pontine nuclei where a synapse occurs. The information is then conveyed from the pontine nuclei to the cerebellum via the middle cerebellar peduncle. Finally, the major outflow from the

cerebellum to the thalamus, and eventually to the cerebral cortex, is via the *superior cerebellar peduncles.* The cerebellum, then, receives, via the inferior cerebellar peduncle, information as to where the limbs are in space, and, via the middle cerebellar peduncle, information as to where they are commanded to be. This information is compared in the cerebellum, and commands are sent out via the superior cerebellar peduncle. The cerebellum also has a strong input from the semicircular canals concerning orientation in space. The cerebellum, then, is involved in the unconscious adjustment of the many body muscles to keep us standing up and to provide a background for appropriate muscle movement.

THE CEREBRUM
(A HORIZONTAL SECTION)

The major structures of the cortex, the outside of the cerebrum, have already been

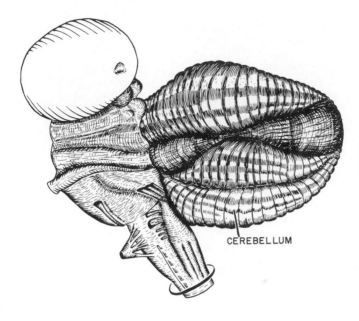

Figure 1–19 The cerebellum and its relationship to the brain stem. These relationships can also be seen in the hemisected brain in Figure 1–13.

CEREBELLUM

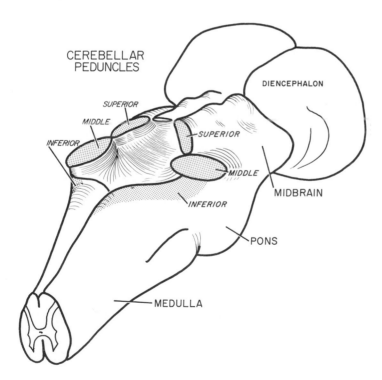

CEREBELLAR PEDUNCLES

DIENCEPHALON

SUPERIOR

MIDDLE

INFERIOR

SUPERIOR

MIDDLE

INFERIOR

MIDBRAIN

Figure 1–20 The three connections between the cerebellum and the brain stem.

PONS

MEDULLA

discussed, although it might be well to review them now. The internal structures are revealed by sectioning the brain.

When a brain is sectioned in a plane parallel with the ear and the nose, as shown in Figures 1–21 and 1–22, it is called a horizontal section, the results of which are seen in Figure 1–23. Several of the structures seen have already been discussed. The thalamus (Fig. 1–22) is buried deep within the cerebrum. The corpus callosum is in the anterior and posterior ends of the section since it has an upward curve in its midportion (Fig. 1–22).

Notice that the cerebrum is divided into white matter (axons) on the inside and gray matter (cells) on the outside. The extensive convolutions on the surface give the brain a much greater surface area for gray matter.

There are two large collections of cell bodies (nuclei) lying between the thalamus and the gray matter of the cortex. They are jointly referred to as *basal nuclei*. The *caudate nucleus* is the more anterior and medial, while the *lenticular nucleus* is more lateral.

Both these nuclei are part of the extrapyramidal motor system. The very simplest voluntary movements, such as opposing the thumb to the little finger, are initiated in the motor cortex on the contralateral precentral gyrus. The signal runs down through the brain stem and spinal cord to the appropriate spinal cord segment and synapses with anterior horn cells. There the signal leaves the central nervous system and runs in the peripheral nerve to the muscle which then contracts. The basal nuclei are a part of a system which modifies rather than initiates movement. Our understanding of the function of this system is so incomplete that it is difficult at this point to spell out specific functions for each part.

The tract (white matter) separating the thalamus and caudate nucleus from the lenticular nucleus is the *internal capsule*. All of the fibers that leave the precentral gyrus and the other motor areas of the frontal lobe flow through this area on their way to the brain stem and spinal cord.

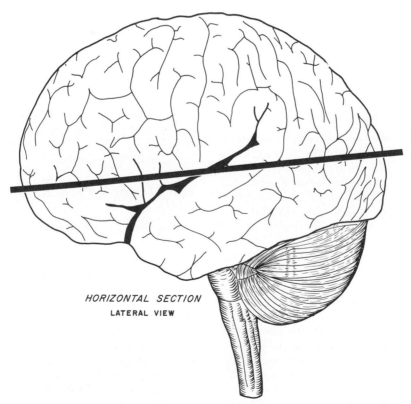

HORIZONTAL SECTION
LATERAL VIEW

Figure 1–21 The plane of section, on the lateral surface, of the horizontal section shown in Figure 1–23.

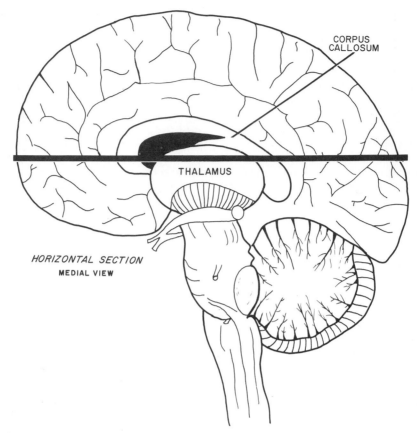

Figure 1–22 The plane of section, on the medial surface, of the horizontal section shown in Figure 1–23.

THE VENTRICULAR SYSTEM

Finally, there are the ventricles, structures that are filled with cerebrospinal fluid; their function is not fully understood. The *lateral ventricles* (Fig. 1–24) lie in the cerebrum and are the largest of the ventricles. The horizontal section (Fig. 1–23) cuts through the lateral ventricles as shown in Figure 1–25. The connection between the anterior and posterior horns lies above the plane of the section. Remember that the lateral ventricles, like the cerebral hemispheres in which they lie, are bilateral. They both connect with a single midline structure, the third ventricle. The *third ventricle* lies between the two halves of the diencephalon and is connected with a midline structure in the brain stem, the *fourth ventricle*, via the cerebral aqueduct. Cerebral spinal fluid is produced in the lateral ventricles and flows through the third and fourth ventricles. Fluid leaves the system through holes in the roof of the fourth ven-

tricle, flows up around the brain, and is reabsorbed by a large venous sinus at the top of the brain. The brain floats in the cerebral spinal fluid surrounding it.

THE BLOOD SUPPLY TO THE BRAIN

The cells of the brain are completely dependent on a continuous supply of glucose and oxygen. They have meager stores of glycogen and do not carry out glycolysis. Brain damage will occur if the oxygen supply is cut off for 4 to 5 minutes or if the glucose supply is cut off for 10 to 15 minutes. Probably the greatest cause of brain damage and neurological disease is the stoppage of blood flow to a region of the brain (a stroke). The cells and axons in the area deprived of blood die and no longer function. If these cells are in the precentral gyrus, voluntary movement of a part of the opposite side of the body is impaired.

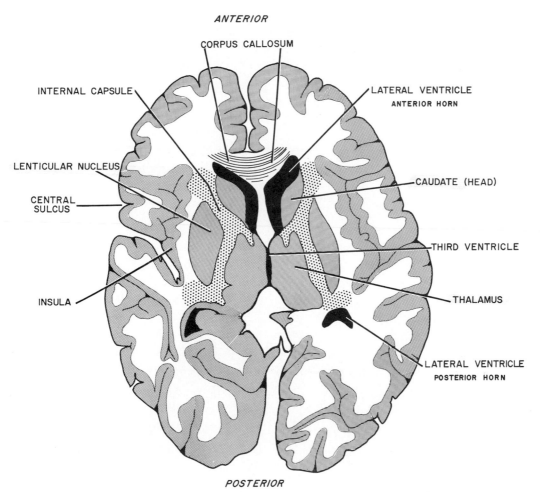

Figure 1–23 A horizontal section of the brain shown from above.

See Filmstrip, Frame 4.

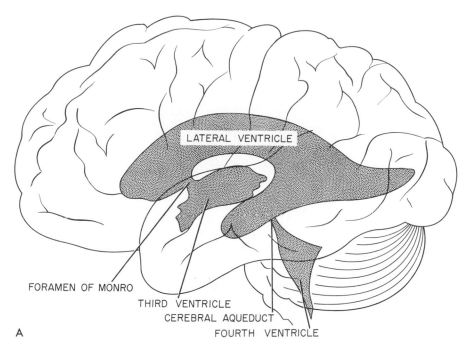

LATERAL VENTRICLE

FORAMEN OF MONRO

THIRD VENTRICLE

CEREBRAL AQUEDUCT

FOURTH VENTRICLE

A

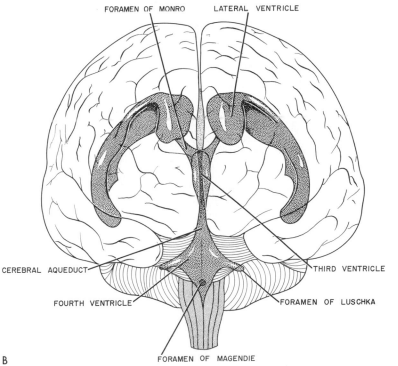

FORAMEN OF MONRO   LATERAL VENTRICLE

CEREBRAL AQUEDUCT

THIRD VENTRICLE

FOURTH VENTRICLE

FORAMEN OF LUSCHKA

B

FORAMEN OF MAGENDIE

Figure 1–24   The ventricular system of the brain shown in (*A*) lateral and (*B*) anterior-posterior views.

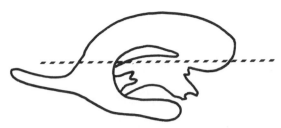

Figure 1–25 The plane of section, through a lateral view of the ventricular system, of the horizontal section in Figure 1–23.

The brain receives blood from four arteries (Fig. 1–26). Two *vertebral arteries* enter the skull (together with the spinal cord) through the *foramen magnum*. These arteries send branches to the medulla oblongata and the cerebellum. More superiorly, they join to form the *basilar artery* which supplies (via branches) the pons, midbrain, and parts of the cerebellum. At its superior end the basilar artery branches to form the *posterior cerebral arteries* which supply the occipital lobes and part of the temporal lobes. This whole system forms the posterior circulation of the brain.

The anterior circulation is supplied by the *internal carotid arteries*. These arteries enter the cranial cavity and almost immediately branch into middle and anterior cerebral arteries. The middle cerebral arteries run laterally through the lateral fissure to supply the lateral surface of the hemispheres. The anterior cerebral arteries run anteriorly and medially to loop over the corpus callosum between the hemispheres, supplying blood to the medial surface of the brain.

The anterior and posterior circulations are connected by the *posterior communicating* arteries (Fig. 1–26). The right and left anterior cerebral arteries are connected by the anterior communicating artery. Since the major arteries at the base of the brain are usually interconnected, a failure in blood supply in one of these major arteries will not usually produce a critical decrease in blood flow in the region supplied by that vessel. The interconnection of these arteries forms a circle that was first described by the eminent English anatomist, Thomas Willis, and is consequently called the *circle of Willis* in his honor.

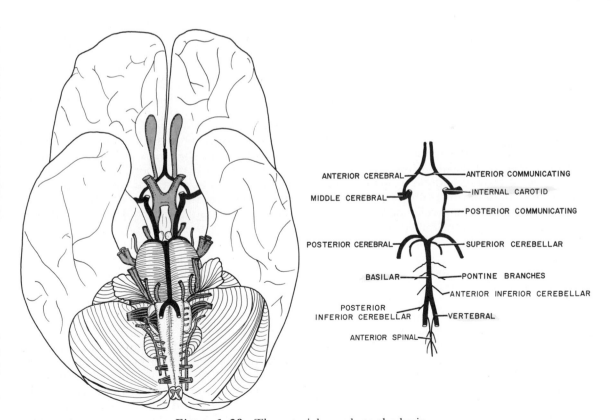

Figure 1–26 The arterial supply to the brain.

2

Neuroembryology

STANLEY JACOBSON

DIFFERENTIATION

The first evidence of the differentiation of the nervous system appears at the end of the second week of gestation. At that time a "heaping up" of ectodermal cells can be noted at the caudal end of the embryonic disc. This accumulation of cells is known as the primitive streak (Fig. 2–1A). As development continues surface ectodermal cells involute through the primitive streak and migrate laterally, forming the intraembryonic mesoderm, interposed between the surface ectoderm and subjacent endoderm. As the intraembryonic mesoderm forms, another thickening of ectodermal cells occurs at the cephalic end of the primitive streak; this is Hensen's node (Fig. 2–1A). Cells migrate inward through this zone and extend between the surface ectoderm and subjacent endoderm, forming the notochord or head process.

On either side of the neural plate is a thin strip of ectoderm known as the neural crest. As development proceeds, the neural plate sinks inward to form the neural groove (Figs. 2–1A and 2–2A). This midline groove continues to deepen until the dorsal lips of the groove meet and fuse, forming the neural tube (Figs. 2–1B, C, and 2–2). The adjacent neural crest separates from the overlying

ectoderm and comes to lie lateral to the neural tube (Fig. 2–2). The central nervous system is derived from the neural tube, the neural crest yields many parts of the peripheral nervous system, and the remaining ectoderm becomes the epidermis (somatic ectoderm) of the embryo.

Prior to the formation of the neural tube the paraxial mesoderm begins to form the somites. Fusion of the dorsal margins of the neural groove begins on about the twenty-second day in the region of somites 4 to 6, forming the neural tube (Fig. 2–1C). Fusion continues in both cranial and caudal directions, and by the twenty-fifth day only the cranial and caudal ends of the neural tube remain open; these are known as the anterior and posterior neuropores respectively. The lumen in the neural tube will become the ventricular system of the central nervous system.

After delineation of the neural and somatic ectoderm, the neural crest cells appear as an almost continuous column of cells along the dorsal surface of the neural tube from the mesencephalic level through all spinal cord levels (Fig. 2–2). The neural crest cells form the primordium of the sensory ganglia, the cranial nerves and the spinal ganglia, the neurilemmal cells, satellite cells, the autonomic ganglia, and probably the pia-arach-

20

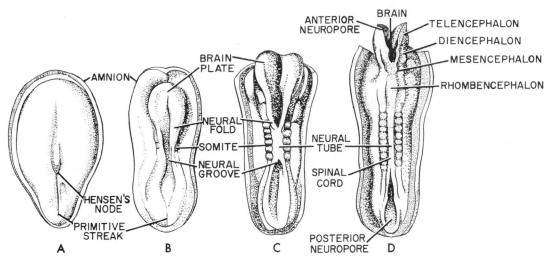

Figure 2–1 Dorsal view of human embryo. *A*, Primitive streak stage (16-day presomite embryo). *B*, Neural plate stage (20-day two somite embryo). *C*, Beginning of neural tube (22-day seven somite embryo). *D*, Brain vesicle stage (23-day ten somite embryo).

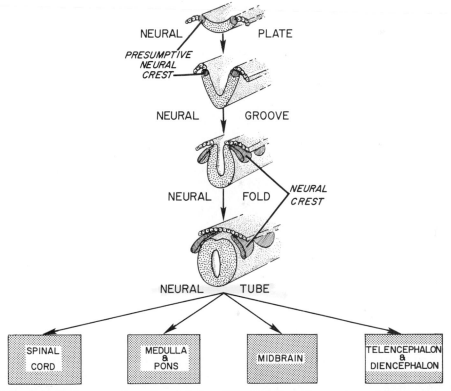

Figure 2–2 Schematic coronal section showing differentiation of neural ectoderm in the neural plate stage, the neural groove stage, the neural fold stage, and the neural tube stage. (Adapted from Ham, A. W., *Histology.* Philadelphia, Lippincott, 1969.)

noid membrane. Shortly after the closure of the neural tube, processes from the neural crest cells enter the spinal cord or brain stem and form the sensory roots of the spinal and cranial nerves.

HISTOGENESIS

The walls of the neural tube throughout the nervous system consist of neural epithelial cells or germinal cells which form a pseudostratified epithelium. After the closure of the neural tube another cell type is found external to the germinal cell layer. This new cell is the *neuroblast*. The neuroblast cells form a new layer, the mantle layer, and external to the mantle layer is seen a cell-free zone, the marginal layer.

Initially the neuroblasts are connected to the lumen by an elongate process, a transient dendrite. As they migrate into the subjacent mantle layer they lose this process and become apolar neuroblasts. Shortly thereafter two new processes appear; one becomes the axon, the other the dendrite. The axonal process elongates and more dendritic branches appear, forming a multipolar neuroblast. There are also some neurons which form only a single process; these are the sensory ganglion neurons and the mesencephalic nucleus of cranial nerve V. Some neurons such as the olfactory receptor cells, rods, and cones of the retina, the bipolar cells in the retina, and the receptor cells in the vestibular and cochlear ganglion will remain bipolar. The axonal process enters the cell-free zone external to the mantle zone, the marginal zone.

It should be noted that the germinal cells will also form the supporting cells in the central nervous system.

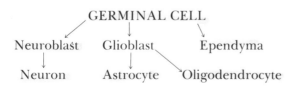

Throughout the central nervous system neurons migrate into the mantle layer to become the definitive structures of the spinal cord, much of the brain stem, and the basal nuclei (Sidman and Miale, 1959; Sidman and Feder, 1959). In these regions the cells in the mantle layer become the gray matter, while their axons form the marginal lamina or white matter. On the other hand, the cerebral cortex and cerebellar cortex are formed by the migration of neuroblasts through the mantle layer into the marginal layer.

The cerebral cortex forms from the inside out. The first layer to form is layer VI and the last to form is layer II (Angevine and Sidman, 1961; Berry and Rogers, 1965). The pyramidal cells in the cerebral cortex appear to mature prior to the stellate cells (Altman, 1966). Formation of the cerebral cortex begins around the seventh week and is completed in the first year of life.

The cerebellum and deep cerebellar nuclei are formed by the migration of cells from the germinal layer through the mantle layer into the marginal layer (Fujita, 1962, 1966). The Purkinje cell layer is the first to form. Other cells migrate externally and form the molecular layer. A little later on cells migrate inward from the more external layers to form the granular layer. In the adult the molecular layer has only a few cells, while the Purkinje layer and granule cell layer have many neurons.

The means by which cells migrate to form the cerebellum and cerebrum and provide the connections that are necessary for the proper function of these structures is not entirely clear.

SPINAL CORD

By the twentieth day two distinct regions can be seen: caudally, a single elongate cylindrical region which will become the spinal cord; and, cranially, a shorter broader region which will become the brain (Fig. 2–1*B*).

Up to the third month the spinal cord fills the vertebral column. However, from then on the cartilage and bone grow faster than the central nervous system, and by birth the coccygeal end of the spinal cord lies at the level of the third lumbar vertebra. In an adult it is found at the level of the first lumbar vertebra.

At the end of the somite period (30 to 35 days) the mitotic divisions in the spinal cord region produce thickened walls and a thin roof and floor, with almost complete obliteration of the central canal (Fig. 2–3). The ventral portion of the lateral walls develops and expands earlier than the dorsal re-

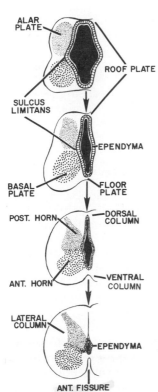

Figure 2-3 Schematic representation of the development of the spinal cord. (After Hamilton, W. J., Boyd, J. D., and Mossman, H. W.: *Human Embryology.* Cambridge, England, Heffer and Sons, 1964.)

gion. The ventral portion is called the *basal plate* and the dorsal portion is called the *alar plate.* Processes from cells in the mantle layer enter the external-most region of the cord, which is called the *marginal zone.*

Axons of developing motor neurons in the basal plate enter the adjoining somites, while sensory roots derived from the adjacent neural crest zone enter the dorsal or alar plate. In the spinal cord (Fig. 2-3) the alar plate will become the dorsal or sensory associative horn, and the basal plate will become the ventral or motor horn. In the medulla (Fig. 2-4), pons (Fig. 2-5), and midbrain (Fig. 2-6) the alar and basal plates are restricted to the floor of the developing ventricular system. The remaining bulk of these zones consists of nuclei and tracts which are related to the head, neck, and special senses.

In the spinal cord the marginal zone also increases in width as axons which form the ascending and descending tract enter (Fig. 2-3). The formation of a dorsal and ventral horn delimits the dorsal, ventral, and lateral columns or funiculae in the marginal zone. An intermediate horn develops dorsal and lateral to the anterior horn in the thoracic and lumbar levels of the spinal cord. These cells are the preganglionic sympathetic neurons.

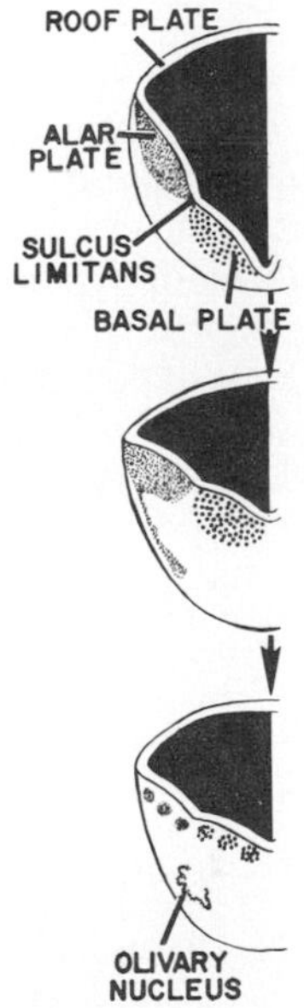

Figure 2-4 Schematic representation of the development of the medulla. (After Hamilton, W. J., Boyd, J. D., and Mossman, H. W.: *Human Embryology.* Cambridge, England, Heffer & Sons, 1964.)

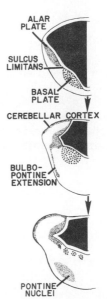

Figure 2-5 Schematic representation of the development of the pons. (After Hamilton, W. J., Boyd, J. D., and Mossman, H. W.: *Human Embryology.* Cambridge, England, Heffer and Sons, 1964.)

BRAIN

The brain starts as a broader zone with three distinct regions appearing early: the prosencephalon, the mesencephalon, and the rhombencephalon. Table 2–1 summarizes the differentiation of these three regions.

MYELENCEPHALON (FIG. 2–4) AND METENCEPHALON (FIG. 2–5)

The metencephalon and myelencephalon are further divided by their relationship to the ventricular system. That portion forming the floor of the ventricle is called the tegmentum, while that forming the roof of the ventricle is called the tectum. In the spinal cord the basal plate was ventral and the alar plate dorsal. In the medulla, pons, and midbrain both basal and alar plates are restricted to that portion of the tegmentum which forms the ventricular floor. The alar or sensory region is lateral, while the motor region is medial. The sulcus limitans on the ventricular floor separates the medial motor region from the lateral sensory region.

The dorsal portion of the alar plate in the metencephalon forms the primordium of the cerebellum. This region, the rhombic lip, thickens and the cerebellum continues to expand laterally and then medially so that a pair of lateral regions, the hemispheres, and a medial zone, the vermis, are now formed. The roof of the lower medulla is formed by the ependymal lining and pia, the tela choroidea.

Added to the anterior surface of the medulla, pons, and midbrain is the basilar region which, in the medulla, consists of the pyramids and, in the pons, consists of the middle cerebellar peduncle and pyramids. In the midbrain it consists of the cerebral peduncles. Other tracts and nuclei form the bulk of the tegmentum of the pons and medulla and midbrain.

The ventricular lumen in pontine and medullary levels is called the fourth ventricle. The neural tube in these zones changes from a tube to a rhomboid-shaped fossa as a result of the broadening of the tegmentum and the overgrowth of the cerebellum.

MESENCEPHALON (FIG. 2–6)

The mesencephalon starts as a widely dilated tube with a conspicuous floor (tegmentum) and a thin roof (tectum). The addition of fibers and nuclei in the mantle zone of the tegmentum, concomitant with the formation of the superior and inferior colliculi in the tectal area, produces a narrow cerebral aqueduct with a large tegmentum and tectum. The tectum consists of neurons which receive input from the cranial nerves which relay auditory (inferior colliculus) and visual information (superior colliculus). The cerebral peduncles form the anterior surface or basis of the midbrain, with the tegmentum located between the basis and tectum. The cerebral peduncles consist of fibers descending from the cerebrum to the brain stem and spinal cord.

FOREBRAIN (FIG. 2–7)

The prosencephalon starts as a dilation of the cranial end of the neural tube (Fig. 2–1C, D). Early in development an optic vesicle (which will become the eye) appears as a lateral diverticulum of the anterior portion of the prosencephalon. In front of and above the optic stalk a pair of cerebral vesicles form. The cerebral vesicles expand superiorly, anteriorly, and posteriorly.

Table 2–1   *Differentiation of Brain*

DEVELOPING BRAIN	MATURE BRAIN	
Prosencephalon	Gross Divisions	Subdivisions
	Telencephalon	Cerebrum, Basal ganglia
	Diencephalon	Thalamus, Hypothalamus, Epithalamus
Mesencephalon	Mesencephalon	
		Midbrain
Rhombencephalon	Metencephalon	
	Myelencephalon	Cerebellum, Pons Medulla

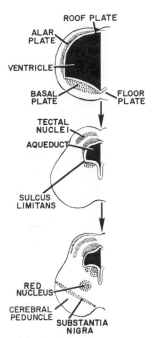

Figure 2-6 Schematic representation of the development of the midbrain. (After Hamilton, W. J., Boyd, J. D., and Mossman, H. W.: *Human Embryology.* Cambridge, England, Heffer and Sons, 1964.)

Diencephalon. The diencephalon originates from the caudal portion of the prosencephalon (Fig. 2-1*D*) and represents the thickened lateral wall of the primordium of the third ventricle. The dorsal half of the diencephalon will become the thalamus and epithalamus, while the floor differentiates into the hypothalamus and neurohypophysis. Fibers to and from the telencephalon will form the lateral limit of the diencephalon. These fibers are the internal capsule.

The deep telencephalic nuclei, the basal ganglia, form at the level of the interventricular foramen of Monro by the migration of cells from the neuroepithelial lining of the prosencephalon. The fibers going to and from the cortex split the developing deep telencephalic nuclei so that the medial portion, the caudate, is separated from the lateral portion, the globus pallidus and putamen, by the internal capsule.

Telencephalon. The telencephalon starts at 10 weeks as paired small smooth telencephalic vesicles; by birth a large, convoluted cerebral cortex is present. The first prominent features seen in the hemisphere are the

formation of the primary sulci or depressions (Figs. 2-8 and 2-9).

Sulci. The first of these sulci appear at about 19 weeks; they are the Sylvian fissure, on the lateral surface (Fig. 2-8), and the parieto-occipital fissure, on the medial surface (Fig. 2-9). By the twenty-fourth week the Sylvian fissure on the lateral surface (Fig. 2-8) is more pronounced and the calcarine fissure on the medial surface is also prominent (Fig. 2-9). Shortly thereafter the other primary sulci—the central, callosal, and hippocampal—appear. After the appearance of the sulci (from about 28 to 30 weeks) there is a rapid increase in the secondary sulci and

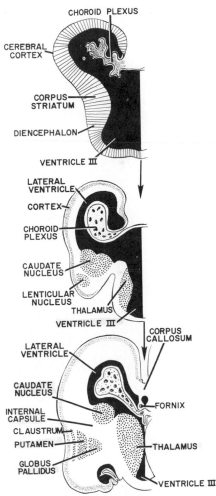

Figure 2-7 Schematic representation of the development of the telencephalon and diencephalon. (After Hamilton, W. J., Boyd, J. D., and Mossman, H. W.: *Human Embryology.* Cambridge, England, Heffer and Sons, 1964.)

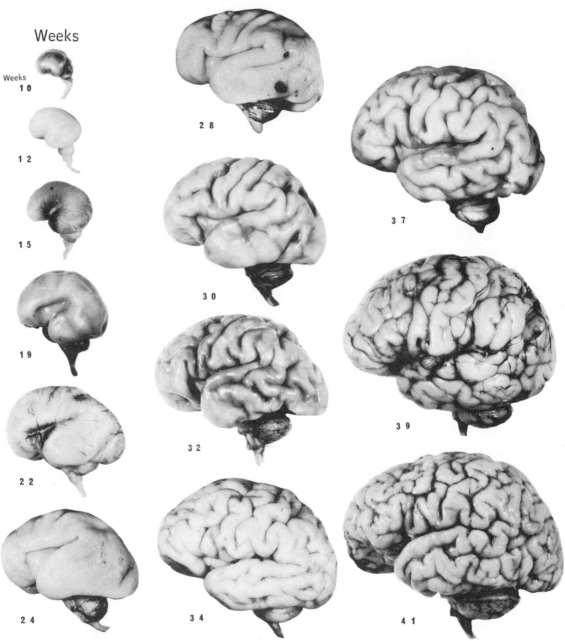

Weeks

Figure 2–8 Development of the lateral surface of the brain during fetal life. Numbers represent gestation age in weeks. (From Larroche, J. Cl.: The Development of the Central Nervous System During Intrauterine Life. *In* Falkner, F. (ed.): *Human Development.* Philadelphia, W. B. Saunders, 1966, p. 258.)

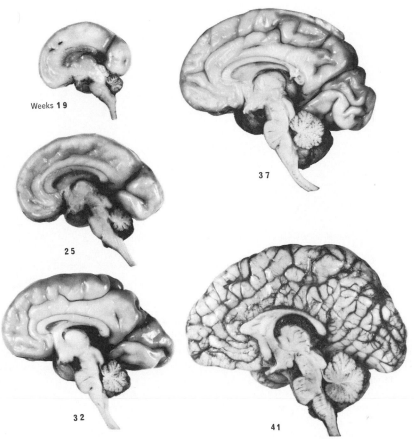

Weeks 1 9

2 5

3 7

3 2

4 1

Figure 2–9 Development of the medial surface of the brain during fetal life. Numbers represent gestation age in weeks (From Larroche, J. Cl.: The Development of the Central Nervous System During Intrauterine Life. *In* Falkner, F. (ed.): *Human Development.* Philadelphia, W. B. Saunders, 1966, p. 259.)

gyri. By term, formation of most of the gyri and sulci is complete. From this time on the gyri increase in bulk as the neurons continue to differentiate.

The telencephalic vesicle rapidly changes shape as the frontal lobe forms and pushes anteriorly, as the temporal lobe then grows inferiorly, and also as the occipital and parietal regions expand. The olfactory bulb forms from the base of the frontal lobe by an evagination of cells which quickly obliterates any trace of the ventricle in the olfactory bulb.

The sulci begin as rather shallow depressions. However, as the neurons continue to form, more and more cells are added and the gyri become larger and the sulci become deeper. In the term and adult brain more than 70 per cent of the cortical surface is hidden from view, deep in the banks of the sulci. Therefore, when we speak of the total surface of the cerebral hemispheres we must include not only the superficial cortex but also the hidden sulcal cortex.

The brain at birth weighs from 300 to 400 grams; by one year it weighs 1000 grams. The brain continues to grow and by late childhood reaches its final weight of approximately 1500 grams.

The development of certain areas is of special importance in understanding the final form of the brain. As the lateral fissure forms, the cortex above and below the lateral fissure overgrows the cortex deep in the Sylvian fissure. This cortex, the insula, soon disappears from view and is covered over by this overgrowth of frontal, parietal, and temporal cortex.

Commissures. The two cerebral hemispheres are interconnected by fiber bundles, called commissures (refer to Fig. 2–10*A, B, C, D*). The anterior commissure intercon-

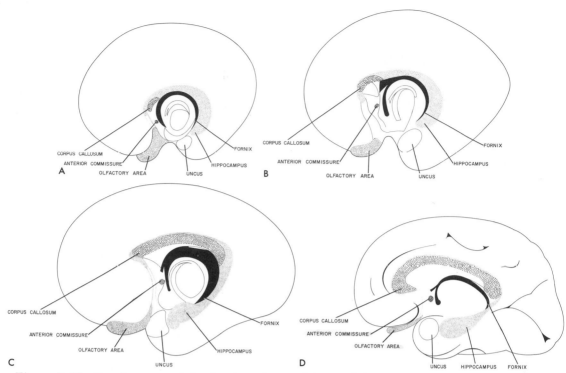

Figure 2-10 Development of the fornix and commissures of the cerebral hemispheres. *A*, 3-month fetus. *B*, 4-month fetus. *C*, Fetus at beginning of 5th month. *D*, Fetus at end of 7th month. (After Keibel, F., and Mall, F. P.: *Manual of Human Embryology*, Philadelphia, Lippincott, 1910–12.)

nects the olfactory bulbs and parts of the temporal lobe. The huge corpus callosum interconnects the remaining portions of the hemisphere. The hippocampal commissure interconnects the hippocampus and adjacent portions of the hippocampal gyrus. These commissures form in the lamina terminalis which marks the site of the closure of the anterior neuropore. The ventral surface of the hemispheres at this place fuse, and the fibers can then cross and interconnect the two hemispheres.

Initially, the anterior commissure, corpus callosum, and fornix (which connects the hippocampus and hypothalamus) are close to one another (Fig. 2–10*A*), but as the brain grows, the corpus callosum expands anteriorly, inferiorly, superiorly, and caudally with only the rostral tip remaining attached to the lamina terminalis.

Fornix. The pathway of the fornix is always perplexing to the student. The fornix initially is just a short fiber tract running from the hippocampus to the hypothalamus (Fig. 2–10*A*). However, as the temporal lobe expands, the hippocampus migrates inferiorly and anteriorly and the fibers of the fornix elongate so that they finally stretch from the hippocampus near the medial surface of the temporal pole to the foramen of Monro (Fig. 2–10*B, C, D*). The fornix runs in the superior wall of the inferior horn of the lateral ventricle. In the body of the ventricle the fornix is attached to the undersurface of the corpus callosum. Near the foramen of Monro it enters the hypothalamus and runs through the mammillary bodies. Only the anterior commissure remains more or less in the same position in the lamina terminalis.

Foramen of Monro. Early in development, the lumen in the paired telencephalic vesicles is continuous with that of the neural tube. As the telencephalon differentiates into cerebral cortex and basal nuclei, the ventricles take up relatively less space. A narrow channel persists between the cerebral ventricles and the third ventricle and is called the interventricular foramen of Monro (Fig. 2–7*B, C*).

Blood Vessels and Connective Tissue. Mesodermal constituents early in development migrate into the central nervous system to form microglia and the blood vessels. The connective tissue of the peripheral nervous system and the skull, vertebral column, and ligaments which support the central nervous system also are formed from mesoderm.

VENTRICULAR SYSTEM

When the neural folds fuse, a neural tube is formed. At the rostral end of the nervous system two lateral dilations appear: the primordia of the cerebral vesicle. This region will grow rapidly, extending anteriorly, inferiorly, and posteriorly as it forms the cerebral hemisphere.

Lateral Ventricle. The cavity in the cerebral vesicle is the lateral ventricle. As the cerebral hemisphere grows by continued outward migration of nerve cells, the ventricle takes up less and less space in the brain and is modified into a C-shaped structure with a spur extending occipitally. The lateral ventricle in its final form is divided into an anterior horn, body, inferior horn, and posterior horn.

Third Ventricle. The cavity in the diencephalon—the third ventricle—narrows as the diencephalon forms. In the midbrain the tectum and tegmentum expand greatly and constrict the lumen so that only the narrow cerebral aqueduct remains.

Fourth Ventricle. In the metencephalon (cerebellum and pons) and myelencephalon (medulla), the tegmentum undergoes a series of flexures and expands laterally concomitant with the overgrowth of the cerebellum, so that the cavity—the fourth ventricle—in its final form is rhomboid-shaped and is continuous with the narrow cerebral aqueduct above and the constricted spinal canal below.

Spinal Canal. In the spinal cord, the expanding gray and white matter nearly obliterate the ventricular cavity so that only the small spinal canal remains.

PERIPHERAL NERVOUS SYSTEM

Peripheral structures are innervated from nuclei in the brain (cranial nerves) and from nuclei in the spinal cord (spinal nerves). The twelve cranial nerve nuclei innervate skin, glands, viscera, striated muscles, and special sense organs (eye and ear) in the head and neck. The spinal nerves innervate skin, glands, and striated muscles in the upper and lower extremities and in the thorax, abdomen, and pelvis.

SPINAL NERVES

The spinal cord demonstrates a segmental arrangement which reflects the somite pattern of the embryo. Each spinal cord segment initially innervates and receives from only one somite. However, as the embryo differentiates, this arrangement becomes somewhat modified. In the gray matter of the spinal cord, neurons are arranged in columns which innervate structures having similar functions.

There are four basic columns in each half of the gray matter of the spinal cord: two motor and two sensory. The somatic afferent and efferent column innervates skin and muscle related to the somites, while the visceral afferent and visceral efferent columns innervate the visceral structures. The somatic efferent cells are the motor neurons in the ventral horn of the spinal cord. The somatic afferent cells are the neurons in the spinal ganglia. The visceral efferent cells consist of sympathetic and parasympathetic neurons. The sympathetic neurons consist of two neurons: (1) the preganglionic visceral neurons in the intermediate column of thoracic and lumbar levels, and (2) the postganglionic visceral neurons in the paravertebral sympathetic chain or in ganglia associated with the visceral organs. The preganglionic parasympathetic innervation originates from the motor neurons in cranial nerves III, VII, IX and X and the sacral spinal cord and innervate ganglia which connect the appropriate organ or gland. Again, these ganglia differentiate very close to the appropriate structure.

In the dorsal or sensory horn of the spinal cord there are sensory neurons which provide connections throughout the spinal cord or brain stem.

The segmental arrangement of the central nervous system stops at the spinomedullary junction which marks the site of transition from the spinal cord to the brain stem. The brain stem and cerebrum are suprasegmental with no evidence of segmentation present. These regions of the central nervous system are specialized to control structures in the head and neck as well as exerting control over the entire body.

Developmentally the spinal cord and the somites lie very close to one another so that the distance the axon must travel to reach its appropriate muscle is very short. There are undoubtedly some chemical factors which help direct the axon to the correct muscle. The sensory fibers also have only a short distance to run from skin or muscle into the central nervous system; again probably under some chemical mediation they establish the connection with the correct dorsal horn cells.

CRANIAL NERVES

A detailed discussion of the cranial nerves can be found in Chapter 10. In this section, the cranial nerves (Fig. 2–11) will be categorized on the basis of the structures they innervate:

1. Muscles of presumptive somite origin—nerves XII, VI, IV, and most of III.

2. Muscles and skin related to the pharyngeal arches—nerves V, VII, IX, X and XI.

3. Preganglionic parasympathetic innervation—nerves IX, X, VII, V, and a small part of III.

4. Special senses nerves I, II, and VIII, and gustatory portions of nerves VII, IX, and X.

Cranial Nerves Innervating Muscles of Presumptive Somite Origin.

Nerve XII (hypoglossal) is a purely motor nerve and innervates the extrinsic and intrinsic muscles in the tongue. The epithelium and general connective tissue of the tongue arises by the fusion of pharyngeal endoderm and branchial mesoderm which are innervated by nerves VII, IX, and X. Occipital myotomes migrate ventrally and form the tongue musculature and are innervated by cranial nerve XII.

Nerve VI (abducens) is a purely motor nerve and innervates the lateral rectus muscle of the eye.

Nerve IV (trochlear) is a purely motor nerve and innervates the superior oblique muscle of the eye. This is the only cranial nerve with rootlets that leave the central nervous system from the posterior surface of the brain.

Nerve III (oculomotor) is a purely motor nerve and innervates the inferior oblique and the medial, superior, inferior recti and levator palpebrae superior muscles. The extrinsic eye muscles develop from mesenchyme in the optic region.

Cranial Nerves Innervating Muscles and Skin in the Pharyngeal Arches

After the beginning of somite formation, five ectodermal grooves appear lateral to the embryonic pharynx and caudal to the stomatoderma (primitive mouth). The grooves are separated from one another by elevations, which gradually elongate and fuse with their mate from the opposite side, and extend laterally and anteriorly around the pharynx, forming arches. In lower vertebrates these arches form the gills, while in vertebrates without gills they are called *pharyngeal arches.* Many of the muscles and bones in the face and neck originate from these arches.

Nerve V (trigeminal) is a mixed nerve (motor and sensory) which innervates the first or maxillary arch and also contains a portion (ophthalmic) which distributes to the skin up to the vertex of the skull. The motor division of this nerve innervates the muscles of mastication derived from the first arch. The sensory division innervates the skin on the face and forehead.

Nerve VII (facial) is a mixed nerve which distributes to the second pharyngeal or hyoid arch. The motor division of this nerve inner-

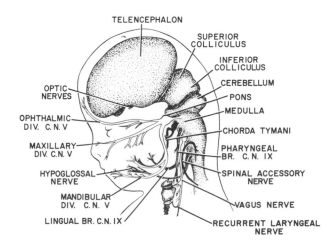

Figure 2–11 Lateral surface of 11-week human embryo demonstrating the cranial and upper spinal nerves. (After Patten, B. M.: *Human Embryology,* New York, McGraw-Hill, 1953.)

vates the muscles of facial expression. The sensory division innervates the taste buds on the anterior two-thirds of the tongue.

Nerve IX (glossopharyngeal) is a mixed nerve which innervates structures associated with the third arch. The motor divisions of this nerve innervate the stylopharyngeus muscles.

Nerve X (vagus) is a mixed nerve which innervates structures associated with the fourth and sixth arches as well as providing afferent and efferent components to the heart, lungs, and much of the gastrointestinal system. The fifth arch regresses.

Nerve XI (accessory) is purely motor and innervates the sternomastoid and trapezius muscles which originate from somatic and branchial mesenchyme in the cervical region.

Preganglionic Parasympathetic Innervation

Nerve III innervates the ciliary ganglion; postganglionic fibers then pass to the sphincter of the iris which constricts the pupil in bright light.

Nerve VII provides innervation to the ganglia associated with the following glands: submaxillary, sublingual, nasal, and lacrimal. *pterygomandibular ganglion*

Nerve IX provides innervation to the parotid gland via the otic ganglion.

Nerve X provides innervation to the heart, lungs, and gastrointestinal system up to the transverse colon.

Special Senses

Nerve I (olfactory): The cell bodies are located in the nasal placode in the upper fifth of each nasal cavity. The neuroblasts in the olfactory epithelium differentiate into olfactory epithelial cells; the axons of these cells grow toward the cerebral hemisphere, pierce the roof of the nasal cavity, and enter the region of the hemisphere which will become the olfactory bulb. The primary fibers synapse in the olfactory bulb. The secondary cell bodies are located in the olfactory bulb and form the secondary olfactory tracts.

Nerve II (optic) originates from a tertiary neuron in the retinae. These axons are really a tract in the central nervous system and do not constitute a peripheral nerve. The axons synapse in the lateral geniculate nucleus of the thalamus. The details of the formation of the eye from the optic vesicle and lens vesicles should be reviewed in a standard embryology text.

Nerve VIII (vestibulocochlear): The primary cell bodies of this nerve are located in the cochlea (auditory division) and vestibule (vestibular division) of the inner ear. The details of the formation of the inner ear from the otic placode should also be reviewed in a standard embryology textbook.

Nerves VII, IX, and X provide innervation to the taste buds on the tongue and pharynx.

ABNORMAL DEVELOPMENT

Many defects in the brain and spinal cord may be seen at birth. Defects may be limited to the nervous system or they may include overlying ectodermal and mesodermal structures (bone, muscle, and connective tissue). Many of the malformations seen are due to genetic abnormalities. Other categories of defects can be acquired from the maternal environment: infections such as syphilis and rubella (measles), drugs, ionizing radiation, metabolic disease. Most of the serious defects produce death, while less severe abnormalities cause impairment of function.

Malformations Resulting from Abnormalities in Growth and Migration.

In the following malformations, neurons or glia have failed to migrate and consequently the brain has only developed up to a point.

Anencephaly. This is a lethal condition in which skull, cerebral hemisphere, diencephalon, and midbrain are absent. The amount of tissue absent can vary from only the cerebrum to all of the diencephalon and telencephalon.

Holoprosencephaly (Fig. 2–12A, B). The brain has failed to form two distinct cerebral hemispheres. Instead, there is a single partially differentiated hemisphere.

Lissencephaly. The brain has failed to form sulci and gyri and corresponds to a 12-week embryo.

Micropolygyria (Fig. 2–13). The gyri are more numerous, smaller, and more poorly developed than normal.

Macrogyria. The gyri are broader and less numerous than in the normal brain.

Microencephaly. This is another abnormal defect in which development of the brain is rudimentary and the individual has a low-grade intelligence.

Porencephaly. There are symmetrical cavities in the cortex due to the absence of cortex and white matter in these sites.

Heterotopias. Displaced islands of gray matter appear in the ventricular walls or

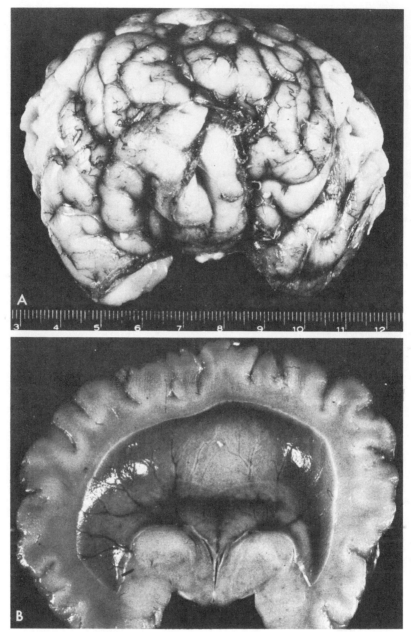

Figure 2–12 Holoprosencephaly. *A*, view of frontal poles. *B*, coronal section. Note the absence of any differentiation of the hemispheres. (Courtesy of Dr. John Hills, New England Medical Center Hospitals.)

white matter due to incomplete migration of neurons.

Agenesis of Corpus Callosum. There is a complete or partial absence of the corpus callosum (Fig. 2–14).

Cerebellar Agenesis. Portions of the cerebellum, deep cerebellar nuclei, and even the pons are either absent or malformed. In some instances portions of the basal ganglia and brain stem and spinal cord may also be malformed or absent.

Malformations Resulting from Defective Fusion of Dorsal Structures

Spinal Bifida. This is the most common malformation in this category; the arches and dorsal spines of the vertebrae are ab-

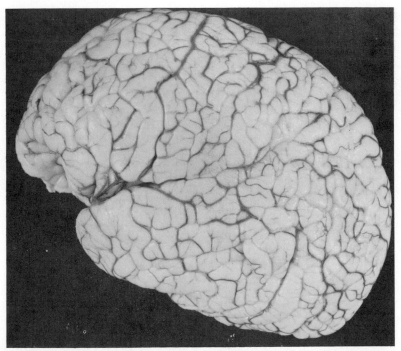

Figure 2–13 Micropolygyria. (Courtesy of Dr. John Hills, New England Medical Center Hospitals.)

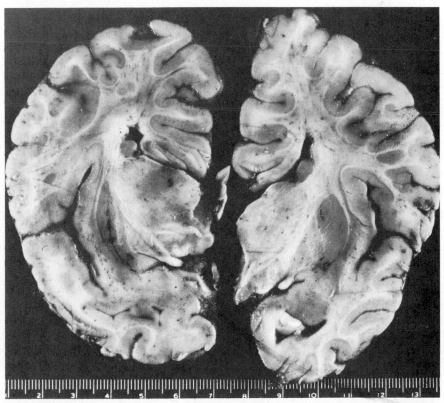

Figure 2–14 Agenesis of corpus callosum. (Courtesy of Dr. John Hills, New England Medical Center Hospitals.)

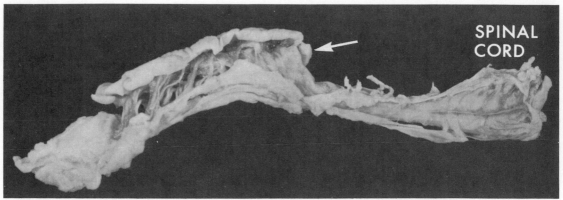

Figure 2–15 Meningomyelocele at sacral level of the spinal cord. Arrow refers to sac, meninges, neural tissue, and overlying skin. (Courtesy of Dr. John Hills, New England Medical Center Hospitals.)

sent. Often the bony deficit alone is present. The spinal cord, however, may be malformed either at one level or at many levels. In some instances the spinal cord, nerve root, and meninges have herniated through the midline defect in the skin and bone — *meningomyelocele* (Fig. 2–15). In other instances only the meninges have herniated through the midline defect — *meningocele.*

Cranial Bifida. This condition is less common and usually occurs only in the suboccipital region. The cranial bones either fail to fuse or do not form. The abnormality may only be restricted to the underlying portion of the cerebrum or it may be accompanied by a herniation of meninges — *meningocele* — or meninges and brain tissue — *encephalocele.* Cranial bifida is commonly associated with hydrocephalus and extensive brain damage.

Arnold–Chiari Malformation. In this condition there is elongation and displacement of the brain stem and a portion of the cerebellum through the foramen magnum into the cervical region of the vertebral canal. Hydrocephalus, spina bifida with meningocele, or meningomyelocele may also be associated with this abnormality, which may be fatal or produce neurological symptoms due to compression of the cervical roots and the overcrowding of the neural tissue in the posterior fossa (Fig. 15–7).

Malformations Resulting from Abnormalities in the Ventricular System

Hydrocephalus. Any abnormality in absorption of cerebrospinal fluid which produces increased cerebrospinal fluid pressure and dilation of the ventricular system is called hydrocephalus. Blockage of the flow in the ventricular system is called noncommunicating hydrocephalus, while blockage of the cerebrospinal fluid in the subarachnoid space is called communicating hydrocephalus.

Noncommunicating hydrocephalus may be due

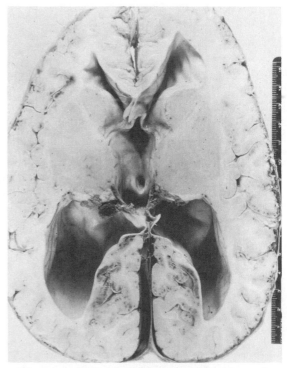

Figure 2–16 Noncommunicating hydrocephalus, Dandy-Walker syndrome. (Courtesy of Dr. John Hills, New England Medical Center Hospitals.)

See Filmstrip, Frames 5 and 6.

either to blockage of flow at the interventricular foramen, the cerebral aqueduct, or in the fourth ventricle or to the malformation of any portion of the ventricular system. The passageways from the fourth ventricle to the foramina of the subarachnoid space (foramina of Luschka and Magendie) may also be blocked or ill-formed (as in the Dandy-Walker malformation, Fig. 2–16).

Communicating hydrocephalus, which results from the inability of fluid to pass from the subarachnoid space into the venous channels (via the arachnoid granulations) or the malformation of the arachnoid villi, produces excess fluid in the subarachnoid space with resultant pressure on the central nervous system. Obliteration of the subarachnoid cisterns or of the subarachnoid channels may produce this syndrome.

Hydrocephalus can produce thinning out of the bones of the skull with a prominent forehead and atrophy of the cerebral cortex and white matter, compression of the basal ganglia and diencephalon, and herniation of the brain into the foramen magnum. Depending on the severity of the brain damage the infant may die or survive with mental retardation, spasticity, ataxia, and other defects. Prior to closure of the sutures such pressure will result in an increase in the size of the head.

References

Adams, R., and Sidman, R. L.: *Introduction to Neuropathology.* New York, McGraw-Hill, 1968.

Altman, J.: Autoradiographic and histological studies of postnatal neurogenesis. J. comp. Neurol., *128:*431, 1966.

Angevine, J. B., and Sidman, R. L.: Autoradiographic study of cell migration during histogenesis of cerebral cortex in the mouse. Nature, *192:*766, 1961.

Berry, M., and Rogers, A. W.: The migration of neuroblasts in the developing cerebral cortex. J. Anat. (Lond.), *99.*691, 1965.

Berry, M., and Rogers, A. W.: Histogenesis of mammalian neocortex. *In* Hassler, R., and Stephans, H. (eds.): *Evolution of the Forebrain.* New York, Plenum Press, 1966, p. 197.

Fujita, S.: Kinetics of cellular proliferation. Exp. Cell Res., *28:*52, 1962.

Fujita, S., Shimada, M., and Nakanura, T.: H³ thymidine autoradiographic studies on the cell proliferation and differentiation in the external and internal granular layers of the mouse cerebellum. J. comp. Neurol., *128:*191, 1966.

Hamilton, W. J., Boyd, J. D., and Mossman, H. W.: *Human Embryology.* Cambridge, England, Heffer and Sons, 1964.

Larroche, J. Cl.: The Development of the Central Nervous System During Intrauterine Life. *In* Falkner, F. (ed.): *Human Development.* Philadelphia, W. B. Saunders, 1966, p. 257.

Sidman, R. L., and Feder, N.: Cell proliferation in the primitive ependymal zone: an autoradiographic study of histogenesis in the nervous system. Exp. Neurol., *1:*322, 1959.

Sidman, R. L., and Miale, I.: Histogenesis of the mouse cerebellum studies by autoradiography with tritiated thymidine. Anat. Rec., *133:*429, 1959.

3

Neurocytology

STANLEY JACOBSON

The nervous system consists of two basic elements: (1) nerve cells or neurons and (2) supporting cells—the glia, ependyma, Schwann cells, and satellites. In addition to these cells, there are blood vessels, fibroblasts, and protective coverings (meninges) associated with the nervous system (Fig. 3–1).

MICROSCOPIC EXAMINATION OF THE NERVOUS SYSTEM

Any investigation of the structure of the nervous system is complicated by the fact that there is no single stain which demonstrates all details of a neuron. However, there are many techniques available for microscopic examination of the nervous system. But before nerve tissues can be examined, they must be preserved (fixed). Neutral formalin is the most common fixative used for light microscopy.

The shapes of neurons and glia can be seen by means of the Golgi method, whereby thick blocks of nervous tissue are incrusted with heavy metals, more specifically silver or mercury. For some unexplained reason, with the Golgi method, only about 1 in every 60 cells stains completely so as to reveal the axon, soma, dendrites, and dendritic spines in full detail. A disadvantage of the Golgi method is that it does not reveal any details

of the internal structure of the neuron. However, the most pronounced organelle in the soma, the rough-surfaced endoplasmic reticulum (the Nissl substance) is demonstrable with basophilic dyes.

Neurons are argyrophilic (silver-lovers). Consequently silver nitrate, preceded by various fixatives and other chemicals, can be used to demonstrate normal neurons and the various organelles within them. These same techniques become even more potent in lesioned material because axons that are degenerating have an even greater affinity for silver; thus we can tell the degenerating axons from the normal axons (Nauta method, 1957; Fink and Heimer method, 1967; Heimer, 1970: Fig. 3–2). The myelin sheath covering the axon is best seen following preservation with potassium dichromate or osmium tetroxide. There is also a stain (the Marchi method) which demonstrates degenerating myelin sheaths (Swank and Davenport, 1935).

These experimental techniques for staining degenerating axons and myelin sheaths can enable the experimenter to trace a tract in the central nervous system and find out where it leads. For instance, if a lesion is made in the cortex, the axons can be traced down into the corpus striatum, the thalamus, and the various parts of the brain stem; degenerating axons can even be found going down into the spinal cord.

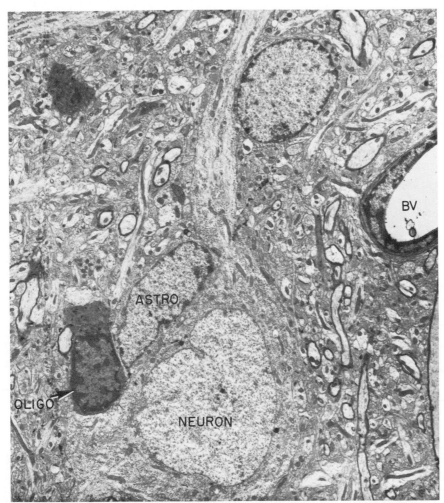

Figure 3–1 Electron micrograph of the cerebral cortex showing the principal cell types in the nervous system: neuron, astrocyte (astro), oligodendrocyte (oligo), and a blood vessel (BV). ×6000.

There is another method of tracing degenerating axons (the Weil or Weigert method) which is more commonly applied to human material. If, after many months following an injury to the brain, a myelin stain is applied to a block of tissue, those regions lacking myelin will be revealed. What has happened here is that the myelin and glia have been phagocytized by supporting cells (Wallerian degeneration) with only glia remaining; thus one can determine where a tract was—a sort of negative image (Fig. 3–3).

Synapses are demonstrable with silver stains; the best example of this is the Rasmussen method (1957). But only examination of tissue with the electron microscope reveals the detailed structure of the synapse, with its pre- and postsynaptic membranes, synaptic vesicles, and intersynaptic filaments.

In addition to the aforementioned techniques, there are the evoked potential methods employed by physiologists and psychologists to determine connections in the central nervous system. There are also chemical, fluorescent, and radiographic and immunological techniques in current use which can supply much information about the central nervous system, its connections, and structure.

THE NEURON

The basic functional unit of the nervous system is the neuron. The *neuron doctrine*,

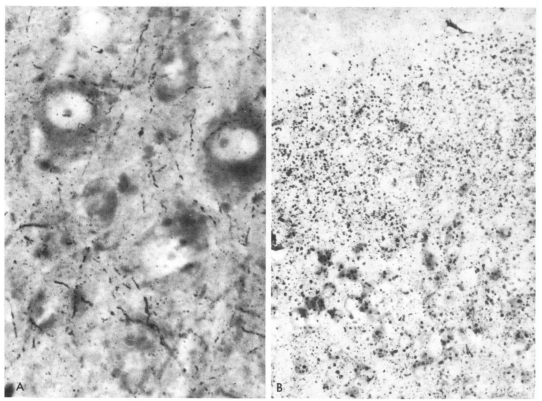

Figure 3–2 Terminal degeneration in the cerebral cortex of the rat. Fink-Heimer silver method. *A*, Axonal degeneration in the cerebral cortex in the cat. *B*, Terminal degeneration in the cerebral cortex of the rat. *A* ×600. *B* ×300.

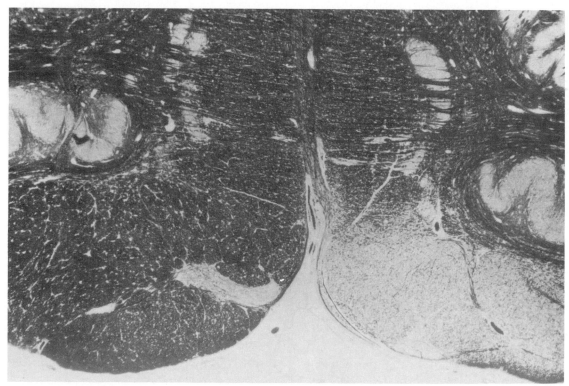

Figure 3–3 *Wallerian Degeneration.* Medullary pyramids in a human some months after a cortical infarct. *Left side,* normal; *right side,* note absence of myelin. ×80. Weigert myelin sheath stain.

38

as presented by Waldeyer in 1891, described the neuron as having one axon which is efferent and one or more dendrites which are afferent. In addition it was noted that the nerve cells are contiguous and not continuous and that all other elements of the nervous system are there to feed, protect, and support them. Although the neurons are not the only cells in the body capable of conducting impulses, (muscle cells can also conduct impulses) neurons, when arranged in networks and provided with adequate in-

formational input can store information and respond in many ways to any stimulus.

Neurons vary in size and shape and may be unipolar, bipolar, or multipolar. Even apolar cells may be found during stages of development. However, the most common neuron is multipolar.

In the adult nervous system the unipolar cells are found in the sensory ganglia of the spinal and cranial nerves and in the mesencephalic nucleus of cranial nerve V. In these cells a single process acts as the axon and

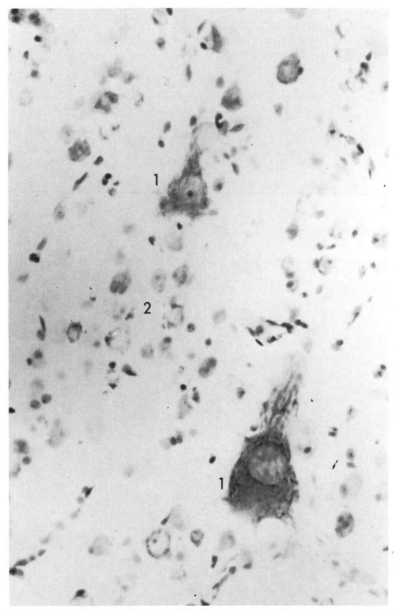

Figure 3-4 Motor cortex of the chimpanzee, demonstrating a pyramidal neuron. (1), Golgi type I cells; (2), a group of Golgi type II cells. Nissl stain, ×150.

dendrite. Bipolar neurons, which are sensory in function, are found in the retina, rods, and cones, in the olfactory neuroepithelial cells, in the olfactory mucosa in the nasal passages, and in the vestibular and auditory receptors in the inner ear.

Multipolar neurons are found throughout the central nervous system and in the sympathetic ganglia of the peripheral nervous system. They convey both sensory and motor impulses. The multipolar neurons vary greatly in size and in the complexity of their axonal and dendritic fields.

Golgi Type I and Golgi Type II Cells.
Neurons are segregated on the basis of the length of their axons: those with long axons are called Golgi Type I cells; those with short axons are known as Golgi Type II cells.

The majority of neurons in the central nervous system are the Golgi Type II cells; they form the internuncial cells of the central nervous system. The axons of the Golgi Type I cells form the tracts and commissures in the central nervous system, as well as the effectors of the peripheral nervous system.

In this section we are going to take as examples different cells found in the cerebral cortex. We will compare a cerebral pyramidal or Golgi Type I cell having a long axon (Fig. 3–4) with a stellate or Golgi Type II cell having a short axon (Fig. 3–5).

The Golgi Type II cell has a small dendrite and axonal field. The axon usually extends only short distances within the cerebral cortex (0.5 mm. to 5 mm.). The Golgi Type II cell has dendritic spines, but they are less numerous than those found on the Golgi Type I cell. Spines, which are common to many neurons, are small knob-shaped structures approximately 1 to 2 microns in diameter (Fig. 3–6*B, C, D*). Their importance stems from the fact that they greatly extend the receptive or synaptic surface of any dendrite.

The Golgi Type I cell or pyramidal cell (Fig. 3–6*A*) has an apical and a basal dendrite, each of which has numerous secondary, tertiary, quaternary branches, with smaller branches then arising from each of these branches. The branches extend into all planes. The spines of the pyramidal cell are absent from the initial segment of the apical and basal dendrite but they become very common farther along the dendritic branches. The axons of pyramidal neurons run long distances within the cortex, but they can also exit from the cortex and distribute to the subcortical nuclei.

PARTS OF THE NEURON

Each neuron has the following parts (Bodian, 1967):

1. The dendritic zone (dendrite and soma)
2. Axon origin (axon hillock)
3. Axon
4. Synaptic telodendria

The dendritic zone receives the input

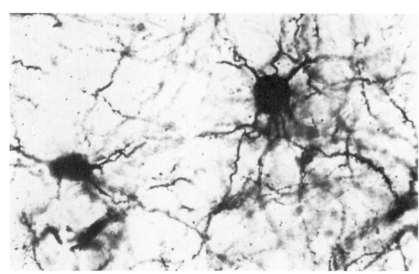

Figure 3–5 Golgi type II cells (neurons with short axons) in the motor cortex of the rat. Golgi neuronal stain, ×450.

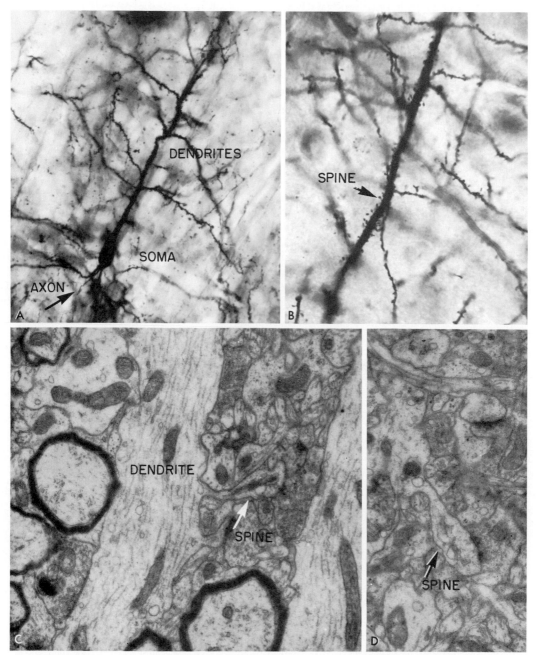

Figure 3–6 Golgi type I cells—neurons with long axons in the motor cortex of the rat. *A* shows entire cell—soma, axon, and dendrite; *B* demonstrates dendritic spines; *C* and *D* are electron micrographs of dendritic spines. *A*, Golgi stain, ×100; *B*, Golgi stain, ×250; *C* and *D*, ×30,000.

See Filmstrip, Frame 8.

which converges from many different sources. The action potential originates at the site of origin of the axon and is transmitted down the axon in an all-or-none phenomenon to the synaptic telodendria where the impulse is transmitted to the dendritic zone of the next neuron on the chain.

DENDRITIC ZONE

Soma. The soma (perikaryon or cell body) of the neuron varies greatly in form and size. Unipolar cells have circular cell bodies; bipolar cells have ovoid cell bodies; and multipolar cells have polygonal cell bodies.

The neuronal *nucleus*, found in the center of the cell body, is large and ovoid (Figs. 3–7 and 3–8). Within the nucleus there is usually only a single spherical nucleolus which stains strongly for RNA (ribonucleic acid). DNA (deoxyribonucleic acid), which can be demonstrated by staining the neuron with the Feulgen method, appears dispersed (heterochromatin) in mature neurons. These cells are very active in metabolizing protein; consequently the DNA is dispersed.

In females the cell body also contains a perinuclear accessory body, the *Barr body* (Fig. 3–9), discovered by Barr. The Barr body may be one of the X chromatins of the female which in this instance is in the euchromatin stage.

In the cytoplasm of the neuron are found the *organelles* which produce the metabolic requirement of the cell: Nissl substance, Golgi apparatus, mitochondria, and inclusions (Fig. 3–10). In addition most of the cytoplasm in the neuron is formed in the soma and flows into the other processes. As long as the soma with a majority of its organelles is intact, the nerve cell can live. Thus it is the trophic center of the neuron. Separation of a process from the soma produces death of that process.

Nissl Substance (Figs. 3–4 and 3–11). The Nissl substance, or the chromidial substance found in the cell bodies, can be demonstrated in the light microscope with basic dyes such as methylene blue, cresyl violet,

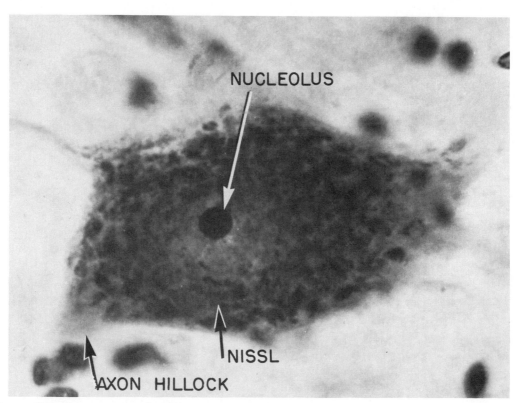

NUCLEOLUS

NISSL

AXON HILLOCK

Figure 3–7 Motor neuron from the ventral horn of a human, demonstrating Nissl substance, axon hillock, and nucleolus. Nissl stain, ×600.

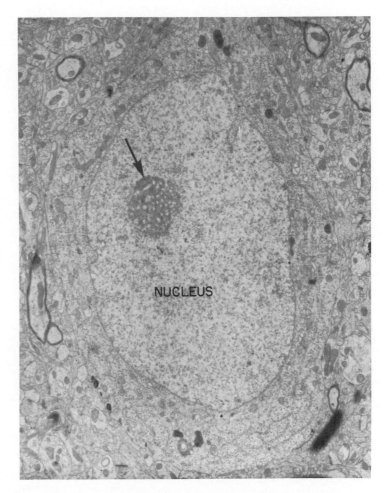

Figure 3-8 Electron micrograph of a neuron in the cerebral cortex of the rat, demonstrating the nucleus and nucleolus (arrow). ×10,000.

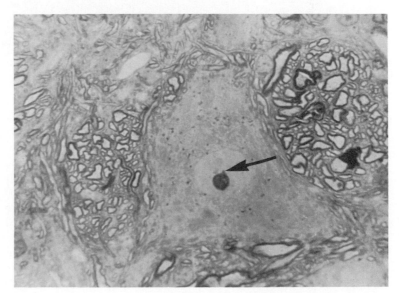

Figure 3-9 Motor neuron from the ventral horn of a squirrel monkey. Note the nucleus, nucleolus, and accessory body of Barr (arrow). One micron epoxy section. ×1400.

See Filmstrip, Frame 7.

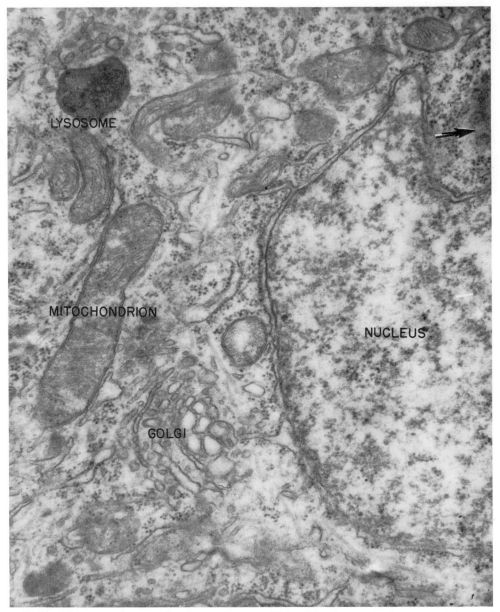

Figure 3–10 Electron micrograph of a small pyramidal cell in the cerebral cortex of the rat demonstrating the following organelles: Golgi apparatus, mitochondria, lysosome, and Nissl substance. Note the nuclear pore (arrow). ×60,000.

and toluidine blue. Its appearance and amount vary from cell to cell. With the electron microscope it is seen to consist of cisterns of parallel rows of interconnecting rough-surfaced endoplasmic reticulum (Fig. 3–11). Ribosomes are attached to the outer surfaces of the membranes.

The Nissl substance is most concentrated in the soma and adjacent parts of the dendrite (Fig. 3–12*A*). It is, however, also found throughout other parts of the dendrite (Fig. 3–12*B*). With the light microscope it was always presumed that the axon hillock was devoid of Nissl substance, but it has now been shown that there are polyribosomes in the region of the axon hillock. The Nissl substance, like the basophilic substance in all cells, is where amino acids are linked together to form proteins.

Golgi Apparatus (Fig. 3–10). The Golgi apparatus is demonstrated in light microscopic sections with osmium and silver. It appears as an irregular network, commonly in a perinuclear location, and is found in all cells. In electron micrographs it is seen to consist of stacks of flattened smooth surface membranes, called saccules.

The protein secretion from the Nissl substance is transferred to the Golgi apparatus where the carbohydrate component is added to the protein and released as secretory vesicles. Current evidence suggests that some of the secretory vesicles may participate in membrane formation throughout the cell.

Mitochondria (Figs. 3–10 and 3–12). These organelles are found throughout the neuron. They are rod-shaped and vary in size from .25 to 10μ in length and .25 to $.5\mu$ in diameter. Mitochondria can be demonstrated in light microscopic tissue, but details of their structure are best seen in electron micrographs. The walls of mitochondria consist of two membranes—an outer and an inner membrane. The inner membrane is thrown into folds called cristae that project into the center of the mitochondrion. The interior of the mitochondria is filled with a fluid which is commonly denser than cytoplasm; cations have been demonstrated in the mitochondrial matrix.

On the inner membrane, enzymes which provide much of the vital role required for the nerve cell have been localized; these respiratory enzymes (flavoproteins and cytochromes) catalyze the addition of a phosphate group to ADP (adenosine diphosphate), forming ATP (adenosine triphosphate) which is broken down to ADP in the cytoplasm, providing the energy required for the metabolic functions in the cell. In the cytoplasm are found enzymes which break down glucose into pyruvic and acetoacetic acid. These substances are taken into the mitochondrial matrix and participate in the Krebs citric acid cycle whereby the mito-

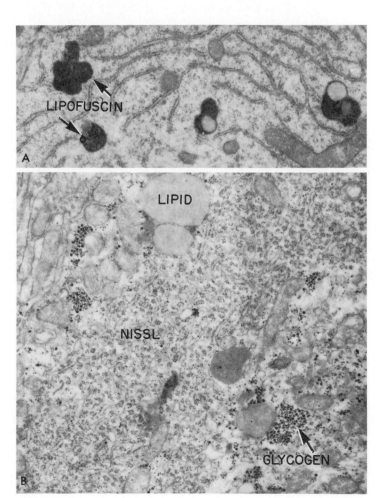

Figure 3–11 Electron micrographs showing (*A*) lipofuscin; (*B*) glycogen, lipid, and Nissl substance. ×20,000.

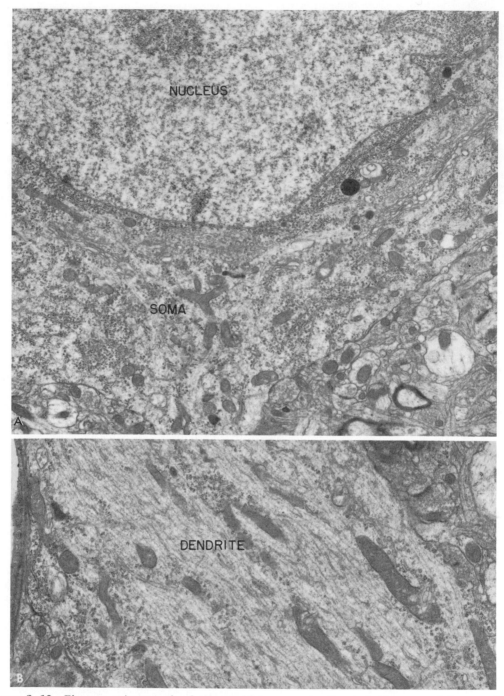

Figure 3–12 Electron micrograph of a pyramidal neuron in the cerebral cortex of the rat: *A*, Soma and nucleus; *B*, Dendrite. Note the large amount of Nissl substance in the soma, while in the dendrite there is less Nissl substance and many microtubules. ×25,000.

chondria metabolize amino acids and fatty acids.

Lysosomes (Figs. 3–10 and 3–14). These are most common in the cell body and appear as a dense body in light and electron microscopy. They are membrane-bound and vary in size from .25 to 2μ in diameter and commonly contain small granules. Hydrolytic enzymes, acid hydrolysates, have been localized in the lysosomes and are capable of breaking down protein, DNA, RNA, and certain carbohydrates. The lysosomes help in the digestion of macromolecules by forming membrane-lined vesicles (deDuve and Wattiaux, 1966).

Centrosomes. Centrioles are seen in the immature, dividing neuroblast and also in the adult neuron. However, the mature neurons are incapable of dividing and therefore it is questionable whether centrosomes have any function in the adult nerve cell.

In silver-stained sections examined in the light microscope a *neurofibrillar* network can be seen in the neurons (Fig. 3–13). In electron micrographs no corresponding network has been seen; instead, *neurotubules*, 200 to 300 Å in diameter, and *neurofilaments*, 100 Å in diameter, are present. It appears that fixation produces clumping of the tubules and filaments into the fibrillar network.

Neurotubules (microtubules) predominate in dendrites and in the axon hillock, while filaments are few in dendrites and most numerous in axons (Fig. 3–16). Current evidence suggests that the neurotubules may be involved in the flow of various substances from the soma into the cell body and axon, while the filaments may form a cytoskeleton

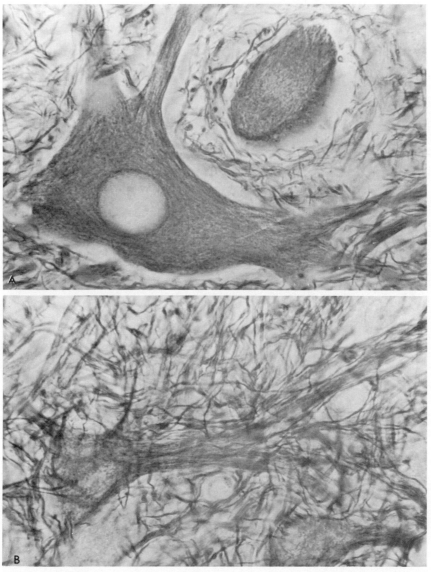

Figure 3–13　Neurofibrillar stain of a ventral horn cell in the cat spinal cord, showing neurofibrillar network in soma and dendrites. (*A*); and in axons (*B*). ×400.

See Filmstrip, Frame 9.

for the nerves. Neurotubules may possibly also participate in the transmission of nerve impulses.

Inclusions. These are substances which are stored in a cell and include pigment, glycogen and lipid droplets. Pigment granules (melanin) are common in certain parts of the brain—the substantia nigra and locus ceruleus (Fig. 3–14). In man *lipochrome* pigment (lipofuscin) (Fig. 3–11*A*) is found in most cells and appears to increase with age. This consists of pigment combined with some fatty material and probably is a metabolic by-product which is not readily disposable. It is commonly referred to as the wear-and-tear pigment. The lipofuscin pigment is probably a result of lysosomal activity.

Glycogen (Fig. 3–11*B*) is a polymer of d-glucose and is commonly seen in electron micrographs of nerve cells and glia. The glycogen appears in the form of electron-dense rosettes much larger than the RNA rosettes, and they are a local source of energy.

Lipid droplets (Fig. 3–11*B*) are seen in the soma and represent a local store of energy as well as a source of carbon chains for membrane formation.

Neurosecretion. Neurons in the supraoptic and paraventricular nuclei of the hypothalamus form neurosecretory material (Bodian, 1963, 1966; Palay, 1957; Scharrer, 1966).

The axons of these cells form the hypothalamic-hypophyseal tract which runs through the median eminence down the infundibular stalk to the neurohypophysis (pars nervosa) where the axons are seen to end in close proximity to the endothelial lining of the blood vessels (Fig. 3–15*A*). The vesicles in these endings are 1200 to 1500 Å in diameter. The secretory granules are 120 to 150 millimicrons in diameter and are found in the tract (Fig. 3–15). They appear to gain in size as one approaches the endothelial end of the axons.

The protein is made in the Nissl substance; the granules are formed in the Golgi apparatus. They are transported by the axons of the hypothalamic-hypophyseal tract to the infundibulum where they are stored in the neural lobe. The places of storage of the neurosecretory granules are called Herring bodies (Fig. 3–15*B*). Interruption of the hypothalamic-hypophyseal tract produces diabetes insipidus. (See Chapter 16.)

AXON AND AXON ORIGIN

The axon contains some elongate mitochondria, many filaments which are oriented parallel or collateral to the long axis of the axon (Fig. 3–16), and some tubules. (A dendrite contains a few filaments and many tubules, all of which are arranged parallel to the long axis of the dendrite.)

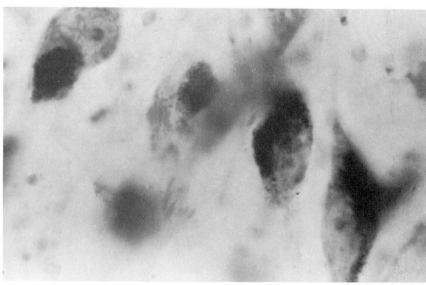

Figure 3–14 Neurons in substantia nigra of the human, demonstrating melanin pigment. ×300.

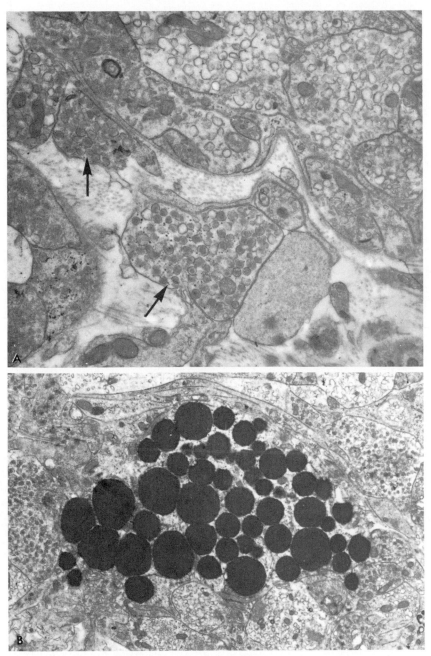

Figure 3–15 Electron micrograph of rat neurohypophysis. *A* shows neurosecretory granules in the axoplasm of fibers of the hypothalamo-hypophyseal tract, ×20,000. *B* demonstrates a Herring body which is a site of storage of neurosecretory material. ×8000.

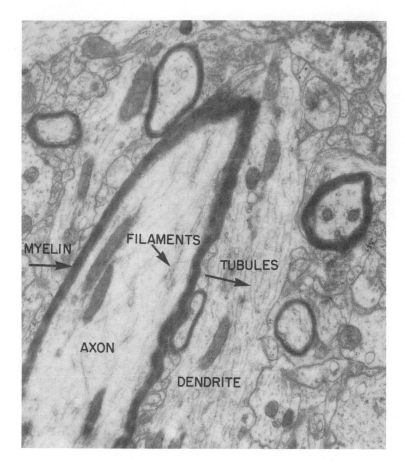

Figure 3–16 Electron micrograph of the rat cerebral cortex demonstrating the difference between a myelinated axon and a dendrite. Note the axon has numerous filaments while the dendrite has numerous microtubules. ×20,000.

Polyribosomes are present, but the highly organized, rough endoplasmic reticulum is absent.

Axon Hillock. The axon hillock is a slender process which usually arises from a cone-shaped process (axon hillock) on the perikaryon (Fig. 3–17A). Axons, however, may also arise from dendritic processes. With the light microscope the axon hillock appears devoid of structure (Fig. 3–17A), while in an electron micrograph, filaments, tubules, and polyribosomes can be seen (Fig. 3–17B). The axonal membrane at the hillock is covered by an electron-dense material.

Myelin. In the nervous system axons may be myelinated or unmyelinated. The myelin is formed by a supporting cell, which in the central nervous system is called the oligodendrocyte and in the peripheral nervous system, the Schwann cell. Thus, the myelin sheath is not a part of the neuron; it is a covering for the axon. Myelin consists of segments approximately .5 to 1 mm. in length. Between these segments are nodes, the nodes of Ranvier; the axon, however, is

continuous at the nodes, and axon collaterals can leave at the nodes.

In the peripheral nervous system, there is usually only one Schwann cell for each length (internode) of myelin. In the central nervous system each oligodendrocyte may form and maintain myelin sheaths on 30 to 60 axons.

The unmyelinated axons in the peripheral nervous system are found in the cytoplasm of the Schwann cell. There can be as many as 12 unmyelinated axons in one Schwann cell. The unmyelinated axons in the central nervous system are usually found in small bundles without any special covering.

Peripheral and Central Nerve Structure.
Peripheral Nerves. The structure of a peripheral nerve is different from that of the fiber bundles in the central nervous system. Peripheral nerves consist of many axons, called a fascicle, held together by connective tissue of mesodermal origin (Fig. 3–19). The outer layer, covering nerve trunks and filling in between the individual fascicles, is called the epineurium which consists of con-

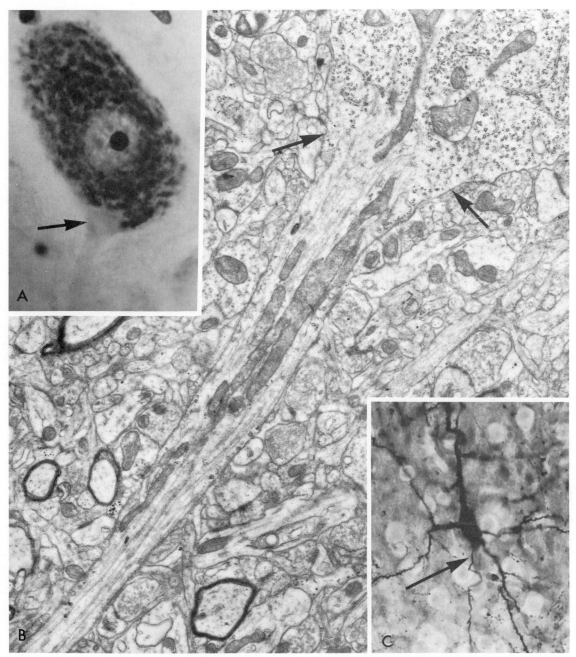

Figure 3–17 Appearance of axon hillock in (*A*) Nissl stain, (*B*) electron micrograph, (*C*) Golgi stain. *A*, ×400; *B*, ×15,000; *C*, ×250.

nective tissue cells, collagen, and some fat cells. Each of the fascicles is wrapped in a dense layer of connective tissue which is called the perineurium. Strands of collagen, fibroblasts, and other cells run between the individual nerve fibers to form the endoneurium. The term endoneurium is also applied to the delicate trabeculum surrounding each nerve fiber. This term is synonymous with the sheath of Key-Retzius. Remember, the peripheral nerve fiber or axon is engulfed in the Schwann cytoplasm (neurilemmal sheath) which also forms the myelin sheath. Large blood vessels are found in the

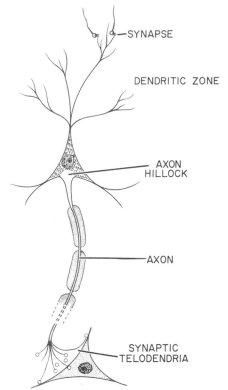

SYNAPSE

DENDRITIC ZONE

AXON HILLOCK

AXON

SYNAPTIC TELODENDRIA

Figure 3–18 Schematic drawing of a multipolar neuron demonstrating dendritic zone (dendrite and soma), axon hillock, axon covered with myelin, and synaptic telodendria.

epineurium and perineurium and capillaries are seen in the endoneurium.

Fiber diameters can vary from less than half a micron up to 22 microns. Depending on size and function the axons can be classified into three groups—types A, B, and C. (See Chapter 5.) The group A fibers are myelinated somatic efferent and afferent fibers, 1 to 22 microns in diameter. They conduct at 5 to 120 meters per second.

The group B fibers are myelinated efferent preganglionic autonomic fibers, 1 to 3 microns in diameter. They conduct at 3 to 15 meters per second.

The group C fibers are unmyelinated afferent or efferent postganglionic sympathetic fibers, .3 to 1.3 microns in diameter. They conduct at .5 to 2 meters per second.

Central Nervous System. Axons in the central nervous system also vary in size ($5-22\mu$), but it is impossible to separate these axons into functional categories based on only axonal diameter.

The axons in the central nervous system run in groups called tracts. These tracts

are enwrapped by processes of fibrous astrocytes. There is, however, no specific covering which corresponds to the endoneurium, epineurium, or perineurium. In the central nervous system each axon is encircled by an oligodendral glial sheath which corresponds to the sheath of Schwann in the peripheral nervous system.

The axonal arborization of neurons is usually not as elaborate as that of the dendrite. Although the surface area of many dendrites may total more than that of an axon, some axons run very long distances, i.e., from cerebral cortex to the motor neurons in the sacral spinal cord or from a motor neuron in the spinal cord out and down a peripheral nerve all the way to a muscle in the foot.

Action Potentials. The axon potentials from other neurons are received on the dendrites and, to a lesser degree, in the soma. The action potential is generated at or near the axon hillock and is then propagated down the axon as an all-or-none phenomenon to the synaptic telodendria. Axons vary in length in a continuous spectrum from the short axons of the Golgi type II cell to the long axons of the ventral horn cells in the spinal cord.

Many axon terminals are found on any one neuron. These terminals come from many sources. The dendrite does not respond in an all-or-none fashion like the axon. Instead, each nerve impulse at a given site on the dendrite produces a change in the electrical activity. The sum total of all of these electrical changes will result in a variation in the threshold in the neuron either below or above the firing level. As previously stated, the axon conducts the action potential, in an all-or-none fashion, to the synaptic telodendria.

SYNAPTIC TELODENDRIA

The synaptic telodendria consists of the axonal ending, which forms the presynaptic side, and the dendritic zone (dendrite and soma), which forms the postsynaptic side. Collectively the pre- and postsynaptic sides are called the synapse.

The synapse is the place where the nervous impulse from one cell is transmitted to another. Synapses vary in size from the large endings on motor neurons (1 to 3 microns) to smaller synapses on the granule and stellate cells of the cortex and cerebellum (much less than one-half micron). Synapses

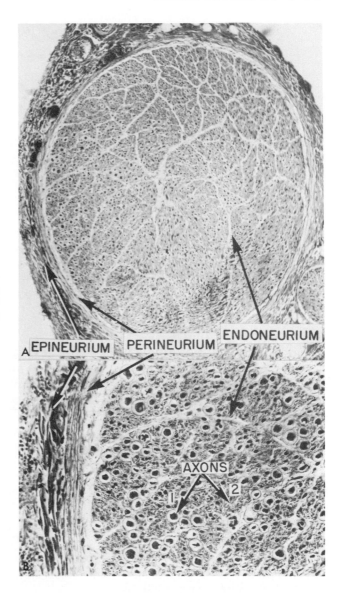

Figure 3–19 Peripheral nerve of the cat. In *B*, 1 demonstrates a large myelinated axon, while 2 points to a small myelinated and unmyelinated axon. Bodian stain: *A*, ×100; *B*, ×350.

primarily occur between the axon of one cell and the dendrite of another cell, and are commonly located on the dendritic spines. Synapses are also seen on the soma and rarely between axons. At the synaptic telodendria the axon arborizes and forms several synaptic bulbs (Fig. 3–20) which are attached to the plasma membrane of the opposing neuron by intersynaptic filaments.

Synaptic Structure. Synapses can be identified in the light microscope, but the electron microscope has revealed many new details in synaptic structure (Bodian, 1966, 1970; Colonnier, 1969; Gray, 1959; Palay, 1967). In an electron micrograph, the pre-synaptic or axonal side contains mitochondria and many synaptic vesicles (Fig. 3–21). Synaptic vesicles are most concentrated near the presynaptic surface with some vesicles actually seen fusing with a membrane, thus suggesting that this is the site of release of the transmitter substance. Neurofilaments are usually absent on the presynaptic side. Pre- and postsynaptic membranes are electron-dense and are separated by a 300 to 400 Å space, the synaptic cleft, which is continuous with the extracellular space of the central nervous system.

Throughout much of the central nervous system, bulbous-shaped dendritic spines are found on the dendrites. In the cerebral cortex a spine apparatus is found within the

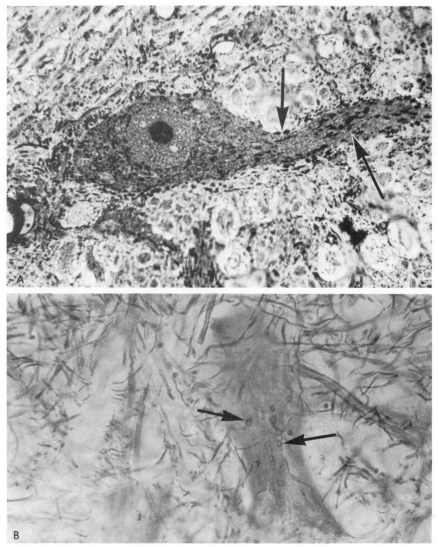

Figure 3–20 Silver stains demonstrating synaptic boutons: *A*, neurons in reticular formation in rat; *B*, ventral horn cells in cat. ×400.

See Filmstrip, Frame 9.

spine. This spine apparatus has been considered to function much as a capacitor, charging up and then discharging when its current load is exceeded (Fig. 3–6).

In the central nervous system, the opposing pre- and postsynaptic membranes are usually thickened. Intersynaptic filaments are seen running through the synaptic cleft connecting the pre- and postsynaptic membranes. A postsynaptic web is formed under the postsynaptic membrane on dendrites; these synapses are called asymmetrical endings (Fig. 3–21), while synapses on the soma are symmetrical (they have no postsynaptic web). Even though the membranes are attached, the cells are contiguous and not con-

tinuous, they are separated by the extracellular space. This is, of course, consistent with the neuron doctrine of Waldeyer.

Synaptic Vesicles. In electron micrographs synaptic vesicles differ in size and shape depending on the fixative used. Synaptic vesicles may be agranular, spherical, flattened, or round with a dense core. The method of fixation will affect the shape of a vesicle. Bodian (1970) has shown that osmium fixation produces only spheroidal vesicles. Aldehyde followed by osmium produces spheroidal and flattened vesicles. The shape of the flattened vesicles may be modified by washing the tissue in buffer or placing the tissue directly from the aldehyde into osmium. The spheroidal vesicles retain their shape regardless of any manipulation.

There are four basic categories of synaptic vesicles (Palay, 1967) which may be described as follows:

1. The most common vesicle is 200 to 400 Å in diameter, is spheroidal, with a clear center, and is found at neuromuscular junctions in skeletal muscle, and throughout the central nervous system (Fig. 3–21). Acetylcholine is presumed to be the transmitter in these synapses.

2. The second category is 400 to 800 Å in diameter, is spheroidal, and has a 280 Å electron-dense granule in the center. These vesicles are found in autonomic endings in the intestine, vas deferens and pineal body.

3. The third type is 800 to 900 Å in diameter and is spheroidal, with a 500 Å electron-dense granule in the center. These vesicles are found at preganglionic sympathetic sites in the autonomic nervous system, at neuro-muscular junctions in smooth muscle, and in part of the hypothalamus, basal nuclei, brain stem, and cerebellum. Catecholamines may be involved with transmission of these sites.

4. The last type is 1200 to 1500 Å in diameter and spheroidal and contains a large droplet which nearly fills the vesicle. These vesicles are characteristic of nerve endings in the neurohypophysis and are found *only* in the soma, axons, and presynaptic endings of nerve cells which form the hypothalamic-hypophyseal tract. Vasopressin (ADH-anti-diuretic hormone) and oxytocin have been associated with these granules (Fig. 3–15*A*).

Synaptic Transmission. Current evidence suggests (McLennan, 1969) that synaptic transmission is a chemically and not

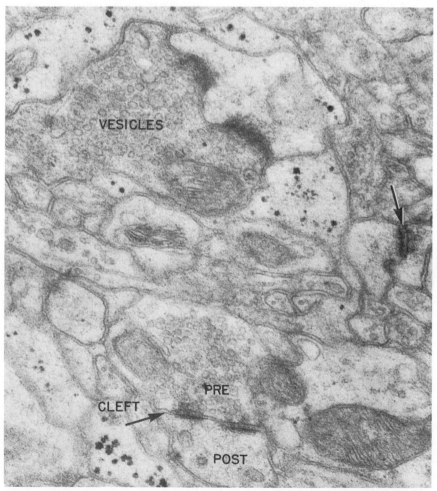

Figure 3–21 Synapse in the cerebral cortex of the rat demonstrating agranular synaptic vesicle (300 to 500 Å) in the presynaptic axonal side. Note the electron dense synaptic membranes and the intersynaptic filaments in the cleft. ×65,000.

electrically mediated phenomenon, based on the presence of (1) a 300 to 400 Å cleft, (2) synaptic vesicles, and (3) appreciable synaptic delay. Various chemical substances have been found which can partake in synaptic transmission.

Acetylcholine is the best documented transmitter in the central and peripheral nervous systems. Acetylcholine has been isolated in synaptic vesicles and acetylcholine esterase has been found throughout the central and peripheral nervous systems and at postganglionic sympathetic endings.

Catecholamines and 5-hydroxytryptamine have also been linked to synaptic transmission in the central nervous system. Noradrenaline has been associated with transmission in the preganglionic sympathetic synapses. Glutamine, glycine, and GABA (gamma-amino butyric acid) have also been shown to participate in nervous transmission. There is still much uncertainty as to whether these aforementioned substances normally participate in nervous transmission. ATP, substance P, histamine, prostaglandin, steroids, and hormones have also been linked to synaptic transmission. It is still uncertain whether these compounds play a direct role in nervous transmission or if they are just related by their importance to the ongoing functions of the entire body.

RECEPTORS AND EFFECTORS

Each peripheral nerve, whether sensory, motor, or secretory, terminates by arborizing in a peripheral structure (Fig. 3–22).

EFFECTORS

The motor or efferent nerves from the *somatic nervous system* end in skeletal muscles and form the motor end plates. In smooth and cardiac muscle and in glands nerve

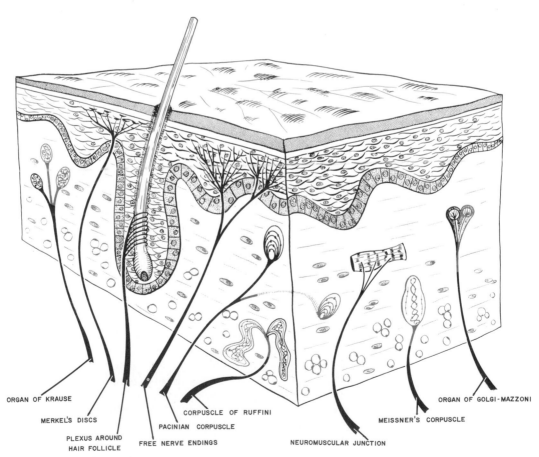

ORGAN OF KRAUSE

MERKEL'S DISCS

PLEXUS AROUND HAIR FOLLICLE

FREE NERVE ENDINGS

PACINIAN CORPUSCLE

CORPUSCLE OF RUFFINI

NEUROMUSCULAR JUNCTION

MEISSNER'S CORPUSCLE

ORGAN OF GOLGI-MAZZONI

Figure 3–22 Stereogram of the skin, demonstrating sensory receptors and effectors. (After Noback, C. R.: *The Human Nervous System.* New York, McGraw-Hill, 1967.)

endings resemble the synaptic endings in the central nervous system.

Visceral motor endings are seen on muscles in arterioles (vasomotor), muscles in hair follicles (pilomotor), and sweat glands (sudomotor).

RECEPTORS

Sensory endings are found throughout the body and are modified according to the functional specialization of the region. Visceral sensory receptors are similar to somatic sensory receptors associated with the somatic nervous system, except that they are located in the viscera and their accessory organs. The sensory endings subserve pain, touch, temperature, vibration, pressure, heat, cold, proprioception in skin, muscles, and viscera as well as the specialized somatic and visceral sensations of taste, smell, vision, audition, and balance.

Free Nerve Endings. Free nerve endings are formed by sensory fibers which arborize in various tissues including stratified epithelium, muscle, tendon, connective tissue, mucous, serous membranes, and joints. These receptors are considered to be pain receptors as they are found in tissues where pain is the primary sensation, i.e., tooth pulp and dentin, and cornea. Crude touch may also be subserved by these receptors.

Free nerve endings are also found in terminal networks around the disc-shaped tactile cells of Merkel and around the hair follicles in the dermal sheath and outer root sheath. These structures appear to subserve touch.

Encapsulated Sensory Endings. In these endings the nerve is surrounded by a specialized connective tissue capsule of varying thickness. These include Meissner corpuscles, Paccinian corpuscles, muscle and tendon spindles, and the cylindrical end bulb of Krause, and the end bulb of Golgi-Mazzoni.

Meissner Corpuscles. Meissner (tactile) corpuscles are presumed to subserve touch. They are elliptical and may have from one to five myelinated nerve fibers arborizing in their lamellated capsule. These end organs are found in dermal papillae, being most numerous in fingertips, soles and palms, lips, glans penis, and clitoris.

Paccinian Corpuscles. These corpuscles resemble a sliced onion bulb with numerous concentric layers built upon the centrally placed axon. They are found throughout subcutaneous tissue and are especially numerous in the hand, foot, mammary glands, clitoris, and penis. These corpuscles are pressure receptors. Herbst's corpuscles are similar to the Paccinian corpuscles but are smaller.

End Bulb of Krause and End Bulb of Golgi-Mazzoni. These endings contain a single extensively ramified axon within their matrix and are found throughout the body. Many variants of this structure have been identified. This organ is presumed to subserve heat and cold.

Muscle and Tendon Spindles. The *muscle spindles* and annulospiral endings in muscles, as well as the *tendon spindles* and free nerve endings in muscles, are proprioceptive endings which transmit information concerning muscular activity and tendon stretching into the central nervous system.

It should be noted that all the sensory endings are the *primary* neurons in the sensory system; their cell bodies are located in the spinal and cranial nerve ganglia and their axons enter the central nervous system. The motor or effector axons represent the *final* neuron in the motor system.

SUPPORTING CELLS

There are billions of neurons in the central nervous system, but the number of nonnervous cells exceeds them by about five or six times. The astrocytes, oligodendrocytes, microglia, and ependyma are the supporting cells or neuroglia (nerve glue) of the central nervous system, while the Schwann cells, satellite cells, and fibroblasts are the supporting cells of the peripheral nervous system. These cells thus form the structural matrix of the central nervous system, but they also play a vital role in transporting gas, water, electrolytes, and metabolites from blood vessels to the neural parenchyma and in removing waste products from the neuron. In contrast to the neuron, the supporting cells in the adult CNS normally undergo mitotic divisions.

Astrocytes (Figs. 3–23, 3–24). There are two types of astrocytes in the central nervous system: fibrous and protoplasmic. The fibrous astrocytes are most common in white matter; the protoplasmic astrocytes are most

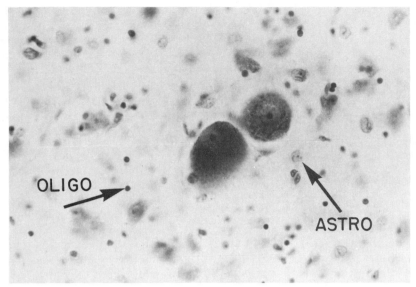

Figure 3–23 Appearance of neuron, astrocyte (astro), and oligodendrocyte (oligo). Nissl stain, ×300.

common in gray matter. All astrocytes are larger and less dense than the oligodendrocytes. The astrocytes form a complete membrane on the external surface of the brain (external glial limiting membrane), surround all blood vessels, and fuse with the ependymal processes to form the internal glial limiting membrane (Fig. 3–25). The processes of these cells intermingle with neuronal processes and tend to separate neuronal processes.

Electron micrographs demonstrate that these cells have many filaments which in places appear to fill the cytoplasm except where the other organelles are seen. There are few microtubules, and the processes appear pale. The nuclei of these cells have some condensed chromatin adjacent to the nuclear membrane. Glycogen is also common in astrocytic processes. In light micrographs the astrocyte appears as a pale cell with little if any detail of the cytoplasm, with the nuclear size being smaller than a neuron but larger and less dense than an oligodendrocyte (Fig. 3–23). Protoplasmic astrocytes have a nucleus which is a little darker than that of a neuron and are similar to the fibrous astrocytes except that they have few filaments.

Functionally, astrocytes not only form the skeleton of the central nervous system, but they also tend to segregate synapses in the central nervous system and also help to form a barrier at the inner and outer surface of the brain and around the blood vessels (outer and inner limiting membrane). In addition, astrocytes may proliferate and form scars following the death of neurons, and in combination with the endothelial cells they help to form the blood-brain barrier.

When disease processes in the central nervous system affect only astrocytes, the reaction is called primary astrogliosis. More commonly the disease process affects nerve cells primarily with the resultant reaction of the astrocytes being called secondary astrogliosis. When an injury occurs to the nerve cell in the central nervous system without any concomitant injury to blood vessels and glia, the nerve cells will be phagocytized and the astrocytes proliferate and replace the neurons forming a glial scar (replacement gliosis). In a more severe injury to the nervous system—an infarct, in which glia, nerve cell, and blood vessels are injured—the astrocytes will proliferate along the walls of the injury and the remainder of the dead nerve cells and glia will be phagocytized, leaving only a cavity covered over with meninges. In all other organs there are enough fibroblasts to proliferate and form a scar, but in the central nervous system there are only a few fibroblasts in relation to blood vessels so that cavitation is a common sequel to extensive destruction.

Oligodendrocytes. In light micrographs the oligodendrocyte has a small darkly stained nucleus surrounded by a thin ring of cytoplasm (Fig. 3–23). In electron micrographs oligodendrocytes are dense cells with many microtubules and few neurofilaments (Fig. 3–24). They have dense clumps of rough endoplasmic reticulum and clusters of polyribosomes which are seen in the cytoplasm. The cytoplasm is denser but scantier than that found in a neuron. The nucleus tends to be located more toward one pole of the cell; the nuclear chromatin tends to be heavily clumped. In electron micrographs (Fig. 3–24) oligodendrocytes can be differentiated from astrocytes because they have a darker cytoplasm and nucleus and more heavily condensed chromatin and few if any filaments.

Oligodendrocytes form and maintain myelin; they also may digest myelin. These cells are also seen in close proximity to the nerve cells even where there is no myelin,

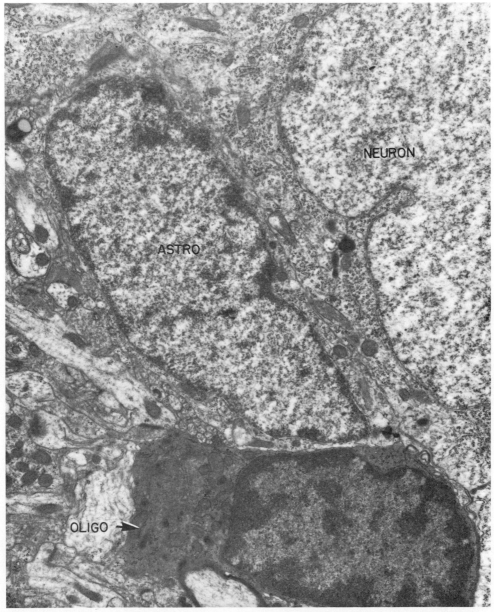

Figure 3–24 Electron micrograph demonstrating appearance of neuron, astrocyte (astro), and oligodendrocyte (oligo). ×18,000.

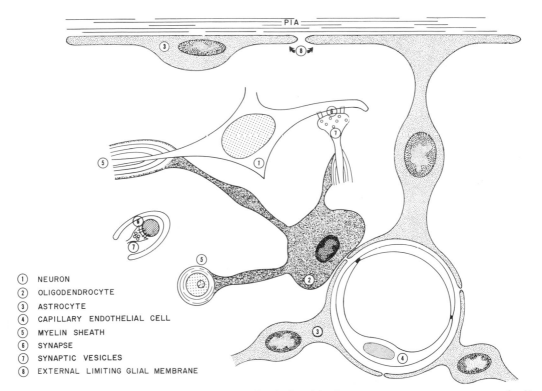

Figure 3-25 Diagrammatic representation of relationship between neuron, astrocyte, and oligo-dendrocyte.

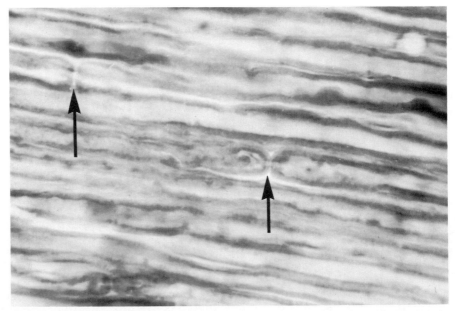

Figure 3-26 Longitudinal section of a peripheral nerve fixed in osmium, demonstrating nodes of Ranvier (arrow). ×1000.

which has suggested some as yet undemonstrated symbiotic relationship between neurons and oligodendrocytes.

The *myelin sheath* is in contact with the axon. In light microscopy it appears as a tube. The myelin sheaths are discontinuous tubes 0.5 to 2 mm. in length, interrupted at the node (Fig. 3–26). The axon is devoid of myelin at the site of origin, at the nodes, and at the axonal telodendria. At the site of origin the axon is covered by an electron-dense membrane, and at the site of the synaptic telodendria the various axonal endings are isolated from one another by astrocytic processes. The lipid and protein layers of myelin are arranged in alternating concentric layers about 170 Å apart. In electron micrographs each myelin lamella actually consists of two-unit membranes with the entire lamella being

130 to 180 Å thick (Fig. 3–27). Myelin is thus seen to consist of a series of light and dark lines. The dark line is called the major dense line. The less dense line is called the interperiod line. The major dense line represents the apposition of the inner surface of the unit membranes, while the interperiod line represents the approximation of the outer surfaces of adjacent myelin membranes.

The *process of myelination* has been followed with the electron microscope. An axon starts with just a covering formed by the plasma membrane of either the Schwann cell or the oligodendrocyte. More and more layers are added until myelination is complete. One theory is that myelin is laid down by the Schwann cell twisting around the axon (Geren, 1956; Robertson, 1955). This may well occur in the peripheral nervous system,

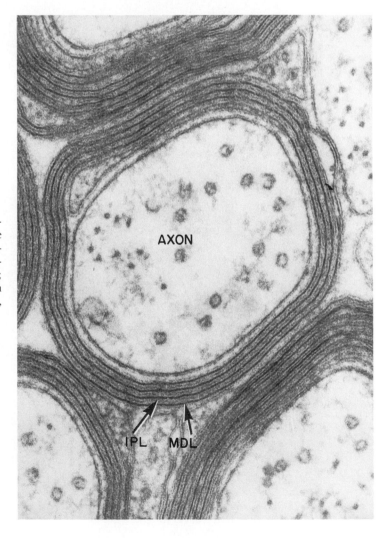

Figure 3–27 Electron micrograph of myelin sheath from the optic nerve of the mouse, demonstrating repeating units of myelin sheath. IPL = interperiod line; MDL = major dense line. (From Peters, A.: J. Cell Biol., *20*:281, 1964).

but in the central nervous system each oligo-dendrocyte enwraps many axons. Thus another method would seem to be suggested. Another possibility is that myelin is laid down in concentric layers by a process which might be similar to the formation of a shell.

Microglia. The nerve cell, astrocyte, and oligodendrocyte are ectodermal in origin while the microglial cell is mesodermal in origin (Fig. 3-28). These ovoid cells are the smallest of the supporting cells. In electron micrographs they are not as electron-dense as the oligodendrocyte and lack the tubules of the oligodendrocyte and the filaments of

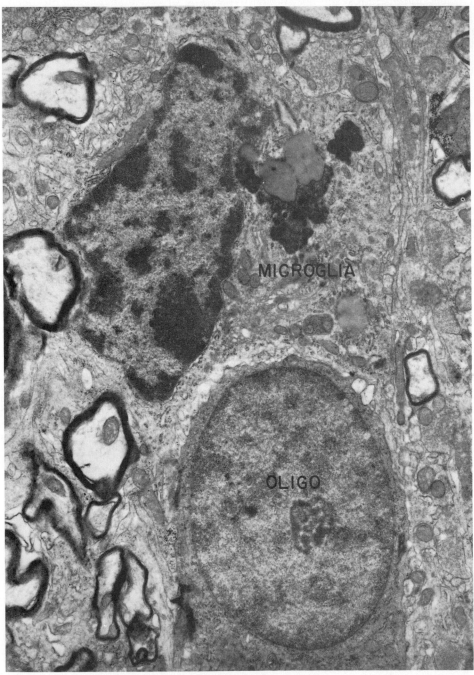

Figure 3–28 Electron micrograph of human cerebral cortex demonstrating differences between microglial cells and oligodendrocyte (oligo). ×20,000.

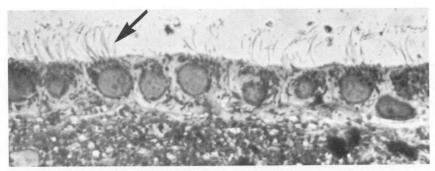

Figure 3–29 Ependymal lining cells in third ventricle of the rat. Note prominent cilia (arrows). ×1400.

the astrocyte. The cytoplasm is denser than that of the astrocyte and contains fat droplets and laminar dense bodies. The granular endoplasmic reticulum consists of long stringy cisterns. This cell has been called a multipotential glial cell since it appears to be able to act as a phagocyte or to become an astrocyte or oligodendrocyte (Vaughn and Peters, 1968).

Mononuclear Cells (Lymphocytes, monocytes and histiocytes). These cells have also been traced in the central nervous system and also seem to act as phagocytes, breaking down the myelin and nerve cells. Myelin destruction always triggers intense macrophage reaction within 48 hours. It should be pointed out that in experimental tissue in electron micrographs astrocytes have also been shown to engulf degenerating myelin sheaths, axonal processes, and degenerating synapses.

Ependymal Cells (Fig. 3–29). These cells line all parts of the ventricular system. They are cuboidal and ciliated and contain filaments and all the other organelles. The process of this cell extends in the central nervous system and fuses with astrocytic processes to form the inner limiting glial membrane. Highly modified ependymal cells are found attached to the blood vessels in the roof of the body and the inferior horn of the lateral ventricles, and the third and fourth ventricles, where they form the choroid plexus which secretes much of the cerebrospinal fluid (Fig. 3–30).

Satellite Cells (Fig. 3–31). Satellite cells are found in sensory and sympathetic ganglia and originate from neural crest cells. Many satellite cells envelop a ganglion cell. Functionally, they are similar to astrocytes although they look more like oligodendrocytes.

Schwann Cells. The Schwann cell in the peripheral nervous system functions like the oligodendrocyte, forming the myelin and neurilemmal sheath. In addition, the unmyelinated axons are embedded in their cytoplasm. The Schwann cell cytoplasm stops before the node, leaving a space between the node and the Schwann cell. In an injured nerve the Schwann cells can form tubes which go through the scar and permit regeneration of the peripheral axon.

DEGENERATION

Neuronal death or atrophy may result as a consequence of trauma, circulatory insufficiency, tumors, infections, metabolic insufficiency, developmental defects, and degenerative and heredodegenerative diseases. These neuropathological processes will produce responses in the nerve cells and glia (Ramon y Cajal, 1928; Young, 1942). The neuronal response to injury will be examined in the cell body and axon.

NEURONAL RESPONSE TO INJURY

Retrograde Changes in the Cell Body. Section of the axon or direct injury to the dendrites or cell body produces the following series of responses in the various organelles in the soma (see Fig. 3–32).

1. The nucleus, cell body, and nucleolus swell. The nucleus becomes displaced from the center of the cell body and may even lie adjacent to the plasma membrane of the neuron.

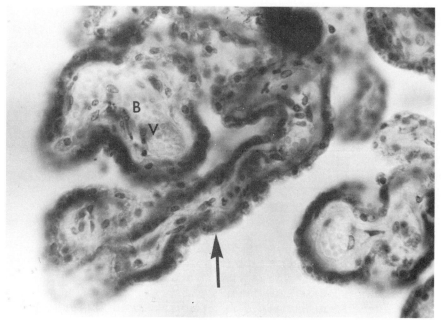

Figure 3–30 Choroid plexus in the fourth ventricle (human). Note the blood vessels (BV) in the center and the cuboidal epithelial cells on the outside. ×200.

2. The Nissl substance begins to dissolve starting centrally and proceeding peripherally until only the most peripherally placed Nissl substance is still intact. This dissolution of the Nissl substance (RNA) occurs in order that the protein manufacturing processes can be mobilized to help the neuron successfully survive the injury.

3. All other organelles in the cell body and dendrites also respond to the injury. The

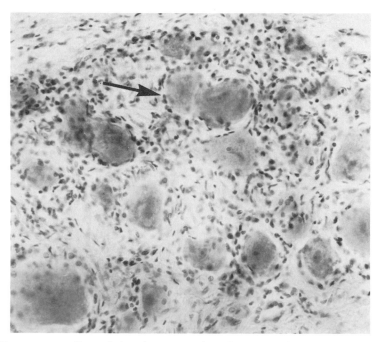

Figure 3–31 Sensory ganglion of the rhesus monkey demonstrating neurons surrounded by satellite cells (arrow). ×300.

mitochondria swell, and the Golgi substance appears to proliferate.

These responses represent the increased energy requirements of the nerve cell and the need to form plasma membrane during the regenerative process. If the cell successfully survives the injury, all organelles return to their normal appearance: the nucleus returns to the center of the cell body, and the soma returns to its pretraumatic size. If the injury is too extensive the nerve cell will atrophy or die.

Atrophic Change. In the instance of atrophic change the nerve cell is too severely damaged to repair itself. Consequently, the cell body shrinks and becomes irregular in profile. The nucleus also shrinks. The neurofibrils become more prominent. This response is similar to the response of a nerve cell when there is an insufficient blood supply, which produces an ischemic neuron.

In necrosis, if a nerve cell is too damaged to survive, the Nissl substance begins to disperse, and by seven days the nucleus has become dark and the cytoplasm eosinophilic. Within a few days these cells will be phagocytized.

Wallerian Degeneration. When an axon is sectioned, the distal part, separated from the trophic center or cell body, degenerates, a process called *Wallerian* or *anterograde degeneration.* At the same time the cell body reacts in a process called *axonal* or *retrograde degeneration.* If the cell body is intact the proximal portion will begin to regenerate. The distal stump will be viable for a few days, but degeneration will already have begun within 12 hour. The axon starts to degenerate before the myelin sheath, within four to seven days the axon appears beaded and is beginning to be phagocytized by macrophages, which probably come in

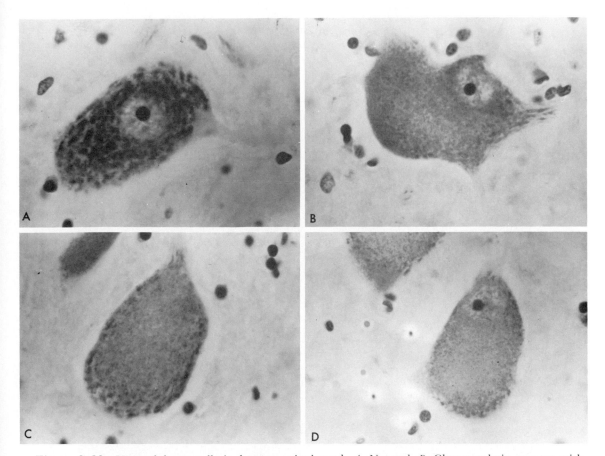

Figure 3–32 Ventral horn cells in human spinal cord. *A,* Normal. *B,* Chromatolytic neuron with eccentric nucleus and some dissolution of the Nissl substance. *C,* Chromatolytic neurons showing a peripheral ring of Nissl substance (peripheral chromatolysis). *D,* Chromatolytic neuron showing eccentric nucleus and only a peripheral ring of Nissl substance. Nissl stain, ×400.

See Filmstrip, Frame 10.

from the circulation. The fragments of degenerating axons and myelin lie in digestion chambers (Fig. 3–33), and it may be several months before all of the degenerating fragments are ingested. In the proximal portion, degenerative changes are noted back to the first unaffected node. The myelin, as it degenerates, is broken up into small pieces so that it can be ingested more easily (Figs. 3–34 and 3–35).

GLIAL RESPONSE TO INJURY

Neuronal death will produce a migration of cells into the region of the dead or dying

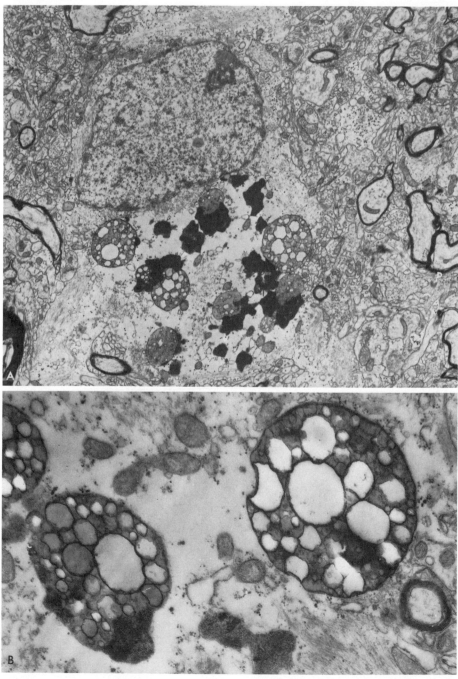

Figure 3–33 Electron micrograph of a reactive astrocyte in the cerebral cortex of a human. Note the prominent digestion vacuoles shown in higher power (*B*). *A*, ×8000; *B*, ×25,000.

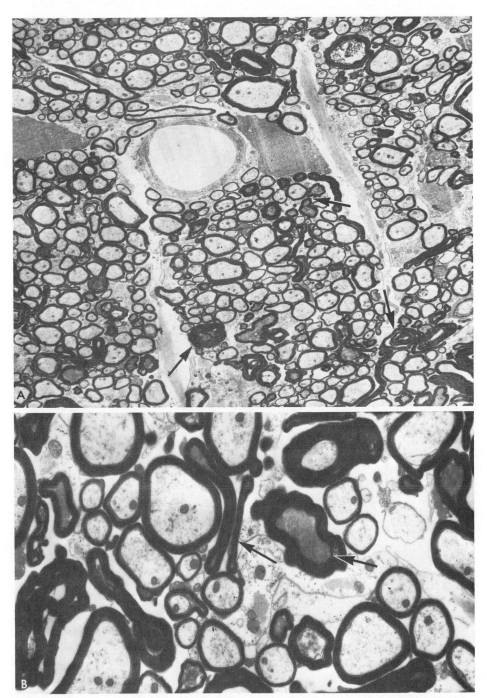

Figure 3–34 Electron micrograph of degenerating axons in the medullary pyramid of a rat 15 days after a cortical lesion. *A*, Arrows point to some degenerating axons. ×8000. *B*, Showing details of degenerating axons. Note the collapsed axons and dense axoplasm and that many axons were unaffected by the lesion. ×20,000.

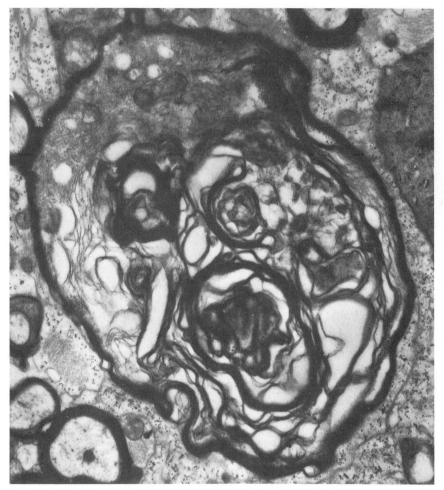

Figure 3–35 Electron micrograph of a degenerating myelin sheath in the medullary pyramid of the rat 30 days after a cortical lesion. Note the unraveling and vacuolization of the myelin. × 20,000.

cells. These phagocytic cells proliferate by mitosis and break down the dying neurons.

Necrosis. Within a few days of an ischemic attack neutrophils are seen at the site of the injury. Shortly thereafter microglial cells and histiocytes will be seen in the region of the dying cells. The blood-brain barrier is affected so that monocytes may now migrate into the parenchyma of the central nervous system. The time it takes for the complete removal of the injured cells depends on the size of the lesion; large infarcts may take several years before phagocytosis is complete. If the lesion is very large i.e., a large infarct in the precentral gyrus, a cavity will form with the edges of the cavity sealed by an astrocytic scar. In small lesions the neurons will be phagocytized and the astrocytes will proliferate and fill in or replace the space occupied by the neurons, a process called replacement gliosis. In organs with numerous fibroblasts, necrotic areas are soon filled in by proliferation of fibroblast, but in the central nervous system there are too few fibroblasts for this, while the astrocytes do not proliferate in sufficient numbers.

NERVE REGENERATION

Peripheral Nerve Regeneration. In the peripheral nervous system, within a few days after section, the proximal part of the nerve starts regrowing. If a wound is clean, i.e., a stab wound, and the nerve ends are sewn together, the regenerating nerves may cross the scar within a week (Fig. 3–36). In certain disease processes in the peripheral nervous system only segmental degeneration occurs as with the diphtheria toxin; the myelin sheath degenerates and the axon remains intact. Phagocytes break down the myelin

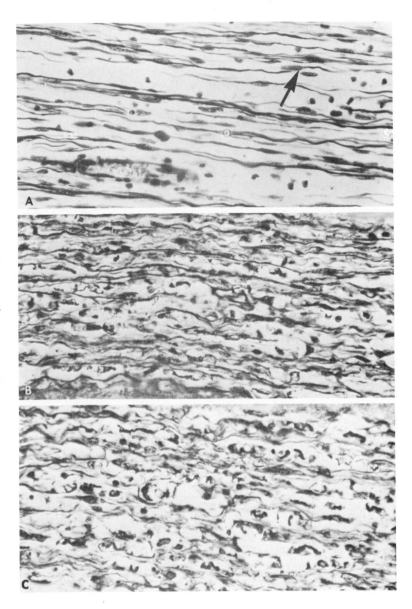

Figure 3–36 Sciatic nerve of a rat demonstrating appearance of regenerating nerves 3 weeks after crushing injury. *A,* At the site of the lesion the nerves look similar to a normal nerve (arrow identifies Schwann cell nucleus). *B,* About 20 mm. distal to site of injury, note some regenerating axons and many axon fragments. *C,* About 25 mm. from site of the crush showing transition from regenerating axons to only degenerating axons. Bodian silver stain, ×500.

and the Schwann cells rapidly re-form myelin. The process of the regenerating nerves crossing the scar is helped by the Schwann cells and fibroblasts which proliferate from the proximal end and, to a lesser degree, from the distal ends, providing tubes for the regenerating axons to grow through.

As the regenerating axons grow the axonal end sprouts many little processes. If one axonal sprout gets through the scar the other sprouts will degenerate and the axon will then follow the path established by the penetrating sprout. If an axon reaches one of the tubes formed by the Schwann cells, it will grow quickly. Once it crosses the scar it will grow down the distal stump at a rate of about 3 or 4 millimeters a day (Jacobson and Guth, 1965; Guth and Jacobson, 1966).

When the motor end plate is reached there is some delay until the axon reinnervates the muscle and reestablishes function, producing an average rate of regeneration of 1–2 mm a day.

Only a small percentage of the nerves reach the effectors or receptors and only chance determines where the regenerating nerve goes. If a sensory fiber innervates a motor end plate it will remain nonfunctional and probably degenerate with the cell body undergoing atrophy. If a sensory fiber reaches a sensory receptor it can become functional, though it may be the wrong receptor. An example of this is a patient, who, after nerve regeneration, complains that rubbing or pressing the skin produces pain. It would appear that a fiber sensitive to pain has reached a tactile or pressure sensitive receptor. A motor fiber can also reinnervate the wrong motor end plate, i.e., a flexor axon innervating an extensor. In such a case the patient will then require retraining in order to learn to use this new arrangement.

Successful regeneration also depends on an adequate blood supply. If a lesion is huge, i.e., a gun shot leaving a large gap, the nerve will attempt to regenerate but will not succeed. If the lesion injures the cell body, regeneration may not occur and the cell may even die.

Central Nerve Regeneration. Following injury, axons, in the central nervous system attempt to regenerate, but the oligodendrocytes and astrocytes do not form tubes. Instead they form a scar which prohibits the axon's growth through the scar. Even if the axons get through the scar by chance, they have no way of reaching the neuron to which they were originally connected and, in fact, seem not to form new synapses.

Regenerating axons in the central nervous system may grow and grow and form a ball — a neuronal ball or neuroma. In time, in the damaged regions of the central nervous system, the dead neurons and axons are phagocytized by the glia and macrophages and the astrocytic scar usually remains behind.

Nerve Growth Factors. Many people are interested in nerve growth factors which would help speed regeneration in the peripheral and central nervous systems. Certain factors have been found but they have never been able to be produced by investigators in large enough quantities (Levi-Montalcini and Angeletti, 1968). Also, attempts have been made to help regeneration in the central nervous system, for instance by placing Teflon tubes through the scarred portion of the spinal cord in the hope that the nerves would grow down these channels. Even though nerves have grown down these channels there has been no functional recovery. Further information is needed as to the chemical nature of the scar which retards the axonal regeneration. Even if the axon grows, the factors which direct the axon seem to be available only in the immature nervous system so that the axon has no direction as to where to go.

BLOOD-BRAIN BARRIER

All vascular branches within the central nervous system are surrounded by a thin covering formed by the processes of astrocytes (Fig. 3 -25). The plasma in the blood vessel is separated from the actual central nervous system tissue by the endothelial lining of the blood vessel and the basement membrane. The extracellular space of the central nervous system lies external to the basement membrane. The astrocyte processes which surround the blood vessel do not fuse with the endothelial lining of the blood vessel or with the processes of other cells. Consequently the extracellular space will be entered once the endothelium is passed. The opposing endothelial plasma membranes form tight junctions so that the capillaries are not perforated. The blood-brain barrier thus consists of the endothelial lining cells and the perivascular processes of astrocytes.

The intravenous perfusion of various dye compounds (trypan blue or proflavine HCl) into the blood-brain barrier demonstrates staining only in the astrocytic processes. In certain places the blood-brain barrier is incomplete and the nervous parenchyma stains with the dye: pineal body, pituitary, area postrema, subfornial organ, choroid plexus, and locus ceruleus (Brightman, 1965; Dempsey and Wislocki, 1955; Wislocki and Leduc, 1952). The intravenous injection of large molecules (ferritin, horseradishes peroxidase) has demonstrated that these molecules will not pass out through the endothelial lining cells (Brightman, 1965, Reese and Karnovsky). When they are injected into the central nervous system they will fill the extracellular spaces between the glia and neurons, but they will not penetrate back into the blood vessels (Reese and Karnovsky, 1968). These studies have shown that the blood-brain barrier is impermeable to certain dye compounds, but substances such as gases, water, glucose, electrolytes (Na^+, K^+, and Cl^+), and amino acids can pass from the plasma into the intracellular space (in neurons and glia) or into the extracellular space between neurons and glia. Acute lesions of the central nervous system usually produce an increase in the permeability of the barrier and cause alterations in the concentration of water, electrolytes, and protein.

Between the cells in the central nervous system there is some extracellular space, measuring between 200 and 400 Å. The amount of extracellular space in the brain is still a matter of controversy. Physiologists speak of a 25 to 40 per cent space, while electron microscopists have calculated a 5 to 15 per cent space. Regardless of the percentage of the extracellular space, solutes can readily pass from the blood plasma through the endothelial lining into the extracellular space. It also appears that a portion of the cerebrospinal fluid is formed by the diffusion of extracellular fluid.

References

Barr, M., and Bertram, R.: A morphological distinction between neurones of the male and female, and the behaviour of the nucleolar satellite during accelerated nucleoprotein synthesis. Nature, *163*:676, 1949.

Bodian, D.: Cytological aspects of neurosecretion in opossum neurohypophyses. Bull. Johns Hopk. Hosp., *113*:57, 1963.

Bodian, D.: Herring bodies and neuroapocrine secretion in the monkey. An electron microscopic study of the fate of the neurosecretory product. Bull. Johns Hopk. Hosp., *118*:282, 1966.

Bodian, D.: Neurons, circuits and neuroglia. *In* Quarton, G. C., Melnechuk, T., and Schmitt, F. O. (eds.): *The Neurosciences: A Study Program.* New York, The Rockefeller University Press, 1967.

Bodian, D.: An electron microscopic characterization of classes of synaptic vesicles by means of controlled aldehyde fixation. J. Cell Biol., *44*:115, 1970.

Brightman, M. W.: The distribution within the brain of ferritin injected into cerebrospinal fluid compartments: I. Ependymal distribution. J. Cell Biol., *26*:99, 1965.

Brightman, M. W.: The distribution within the brain of ferritin injected into the cerebrospinal fluid compartments: II. Parenchymal distribution. Am. J. Anat., *117*:193, 1965.

Colonnier, M.: Synaptic patterns on different cell types in the different laminae of the cat visual cortex: An electron microscopic study. Brain Res., *9*:268, 1969.

deDuve, C., and Wattiaux, R.: Functions of lysosomes. Annual Rev. Physiol., *28*:435, 1966.

Dempsey, E. W., and Wislocki, G. B.: An electron microscopic study of the blood-brain barrier in the rat, employing silver nitrate as a vital stain. J. biophys. biochem. Cytol., *1*:245, 1955.

Fink, R. P., and Heimer, L.: Two methods for selective silver impregnation of degenerating axons and their synaptic endings in the central nervous system. Brain Res., *4*:369, 1967.

Garrison, F. H.: *An Introduction to the History of Medicine.* Philadelphia, W. B. Saunders, 1960.

Geren, B. B.: Structural studies of the formation of the myelin sheath in peripheral nerve fibers. *In* Rudnick, D. (ed.): *Cellular Mechanisms in Differentiation and Growth.* Princeton, Princeton University Press, 1956.

Gray, E. G.: Axosomatic and axodendritic synapses of the cerebral cortex: an electron microscopic study. J. Anat., *93*:420, 1959.

Guth, L.: Regeneration in the mammalian peripheral nervous system. Physiol. Rev., *36*:441, 1956.

Guth, L., and Jacobson, S.: The rate of regeneration of the cat vagus nerve. Exp. Neurol., *14*:439, 1966.

Heimer, L.: Bridging the gap between light and electron microscopy in the experimental tracing of fiber connections. *In* Nauta, W. J. H., and Ebbeson, S. O. E. (eds.): *Contemporary Research Methods in Neuroanatomy.* New York, Springer-Verlag, 1970.

Heimer, L.: Selective silver impregnation of degenerating axoplasm. *In* Nauta, W. J. H., and Ebbeson, S. O. E. (eds.): *Contemporary Research Methods in Neuroanatomy.* New York, Springer-Verlag, 1970.

Jacobson, S., and Guth, L.: An electrophysiological study of the early stages of peripheral nerve regeneration. Exp. Neurol., *11*:48, 1965.

Levi-Montalcini, R., and Angeletti, P. U.: Biological aspects of the nerve growth factor. *In* Wolstenholme, C. E., and O'Connor, M. (eds.): *Growth of the Nervous System.* Boston, Little, Brown and Company, 1968.

McLennan, H.: *Synaptic Transmission.* Philadelphia, W. B. Saunders, 1970.

Nauta, W. J. H.: Silver impregnation of degenerating axons. *In* Windle, W. F. (ed.): *New Research Techniques of Neuroanatomy.* Springfield, Illinois, Charles C Thomas, 1957.

Palay, S. L.: The fine structure of the neurohypophysis, *In* Waelsek, H. (ed.): *Progress in Neurobiology: II. Ultrastructure and Cellular Chemistry of Neural Tissue.* New York, Paul B. Hoeber, 1957.

Palay, S. L.: Principles of cellular organization in the nervous system, *In* Quarton, G. C., Melnechuk, T, and Schmitt, F. O. (eds.): *The Neurosciences: A Study Program.* New York, The Rockefeller University Press, 1967.

Peters, A.: The fixation of central nervous tissue and the analyses of electron micrographs of the neuropil, with special reference to the cerebral cortex. *In* Nauta, W. J. H., and Ebbeson, S. O. E. (eds.): *Contemporary Research Methods in Neuroanatomy.* New York, Springer-Verlag, 1970.

Ramon y Cajal, S.: *Histologie du Systeme Nerveux de l'homme et des vertebres.* Paris, A. Maloine, 1909.

Ramon y Cajal, S.: *Degeneration and Regeneration of the Nervous System.* London, Oxford University Press, 1928.

Rasmussen, G. T.: Selective silver impregnation of synaptic endings. *In* Windle, W. F. (ed.): *New Research Techniques of Neuroanatomy.* Springfield, Illinois, Charles C Thomas, 1957.

Reese, T. S., and Karnovsky, M. J.: Fine structural localization of a blood-brain barrier to exogenous peroxidase. J. Cell Biol., *34*:207, 1968.

Robertson, J. D.: The ultrastructure of adult vertebrate peripheral myelinated nerve fibers in relation to myelin agenesis. J. biophys. biochem. Cytol., *1*:271, 1955.

Scharrer, E.: *Endocrines and the Central Nervous System.* Baltimore, Williams and Wilkins, 1966.

Sidman, R. L.: Autoradiographic methods and principles for study of the nervous system with thymidine-H^3, *In* Nauta, W. J. H., and Ebbeson, S. O. E. (eds.): *Contemporary Research Methods in Neuroanatomy.* New York, Springer-Verlag, 1970.

Swank, R. L., and Davenport, H. A.: Chlorate-osmic-formalin method for staining degenerating myelin stain. *Techn.*, *10*:87, 1935.

Vaughn, J. E., and Peters, A.: A third neuroglial cell type: An electron microscopic study. J. Comp. Neurol., *133*:269, 1968.

Wislocki, G. B., and Leduc, E. H.: Vital staining of the hematoencephalic barrier by silver nitrate and trypan blue and cytological comparisons of neurohypophysis, pineal body, area postrema, intercolumnar tubercle and supraoptic crest. J. Comp. Neurol., *96*:371, 1952.

Young, J. Z.: Functional repair of nervous tissue. Physiol. Rev., *22*:318, 1942.

4

Cell Physiology

BRIAN CURTIS

Cell physiology is the study of the function of individual cells. In this chapter we will consider the cells of the nervous system. Research has demonstrated four very important and interesting properties of such cells:

1. There are gross inequalities of chemical concentration between the inside and outside of the cells. For example, in the human, the concentrations of Na, K, and Cl are as follows:

ION	SERUM	MUSCLE
Na	145 mM	12 mM
K	4 mM	155 mM
Cl	120 mM	4 mM

2. The solution inside the cell is electrically negative with respect to the outside solution.
3. Some ions move through the cell membrane more easily than others.
4. The ease with which certain ions move through the cell membrane can vary in time. These four properties are interrelated and form the basis of all cell function in the nervous system.

To understand the interrelation of the properties and how these properties interact in nerve function, the student must first have a modest understanding of the behavior of ions in solution and of the equations that describe this behavior. Although a detailed discussion of the physical chemistry of solutions may seem a digression, such physical chemistry forms a basis for our present understanding of nerve function, nerve-muscle junction activity, and the integrative activity of a motor neuron of the spinal cord. Further, many other phenomena in medicine rest on the same basis of solution theory.

Both an intuitive approach and a more rigorous approach to the derivation and consequences of a few simple equations will be given, the former appearing in large type, the latter in smaller type at appropriate places in the discussion. The discussion in small type will assume a modest knowledge of calculus and thermodynamics.

ENERGY

We know intuitively that a reservoir full of water contains a certain amount of energy; it has the potential to do some work as it flows from the reservoir. Whether this work is the frictional heat of water falling on rock or the rotation of the turbine of an electric generator is largely a measure of the cunning of the engineer. We know, however, that the energy of the reservoir is conserved; it goes somewhere and is turned into some kind of work.

Energy can be defined in terms of heat and pressure-volume work.

$$dU = q - w \qquad (4-1)$$

where U = the internal energy,
  q = heat absorbed by the system, and
  w = work done by the system.

The first law of thermodynamics states that the internal energy of a system is conserved.

The second law defines the elusive measure of energy, entropy:

$$dS = \frac{q}{T} \qquad (4-2)$$

where S = entropy
  q = heat absorbed
  T = temperature

Adding this relationship to the statement of the first law we obtain

$$dU = TdS - dw \qquad (4-3)$$

or since

$$dw = PdV$$

$$dU = TdS - PdV \qquad (4-4)$$

This energy function is not very convenient for use in biological systems. An energy function derived by the American, J. Willard Gibbs (1876), is much easier to handle, both experimentally and conceptually. It is defined as

$$G = U + PV - TS \qquad (4-5)$$

On differentiation:

$$dG = dU + PdV + VdP - TdS - SdT \qquad (4-6)$$

When the expression for dU shown in (4-4) is substituted into (4-6), then

$$dG = SdT + VdP \qquad (4-7)$$

The Gibbs free energy function is of great value because at constant temperature the troublesome entropy factor drops out.

If water flows from a reservoir, the distance the water falls is the *potential* of the system to do work. The amount of work done is basically dependent on the size or *capacity* of the reservoir. The total extractable work, the energy of the system, is proportional to the distance (i.e., potential) the water can fall and the amount (i.e., capacity) of water available to fall.

Similarly, the total energy of *any system* is equal to the product of a *potential factor* and a *capacity factor*. Several examples are given in the following table:

TYPE OF ENERGY	POTENTIAL (or Intrinsic) FACTOR	CAPACITY (or Extrinsic) FACTOR
Gravitational	Height	Weight
Expansion	Pressure	Volume
Electrical	Voltage	Current
Heat	Temperature	Caloric content

It is the potential factor that determines whether any work will proceed at all. We can get work from two reservoirs of water only if they are at different heights. Heat will flow between two bodies only if they are of different temperatures. The idea of a difference in potential is crucial to an understanding of the direction in which a system can go. Of its own accord, a stone can only roll downhill.

THE CHEMICAL POTENTIAL

Cells exist in aqueous solutions. Consequently, it is the energy of aqueous systems and their potential for doing work that are of interest to us in the study of cell physiology. The potential factor, called the *chemical potential,* is analogous to all the other potential factors, such as height, temperature, pressure, or voltage. The capacity factor is the number of moles involved in the reaction.

Metallic sodium reacts with water to form sodium hydroxide, hydrogen, and heat. The chemical potential of pure sodium is greater than that of sodium hydroxide. Consequently, the reaction proceeds spontaneously and energy is liberated. The reaction proceeds from a state of higher chemical potential to a state of lower chemical potential; all spontaneous reactions do. The reactants have a higher chemical potential than do the products. The total amount of energy liberated, as you might expect, depends on the number of moles of sodium that react.

It turns out that the chemical potential (μ_i) of a simple reactant is, to a first approximation, a very simple function of concentration,

$$\mu_i = \mu^0_i + RT \ln C_i$$

where μ^0_i = standard state chemical potential
   R = a constant
   T = absolute temperature of the solution
   C_i = molar concentration of the reactant

μ^0_i is the chemical potential of a 1 molar solution of the reactant at $273°K$ ($0°C$) and 760 mm. Hg pressure. It enters the equation because of the units chosen for concentration. Note that when $C_i = 1$, $\mu = \mu^°$, because ln 1 = 0.

The Gibbs free energy (G) can be a function of many properties of a system. The one of greatest interest to us is the number of moles of substance in the system. A function, the chemical potential, is defined as

$$\mu_i = \frac{\delta G}{\delta n_i}\bigg]_{T, P, n_j} \tag{4–8}$$

where μ_i = chemical potential
   n_i = number of moles of the i species and T, P, and n_j are constant

Since biological systems operate at constant temperature and pressure, the equation

$$dG = -SdT + VdP + \sum_{i=1}^{c} \mu_i \, dn_i \tag{4–9}$$

becomes

$$dG = \sum_{i=1}^{c} \mu_i \, dn_i \tag{4–10}$$

We see that μ_i and n_i become the sole determinants of the free energy of the system. The energy of a system containing one substance at constant T and P is

$$G = n_\gamma \, \mu_\gamma$$

For more than one substance, the energy of a system at constant T and P is

$$G = n_\delta \, \mu_\delta + n_\beta \, \mu_\beta + n_\alpha \, \mu_\alpha + \ldots + n_g \, \mu_g$$

In the study of the movement of a substance through cell membranes, an important factor is the difference, if any, in chemical potential between the inside of the cell and the outside solution. Unless this is known, only conjectures can be made about the nature of the process by which the substance enters the cell. If the substance is moving from a region of low chemical potential to one of high chemical potential we know immediately that energy must be expended.

To sum up, the chemical potential is, as the name implies, a potential function. We expect that energy will flow from a phase of greater chemical potential to a phase of lower chemical potential. This principle is the cornerstone of thermodynamics. The maximum work we can get from a system is equal to the product of the chemical potential times the number of moles involved.

If, however, the chemical potential is equal in two phases, we do not expect energy to flow. Two phases are, by definition, in equilibrium when the chemical potentials of the two phases are equal.

DIFFUSION

The flow of mass is one form of work in which energy can be expended. All of you have seen the classic demonstration of a crystal of potassium permanganate dropped into a cylinder of water. The purple color gradually spreads throughout the cylinder. The color change indicates that permanganate ions are spreading through the water by the mechanism of diffusion. The potassium and permanganate ions are moving from a region of high chemical potential to a region of low chemical potential.

Diffusion is an irreversible process and as such is not included under the heading of thermodynamics. Thermodynamics describes the condition of unequal chemical potential which leads to diffusion; it also describes the condition of equal chemical potential, of final equilibrium. Thermodynamics does not, however, describe the kinetic pathway between the two states. Diffusion is described by the equation

$$\frac{\Delta \text{ moles}}{\Delta t} = -DA \frac{\Delta c_i}{\Delta x}$$

where
Δt = time   A = area available for
D = constant   diffusion
              $\Delta c_i / \Delta x$ = concentration
                        gradient

The number of moles of glucose that will flow per minute from a solution of 2 molar glucose to a solution of 1 molar glucose is dependent on the area of contact between the two solutions. Clearly, the greater the area exposed, the greater the flow. The diffusion constant, D, varies inversely as the molecular weight of the diffusing particle, usually as the square root of the molecular weight. It is also inversely proportional to the viscosity of the fluid.

Specific solutions to the diffusion equation for various boundary conditions (physical situations) are fairly difficult to derive and harder to solve. There is an excellent book, *Diffusion Processes* by M. H. Jacobs, which clearly discusses the problem. It is more profitable for us to look at three specific examples.

Linear Diffusion. When a substance is diffusing in an infinitely long tube, the rate of diffusion is proportional to the square of the distance. After diffusion has progressed a while, the log of the concentration at any point along the tube will be proportional to the square of the distance from the original interface.

$$\ln(C)_2 = -\frac{X_2^2}{4Dt}$$

where
$(C)_2$ = concentration at any point
X_2 = distance to that point from the original interface
D = diffusion coefficient
t = time elapsed

The diffusion equation was derived by Einstein from first principles (see, for example, Jacobs, p. 12), and D, the diffusion constant, can be written as

$$D = \frac{RT}{N} \cdot \frac{1}{6\pi\eta r} \qquad (4-11)$$

where R, T, and π have their usual meaning, and

N = Avogadro's number = 6.06×10^{23}
η = viscosity of solution
r = radius of the spherical, uncharged particle diffusing

Since all the terms on the right are known except r, r can be calculated from the diffusion constant. The molecular weight of a large particle can

be calculated from experimentally obtained values of r and the specific gravity:

$$m = \frac{4}{3}\pi\delta^3 gN \qquad (4-12)$$

An example of linear diffusion is shown in the following table. One million sugar molecules were concentrated in a very fine layer at the bottom of a graduated cylinder. One hour later the distribution was:

DISTANCE	NUMBER OF MOLECULES
0–1 mm.	453,000
1–2 mm.	319,000
2–3 mm.	157,000
3–4 mm.	55,000
4–5 mm.	13,000
5–6 mm.	2000
6–7 mm.	170
Over 7 mm.	20

As you can see, almost half the molecules have not moved 1 mm. from the starting position. A handy rule of thumb for simple electrolytes in water is that it will take 1 millisecond for a substance to diffuse 1 μ; further times for diffusion will be proportional to the square of the distance.

Northrop and Anson (1929) used the diffusion method to measure the molecular weight of hemoglobin. The diffusion constant for hemoglobin is 0.0420 cm.^{2}/day and the following values were used to calculate r:

$$R = 8.3 \times 10^7, N = 6.06 \times 10^{23},$$
$$T = 278° K, n = 0.01519.$$

Substituting these values into (4–11) gives r = 2.73×10^{-7} cm. The specific gravity of hemoglobin is 1.33 and the calculated molecular weight equation (4–12) is 68,500 ± 1000.

Today the analytical ultracentrifuge gives values faster and somewhat more accurately, but Northrop and Anson's value is very close to the presently accepted value of 66,000.

Diffusion into a Cylinder. The second case concerns the diffusion of nitrogen into a cylindrical muscle fiber. Consider, for example, that pure nitrogen is suddenly bubbled into the fluid surrounding a muscle fiber.

How long will it take before the concentration in the center of the fiber is equal to the concentration at the membrane? Infinitely long, since the final concentration is reached asymptotically. How long will it take before the concentration reaches 90 per cent of its final value? That depends on the diameter of the cell. Values for both 50 per cent and 90 per cent of the value at the surface for cylindrical cells of varying diameter are given in the following table:

DIAMETER	TIME (sec.) FOR 50 PER CENT SATURATION	TIME (sec.) FOR 90 PER CENT SATURATION
20μ	0.008	0.044
40μ	0.034	0.177
100μ	0.213	1.11
200μ	0.852	4.44
1000μ (1 mm.)	21.3	111
2000μ (2 mm.)	852	4400

Since the situation for other small molecules is similar, it can readily be seen that large cells are at a considerable disadvantage since they must obtain all their nutrients and excrete all their waste products by diffusion. The time in which it takes the large cell to move even small quantities of these substances is so long that they cannot metabolize at a reasonable rate. For that reason large (>200μ) cells are very rare.

Furthermore, calculations such as these show that the distance between a cell and the nearest capillary must be fairly short to provide rapid diffusion and "good service."

Diffusion and Consumption in a Cylinder. The previous calculation was for a substance that was not being consumed. When the case for oxygen, which is metabolized, is considered, solving the equations becomes very complex. A generalized solution for a cell using a metabolite has been worked out by Rashensky and is shown in Figure 4–1.

The diffusion equation can also be derived from a statistical basis, the random walk approach. Indeed, this is the molecular basis of diffusion, the probability that a particle will move toward more particles (up the macroscopic concentration gradient) is lower than the probability that it will move away from these particles (down the macroscopic concentration gradient). For a derivation see Rashensky, *Mathematical Biophysics,* University of Chicago Press, 1948.

CALCULATION OF CHEMICAL POTENTIALS

The Chemical Potential of a Gas. The chemical potential of a gas is described by

$$\mu_g = \mu_g^\circ + RT \ln P_g$$

where P is the pressure of the gas, and μ_g° is a standard-state chemical potential at 0°C. at 1 atmosphere pressure. Where R = gas constant and T = absolute temperature. This relationship is shown in Figure 4–2. Let us consider a bottle half full of water and half full of oxygen under 1 atmosphere pres-

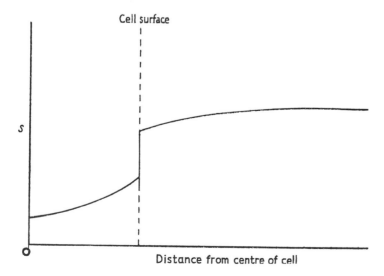

Figure 4–1 The concentration of a substance metabolized by the cell as a function of distance from the cell membrane. (After Rashevsky: *Mathematical Biophysics,* 3rd Edition, Chicago, University of Chicago Press, 1960, Chapter 2, p. 33.)

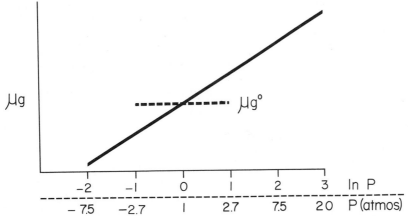

Figure 4–2   The variation of the chemical potential of a mole of gas with pressure.

sure at 20°C. After the contents are mixed, some of the oxygen will be dissolved in the water. An equilibrium situation will be established; as many molecules of oxygen will leave the water as will enter. An equilibrium is reached when there is no net energy flow between the two phases—no net mass transfer. To achieve this, the chemical potentials of oxygen in the two solutions must be equal, since then there will be no potential force to move mass from one phase to another. We write μO_2 gas $= \mu O_2$ liquid.

In a gas phase the number of molecules of gas in a given volume determines the pressure. $PV = nRT$. Therefore, we expect that the chemical potential will change with pressure. Returning to equation (4–7), $dG = SdT + VdP$,

$$\frac{\delta G}{\delta P} = V \text{ at constant } T$$

for a perfect gas $V = \dfrac{nRT}{P}$

and

$$\frac{\delta G}{\delta P} = \frac{nRT}{P}$$

or

$$dG = nRT\,\frac{dP}{P}$$

Starting from one mole ($n = 1$), very small changes in the number of molecules will lead to very small reversible pressure charges. Under these circumstances

$$d\mu = dG$$

and

$$d\mu = nRT\,\frac{dP}{P}$$

Let μ°_g be the chemical potential of 1 mole, P_o is then one atmosphere

$$(P_0 = 1)$$

and

$$\int_{\mu^{\circ}_g}^{\mu_g} d\mu = RT \int_{P_0}^{P} \frac{dP}{P}$$

$$\mu_g - \mu^{\circ}_g = RT \ln \frac{P}{P_0}$$

or

$$\mu_g = \mu^{\circ}_g + RT \ln P$$

Now,

$$\mu O_2 \text{ gas} = \mu_g^{\circ} + RT \ln P_{O_2}$$

and

$$\mu O_2 \text{ liquid} = \mu_1^{\circ} + RT \ln [O_2]$$

At equilibrium

$$\mu_g = \mu_1;$$

so

$$\mu_g^{\circ} + RT \ln P_{O_2} = \mu_1^{\circ} + RT \ln [O_2]$$

$$RT \ln Po_2 - RT \ln [O_2] = (\mu_1^\circ - \mu_s^\circ)$$

$$\ln \frac{Po_2}{[O_2]} = \frac{\mu_1^\circ - \mu_g^\circ}{RT}$$

$$\frac{Po_2}{[O_2]} = e^{\frac{(\mu_1^\circ - \mu_g^\circ)}{RT}}$$

Since all the right-hand terms are constants, they can be replaced by a single constant conveniently designated as 1/k

$$\frac{Po_2}{[O_2]} = \frac{1}{k}$$

$$[O_2] = kPo_2$$

This relationship, known as *Henry's law*, states that the amount of a gas dissolved in solution is directly proportional to the pressure of gas above the liquid. It should be kept in mind that the value of k, the solubility coefficient, varies with temperature. For example, at 37° C., 0.003 ml. O_2 will dissolve in 100 ml. of water or blood per millimeter pressure. Therefore in a pure O_2 atmosphere 100 ml. of H_2O would contain 0.003 ml. O_2/mm. Hg × 760 mm. Hg = 2.280 ml. O_2/100 ml. blood. When a patient is placed in a hyperbaric chamber at 3 atmospheres O_2 pressure, his blood will contain 0.003 ml. O_2/100 ml. blood/mm. Hg × 2280 mm. = 6.84 ml. O_2/100 ml. blood. By the same token, water vapor in the gas is in equilibration with the liquid water. Henry's law is used extensively in all situations of respiration when a gas is in contact with a liquid.

The Chemical Potential of an Ion in Solution. The chemical potential of an ion in solution is

$$\mu_i = \mu_i^\circ + RT \ln c_i + Z_i F\psi_i$$

where Z_i is the valence, F the Faraday, and ψ_i the absolute electrical potential of solution, μ_i° = standard-state chemical potential, R = gas constant, and T = absolute temperature. The last term, $Z_i F\psi_i$, is added to account for the attraction between an ion and an electrical potential, that is, a charge difference. Let us consider a system in equilibrium that consists of two potassium acetate solutions separated by a membrane through which only potassium can pass. When the system has reached equilibrium, by defini-

tion, $\mu_{k_\alpha} = \mu_{k_\beta}$ where α and β are the two sides of the membrane. Consequently $\mu_k^\circ + RT \ln K + Z_k F\psi_\alpha = \mu_k^\circ + RT \ln [K]_\beta + Z_k F\psi_\beta$.

The μ_k°'s are usually equal or very nearly equal; canceling the μ_k°'s and rearranging

$$Z_k F(\psi_\alpha - \psi_\beta) = RT \ln [K]_\beta - RT \ln [K^+]_\alpha$$

$$E = (\psi_\alpha - \psi_\beta) = \frac{RT}{Z_k F} \ln \frac{[K^+]_\beta}{[K^+]_\alpha}$$

where E is the electrical potential between the two sides of the system. We see at once that any difference in the concentration of potassium between the two sides will result in an electrical potential difference. This is known as the *Nernst equation*; it also describes with considerable accuracy the electrical potential across the membrane of a nerve or muscle fiber.

An intuitive view of why an electrical potential is generated can be obtained by considering a porous membrane of finite thickness. The pores are larger than the diameter of the hydrated potassium ion and water molecules, but smaller than the acetate ion (see Fig. 4–3).

Since there is a difference in the chemical potential of the potassium on the two sides due to the concentration difference, potassium will diffuse out through the holes. As potassium ions enter the holes they be-

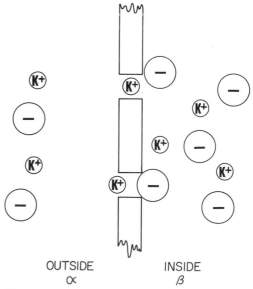

OUTSIDE
α

INSIDE
β

Figure 4–3 A model of a porous membrane showing permeability only to potassium.

come separated from the acetate ions, which cannot enter the holes. Since voltage is defined as a separation of charges, this charge separation produces the measured voltage.

There are two equal but opposite forces at work on the potassium ion. Diffusion forces the potassium out and an electrostatic force holds it in. There is an attraction between the positively charged potassium ion and the negatively charged acetate ion it is leaving behind.

The experiment shown in Figure 4–4 plots E, the potential, across the membrane of a muscle fiber, against the log of the external potassium concentration. The internal potassium concentration does not change during the experiment. The line has a negative slope of 58 mv. per ten-fold change in potassium concentration. This slope is arrived at by substituting values for R, T, Z, and F in the Nernst equation and changing from natural to base 10 logarithm.

$$E = 58 \log \frac{K_o}{K_i} \quad \text{or} \quad E = -58 \log \frac{K_i}{K_o}$$

For a noncharged solute such as glucose, $Z = 0$ and the chemical potential is

$$\mu = \mu° + RT \ln C$$

These equations are valid when there is no solute-solute or solute-solvent interaction. Very dilute solutions (0.001 M) meet these requirements reasonably well. For more concentrated solutions activity coefficients should be used. They are not used extensively in biological work for two reasons. Concentrations often appear as ratios, so the activity coefficients cancel. We are uncertain of the activity coefficient to use in the protein-rich cytoplasm.

Remember that T and Z can change. At mammalian body temperature, 37° C., there is a 61 mv change for every ten-fold increase in concentration difference. For Cl⁻ the ratio is reversed because Z is negative for chloride.

$$E = 58 \log \frac{Cl_i}{Cl_o}$$

All these equations use the common convention that the solution outside the cell has zero absolute potential. As can be seen in Figure 4–4 the Nernst equation very adequately describes the relation between the transmembrane potential and the ratio of the potassium concentrations.

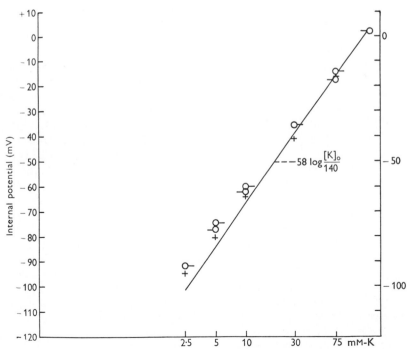

Figure 4–4 The relationship between the external potassium concentration and the resting membrane voltage. (From Hodgkin, A. L.; and Horowicz, P.: J. Physiol., *148*:127, 1959.)

We find electrical potentials across the membranes of most types of cells, and most of these potentials can be described to a first approximation by the Nernst equation. This principle is also used in glass electrodes for measuring hydrogen ion concentration. The tip of the electrode is made of a special glass through which only the hydrogen ion can pass. The potential developed is proportional to the log of the concentration in the solution.

OSMOTIC PRESSURE

When we think of the solution that surrounds cells, we usually concentrate on the salts and the organic components and forget about the water in which all of them are dissolved. Yet the water is extremely important because it makes up a major portion of the volume of most cells; for example, consider a wilted (dehydrated) cucumber slice. The equation for chemical potential is just as applicable to solvent (water) as solute (sodium chloride). At equilibrium, the chemical potential of the solvent must be equal throughout the system.

Consider a system containing two phases, one of pure solvent (α), and one of solvent diluted by sodium chloride (β), separated by a membrane through which only water will pass. Remembering that $\mu = \mu^\circ + RT \ln c_i$, the chemical potential of the water on side α will be greater than on side β since the water on side β is in lower concentration because of the dilution of the water by the sodium chloride. Remember that the reverse is true of sodium chloride. Since the chemical potential of water is higher on side α, water will flow through the membrane. Rather than an equilibrium situation, we have unequal chemical potentials and mass flow.

The chemical potential of water is a function of pressure and increases with increasing pressure. Therefore the application of pressure to side β will increase the chemical potential of the water. Equilibrium is reached when the pressure on side β increases to the point at which $\mu_\alpha = \mu_\beta$. The additional pressure is known as the osmotic pressure and is often applied as a column of water. The osmotic pressure of a solution equilibrated against pure water is: $\pi = RTC_a$, where π = osmotic pressure, R = gas constant, T = absolute temperature, and C_a = solute concentration.

Just as there are activity coefficients to describe the nonideal behavior of electrolytes in other types of solution theory, there are osmotic coefficients to describe nonideal behavior in osmotic situations. For some solutes they are very concentration-dependent, and tables of osmotic coefficients should be consulted before any type of precise calculations is made.

Osmotic pressure can be measured directly by the method shown in Figure 4–5. At the beginning, the water level in the tube and the beaker are even. As water flows into the chamber, the water level rises and creates pressure. As the pressure rises the chemical potential of the water inside increases until the chemical potential of the water inside is equal to the chemical potential of the pure water outside.

It is very unusual for animal cells to exist in pure water although plant and bacteria cells do so readily. The reason is quite simple; animal cells have very fragile membranes and swell up and burst when placed in pure water. They cannot generate pressure within to elevate the chemical potential of the water within the cell. Plant and bacteria cells on the other hand have a rigid cell wall against which the membrane can expand. Many plants remain rigid as a consequence of the osmotic pressure exerted on the cell wall by the semipermeable membrane.

If the membrane between two phases is permeable to salts and water, but impermeable to larger protein molecules, a colloid osmotic pressure is said to exist. We speak of a membrane being permeable to a substance if the substance can move through the membrane. The substance is described as permeant. In most cases permeability is not an all or nothing proposition, but the membrane may be more permeable to some substances than to others. Since the salt is permeable, it will readily diffuse through the membrane and dilute the water to the same degree on each side; the protein cannot diffuse and will reduce the chemical potential of the water inside. Equilibrium is not reached until the pressure inside is elevated to increase the chemical potential of the water inside.

We speak so often of the osmolarity of a solution in terms of the solute that is diluting the water

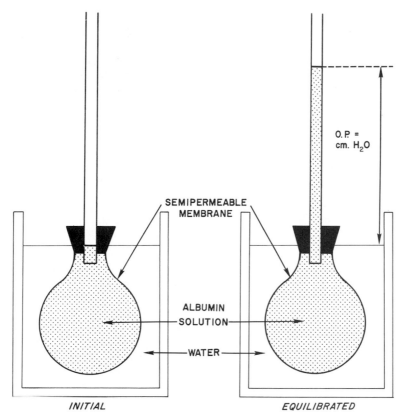

O. P. =
cm. H_2O

SEMIPERMEABLE
MEMBRANE

ALBUMIN
SOLUTION

WATER

INITIAL   *EQUILIBRATED*

Figure 4–5   A direct method for measuring osmotic pressure.

that we forget that osmotic pressure is a function of the chemical potential of water. The calculation of osmolarity does little to alter this tendency. The osmolarity of a solution is calculated as the sum of the concentration of the uncharged species plus the sum of the concentration of each ion. A solution containing 0.1 M glucose+0.1 M KCl has an osmolarity of 0.3. Described in milliosmoles, the above solution is 300 mOsm.

The pressure necessary to raise the chemical potential of diluted water to make it equal to the chemical potential of pure water can easily be derived. When we are dealing with the solvent it is more convenient to use the mole fraction (X_s) rather than concentration. If a solution contains 52 moles of water and 2 moles of sodium chloride, the mole fraction of water is $52/52 + 2 = 52/54 = 0.963$. The expression for the chemical potential is

$$\mu = \mu^\circ + RT \ln X_s$$

where μ° is the chemical potential of the pure solvent, when $X_s = 1$. If very small charges in pressure are applied to the solution, the variation in chemical potential is described by

$$d\mu = \overline{V}_s dP + RT \, d\ln X_s$$

where $\overline{V}_s$ is the partial molar-volume. When the two sides are in equilibrium, $d\mu = 0$, $-V_s \, dP = RT \, d\ln X_s$ integrating between the limits $(P_\alpha; X_s = 1)$ and $(P_\beta; X_s = X_{s\beta})$

$$\int_{P_\alpha}^{P_\beta} \overline{V}_s \, dP = RT \int_1^{X_{s\beta}} d \ln X_s$$

To integrate the left hand side we assume $\overline{V}$ is not a function of pressure; the liquid is incompressible.

$$\overline{V}_s(P_\beta - P_\alpha) = RT \ln X_{s\beta}$$

we define $P_\beta - P_\alpha$ as the osmotic pressure π

$$\frac{\pi \overline{V}_s}{RT} = \ln X_{s\beta}$$

Now $X_{s\beta} = 1 - X_A$ where X_A is the mole fraction of solute. We can expand the log term,

$$\ln (1 - X_A) = -X_A - \frac{X_A^2}{2} - \frac{X_A^3}{3}$$

since X_A is very small to begin with, typically 0.1

to 0.3 M, subsequent terms are insignificant, and when dropped we obtain upon substitution,

$$\pi = \frac{RT}{\overline{V}_s} X_A$$

at these dilute concentrations

$$X_A = \frac{N_A}{N_A} + N_S \sim \frac{N_A}{N_S}$$

where N_A = number of moles of A
N_S = number of moles of solvent

since $N_S \overline{V}_s$ = volume

$$\pi = RT \frac{N_A}{V} = RT\ C_A$$

Since animal cells have very fragile membranes and cannot withstand pressure differences, they must exist in conditions in which the chemical potential of water is equal on both sides of the membrane. The water must be diluted equally on both sides of the membrane. Inside the cell there are permeable salts in equilibrium across the membrane and many types of impermeable proteins that are essential to cell function. Outside the cell there are permeable salts in low concentration and there must be an impermeable substance. This is often the sodium ion. If the chemical potential of the water outside a cell is altered, equilibrium will not be reached until water has moved across the membrane. The force moving the water is the unequal chemical potential of water. Water will flow from higher to lower chemical potential. Since water makes up the major portion of the cell volume, water movement results in changes in the cell volume.

We speak of the osmotic pressure of a solution as a measure of the chemical potential of water in it. We can calculate with considerable accuracy the osmotic pressure from the concentration of salts in the solution. The only time a physical pressure is measured is when the solution is placed in an apparatus as shown in Figure 4–5. Changes in the volume of an animal cell with changes in the concentration of the solution surrounding it can readily be described by the simple van't Hoff equation:

$$V = \frac{RTn_i}{\pi_0}$$

where π_0 is equal to the osmotic pressure of the solution outside the cell, V is the volume of the cell, R and T have their usual meaning, and n_i is the number of moles of impermeable solution inside the cell. An example of this behavior is elegantly shown in Figure 4–6. The outlines are optical cross sections of a single muscle fiber. The cell volume was determined by measuring the area at ten places along the length of the fiber, averaging them, and multiplying by the length.

The principle that cells will shrink when placed in a medium of greater salt concentration, i.e., hypertonic solution, is used, for example, to combat increased intracranial pressure. Since the brain is completely enclosed in the nonexpandable skull, an increase in volume will cause an increase in the intracerebral pressure. Continued pressure will destroy brain cells. The infusion of large colloidal particles into the blood will shrink the brain cells and lower the intracranial pressure. An example is shown in Figure 4–7.

We speak of a solution that will allow a cell to maintain its *in vivo* volume as isotonic. An isotonic solution usually has the same osmotic pressure as do the salt constituents of plasma, since interstitial (around cells) fluid is largely protein-free. A hypotonic solution has a lower osmotic pressure and causes cells to swell. Hypertonic solution has a higher osmotic pressure and causes cells to shrink.

The astute student will no doubt have already realized that osmotic pressure is a function of the number of particles that are diluting the water. This brings osmotic pressure into the class of properties called colligative properties, such as vapor-pressure lowering, freezing-point depression, and boiling-point elevation. Biologists use this similarity to measure osmotic pressure. The standard commercial osmometer really measures freezing point depression, but is calibrated in milliosmoles.

GIBBS-DONNAN EQUILIBRIUM

Let us now consider a specific system that resembles a cellular system. First, 40 gm. of albumin are placed inside a cellophane tube and the ends are tied so that the total volume inside is very close to 1 liter. The cellophane is impermeable to albumin. The bag is immersed in a very large volume of 10 mM KCl. What are the conditions of equilibrium?

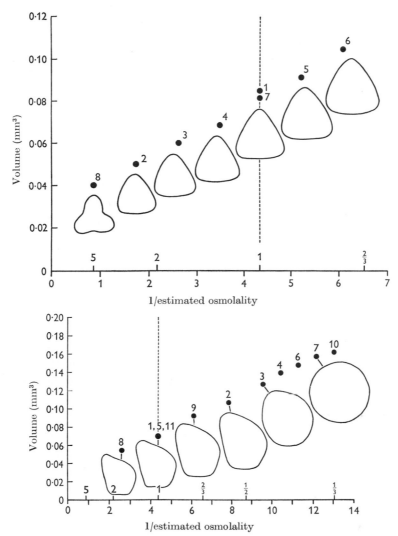

Figure 4-6 The influence of osmotic strength of the bathing solution on the cross-section area and volume of two isolated single muscle fibers. (From Blinks, J.: J. Physiol., *177*:42, 1965.)

Both salt and water can pass through the cellophane, so at equilibrium the chemical potentials of each species must be equal.

$$\mu H_2 O_{(O)} = \mu H_2 O_{(i)}$$

$$\mu K^+_{(O)} = \mu K^+_{(i)}$$

$$\mu Cl^-_{(O)} = \mu Cl^-_{(i)}$$

Second, there must be electroneutrality on both sides; the number of positive and negative charges must be equal in any microscopically definable region.

For the outside solution (neglecting H^+ and OH^-):

$$(K^+)_o = (Cl^-)_o$$

For the inside solution we must take into account the albumin which has Z_p negatively charged sites per molecule:

$$(K^+)_i = (Cl^-)_i + Z_p(Alb^-)_i$$

Third, whatever electrical potential exists across the membrane, it affects all permeant ions.

$$E_{K^+} = E_{Cl^-}$$

or

$$E_{K^+} = \frac{RT}{ZF} \ln \frac{K_o}{K_i} = E_{Cl^-} = \frac{RT}{-ZF} \ln \frac{Cl_o}{Cl_i}$$

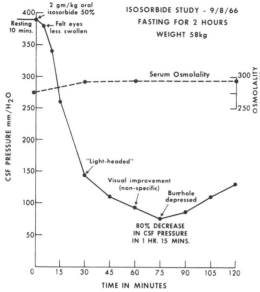

Figure 4-7 The effect of increased serum osmolarity (dashed line) on intercranial pressure (solid line). (From Wise, B. L., and Mathis, J. L.: J. Neurosurg., *28*:124, 1968.)

Remember that Z is positive for potassium and negative for chloride. Consequently,

$$\ln \frac{K_o}{K_i} = -\ln \frac{Cl_o}{Cl_i} = \ln \frac{Cl_i}{Cl_o}$$

Raising both sides to the power e

$$\frac{K_o^+}{K_i^+} = \frac{Cl_i^-}{Cl_o^-} = r$$

This is the basic Gibbs-Donnan equation or condition. If another cation, such as sodium, were permeable, then

$$\frac{K_o^+}{K_i^+} = \frac{Na_o^+}{Na_i^+} = r$$

If a divalent cation, such as calcium, were present then

$$\frac{(Ca_o)^2}{(Ca_i)^2} = \frac{K_o}{K_i}$$

In every case, the ratio is called the Gibbs-Donnan ratio, and is variously labeled r or g. Returning to the electroneutrality condition

$$(K)_i^+ = (Cl)_i^- + Z_p (Abl^-)_i$$

Let us divide through by $(K)_o$ on the left

and (Cl_o) on the right, since by electroneutrality these must be equal $[(K)_o = (Cl)_o]$

$$\frac{K_i}{K_o} = \frac{Cl_i}{Cl_o} + \frac{Z_p(Abl^-)_i}{Cl_o}$$

which gives

$$\frac{1}{r} = r + \frac{Z_p(Alb)}{Cl_o}$$

We can solve for r by rearranging:

$$1 = r^2 + Z_p\, r\, \frac{(Alb)}{Cl_o} \text{ or } r^2 + r\left[Z_p \frac{(Alb)}{Cl_o}\right] - 1 = o$$

$$r = \left[\frac{Z_p\, Alb}{2Cl_o}\right] + \left[\frac{(Z_p\, Alb)^2}{2Cl_o} + 1\right]$$

This can be simplified when Z_p Alb $\ll Cl_o$ to

$$r \cong 1 + \frac{Z_p\, Alb}{2Cl_o}$$

Both the equations note that the asymmetry (r) of concentration on each side of the cellophane of the permeant ions increases as the amount of protein increases or the charge on the protein increases. At the isoelectric point of the protein, the charge becomes zero, r becomes one, and there no longer is an asymmetry of distribution of the permeant ions.

The electrical potential across the membrane is

$$E = \frac{RT}{ZF} \ln r$$

so it too depends on the presence of a charged protein inside the cellophane. The pressure developed across the cellophane is

$$\pi = RT[(r - 1)2K_o + (1 - Z_p)(Alb)]$$

When $Z_p = 0$, r = 1, so

$$\pi = RT [(0) + (Alb)] \\ = RT (Alb)$$

An osmotic pressure exists due to the concentration of unchanged albumin alone. As Z_p increases, r increases, and so does π.

We should note that the Gibbs-Donnan equation describes an equilibrium condition. The electrical, chemical, and pressure differences all contribute in differing proportions to the chemical potentials of each side of the membrane to give $\Delta\mu$ and $\Delta G = 0$.

To return to our specific example, let us calculate r, E, and π.
At equilibrium

$$\frac{K_i}{K_o} = \frac{Cl_o}{Cl_i}$$

$$K_o = Cl_o = 10 \text{ mM},$$

therefore,

$$K_o \times Cl_o = K_i \times Cl_i = 100 \text{ mM}$$

Now,

40 gm. albumin with MW = 66,000

$$\frac{40 \text{ gm.}}{66,000 \text{ gm./mole}} = 0.606 \text{ mM}$$

Assume 20 negative charges/molecule, hence there is the equivalent of 12.12mM impermeant ions.
Now, $12.12\text{mM} + Cl_i = K_i$ and $K_i \times Cl_i = 100$ mM.
Substituting

$$Cl_i = \frac{100 \text{mM}}{K_i},$$

$$12.12 + \frac{100}{K_i} = K_i \text{ or } K_i^2 - 12.12 \, K_i - 100 = 0$$

$$K_i = \frac{12.12 \pm \sqrt{146.89 + 400}}{2}$$

$$= \frac{12.12 + 23.38}{2} = 17.75 \text{mM} = K_i$$

and

$$Cl_i = \frac{100}{17.75} = 5.63 \text{mM} = Cl_i$$

$$r = \frac{Cl_i}{Cl_o} = \frac{5.63}{10} = 0.56$$

$$r = \frac{K_o}{K_i} = \frac{10}{17.75} = 0.56$$

The electrical potential:
Now at 20° C.

$$E = \frac{RT}{F} \ln r = 58 \log 0.565 = -58 \log \frac{1}{0.565}$$

$$= -58 \log 1.775 = -58 \, (0.2490)$$

$$= -14.5 \text{mV} = E$$

The osmotic pressure:

$$\pi = RT\Delta C$$
$$c_i = 0.606 + 17.75 + 5.63 = 23.99$$
$$C_o = 20$$
$$\Delta C = 3.99 \text{mM}$$

$\pi = RT \, (3.99\text{mM}) = 8.2 \times 10^{-2} \times 2.93 \times 10^2 \times 3.99 \times 10^{-3} = 0.095$ Atm or 72 mm. Hg. There will be a physical pressure equivalent to 72 mm. Hg on the cellophane bag.

The situation in cells is not quite so simple. First of all animal cells cannot maintain a pressure difference across their membranes as the cellophane bag can. If sodium is treated as impermeable, then a Gibbs-Donnan equilibrium is set up in which there is no pressure difference, but there is an electrical potential difference. The red blood cell is one of the best studied cells. When the anion distribution is very carefully measured, it is clear that the anions distribute across the membrane as predicted by the Gibbs-Donnan principle.* For example, at pH 7.4,

$$\frac{H_s^+}{H_c^+} = 0.92 \frac{[Cl_c^-]}{[Cl_s^-]} = 0.93 \frac{[HCO_3^-]_c}{[HCO_3^-]_s}$$

PROBLEMS

One of the greatest contributions the biophysicists and the physical chemists have made to biology and medicine is the introduction of quantitative analysis. These problems are examples of the application of the principles just discussed and serve to help you evaluate your understanding of the theory.

1. (a) Calculate the plasma colloid osmotic pressure of a cirrhotic (liver diseased) patient with a serum albumin of 1.5 gm./100 ml. blood and a serum globulin of 3 gm./100 ml. blood when equilibrated against a 0.14 M NaCl solution. Assume 18 negative sites per molecule of serum albumin (m.w. 69,000) and 20 per serum globulin (average m.w. 175,000). This approximates the distribution across the capillary membrane at zero blood

---

*Fitzsimons, E. J., and Sendroy, J. Jr.: Distribution of electrolytes in human blood. J. biol. Chem., *236*:1595, 1961.

pressure. Carry your calculations to 6 decimal places.

(b) In relationship to albumin, how important is the globulin in the generation of the colloid osmotic pressure?

(c) What would be the effect on colloid osmotic pressure of a genetic mutation lowering the net charge of albumin to -2? Use $R = 0.082$ liter-atmosphere/mole-degree.

2. If the pH of a muscle cell is 7.0 and of the interstitial fluid 7.4, is the H^+ ion in equilibrium at the resting membrane potential of $-90mV$?

3. The muscle fiber shown in Figure 4–6 (upper) has a volume of 0.85 mm^2 in 0.12 M NaCl. When placed in 0.24 M NaCl the fiber shrinks to a volume of 0.56 mm^2. What volume would you expect if the muscle were placed in 0.24 M sucrose solution, in 0.12 M $AlCl_3$ solution?

4. The internal potassium concentration of the squid giant axon is 369 mM. Calculate values for the potassium equilibrium potential (E) when the potassium in the fluid surrounding the axon contains: 13 (normal sea water), 50, 200, and 500 mM K^+. The curious student may wish to compare these values for E with the experimental values to be found in: A. L. Hodgkin and R. D. Keynes, J. Physiol., *128*:61, 1955.

5. Cerebral spinal fluid is formed in the choroid plexus of the lateral and fourth ventricles and is protein free. For many years it was thought to be an ultrafiltrate of plasma; that is, all of the small molecules and water are forced through a membrane leaving the proteins behind (the fluid of the glomerular filtrate is formed this way). You now have the theoretical data to test this hypothesis. The value for r between human plasma and a protein free solution is 0.96. Which of the following ions are distributed as predicted by the Gibbs-Donnan theory?

	plasma	*CSF*	(m equiv/by H_2O)
Na^+	148	149	
K^+	4.3	2.9	
Cl^-	106	130	
Glucose	8.3	5.35	

Are the experimental results compatible with the theory that cerebrospinal fluid (CSF) is an ultrafiltrate of plasma?

References

Baylis, L. E.: *Principles of General Physiology*. New York, John Wiley & Sons, 1959.

Davson, H.: *A Textbook of General Physiology*, 3rd Edition. Boston, Little, Brown, and Company, 1964.

Jacobs, M. H.: *Diffusion Processes*. Berlin, Springer-Verlag, 1967.

Katchalsky, A., and Curran, P. F.: *Nonequilibrium Thermodynamics in Biophysics*. Cambridge, Massachusetts, Harvard University Press, 1965.

Northrop, J. H., and Anson, M. L.: A method for the determination of diffusion constants and the calculations of the radius and weight of the hemoglobin molecule. J. Gen. Physiol., *12*:543, 1929.

Snell, F. M., Sholman, S., Spencer, R., and Moos, C.: *Biophysical Principles of Structure and Function*. Reading, Massachusetts, Addison-Wesley Publishing Company, Inc., 1965.

5

Nerve Physiology

BRIAN CURTIS

When an electrode is placed inside a nerve axon, the axoplasm is found to be 70 to 90 millivolts (0.07 to 0.09 volts) negative, with respect to the bathing fluid. This negative potential is called the resting potential. When the distal end of the axon is stimulated, usually by an electric current, the potential suddenly becomes 40 mV positive and just as suddenly (1 to 2 milliseconds) returns to the resting level. This transient change in potential, called an action potential, is shown in Figure 5–1.

The action potential always has the same duration and magnitude, no matter where it is measured in the nervous system. When the action potential is measured at several places, each successively farther away from the stimulating electrode, the potential change occurs at successively greater intervals after the stimulus occurs; the action potential is propagated down the axon at a finite velocity. Conduction velocities range from 1 to 100 meters per second.

Since the action potential always has the same magnitude and duration, there must be many "repeater stations" along the nerve. At each of these stations the action potential is renewed.

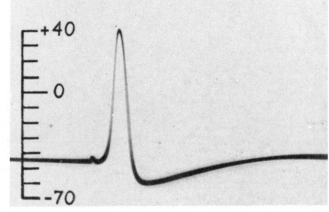

Figure 5–1 An intracellular record-ing of an action potential from a squid giant axon. The electrical sign is in respect to the bathing solution, which is con-sidered to be at zero potential. (From Hodgkin, A. L., and Huxley, A. F.: J. Physiol., *104*:176, 1945.)

A single action potential traveling into the central nervous system along a single nerve can inform the system of its presence or occurrence. More complex messages can be carried only by varying the interval between action potentials. The interval between action potentials is the reciprocal of frequency; an interval of 200 msec. between action potentials gives a frequency of 5/sec. An example of a frequency-coded message is shown in Figure 5–2, where the action potential frequency of a pressure-sensitive receptor in the carotid sinus is plotted as a function of pressure.

MEASUREMENT OF THE ELECTRICAL POTENTIAL OF CELLS

The electrical potential across a cell has been measured in two ways: by passing a tube into the cut end and by puncturing the membrane with a very fine pointed tube. The first method is applicable only to very large ($>300\ \mu$) axons such as the squid giant axon. The action potential record in Figure 5–1 was obtained by this method.

The second method, called the microelectrode method, uses a tube with a pointed tip of less than $0.1\ \mu$ diameter. Microelectrodes seal into the membrane and do re-

markably little damage to the cell. They are very widely used in all studies of the nervous system. Both electrode types are filled with a conducting solution of 3 M KCl. The potential is measured between two Ag–AgCl electrodes, one in the electrode tube, the other in the bath.

RESTING POTENTIAL

As was described in the last chapter, the resting potential (E) of excitable tissue can be described by the Nernst equation for potassium, the potassium equilibrium potential.

$$E = -\frac{RT}{F} \ln \frac{K_i}{K_o}$$

where R = gas constant, T = absolute temperature, F = Faraday, and K_i and K_o are the internal and external potassium concentrations. At $20°$ C. the equation becomes

$$E = -58\,(mV),\ \log \frac{K_i}{K_o}$$

Because the resting potential is described by the Nernst equation we assume that potassium is in equilibrium across the membrane; there is no net force tending to move potassium across the membrane.

When we examine the fit of the data to the Nernst equation in Figure 5–3, we see that the fit is good for high K_o but poor for low values of K_o. This discrepancy comes about because of the very small quantity of sodium that leaks into the cell.

Sodium is far from being in equilibrium across the membrane. $E_{Na} \cong +50$ mV for most nerves. For sodium to be in equilibrium at a resting potential of -90 mV the internal concentration would have to be about 8 molar, which is clearly impossible. Sodium is drawn into the cell by both an electrical gradient (a positive ion attracted to a negative region) and a chemical gradient. The sodium ions are moving down an electrochemical gradient. The influx, the number of ions moving in per unit membrane area, is small because the membrane is not very permeable to sodium: it resists the flow of sodium ions through it.

Since the dilution of water inside the cell remains constant, for each sodium ion that enters, a potassium ion must leave. This swap

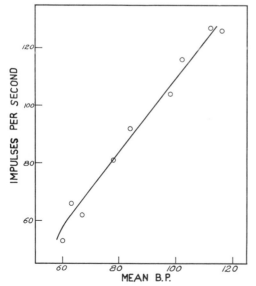

Figure 5–2 The relationship between the frequency of discharge from a pressure receptor in the carotid sinus and the endosinusoidal pressure. (From Bronk and Stella: J. cell. comp. Physiol., *1*:113, 1932.)

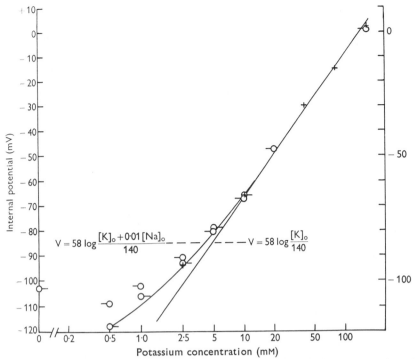

Figure 5–3 The data points are resting potential values for frog single muscle fibers in solutions of varying potassium concentration. Note that the potassium concentration is plotted on a log scale. The normal values for frog muscle are $Na_o = 120$ mM/L, $Na_i = 20$ mM/L, $K_i = 140$ mM/L, and $K_o = 2.5$ mM/L. (From Hodgkin, A. L., and Horowicz, P.: J. Physiol., *148*:127, 1959.)

of cations maintains both the dilution of water and electroneutrality. The other alternative is the movement of an anion, such as chloride, into the cell along with the sodium ion. This would preserve electroneutrality but would dilute the water inside the cell. While the number of sodium ions entering the cell is small, they must be removed to maintain a steady-state sodium concentration. This removal process requires the expenditure of energy since the ions are being moved up on an electrochemical gradient.

The constant field or Goldman equation was derived to describe the electrical potential across a membrane when more than one ion is permeable. It does not have as firm a thermodynamic basis as does the Nernst equation, but has proved very useful over the last 25 years,

$$E = \frac{RT}{F} \ln \frac{P_K[K]_o + P_{Na}[Na]_o + P_{Cl}[Cl]_i}{P_K[K]_i + P_{Na}[Na]_i + P_{Cl}[Cl]_o}$$

where R = gas constant, T = absolute temperature, F = Faraday, P_K, P_{Na}, P_{Cl} are the

potassium, sodium, and chloride permeabilities, and $[K]_o \ldots$ are the concentrations of the ions on either side of the membrane. The equation states that the equilibrium potential of an ion will have an influence on the final potential of the membrane in proportion to the ease in which that ion can move across the membrane (its permeability).

Since chloride is, by and large, in equilibrium across the membrane ($E_{Cl} = E$), we can ignore the chloride ions' contribution except in transient responses.

The second curve in Figure 5–3 is calculated from the Goldman equation, in which 0.01 as the experimentally measured ratio of sodium to potassium permeability is used. When we ignore chloride, the Goldman equation can be rewritten:

$$E = \frac{RT}{F} \ln \frac{K_o + P_{Na}/P_K \, Na_o}{K_i + P_{Na}/P_K \, Na_i}$$

It can be seen that the new curve fits the data points very nicely.

The resting potential is basically a potassium equilibrium potential and as such the cell does not need to expend energy to maintain it. Indeed, the resting potential of a cell is affected very little when the energy supply to the cell is cut off by metabolic poisons or cooling. The one troublesome aspect is the small sodium leak with its consequent potassium exchange. That will be discussed later in the section on active transport.

The resting potential originates when a very small number of potassium ions move from the axoplasm into the membrane, thus separating them from the negative ions inside the membrane. In a 1 cm. length of a squid giant axon, 9×10^{-14} moles of potassium move into the membrane in comparison with 1×10^{-6} moles of potassium in the axoplasm. These ions, since they have mass, take time to move into the membrane and, of course, will take time to move if the equilibrium condition is upset.

PASSIVE PROPERTIES OF THE MEMBRANE

When a microelectrode is introduced into an axon and a voltage is applied to the tip of the electrode ions will be forced into the cell and across the cell membrane. These ions meet resistance as they pass through the cell membrane and produce a voltage difference, which is described by Ohm's law:

$$E = IR,$$

where E is the voltage, I is the ionic current, and R the total resistance of the membrane to the passage of ions. When ions are injected into an axon some of them will pass out through the membrane directly under the electrode. Others will flow down the axon core and pass out farther away from the electrode. Wherever they pass out through the membrane, they will cause a voltage change across the membrane. This is illustrated in Figure 5–4. It will be seen that the change of membrane voltage decreases rather quickly as the recording electrode is moved further away from the current passing electrode. The current pulse that caused these changes had a rectangular form, yet the induced voltage did not. This is due to the time it takes for the ions to move physically through the membrane.

Electrically, the passive characteristics of the axon can be described by three properties: an axoplasmic resistance, a membrane re-

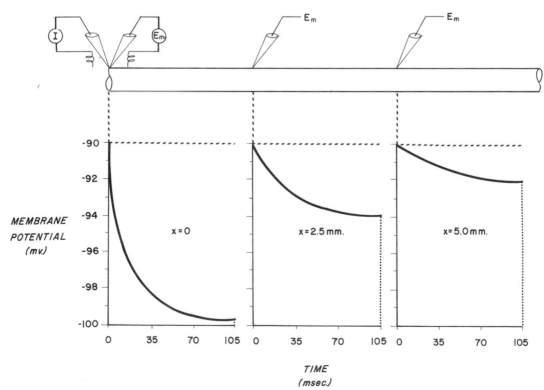

Figure 5–4 Cable properties of a membrane.

sistance, and a membrane capacity. These same properties describe the passage of current through and the leakage of current from a telegraph cable under the ocean. The equations that describe the electrical properties of submarine cables were worked out by Lord Kelvin in the last half of the 19th century and were applied to axons by Hodgkin and Rushton. Thus, the passive properties of axons are often referred to as cable properties.

It is worth noting that a local disturbance at X = 0 will die out very quickly, so that 5 mm. away there will be very little voltage change. This is in contrast to the action potential, which has the same amplitude everywhere along the axon. The difference is that work is being done everywhere along the axon during the propagation of an action potential, but only at one place, the current-passing electrode, during the measurement of cable properties.

ACTIVE MEMBRANE RESPONSES

Threshold. As long as current pulses make the potential on the membrane more negative (hyperpolarization), the membrane continues to react as a cable; this is shown in the lower set of curves in Figure 5–5. When the direction of the current flow is reversed and the membrane is made less negative (depolarization) the membrane reacts as a passive cable for only small depolarizations. As can be seen in Figure 5–5, when the potential on the membrane reaches a critical point, the response no longer bears any resemblance to the stimulus. The responses c to k are all directly proportional to the intensity of the stimulus—to the amount of current (the number of ions) passing through the membrane. The external current is doing work on the membrane. As soon as a critical membrane potential is reached, the response, an action potential, no longer bears any resemblance to the stimulus. Work is being done on the membrane by some other source.

The threshold potential is very constant from axon to axon and is very close to −55 mV for all excitable tissues. At all potentials more negative than threshold, the membrane behaves as a passive cable; at potentials less negative, it has active properties of its own, the action potential.

The Action Potential. Just as the resting potential of the cell is dominated by the

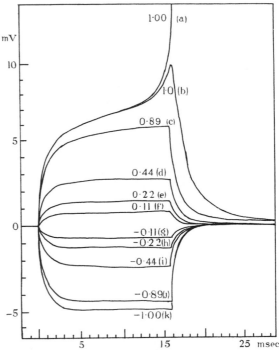

Figure 5–5 The response of a crab axon of 80μ diameter to current passage. The experiment is conducted in much the same manner as the one shown in Figure 5–4. The 0 point is the resting membrane potential of about −65 mV. Depolarization is shown as the upward deflection. The numbers beside each trace give the current strength relative to the threshold current. The upstroke seen in (a) is the beginning of an action potential similar to the one seen in Figure 5–1. (From Hodgkin, A. L., and Rushton, W. A. H.: Proc. Roy. Soc., *B133*:444, 1946.)

potassium ion, so the action potential is dominated by the sodium ion. The upswing of the action potential represents a brief change in the properties of the membrane, so that sodium is the dominantly permeable ion. Since the membrane potential is controlled by the dominantly permeable ion, the potential moves toward the sodium equilibrium potential of +40 to 50 mV. For some reason the increased sodium permeability turns off very soon after its onset and the potential, in consequence, returns to the resting level.

When we consider the Goldman equation, the role of the sodium permeability becomes clearer:

$$E = \frac{RT}{F} \ln \frac{P_K K_o + P_{Na} Na_o}{P_K K_i + P_{Na} Na_i}$$

If both top and bottom of the ln term are multiplied by $1/P_K$ we obtain

$$E = \frac{RT}{F} \ln \frac{K_o + P_{Na}/P_K \, Na_o}{K_i + P_{Na}/P_K \, Na_i}$$

Since R, T, F, K_o, K_i, Na_o, and Na_i do not change under normal circumstances, the only way that the potential, E, can change is by altering the ratio of P_{Na} to P_K. At rest P_{Na}/P_K is approximately 0.01 and the membrane potential is very close to E_K, the potassium potential, of ~ -100 mV. At the peak of the action potential, $P_{Na}/P_K = 20$ and the potential is very close to E_{Na}, $\sim +50$ mV.

There are two major lines of evidence which give qualitative support to the sodium hypothesis. The peak voltage should never be greater than E_{Na}. There should be an influx of sodium during the action potential.

We find experimental proof of the first point in Figure 5–6. As the concentration of sodium in the external solution is reduced so is the magnitude of the peak of the action potential. When the sodium is removed from the bathing solution, there is no action potential; there is no E_{Na} to move toward.

The second line of evidence is obtained from experiments with radioactive sodium. The influx of sodium increases many times with stimulation. It is fairly simple to calculate that a transfer of this number of ions will discharge the membrane capacity and swing the potential to about $+40$ mV. These ions displace the potassium ions in the membrane.

The Sodium Carriers. We can describe the action potential by saying that the potential change represents a brief condition of high sodium permeability. There is still no good explanation of why the sodium permeability turns off so rapidly.

The increase in the ease with which ions cross the membrane during the action potential can be measured. Such a measurement is shown in Figure 5–7 and indicates that there is a great increase in the ease with which ions can cross the membrane during the action potential.

A model has been devised to describe the phenomenon. The model postulates "carriers" which reside in the membrane and which are responsible for carrying sodium ions from the outside solution, across the membrane, and into the cell. When the cell is depolarized, the carriers, with sodium ions attached, move from the outside to the inside of the membrane. The carriers cannot move back to the outside until the membrane is repolarized. Since there are a limited number of carriers available, the number of sodium ions which can move across the membrane is limited, and the period of sodium influx is also limited. When the carriers are all on the inside of the membrane, sodium is once again impermeable and the membrane potential returns to E_K. These postulated carriers are thought to be entirely separate from other carriers which are thought to participate in active transport.

The Hodgkin-Huxley Equations. The evidence presented so far in favor of the ionic basis of the action potential has been qualitative. All the experimental effects have been in the "right direction." Hodgkin and Huxley were able to show quantitatively that the action potential could be described by changes in ion permeability. Their description was one of the very first such proofs in biology; proofs of this type are common in physics and chemistry. Their elegant series of papers led to the Nobel Prize for Medicine in 1963. Their analysis was based on the ability

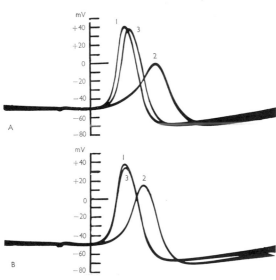

Figure 5–6 The effect of low sodium solutions on the action potential. Records 1 and 3 were taken with the axon in normal sea water. Record 2A was taken with the axon in $1/3$ sea water, $2/3$ dextrose, while 2B was taken in $1/2$ sea water, $1/2$ dextrose. Note that the peak voltage of the action potential is reduced in 2.

E_{Na} for 1 and 3 = 58 log 460/50 = +56 mV
E_{Na} for 2A   = 58 log 153/50 = +28 mV
E_{Na} for 2B   = 58 log 230/50 = +38 mV

(From Hodgkin, A. L., and Katz, B.: J. Physiol. *108*:37, 1949.)

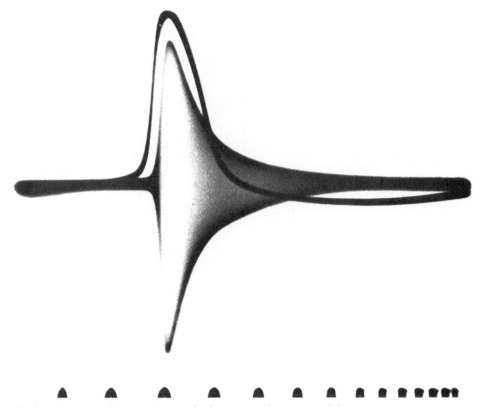

Figure 5-7 The impedance change during an action potential. Two superimposed records are shown. The thin line is an action potential of a squid giant axon and the continuous curve is a measure of the ease with which ions can pass across the membrane (impedance). (From Cole, K. S., and Curtis, H. J.: J. gen. Physiol., *22*:649, 1938.)

to sort out the ionic currents of the action potential and to determine their time course. The method used is called the voltage clamp.

The general theory of clamping experiments is of sufficient interest for it to be explained thoroughly here. The theory can be grasped somewhat more easily if it is explained first in chemical and then in electrical terms.

We know that the glucose concentration of circulating blood is maintained at a constant level by a variety of forces. We can study these forces by injecting various amounts of glucose into an animal and studying the changing level of blood glucose as shown in Figure 5-8a. We can calculate the initial change in the blood glucose concentration by dividing the number of added moles of glucose by the blood volume of the experimental animal. (Here, 900 mg./1 L. or 90 mg./100 ml. in addition to the 90 mg./100 ml. there.) The rate of disappearance of glucose is a function of the control system. In the experiment shown in Figure 5-8a we are not studying the response to a single blood glucose level but the response to a whole series of decreasing blood glucose levels.

We can arrange our apparatus so that we can maintain a constant, elevated blood glucose level as is shown in Figure 5-8b. Here the blood glucose level is constant and the initial amount of glucose added (α) is, as before, a measure of the size or capacity of the system, while the steadily added glucose (β) is equal to the amount of glucose removed by the control system. Since the glucose concentration is not changing, the amount added per minute must be equal to the amount removed per minute. We are "clamping" or fixing the blood glucose concentration at a predetermined level and keeping it there by adding more glucose. This experiment can be done at several blood glucose levels; the hypothetical results are seen in Figure 5-8c.

We can calculate the natural response of this system to the injection of any amount of glucose, say, 900 mg. First, we must determine the initial concentration of glucose by dividing the added amount by the blood volume (900 mg./1 L. + 90 mg./100 ml. = 180 mg./100 ml.). Then we can read from the graph in Figure 5-8c the rate of removal for that concentration (7 mg./min.). Five minutes later the control system will have removed

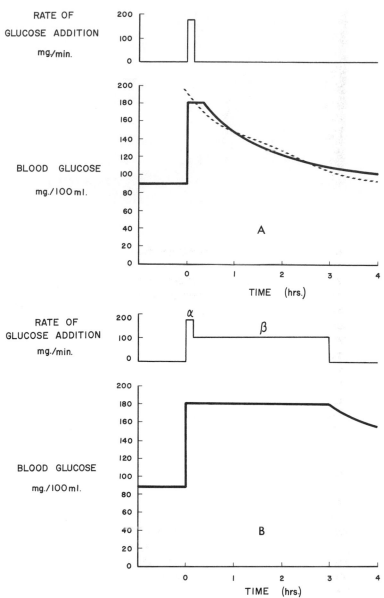

Figure 5–8 *A* and *B*, An illustration of the theory of clamping experiments, using a chemical example. *A* shows the actual (solid line) and calculated (dashed line) decline in blood-glucose concentration following a single glucose injection. *B* shows the amount of glucose which must be added to maintain a constant glucose concentration.

some glucose (35 mg.) and the concentration will be reduced (180 mg./100 ml. × (10–35)/10). Now the rate of removal will be reduced, so we must recalculate the amount removed in the next 5 minutes, and so on for each 5-minute interval.

The dashed curve in Figure 5–8*a* shows the final calculation, which is very close to the "real" curve. Consequently, we can say that the curve in Figure 5–8*c* describes the **rate of removal** as a function of concentration.

The situation with the axon is very similar; we wish to maintain the membrane potential at a predetermined level. To do this we must force ions through the membrane in a magnitude equal to, but in a direction opposite from, the natural flow of ions. The membrane potential is analogous to the glucose concentration and the forced ion flow is analogous to the injection of glucose.

A record is shown in Figure 5–9. The membrane is suddenly depolarized to −10

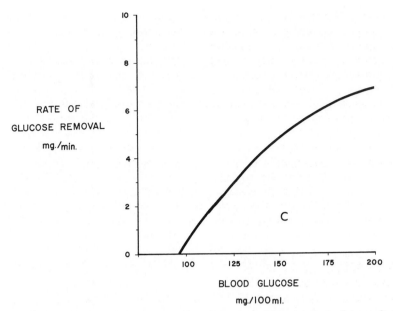

Figure 5-8 *(Continued.)* C shows the rate of glucose removal at constant glucose levels. These data are obtained from a series of experiments similar to the one shown in *B*. Since the glucose concentration is not changing, the rate of addition must be equal to the rate of removal.

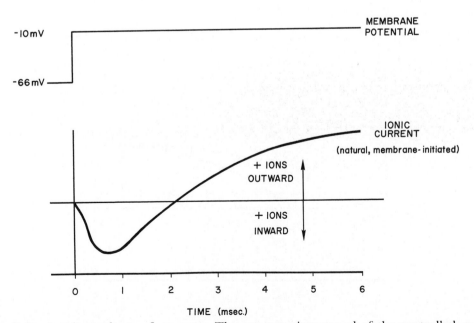

Figure 5-9 A voltage clamp of an axon. The top trace is a record of the controlled membrane voltage. The lower trace is a record of the ionic current which the control unit passed across the membrane to maintain the membrane potential at −10 mV. The current that the membrane generated is of equal magnitude but opposite sign, and the lower curve is labeled as membrane current.

mV and held there. Remember, the axon would fire an action potential if it were not clamped. These experiments differ somewhat from the glucose experiment in that we can pass ions in either direction across the membrane—the equivalent to injecting and withdrawing glucose.

The record of the ions passed through the membrane is shown in the lower half of Figure 5–9. For the first millisecond or so, the control system had to pass positive ions out through the membrane to maintain the potential; therefore, the natural, membrane-initiated flow is inward. At about 2 msec., the control system had to pass positive ions in through the membrane, corresponding to a natural flow outward. The concept of the control system passing ions through the membrane is a simplification. Actually the system removes them from one side of the membrane and replaces them on the other side.

While this experiment will measure the magnitude of the ionic flow, it will not differentiate between sodium and potassium. To do that we can replace the sodium outside the cell with sucrose or choline and obtain the set of records shown in Figure 5–10. The voltage record is the same as in Figure 5–9, as is the solid ionic flow record. The heavy dashed line shows the ionic current when the

axon is bathed in sodium-free solution; remember, the axon cannot fire an action potential under these conditions. This time the membrane-initiated ionic flow is in the form of positive ions moving outward. These are postassium ions leaving the cell. When the heavily dashed line is subtracted from the solid record, the dotted record is obtained. It shows the inward flow of sodium ions.

The ionic flow across the membrane, then, can be broken up into two flows: an inward sodium flow soon after depolarization and an outward potassium flow which begins after a short delay and continues as long as the membrane is depolarized.

This experiment was then repeated at a number of different membrane potential values and the ionic flow separated into an inward sodium flow and an outward potassium flow. Ionic flow is a function of two factors: the force pushing the ion through and the ease with which the ion will pass through the membrane. This is stated as follows:

$$g_{Na} = \frac{I_{Na}}{V_m - V_{Na}}$$

where g_{Na} = sodium conductance
I_{Na} = ionic flow
V_m = membrane potential
V_{Na} = sodium equilibrium potential

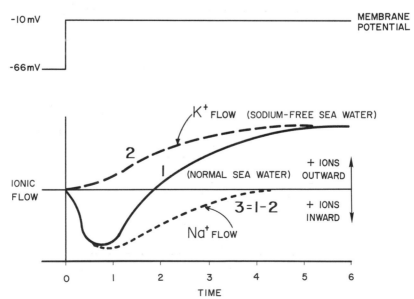

Figure 5–10 Two ionic current tracings from voltage clamp experiments. The first, solid record (1) is taken in normal sea water. The dashed record (2) is taken in sodium-free sea water. The dotted line (3) is obtained by subtracting the sodium-free tracing from the normal tracing. (Data from Hodgkin, A. L., and Huxley, A. F.: J. Physiol., *116*:449, 1952.)

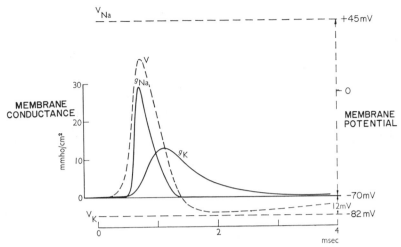

Figure 5–11 Theoretical solution for a propagated action potential (dashed line) and the calculated ionic conductances (solid lines). (From Hodgkin, A. L., and Huxley, J.; J. Physiol., *117*:500, 1952.)

When $V_m = V_{Na}$ no sodium flow would be expected, since there is no driving force; indeed, none is measured. Conductance is a property of the membrane and is a more general property than ionic flow; consequently, all further development will be in terms of conductance.

A series of experimental curves was obtained—one for potassium conductance as a function of membrane potential and time, one for sodium conductance as a function of membrane potential and time, and one for sodium carrier availability as a function of membrane potential and time. These three curves plus a description of the cable properties of the nerve should be sufficient to calculate an action potential, given the initial conduction of a threshold stimulus; indeed they do, as is shown in Figure 5–11. It can be and has been concluded that the action potential can be completely explained in terms of changes in the membrane's conductance of sodium, and later of potassium.

In addition to showing the calculated action potential, Figure 5–11 also depicts the conductance changes for sodium and potassium. The rapidly rising sodium conductance brings a rush of sodium ions into the membrane; these ions displace the potassium ions there and drive the potential across the membrane close to E_{Na}. This sodium conductance rapidly falls as a result of a lack of carriers, and the membrane begins to return to E_K. Repolarization is speeded by the delayed increase in potassium conductance, a condition that hastens the process of removing sodium ions from the membrane and replacing them with potassium ions needed to regain the resting state. An excellent discussion of this material can be found in Hodgkin's Cronian Lecture, Proc. Roy. Soc., B148, 1, 1958.

The Perfused Axon. The previous discussion has assumed that all active processes in the nerve take place at the membrane. While earlier researchers knew that the membrane was very susceptible to injury and that membrane injury correlated with axon dysfunction, it was Baker, Hodgkin, and Shaw who showed that the axoplasm could be squeezed out of an axon and replaced by isotonic potassium sulfate, and that the axon would still conduct an action potential. The perfused axon allows study of the membrane properties with alteration of the internal solution; such an experiment is shown in Figure 5–12.

Action Potential Propagation. The preceding discussion was concerned with the properties of a single patch of membrane immediately under the tip of the recording electrode. The mechanism by which the action potential spreads down the axon is simply current spread from the active to the inactive regions (Figure 5–13). The potential of the active region is very close to the sodium equilibrium potential, whereas the potential of the resting region, a little further down the axon, is close to the potassium equilibrium potential. Ions will flow between these two regions of unequal potential. When the ionic

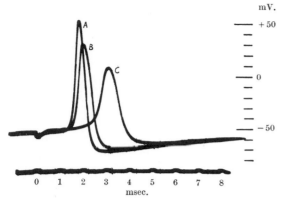

Figure 5–12 Action potentials recorded across the membrane of a squid giant axon whose axoplasm has been squeezed out and replaced with an artificial solution. In record *A* the solution is isotonic potassium sulfate, 600 mM K^+. In record *B* the internal solution is 3/4 K^+, 1/4 Na^+, 450 mM K^+. In record *C* the internal solution is 1/2 K^+, 1/2 Na^+. The Na in the sea water is 460 mM. (From Baker, P. F., Hodgkin, A. L., and Shaw, T. I.: Nature, *190*:885, 1961.)

flow crosses the membrane of the resting region, it depolarizes the membrane to threshold, the sodium permeability increases, resulting in further depolarization, and an action potential is generated in this previously resting region. This process continues on in each thin region of the axon. As can be seen in Figure 5–13, there is a short time delay between the peak of the action potential at A and B. The conduction velocity is obtained by dividing the distance, ΔX, by the time, Δt. The conduction velocity of nonmyelinated nerves is roughly proportional to the square of the diameter and varies from 0.3 meters/sec. for a 0.7 μ axon to 25 meters/sec. for a 500 μ squid giant axon.

Saltatory Conduction. In unmyelinated nerves, increased conduction velocity is achieved by increasing the diameter of the axon. Nature has found another way to achieve this—by increasing the distance between active regions along the nerve fiber. The time, Δt, between successive peaks of the action potential is little affected by the distance between the active regions. Consequently, the conduction velocity will increase as the distance between active regions increases. The myelin sheath around many nerves prevents ions from moving across the membrane, and therefore only the spaces between successive myelin sheaths, the nodes

of Ranvier, are used for ionic movement. Consequently, the action potential jumps from node to node, about 1 mm. at a jump. Conduction velocities in myelinated nerves run from 10 meters/sec. for a 2 μ fiber to 100 meters/sec. for a 20 μ nerve.

Refractory Period. Immediately after an action potential, the axon is incapable of carrying a second action potential. This period lasts for about the duration of the action potential, 1 to 2 msec. This absolute refractory period is followed by a relative refractory period during which a supranormal stimulus is necessary to evoke an action potential. This period lasts for another 2 to 3 msec. These two refractory periods put an upper limit of the nerve's frequency response at about 200 per second.

Active Transport. As was previously discussed, sodium is very far from electrochemical equilibrium across the axon membrane. A small efflux of sodium can be measured; sodium ions are moving up their electrochemical gradient. This process must require energy since work is being done. This conclusion is confirmed by the almost complete cessation of sodium efflux when the metabolic processes of the axon are shut off by poisons such as cyanide or DNP, as seen in Figure 5–14. It can also be seen in Figure 5–14 that injection of ATP will increase the sodium efflux for a short time. The ATP is broken down in the sodium transport.

The efflux of one sodium ion is coupled with the influx of one potassium ion. In this way the number of cations in the cell remains constant as does the number of particles in the cell. When potassium is removed from around the axon, the sodium efflux falls to very low values. In other systems the sodium is actively transported in conjunction with an anion, thereby preserving electroneutrality. In other systems only the sodium is actively transported and the accompanying ion is "dragged" through the membrane by an increased potential across the membrane.

In the nerve, active transport is a relatively slow continuous process that increases slightly after a large number of action potentials. Active transport maintains the ionic gradients on an hour to hour basis. It is not necessary to pump out the sodium that enters during a single action potential before a second action potential will fire. In fact, the average nerve will conduct thousands of action potentials while poisoned.

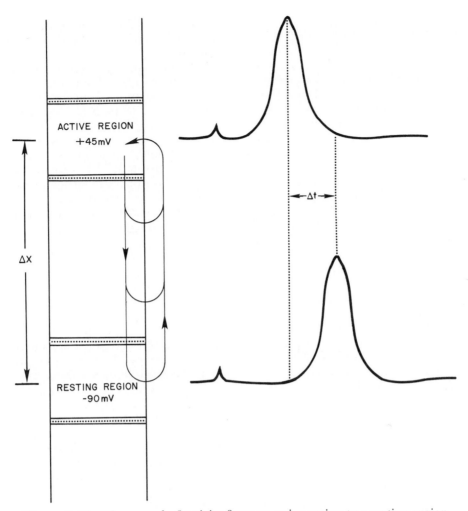

Figure 5–13 The spread of activity from an active region to a resting region.

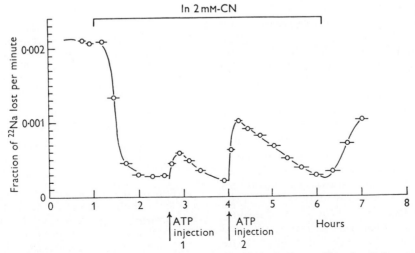

Figure 5–14 The effect of the metabolic poison, cyanide, on sodium efflux from the squid giant axon. Note that after ATP injection into the axon the Na⁺ efflux is briefly restored. (From Caldwell, P. C., Hodgkin, A. L., Keynes, R. D., and Shaw, T. I.: J. Physiol., *152*:561, 1960.)

MECHANISMS OF MEMBRANE PERMEABILITY AND SELECTIVITY

One of the earliest observations on the differences among molecules with different permeabilities was the high lipid solubility of highly permeable molecules. This is not too surprising in view of the high lipid content of membranes. These molecules apparently enter the cell by first dissolving in the lipid phase of the membrane.

Many substances of great importance to the cell, water and ions for example, are only very slightly soluble in lipid. These substances may enter the cell through pores in the membrane. It is fairly simple to develop equations to predict the size of these postulated pores (see Stein, 1967) from data on the movement of water into red blood cells under hydrostatic or osmotic gradients—data which is in good agreement with values for tritiated water flow under conditions of no net water flow. The calculated value of pore diameter is about 3.5Å. There are, however, many molecules of this radius, both charged and uncharged, which are not nearly as permeable as the theory of plain membrane pores would suggest. To be tenable, the pore hypothesis must assume some interaction between the pore and the penetrating substance. Much the same conclusions are reached in the study of water and electrolyte permeability in the toad bladder.

All the studies of charged ions point to a variety of patterns in ease of permeability. A recent and intriguing theory of ionic selectivity is presented by Diamond and Wright (1969). For one type of selectivity, they consider the first step in the entrance of an ion to the cell to be an interaction between a charged membrane site and a hydrated ion. There are two forces acting on the hydrated ion. One is the electrostatic attraction between ion and site. For ion-site binding to occur, however, the hydrated ion must be pulled away from its shell of water molecules. The latter requires a force equal to the energy of hydration. Since ions of small radius have a high charge density, they have a high energy of hydration and will require an intense ion-site attraction to pull them away from their water shell. This kind of intense ion-site attraction for a small ion is provided by a small, highly charged site. Such a site will have little attraction for a large, poorly hydrated ion and the attraction ratio and

hence permeability ratio will be $Li^+ > Na^+ > K^+ > Rb^+ > Cs^+$. On the other extreme a site of very low charge density will attract primarily large ions since these have very little water of hydration and large radii.

Even this brief summary should make it clear that membrane permeability and selectivity are very poorly understood. Since these mechanisms are central to the life of the cell and, consequently, the organism, they are being actively pursued, and an understanding of these mechanisms will, hopefully, soon be forthcoming.

Local Anesthetics. Local anesthetics are widely used to block nerve conduction in the peripheral nervous system. Their mechanism of action is well illustrated in the voltage clamping curves shown in Figure 5–15. The local anesthetic, procaine in this case, specifically blocks the increase of P_{Na} with voltage. Since the sodium permeability does not increase, the axon remains as a passive cable and will not conduct a nerve impulse. As can be seen in Figure 5–15, the potassium current, for the same depolarization, is reduced; the membrane resistance has increased. Local anesthetics do not change the resting membrane potential.

Local anesthetics affect small nerve fibers before affecting large nerve fibers. Consequently pain fibers are blocked before motor fibers. As the anesthesia wears off, the small fibers are the last to recover.

There are two main groups of local anesthetics, one based on the chemical formula

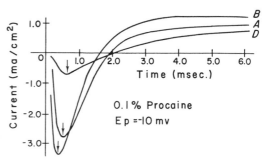

Figure 5–15 The effect of 0.1% procaine at pH 7.9 on the membrane currents following a depolarizing step. *B*, before; *D*, during; and *A*, after the application of procaine. Arrows indicate the time of the peak inward current. Axon 57–60, 12.5° C. (From Taylor, R. E.: Am. J. Physiol., *196*:1071, 1959.)

of procaine

$$H_2N \langle \bigcirc \rangle \overset{\overset{\displaystyle O}{\|}}{C}-O-(CH_2)_2-N \overset{\displaystyle C_2H_5}{\underset{\displaystyle C_2H_5}{\diagdown}}$$

and the other on lidocaine

$$\underset{CH_3}{\overset{CH_3}{\diagdown}} \langle \bigcirc \rangle -NH-\overset{\overset{\displaystyle O}{\|}}{C}-CH_2-N \overset{\displaystyle C_2H_5}{\underset{\displaystyle C_2H_5}{\diagdown}}$$

There are so many effective variants on these two themes that it is unlikely that the local anesthetics have any specific effect on a single chemical reaction.

Since there are so many local anesthetics available, the practitioner has the luxury of choice in what drug to use. The perfect local anesthetic would be effective in low dose and nonirritating to tissues, and the nerve block would be completely reversible. This perfect drug would have no effects on other systems of the body and would have a short latency of onset and its duration of action could be controlled. As one has come to expect in the real world, no drug is perfect. All of the local anesthetics available today cause a block which has a rapid onset and is completely reversible and do not irritate tissues. Unfortunately local anesthetics with a duration of action of greater than one hour are not presently available.

The major problem with local anesthetics is their systemic effects. The drug leaves the site of injection, enters the blood stream and will, in moderate serum doses, affect the central nervous system. The patient first becomes excitable and restless, and may have convulsions, but soon goes into a state of massive central nervous system depression, often leading to a cessation of breathing. These toxic effects are so severe that each potential local anesthetic must be examined to determine its toxic dose. In particular, we are looking for the drug which will have the widest margin between the effective blocking dose and the toxic dose.

The systemic toxicity of local anesthetics can be reduced by keeping the drug at the injection site. This is accomplished by the addition of a peripheral vasoconstrictor which will reduce the blood flow and keep the local concentration higher for longer periods of time; therefore less drug will need to be injected.

Most local anesthetics are broken down in the liver. A patient with poor liver function will often obtain very high serum drug levels because the rate of destruction is reduced, even though normally safe amounts of the drug are injected.

PROBLEMS

1. a. Values of the membrane potential at various external potassium concentrations are shown below for a cell at 20° C. with an internal potassium concentration of 140 mM.

K_o	Membrane Potential
1.0 mM	−102 mV
2.5	−92
5	−80
10	−66
20	−47
40	−30
80	−15
140	+2

Calculate the value of the potassium equilibrium potential in each case. Do all the data points agree with the values of the potassium equilibrium potential? One of the assumptions of the Nernst equation was that only one ion be permeant. As judged by the preceding data, under what circumstance is this most true for the cell membrane? Least true?

b. After an overnight soak in a high potassium solution, the same cell now has an internal potassium concentration of 200 mM. What is the expected membrane potential immediately after placing it in 2.5 mM potassium Ringer solution?

c. The Goldman equation was developed to describe the situation in which more than one ion is permeant. Use it to fit the data for 1.0 and 40 mM K_o. Try ratios of P_{Na} to P_K of about 0.01.

2. a. Now let us stimulate the cell and record the action potential with an intracellular microelectrode. Typical results are shown in Figure 5–16. What is the sodium equilibrium potential in each case? Does the peak of the action potential reach E_{Na}? Can you give a reason for your answer?

b. Measure the slope of the steepest part of the rising phase of the action potential. Has it changed? Can you give a reason for your answer?

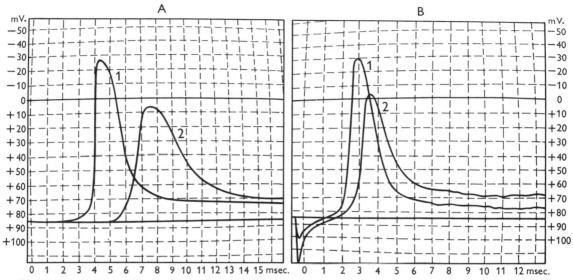

Figure 5–16 Four intracellular recordings from a single frog muscle fiber. Records 1 in *A* and *B* were taken in 120 mM Na^+ Ringer's fluid. Record 2 in *A* was taken in 24 mM Na^+ Ringer's fluid. Record 2 in *B* was taken in 36 mM Na^+ Ringer's fluid. The internal sodium may be taken as 20 mM. (From Nastuck, W. L., and Hodgkin, A. L.: J. cell. comp. Physiol., *35*:39, 1950.)

c. The fiber was stimulated at zero time by an electrode 2.5 mm. away from the recording electrode. What is the conduction velocity in each case? Can you think of a reason why it might change?

3. The average sodium influx per action potential is 4×10^{-12} moles per impulse per cm.² of surface area. The giant squid axon is 800×10^{-4} cm. in diameter and contains 20 mM/L of Na at rest. After the axon conducts 10,000 impulses, what will be the percentage increase in the internal sodium concentration if no active transport of sodium occurs? Small unmyelinated nerves are about 5×10^{-4} cm. in diameter; what is the percentage increase under the same circumstances?

4. A gallbladder of a rabbit was excised and filled with a solution containing 110 mM NaCl and a tiny amount of a neutral, impermeable dye, phenol red. It was suspended in a solution of 110 mM NaCl with an identical osmotic pressure and the following data obtained:

	$t = 0$	$t = 120$ min.
weight	2700 mg.	2220 mg.
Na_i	110 mM/L	110 mM/L
phenol red inside	0.2 μgm./ml.	0.25 μgm./ml.

The solution outside the gallbladder did not contain any phenol red, which is a large colloidal particle.

a. Assume that 200 mg. of the initial weight was tissue weight; what was the volume of solution inside the gallbladder at $t = 0$?

b. What was the *volume* after 120 minutes?

c. Has the *amount* of sodium inside the cell changed? By how much?

d. Has the *amount* of phenol red inside the gallbladder changed during this time?

e. There is no electrical potential difference across the gallbladder wall. Are Na^+ and Cl^- in equilibrium across the membrane? Are there any passive forces that could cause this movement?

f. When the preparation is treated with 3 mM CN^- and 3 mM iodoacetate, the weight remains constant. What causes the weight loss in the nonpoisoned gallbladder?

g. When sucrose is added to the inner solution, the following data is obtained (Fig. 5–17). Why has the rate of water loss decreased as the sucrose inside the gallbladder increased?

h. If a gallbladder containing 80 mM sucrose, in addition to the usual salts, were poisoned with CN^- and iodoacetate, what would the rate of weight change be?

5. A recent expedition studied a curious annelid (worm), *Porcellus terristrus*, which lives in a lithium-rich lake. The lake water

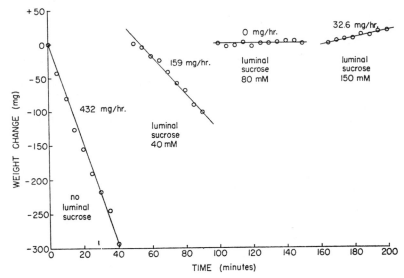

Figure 5-17 The effects of osmotic gradients upon fluid transport by rabbit gallbladder. (From Diamond, J. M.: J. gen. Physiol., *48*:1, 1964.)

contained 246 mM/L Li and 2 mM/L Rb; the anion was bromide (248 mM/L).

The interstitial fluid of this curious beast contains the same concentrations of Li, Br, and Rb as the lake water.

There is 190 μ nerve fiber in the ventral nerve cord, which is easily dissected. Within the axoplasm the concentrations were Rb, 200 mM/L, Li, 40 mM/L and Br, 2.5 mM/L. The membrane potential of the freshly dissected axon was −147 mV. All experiments were carried out at 20° C.

a. Calculate E_{Rb}, E_{Li}, and E_{Br}.

b. Does the membrane potential appear to be an equilibrium type potential of any of these ions?

c. The lithium influx was 18×10^{-12} moles/cm.²/sec. Since the axon was neither gaining nor losing Li, what was the Li efflux?

d. When the axon was poisoned with cyanide the membrane potential fell immediately to −95 mV and the Li efflux fell to 0.2×10^{-12} moles/cm.²/sec.

When Rb_o was altered, the following data was obtained from the poisoned axon:

Rb_o	V_m
40	−43
60	−30
80	−22
120	−12

Calculate E_{Rb} for each case. Now does the membrane potential of the poisoned axon appear to be an equilibrium potential?

e. When the same experiment was carried out on the intact axon this data resulted:

Rb_o	V_m
20	−115
40	−88
60	−82
80	−69
120	−61

Does the membrane potential in this case relate to the E_{Rb} values calculated earlier?

f. Can you divide the normal resting membrane potential into two parts?

References

Cole, K. S.: *Membranes, Ions and Impulses.* Berkeley, University of California Press, 1968.

Diamond, J. M., and Wright, E. M.: Biological membranes: the physical basis of ion and nonelectrolyte selectivity. Ann. Rev. Physiol., 1969.

Hodgkin, A. L.: Ionic movements and electrical activity in giant nerve fibres. Proc. Roy. Soc., *B148*:1, 1958.

Hodgkin, A. L.: *The Conduction of the Nerve Impulse.* Springfield, Ill., Charles C Thomas, 1964.

Hodgkin, A. L., and Huxley, A. F.: Resting and action potentials in single nerve fibers. J. Physiol., *104*:176, 1945.

Hodgkin, A. L., and Rushton, W. A. H.: The electrical constants of crustacean nerve fibers. Proc. Roy. Soc., *B133*:444, 1946.

Stein, W. D.: *The Movement of Molecules Across Cell Membranes.* New York, Academic Press, 1967.

6

Muscle and Nerve-Muscle Junction

BRIAN CURTIS

STRIATED MUSCLE

The major ending of the efferent branch of the central nervous system consists of the skeletal muscles. We work our will upon the outside world through these muscles. Skeletal muscles occupy about 80 per cent of the total weight of the body. They use about 10 per cent of the resting oxygen consumption; after strenuous exercise they may use as much as 70 per cent of the oxygen consumption. Each muscle is delimited by strong fascial sheets and has a characteristic origin and insertion. The basic unit of the muscle is the muscle fiber or cell that runs from one end of the muscle to the other end and has a diameter of 50 to 100 μ.

The structure of a group of fibers is shown in Figure 6–1. The muscle is subdivided anatomically into bundles of many fibers. Groups of fibers are delimited functionally by their nervous innervation. As the diagram shows, the muscle or motor nerve branches and innervates a number of muscle fibers. The muscle fibers which are innervated by a single motor nerve are called a motor group. All these fibers act in the same manner since they are controlled by a single nerve. The number of muscle fibers in a motor group varies from 300 to 400 in the gastrocnemius (calf) muscle to 4 to 6 in the extraocular muscles. In general, the size of the muscle group is proportioned to the sensitivity of the movement required. The extraocular muscles make very small, fine adjustments; the gastrocnemius muscle, coarse, powerful movements.

When the motor nerve is stimulated, an action potential travels down the axon until it reaches the end-plate region, where it releases a chemical transmitter, acetylcholine. The acetylcholine diffuses to a specialized portion of the muscle surface, the motor end plate, and initiates a second action potential there. We will discuss this step in greater detail later in the chapter.

The action potential travels out along the muscle surface from the end-plate region with a conduction velocity of about 1 meter/sec. The muscle action potential and its propagation are essentially similar to the nerve action potential which we discussed in the previous chapter. After a delay of 5 to 10 msec. the muscle generates tension. We study this tension with the muscle pulling either at constant length (isometrically) or at constant load (isotonically).

A single contractile event takes approximately 50 msec. and is shown graphically in Figure 6–2A. The response to a single stimulus, either to the motor nerve or to the muscle surface, is called a *twitch* and is relatively uncommon in the intact animal.

Muscular activity usually occurs in response

104

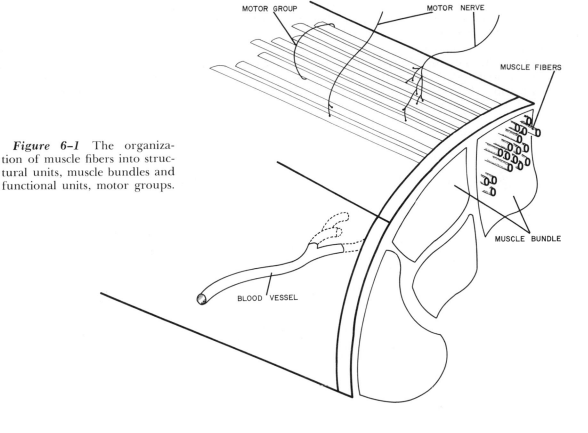

Figure 6–1 The organization of muscle fibers into structural units, muscle bundles and functional units, motor groups.

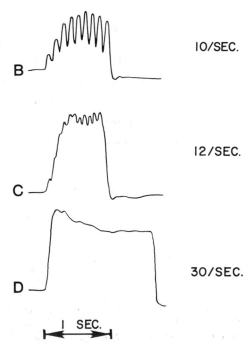

Figure 6–2 Isometric tension in response to stimuli of constant voltage and a varying frequency. Note that the total tension is greater when the frequency of stimulation is increased until a maximum (tetanus) tension is reached. Record from a human flexor carpi radialis muscle *in situ*. The subject's arm was held to a table with adhesive tape; stimulation was via a carbon electrode over the muscle mass in the upper forearm and a large ECG electrode at the wrist. The tension transducer was in contact with the styloid process on the wrist below the base of the thumb. Both wrist and finger flexors can be stimulated by this method.

to a series of action potentials, a partial or complete tetanus as illustrated in Figure 6–2*B, C, D*. It can be seen that increasing the frequency of stimulation to a muscle can increase the tension generated. Since motor units are in parallel, the tension from each adds up to give the final tension. The total tension a muscle produces is primarily a function of the number of motor units activated.

When we study the structure of the muscle fiber, the mechanism of contraction becomes clearer. Figure 6–3 shows the structure of a 100μ diameter muscle fiber and its component 1μ myofibrils. The banded pattern is clearly seen in the light microscope in

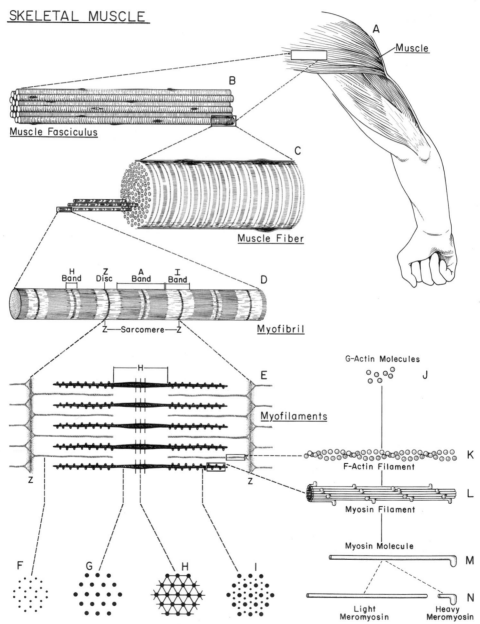

SKELETAL MUSCLE

Figure 6–3 Diagram of the organization of skeletal muscle from the gross to the molecular level. F, G, H, and I are cross sections at the levels indicated. (Drawing by Sylvia Colard Keene from Bloom and Fawcett: *A Textbool of Histology.* Philadelphia, W. B. Saunders, 1968.)

either single living fibers or fixed and stained material. The principal bands are a dark *A band* alternating with a light *I band*. The I band is bisected by a thin, dark *Z line*. The typical *sarcomere length* (Z line to Z line) is 2.5 μ. The basic contractile unit is a length of myofibril from Z line to Z line; after isolation, this unit, 1 μ in diameter and 2.5 μ long, will still contract. At higher magnification, in the electron microscope, it is clear that the bulk of the muscle structure is made up of two sets of filaments. The larger of these filaments, the thick filament, is 100 Å in diameter and 1.5 μ long and is located entirely within the A band. Indeed all of the properties of the A band can be attributed to these filaments. The thin filaments are 40 Å in diameter and 1.0 μ long and run from the Z line various distances into the A band. They are shown diagrammatically in Figure 6–3.

SLIDING FILAMENT HYPOTHESIS

Shortening of muscle fiber occurs as the result of thin filaments sliding past thick filaments. In this manner the distance between individual Z lines (sarcomere length) decreases, and the muscle length decreases as the product of the decrease per sarcomere times the number of sarcomeres per muscle. The exact mechanism of the interaction between the two sets of filaments is not clear at the moment, yet there is little doubt that the interaction exists. There are four major lines of evidence which lead to this mechanism. They were primarily developed by two Englishmen, Hugh E. Huxley and Andrew F. Huxley.

Cross sections through the array of thick and thin filaments are shown in Figure 6–3. Each set of filaments is arranged in a basically hexagonal array. In the region of overlap, section I, each of the thin filaments is related to three thick filaments and each thick filament is related to six thin filaments. Contact between these filaments is made by bridges as seen in Figure 6–4. These bridges stick out from the thick filaments and are arranged in a six-fold helix, like the treads on a spiral staircase. In this case, the stairs make a complete revolution in six steps.

When resting muscle is fixed at various sarcomere spacings, the length of each set of filaments remains constant as does the diameter. The amount of overlap between the thick and thin filaments varies in direct proportion to sarcomere length.

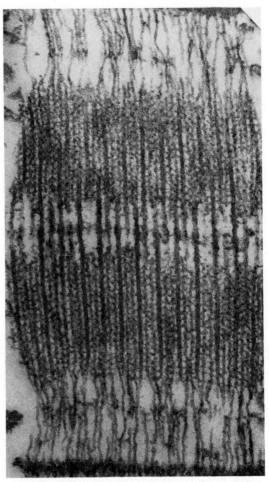

Figure 6–4 A view of the central region of the A band at 600,000 × magnification. The projections from the thick filaments, the bridges, are the site of interaction between the thick and thin filaments. (From Huxley, H. E.: J. Biophys. biochem. Cytol., *3*:631, 1957.)

Since the sliding filament model postulates that the filament lengths remain constant, the A band length should remain unchanged during contraction; two types of experiment have shown this to be true. Observation of living single muscle fibers with the interference microscope shows the A band width to remain constant during contraction. Only at very short sarcomere spacings does the A band width decrease. Experiments with contracting isolated fibrils observed with the phase contrast microscope show the same constancy of the A band width with the I band decreasing in width with decreasing sarcomere spacing.

It is the interaction between the two filament arrays that produces tension; the bridges (Fig. 6–4) of the thick filaments "hook on" to the thin filaments. The tension production, then, should be related to the number of bridges connected to thin filaments, to the degree of overlap, and to the sarcomere spacing. When the sarcomere spacing is just greater than the sum of the lengths of the A and I band filaments (3.6μ) there should be no overlap, no bridge interaction, and consequently no tension production. This is shown as point A of Figure 6–5A. As the sarcomere spacing decreases, the number of bridges increases and so does the tension. The number of bridges and the tension increase until length B is reached. At this point all of the bridges are attached since there are no bridges in the center of the A band, as can be seen in Figure 6–4.

Further shortening gives no increase in tension since there are no more bridges to interact, lengths B to C. In fact further shortening leads to decreased tension since one thin filament must force its way past its opposite filament, probably disturbing the bridge filament interaction, lengths C to D. Further shortening comes at the cost of compressing the A filaments so that most of the tension produced goes to compress the thick filaments. These then are the major lines of evidence favoring the sliding filament model which is almost universally accepted.

ACTIVE STATE

When the bridges from the thick filaments interact with the thin filaments, they develop tension 3 to 5 msec. after the action potential runs along the surface. Tension cannot, however, be measured in the tendon for 10 to 20 msec. following stimulation. What causes the delay? Between the tension-generating elements (the bridges) and the tendon there is a great deal of elastic material in series with the tension-generating element. The tension produced by the bridges must first stretch the elastic material before tension can be transmitted to the tendon and the load. Consider for a moment a man pulling on a rope which is attached, with a spring, to a large rock. When he begins pulling, the spring stretches until it transmits the full force of his pull. Remember that for each force placed on a spring, the spring will extend to a characteristic length and no further.

Let us return to the case of the muscle. Following a single stimulus, the bridges gen-erate tension for a very short time (Fig. 6–6). This tension is mainly expended in stretching the series elastic element; about one-half of the bridge tension appears as tendon tension. If a second stimulus follows soon after the first, the renewed bridge tension pulls on a partially extended elastic element and consequently must do less work on it to transmit tension to the tendon; more of the bridge tension is applied to the tendon. This is best demonstrated in the form of a diagram (Fig. 6–6). If a third stimulus follows the first two, the work the bridges do on the series elastic element is reduced. Consequently, the work done and tension produced on the tendon is increased (Fig. 6–2).

In the years before the sliding filament model was developed, the interaction between the bridges and the thin filaments—the basic work-producing reaction—was known as the active state. The duration of the active state has been measured in a number of ways. If the muscle is suddenly stretched with a load equal to tetanus tension very soon after stimulation, it will not lengthen. Clearly, there must be a force equal to the tetanus tension being generated within the muscle to resist the stretch. Since this force can be measured by the stretching technique long before the peak of tension, it must exist but is usually masked by the series elastic element. In this case the experimenter is extending the series elastic element so that the bridge tension can be transmitted to the force transducer.

A great deal of information about active state has been obtained by releasing the muscle after it has developed isometric tension. If the muscle is allowed to shorten 10 per cent of its length at the time of peak of twitch tension, the tension falls to zero and then is redeveloped but at a slower rate and reaching a lower peak. Clearly, the bridges are not working as hard at this time as they were earlier. By altering the time of release, the intensity of the active state can be plotted. This curve agrees quite well with the curve obtained by the quick stretch experiments.

FORCE-VELOCITY CURVE

We have concentrated so far on the generation of tension; to do useful work the muscle must shorten. When a muscle shortens against a very light load (weight) it shortens very quickly. As the load increases, the velocity decreases. A force-velocity curve is

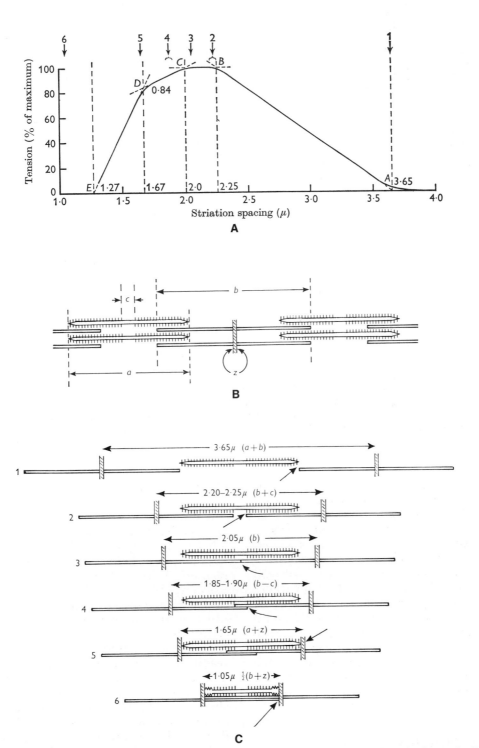

Figure 6–5 The length-tension diagram (*A*) for single muscle fibers and its basis (*B* & *C*) in the molecular structure of the thick and thin filaments. (From Gordon, A. M., Huxley, A. F., and Julian, F. J.: J. Physiol., *184*:170, 1966.)

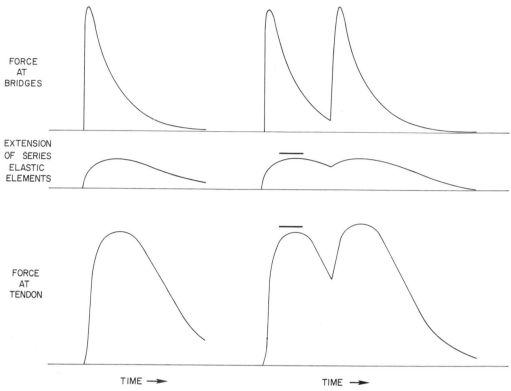

FORCE
AT
BRIDGES

EXTENSION
OF SERIES
ELASTIC
ELEMENTS

FORCE
AT
TENDON

TIME ⟶   TIME ⟶

Figure 6–6 Calculated values for bridge tension, length of series elastic component, and tension. Note especially that a second stimulus can capitalize upon extension of the series elastic element and thereby increase the tension at the tendon. (These records were kindly supplied by Dr. F. J. Julian. For further details of the computation, see Julian, F. J.: Biophysical J. *9*:547, 1969.)

shown in Figure 6–7. It was made with the human forearm lifting increasingly heavy weights. The same curve can be obtained with an isolated muscle; maximum tension and maximum speed will vary, however, from muscle to muscle.

The curve has been fitted by A. V. Hill with the equation $(P + a)(V + b) = (P_0 + a)b$, where P is the force, P_0 is the isometric tetanic force, V is the velocity of shortening, and a and b are constants. The constants, a and b, can be fitted uniquely and are a major goal for theoretical models of muscle function. One such model has been very successfully developed by A. F. Huxley and expanded by F. Julian (1969), see Figure 6–6.

MUSCLE PROTEINS

Three major proteins have been extracted from skeletal muscle: actin, myosin, and tropomyosin. The first two are the major protein constituents; the third is a relatively small fraction. Figure 6–3 shows the packing

of the myosin molecules into the thick filaments.

Myosin has a molecular weight of 420,000 and can be readily divided into two subunits — heavy and light meromyosin. The heavy meromyosin retains the adenosinetriphosphatase (ATP) activity of the intact myosin. This fragment, which is thought to form the bridges, is the site of the degradation of ATP which is the immediate energy source for contraction.

Actin has a molecular weight of 60,000 and readily forms long chains of a fibrous protein. Two chains of F-actin, wound around each other, form the thin filaments. Tropomyosin alters the ATPase activity of myosin so that calcium ions are required for ATP breakdown and consequently for muscle activity.

Both actin and myosin can be brought into solution in 0.7M KCl and a thread of actomyosin can be formed when they are squirted out of a hypodermic needle into 0.1M KCl. This thread will contract when ATP is added to the solution. In fact, the tension for each

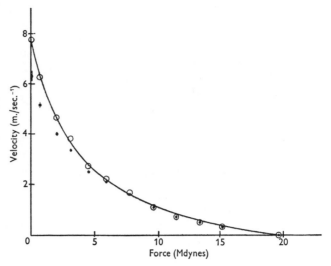

Figure 6-7 The relationship between the velocity of movement and the force of contraction of the human forearm. The force at zero movement is the maximum, presumably tetanic, isometric tension. (From Wilkie, D. R.: J. Physiol., *110*:249, 1949.)

cross sectional area is about that of intact muscle. Since the actomyosin threads have no apparent structure, it is clear that the regular structure of the striated muscle is not absolutely necessary for contraction. Indeed, smooth muscle shows no regular internal structure.

ENERGY FOR CONTRACTION

The immediate energy source for contraction is ATP. Experiments with model systems such as actomyosin threads have shown this beyond a doubt. Intact muscle contains rela-

tively large quantities of creatine phosphate. When all other sources of energy are cut off by treatment with nitrogen and iodoacetate, the fall in creatine phosphate content is directly proportional to the work done and the heat generated by the muscle. We are aware subjectively that muscular work produces heat in our muscles. In fact, this is one of the most important sources of heat for warm-blooded animals. Shivering is a manifestation of underlying muscular activity to produce heat. The relationship between creatine phosphate breakdown and work can be seen in Figure 6-8.

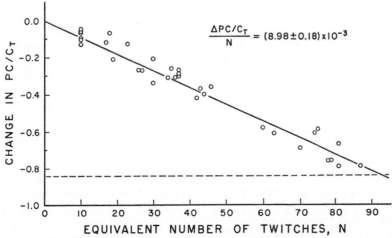

$$\frac{\Delta PC/C_T}{N} = (8.98 \pm 0.18) \times 10^{-3}$$

Figure 6-8 A plot of the change in creatine phosphate (normalized to the total creatine) versus the number of isometric twitches the muscle performed. The dotted line is the average maximum change in PC/C_r if all the creatine phosphate were split. (From Carlson, F. D., and Siger, A.: J. Gen. Physiol., *44*:33, 1960.)

The heat produced by muscle during activity has been measured by A. V. Hill using very sensitive instruments. He has been able to describe the heat produced by three components: (a) heat of activation, (b) heat of shortening, and (c) work. Attempts to correlate creatine phosphate breakdown with the heat of shortening have not yet been successful.

EXCITATION-CONTRACTION COUPLING

Skeletal muscle has a very enlarged and specialized reticular network which is shown in Figure 6–9. It can be subdivided into two portions: (1) transverse tubules or T system and (2) a longitudinal or sarcoplasmic reticulum. The T system is a tubular network which is continuous across the whole fiber and contains extracellular fluid. If a perfect cross section were cut across the fiber, the T system would look like a chicken wire fence with the fibrils running through the holes in the wire.

The elegant experiments by A. F. Huxley and his collaborators have shown that this system conducts the surface electrical activity inwards to cause contraction. By stimulating very small patches of the surface membrane they showed that the location of sensitive areas corresponded to the longitudinal location of the T system. This location varies; it is at the Z line in the frog and at the A-I junction of the lizard and many mammals. The inward conduction is probably by passive cable properties of the tubular wall.

After the surface depolarization travels inward, the next few steps are very cloudy. They result in the ultimate release of Ca^{++} from the longitudinal reticulum. This Ca^{++} diffuses to the contractile elements, activates the ATPase and brings about tension production. The Ca^{++} is then actively transported back into a different portion of the longitudinal reticulum causing relaxation. Successive stimuli release successive aliquots of Ca^{++} and result in the continued contraction seen in tetanus.

It should be noted that the highly regular structure of the skeletal or cross-striated muscle apparently has its major significance in the control of contraction rather than in the molecular organization of the contractile elements. The skeletal muscle is highly specialized to contract and relax quickly.

SMOOTH MUSCLE

Smooth muscle cells are spindle-shaped, have an average diameter of 10μ, and are 20 to 70μ long. They have little internal structure but contain actomyosin. They have none of the ordered reticular structure of the skeletal muscle. They are always found as part of a complex tissue—the intestines and blood vessels, to name a few. Typically the smooth muscles are rhythmically active, and control, via the autonomic nervous system, serves to regulate the general level of activity rather than to initiate each contraction. Since the cells are small, intracellular recording is difficult. Figure 6–10 shows both the electrical and contractile activity of a smooth muscle strip. Notice that the membrane potential slowly depolarizes until the threshold is reached and a train of action potentials is fired. Tension rises slowly following the action potentials.

Coordination between individual cells is by low resistance bridges, called the nexus. An example of one is shown in Figure 6–11. Action potentials are transmitted by electrical conduction from one cell to another by way of these specialized connections. The whole mass of cells acts as a single cell, a syncytium. If two microelectrodes are placed into a sheet of cells taken from the intestine, cable properties can be measured. The resistance between cells is considerably higher in the transverse direction than the longitudinal. Consequently, the action potential will spread from cell to cell faster in the longitudinal, down the tube, direction than in the circular direction.

The syncytial nature of smooth muscle makes study of the electrical properties much more difficult. It would appear that the ionic basis of the resting and action potentials is much the same as in nerve tissue. The slow depolarization preceding the action potentials is thought to represent a slow increase in P_{Na}. The only significant difference in the mechanism of contraction is in the origin of the Ca^{++} for activation. It would appear that Ca^{++} moves in through the membrane during the action potential and is subsequently pumped out, causing relaxation. There are no well-developed end plates; the nerve runs through the mass of smooth muscle cells. Each cell is not necessarily in contact with a nerve fiber. The nature of the nervous control will be discussed in Chapter 16.

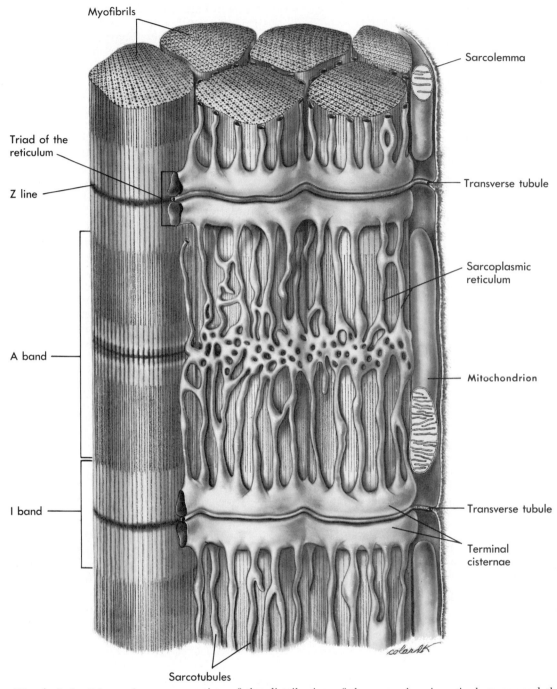

Figure 6–9 Schematic representation of the distribution of the sarcoplasmic reticulum around the myofibrils of skeletal muscle. The longitudinal sarcotubules are confluent with transverse elements called the terminal cisternae. A slender transverse tubule (T tubule) extending inward from the sarcolemma is flanked by two terminal cisternae to form the so-called triads of the reticulum. The location of these with respect to the cross-banded pattern of the myofibrils varies from species to species. In frog muscle, depicted here, the triads are at the Z line. In mammalian muscle there are two to each sarcomere, located at the A-1 junctions. (Modified after L. Peachey, from Fawcett, D. W., and McNutt, S.: J. Cell Biol., *25*:209, 1965. Drawn by Sylvia Colard Keene.)

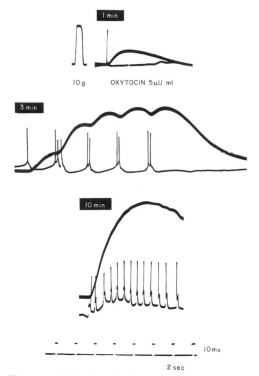

Figure 6–10 Intracellularly recorded action potentials and tension in a strip of uterus stimulated by oxytocin. The intracellular action potential is from a small group of cells; the tension is from the whole strip containing many thousands of cells. The average resting potential was −48 mv. (From Csapo, A. I., and Kuriyama, H.: Endocrinology, *68*:1010, 1961.)

NERVE-MUSCLE JUNCTION

To return to the control of skeletal muscle contraction, the motor nerve enters the muscle, branches, and forms a very close attachment (a synapse) with the center of the muscle fiber. The axon (presynaptic) and muscle (postsynaptic surface) remain two distinctly separate cells. The structure of the region is shown in Figure 6–12. Transmission between the axon and muscle is by the chemical, acetylcholine. The diagram clearly shows the specialization of the end plate to give a much larger postsynaptic than presynaptic surface. This arrangement, by itself, strongly suggests the release of a chemical, a transmitter, from the nerve which activates the postsynaptic surface.

To be considered as a transmitter, a substance must meet four criteria: (a) it must be effective at the postsynaptic surface, (b) it must be liberated by the presynaptic surface in response to and in proportion to nerve stimulation, (c) there must be an enzyme system for destroying liberated transmitter, and (d) there must be an enzyme system for synthesizing the transmitter.

Each of these criteria has, at the nerve-muscle junction, been met by acetylcholine. The idea of a chemical transmitter between nerve and muscle came from experiments by Otto Loewi on the slowing of the heart when the vagus nerve was stimulated. He noticed that fluid dripping over a slowed heart caused a second heart to slow as well. The only link between the two hearts was the Ringer's solution. Vagal stimulation liberated some substance into the solution which affected the second heart. It was soon clear that the substance was acetylcholine which had been studied earlier by H. H. Dale. Acetylcholine can be collected in small veins from stimulated muscles and from perfused preparations.

Acetylcholine is effective in stimulating contraction if it is injected very close to the muscle. When acetylcholine is microinjected onto an excised muscle, it elicits contraction only when perfused at the end-plate region. The rest of a normal muscle does not have ACh receptors. Both biochemical and histochemical studies show the presence at the

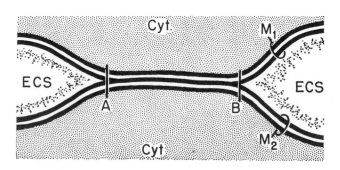

Figure 6–11 A drawing of a nexus. (*Cyt*) cytoplasm of the smooth muscle cells; (*ECS*) extracellular space; (*M₁*) and (*M₂*) plasma membranes; (*A*) to (*B*), nexus. (From Dewey, M. M., and Barr, L.: Science, *137*: 670, 1962. See also J. Cell. Biol., *23*:553, 1964.)

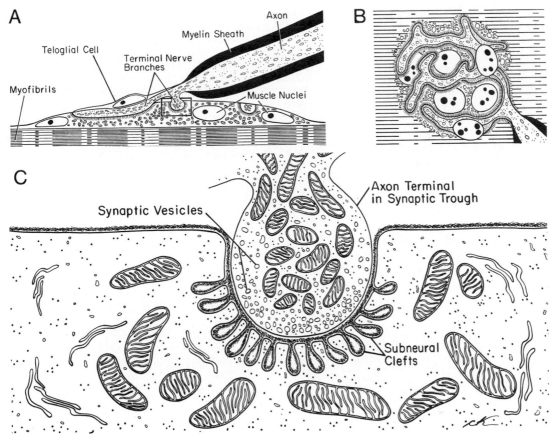

Figure 6–12 Schematic representations of the motor end plate as seen by light and electron microscopy. *A,* End plate as seen in histological sections in the long axis of the muscle fiber. *B,* As seen in surface view with the light microscope. *C,* As seen in an electron micrograph of an area such as that in the rectangle on A (After R. Couteaux. From Bloom and Fawcett: *A Textbook of Histology.* Philadelphia, W. B. Saunders, 1968.)

myoneural junction of an enzyme, acetylcholine esterase. It is present in the postsynaptic surface in the subneural folds and on the presynaptic side. It is also present in fairly high concentration in the blood which explains the general ineffectiveness of acetylcholine when injected intra-arterially.

The enzyme, choline acetylase, is present to reconstitute the transmitter. It would appear that the acetylcholine is packaged in the synaptic vesicles. Synaptic vesicles from the hypothalamus have been obtained by osmotic lysis; they look very similar to intact vesicles and contain acetylcholine. The vesicles are produced in the nerve cell body or under its direct control, since the number of vesicles decreases rapidly after section of the motor nerve.

Acetylcholine acts upon the postsynaptic membrane and destroys its selective permeability to all small ions as shown by an equilibrium potential of zero millivolts. This potential is, of course, never reached, but would be if acetylcholine were continuously applied to the end plate. The large concentration of acetylcholine esterase prevents such a large concentration from occurring. The depolarization brought about by the usual amount of acetylcholine causes a current to flow to the surrounding area. As the current flows through the peripheral membrane it depolarizes that membrane and sets up a propagated action potential. The end-plate region itself is not electrically excitable; current must flow to the surrounding area.

End-plate Potentials. When a microelectrode is inserted into the end-plate region, the usual resting membrane potential is recorded. When the motor nerve is stimulated the microelectrode records an action potential as shown in the lower traces of Figure 6–13. Careful examination of the left

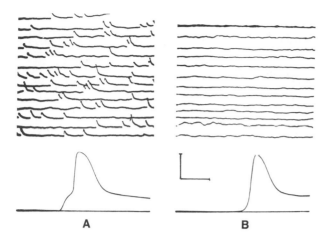

Figure 6–13A, Intracellular electrical events at the end-plate region, and *B*, 2mm. away. The upper traces are at high gain 3.6 mv and slow time scale, 47 msec. In *A* the miniature end-plate potentials (minis) are clearly shown, whereas in *B* they are almost nonexistent. The two bottom traces are at low gain, 50 mv and fast time scale, 2 msec. Note the end-plate potential at the leading edge of the action potential in *A*. (From Fatt, P., and Katz, B.: J. Physiol., *117*:109, 1952.)

hand action potential will reveal a lump on the leading edge of the action potential. This lump is the first part of the end-plate potential caused by the release of acetylcholine. It is a local change in the end-plate region; no end-plate potential is seen 2mm. away (B). The end-plate potential can be seen more clearly when curarine is applied to reduce the effectiveness of the acetylcholine and to produce a subthreshold depolarization.

Small depolarizations are recorded at times when the motor nerve is quiet (Fig. 6–13). They originate in the end-plate region and can be recorded only very close to it. These miniature end-plate potentials ("minis") are quantized in occurrence and in amplitude, although they rarely exceed 5 mV. These miniature end-plate potentials represent the release of several small pockets of acetylcholine; the smallest may very possibly represent the release of a single vesicle. The amplitude of these potentials increases as more pockets or vesicles are released. Each pocket or vesicle releases 10^{-17} moles of acetylcholine which results in a depolarization of 0.4 mV. An action potential arriving at the presynaptic terminal causes an increase in the rate of vesicle release so that about 100 vesicles discharge their acetylcholine over a very short interval; this amount of acetylcholine is sufficient to initiate an action potential on the muscle surface.

DRUGS ACTING ON NERVE-MUSCLE JUNCTION

D-tubocurarine competes for the same postsynaptic site as does acetylcholine; it binds more strongly to the site and does not bring about a permeability change. Conse-

quently, neuromuscular transmission is blocked since the acetylcholine cannot get to the sites to cause a permeability change. Hexamethonium and tetramethylammonium (TEA) also block by competitive antagonism. Gallamine (Flaxedil) is a synthetic d-tubocurarine. These drugs are slowly broken down and paralysis wears off.

Continued application of acetylcholine, and continued depolarization, does not result in continued skeletal muscle activity since the action potential mechanism of the muscle surface must be reset by repolarization after the first action potential. Any drug which acts by producing a continual depolarization at the end-plate produces a depolarization block. Consequently, nerve-muscle block and muscle relaxation should be achieved by infusing large quantities of acetylcholine; this method is very inefficient as the acetylcholine is broken down rapidly. Succinylcholine will bind to the postsynaptic surface and cause a permeability change but is slowly broken down by the esterase. Consequently, it produces a long-lasting depolarization. Since it depolarizes the muscle membrane, the muscle contracts once and then relaxes. Decamethonium also acts in this manner.

Drugs which block the nerve-muscle junction are often used in conjunction with anesthetics to achieve muscle relaxation during surgery. It should always be borne in mind that the respiratory muscle will also be blocked so that the patient must be artificially ventilated.

The end-plate can also be blocked by prolonging the action of the released acetylcholine by blocking the esterase activity. The anticholinesterases, such as neostigmine, edrophonium (Tensilon), eserine, and diisopropyl fluorophosphate (DFP), all combine with acetylcholine esterase and prevent it from destroying the acetylcholine, so that it continues to depolarize the end-plate region and to block transmission.

EFFECTS OF MOTOR NERVE ON MUSCLE

From the discussion so far, it would appear that the motor nerve supplies only the stimulus to contract; this is far from the case. When the motor nerve is cut, the muscle rapidly atrophies, its volume and strength of contraction decrease—all the fibers decrease in size as does the total muscle bulk. After three months, the muscle bulk may have decreased to as little as 25 per cent of its original size. This is not due to muscle disuse alone since disuse, such as that caused by immobilization, will result in atrophy to not more than 70 to 75 per cent of the original size. An intact motor nerve is necessary for continued survival of the muscle fiber. It would appear that the continued release of acetylcholine from the nerve, to cause either end-plate potentials or miniature end-plate potentials, is the agent responsible for this trophic influence.

Denervation Sensitivity. When the muscle is denervated the entire surface of the muscle fiber slowly becomes sensitive to acetylcholine. After several weeks, application of ACh anywhere on the surface will result in an action potential and contraction. Patients who have had a motor nerve severed show very great sensitivity to injected ACh for this reason.

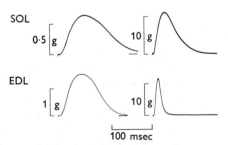

Figure 6-14 Twitch time in a fast, extensor digitorum longus (EDL) and a slow, soleus (SOL) muscle. At birth (left) the difference in twitch time is not striking, yet 5 weeks later (right) the difference is very pronounced. (From Close, R.: J. Physiol., *180*:542, 1965.)

Reinnervation. If the cut ends of a motor nerve are rejoined, sprouts of the central end will grow down the tube left by the degenerated axon. If the distance between the cut and the muscle is short and the cut ends are well aligned, the nerve will make contact with the muscle. A new end plate will form, and muscle function will be restored. Passive exercise of the muscle during regrowth is helpful to prevent disuse atrophy.

Slow and Fast Muscles. It is apparent on gross inspection that there are two sorts of mammalian skeletal muscle: red and white. The red ones have a much darker red cast than do the white ones. The best known example of this difference is in the white and dark meat of a chicken; the same qualitative differences carry over to mammals.

Figure 6-14 shows twitches from a red and a white muscle. Red muscle is characterized by a long twitch time, and concomitantly a low frequency of stimulation will result in tetanus. These muscles are primarily antigravity or postural muscles; their movements are characterized by long-sustained contractions. The red color is caused by enzymes of oxidative metabolism. The white muscles, on the other hand, have short twitch times and are used for quick phasic movements (a fast muscle).

The speed of contraction is determined by the pattern of activity in the motor nerve. When nerves from fast and slow muscles are crossed, the fast muscle slows down and the slow muscle speeds up. When a limb is immobilized, the activity to a slow muscle, which is usually intense, decreases; after several weeks the speed of contraction has increased markedly. It is not clear how the pattern of activity alters the biochemical control mechanisms and the contractile properties of a muscle.

COMMON DISEASES OF MUSCLE AND NERVE-MUSCLE JUNCTION

It should now be very clear that motor nerves have a profound effect on skeletal muscles. If the nerve is injured and dies, the muscle will be paralyzed and will atrophy. A discussion of this whole class of lower motor neuron diseases will be put off until after the spinal cord has been discussed. There are two major diseases of these tissues which will be covered here.

Myasthenia Gravis. The disease is characterized by progressive muscular weakness during activity. If the affected muscle is in the flexor of the hand, the first squeeze of a ball will be quite forceful, but the next few will rapidly decrease in power, until after a dozen squeezes there will be hardly any power left. The strength will return with rest. The condition is diagnosed by the characteristic history and by improvement with anticholinesterase therapy. The disease is limited to the end-plate region, yet its specific locus therein is uncertain.

Three major hypotheses as to the pathophysiology exist with some evidence suggesting each.

(1. The amount of acetylcholine released is less than normal and the anticholinesterase enhances the effectiveness of that which is released.

(2. There is a circulating factor, possibly an antibody produced by the thymus, which has a curarine-like effect. Babies born of myasthenic mothers show symptoms of myasthenia for several weeks after birth. Thymectomy, in adults, often relieves the severity of symptoms.

(3. There is some alteration in the postsynaptic membrane which makes it less sensitive to the acetylcholine released.

Any of these three possibilities would be compatible with improvement during anticholinesterase therapy. The second one is the favorite in 1971.

Not all muscles are uniformly affected by the disease. About one-third of the cases begin with weakness of a few muscles of the trunk or the extremities. These cases, as well as the others, generally have an insidious, gradual onset with no obvious cause. Indeed, the cause is unknown. This class shows dramatic improvement with the anticholinesterase drugs. Edrophonium (Tensilon) is a short-acting drug which must be injected; it is used for diagnostic purposes. Neostigmine, pyridostigmine (Mestinon), and ambenonium (Mytelase) can be given orally and have obvious advantages for long-term therapy. The dosage and schedule must be worked out for each patient and will change from time to time. This group has an excellent prognosis for adequate regulation by continued drug therapy.

Double vision, diplopia, is the most common presenting symptom, occurring in approximately one-half the cases. This is the result of involvement of the extraocular muscles. This group often responds poorly to anticholinesterase therapy.

Weakness of the muscles involved in chewing and swallowing constitutes the last major group. When these patients start a meal, they have no trouble chewing, but with each successive mouthful, chewing becomes labored and the patient is finally unable to swallow. Strength returns with rest. The prognosis of this group is often poor since they do not respond well to anticholinesterase therapy and often develop upper respiratory tract infections.

No matter where the disease starts, it slowly spreads to other muscles. The course is punctuated by remissions and exacerbations which require readjustment of drug dose. In a recent series of 1355 patients (Perlo et al., 1966) four-fifths of the patients had died within 10 years of the onset of the disease, which usually starts in the second to fourth decade and is more common in females.

Progressive Muscular Dystrophy. This is the most common disease of skeletal muscle. It is characterized by profound weakness of a muscle or muscle group. This class can be divided at once into hereditary and non-hereditary groups. Only the hereditary group will be considered here; the other types are rare and there are too many subclasses to be discussed in an introductory text. The hereditary dystrophies have been broken down into three groups.

1. The *Duchenne* type occurs almost exclusively in males and is inherited as a sex-linked recessive trait. More than half the cases begin before the boy is 3-years-old; almost all by 10 years. The muscles of the pelvic girdle are always affected first. Their weakness leads to a clumsiness in walking, frequent falling, and difficulty in climbing stairs and in getting up from the floor. The disease progresses rapidly so that 5 years after the onset the child is confined to a wheelchair and the disease has usually spread to the shoulder girdle as well.

During this time several of the muscles which are very weak look enlarged, the calf muscles in particular. This enlargement is not by muscle tissue but by fat invading the muscle and is known as pseudohypertrophy. In general, the muscle bulk is much larger than would be expected by the strength of the muscle. The course of the disease is downhill, and death of heart or respiratory failure usually occurs 15 to 20 years after the onset. The heart is often involved in the pathological process.

A muscle biopsy taken soon after onset

shows a much larger range of fiber size than usual. Many of the fibers are twice normal size while some are atrophied to very small size. Fat and connective tissue have already replaced some of the muscle substance. Later in the disease the muscle biopsy shows very small fibers and large quantities of fat and connective tissue.

2. The *limb-girdle* type of progressive muscular dystrophy is a more variable and less certain category. The disease usually begins in the shoulder girdle during the second or third decade of life. Weakness in lifting the arms and winging (protrusion) of the scapula are common. The progression of the disease is similar to the Duchenne type but is much slower. There are various modes of inheriting the disease; the most common is as an autosomal recessive trait. The severity of the disease is variable, yet it is not uncommon for a patient to be working 20 years after onset. The life span is probably reduced.

3. The *facioscapulohumeral* group is the third classification. The disease usually begins in the facial muscles during adolescence and spreads to the shoulder girdle. It is usually transmitted as a dominant trait. Its progression is very slow; many patients have only a few muscles involved years after onset. The life span is normal. The pathology is similar to the Duchenne type.

These three categories are by no means exhaustive and distinct; many borderline cases exist. Their major advantage is one of prognosis. The underlying cause is unknown, and there is no known treatment.

Diagnosis: Electromyography. A sterile electrode, in the form of a needle, can be inserted into a muscle and used for making electrical recordings which have considerable value in the differential diagnosis of several types of diseases which cause muscle weakness. When the patient is asked to contract the muscle containing the electrode, large (500 mv) potentials, the synchronized action currents from many muscle units, are recorded. There are no spontaneous potentials in a normal recording. When there is disease of the motor nerves, spontaneous potentials are recorded which are smaller (100 mv) yet still synchronous.

These are often accompanied by visible twitchings beneath the skin which are called *fasciculations*. Fasciculations usually indicate disease in the motor nerve or its cell body, the anterior horn cell, in the central nervous system (CNS). When single muscle fibers contract spontaneously, very small (<50 mv), very rapid, spontaneous potentials are recorded and are termed *fibrillations*. They are rarely accompanied by visible twitching beneath the skin.

References

Adams, R., Denny-Brown, D., and Pearson, C.: *Diseases of Muscle.* New York, Hoeber, 1962.

Bulbing, E., Brading, A., Jones, A., and Tomita, T.: *Smooth Muscle.* Baltimore, Williams and Wilkins, 1970.

Davson, H.: A Textbook of General Physiology, 3rd Edition. Boston, Little, Brown, and Company, 1964.

Eccles, J. C.: *The Physiology of Synapses.* New York, Academic Press, 1964.

Hill, A. V.: *First and Last Experiments in Muscle Mechanics.* Cambridge, Cambridge University Press, 1970. (Contains a short history of much of muscle physiology.)

Hubbard, J., Llinas, R., and Quastel, D.: *Electrophysiological Analysis of Synaptic Transmission.* Baltimore, Williams and Wilkins, 1969.

Peachey, L. D.: Muscle *In* Annual Review of Physiology, Vol. 30, Palo Alto, California, Annual Reviews, 1968.

Perlo, V. P., Poskanzer, D. C. Schwab, R. S., Viets, H. R., Osserman, K. E., and Genkins, G.: Myasthenia gravis: evaluation of treatment in 1355 patients. Neurology (Minn.), *16*:431–439, 1966.

Podolsky, R. J. (ed.): *Contractility of Muscle Cells and Related Processes.* Englewood Cliffs, New Jersey, Prentice-Hall, 1971.

Riker, W. F. Jr., and Ramoto, M.: Pharmacology of Motor Nerve Terminals, *In* Annual Review of Pharmacology, Vol. 9, Palo Alto, California, Annual Reviews, 1969.

7

Spinal Cord

BRIAN CURTIS

Since the spinal cord is the best understood and least complex of the major elements of the central nervous system, it is appropriate to begin the discussion of the CNS with it. The spinal cord has two fairly distinct functions. It conducts action potentials to and from the brain and it relates to "its" segment.

The spinal cord is segmented, one segment per vertebra, and in the less complex nervous system of fish, the region of the body relating to each segment is a cylindrical band the width of the vertebra. Into this spinal cord segment flows all of the sensory information from the body segment: information on pain, temperature, position of the muscles, touch, and vibration. The axons which innervate the muscles of the body segment have their nuclei in the spinal cord segment.

In the human there is only a general relationship between the sensory segments and muscles innervated by the same segment of the cord. The size and shape of the regions vary considerably, but the principle remains the same—that of relating, in sensory reception and motor control, to a delimited region. The spinal cord also processes the sensory information and can initiate stereotyped motor activity.

In addition to relating these functions to specific regions, the spinal cord processes incoming sensory information and sends some of it on to the brain. This is a second and basically distinct function of the spinal cord: conduction to and from the brain. These two functions are anatomically separated. Inspection of cross section of an unstained spinal cord shows a white band surrounding a gray, butterfly-shaped interior (Fig. 7–1). The myelin sheaths of the thousands of axons running up and down in the white matter produce the white color. The thousands of cell bodies in the center give

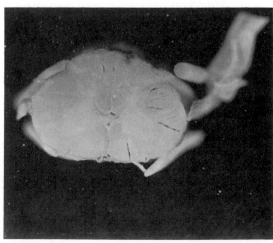

Figure 7–1 A photograph of an unstained cross section of a human spinal cord.

120

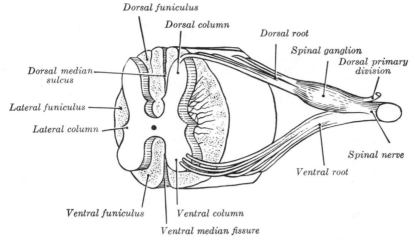

Figure 7–2 The dorsal and ventral roots in relation to the spinal cord. (From Gross, C. M. (ed.): *Gray's Anatomy.* Philadelphia, Lea and Febiger, 1966.

that region a gray appearance. We speak, then, of gray matter, which contains synapses relating to the sensory and motor activities of the segment, and of white matter, which contains axons running to and from the brain.

Each spinal cord segment has four nerve roots attached to it (Fig. 7–2). The two *anterior* or *ventral roots*, which carry axons to innervate muscles, are known as motor axons. The two *posterior* or *dorsal roots* carry sensory information into the spinal cord. The cell bodies of all of the sensory fibers are in the posterior root ganglion. The two roots on each side join to form a *spinal nerve* to the same side of the body. Damage to the right anterior root will paralyze a few muscles on the right side of the body. Damage to the left posterior root will interrupt *all* modalities of sensation from a small region on the left side of the body.

GROSS ANATOMY OF THE SPINAL CORD

The gross anatomy of the spinal cord is well illustrated in Figure 7–3. The cord runs through the spinal canal of each vertebra, as is shown in Figure 7–4, and is protected by a number of layers of meninges. The pia mater is closely adherent to the cord. Immediately surrounding the pia mater in the *subarachnoid space* is cerebrospinal fluid. The arachnoid lies inside the thick, tough *dura*, which is in close contact with the vertebra.

The denticulate ligaments anchor the spinal cord to the dura.

The spinal cord and, more importantly, the spinal roots, are named in relation to the vertebral column. In man there are 8 *cervical*, 12 *thoracic*, 5 *lumbar*, and 5 *sacral* segments. They are shown in relation to the vertebral column in Figure 7–3. Older books and neurologists refer to the thoracic spine as the dorsal spine and abbreviate it *D*.

During development and growth, the vertebral column grows faster than the spinal cord it contains so that, in the adult, the spinal cord does not extend the length of the vertebral column (Figure 7–3). As a result the spinal nerves run inferiorly before they leave the spinal canal. The spinal cord ends at the first or second lumbar vertebra, and below this level the spinal canal contains only spinal nerves. This mass of nerves reminded early anatomists of a horse's tail, so it was named *cauda equina*. The nerve roots run through the subarachnoid space, which is filled with cerebrospinal fluid. When a needle is inserted through the space between the fourth and fifth lumbar vertebra (Fig. 7–5), the point penetrates the dura and pushes aside the spinal roots. If the needle were inserted above L2 there would be danger of damaging the spinal cord. Samples of cerebrospinal fluid can be taken through this needle, and pressure can be measured or anesthetic agents injected at this point.

The spinal nerves exit from the vertebral column through recesses in the posterior process of each vertebra, as is shown in Fig-

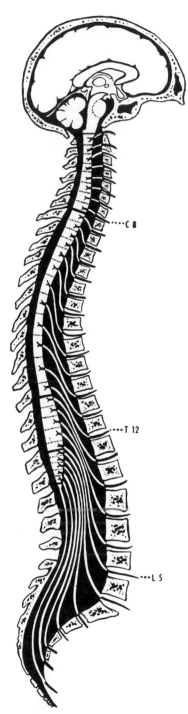

Figure 7-3 Diagrammatic representation of the brain and spinal cord to show the relation of cord, spinal nerves, and vertebrae. The anterior and posterior roots are shown as single nerves emerging from each segment. (From Gardner, Gray, and O'Rahilly: *Anatomy.* Philadelphia, W. B. Saunders, 1969.)

ure 7-6. The canal, the intervertebral neural foramina, is only a little larger than the nerve so that any swelling of the nerve or diminution of the diameter of the canal will pinch the nerve. It is not uncommon for the intervertebral disc to rupture posteriorly or laterally and press on a spinal nerve as it exits. The very intense pain this pressing causes is referred to the area of the skin where the nerve began. A frequent site where the nerve roots are pinched is the area between L2 and S1, which gives rise to the sciatic nerve. The pinched nerve gives the patient the impression that a hot knife is being dragged up the posterior aspect of his calf.

The cross sections of the spinal cord vary with the level (Fig. 7-7) as a result of the change in the white and gray matter. The white matter decreases in bulk as the sections are taken further from the brain. Motor tracts from the brain leave the white matter to enter the gray matter and synapse with motor neurons. Sensory fibers entering the cord, section by section, also form the white matter.

A section of the cervical cord contains sensory fibers running up to the brain from the thoracic, lumbar, and sacral sections. It also contains motor fibers running down to innervate motor axons of the thoracic, lumbar, and sacral sections. The white matter of a section of the lumbar cord, however, contains fibers to and from the lumbar segments inferior to it and the sacral segments. The white matter columns have the shape of thin pyramids with their bases at the foramen magnum and their tips at the last sacral section.

The situation in the gray matter is quite different. Since the gray matter innervates a segment, the size of the gray matter (the number of cells it contains) is related to the complexity of the segment. The hand, for example, is innervated by cervical segments 5, 6, 7, and 8 (C5, C6, C7, and C8). The hand has the highest concentration of sensory receptors of any region of the body. All of these receptors send their axons into C5 to C8 where they synapse, thus increasing the girth of the gray matter. The muscles of the hand can carry out very fine and intricate movements. They are innervated by nerves having their cell bodies in the gray matter of C5–C8. Such movements require many motor nerves and many cell bodies in the gray matter. Consequently, the cord is enlarged at C5 – C8.

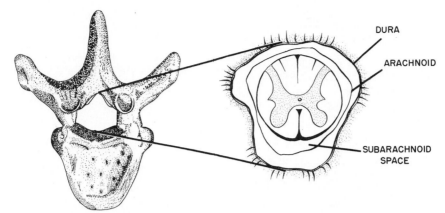

DURA

ARACHNOID

SUBARACHNOID
SPACE

Figure 7-4 The relationships of the vertebral column, the meninges, and spinal cord.

Two regions of the spinal cord—the cervical and the lumbar regions—have large masses of gray matter. The cervical segments innervate the arm, and the lumbar segments innervate the leg. The thoracic segments and the sacral segments, on the other hand, have very small gray matter areas since they innervate only a few muscles.

Segments can be recognized, then, by the amount of gray and white matter relative to the whole cross section. In the cervical segments the section is large, and white matter and gray matter are nearly equal. The tho-racic segments have much more white matter than gray matter. The lumbar have more gray matter than white matter, and the sacral segments are very small and have much more gray matter than white matter. The segments can also be recognized by the shapes of the gray matter. A careful review of Figure 7-7 and Figures 29-1 to 29-4 should provide a basis for recognizing the segmental levels of spinal cord sections.

The area of the body which sends sensory fibers into a given spinal cord segment is called a *dermatome*. These have varying shapes

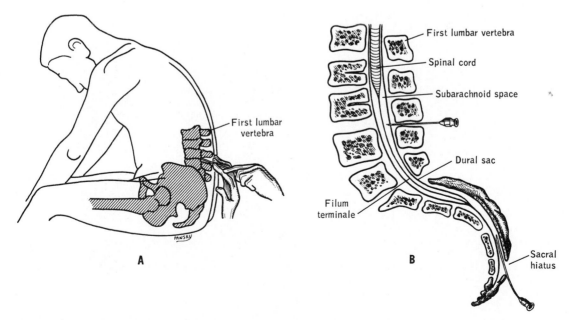

First lumbar
vertebra

First lumbar vertebra

Spinal cord

Subarachnoid space

Dural sac

Filum
terminale

Sacral
hiatus

A

B

Figure 7-5 The technique of lumbar puncture. (From House and Pansky: *A Functional Approach to Neuroanatomy.* New York, McGraw-Hill, 1960.)

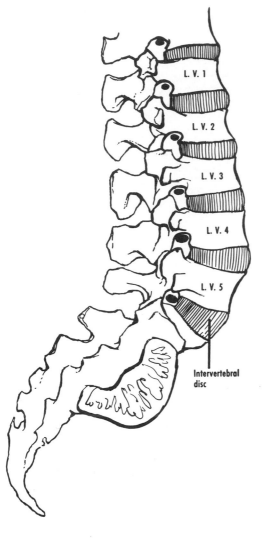

L.V. 1

L.V. 2

L.V. 3

L.V. 4

L.V. 5

Intervertebral
disc

Figure 7–6 The emergence of the right lumbar spinal nerves through the intervertebral foramina. (From Gardner, Gray, and O'Rahilly: *Anatomy.* Philadelphia, W. B. Saunders, 1969.)

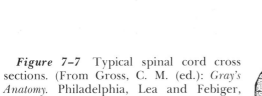

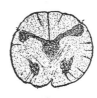

C.1.

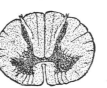

C.2.

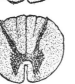

C.5.

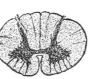

C.8.

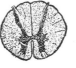

Th.2.

Th.8.

Th.12.

L.3.

S.2.

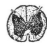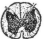

Coc.

Figure 7–7 Typical spinal cord cross sections. (From Gross, C. M. (ed.): *Gray's Anatomy.* Philadelphia, Lea and Febiger, 1966.)

See Filmstrip, Frame 11.

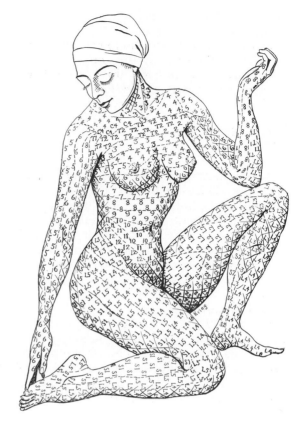

Figure 7–8 The distribution of the dermatomes over the body surface. (From Krieg: *Functional Neuroanatomy*, 3rd Ed. Brain Books, 1966.)

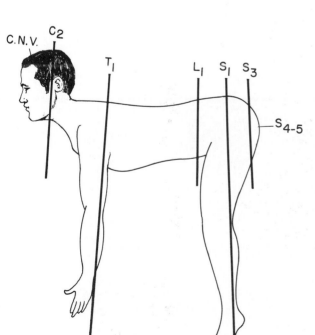

Figure 7–9 Key dermatome boundaries in man.

and sizes. Their distribution can be seen in Figure 7–8.

Figure 7–9 may help you to remember the general area served by the cord segments. The muscles underlying these areas have essentially the same innervation.

SEGMENTAL FUNCTION OF THE SPINAL CORD

To understand the function of the spinal cord as a whole, it is best to begin with a discussion of the function of the gray matter in a single segment. The fibers in the anterior or motor root are axons from large cell bodies (20 μ in diameter) which are located in the anterior horn of the gray matter (Fig. 7–10). These cells are known as *anterior horn cells*.

Each anterior horn cell gives rise to one large (8 to 12 μ) axon, called an alpha motor neuron, which innervates a muscle group containing from 10 to 200 individual muscle fibers. There is only one motor end plate on each muscle. Therefore, for a motor group to contract, the anterior horn cell on the proximal end of the axon must fire an action potential. The muscle group is chained to its anterior horn cell. It contracts only if the anterior horn cell fires. This anatomical relationship is often called the *final common pathway*. Activation of a specific anterior horn cell must precede activity of a motor group. There are many ways to activate this anterior horn cell.

All the motor cells are located in the anterior horn from which their axons innervate muscles on the same side of the body. The general relationship of the position of the anterior horn cell to the body location of its motor group is shown in Figure 7–11.

REFLEXES OF A SINGLE MUSCLE

All of the sensory axons entering the posterior roots are bipolar cells having their cell bodies in the posterior root ganglion. The axons can be divided into many classes by the sensory modality they carry. As far as we know, each axon carries information about only one modality, such as pain. The intensity of the pain or other sensation is coded as action potential frequency. Later in this chap-

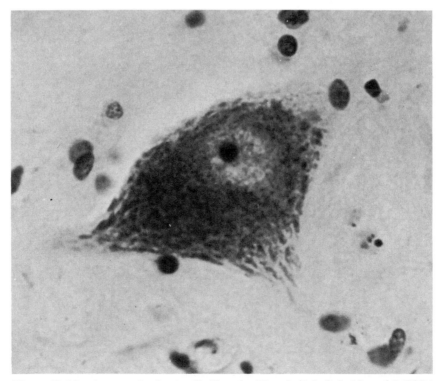

Figure 7–10 An anterior horn cell. (See also Figs. 3–7, 3–9, 3–13, and 3–20*B*.)

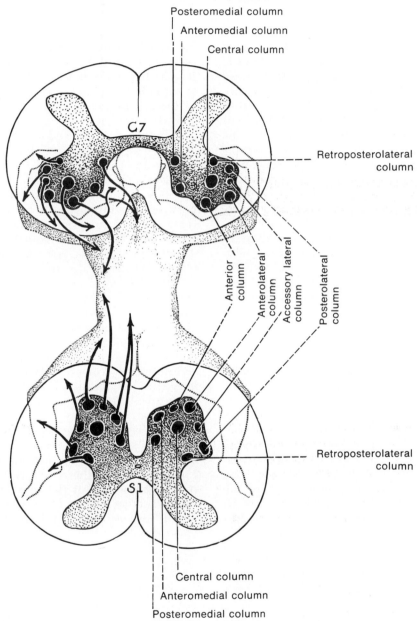

Figure 7–11 Functional localization within the anterior horns. (From Bossy: *Atlas of Neuroanatomy.* Philadelphia, W. B. Saunders, 1970.)

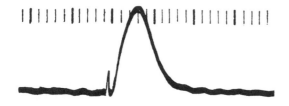

Figure 7–12 A brief stretch reflex recorded from the quadriceps tendon. The initial small, sharp response is the quick stretch which initiated the large response. The time marks are 20 msec. apart. (From Ballif, et al.: Proc. Roy. Soc., *B98*, 589, 1925.)

ter, the various modalities will be discussed in detail. For the present, two modalities will suffice for examples: stretch reflexes and pain. Pain is carried by very small axons, many of them unmyelinated, which have slow conduction velocities. The stretching of muscles, on the other hand, leads to a barrage of action potentials in large, heavily myelinated nerve fibers. These axons have low thresholds and rapid conduction velocities.

Stretch Reflexes. The classic stretch reflex is the *knee jerk*, produced by tapping the patellar tendon. This simple involuntary response is such a familiar part of the physical examination and has been used so frequently in medical humor that precise description seems unnecessary. This simple test can give the astute examiner many clues to the function and dysfunction of the nervous system.

The knee jerk is described quantitatively by Figure 7–12, which is taken from the early work of the great English physiologist Sir Charles Sherrington. As the figure indicates, after a brief stretch, the muscle contracts with a delay of about 10 msec. It can readily be shown that this is a response mediated by the spinal cord. When the nerve to the muscle is cut the response is abolished. When the spinal cord is severed from the rest of the nervous system, the response remains.

The pathway of this response is very simple (see Fig. 7–13). The axon from the stretch receptor runs in the posterior root, and while it branches many times in the gray matter, it eventually synapses directly on the dendrites of the anterior horn cells. The stretch reflex is often referred to as a monosynaptic reflex. The only muscle affected is the one stretched. The reflex continues for as long as the muscle is stretched (see Fig. 7–14).

There are stretch reflexes in all muscles, but they are much stronger in the antigravity muscles. In addition to the familiar knee jerk from the quadriceps group, brisk stretch reflexes can be elicited from the ankle (the Achilles tendon), the jaw, and the biceps and triceps muscles in the arm.

Although the reflex loop is completed within a few segments of spinal cord, the magnitude of the response can be drastically altered by input from other levels. For example, grasping the hands together and pulling will greatly enhance the knee-jerk response (reinforcement). As will be discussed later, the magnitude or briskness of the response can give many clues to pathological processes.

Reflexive Response to Pain. The majority of spinal cord responses have more flexibility than the monosynaptic response, as can be seen in the reflex withdrawal from pain. This is one of the most important of the protective reflexes of the spinal cord. The flexors are activated and the injured limb

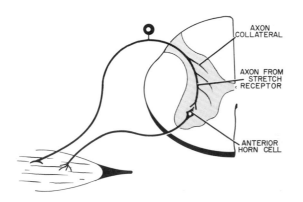

AXON COLLATERAL

AXON FROM STRETCH RECEPTOR

ANTERIOR HORN CELL

Figure 7–13 The pathway for the monosynaptic stretch reflex.

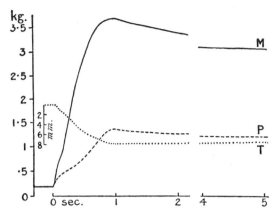

Figure 7–14 A long lasting stretch reflex. *M*, Tension developed in innervated quadriceps muscle; *T*, Extension of tendon; *P*, Tension developed by denervated muscle. (From Liddell and Sherrington: Proc. Roy. Soc., *B96*, 212, 1924.)

withdrawn. Figure 7–15 shows the responses of the ankle flexor muscle, the tibialis anterior, to stimulation of the nerve branches leading to the skin—branches which contain predominantly pain fibers. It can immediately be seen that the combined response is considerably greater than the sum of the two. This augmentation of response is known as *facilitation* and is one of the most basic integrative responses of the nervous system. The reaction is graded in response to the intensity of the stimulus and the area stimulated.

The mechanism of facilitation is shown in Figure 7–16. Stimulation of nerve A excites two anterior horn cells to threshold. Two more are excited in a subthreshold manner; they do not fire an action potential. Nerve B stimulates two totally different anterior horn cells to threshold and the same two to just below threshold. Simultaneous activation of nerves A and B brings all six cells

to threshold and elicits a greater tension from the muscle.

THE RECIPROCAL INNERVATION OF A JOINT

When the biceps femoralis muscle contracts, the opposing muscle, the quadriceps, is stretched because both muscles are connected to the tibia (Fig. 7–17). The quadriceps group has a strong stretch reflex which is not elicited when the biceps femoralis contracts. Only when the quadriceps tendon is stretched does tension develop (Fig. 7–18). The tension is maintained until the biceps tendon is stretched; then the tension abruptly drops. The diminution or abolition of a stretch reflex, called *inhibition*, is, together with facilitation, the keystone of the integrative action of the spinal cord and probably the entire nervous system.

The pathway for the inhibitory response is shown in Figure 7–19. A collateral (branch) of the stretch receptor nerve from the quadriceps muscle runs to an interneuron, which in turn synapses on the anterior horn cells of the biceps. As far as we know, all inhibitory responses are carried out through at least one interneuron (see p. 137). The endings of one nerve, such as the stretch receptor nerve, all have the same effect, either facilitation or inhibition. For the nerve to exhibit the other type of function, an interneuron must intercede.

THE MEMBRANE BASIS OF INTEGRATION AT THE SPINAL CORD LEVEL

When a microelectrode is inserted into the anterior horn of the spinal cord, the tip, with luck, eventually penetrates an anterior horn cell. This penetration is signaled by the abrupt jump of potential between the tip and

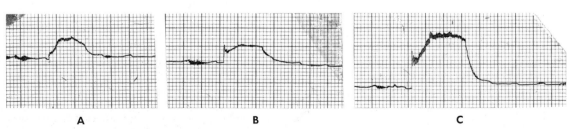

A   B   C

Figure 7–15 Tension response in the tibialis anterior to stimulation of the skin of (*A*) the ipsilateral foot, (*B*) calf, or (*C*) both. Spinal rabbit. (From unpublished experiments of B. A. Curtis, M. C. Fleming, and E. M. Marcus.)

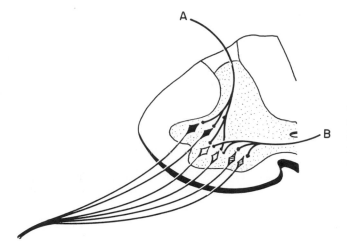

Figure 7-16 A mechanism of summation. Stimulation of A fires the solid anterior horn cells and excites the clear cells. Stimulation of B excites the lined cells to fire and excites the clear cells. Stimulation of both nerves fires all of the cells.

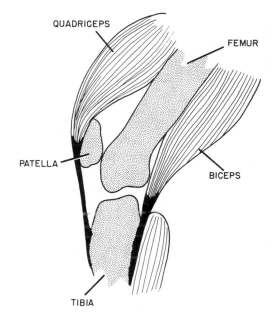

Figure 7-17 Antagonistic muscles at the knee joint.

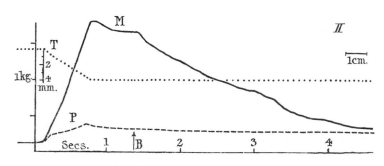

Figure 7-18 Inhibition of a stretch reflex in an extensor muscle, quadriceps, by stretch, at B, of a flexor muscle, biceps. (From Liddell and Sherrington: Proc. Roy. Soc., *B97*. 267, 1925.)

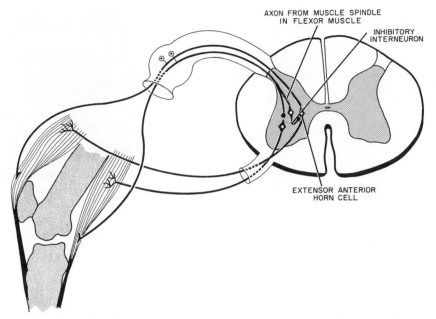

Figure 7–19 The pathway for the inhibition shown in Figure 7–18.

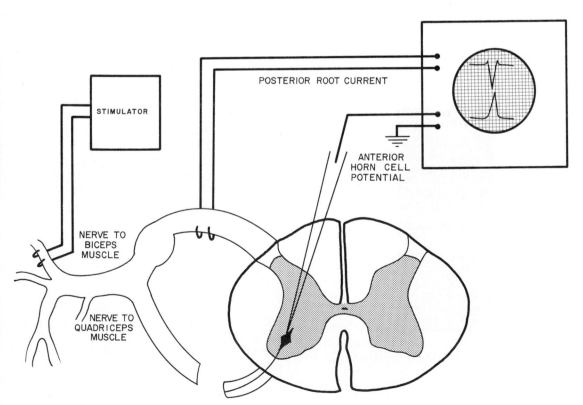

Figure 7–20 A typical experimental setup to study anterior horn cells with intracellular micro-electrodes.

the extracellular fluid from 0 to 70 mV. The recording setup is shown in Figure 7–20. (Almost all of this intracellular work to be described was done by Sir John Eccles and his collaborators and is discussed at length in his book, *The Synapse.*)

In this experiment the anterior roots are cut to prevent action potentials from traveling up the motor axons antidromatically (backwards). The extracellular recording from the posterior root gives a signal proportional to the number of axons stimulated. After the cell is penetrated it must be identified; it is almost certain to be an anterior horn cell because of their large size. Other cell bodies and glia cells are so small that penetration is very unlikely. The destination of its axon is determined by using the stretch reflex pathway. Each muscle nerve is stimulated in turn until a short latency, all or nothing, spike (action potential) response is obtained. This is the equivalent of a monosynaptic stretch reflex. A spike response recorded from an anterior horn cell is the counterpart of muscle tension.

EPSP. When a flexor anterior horn cell has been located, the record in Figure 7–21 is obtained by stimulating a cutaneous nerve to mimic pain. When the nerve is stimulated at high voltage, many small pain fibers are stimulated. The response in the anterior horn cell is the firing of an action potential, *A*.

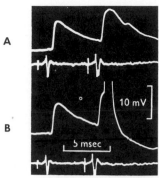

Figure 7–22 The summation of two EPSP's to fire an action potential. In B the second EPSP followed sooner and added upon the first to achieve a threshold depolarization, initiating an action potential. (From Brock, Coombs, and Eccles: J. Physiol., *117*, 431, 1952.)

This response is the electrically recorded counterpart of the reflexive withdrawal from a painful stimulus, as shown in Figure 7–15. When the stimulus intensity is reduced (B to D), an intensity is reached when no action potential is produced, yet the cell body still responds. The response is a subthreshold depolarization of the anterior horn cell called an *excitatory postsynaptic potential,* known as EPSP. This response brings the anterior horn cell closer to threshold, that is, closer to firing an action potential that would cause contraction of a motor group. The EPSP is localized to the cell body and a few dendrites. The axon is unaffected. In contrast to the action potential, it is a graded response.

The EPSP's can add up until threshold is reached and an action potential is fired as is shown in Figure 7–22. Note that the second EPSP in *A* is larger (greater depolarization) than the first. The effect of the first had not yet "worn off" and the second could add on top of it. In *B* the second EPSP follows sooner and adds up to a threshold depolarization, initiating an action potential.

This is the basic mechanism of facilitation. The two classic types of facilitation, temporal and spatial, are the same in terms of a membrane response: the EPSP's add up. Spatial response refers to the EPSP's generated as a result of the activation of two different nerves. Temporal summation, as illustrated in Figure 7–22, means summation in time; its membrane basis depends upon the time course of the EPSP. The membrane repolarizes slowly following the initial rapid

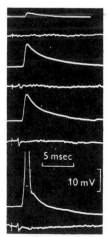

Figure 7–21 EPSP's: The upper trace of each pair is an intracellular record from a biceps anterior horn cell. The lower trace of each pair is from the posterior root. The rest of the action potential of the lower record is off the scale. The average resting potential is −70mV. (From Brock, Coombs, and Eccles: J. Physiol., *117*, 431, 1952.)

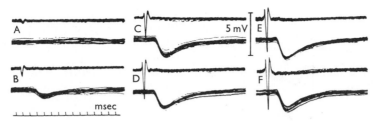

Figure 7–23　The response (an IPSP) of a biceps anterior horn cell to stimulation of the quadriceps nerve. The upper trace of each pair is the action current from the posterior root; the lower is the intracellular record. (From Coombs, Eccles, and Fatt: J. Physiol., *130*, 396, 1955.)

depolarization of an EPSP and a second EPSP can add upon the first. Frequently this "added boost" will bring the cell membrane to the threshold for firing an action potential in the axon.

There is a delay of approximately 0.8 msec. between the arrival of an action potential from a stretch receptor axon and response of an anterior horn cell. This delay and other features strongly support chemical transmission at the synapses on the anterior horn cell. The identity of the transmitter is still not entirely clear although there is a great deal of evidence to suggest that acetylcholine is the transmitter for many of the excitatory synapses in the spinal cord.

Acetylcholine destroys the selective permeability of the postsynaptic membrane, just as it does at the myoneural junction. The equilibrium potential is then zero millivolts. The membrane never reaches zero under the influence of acetylcholine since the acetylcholine is destroyed rapidly. However, at the anterior horn cell membrane, unlike the myoneural junction, the amount of acetylcholine released is not always sufficient to depolarize the cell body to threshold.

IPSP.　When the nerve leading to the quadriceps is stimulated, the membrane of a flexor anterior horn cell hyperpolarizes, as shown in the recordings in Figure 7–23. This hyperpolarizing response, called an *inhibitory postsynaptic potential (IPSP)*, moves the membrane further from threshold, making it more difficult to fire an action potential. The IPSP is the membrane equivalent of inhibition. As noted earlier, inhibition is effected through an interneuron (Fig. 7–19).

In spite of a great deal of experimentation, the transmitter substance responsible for the IPSP is unknown. Whatever the transmitter or transmitters are, they specifically increase the chloride conductance of the anterior horn cell. The membrane potential at rest is −74 mV, a fact which indicates that there is considerable sodium conductance in relationship to potassium and chloride conductances. The calculated values for potassium, chloride, and sodium equilibrium potentials are:

$$E_K = -90 \text{ mV}, E_{Cl} = -80 \text{ mV and } E_{Na} = +45 \text{ mV}.$$

A large increase in chloride conductance will result in a membrane potential of −80 mV and this is the equilibrium potential at the height of the IPSP.

Summation of IPSP's and EPSP's can occur as shown in Figure 7–24. The microelectrode is recording from a biceps cell (a flexor). When the nerve to the biceps is stimulated (Fig. 7–24*A*), an action potential fires; this is the stretch reflex. When the nerve to the quadriceps is stimulated (Fig. 7–24*B*), a large IPSP is recorded; this is the inhibition of a stretch reflex of an opposing muscle. When both nerves are stimulated, the membrane depolarizes but does not reach threshold (Fig. 7–24*D*).

The only other major variants seen when recording from anterior horn cells are long-lasting (30 to 40 msec.) responses. These are thought to involve many interneurons possibly arranged in a circular path so that an action potential "chases its tail" around the circuit for several revolutions, stimulating the anterior horn cell on each revolution.

Slow Potential Theory.　Action potentials in axons making synaptic contact with the dendrites or cell body of an anterior horn cell are expressed within the anterior horn cell as depolarizations (EPSP's, a very few of which will, by themselves, fire the cell) and hyperpolarization (IPSP's, which inhibit firing). The membrane potential of the cell is constantly changing under the influence of

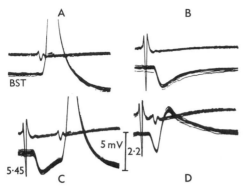

Figure 7-24 Summation of an IPSP and an EPSP. The lower trace of each pair is an intracellular recording from a biceps anterior horn cell. The upper trace is the action current in the posterior root. In *A* the nerve to the biceps was stimulated and an action potential evoked; this is the intracellular equivalent of a stretch reflex. In *B* the nerve to quadriceps was stimulated and an IPSP was evoked. In *C* the two were stimulated 45 msec. apart and a spike resulted. In *D* the two were stimulated 2.2 msec. apart and no action potential resulted; the IPSP generated by the quadriceps stimulus inhibited the biceps anterior horn cell. In *C* the hyperpolarization effect of the IPSP had declined by the time the second nerve was stimulated. (From Coombs, Eccles, and Fatt: J. Physiol., *130*, 396, 1955.)

these two types of input. Whenever the membrane potential reaches the firing level of the axon (−55mV), action potentials are generated with a frequency proportional to the depolarization past threshold. For the purposes of transmission, depolarization, more positive than threshold, is coded as frequency. When these action potentials bombard another cell they are once again decoded into changes in the membrane potential of that cell body.

It is not clear why the EPSP's and IPSP's recorded from the cell body are of different amplitude. This may be due to alterations in the amount of transmitter released or may be due to the location of the synapse on the cell. Since the dendrites, like the cell body, conduct potential disturbances in a decremental, cable fashion, synapses close to the cell body will have a greater influence on the membrane potential.

Presynaptic Inhibition. It is possible to show inhibition of firing of anterior horn cells without any change in the resting membrane potential; no IPSP precedes the inhibition. The inhibition is thought to take place presynaptically, either at a nearby unidentified interneuron or more probably in the junction region between the axon and the dendrite.

STRETCH RECEPTORS

The Gamma System. In the previous discussion of spinal reflexes, reference to stretch receptors was very general. The major dynamic stretch receptor is the *muscle spindle.* This is a bundle of modified muscle fibers that lie parallel to the rest of the muscle fibers. Its structure is shown in Figure 7–25; it is composed basically of three to five small muscle fibers that contain a specialized, nonstriated region in the center. The ends of the muscle fibers can contract and are innervated by small, gamma motor neurons. These gamma motor neurons have cell bodies in the anterior horn, just as do the large alpha fibers which innervate the bulk of the muscle. The small muscle fibers in the spindle are called *intrafusal fibers,* and the large muscle fibers that make up the bulk of the muscle are called *extrafusal fibers.*

There are two sensory nerves which take origin from the unstriated center region of the muscle spindle. The largest (12 μ), classified Ia, comes from the center of this sensory region. The unmyelinated ends of the nerve wrap around each of the muscle fibers and are called *annulospiral endings.* From these endings arise the action potentials that stimulate the stretch reflexes. This axon gives off many collaterals within the gray matter of the cord which then travel up and down the cord for several segments.

The second ending gives off a smaller nerve, classified IIa, from specialized, flower-spray endings on either side of the annulo-spiral ending. The destination and function of these nerves are not clear. They apparently play no part in the stretch reflex.

The basic function of the stretch receptor is to fire when the muscle is stretched. The response of the annulospiral ending is of short latency. The frequency of firing is at first high; it then slows down, but never adapts completely.

The function of the intrafusal muscle fibers is more difficult to understand. The first function is to keep the muscle spindle tight as the extrafusal fibers contract; Figure 7–26 shows this. At the rest length (*A*) the spindle is stretched. Any further stretch will

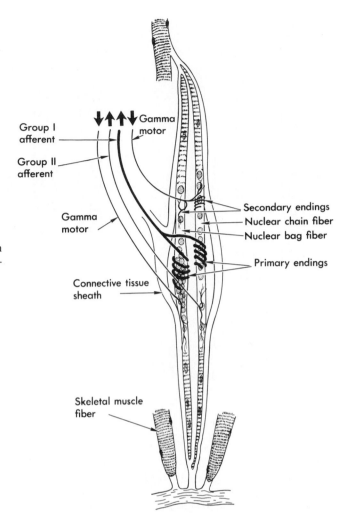

Figure 7-25 A muscle spindle. (From Gardner: *Fundamentals of Neurology.* Philadelphia, W. B. Saunders, 1968.)

set up a volley of action potentials in the Ia sensory nerve that will lead to a stretch reflex—contraction of the extrafusal fibers. When the extrafusal fibers contract because of firing in the alpha motor neuron, the spindle goes slack (as in *B*) and is no longer responsive to stretch. Indeed the muscle would have to be pulled out slightly further than the rest position for the spindle to react. To rectify this situation, the gamma motor neuron fires, thus contracting the intrafusal fiber, and the spindle is tight again (*C*). Through the mechanism of the gamma motor neurons the sensitivity of the stretch reflex is maintained throughout the entire range of the limb movement. For example, the knee-jerk reflex can be elicited in many positions of the lower leg.

Another function of the intrafusal fibers is to change the sensitivity of the annulospiral ending. This is shown in Figure 7-27. It can easily be seen, in the last column, that the response to 20 gm. tension or an equivalent stretch can be drastically altered by activity of the intrafusal fiber. Apparently the annulospiral ending reacts to stretch or deformation whether it is from without, as in stretch, or from within, as in intrafusal muscle fiber activity.

Probably the most important function of the intrafusal fibers is to initiate contraction of the extrafusal fibers via the stretch reflex. It is clear from Figure 7-27 that activation of the gamma fibers and subsequent contraction of the intrafusal fibers sets up a response in the Ia sensory fibers which is indistinguishable from the response to stretch (compare response A3 and D1 in Figure 7-27). This activation of the Ia sensory fiber leads to contraction of the extrafusal fibers. This

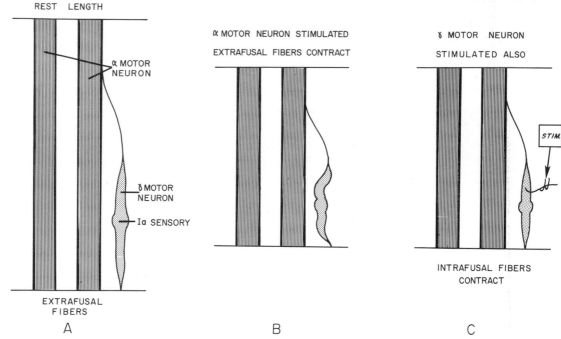

REST LENGTH

α MOTOR NEURON

γ MOTOR NEURON

Ia SENSORY

EXTRAFUSAL FIBERS

A

α MOTOR NEURON STIMULATED
EXTRAFUSAL FIBERS CONTRACT

B

γ MOTOR NEURON
STIMULATED ALSO

STIM.

INTRAFUSAL FIBERS CONTRACT

C

Figure 7–26   The effect of gamma activation upon maintenance of "tone" in the muscle spindle.

is probably best shown by the accompanying sketches (Figs. 7–28 and 7–29).

In Figures 7–28 and 7–29 at *A* the gamma fiber is suddenly activated. During the period *B*, the intrafusal fibers are contracting, stretching the annulospiral ending and altering the sensitivity of the primary stretch receptor to the dashed line. The Ia ending increases its rate of firing and causes reflexive shortening of the extrafusal fibers and shortening of the muscle as a whole, as is happen-

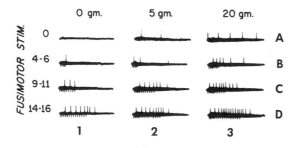

Figure 7–27   The response of a Ia fiber from an annulospiral ending to stretch and gamma activity. Notice that the number of action potentials fired increases with stretch (weight) and gamma activation. The downward deflections are stimulus artifacts of gamma stimulation. (From Kuffler, et al.: J. Neurophysiol., *14*, 29, 1951.)

ing in *C*. This process continues in *D* until point *E* is reached. At *E* the muscle as a whole has contracted sufficiently to decrease the stress on the center region and reduce the rate of firing of the Ia fiber to threshold for the stretch reflex. Remember that during this entire time the gamma system has been activated by the brain.

The shortening and subsequent maintenance of muscle length and, consequently, of the joint angle was brought about by a constant gamma activation. The rate of firing of the gamma system, initiated by the brain, has not changed during the entire time. The new position (*E*) is not affected by the load the muscle had to move. If the load is light, the new position is reached quickly; if the load is heavy the new position is reached slowly. In any event, the new position is reached without further judgment from the motor centers of the brain. The idea that the gamma system acts as a feedback loop was proposed by Merton (1953), and while it has gained some acceptance it is far from proven.

Let us digress a moment and consider the simplest type of muscle movement—opposing the thumb to the palm. Cells in the anterior horn are activated by fibers from a large descending tract, the pyramidal tract, a direct pathway, of which more will be said later. The intensity of stimulation and the number of motor groups activated are determined by the motor cortex. The motor cortex basically sets the tension which is to be developed. The distance moved is a function of the resistance to movement and the duration of the stimulus. The extent of movement is visually controlled; when the thumb reaches the desired position, the motor cortex stops stimulating the anterior horn cells.

In contrast to this type of movement, which requires constant attention if the desired position is to be achieved, many of our movements, such as walking, require no such attention. These movements are probably carried out through mediation of the gamma system, which allows the brain to set a desired position and then forget about it. Compare, then, a pyramidal system, which produces a force, and a second system, the gamma system, which produces a new position. Although it is not completely clear at this time, it would appear that the gamma anterior horn cells are innervated by the extrapyramidal motor system. This system is controlled by neurons in the brain stem; the reticular formation.

Golgi Tendon Organs. Golgi tendon organs are a second type of stretch receptor found in the tendinous insertion of muscles. This receptor is in series with the muscle fibers and has a high threshold for activation. It contains no muscle fiber system. Activation of the sensory fibers from the tendon organ causes an inhibition of the contraction of the muscle. The function of the tendon organ is to protect the insertion of the muscle from too great a stress which might tear the insertion from the bone.

INTERNEURONS

Only a very small portion of the cells of the gray matter of the spinal cord are anterior horn cells; the vast majority are interneurons—small cells with short dendrites and axons. These cells interconnect incoming sensory axons and descending spinal cord tracts with each other and with anterior horn cells.

One such interneuron is the *Renshaw cell* that must be studied in a somewhat roundabout fashion. After the posterior (sensory) roots have been cut, stimulation of a muscle nerve (for example, to the gastrocnemius) will result in action potentials traveling back up the motor nerve (antidromic) and entering the spinal cord. An extracellular electrode records a burst of high frequency action potentials from the Renshaw cell in response to a single volley of action potentials (Fig. 7–30A1). These cells have been localized by electrophoresing dye from a recording electrode. After a Renshaw cell has been characterized physiologically by its response to antidromic stimulation, dye is deposited at the tip of the electrode by passing current through the microelectrode. An example of this widely used technique is shown in Figure 7–31A. When many such dots are placed together on a spinal cord cross section (Fig. 7–31B), they all appear in the most anterior portion of the anterior horn. This is the same region in which the axons from the anterior horn cells branch.

The Renshaw cell is activated by the firing of anterior horn cells. Studies of a Renshaw cell show it to be activated by antidromic stimulation of any of a great many motor nerve fibers; even from different muscles. These muscles, however, usually belong to a single functional grouping, such as knee flexors or ankle extensors. The effect of Renshaw cell activation upon other anterior horn cells is inhibitory; it depresses or totally inhibits firing. This is shown diagrammatically in Figure 7–32. Activity in anterior horn cell 1 will inhibit, via the Renshaw cell, anterior horn cell 2. This inhibition is usually to opposing muscle groups. The Renshaw cell itself can be inhibited by a variety of pathways, such as squeezing the ipsilateral toes and stimulating the muscle nerve on the contralateral side (Fig. 7–30 A, B). Note that in each case the response to the antidromic stimulation is much reduced.

Since the Renshaw cell is inhibitory to anterior horn cells, inhibiting the Renshaw cell will remove inhibition from the anterior horn cell 2 in Figure 7–32. The effect of inhibition of an inhibitory cell is called disinhibition. This doesn't mean that anterior horn cell 2 will fire, since that requires a facilitatory stimulus, but it does mean that no inhibition is being applied via that particular Renshaw circuit. This phenomenon of disinhibition is quite common in the nervous system. It was first described in the lateral eye of *Limulus* by Hartline and Ratliff (1957).

The interactions possible between the elements shown in Figure 7–32 are very diverse

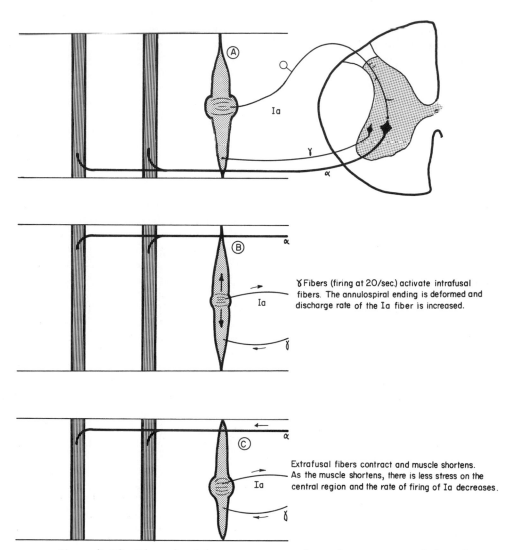

Ia

Ⓐ

Ia

Ⓑ

α

γ Fibers (firing at 20/sec.) activate intrafusal fibers. The annulospiral ending is deformed and discharge rate of the Ia fiber is increased.

Ia

γ

α

Ⓒ

Ia

γ

Extrafusal fibers contract and muscle shortens. As the muscle shortens, there is less stress on the central region and the rate of firing of Ia decreases.

Figure 7–28 The role of the gamma system in setting a new muscle length. The letters inside the circles refer to Figure 7–29.

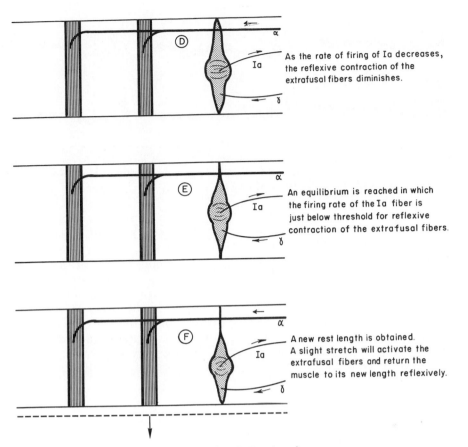

As the rate of firing of Ia decreases, the reflexive contraction of the extrafusal fibers diminishes.

An equilibrium is reached in which the firing rate of the Ia fiber is just below threshold for reflexive contraction of the extrafusal fibers.

A new rest length is obtained. A slight stretch will activate the extrafusal fibers and return the muscle to its new length reflexively.

Figure 7–28 (Continued)

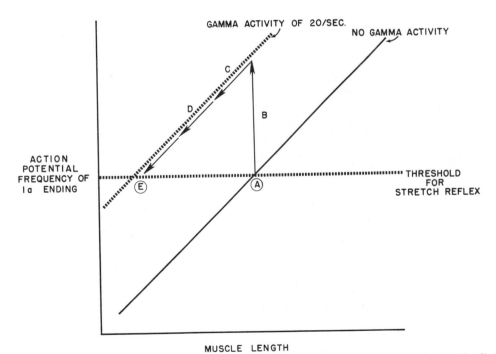

Figure 7–29 The relationship between gamma activity and muscle length. (Refer to Fig. 7–28 and the text for discussion.)

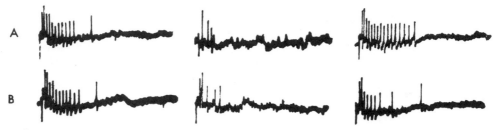

Figure 7-30 Inhibition of Renshaw cell activity by (*A*) a squeeze of the ipsilateral toes and (*B*) by stimulus to the contralateral biceps semitendonosis nerve. 1 and 3 are control responses produced by stimuli to the ventral root and conducted antidromically; 2 is the experimental response. (From Wilson, Talbot, and Kato: J. Neurophysiol., *27*, 1063, 1964.)

and offer rich possibilities for subtle interaction between neural elements—so rich as to defy elucidation. A bit of study of Figure 7-32 may give some impressions of the problems faced by the scientist who tries to describe behavior in terms of single cell action.

There have been many speculations, and as yet little proof, as to the function or functions of Renshaw cells. Probably they act to coordinate muscle movement.

TRACTS OF THE SPINAL CORD

The white matter of the cord contains axons which run up and down the spinal cord connecting segment to segment and the segments to the brain. The white matter is divided into three areas: the posterior funiculus, the lateral funiculus, and the anterior funiculus (Fig. 7-33).

The *posterior funiculus* carries a single as-

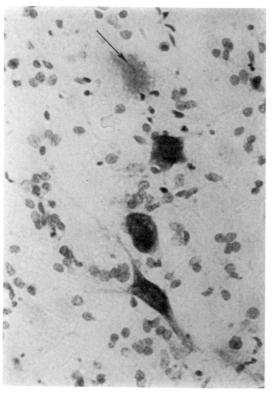

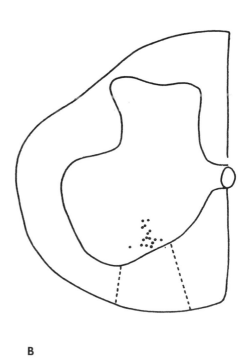

A

B

Figure 7-31 Localization of the Renshaw cells by the method of dye electrophoresis from the recording electrode. *A,* The dye spot among the anterior horn cells. The dye spot is an azure blue while the cells are purple. *B,* The location of a number of dye spots superimposed upon a tracing of a lumbar spinal cord segment. (From Thomas and Wilson: Nature, *206*:211, 1965.)

See Filmstrip, Frame 13.

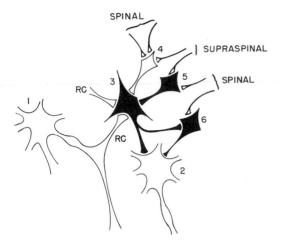

Figure 7–32 The major classes of input to a Renshaw cell. The white cells and synapses are excitatory; the black cells are inhibitory. 1 and 2 are anterior horn cells; 3 is the Renshaw cell; and 4, 5, and 6 are interneurons.

location of individual tracts can be determined is to section the fibers of the tract and look at sections beyond the cell bodies. Remember that, in general, only the part of the axon cut off from the cell body degenerates. If the descending corticospinal tract is severed at T1, only the sections below T1 will degenerate and show loss of myelin. The cervical sections will look normal. The reverse will be true of ascending tracts. An example of a degenerating tract will be given shortly.

The *anterior funiculus* likewise carries many tracts and has no anatomical subdivisions. The location of the tracts must be determined by observing any degeneration caused by discrete lesions.

DESCENDING TRACTS

Corticospinal Tracts. Commands for voluntary movement travel from the brain and through the spinal cord in the corticospinal tract. This tract has its origin in the cerebral cortex, most prominently from the motor and premotor cortex of the frontal lobe (Fig. 1–9). The fibers come together in the internal capsule and run through the brain stem. At the junction between the medulla and the spinal cord (the level of the foramen magnum) most of the fibers cross the neuraxia, decussate, and move laterally and posteriorly to form the lateral corticospinal tract (Fig. 7–34). About 15 per cent

cending tract, the posterior columns, which will be discussed shortly. The *lateral funiculus* has its anterior boundary at the anterior lateral sulcus which is the groove through which the anterior or motor roots leave the cord. Consequently, the lateral funiculus lies between the posterior and anterior roots.

The lateral funiculus is a solid mass of nerve fibers containing many tracts and having no anatomical subdivisions observable in the normal section. The only way that the

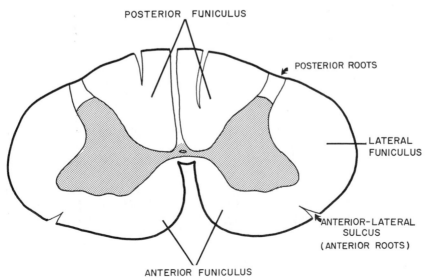

Figure 7–33 The three funiculi of the spinal cord.

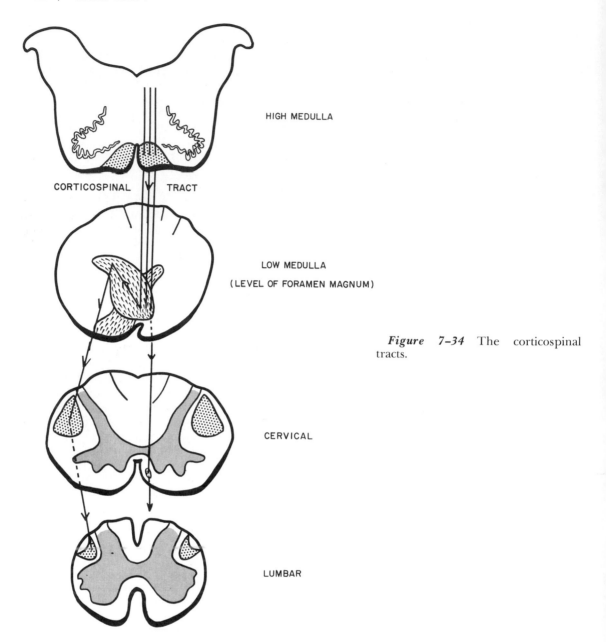

HIGH MEDULLA

CORTICOSPINAL   TRACT

LOW MEDULLA

(LEVEL OF FORAMEN MAGNUM)

Figure 7–34 The corticospinal tracts.

CERVICAL

LUMBAR

of the fibers continue on uncrossed to form the anterior corticospinal tract. Further discussion of the order of decussation will be found in Chapter 11.

The location of the corticospinal tract is easily determined by examining spinal-cord sections from a monkey or chimp following medullary pyramid section. The location in the human is determined by analyzing cord sections obtained at autopsy from cases where massive cortical destruction has occurred in the motor areas of the precentral gyrus or in the internal capsule. The most common cause of such degeneration is occlusion of the middle cerebral artery (a stroke). Since the cell bodies of these axons are in the cerebral cortex, the axons degenerate following death of the cell body. Such a spinal-cord cross section is shown in Figure 7–35.

The Anterior Corticospinal Tract. This tract is uncrossed and contains about 15 per cent of the fibers in the original pryamidal tract. It rarely extends below the cervical levels and occasionally does not appear at all. It is

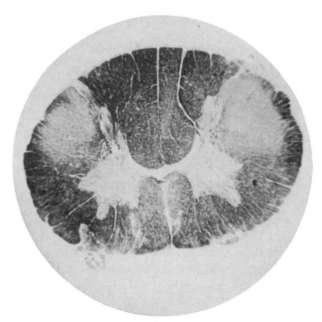

Figure 7-35 The location of the cortico-spinal tracts as shown by degeneration caused by a lesion in the internal capsule. (From Wechsler, I. S.: *Clinical Neurology.* Philadelphia, W. B. Saunders, 1963.)

See Filmstrip, Frame 12.

thought that when axons leave the tract they cross the midline before synapsing, making synaptic contact with anterior horn cells.

The Lateral Corticospinal Tract. This is the major tract for voluntary control of skeletal muscle. Destruction of this tract leads to paralysis of skeletal muscle and the loss of voluntary movement. This paralysis is usually total distally, in the hand, and somewhat less severe in the trunk musculature. If the right tract is severed at C1, a paralysis of both the right arm and leg will result. *Hemiplegia* is the paralysis of the arm and leg on the same side. *Monoplegia* is the paralysis of a single limb.

The axons leave this tract and synapse with anterior horn cells. Axons controlling finger movement probably go there directly but most other axons go there via one or two interneurons. The tract decreases in size as it descends; almost half of the fibers end in the cervical segments, about one-fourth in the thoracic segments and the rest in the lumbosacral region.

The corticospinal tract does not completely myelinate until the second year. In many of the studies of the tract performed on still-born infants, the unmyelinated corticospinal tract contrasts with the rest of the tracts which have already myelinated. This late myelination is no doubt correlated with the late appearance of motor skills in the human infant.

Extrapyramidal Tracts. A variety of tracts descend from various nuclei in the

brain stem and undoubtedly have a very important function in motor control. Our present level of knowledge does not permit any specific allocation of function to these tracts. Consequently, they will be lumped together here and called extrapyramidal tracts. Their location is shown in Figure 7–36 in relationship to the corticospinal tracts. Their functions will be discussed in the chapter on integration of motor movement.

On gross neurological examination, it is difficult to separate the results of damage to the pyramidal and extrapyramidal systems. This is partially because our knowledge of their separate functions is limited and partially because they run close together in the brain stem and spinal cord. Consequently at this level of sophistication it is best to discuss the descending motor system and leave the finer points to the chapter on the motor system.

Loss of muscle movement and the presence of muscle weakness can be grouped functionally into two categories. If the difficulty is located in the corticospinal or other descending motor tract the problem is called an upper motor neuron lesion or paralysis. If the problem is in the anterior horn cell, its axon, or its motor group, the problem is called a lower motor neuron lesion.

The *upper motor neuron syndrome* is characterized by weakness, hyperreflexia, the Babinski sign, and a type of increased resistance to passive movement at a joint,

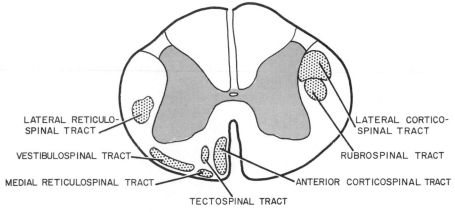

LATERAL RETICULO-
SPINAL TRACT

VESTIBULOSPINAL TRACT

MEDIAL RETICULOSPINAL TRACT

TECTOSPINAL TRACT

LATERAL CORTICO-
SPINAL TRACT

RUBROSPINAL TRACT

ANTERIOR CORTICOSPINAL TRACT

Figure 7–36 The major descending tracts in man.

spasticity. The increased tone is easily demonstrated by passively moving or rotating the ankle, knee, hip, shoulder, elbow, or wrist joints. In the normal individual, the joints all move easily. When spasticity is present, the joint is easy to move for a short interval, then resistance to movement increases rapidly; upon further pressure, the resistance suddenly gives way. This latter phenomenon is often referred to as a clasp-knife reflex. In the leg, spasticity is greatest in the extensors, whereas in the arm the flexors are more affected.

Descending motor tracts normally exert an inhibitory effect on spinal cord reflexes. *Hyperreflexia* is a sure sign of decreased corticospinal function. Decreased function of the corticospinal tract also effects a curious reflex of the foot. If a moderately sharp object, such as a key, is drawn over the lateral boundary of the sole of the foot, the toes of an adult flex (curl up). In very young children and in adults with corticospinal tract destruction, the toes extend and fan out as shown in Figure 7–37.

The *lower motor neuron syndrome* is characterized by weakness, loss of reflexes, extreme muscle wasting, and a flaccid tone to the muscles. The reasons for the weakness and muscle wasting are discussed in Chapter 6 and relate to the loss of the anterior horn cell or the motor axon. The loss of reflexes and the flaccid tone of the muscles relate to the loss of the stretch reflex pathway. Often, it is possible to observe spontaneous twitching of the muscle (fasciculation).

Contrast, then, the two causes of muscle weakness and eventual paralysis as follows:

Upper Motor Neuron Dysfunction
    Spasticity
    Hyperreflexia
    Babinski sign
    Very little atrophy
Lower Motor Neuron Dysfunction
    Flaccidity
    Hyporeflexia
    Fasciculation
    Severe muscle atrophy

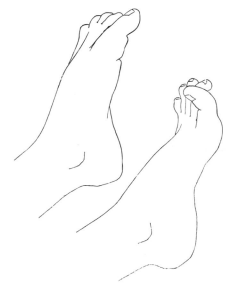

Figure 7–37 The Babinski response. *Upper,* The normal adult response to stimulation of the lateral plantar surface of the foot. *Lower,* The normal infant and abnormal adult response. (From Gardner: *Fundamentals of Neurology.* Philadelphia, W. B. Saunders, 1968.)

ASCENDING TRACTS

Spinothalamic Tracts. The spinothalamic tracts, like the corticospinal tracts, can be divided into lateral and anterior tracts.

The Lateral Spinothalamic Tract. This tract carries information on pain and temperature sensations from the segmental levels of the spinal cord to the thalamus (Fig. 7–38). Pain modality is tested by pinprick. The pain and temperature fibers are usually very small, myelinated or unmyelinated fibers. The sense endings for pain sensation are unmyelinated, naked nerve endings.

These fibers enter the posterior root and branch extensively, as shown in Figure 7–38. The branches run several segments up and down the spinal cord in the most lateral position of the posterior gray horn (Lissauer's fasciculus) before synapsing in the posterior horn, usually in the apical zone. Branches of the entering axons also enter the posterior horn and synapse with the segment of entry. All of these fibers synapse in the posterior gray and send axons of second order neurons across the midline, through the anterior commissure, to the anterior lateral portion of the lateral funiculus, forming the lateral spinothalamic tract.

The fibers join the tract from the opposite

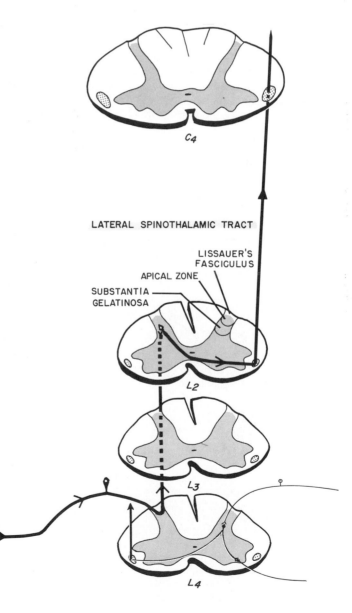

Figure 7-38 The lateral spinothalamic tract.

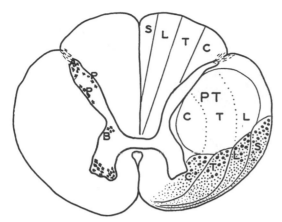

Figure 7–39 The lamination pattern of the major tracts of the spinal cord. (From Walker: Arch Neural. Psychiat. (Chicago), *43*:284, 1940.)

four segments above their entry into the spinal cord.

Patients suffering from severe intractable pain from a disease such as cancer often elect to have the spinothalamic tract cut (an anterolateral chordotomy) when the pain cannot be controlled by drugs. Since the lateral spinothalamic tract is close to the surface a knife is inserted in the lateral surface and swept anteriorly to severe the axons in the tract (Fig. 7–40). This, of course, destroys all of the axons from dermatomes two to four segments below the section on the opposite side of the body, causing analgesia on the affected area. Occasionally, several years after the chordotomy, pain and temperature sensation returns to the previously analgesic region. Apparently, a multisynaptic pathway develops in Lissauer's tract which bridges the area of damaged axons and eventually reaches the thalamus. Since this pathway is multisynaptic, it is virtually impossible to map it by degeneration experiments since degeneration extends only to the next synapse. In addition, there is some evidence that uncrossed pain pathways exist.

Pain and temperature are carried almost exclusively in the lateral spinothalamic tract and since these modalities are easy to test and have localizing significance they are an extremely valuable aid to the neurologists. No examination of the nervous system is complete without a check on the presence of pain sensation. Curiously, the patient may be un-

side of the cord and push the fibers from more inferior segments further laterally and posteriorly. Consequently there is a lamination pattern in the spinothalamic tract. The axons from the sacral segments are usually the most lateral and posterior, and those from the cervical segments are more medial and anterior, as seen in Figure 7–39. There seems to be no fixed arrangement of pain fibers and temperature fibers within each region; there is considerable variation in location. All of the pain fibers and temperature fibers from a posterior root do not enter the tract until they have traveled three or

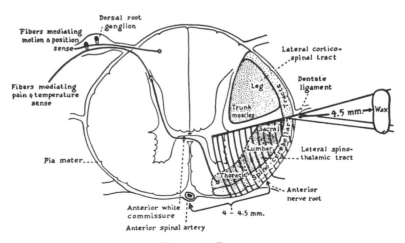

Thoracic II.

Figure 7–40 Diagram illustrating a chordotomy. The cross section of the spinal cord shows the lamination of the spinothalamic tract, the position of the pyramidal tract in relation to it, and the presence of other tracts in the lower quadrant. A piece of bone wax is mounted 4.5 mm. from the tip of the knife as a depth gauge. Heavy curved lines in the ventral quadrant indicate the sweep of the knife. Note that a desire to spare the lateral corticospinal tract would result in sparing the sacral dermatomes. (From Kahn and Rand: J. Neurosurg., *9*:611–619, 1952.)

aware of the loss of this sensation over a considerable area of the body, although he is rarely unaware of this loss in the fingers. One word of caution—a pinprick tests the entire conduction system: the peripheral nerve, the posterior root and ganglion, the spinothalamic tract, and the thalamus and postcentral gyrus. You must decide from other evidence which of these structures is involved. If, for example, all modalities of sensation are lost equally, the peripheral nerve is suspect, especially if there is a lower motor neuron type weakness.

The Anterior Spinothalamic Tract. This pathway carries touch sensation from the spinal segments to the thalamus, but it is not the only pathway by which touch sensation

reaches the consciousness level; touch sensation is also carried in the posterior columns. The anterior spinothalamic tract is a predominantly crossed tract and lies in the lateral boundary of the anterior fasciculus near the emergence of the anterior roots. Since touch is carried by other pathways as well, this pathway has little localizing significance.

Posterior Columns. The posterior columns carry the axons for conscious position sense and vibration. This tract also carries the information that higher centers need to discriminate size and shape. The axons enter the posterior root, then branch and enter the posterior fasciculus (Fig. 7–41). They synapse in the lower medulla and cross to the other side of the neuraxis. The axons

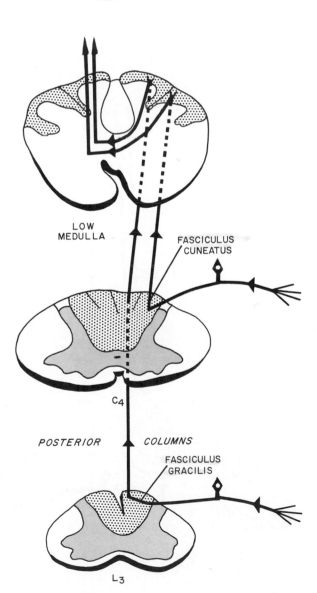

Figure 7–41 The posterior columns.

from the lower limbs (from the sacral and lumbar segments) lie in the medial position, the fasciculus gracilis. The axons from the upper limbs (from the thoracic and cervical segments) run in the more lateral fasciculus cuneatus.

Vibration sense is tested by placing a tuning fork on the bony eminences of the ankle, knee, hip, elbow, and wrist. Conscious position is tested by asking the patient to close his eyes and indicate which way a joint, such as a finger, is being moved. Since the axons subserving the sense of vibration and con-

scious position travel almost exclusively in the posterior columns, these modalities also have excellent localizing value. The posterior columns end in the same region of the thalamus as does the spinothalamic tract. The information is then projected to the postcentral gyrus for perception and sensory discrimination.

Spinocerebellar Tracts. These are two different pathways from the posterior roots to the cerebellum. Both pathways carry information on unconscious position sense. The cell bodies of the primary sensory neu-

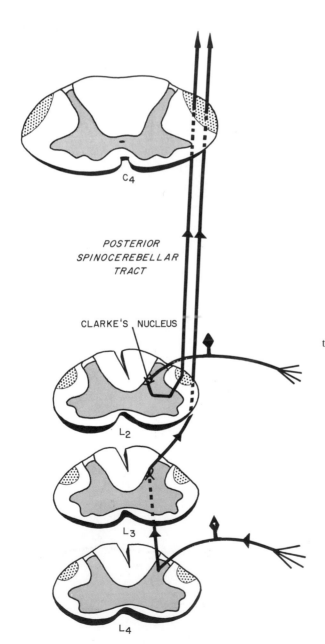

Figure 7–42 The posterior spinocerebellar tract.

rons are located in the posterior root ganglia. The posterior spinocerebellar tract is composed of large axons whose cell bodies are found in Clarke's nucleus or column which is located in the posterior and medial region of the gray matter in the segments above T4 to T6 and runs up to C7 to C8 (Fig. 7–42). These axons leave Clarke's column and run laterally and superiorly to lie on the lateral aspect of the spinal cord just anterior to the sensory roots and lateral to the corticospinal tract (Fig. 7–40). From there the fibers run up to the cerebellum via the inferior cerebellar peduncle (Fig. 1–20). The tract is uncrossed all the way to the cerebellum.

The origin of the axons that synapse in Clarke's column is less clear, but it may be in the Golgi tendon organs and muscle spindles. The posterior tract carries fibers related to segments lower than T4 to T6, but the pathway from the posterior root to Clarke's column is unclear. Fibers which enter the cord above C7 to C8 and are destined for the cerebellum synapse in a nucleus in the low medulla, the external cuneate nucleus.

The anterior spinocerebellar tract receives fibers predominantly from the sacral and lumbar regions; these fibers synapse in the gray matter on the same side and then cross the cord to lie on the lateral boundary of the lateral fasciculus. They continue superiorly and enter the cerebellum via the *superior cerebellar peduncle,* crossing again as they enter the cerebellum.

These two tracts are clinically indistinguishable in the spinal cord; indeed, it is difficult to associate any specific clinical picture with an interruption of these tracts in the spinal cord.

Intersegmental tracts. Intersegmental tracts connect the individual segments of the cord. Lissauer's fasciculus or tract carries branches of incoming sensory fibers up and down the cord. Pain fibers from the foot, for example, travel several segments up and down the cord before they enter the gray matter and synapse with the flexor anterior horn cells to subserve the reflex withdrawal from pain. There are thin layers of fibers on the inner surface of the white columns, the fasciculus proprius, which also interconnect segments.

References

Eccles, J. C.: *The Physiology of Synopsis.* New York, Academic Press, 1964.

Hartline, H. K., and Ratliff, F.: Inhibitory interaction of receptor units in the eye of Limulus. J. gen. Physiol., *40*:357, 1957.

Merton, P. A.: *In* Wolstenholme, G. E. (ed.): *The Spinal Cord.* A Ciba Foundation Symposium. London, Churchill, 1953.

8

Clinical Considerations
of the Spinal Cord

ELLIOTT M. MARCUS

**DIFFERENTIATION OF LESIONS
OF MUSCLE, PERIPHERAL NERVE,
NERVE ROOTS, AND SPINAL CORD**

In this chapter the student will begin his study of the various disease processes affecting the central and peripheral nervous system. In this undertaking, he will be learning certain principles of differential diagnosis. An understanding of neurological differential diagnosis requires a knowledge of the basic anatomical and physiological information which has been studied in the preceding chapters.

In approaching the patient who has neurological disease, we seek, from a diagnostic standpoint, to answer two basic questions:
1. What is the location of the disease process (the lesion) causing the patient's symptoms?
   a. By location we mean where is the disease process located as regards the central nervous system as opposed to the peripheral nervous system, as opposed to muscle?
   b. By location we mean where is the disease process located in the rostral caudal extent of the neural axis?
   c. By location we mean how extensive

is the disease process at a particular level of the neural axis? What is its transverse extent at a given rostral caudal segment? Is the process focal, multifocal or diffuse?
2. Having established the location of the disease process, we then ask the second question: what is the pathological nature of the lesion?

LOCATION OF DISEASE PROCESS

Let us first consider the problem of the location of the disease process. Patients with neurological disease come to medical attention because of certain symptoms (complaints) and signs (findings on examination). These symptoms and signs fall into several large general areas.
1. Disturbance of mental status.
2. Disturbance of cranial nerve function.
3. Disturbance of motor strength.
4. Disturbance of motor control: coordination and reflex function.
5. Disturbance of sensation.
6. Pain, including headache.

In considering the differentiation of disease of muscle, peripheral nerve, and central nervous system, the following initial generalizations may be made.

150

Muscle Disease. Patients with disease of muscle do not show evidence of damage to the long fiber systems involved in transmitting motor and sensory information within the central nervous system. They do not have involvement of mental status. They do not have sensory symptoms or signs.

These patients, however, have significant weakness accompanied by a significant degree of atrophy. The form of voluntary movement is intact; spasticity is not present. In general, the more common types of myopathy involve proximal muscles, e.g., the pseudohypertrophic form (Duchenne-Erb) of muscular dystrophy and polymyositis. (See Chapter 6, p. 118.) In general, there is some preservation of reflex function, since the neural apparatus is intact and not all muscle fibers are severely affected in the early stages of the disease. Fasciculations (twitching of the muscles), which are indicative of disease of the anterior horn cells, are usually not noted in muscle disease.

Peripheral Nerve Disease. In contrast, diseases involving the peripheral nerves have a combination of motor and sensory symptoms and signs. Lower motor neuron findings are present with a flaccid type weakness and atrophy. Sensory findings (involving to some extent all modalities of sensation) are present within the same distribution as the motor findings. These patients, however, do not show evidence of damage to the long fiber systems involved in transmitting information within the central nervous system.

In general, mental status and cranial nerves are intact. Deep tendon reflexes and superficial reflexes (response to plantar stimulation) are absent within the distribution of the involved peripheral nerves. Fasciculations may be present within the distribution of the involved peripheral nerves. Damage to the sympathetic fibers, traversing the peripheral nerves, may result in alterations in sweating and skin temperatures.

As will be discussed later in greater detail, diseases of peripheral nerves are essentially of two types: (a) symmetrical polyneuropathies—usually distal and usually due to a metabolic disturbance involving many nerves, and (b) localized mononeuropathies involving a single peripheral nerve, often due to trauma or compression. Less often, there has been an occlusion of blood supply.

In a mononeuropathy, the weakness and sensory signs and symptoms are clearly within the distribution of a specific peripheral nerve, e.g., sciatic, radial, median, and ulnar. Common sites of compression include the radial nerve at the radial (or spiral) groove of the humerus, the ulnar nerve at the olecranon process of the elbow, the median nerve in the carpal tunnel, the brachial plexus at the thoracic outlet, and the peroneal nerve in the popliteal fossa.

Nerve Root or Spinal Nerve Disease. In contrast, diseases involving nerve roots or spinal nerves produce pain, with atrophy, flaccid weakness, sensory symptoms and signs within the segmental (i.e., dermatomal) distribution of the involved nerve root. All sensory modalities are involved. Unless associated involvement of the spinal cord is present, these patients do not have evidence of damage to the long fiber systems involved in transmitting motor and sensory information within the spinal cord (the corticospinal tracts, the lateral spinothalamic tracts, and the posterior columns).

Mental status is unaffected. Deep tendon and superficial reflexes are absent or depressed within the segmental distribution of the involved roots. Fasciculations are often present within the distribution of the involved nerve root.

The student should refer to the diagrams (Figs. 8–1, 8–2, and 8–3) and contrast the root (or segmental or dermatomal) sensory distribution with the sensory distribution of the peripheral nerves. The following sensory segments should be remembered by the student:

1. C2—compared to trigeminal
2. C6, C7, C8—in the hand
3. T1—axilla
4. T5, T6—xyphoid process
5. T10—umbilicus
6. T12—above inguinal ligament
7. L5—medial aspect foot
8. S1—lateral aspect foot
9. S3, S4, S5—perianal area

The radicular sensory pattern of Figure 8–1 is based on the work of Keegan and Garrett who studied the area of hypesthesia, following rupture of an intervertebral disc. The actual area supplied by a single nerve root is more extensive than the areas indicated in this diagram. This can be demonstrated by using the method of remaining sensibility devised by Sherrington (Fig. 8–4). In studies of the monkey, Sherrington sectioned three roots above and three below the intact root to be studied. An area of intact sensation

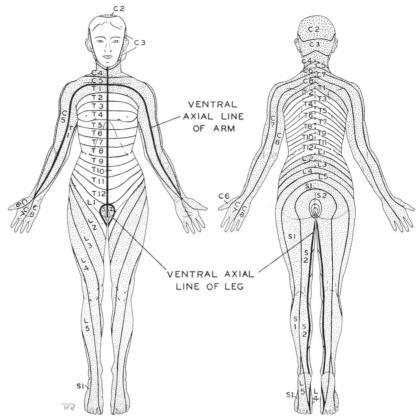

Figure 8–1 Dermatome charts of the human body determined by the pattern of hypalgesia following rupture of an intervertebral disk. (From Keegan, J. J., and Garrett, F. D.: Anat. Rec., *102*:411, 1948.)

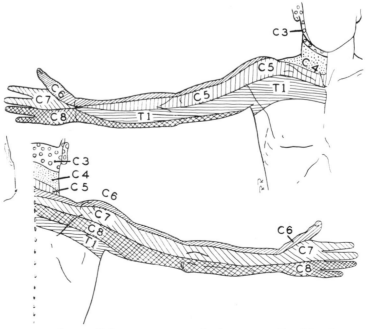

Figure 8–2 Dermatome charts of the upper extremity in man outlined by the pattern of hypalgesia, following rupture of an intervertebral disk. (From Keegan, J. J., and Garrett, F. D.: Anat. Rec., *102*: 417, 1948.)

surrounded by an area of anesthesia resulted. Using a similar method in man, Foerster found the dermatomes illustrated in Figure 8–5.

In considering radicular segments, the student should keep in mind the following muscle innervations:

1. Shoulder muscles, e.g., supraspinatus, deltoid, and infraspinatus—C4, C5, C6
2. Biceps—C5, C6
3. Triceps—C6, **C7, C8**
4. Finger muscles, e.g., abductor pollices longus and brevis, opponens, flexors, and extensors—C7, C8, T1
5. Quadriceps—L2, **L3**, L4
6. Gastrocnemius—L4, L5, **S1**, S2
7. Dorsiflexors of foot (peroneal)—L4, L5, S1

For deep tendon reflexes the following segmental levels should be recalled:

1. Jaw—cranial nerve V, pons
2. Biceps—C5, C6
3. Triceps—C6, **C7, C8**
4. Radial periosteal—C5, C6, C7
5. Quadriceps—L2, **L3**, L4
6. Achilles—L4, L5, **S1**, S2

For superficial reflexes the following segments are involved:

1. Upper abdomen—T7, T8, T9, T10
2. Lower abdomen—T10, T11, T12
3. Plantar—S1, S2

The most common cause of symptoms involving the nerve roots is rupture or degeneration of the intervertebral discs. The most common sites of rupture are in the cervical and lumbar areas. In the cervical area, most lateral, disc protrusions occur at C5–C6 interspace (compressing C6 nerve root) and C6 to C7 interspace (compressing C7 nerve root). In the lumbar area the favorite sites are the L5–S1 interspace, involving **S1** or L5 nerve roots or L4–L5 involving L4 or **L5** nerve roots. The relation of nerve roots to intervertebral disc space is shown in Figure 8–6.

Spinal Cord Disease. In contrast to the levels of disease process previously considered, lesions of the spinal cord involve the long sensory and motor fiber systems within the central nervous system. When the motor fiber system is involved the signs of an upper motor neuron lesion are produced: spastic paralysis, increased deep tendon reflexes, and the sign of Babinski. Involvement of the sensory system produces selective involvement of sensory modalities, e.g., the posterior columns (position and vibration) and the lateral spinothalamic tract (pain and temperature).

The fact that the spinal cord is involved rather than a higher level in the central nervous system can be determined by noting that there is no involvement of mental status and cranial nerves.

Essentially, two types of spinal cord lesions must be considered: (a) transverse or segmental lesions, and (b) system lesions which involve neuron or fiber systems over a number of segments.

Transverse segmental lesions are more often extrinsic than intrinsic. By *extrinsic*, we mean arising outside the substance of the spinal cord and compressing the spinal cord. Extrinsic lesions can often be surgically removed with a recovery of some or all functions. By *intrinsic*, we mean arising within the substance of the spinal cord.

In considering segmental lesions, the following determinants of "level" are used:

1. Local anterior root or anterior horn level, indicated by segmental atrophy and segmental flaccid weakness.
2. Local segmental sensory level, indicated by segmental (radicular) loss of all modalities of sensation.
3. Local segmental loss or depression of deep tendon reflexes due to interruption of the stretch reflex arc. This may occur because of damage to the efferent limb of the reflex arc (anterior root or anterior horn) or damage to the afferent limb of the reflex arc (posterior root or posterior horn).
4. Segmental long motor tract level, indicated by increased deep tendon reflexes below this level.
5. Segmental long sensory tract levels, indicated by posterior column and lateral spinothalamic deficits below this level.

LOCAL DISEASES OF NERVE ROOTS

Before examining in greater detail the diseases involving the spinal cord, we will consider several of the more common problems of the nerve root.

LATERAL RUPTURE OF THE INTERVERTEBRAL DISC WITH NERVE ROOT COMPRESSION

Case History 1. NECH #179–753. Date of admission: 6/6/66.

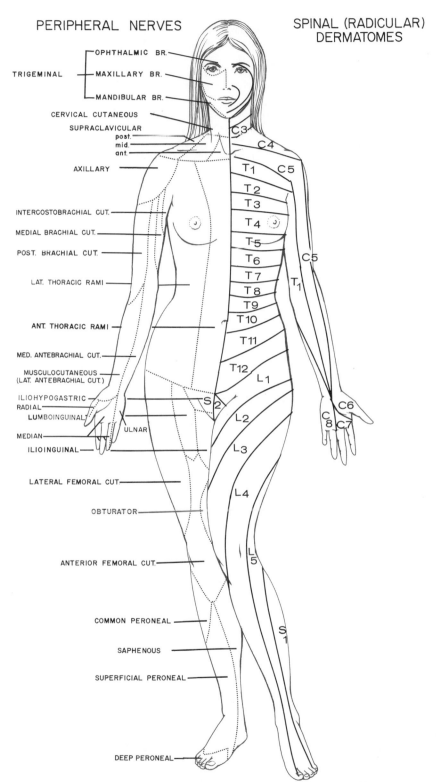

PERIPHERAL NERVES

SPINAL (RADICULAR) DERMATOMES

OPHTHALMIC BR.

TRIGEMINAL — MAXILLARY BR.

MANDIBULAR BR.

CERVICAL CUTANEOUS

SUPRACLAVICULAR
post.
mid.
ant.

AXILLARY

INTERCOSTOBRACHIAL CUT.

MEDIAL BRACHIAL CUT.

POST. BRACHIAL CUT.

LAT. THORACIC RAMI

ANT. THORACIC RAMI

MED. ANTEBRACHIAL CUT.

MUSCULOCUTANEOUS
(LAT. ANTEBRACHIAL CUT.)

ILIOHYPOGASTRIC
RADIAL

LUMBOINGUINAL

MEDIAN

ILIOINGUINAL

ULNAR

LATERAL FEMORAL CUT.

OBTURATOR

ANTERIOR FEMORAL CUT.

COMMON PERONEAL

SAPHENOUS

SUPERFICIAL PERONEAL

DEEP PERONEAL

C3
C4
C5
T1
T2
T3
T4
T5
T6
T7
T8
T9
T10
T11
T12
L1
L2
L3
L4
L5
S1
S2
C5
T1
C6
C7
C8

Figure 8–3 Comparison of radicular (dermatome or segmental) and peripheral nerve innervation.

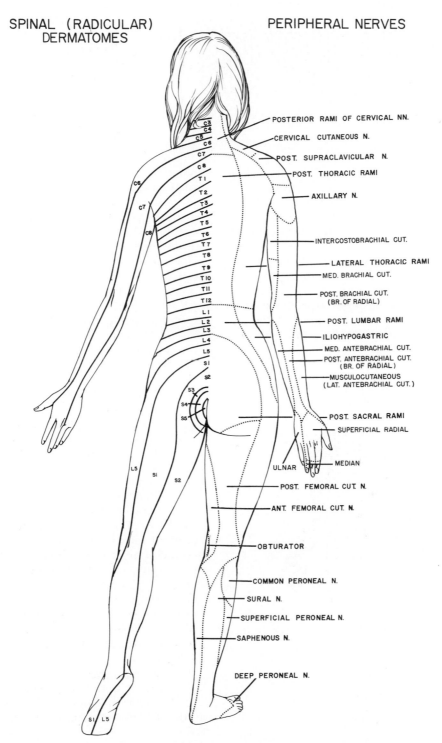

SPINAL (RADICULAR) DERMATOMES

PERIPHERAL NERVES

POSTERIOR RAMI OF CERVICAL NN.

CERVICAL CUTANEOUS N.

POST. SUPRACLAVICULAR N.

POST. THORACIC RAMI

AXILLARY N.

INTERCOSTOBRACHIAL CUT.

LATERAL THORACIC RAMI

MED. BRACHIAL CUT.

POST. BRACHIAL CUT.
(BR. OF RADIAL)

POST. LUMBAR RAMI

ILIOHYPOGASTRIC

MED. ANTEBRACHIAL CUT.

POST. ANTEBRACHIAL CUT.
(BR. OF RADIAL)

MUSCULOCUTANEOUS
(LAT. ANTEBRACHIAL CUT.)

POST. SACRAL RAMI

SUPERFICIAL RADIAL

ULNAR   MEDIAN

POST. FEMORAL CUT. N.

ANT. FEMORAL CUT. N.

OBTURATOR

COMMON PERONEAL N.

SURAL N.

SUPERFICIAL PERONEAL N.

SAPHENOUS N.

DEEP PERONEAL N.

Figure 8–3. *Continued.*

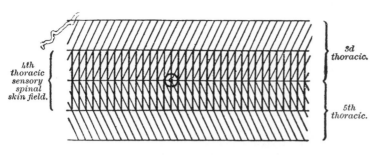

Figure 8–4 Method of remaining sensibility to demonstrate the sensory skin field of a nerve root. Sherrington sectioned three roots above and three below the intact root to be studied. In this diagram the overlap of the third and fifth thoracic spinal roots is demonstrated. (From Ransom, S., and Clark, S.: *The Anatomy of the Nervous System,* 10th Edition. Philadelphia, W. B. Saunders, 1959, p. 129.)

This 42-year-old, Roman Catholic priest (Reverend Z) sustained a minor injury to his lumbosacral area 2 months prior to admission when he slid into third base while playing baseball. Shortly thereafter, he noted dull pains in the lumbosacral area in the mornings. Three weeks prior to admission the patient had the onset of electric shock type pain beginning in the right buttock area and shooting down the posterior aspect of the leg to the foot. This pain was precipitated by coughing, sneezing, straining, and bending.

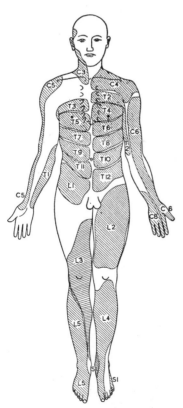

Figure 8–5 Dermatomes in man demonstrated by the method of remaining sensibility. (From Lewis, T.: *Pain.* New York, Macmillan, 1942, p. 20, after Foerster.)

Sharp movements of the neck would also precipitate the pain. During this same time, the patient had noted occasional tingling paresthesia of the right posterior calf, and occasional "spasms" of the back muscles and leg. He had experienced no weakness.

PAST HISTORY: No significant events had occurred.

GENERAL PHYSICAL EXAMINATION: Negative.

NEUROLOGICAL EXAMINATION:
1. *Mental status:* Intact.
2. *Cranial nerves:* Intact.
3. *Motor system:* Intact.
4. *Reflexes:*
   a. Deep tendon reflexes were intact in the upper extremities. Right Achilles tendon reflex was absent (0) compared to a normal (2+) response on the left. Right quadriceps tendon reflex was decreased to a minimal degree compared to left.
   b. Plantar responses were flexor.
5. *Sensation:* All modalities were intact.
6. *Back:* Marked spasm of the right paravertebral muscles was present. There was a marked limitation of flexion of the lumbosacral spine. Local tenderness was present at the L5–S1 area.
7. *Local pain* was present on palpation of the sciatic nerve in the right buttock.
8. *Straight leg raising* was limited to 30 degrees on the right (compared to normal of 90 degrees).

LABORATORY DATA:
1. Lumbar spine x-rays were normal.
2. Lumbar myelogram revealed a defect at the L5–S1 interspace on the right (Fig. 8–7).

HOSPITAL COURSE:
The patient had a 12-day period of complete bed rest during which a bed board was used. When symptoms persisted, a myelogram was performed with the results in-

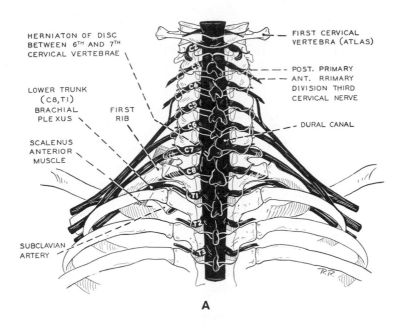

A

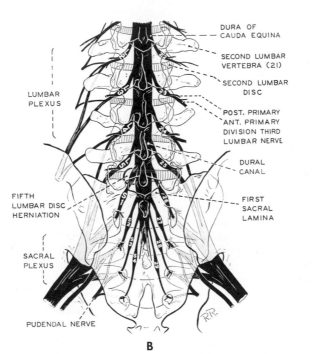

B

Figure 8–6 The relationship of nerve roots to the vertebrae and the intervertebral disc spaces. *A*, Posterior view of the cervical and upper thoracic vertebrae and spinal cord. A lateral herniation of a disc at C6–C7 interspace compressing the C7 nerve root is demonstrated. The composition and relationships of the brachial plexus are also demonstrated.

B, Posterior view of the lumbar sacral vertebrae and spinal cord. A lateral herniation of a disc at L5–S1 interspace compressing the S1 nerve root is demonstrated. The composition and relationships of the lumbar and sacral plexus are also demonstrated. (From Keegan, J. J., and Garrett, F. D.: Anat. Rec., *102*:414, 416, 1948.)

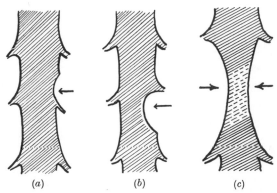

Figure 8-7 Lumbar disc protrusions as shown at myelography: *a* and *b*, lateral; *c*, midline (central). (From Sutton, D.: *In* Brain, Lord: *Recent Advances in Neurology and Neuropsychiatry*, 7th Edition. London, J. A. Churchill, 1962, p. 272.)

dicated above. On June 21, 1966 a laminectomy was performed by Dr. Robert Yuan, and a bulging intervertebral disc was removed at the L5–S1 interspace (similar to that demonstrated in Fig. 8–6B). The patient had an uneventful recovery with relief of pain. He was discharged from the hospital 10 days after surgery. Examination 1 month later indicated continued absence of the right Achilles tendon reflex. A minimal decrease in pain sensation over the lateral border of the right foot, apparently present since surgery, was also noted.

COMMENT:

The patient presented a description of radicular pain (electric shock shooting type precipitated by coughing, straining) that was clearly in the S1 distribution of the right lower extremity. The involvement of the S1 root was also suggested by the paresthesia involving the S1 dermatome. The selective involvement of the Achilles tendon reflex is also consistent with such a level of involvement. Weakness was not present in this case. Had weakness been present, the dorsiflexors of the toe and ankle might well have been involved.

As regards treatment, in the majority of acute lateral disk protrusions the root compression symptoms will lessen and disappear with a period of strict bed rest. Surgery is indicated in those cases where such a period of bed rest has failed to eliminate radicular symptoms or where there is a reasonable expectation that severe radicular symptoms may recur at frequent intervals in future years (e.g., a young adult engaged in heavy labor).

Most disk protrusions in the lumbar area are lateral in location. Occasionally, midline protrusions will occur with compression of the S2, S3, and S4 roots in the cauda equina supplying the bladder. Such midline disks may be the cause of an atonic distended bladder and will, in general, require surgical removal.

As we have previously indicated, rupture of the intervertebral disk also occurs commonly in the cervical area at C5–C6 and C6–C7 interspaces. This problem will be discussed later in relation to the process of cervical cord compression secondary to degeneration and protrusion of the cervical intervertebral disk (cervical spondylosis).

LOCAL INFECTION OF DORSAL ROOT GANGLIA BY HERPES ZOSTER (SHINGLES)

The herpes zoster virus invades the dorsal ganglia of the spinal and cranial nerve roots. Usually symptoms and signs are confined to one or two adjacent sensory roots. The thoracic area is the most frequent location. In about 20 per cent of the cases, the process involves the cranial nerves (V and VII).

The initial symptom is that of sharp burning, lancinating (neuralgic), radicular pain. Within 3 to 4 days, the involved dermatome becomes red and a vesicular eruption appears in a segmental distribution (Fig. 8–8). The herpes zoster virus is closely related to the virus of chickenpox (varicella). The local cutaneous eruption of herpes zoster resembles the generalized eruption of chickenpox.

There is some evidence that cases of herpes zoster may occur in individuals who have had previous immunity to chickenpox and who, in later years, are exposed again to the chickenpox virus. There is also evidence that diseases that alter immune mechanisms, such as infections, lymphomas (generalized tumors of the lymphatic-reticuloendothelial system), or metastatic carcinomas may also predispose to development of herpes zoster infection. In some cases, the primary neoplastic process has arisen in organs in close relationship to the involved dermatome. In some cases, local irritation of the involved nerve root has been previously present, serving in a sense to activate the viral infection.

Although the symptoms are usually re-

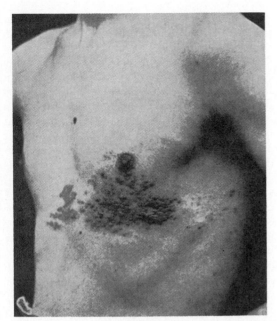

Figure 8–8 Herpes zoster in dermatomes T5 and T6. (From Haymaker, W.: *Bing's Local Diagnosis in Neurological Disease*, 15th Edition. St. Louis, C. V. Mosby, 1969, p. 88.)

lated to the involvement of the dorsal root ganglia, occasionally significant local segmental weakness and atrophy may also be present, indicating involvement of the anterior root or anterior horn. No specific therapy is available. The disease is usually self-limited with the patient recovering completely.

In the few cases that have come to autopsy, inflammatory changes have involved the spinal cord to a minor degree, in addition to the expected involvement of the dorsal root ganglia. In rare instances, patients have demonstrated actual clinical signs of spinal cord or cerebral involvement (herpes zoster encephalomyelitis). In some patients, pain (postherpetic neuralgia) may persist for months or years after the skin lesions have disappeared.

OTHER DISEASES INVOLVING NERVE ROOTS

Several of the disease processes to be discussed under the topic of peripheral neuropathies may also involve the nerve roots, producing a radiculopathy in addition to a polyneuropathy. The dorsal root and dorsal root ganglia may also be involved over a wide area in the late stages of syphilis (tabes dorsalis), but this will be discussed under

system diseases. The nerve roots may also be torn by traumatic injuries.

DISEASES OF THE SPINAL CORD

We will consider diseases of the spinal cord under two essential categories.

Extrinsic: Essentially compressive or traumatic lesions. All are segmental, i.e., transverse type lesions.

Intrinsic: May be (a) localized (usually involving several segments) or (b) system type lesions.

These two major types of disease processes, the extrinsic and the intrinsic, must be clearly differentiated, from a diagnostic standpoint, since the therapeutic implications are quite different. The extrinsic compressive lesion usually represents an acute neurosurgical problem requiring immediate decompression of the spinal cord. The intrinsic disease process, if localized, may require neurosurgical therapy but the aims of such therapy have a somewhat different purpose as will be evident in the case histories that follow. The system category of intrinsic disease in some instances represents varieties of diseases for which an established, specific therapy exists, e.g., vitamin B12 for combined system disease. In other instances, these system diseases represent degenerative processes for which no known treatment exists.

In general terms, the following differential points may be used in distinguishing extrinsic from intrinsic lesions. Extrinsic lesions as we have indicated are segmental lesions with segmental characteristics as regards local motor level, local sensory level, local reflex level, long tract motor level, and long tract sensory level. In general, one or more signs or symptoms of the local segmental level will be present, in addition to the long tract signs. Extrinsic compressive lesions when fully developed tend to involve the spinal cord at a given level in a relatively complete bilateral manner or in a complete hemisectional manner. In contrast, intrinsic lesions tend to involve parts or systems of the spinal cord in a selective or disassociated manner. Even when localized, these processes tend to involve several segments and not a single segment, e.g., syringomyelia (a central cavity or cyst) and glioma (a tumor arising from glial elements). When extrinsic lesions involve the lateral spinothalamic tracts, pain sensation over the sacral segments is involved early in the disease course because this tract is laminated with fibers derived from sacral segments placed most laterally. When intrinsic lesions, such as a syrinx, involve these tracts, sacral sensation is spared since more medial structures are involved first while fibers from the sacral segments are affected late in the disease course.

EXTRINSIC LESIONS OF THE SPINAL CORD

The following outline presents a summary view of extrinsic lesions of the spinal cord.
A. Traumatic related lesions
  1. Direct lacerations with partial or total transections
  2. Direct cord compressions due to fracture dislocations
  3. Indirect cord damage, vascular infarction, and hematomyelia
B. Extradural compressive lesions
  1. Ruptured midline disc or osteophytes of cervical spondylosis
  2. Metastatic carcinoma extending to vertebrae and epidural space
  3. Regional spread of lymphoma to epidural space
  4. Epidural abscess
  5. Metastatic tuberculosis extending to intervertebral disc space and vertebral body, with collapse of vertebra and subsequent cord compression
C. Intradural extramedullary lesions
  1. Meningioma
  2. Neurofibroma

Extrinsic compressive diseases of the spinal cord may produce a variety of clinical effects depending on the rapidity and degree of compression. Thus, acute compressive lesions, e.g., fracture dislocations, tend to produce acute, complete transection syndromes. Chronic compressions from slowly growing tumors produce a less marked syndrome of gradual onset.

Acute Cord Compression with Functional Transection. Let us first consider the effects of acute cord compression with functional transection. The immediate effects of transection reflect both "spinal shock" and the release of the function of lower structures from higher (cortical and brain stem) control. In man, the effects of spinal shock predominate.

Spinal shock may be defined as a loss or depression of segmental reflex activities (stretch reflexes, deep tendon reflexes) following spinal cord transection. Its nature is still uncertain. It is progressively more profound in higher animal forms. In the frog, it is a fleeting phenomenon. In the cat, its duration is a matter of minutes to hours; in the dog, a matter of several hours; in the monkey, it is a matter of days to weeks. In man, a duration of several weeks is usual.

At the level of the alpha motor neuron, spinal shock is characterized by hyperpolarization of the neuronal membrane. It is uncertain whether this hyperpolarization derives from withdrawal of facilitation or from increase in tonic inhibition (that is, an increase in IPSP). It is also uncertain whether the source of the hyperpolarization is supraspinal or segmental. In the cat and dog, spinal shock appears to relate primarily to section of or damage to the vestibulospinal and ventral reticulospinal tracts. In primates, the occurrence of spinal shock depends much more upon corticospinal tract damage.

It is important to note that the depth and duration of spinal shock will depend on (a) the rapidity and completeness of spinal cord section (slowly evolving chronic cord compressions are not characterized by spinal shock) and (b) fever, infection, and nutritional status. Thus fever and infection will prolong the duration. Moreover, once recovery has started, fever and infection may cause the patient to regress to an earlier stage with a reappearance of spinal shock.

In man, then, the immediate effect of transection is a complete loss of stretch reflexes. Thus the paralysis below the level of transection is a flaccid paralysis and there is no resistance to passive motion. The deep tendon reflexes are depressed and usually absent since these reflexes are the phasic component of the stretch reflexes. The segmental reflexes at the sacral level involved in reflex evacuation of the bladder and bowel in response to distension are depressed with a resultant retention of urine and feces. The bladder is referred to as "atonic" (although the smooth muscles of the bladder and bowel do, in a strict sense, retain some tone). The skin is dry because of a loss of autonomic control and of sweating below the lesion. There is a complete loss of sensation below the level of the lesion.

If overdistension of the bladder and an

infection have been avoided, recovery of reflex function in man will become evident within 1 to 5 weeks. The flexion reflex (withdrawal of the leg on painful stimulation) is the initial reflex to reappear, and it remains prepotent. The flexion reflex is polysynaptic with the afferent end of the reflex arc mediated by type III and IV fibers from free nerve endings. Initially, the withdrawal involves abduction of the thigh, then withdrawal of the entire limb. The sign of Babinski occurs in man as one component of this flexion response.* In the spinal cat or dog, a *local sign* very rapidly becomes evident; that is, a differential movement occurs to a different location of stimulus, e.g., a painful stimulus to the inner border of the foot leads to flexion eversion and abduction; a painful stimulus to the outer border of the foot leads to flexion inversion and adduction.

In man, however, the *mass reflex* is usually quite prominent for some time prior to the development of a local sign. In its fully developed form, this mass reflex consists of generalized reflex flexor spasms of the muscles of the trunk and lower extremities, accompanied by sweating, emptying of the bladder, penile erection, and ejaculation. The receptive field for triggering this response is quite extensive, involving any tactile or nociceptive stimulus to the foot, leg, abdomen, or thorax. With the passage of time, the mass reflex becomes less prominent and a local sign develops. However, the mass reflex is likely to return if fever or infection occurs.

With the development of a local sign, there is usually some return of deep tendon reflexes. Extensor postures and reflexes may then return. If transection has been complete, a year may pass before these return. The extensor capacities in man may include, in addition to hyperactive deep tendon reflexes: (a) crossed extension, (b) alternate flexion-extension and alternate stepping. Crossed extension involves extension of the contralateral hind limb at a time when the ipsilateral limb is responding by flexion to a painful stimulus. With marked extensor tone, a partial capacity for brief periods of standing may return.

*It is important to note that the sign of Babinski, taken in isolation, does not indicate disease of the spinal cord per se but rather signifies the release in man of spinal cord reflex activity ·from that higher cerebrocortical control mediated by the corticospinal tract.

Bladder emptying and bowel evacuation reflexes usually return 3 to 4 weeks after injury. The initially atonic bladder then becomes a spastic bladder.

Sweating below the level of transection may not return for 2 to 3 months.

The Hemisection Syndrome of Brown-Séquard. This syndrome will be noted in several of the case histories presented later. It may be seen in traumatic lacerations of the spinal cord (knife wounds) in which a hemisection has occurred. In addition, this syndrome may be noted in chronic cord compressions caused by laterally placed meningiomas in the thoracic area. The particular syndrome may be seen in intrinsic diseases, such as multiple sclerosis, where a large area of demyelination has involved one half of the cord.

From a theoretical standpoint, the hemisection lesion is extremely valuable for the clinical study of spinal cord fiber systems and provides a clear indication of the various determinants of segmental level. Thus, at the level of the hemisection, an ipsilateral segmental area of atrophy and reflex loss will be present corresponding to the segmental destruction of the anterior root and anterior horn. This same ipsilateral segment at the level of injury will be characterized by total destruction of the ipsilateral posterior horn, posterior root, and posterior root entry zone. There will be a corresponding segmental ipsilateral band of complete absence of sensation. Below the level of the hemisection there will be an ipsilateral loss of position and vibratory sensation from damage to the ipsilateral posterior column. There will be, in addition, an ipsilateral spastic paralysis of all segments below the level of the hemisection with an ipsilateral increase in deep tendon reflexes and an ipsilateral Babinski sign from damage to the ipsilateral lateral corticospinal tract (and related motor pathways of the lateral column).

On the side contralateral to the hemisection, beginning two to three segments below the level of the hemisection there will be a loss of pain and temperature sensation from damage to the ipsilateral lateral spinothalamic tract. Touch below the level of the lesion will be intact since this modality of sensation is conveyed in both a crossed (ventral spinothalamic tract) and uncrossed manner (posterior column). A hemisection, then, interrupts only one of these pathways. From a clinical standpoint the long fiber systems previously considered are the significant pathways in the spinal cord. Other tracts, such as the tectospinal, olivospinal, vestibulospinal, and so forth, do not have specific clinical significance.

The Chronic or Subacute Anterior Midline Compression Syndrome. This syndrome occurs as a clinical entity with midline protrusion of a cervical disc. Tumors metastatic to the thoracic vertebrae with collapse of the vertebrae or invasion of the adjacent epidural space may also produce this syndrome. The syndrome has been the subject of extensive experimental investigation by Tarlov (1957). In these studies, small balloons were implanted in the epidural space of the dog anterior to the thoracic spinal cord and gradually inflated. As the balloon was inflated, the spinal cord was displaced backwards against the hard posterior wall of the bony spinal canal, and as the degree of compression increased, the cord was deformed. The compression also to some extent may have acted to occlude the arteries supplying the spinal cord and the resultant ischemia may have added to the damage. (This factor is apparently less significant than the direct compression of neural tissue.) With relatively acute compressions, however, veins may also be occluded with the development of venous stasis and subsequent hemorrhage into the substance of spinal cord.

This preparation is of interest because with gradual (subacute) progressive cord compression, the initial neurological findings relate to posterior and lateral column findings in the lower extremities (deficits in placing of limbs and progressive spastic paraplegia). With progression of the compression, deficits in pain and temperature sensation occurred with an ascending long tract sensory level. With relief of the compression, a significant recovery occurred in many of the animals. In general, pain sensation returned first (normally by 4 to 6 days) and then motor function (normally by 25 to 170 days). Position sense returned very slowly. A complete recovery of sensory and motor function was, however, possible even in dogs in whom gradual compression had been increasing for 48 hours (to the point of complete loss of sensory and motor function in the lower extremities) and in whom the compression had then been maintained for one week.

Beyond one week, the paralysis was irreversible. If the gradual compression was more rapid, e.g., over 20 hours to complete paralysis, the time limit tolerated for this degree of compression was shorter (80 to 90 hours).

The explanation for the greater vulnerability of the posterior and lateral columns to compression is not certain. This may represent a selective vulnerability effect on the large diameter, heavily myelinated fibers of these systems compared to the thin, poorly myelinated fibers involved in the conduction of pain impulses within the spinal cord. Other explanations relate to the possible role of the dentate ligaments.

SPECIFIC EXTRINSIC LESIONS

TRAUMATIC LESIONS OF THE SPINAL CORD

Direct Lacerations with Partial or Total Transections. These lesions are a result of knife or bullet wounds of the spinal cord. Although we have classified these as extrinsic in the sense that the etiology is extrinsic, in reality the actual intrinsic structure of the spinal cord has been lacerated. The effects of the transection and the pattern of recovery of reflex function have already been discussed.

Fracture Dislocations. In civilian life, most injuries to the spinal cord do not represent actual lacerations of the cord but are rather a result of crush injuries from fracture dislocations in the cervical or thoracic areas (see Fig. 8–9). People frequently fall in a manner which transmits force to the thoracic vertebrae; compression fractures of thoracic vertebrae may result with collapse of the vertebrae and sharp angulation of the axis of bony support. A similar compression and collapse may also occur from other nontraumatic causes, e.g., tuberculosis of the spine (Pott's disease), metastatic carcinoma, and osteoporosis. Injuries to the cervical spine resulting from fracture dislocation are common in auto accidents and in diving accidents.

It is important to note that fractures of the vertebrae may occur without a marked degree of dislocation. In such cases, care must be taken when moving these patients. Thus in fractures of the cervical spine, the patient

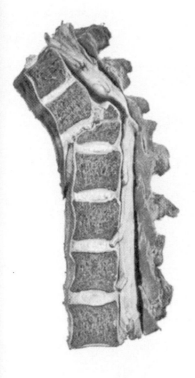
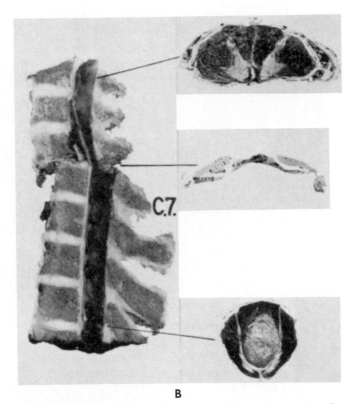

A   **B**

Figure 8–9   Traumatic lesions of the spinal cord: *A,* Fracture dislocation of thoracic vertebra has crushed and almost transected the thoracic spinal cord.

B, A fracture dislocation of the cervical spine (due to an auto accident 2 weeks prior to death) has produced an almost complete transection of the spinal cord at the C7 level. (From Blackwood, W., Dodds, T. C., and Somerville, J. C.: *Atlas of Neuropathology,* 2nd Edition. Baltimore, Williams and Wilkins, 1964, p. 147.)

should remain supine with the neck immobilized (by sand bags placed at the sides of the head or by a makeshift collar prepared from rolled newspaper, if necessary) to avoid flexion and extension during transportation because such movements will tend to exacerbate any dislocation. Once the patient arrives at a treatment center, additional measures, such as traction or spinal fusion, may be considered.

Once crush injury has occurred, a partial or complete functional transection results with the clinical effects and course as previously discussed. The descending and ascending degeneration following such a crush injury are demonstrated in Figure 8–10.

Indirect Effects of Trauma to the Spinal Cord.   As previously indicated acute compression of the spinal cord may produce indirect vascular effects with infarction resulting from anterior spinal artery occlusion or with hemorrhage into the substance of the spinal cord (hematomyelia) as a result of venous compression.

EXTRADURAL COMPRESSIVE LESIONS

Cervical Spondylosis with Cord Compression.   This is probably the most common cause of nontraumatic cord compressions. The term cervical spondylosis refers to degenerative disease of the cervical intervertebral disc. Several processes are involved. Acute lateral or midline ruptures of disc material (the nucleus pulposus) may occur, as in the lumbar area in relation to trauma. More often, however, as the disc degenerates with increasing age, the disc material begins to bulge, the disc space narrows, and secondary formation of osteophytes (bone spurs) occurs. These protrusions and osteophytes may bulge into the neural foramina, producing nerve root compression, or may be located in a midline

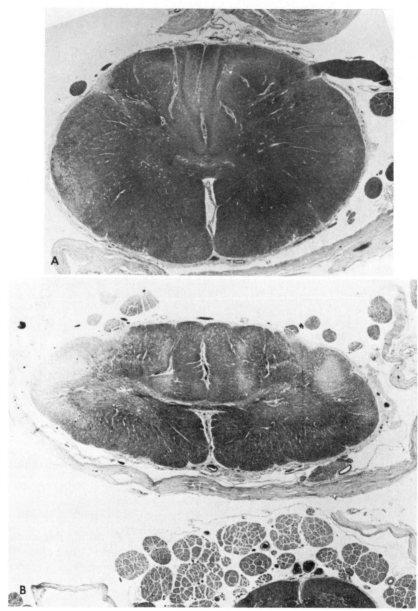

Figure 8–10 Ascending and Descending Degeneration: Cervical Spondylosis with Spinal Cord Compression. This 64-year-old male expired after a six-year history of progressive spastic paraparesis, with bilateral corticospinal and posterior column findings in lower extremities. A deficit in pain sensation was present below the level of T10. Atrophy and fasciculations were present at C4–C8. At autopsy, softening of the spinal cord was present at C7.

A, Myelin stain of upper cervical spinal cord above level of compression, demonstrating ascending degeneration predominantly in posterior columns.

B, Myelin stain of cervical cord just below area of softening, demonstrating descending degeneration predominantly in lateral columns. (Courtesy of Dr. Jose Segarra, Boston Veterans Administration Hospital.)

location, producing spinal cord compression (Fig. 8–11). The following case histories indicate the nature of this problem.

Case History 2. NECH #74–87–95. Date of admission: 1/20/69.

This 30-year-old, white, male sociologist (Mr. G. C.) was referred to Dr. Huntington Porter because of loss of sensation in three fingers of each hand. Approximately 5 years previously, the patient had become aware of pain and stiffness in his neck over the left posterior aspect. He also noted a snapping sound, heard and felt, on turning to the extreme left or right. This condition remained relatively static with, if anything, some improvement of the neck pain until 4 months prior to admission. At that time, the patient noted that extension of the neck would produce numbness of a tingling quality in the three ulnar fingers of both hands. He also noted that extending his neck produced a numbness of the toes of both feet. At the same time, he noted slight weakness of both hands with a loss of coordination in writing and a slight weakness and incoordination of both legs. He believed that the weakness of the legs had increased somewhat over the following 2 months as it became more difficult to climb stairs. The weakness in upper extremities had not progressed over the last 2 months.

NEUROLOGICAL EXAMINATION:

1. *Mental status:* intact.
2. *Cranial nerves:* intact.
3. *Motor system:*
   a. There was weakness of the left triceps and of the extensors of the left wrist. In addition there was some weakness of abduction of the fingers. In the lower extremities there was slight weakness in dorsiflexion of the toes bilaterally.
   b. Gait was slightly spastic and ataxic with a slight tendency to circumduct the left leg. (Circumduction, usually seen in hemiplegia, is characterized by the leg swinging in a lateral arc in walking—related to external rotation at the hip and failure of flexion at the hip, knee, and ankle.)
4. *Reflexes:*
   a. *Deep tendon reflexes:* The left biceps and radial deep tendon reflexes were selectively decreased to 1+ compared to a normal of 2+ on the right. The triceps was increased bilaterally to 3+; that on the left was slightly greater than that on the right. The finger jerks were increased bilaterally. Quadricep reflexes, and Achilles tendon reflexes were increased— quadriceps 3+, Achilles 4+ (the left greater than the right with unsustained ankle clonus bilaterally).
   b. Plantar responses were extensor bilaterally.
5. *Sensation:*
   a. Vibration was absent in the toes and over the lumbar spine up to the midthoracic spine with some decrease to the lower cervical spine. Vibration was also markedly decreased in the fifth finger of both hands and to a lesser extent in the ring and middle fingers, with the loss appearing most marked on the right hand.
   b. Position sense was poor in the right toes, but intact in the left toes.
   c. Pain sensation was slightly decreased over the fifth fingers bilaterally.
6. Extension of the neck produced a tingling numbness in the three ulnar fingers of both hands.

LABORATORY DATA:

Myelogram: Anterior indentations in the dye column were seen in the lateral view of the cervical spine. This was felt to be consistent with an anterior extradural compressive lesion as could be found with extruded discs at C4–C5 and C5–C6 levels.

HOSPITAL COURSE:

On February 11, 1969 a laminectomy was performed by Dr. Robert Yuan, and a soft, ruptured, midline disc at the C4–C5 interspace was removed. The postoperative course was uneventful. At the time of hospital discharge on February 23, the patient's neurological examination revealed no disability. Follow-up evaluation approximately 40 days after surgery indicated that strength and gait were normal. Evaluation 1 year after surgery indicated only minor pyramidal tract signs without significant disability.

COMMENT:

The presence of degenerative disease involving the cervical intervertebral discs was suggested in this case by the 5-year history of pain and stiffness and the noise heard on rotation. Such neck symptoms are not uncommon and do not necessarily indicate that any neurological disease is present. In this case, however, an ominous neurological clue was introduced when mechanical alterations

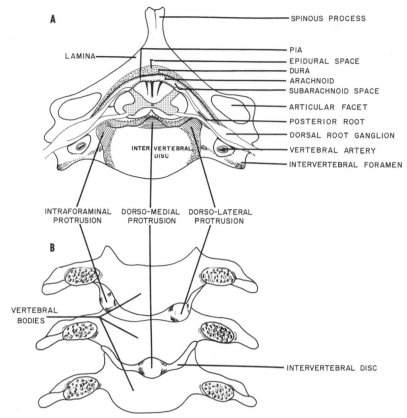

A

SPINOUS PROCESS

LAMINA

PIA
EPIDURAL SPACE
DURA
ARACHNOID
SUBARACHNOID SPACE
ARTICULAR FACET
POSTERIOR ROOT
DORSAL ROOT GANGLION
VERTEBRAL ARTERY
INTERVERTEBRAL FORAMEN

INTERVERTEBRAL DISC

INTRAFORAMINAL PROTRUSION   DORSO-MEDIAL PROTRUSION   DORSO-LATERAL PROTRUSION

B

VERTEBRAL BODIES

INTERVERTEBRAL DISC

Figure 8–11 Anatomic Relationships of the Cervical Spinal Cord and the Cervical Intervertebral Discs. Lateral and midline disc protrusions are indicated. (Modified after Frykholm, Acta. Chir. Scand. *101*:345, 1951.)

Illustration continued on opposite page.

in posture of the neck began to produce definite neurologic symptoms. Thus, extension of the neck produced numbness of the toes, suggesting spinal cord compression. The numbness in the C7 and C8 dermatomes of the hands may also have related to spinal cord compression with involvement of the posterior columns. Posterior root compromise may also have produced this symptom. However, in the present case, the actual level of compression was higher than the C7 and C8 nerve roots. Moreover, such posterior root compression if present should also have produced radicular type pain (segmental burning type pain).

At the time of the patient's neurological evaluation, evidence of spinal cord compression was present with signs of bilateral involvement of the corticospinal tract (bilateral extensor plantar responses, spastic paraplegic gait, and bilateral ankle clonus)

and involvement of the posterior columns (impairment of vibration in both lower extremities). The actual level of involvement of these long fiber systems is suggested by the fact that the upper level of increased reflex activity began at the triceps and finger deep tendon reflexes (C6, C7, and C8). Vibratory sensation was to a variable degree decreased up to the ring and middle fingers (C7 segmental level). The actual level of spinal cord compression must then be somewhat above the C7 segment.

A local lower motor neuron level was not evident in the present case as regards atrophy and fasciculations. The weakness in the triceps and wrist extensor muscles of the left upper extremity presumably reflected local anterior horn or anterior root involvement at the level of compression. The depression of biceps and radial periosteal deep tendon reflex in the left upper extremity did provide

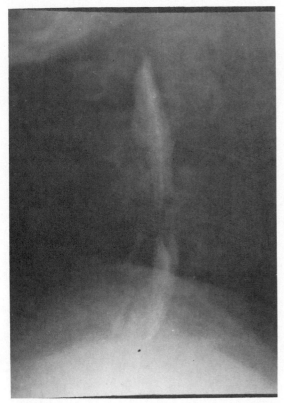 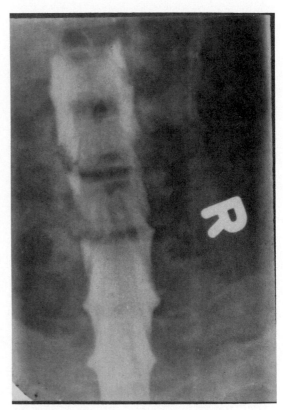

Figure 8–11a: Cervical Spondylosis. Case History #3: Myelographic appearance of midline spurs (osteophytes), narrowing anterior-posterior diameter of spinal canal and compressing spinal cord. *Left,* lateral view; *right,* anterior-posterior view. (Courtesy of Dr. John Sullivan, New England Medical Center Hospitals.)

A myelogram is performed by injecting into the subarachnoid space at the time of a lumbar puncture (Fig. 7–5) a radiopaque substance (a nonwater soluble iodinated oil). The oil which is heavier than cerebrospinal fluid is removed at the conclusion of the procedure.

a local segmental reflex level (C5 and C6). A definite local segmental sensory level in the sense of a segmental (radicular) loss of all modalities of sensation was not present in this case. The slight decrease in pain sensation in the fifth fingers did suggest a possible C8 level of involvement. Such a suggestion was, however, inconsistent with the firm major clinical findings. It is of interest that the long tract findings in this case, showing a midline mass anterior to the spinal cord, were limited to the posterior columns and motor pathways of the lateral columns. There was no definite evidence of involvement of pain and temperature pathways. This clinical pattern corresponds to the experimental situation discussed previously.

In the present case, progression of symptomatology and of disability was prevented by the cervical laminectomy and removal of the soft ruptured disc. In many cases, a soft ruptured disc is not present; instead the spinal cord compression has resulted from an old calcified, ruptured disc or a midline osteophyte (or spur) of bone. In such cases, the surgical procedure may be limited to a laminectomy. Such a procedure allows greater room for the spinal cord by removing the posterior wall of the bony canal. Considerable damage to the spinal cord might follow if an attempt was made to remove bony spurs anterior to the spinal cord from the posterior approach of the laminectomy.

The student should be alert to the possibility of spinal cord compression resulting from cervical spondylosis even when neck pain and radicular symptoms are not present. Many cases, of course, will have a long history of repeated episodes of neck pain and stiffness, with definite cervical radicular symptoms in the C5, C6, or C7 distribution, e.g., root pain, segmental weakness, and segmental sensory deficit. In many cases, however, these symptoms and signs will be lacking and the patient will present with long tract symptoms only, or with long tract symptoms plus minor segmental radicular symptoms.

Case History 3. NECH #126–760. Date of admission: 5/8/59.

This 56-year-old, white male (Mr. H. G.) was referred for evaluation of progressive weakness of the legs. The problem had begun approximately 1 year previously when he noted difficulty in climbing stairs. The disability was progressive but was not associated with lower extremity sensory symptoms. A definite stiffness of gait, however, had developed in the month prior to admission.

For 6 months, the patient had noted burning pains in the hands bilaterally. The actual distribution was not more specifically described. A minor degree of weakness had been noted in the left hand.

The patient denied bladder or bowel symptoms. Neck pain had not been present and there was no history of an injury to the neck.

PAST HISTORY: There was no remarkable feature except for a family history of diabetes mellitus.

GENERAL PHYSICAL EXAMINATION: No remarkable abnormalities were present.

NEUROLOGICAL EXAMINATION:

1. *Mental status:* Intact.
2. *Cranial nerves:* Intact.
3. *Motor system:*
   a. There was a mild weakness of the left triceps muscle (60 per cent of normal strength) accompanied by a minor degree of atrophy and occasional fasciculations. In addition, weakness of the left wrist extensor was present.
   b. A spastic paraparesis was present with a characteristic gait (bilateral spastic weakness as regards voluntary movements in the lower extremities).
   c. A spastic resistance to passive motion was present at the knees and ankles.
4. *Reflexes:*
   a. Deep tendon reflexes were active in the upper extremities with the exception of the left triceps which was relatively decreased. Deep tendon re-

flexes were hyperactive in the lower extremities.
   b. Bilateral Babinski signs were present. Abdominal reflexes were absent.
5. *Sensation:* All modalities were intact.

LABORATORY DATA:

1. *Glucose tolerance test* indicated a diabetic curve with a 2½-hour value elevated to 141 mg./100 ml.

2. *Cervical spine x-rays* showed marked degenerative spurring present at the C5–C6 and C6–C7 interspaces. The spurs projected posteriorly into the spinal cord and laterally into the neural foramina.

3. *Cervical myelogram* revealed midline bony spurs at C3–C4, C4–C5, and C5–C6 interspaces with impairment of dye flow over the C5–C6 interspace (Fig. 8–11*A*). In addition, there was impingement on the neural foramina at C5–C6 on the left.

HOSPITAL COURSE:

A total laminectomy at C3, C4, C5, and C6 was performed on June 3, 1959 by Dr. Samuel Brendler. When the dura was opened, the spinal cord *per se* appeared normal. The dentate ligaments at these four levels were sectioned. A large spur could be palpated, projecting into the surface of the spinal cord at the C3–C4 level. A smaller spur could be palpated at the C5–C6 level. Postoperatively there was increased weakness in the left upper extremity. By the time of discharge on June 16, 1959 the left upper extremity had returned to preoperative level. The lower limbs had shown a significant improvement in motor function. Examination in February 1960, 8 months after surgery, revealed continued improvement in strength; only a minor degree of weakness now was present at the left wrist. Spasticity was no longer present in the lower extremities. Right plantar response was flexor and the left questionably extensor.

COMMENT:

In this case the major symptoms related to bilateral compression of the lateral columns. The burning pain in the hands may have suggested involvement as well of the C6, C7, or C8 nerve roots. The minor weakness and atrophy in the triceps also suggested involvement of these nerve roots on the left. The myelogram confirmed the presence of spinal cord compression and of the C6 root compression at the C5–C6 interspace. In addition, the x-ray studies demonstrated additional midline spurs at C3–C4 and C4–

C5 levels. It is to be noted that when degenerative disc disease is present with osteophyte formation, the bony spurs are usually found at multiple cervical interspaces, as in the present case. Neck pain and local neck tenderness were absent and there was no limitation of cervical spine mobility. In many cases of severe cervical disc degeneration, these local neck findings are present (and are usually included among the symptoms of chronic cervical spine disease). The patient was diabetic as are many patients with cervical spondylosis. The explanation for this relationship is not certain.

The student may perhaps be puzzled by the fact that the dentate ligaments were sectioned in this case. The *dentate ligaments* are lateral extensions of the pia which attach to the inner surface of the dura. These ligaments, in a sense, anchor the spinal cord to the dura. Section of the ligaments then allows, to a certain extent, greater mobility of the spinal cord. Of course, it should be realized that an extradural compressive lesion displaces both the dura and the spinal cord.

Metastatic Carcinoma. Carcinoma may involve, in a metastatic manner, the bodies of the vertebrae. Subsequent collapse may then lead to spinal cord compression. Alternatively, spread may occur to epidural space without actual collapse. The result in each case is extrinsic epidural cord compression. The majority of these cases involve the thoracic vertebrae. Common sites of primary disease are the breast, lung, kidney, prostate, and gastrointestinal tract.

Case History 4. NECH #74–43–26. Date of admission: 3/5/69.

This 55-year-old, white housewife (Mrs. M. P.) was transferred from her community hospital with a 3-month history of slowly progressive weakness of both lower extremities. In October 1968 the patient first noted intermittent pain in the right scapular area. One month previously, the patient had been able to walk into the local hospital, complaining of bilateral leg weakness. Over the next two weeks, she had become completely bedridden, totally unable to move her legs or even to wiggle her toes. During the last two weeks prior to admission, the patient had trouble with bowel movements and urination. She would be unable, for hours at a time, to start her stream in the process of voiding.

During this period she also noted a pins-and-needles sensation involving both lower extremities. This had progressed to the point where her lower limbs felt dull and were without sensation. While these symptoms had been developing, a dull aching pain had been present in the scapular area.

Past History: A left radical mastectomy had been performed in 1954 (15 years previously) for an infiltrating carcinoma of the breast with regional lymph node involvement. A hysterectomy had also been performed at that time.

Neurological Examination:
1. *Mental status:* Intact.
2. *Cranial nerves:* Intact.
3. *Motor system:* A marked relatively flaccid weakness of both lower extremities was present with retention of only a flicker of flexion at the left hip. The upper extremities were intact.
4. *Reflexes:*
   a. Deep tendon reflexes were increased at quadriceps bilaterally with a 3+ response. Achilles jerks were 1+ bilaterally.
   b. Superficial plantar responses were extensor bilaterally (bilateral Babinski sign). Abdominal reflexes were absent bilaterally.
5. *Sensation:*
   a. Position sensation was absent at toes, ankles, and knees bilaterally and impaired at the hip.
   b. Vibratory sensation was absent below the iliac crests.
   c. Pain and touch sensation was absent below the D6–D7 (T6–T7) dermatomes bilaterally. No sacral sparing was present.
6. *Back:* Tenderness to percussion was present over midthoracic vertebrae (T4, T5 spinous processes).

Laboratory Data:
1. *Chest x-rays:* Multiple nodular densities were present in both hilar regions.
2. *Dorsal spine x-rays:* The T4 and T5 vertebrae were involved by destructive (lytic) metastatic lesions.
3. *Metastatic bone series:* Lytic lesions of the head and neck of the left femur were demonstrated.
4. *Myelogram:* A complete block to the flow of dye was present at the T5 level. An extradural lesion was displacing the spinal cord to the left. The myelographic appearance of the various types of tumors involving the spinal cord is diagrammed in Figure 8–12.

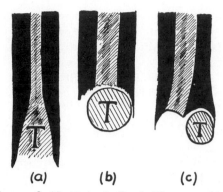

(a)　　　**(b)**　　　**(c)**

Figure 8–12 Spinal Cord Tumors. Myelographic appearance of (*a*) intramedullary tumor, (*b*) extramedullary-extradural tumor, and (*c*) extramedullary-intradural tumor. (From Sutton, D.: *In* Brain, Lord: *Recent Advances in Neurology and Neuropsychiatry*, 7th Edition. London, J. A. Churchill, 1962, p. 273.)

HOSPITAL COURSE:

On March 5, 1969 a thoracic (T3–T6) laminectomy was performed by Dr. Peter Carney for the purpose of decompression. This revealed, in the epidural space, a gelatinous and vascular tumor which was displacing the spinal cord to the left. A metastatic tumor was removed from the vertebral process laminae and epidural space. Histological examination revealed an adenocarcinoma replacing bone (presumably metastatic from the original breast lesion).

Postoperatively, a slow but progressive improvement occurred. Examination 3 weeks after surgery indicated that movement in the lower extremities had returned to 30 per cent of normal. Some pain sensation had also returned to the lower extremities. Vibration was still moderately decreased below the iliac crests and position sensation was absent at the toes. Radiation therapy was started at this time.

COMMENT:

This patient presents a typical story of an epidural compressive lesion. The initial complaint was of back pain, and there was significant local tenderness on percussion of the vertebrae. The back pain may have related to the metastatic spread of the tumor to these thoracic vertebrae. With spread of the tumor to the epidural space and the production of cord compression, the progressive weakness and segmental sensory level soon evolved. The retention of urine probably reflected the rapidity of spinal cord compression with the development of the atonic bladder of spinal shock. The relative flac-

cidity of the paraplegia also undoubtedly reflected spinal shock. The patient's total paralysis in the lower extremities had been present for at least two weeks before the patient had been transferred to an acute neurological facility. A lesser but progressive degree of weakness had been present for 3 months prior to the total paralysis. Only a minor recovery of function could be expected when such a total paraparesis from cord compression has persisted for this length of time. Diagnosis and decompression should *not* have been delayed for this length of time.

The student may inquire as to why decompression of the spinal cord is performed in such cases of advanced malignant disease with metastatic spread to multiple organs. There are several obvious answers. Even though malignant disease has spread to multiple sites in the bone, the case is not terminal and hopeless. Thus in carcinoma of the breast, alterations in the output of gonadal steroids by removing the ovaries or by administering estrogens or testosterone may result in considerable benefit. Moreover, even if one assumed that the patient had only a period of several months of life remaining, one would wish those last months to be comfortable and free of the heavy burden and disability which a total paraplegia imposes on the patient, the family, and nursing personnel. Spinal cord compression, then, is to be avoided under such circumstances and requires prompt diagnosis and surgical decompression.

The long interval between the radical mastectomy and the appearance of widespread metastatic disease is not unusual in carcinoma of the breast. Even when regional lymph node involvement is not evident at the time of mastectomy, such patients remain long-term candidates for metastatic disease.

Regional Spread of Lymphoma to the Epidural Space. Lymphomas are a group of tumors which arise from the reticuloendothelial tissue found in lymph nodes and the spleen and liver. Several histological types have been distinguished: Hodgkin's disease, lymphosarcoma, giant follicular lymphoma, and reticulum cell sarcoma. Related diseases are lymphatic leukemia, in which tumor cells appear in the blood, and multiple myeloma, in which plasma cells proliferate. Neurological symptoms develop in a considerable percentage of cases (12 per cent). Direct metastases to the brain or spinal cord are rare; regional spread of enlarged lymphoid tissue, resulting in compression of peripheral nerve plexus, nerve roots, and spinal cord, is frequent. A particularly common pattern is for spread to take place into the thoracic or lumbar epidural space from the involved thoracic and abdominal lymph nodes, resulting in root and spinal cord compression. In addition to direct compression effects on the spinal cord, indirect effects may also occur from compression of the intercostal blood supply. In some cases, invasion of the thoracic vertebrae may result in collapse of these vertebrae with subsequent angulation of the vertebral column and spinal cord compression.

The lymphomas are often very radiosensitive, demonstrating a marked reduction in mass when subjected to x-ray therapy. Compression of the nerve roots by a lymphoma can often be treated by this method. Spinal cord compression, however, as in the following case, will usually require decompression in addition to radiation therapy.

Case History 5. NECH #146–310. Date of admission: 5/22/67.

This 24-year-old, white laboratory technician (Miss. V. L.) had become ill in 1961 when enlargement of lymph nodes in the neck had been noted. Biopsy revealed Hodgkin's disease. A left radical node dissection and local irradiation was performed. In 1962, 1963, 1964, 1965, and 1966 lymphadenopathy in the axilla, mediastinum, and aortic-iliac regions and involvement of vertebrae D4 and D5 had been treated with x-radiation or cytotoxic agents such as nitrogen mustards or Cytoxan. In March of 1966, fusion of the vertebrae D2–D7 was performed because of the destructive effects of the lymphoma on the bodies of the upper dorsal vertebrae.

In February 1967 the patient had the recurrence of interscapular pain. In April 1967 a band of numbness in the D7 dermatome developed, first on the left side, then becoming bilateral. The numbness was accentuated by coughing or sneezing. Several weeks later, a vague numbness of the left thigh had been noted in addition to some instability in walking. Examination by Dr. John Hills on April 24, 1967 revealed a decrease in pain sensation over the D2–D4 and D6–D8 dermatomes on the right and over D2–D8 on the left in addition to L3–L4 on the left. Chest x-ray revealed a destructive lesion in the right eighth rib in the paravertebral region, associated with a soft tissue mass of tumor tissue. On May 1, 1967 the patient now reported a numbness involving both lower extremities below the D12 level. By May 22, 1967 a detectable bilateral deficit to pain and hot and cold was present below the D7 level. There was no evidence of sacral sparing. Bilateral Babinski signs were now also present.

NEUROLOGICAL EXAMINATION:

1. *Mental status:* Intact.
2. *Cranial nerves:* Intact.
3. *Motor system:*
   a. Strength was intact.
   b. Gait was slightly spastic.
4. *Reflexes:*
   a. Quadriceps deep tendon reflexes were hyperactive (4+) bilaterally.
   b. Bilateral extensor plantar responses were present. Abdominal reflexes were absent.
5. *Sensation:*
   a. Pain and temperature sensation were diminished below D6 on the right and T8 on the left. There was no sacral sparing.
   b. Position sense was intact. There was a minimal decrease in vibratory sensation at the toes.
6. Tenderness was present on percussion over D3.

LABORATORY DATA:

1. Hematocrit was reduced to 28%.
2. Sedimentation rate was elevated to 70 mm.
3. Myelogram revealed an extensive extradural tumor extending from D2–D7 with some decrease in flow of dye as high as C7 and as low as D9.

HOSPITAL COURSE:

A laminectomy from D2–D9 was performed on May 24, 1967 by Dr. Robert Yuan revealing extensive epidural deposits of a granulomatous and necrotic tumor mass encasing the spinal cord and extending laterally about the nerve roots D2–D6 into the mediastinum. Histological examination of this tissue which was partially removed revealed the giant cell forms found in Hodgkin's disease.

Following surgery, the patient developed increased weakness of the legs and also the arms, including muscle groups supplied by C4–C5 segments. The laminectomy was therefore extended from C2–T2. Surgery was followed by local x-ray therapy. The patient had a progressive return of strength in her extremities. By the time of discharge on July 15, 1967, she could ambulate with the aid of a walker. The patient continued to experience weakness in her lower extremities.

Chest x-ray in January, 1968, revealed additional destruction of the vertebral end of the ribs on the left side with progression of the spinal cord compression at the time of her terminal hospitalization in March 1968. This stage of her illness was also characterized by a herpes zoster infection over the D6 and D7 dermatomes on the left side of the chest. Death occurred on April 1, 1968. Postmortem examination of the spinal cord revealed tumor involving the dura, surrounding, compressing, and destroying the thoracic spinal cord. Blood vessels were occluded and infarction had occurred.

COMMENT:

The initial neurological complications in this case suggested involvement of the nerve roots of D7, first on the left, then bilaterally. This level, in general, corresponded to the area of right paravertebral rib destruction. Tumor tissue could have easily extended through the neural foramina into the epidural space, filling this space and compressing the spinal cord. This lymphoma of course could have spread also into the epidural space after involving the vertebral bodies.

In this case the pattern of lateral spinothalamic involvement was consistent with an extrinsic lesion. There was no sacral sparing as regards pain and temperature loss. This should be compared to the pattern in an intrinsic lesion where sacral segments located outermost in the lateral spinothalamic tract are least affected.

In many lymphoma cases, the surgical therapy of the spinal cord compression is limited to a decompressing laminectomy. Attempts at total removal of the epidural deposits may often result in damage to the radicular arteries which extend to the anterior spinal artery and which are likely to be surrounded by the tumor tissue. Decompressive laminectomy may sometimes be performed as a precautionary safety valve prior to irradiation of a tumor in the spinal epidural space in cases where actual paraplegia is not yet present. Irradiation often produces temporary swelling (edema) of the tumor. The added factor of edema in the relatively tightly limited compartment provided by the bony spinal canal could, without a laminectomy, result in a considerable degree of spinal cord compression.

Acute Epidural Abscess. The dura of the spinal cord is separated from the periosteum of the surrounding bony canal by a narrow space containing fatty tissue (the epidural space). This space may be the site of an acute local infection as a result of direct extension of organisms from abscess sites in adjacent tissue, e.g., skin ulcers or carbuncles. More often the infection has spread in a metastatic manner from a focus of infection elsewhere in the body.

The adjacent bone of the vertebrae is often also involved by the infection (osteomyelitis). The responsible organism is usually Staphylococcus aureus. The usual site is midthoracic. The epidural abscess is rare when compared to the epidural tumors just considered and rare when compared to meningitis and brain abscess. Nevertheless, early recognition is essential. The need for prompt drainage and decompressive laminectomy by the neurosurgeon attaches an importance to the problem beyond its low frequency of occurrence.

The early symptoms of severe back pain and fever are followed by the rapid development of the signs of acute spinal cord compression. If treatment is delayed, a functional transection of the spinal cord is the usual outcome. The transection reflects the direct effects of compression and the indirect effects of compression of blood supply and the involvement of blood vessel walls by the infectious process with infarction of the spinal cord.

The diagnosis is established by aspiration of pus from the epidural space and by the demonstration on myelogram of blockage of the subarachnoid space by an epidural mass.

Spinal Cord Compression Secondary to Tuberculous Involvement of Vertebrae. Tuberculous involvement of joints (tuberculous arthritis) was once a not uncommon complication of tuberculosis in children. The most common site of involvement is the dorsal spine. The disease process (Pott's disease or tuberculous spondylitis) results in destruction of the body of the vertebra and of the intervertebral disc. Collapse of the vertebrae and severe angulation of the bony canal occur. The chronic infection may spread into the epidural space as a local mass of infection or may accumulate as a mass under the ligament posterior to the vertebral body. All of these factors may contribute to spinal cord compression. Treatment consists of drainage of any mass pockets of infection compressing the spinal cord, antituberculous chemotherapy, immobilization, and possible fusion of the spine.

INTRADURAL EXTRAMEDULLARY TUMORS

This category of extrinsic tumor, internal to dura but external to substance of the spinal cord, accounts for the largest percentage of neoplasms involving the spinal cord. Thus, among 567 cases collected from the literature by Merritt, 59 per cent were intradural extramedullary, while 25 per cent were extra-(epi-) dural and 11 per cent were intramedullary. The majority of extradural tumors were considered previously in relation to metastatic carcinoma and regional spread of lymphoma. The intramedullary lesions are considered later under intrinsic lesions: gliomas and ependymomas. In general, tumors of the spinal cord are less frequent than intracranial tumors. Essentially two tumors constitute, in a relatively equal proportion, all of the intradural lesions: meningiomas and neurofibromas. Both types are benign in the sense that they are not locally invasive of neural tissue; they have a relatively uniform histological appearance and do not spread to distant sites.

Meningiomas. These tumors arise from arachnoidal cell clusters. Since the more common location occurs in relation to the cerebral hemisphere, a more complete discussion of histological types will be found in the chapter on Diseases of the Cerebral Hemispheres. The typical gross appearance of this tumor in relation to the spinal cord is shown in Figure 8–13. The typical myelographic appearance of intradural tumors is shown in Figure 8–12. Spinal cord meningiomas occur most frequently in middle-aged females. The most frequent location is the thoracic portion of the spinal cord, in part because the thoracic segments constitute the longest extent of the spinal cord. Other areas, however, are not immune; in the upper cervical area, these tumors may arise in relation to the foramen magnum, producing both lower brain stem and upper cervical cord symptoms. The symptomatology and course of a typical meningioma in relation to the thoracic spinal cord is illustrated in the following case history.

Case History 6. NECH #173–926. BD #58–28–22. Date of admission: 10/19/65. This 58-year-old, white housewife (Mrs.

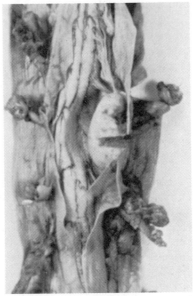

Figure 8–13 Gross appearance of meningioma compressing the ventrolateral aspect of thoracic spinal cord. (From Russell, D. S., and Rubinstein, L. J.: *Pathology of Tumors of the Nervous System,* 2nd Edition. Baltimore, Williams and Wilkins, 1963, p. 45.)

R.W.) presented with a 7-month history of throbbing midthoracic back pain which at times would radiate to the anterior chest and was aggravated by coughing or by straining at stool. Two months prior to admission, numbness of the right foot was noted which gradually spread up the leg so that within a 6-week period a level just below the breast anteriorly and just below the scapula posteriorly was involved. Six weeks prior to admission, a similar ascending numbness of the left foot developed. One month prior to admission, weakness of both lower extremities was noted, the right being weaker than the left. For 2 months, difficulty in urination had been present, primarily a problem in starting stream.

NEUROLOGICAL EXAMINATION:
1. *Mental status:* Intact.
2. *Cranial nerves:* Intact.
3. *Motor system:*
   a. Bilateral decrease in strength was present at hip, knees, and ankles.
   b. Gait was shuffling, possibly spastic.
4. *Reflexes:*
   a. Deep tendon reflexes were active in the upper extremities, possibly related to a significant degree of anxiety. The quadriceps reflexes were markedly hyperactive (4+).

b. Plantar response was markedly extensor on the left, borderline extensor on the right.
5. *Sensation:*
   a. Pain and temperature were decreased bilaterally below the xiphoid-sternum anteriorly and the T6 spinous process posteriorly. The degree of impairment was greater on the right than left side.
   b. Position sensation was absent at the left toes.
   c. Vibratory sensation was absent at the left toes and decreased at the left ankle and knee.
6. Vertebral location tenderness was present over the T3–T5 spinous processes.

LABORATORY DATA:

1. Thoracic spine x-ray was negative.
2. Thoracic myelogram revealed an intradural extramedullary lesion suggestive of a meningioma at the D4–D5 level.
3. Cerebrospinal fluid protein was increased to 57 mg./100 ml.

HOSPITAL COURSE:

On October 22, 1965 a thoracic laminectomy was performed by Dr. Robert Yuan and a meningioma removed at the D4–D5 level. Removal required section of one posterior root on the left.

The patient had a significant improvement in symptomatology. Follow-up examination in June 1966 indicated no significant motor or sensory deficits. Plantar responses were now flexor.

COMMENT:

The early symptoms in this case were, in general, nonspecific. Certain aspects of this complaint, however, raise the question of a more significant neurological problem. The aggravation of the pain by coughing or straining at stool and the radiation of pain to the anterior chest suggest a possible nerve root compression. It should be noted that in this case the classic radicular symptoms of a shooting, toothache like pain with radicular paresthesias were not present. There then developed, beginning two months prior to admission, the symptoms of a progressive cord compression with numbness that ascended to approximately the level of the midthoracic back pain. The information obtained on history, then, suggested a single compressive level lesion of the midthoracic spinal cord.

The findings on neurological examination suggested a modified Brown-Séquard syndrome. The Babinski sign, signifying pyramidal tract involvement, was clearly more marked on the left. The posterior column deficits in position and vibratory sensation were present in the left lower extremity. The deficits in pain and temperature, although bilateral, were clearly more marked on the right. The findings at surgery of a lesion situated more on the left than the right were consistent with these findings.

As regards the actual level of involvement, the upper level pain-temperature impairment was approximately the D6 dermatome. Since the pain fibers entering the lateral spinothalamic tract ascend for approximately 2 segments before decussating, the approximate level of compression could be assumed to be D4. The level, of course, is also provided by the finding of local tenderness over the T3, T4, and T5 spinous processes. Local pain on percussion over the spinous processes in the presence of spinal cord compression may indicate an epidural lesion or an intradural lesion in contact with the meninges. Such local tenderness is usually not found in intrinsic lesions.

Meningiomas compressing the spinal cord require early neurosurgical intervention to avoid progression to a chronic paraplegic state. When compression is promptly relieved, a significant improvement in neurological status may be expected.

Neurofibromas. These benign tumors arise from the Schwann cells of the nerve sheath. These tumors may arise in relation to peripheral nerves, cranial nerves, or nerve roots. Those which arise in relation to nerve roots may be located within the spinal canal, outside the spinal canal, or both within and outside (so called dumb-bell or hourglass-shaped tumors). The location will determine whether the symptoms are those of root compression or of both spinal cord and root compression.

The gross appearance of a neurofibroma is shown in Figure 8–14. The myelographic appearance is demonstrated in Figure 8–12C. The following case history illustrates the symptomatology and course of a solitary spinal cord neurofibroma.

Case History 7. NECH #196–618. Date of admission: 8/21/68.

This 15-year-old white female (Miss L.C.) was referred for evaluation of progressive weakness of the legs which had developed

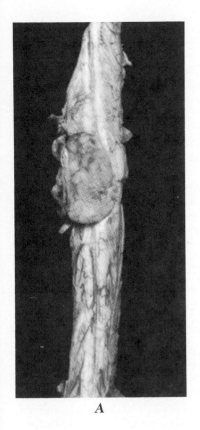

A

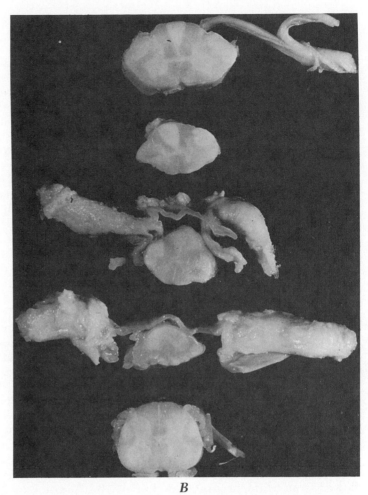

B

Figure 8–14 Neurofibromas. *A*, Neurofibroma compressing spinal cord. (From Kernohan, J. W., and Sayre, G. P.: *Tumors of the Central Nervous System.* Washington D.C., Armed Forces Institute of Pathology, 1952, p. 79.)
B, Multiple neurofibromas arising in relation to and producing marked enlargement of the nerve roots predominantly in the thoracic area. (Courtesy of Dr. Emanuel R. Ross.)

over a 2-week period. Approximately 2 years prior to admission, the patient had the onset of pain between the shoulder blades which radiated into the left arm extending to the middle fingers of the left hand. The pain would be acutely accentuated by coughing, sneezing, or laughing. At the same time, some smallness of the left upper extremity was first noted. The pain in the arm was in large part relieved by manipulation of the spine; the back pain, however, persisted.

Two weeks prior to admission, the patient had the painless onset of weakness of the left leg accompanied by some numbness of this leg. The weakness slowly progressed. On the day prior to admission, weakness and numbness of the right leg was noted. For several days prior to admission, a hesitancy

or difficulty in starting urinary stream had been noted.

PAST HISTORY. Otherwise not remarkable.

GENERAL PHYSICAL EXAMINATION: Not remarkable.

NEUROLOGICAL EXAMINATION:

1. *Mental status:* Normal.
2. *Cranial nerves:* Intact.
3. *Motor system:*
   a. Strength: A minimal degree of weakness was present in the left upper extremity at wrist dorsiflexion. Voluntary movement was markedly decreased in the lower extremities, being 10 per cent of normal on the left and 30 per cent of normal on the right.
   b. Resistance to passive motion: In-

creased at knee and ankle joints with clonus present at these joints bilaterally.

c. Gait: The patient was unable to walk without assistance.

4. *Reflexes:*

a. Deep tendon reflexes: The biceps and radial periosteal reflexes were decreased in the left upper extremity. The quadriceps (knee jerk) and Achilles tendon (ankle jerks) were markedly increased bilaterally, being 4+.

b. Superficial reflexes: Both plantar responses were extensor (bilateral Babinski signs). Abdominal reflexes were absent bilaterally.

5. *Sensory system:*

a. Pain sensation was decreased to the level of the T8 segment bilaterally.

b. There was a marked decrease in position and vibration sensation in the lower extremities, approximately 30 per cent of normal on the right and 10 per cent of normal on the left. There was an apparent vibratory level at the D8 spinous process.

c. Light touch was decreased to approximately the level of D8.

LABORATORY DATA:

1. *Myelogram* demonstrated a complete block at the level of the T1 vertebra. The dye flowed from below up to this level where the inferior margin of an intradural extramedullary lesion could be defined. The upper margin could not be defined.

2. *Complete blood count* was within normal limits.

HOSPITAL COURSE:

On August 21, 1968, following the myelogram, an emergency laminectomy C5–T2 was performed by Dr. Peter Carney. On palpation of the dura, a firm mass was palpated along the left lateral aspect of the spinal cord. On opening the dura, an encapsulated sausage-shaped, 2-inch-long, gray tumor was found in the subarachnoid space at this location, arising from and adherent to the dorsal root of left C6. Significant compression of the left C5 and C7 roots had occurred. Moreover, the tumor had compressed and produced deviation of the spinal cord to the right. Histological examination of the tumor confirmed the operative impression of neurofibroma (schwannoma). There was a hemorrhagic, cystic area in the center of the tumor.

Postoperatively the patient demonstrated a significant improvement. At the time of discharge, 1 month after surgery, a minimal weakness was still present in the left ankle dorsiflexor. The patient was able to walk but required a cane because of a certain degree of unsteadiness. A Babinski sign was still present on the left side with increased deep tendon reflexes bilaterally but more marked in the left lower extremity. Position sense was still defective at the left toes and foot and to a lesser degree at the right toe. Pain and touch were everywhere intact.

Examination, 2 months after surgery, indicated the continued presence of a broad-based gait; the patient had to look to see where she had placed her feet. As previously, increased deep tendon reflexes were present.

Follow-up evaluation at 5 months and at 1 year after surgery revealed no motor or sensory deficit in the lower extremities although deep tendon reflexes were hyperactive in the left lower extremity. Plantar responses were flexor. The patient had no actual disability and was able to dance well.

COMMENT:

The early symptoms in this case certainly indicated radicular pain in the left upper extremity, presumably in the C7 distribution. A diagnosis of a ruptured cervical disc was considered. Ruptured discs do occur in this age group although they are not common. The radicular symptoms then resolved, and when symptoms again appeared, these were the symptoms of spinal cord compression. There was evidence of bilateral disease of the corticospinal tracts, posterior columns, and lateral spinothalamic pathways. That the disease of the spinal cord was extrinsic was suggested by the rapid progression of bilateral long tract signs and by the previous history of radicular pain. As regards the level of the lesion, the pain level at T8 need not indicate the actual level of spinal cord involvement. Most likely, had operation been delayed, the pain, touch, and vibratory sensory levels would have ascended to higher levels, e.g., T1. The actual level of spinal cord involvement was suggested by the residual segmental findings of depression of deep tendon reflexes supplied by the left C5, C6, and C7 segments—the biceps and radial periosteal tendon reflexes. As regards an explanation for the relatively rapid process of spinal cord compression after a relatively quiescent period of 1 to 2 years, this may relate to the hemorrhage and necrosis within the tumor, with a relatively rapid increase in its mass and a significantly rapid rise in the degree of spinal cord compression. The myelographic findings in this case were consistent with the operative findings.

The prompt decompression of the cervical spinal cord with total removal of the extrinsic lesion was rewarded in this case by a significant recovery of function. The pattern of recovery followed the sequence suggested by the studies of Tarlov; the disability relevant to posterior column function was the slowest to recover. (The patient still had deficits in position sense and proprioception at a time when strength and pain sensation had returned to normal.)

Neurofibromatosis (von Recklinghausen's disease) is characterized by multiple neurofibromas, in addition to various anomalies of the skin and skeletal system. Occasionally, patients also manifest intrinsic glial tumors of the optic nerve, brain, or spinal cord.

INTRINSIC DISEASES OF THE SPINAL CORD

Intrinsic lesions of the spinal cord may be categorized according to the following outline.

A. Local intramedullary (semisegment) lesions (involving several adjacent segments)
1. Syringomyelia
2. Intrinsic tumors: (gliomas) astrocytomas and ependymomas
3. Vascular disease: anterior spinal artery occlusion

B. System disease (selective involvement of one or more fiber or cell systems)
1. Selective involvement of anterior horn cells
   a. Poliomyelitis
   b. Amyotrophic lateral sclerosis with predominant anterior horn cell involvement (progressive muscular atrophy)
   c. Werdnig-Hoffmann disease
2. Selective involvement of posterior root ganglion with secondary posterior column degeneration: tabes dorsalis
3. Posterior-lateral column sclerosis
   a. Combined systems disease of vitamin B12 deficiency
   b. Other causes
4. Selective lateral column disease
   a. As variant of amyotrophic lateral sclerosis: primary lateral sclerosis
   b. Familial spastic paraplegia

5. Spinal forms of spinocerebellar degeneration
   a. Friedreich's ataxia (posterior columns, corticospinal and spinocerebellar pathways)
   b. Familial spastic paraplegia
   c. Other variants

C. Multifocal disease
1. Multiple sclerosis
2. Postinfectious encephalomyelitis
3. Acute necrotizing myelopathy
4. Multifocal vascular diseases

This outline of intrinsic diseases of the spinal cord is not meant to be all inclusive. Congenital malformations are considered separately in Chapter 2. Several disease entities appear to be listed under more than one category. Not all human disease processes fit neatly into specific baskets. Thus the student will have noted that although we had indicated earlier in the introduction that intrinsic diseases were either local or system in type, we have now introduced a third category—multifocal. Multifocal diseases involve the nervous system at more than one level or site. In contrast to system diseases, they do not produce selective involvement of particular systems. Thus, in multiple sclerosis, multiple areas of demyelination are noted. In a given area of myelin loss, however, portions of several fiber systems may be involved without regard to their anatomical border. Thus one patch of demyelination might involve part of the dorsal spinocerebellar pathway and an adjacent sector of the lateral corticospinal pathway.

SPECIFIC INTRINSIC DISEASES OF THE SPINAL CORD

LOCALIZED INTRAMEDULLARY LESIONS INVOLVING SEVERAL ADJACENT SEGMENTS

Syringomyelia. This disease usually affects the cervical portion of the spinal cord. The basic pathology involves the formation of an irregular cavity (syrinx) in a central or paracentral location (Fig. 8–15). The cavity is surrounded by a border of gliosis (an area of proliferation of astrocytes with the production of glial fibers). The syrinx is not lined by ependyma. Although usually distinct from the central canal, the syrinx may extend into the ependymal lined canal.

As the cavity forms and enlarges, in a relatively central position, the initial damage involves those fibers crossing the midline in

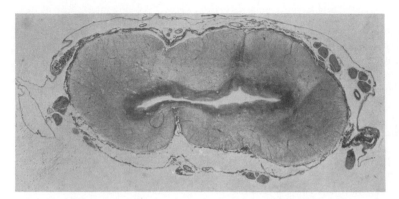

Figure 8–15 Syringomyelia. The large syrinx in this case has enlarged the diameter of the cervical spinal cord, destroying the anterior white commissure and the anterior horn. A dense border of gliosis is evident around the cavity. (Holzer stain for glia.) (Courtesy of Dr. E. Ross.)

the anterior white commissure. Thus the initial symptoms relate to a loss of pain and temperature sensation in the cervical and upper thoracic segments. The patient often reports painless burns and painless trauma to hands and arms. This relative selective damage to the pain and temperature fibers about to enter the lateral spinothalamic tracts results in what is termed a dissociated sensory loss. In the dermatomes affected at this stage of the disease, touch, position, and vibratory sensation are usually intact.

As the syrinx enlarges, the anterior horns are often affected, resulting in local atrophy, fasciculations, local flaccid paralysis of appropriate muscles of the upper extremity, and segmental loss of deep tendon reflexes. With continued expansion of the cavity, there occurs destruction or compression of adjacent posterior horns (with resultant segmental loss of sensation) and of posterior and lateral columns (with resultant long tract motor and sensory findings).

The basic etiology of this primary cavitation remains unknown. In some cases, there is an association with intramedullary tumors of the spinal cord; in other cases, with various congenital malformations involving central nervous system or adjacent bony structures. The cavity of syringomyelia often extends in an irregular manner into the medulla. There the disease process is labeled *syringobulbia.*

The progressively enlarging cyst of syringomyelia should be distinguished from the nonprogressive cavities, which may follow hemorrhages (hematomyelia) or infarcts involving the spinal cord, and from the nonprogressive simple dilatation of the central canal (hydromyelia). The following case history illustrates some of the findings in a patient with syringomyelia.

Case History 8. NECH #146–969. Date of admission: 2/18/62.

This 60-year-old white female (Miss D.R.) first noted numbness of all fingers of the right hand 2½ years prior to admission. Clumsiness of the right hand developed shortly thereafter with dropping of small objects and difficulty in writing. Defective appreciation of temperature with the right hand had been noted 1½ years prior to admission. Seven months prior to admission, a similar numbness of all fingers of the left hand had developed. At the same time, a stiffness of both lower extremities was noted accompanied by an unsteadiness on rapid turning.

Neurological Examination:

1. *Mental status:* Intact.
2. *Cranial nerves:* Intact.
3. *Motor system:*
   a. Fasciculations and a minor degree of atrophy were present in muscles about both shoulders (deltoids). No fasciculations were present in the lower extremities.
   b. Strength was decreased bilaterally as follows: shoulder abductors (60 to 70 per cent of normal); elbow flexors and extensors (80 per cent of normal). There was a marked weakness of intrinsic hand muscles (30 to 40 per cent of normal). The lower extremities were relatively intact (90 per cent of normal).
   c. Spasticity was noted on passive motion in all extremities with the left greater than the right.
   d. Gait was wide-based and spastic. The Romberg test was positive.
   e. Coordination of hand and finger movements with eyes closed was markedly defective.

4. *Reflexes:*
   a. Deep tendon reflexes of the upper and lower extremities were increased bilaterally (at biceps, triceps, quadriceps, Achilles) and were greater on the left than on the right.
   b. Superficial reflexes: Plantar responses were extensor bilaterally (sign of Babinski). Abdominal reflexes were absent.
5. *Sensation:*
   a. Pain and temperature were decreased C3–T2 bilaterally, with total loss in the right hand and lower arm (Fig. 8–16). In these segments touch sensation was intact.
   b. Touch was decreased below the knees bilaterally.
   c. Vibration sensation was absent below C3 bilaterally.
   d. Position sense was absent at fingers and wrists but present in lower extremities and in arms at shoulders.
6. *Vertebrae:* There was no local tenderness.

LABORATORY DATA:

1. Complete blood count was normal.
2. Cervical myelogram revealed widening of the entire cervical spinal cord, most markedly at the C3–C4 level. Partial obstruction to the flow of dye in the subarachnoid space, beginning at C5–C6, was noted. When compared to films of a myelogram per-

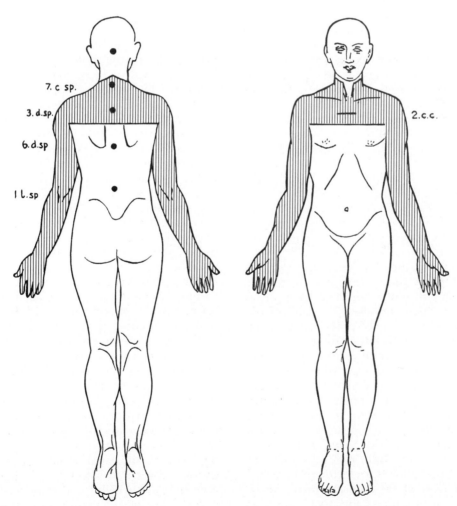

Figure 8–16 Syringomyelia from Case History #8. The cape-like distribution of pain and temperature deficit over the upper extremities is demonstrated. Marked hypalgesia was present in the hands and arms (total analgesia right hand) with a lesser defect over the shoulders.

formed two years previously, little change was noted, suggesting that a rapidly progressive lesion was not present.

HOSPITAL COURSE:

On February 26, 1962, a C2–C6 laminectomy was performed by Dr. Robert Yuan with section of the dentate ligaments. The spinal cord was found to be swollen from C5–C6 upwards to the limit of the surgical exposure (C1). A cystic cavity was evident on the right posterior aspect of the spinal cord. This was punctured and yielded a deep yellow fluid with a high protein content of 4.3 gram/100 ml. A 3 mm. incision was made to drain this cavity.

Immediately following surgery there was a transient increase in the extent of sensory deficit. However, by the time of hospital discharge on March 17, 1962, the patient reported less numbness in her hands, and examination revealed that strength in her hands had improved. Coordination and position sense in the hands had improved and the gait was less ataxic. The patient was able to walk without assistance. Babinski signs were now absent bilaterally. The deficits in pain and temperature in the C3 – T2 area were relatively unchanged with total loss of pain sensation in the right hand and lower arm.

The patient's condition remained relatively unchanged until the sudden development of a total paraplegia following an accidental fall in 1964. No improvement occurred and she expired in 1965.

COMMENT:

The usual textbook patient with syringomyelia presents with a cape-like dissociated loss of pain and temperature and atrophy of the intrinsic hand muscles. The clinical picture presented in this case deviates to a certain extent from this classic stereotype. This variation reflects several factors. The cavity in syringomyelia varies in its shape from one patient to the next (as demonstrated in Fig. 8–15). In some patients a symmetrical central cavity is present. In some, an asymmetrical paracentral cavity is present. In some the cavity extends into the anterior horns; in others, it extends into the posterior columns and posterior horns with relative lack of involvement of the anterior horns. Moreover, in a given patient, the cavity may vary in its shape in a rostral caudal extent, with irregular wedges extending into the anterior horn or posterior column at one level but not present at an adjacent level.

The clinical state in syringomyelia moreover is not static. Had this patient been examined at the onset of symptoms 2½ years prior to her hospitalization, the sensory findings might have been limited to a dissociated sensory loss. The present case might not have shown even this, since the symptoms of clumsiness of the hand suggests a position sense deficit in the hand at that time. The improvement in hand coordination following surgery does suggest a compressive rather than a direct destructive effect as regards the posterior columns.

The central consideration for syringomyelia in terms of an anatomical syndrome is the segmental loss of pain and temperature sensation in the upper extremities, out of proportion to any deficits in light touch involving the upper extremities.

In this particular case, we may presume, based on the clinical findings and on the findings at surgery, that the syrinx in addition to destroying the anterior white commissure involved primarily the posterior columns. The anterior horns at the C4 and C5 levels may have been involved to a minor degree to produce the fasciculations in the deltoid muscles. However, the lack of significant atrophy in the upper extremities and the preservation of hyperactive deep tendon reflexes at the biceps and triceps would argue against any significant destruction of the anterior horns at C5, C6, C7, and C8.

It should be noted also that the usual case of syringomyelia begins somewhat earlier in life, at age 20, 30, and 40. Onset at age 57 is less common but not rare.

Surgery in syringomyelia has several aims. Confirmation of the diagnosis is allowed. The syringomyelia syndrome could be a result of other lesions in relation to the central canal, e.g., a glioma. A patient with a glioma might demonstrate considerable improvement in symptomatology following radiation therapy. Little benefit follows x-ray therapy in syringomyelia. Moreover surgery does serve to provide a decompressive laminectomy, allowing greater room for expansion of the cervical cord without compression against the bony canal. Finally, surgery in occasional cases may allow for drainage of an accessible cyst which has distended the spinal cord. The present example does suggest that using this procedure in selected cases may possibly result in a degree of clinical improvement.

Intrinsic Tumors. Intrinsic tumors affecting the spinal cord with rare exceptions belong to the glial series. More particularly, these tumors are either astrocytomas or ependymomas. Astrocytomas are derived from the astrocytic series; ependymomas are from the type of ependymal cells found lining the central canal. Astrocytomas occur primarily in the cervicothoracic area. Ependymomas, in contrast, arise primarily at the lower end of the spinal cord—the conus medullaris. Both types of intrinsic tumor are relatively rare compared to intrinsic tumors of the cerebral hemispheres and extrinsic tumors involving the spinal cord.

Ependymomas are often relatively localized and are to some extent discrete from the surrounding neural tissue.

Astrocytomas, on the other hand, tend to infiltrate the surrounding tissue without any particular limiting border. Many adjacent segments may thus be involved by the tumor. Grossly, the spinal cord is increased in diam-

eter (Fig. 8–17). This is reflected in plain films of the spine where an increase in the distance between pedicles may be seen over several segments. This increase in diameter or width of the spinal cord is also reflected in the typical myelographic appearance (Fig. 8–12A). From a histological standpoint, the spinal cord astrocytoma is usually of a uniform appearance with a relatively moderate grade of malignancy. This is usually reflected in the clinical course which extends over a period of several years. This is in contrast to the astrocytoma infiltrating the cerebral hemispheres.

Case History 9. NECH #144–578. Date of admission: 10/20/61.

This 21-year-old, single, white female (Miss J. D.) was admitted to the hospital because of progressive difficulty in walking. In January 1958, the patient first noted a relatively rapid onset of weakness in the left

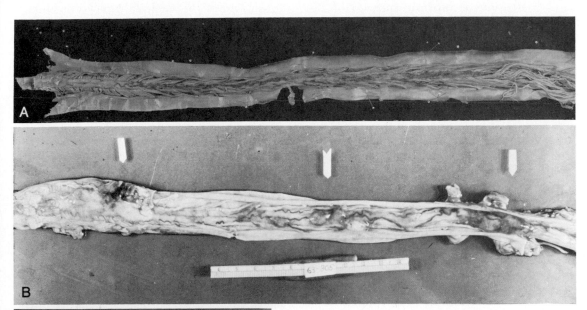

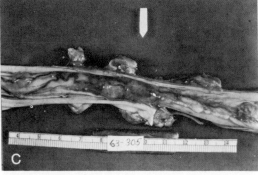

Figure 8–17 Glioma of the Spinal Cord. *A,* Normal spinal cord for comparison of diameter and relationship to dural coverings. *B,* In this case a highly malignant glioma has arisen at multiple foci, producing several areas of marked enlargement of the substance of the spinal cord, most marked in cervical area, but also evident in thoracic and lumbar areas. *C,* Enlargement of lower thoracic—upper lumbar area of the pathological specimen. (Courtesy of Dr. Emanuel R. Ross.)

hand, and in April 1958, she noted a throbbing pain in the neck that radiated into the left arm and left hand and was accompanied by some numbness (paresthesias) of the fingers of the left hand. Weakness of the left upper extremity slowly progressed and was accompanied by atrophy. In June 1961, a more rapid progression of left arm symptoms was noted and weakness of both lower extremities began, initially on the left and to a greater extent there than the right. In October 1961 weakness of the right upper extremity was noted. Bladder symptoms had not been present.

NEUROLOGICAL EXAMINATION:

1. *Mental status:* Intact.
2. *Cranial nerves:* Intact.
3. *Motor system:*
   a. Severe atrophy of all muscles of the left upper extremity was present with flexion (claw-hand deformity) contracture. Fasciculations were present in almost all of the left upper extremity muscle groups. Mild atrophy of intrinsic muscles of the *right hand* also was noted.
   b. There was weakness of the muscles of the *left upper extremity,* most marked distally but also involving the shoulder girdle, with a lesser weakness of the muscles of the *right upper* extremity. Both lower extremities were weak, the left more so than the right.
   c. Spasticity was present bilaterally on passive movement at the knees and ankles.
4. *Reflexes:*
   a. Deep tendon reflexes were depressed in the left upper extremity. The biceps was absent; the triceps and radial periosteal were hypoactive (1+). In the right upper extremity the biceps was depressed (1+), whereas the triceps was 2+. In the lower extremities, the quadriceps and Achilles were hyperactive to a marked degree (4+).
   b. Superficial reflexes: Plantar responses were extensor bilaterally. Abdominal reflexes were absent.
5. *Sensation:*
   a. Pain and temperature were intact.
   b. There was a slight distal decrease in vibratory sensation at the toes.
6. *Cranium and vertebral:* No local tenderness or abnormalities were present.

LABORATORY DATA:

1. Cervical spine x-rays showed bony changes. Widening of the spinal canal in anteroposterior and lateral diameters was noted.
2. Thoracic spine x-rays showed that kyphoscoliosis (curvature) was present.
3. Cerebrospinal fluid protein was increased to 150 mg./100 ml.
4. Myelogram revealed an extensive intramedullary lesion extending throughout the cervical region and into the thoracic region down to the level of D10. The widest point was at C7 where the spinal cord measured 40 mm. The maximum width of the spinal cord at this level is usually less than 20 mm.
5. Complete blood count and sedimentation rate were normal.

HOSPITAL COURSE:

Cervicothoracic laminectomy (C1–T7) was performed on November 1, 1961 and on November 21, 1961 by Dr. Samuel Brendler. A diffuse widening of the cervical and thoracic spinal cord was noted, most markedly in the cervical area extending on up to the lower end of the medulla. No cyst or hemorrhage was present. Despite an extensive laminectomy and postoperative x-ray therapy (3300 roentgens), steady progression of neurological symptoms occurred until death on April 26, 1962.

COMMENT:

This patient presents a 3½-year history which suggested severe involvement of the anterior horn cells or anterior roots over a wide area on the left side of the spinal cord. The occurrence of neck pain early in the course of the disease and of paresthesias in the fingers of the left hand shortly after onset of symptoms meant that the process was not simply limited to the anterior horn cells. Thus, a system-type disease of the anterior horn cell, such as amyotrophic lateral sclerosis or poliomyelitis, could be excluded. The latter diagnosis would in any case be unlikely in view of the progressive nature of the weakness and atrophy.

With progression of symptomatology, evidence of spinal cord involvement emerged. In considering this problem from the standpoint of differential diagnosis, one would certainly wish to exclude remediable extrinsic disease. There are, however, several points which would make extrinsic disease unlikely. A young lady of age 18 would be an unlikely candidate for extensive cervical spondylosis; although, of course, rupture of a disc could occur at this age in relation to trauma. A single disc protrusion would, however, be unlikely to produce widespread atrophy of the entire upper extremity. The 3½-year history and the absence of systemic disease would make unlikely the possibility of an epidural compressive lesion secondary to metastatic carcinoma or regional spread of lymphoma. An intradural lesion such as a neurofibroma or meningioma would be unlikely to selectively involve the extensive number of anterior roots C4–C8 on the left side of the spinal cord prior to producing spinal cord compression. If one postulated that such an extensive extrinsic intradural lesion existed in this case one would have expected some amount of posterior column symptomatology. Moreover, such a large mass, extrinsic to the spinal cord in a lateral location, would have been expected to produce a more classic spinal cord compression picture, e.g., a Brown-Séquard hemisection syndrome or a transection-type syndrome. Instead, the long tract findings were limited to the corticospinal pathways. One would also have to explain how this extrinsic compressive syndrome was also producing involvement of the anterior horn cells or anterior roots supplying the opposite upper extremity.

At this age, then, an intrinsic lesion of the cervical spinal cord is the most likely diagnostic possibility. The student must then note that in differential diagnosis, the age of the patient is an important factor to be considered. In a man of 50 or 60, with a long history of multiple trauma to the neck, a similar clinical picture could possibly be seen resulting from multiple bony spurs narrowing the neural foramina and also producing spinal cord compression.

In this case, however, the age of the patient and x-rays of the cervical spine showing an increase in size of the bony canal all suggested intrinsic local disease. Since pain and temperature sensation in the upper extremities was intact, indicating that the anterior white commissure was not involved (at a time when bilateral anterior horn cell involvement was present), the diagnosis of syringomyelia is unlikely. An infiltrating glioma remains the most likely possibility.

The basic therapy in these cases is to provide additional room for the expanding spinal cord by means of an extensive laminectomy. This reduces the direct compressive effects and the indirect vascular compression effect which an expanding spinal cord would encounter against the bony walls of the spinal canal. Drainage of a large cystic area within the tumor may produce improvement since the compressive effects of an expanding cyst are then reduced. Some cases present an association of glioma and syringomyelia. Radiation therapy is usually employed with a significant temporary reduction in neurological disability in some patients.

Focal Vascular Disease. Primary vascular syndromes of the spinal cord are not common although a secondary vascular component may be present in many compression syndromes involving the spinal cord, e.g., in cervical spondylosis, epidural carcinoma, epidural lymphoma, and epidural abscess. Processes such as tuberculous meningitis or meningovascular syphilis often produce an inflammation of blood vessel walls with secondary occlusion of these blood vessels.

An understanding of the clinical syndrome found in primary vascular disease of the spinal cord is dependent on a knowledge of the anatomy of the arterial blood supply and of the underlying pathology.

The major artery of the spinal cord is the *anterior spinal artery,* located in a midline position at the entry to the anterior median fissure. This single midline vessel has a bilateral origin from the intracranial portion of each vertebral artery. The arterial flow, as this vessel descends, is dependent on additional supply from the radicular arteries. These radicular arteries pass through the intervertebral foramina, and are derived from the cervical portion of the vertebral artery and the inferior thyroid artery and from the aorta as the intercostal, lumbar, and sacral arteries. Most of the radicular arteries do not contribute a significant supply. The critical sources are the radicular arteries to segments C6, T10, and L2. Border zones of blood supply, then, in a rostral caudal extent would be areas located between these segments of major supply. The actual border zones of circulation have been found to be segments T4 and L1. When the transverse anatomy is considered the anterior spinal artery is found to supply the anterior and lateral columns and almost all of the gray matter except the posterior horns. The posterior horns and the posterior columns are supplied by the *posterior spinal arteries,* paired vessels each derived from the intracranial segment of the vertebral artery. These posterior spinal arteries also receive contributions from the posterior branches of the radicular arteries. Moreover, at each level, coronal arteries at the periphery of the spinal cord interconnect the anterior spinal artery and the posterior spinal arteries. These anastomotic vessels at the periphery of the spinal cord also serve to interconnect the blood supply of adjacent segments.

Since the largest area of the spinal cord is supplied by a single anterior spinal artery (whereas there are two posterior spinal arteries which, in total, supply a much smaller area of the spinal cord), it is evident that most vascular disease involving the spinal cord is manifested as the *syndrome of the anterior spinal artery.* This syndrome involves infarction (destruction of tissue resulting from a lack of blood supply) of the territory supplied by the anterior spinal artery (Fig. 8–18). The resultant softening of the tissue is termed myelomalacia. (The process of infarction is discussed in greater detail in Chapter 22.)

In contrast to the cerebral blood vessels, occlusion of the spinal arteries due to deposits of atheromatous material (cholesterol, and so forth) is rare. The cause of the anterior spinal artery syndrome will usually be found in relation to diseases of the aorta or in relation to surgical procedures involving the heart, aorta, or related vessels. Thus, clamping of the upper aorta in relation to surgical treatment of aneurysm (dilated, weakened wall) of the aorta may result in a decreased blood flow in the critical intercostal branches supplying the spinal cord. A dissecting aneurysm of the aorta (a tear within the wall with blood under high pressure dissecting down the media of the wall) often results in the occlusion of intercostal and other vessels arising from the aorta. Arteries arising from the arch of the aorta, such as vertebrals, carotids, and renals, may also be occluded. In other instances the occlusion of intercostal branches, particularly T10, may occur during surgical procedures on the kidney or lumbar sympathetic ganglia.

The resultant neurological syndrome is usually acute in onset, manifested by the flaccid paraplegia of spinal shock and a bilateral deficit in pain and temperature below the level of lesion, with a preservation of position and vibratory sensation. With recovery from spinal shock, a spastic paraplegia may evolve if the anterior horns supplying the lower extremities have not been infarcted. As we have indicated, the anterior

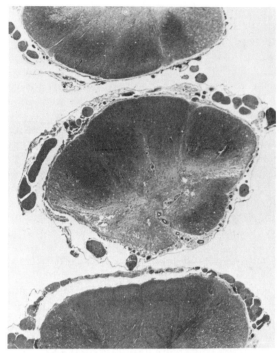

Figure 8–18 Infarction of spinal cord in distribution of anterior spinal artery secondary to occlusion of radicular artery at T6. This 71-year-old man had the acute onset of a flaccid paraplegia with absence of deep tendon reflexes and a sensory level at T7–T8. The patient expired shortly thereafter of a urinary tract infection. In this myelin-stained section relative preservation of posterior columns in contrast to anterior columns, lateral columns, anterior horns, and central canal area is evident. (Courtesy of Dr. Jose Segarra, Boston Veterans Administration Hospital.)

horns are supplied by the anterior spinal artery so that if the anterior lumbar sacral segments are involved, recovery of deep tendon reflexes may never occur. Instead, atrophy and a continued flaccid paralysis will be found in the lower extremities. The prognosis for a significant degree of recovery is usually poor.

In distinguishing other acute processes producing paraplegia, the rapidity of onset and the anatomical pattern of involvement seen in occlusion of the anterior spinal artery should be considered. Other processes, such as trauma or hemorrhage into the spinal cord (hematomyelia) from rupture of a malformed blood vessel, may produce an acute syndrome, but the history or cerebrospinal fluid findings or the anatomical distribution will be distinguishing factors. Epidural compressive lesions, such as acute epidural abscess, epidural carcinoma, or lymphoma, will often produce a relatively acute onset of symptoms. The history or anatomical pattern of symptoms will be the distinguishing features. The student, however, should recall that epidural lesions of this type often have a secondary vascular component. When a history of prior surgical procedure or of aortic aneurysm is absent, myelography may be performed to rule out a treatable compressive epidural lesion. Multiple sclerosis also may produce a relatively acute onset of symptoms, but the anatomical pattern will differ and lesions will usually be present elsewhere in the nervous system.

SYSTEM DISEASES OF THE SPINAL CORD

These are diseases in which there is a relatively selective involvement of particular fiber systems or cell groups. At times, several related cell or fiber systems are involved. The term, relative, is included because from a strict standpoint there is often minor involvement of other cell groups or fiber systems. System diseases are not of a uniform etiology. Nutritional deficiencies (e.g., vitamin B12), infections (e.g., poliomyelitis and syphilis), and degenerative diseases are found in this category.

DISEASES OF THE ANTERIOR HORN CELL

Acute Anterior Poliomyelitis. This disease is caused by a filtrable virus which invades the central nervous system. The virus spreads from the gastrointestinal tract by means of a viremia or by the axis cylinders of autonomic nerve fibers. On invading the central nervous system, the virus involves preferentially the large motor neurons of the spinal cord and brain stem, resulting in damage, degeneration, or death of these nerves and inflammatory changes in the surrounding tissue (Fig. 8–19). Neurons in the posterior horns and elsewhere in the central

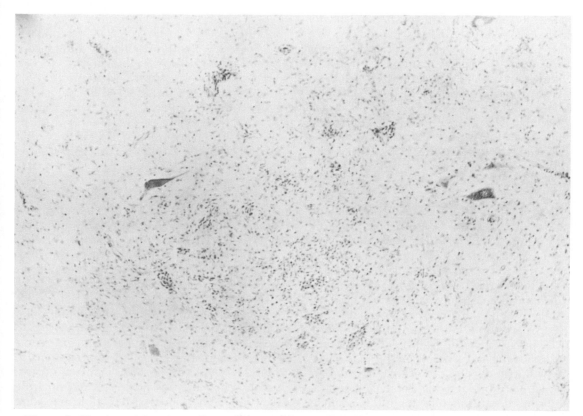

Figure 8–19 Acute anterior poliomyelitis. In this cresyl violet stain of the lumbar spinal cord, a loss of large motor neurons has occurred in the anterior horn. Many clusters of mononuclear cells are present, often apparently located so as to outline the former location of motor neurons. (×100) (Courtesy of Dr. Jose Segarra, Boston Veterans Administration Hospital.)

nervous system are, to a lesser degree, often involved in the acute stage. (The histological features are discussed in greater detail in Chapter 22, p. 588.)

The correlated clinical phenomena consist of a prodromal period of fever, malaise, headache, and gastrointestinal and upper respiratory symptoms, followed by a stage of meningeal irritation, and then the development of a flaccid paralysis. This involves, in an irregular manner, many of the muscles of the extremities and trunk (spinal form) or the muscles supplied by the bulbar nuclei (bulbar form): facial, palatal, and pharyngeal. Respiratory paralysis with the danger of death may occur in severe cases from the involvement of the motor nuclei of the diaphragm and intercostal muscles or from damage to the respiratory centers in the medulla.

The majority of patients with poliomyelitis virus infection make a complete or significant recovery. (A certain proportion may actually be labeled as nonparalytic cases in the sense that significant paralysis fails to develop even in the acute stage.) An estimated 20 to 30 per cent of all cases have a significant residual deficit or disability. We may presume, however, that many neurons invaded by the virus manifest a transient dysfunction but are not destroyed.

With the development of the Salk and Sabin vaccines, infections with the poliomyelitis virus are now rare in the United States. The following case history illustrates the course of the infection in a nonvaccinated adult.

Case History 10. NECH #195–143 and # 73–92–69. Date of admission: 6/14/68.

This 54-year-old, white housewife (Mrs. G.H.) developed a poorly defined illness characterized by malaise, nausea, loss of appetite, headache, and fever, on June 4, 1968. Approximately 5 days later she noted an aching sensation in her right leg and then rapidly developed a weakness and subsequent paralysis of the right lower extremity. The following day the left leg became weak. She was unable to get out of bed, to stand, or to walk. No numbness was present; there was no localized or radicular pain. The patient had difficulty voiding. She had to compress her abdomen in order to void. A fever of 101° was noted. No sensory symptoms had been

present. The patient had never received polio immunizations. She was admitted to the Goddard Memorial Hospital.

NEUROLOGICAL EXAMINATION:

1. *Mental status:* Intact.
2. *Cranial nerves:* Intact.
3. *Motor system:*
   a. Strength: The right biceps showed slight weakness (80 per cent normal strength). The right triceps showed more marked weakness (20 per cent normal strength). Hand muscles were, however, strong. In the lower extremities, there was a virtual total paralysis of the right leg except that the patient was able to wiggle the toes slightly on the right. There was a marked weakness of the left lower extremity. The patient was unable to lift the left leg off the bed and had marked weakness of the proximal thigh muscles. However, the dorsiflexors of the foot and toe and the invertors and evertors of the left foot contracted strongly.
   b. Fasciculations were present in the thigh muscles bilaterally.
4. *Reflexes:*
   a. Deep tendon reflexes: The biceps and radial were normal (2+). The triceps was absent on the right, normal (2+) on the left. The quadriceps and Achilles reflexes were absent bilaterally.
   b. Plantar responses: The left plantar response was flexor; the right showed no response.
5. *Sensation:* Pain, position, temperature, vibration, touch all were intact.
6. *Neck:* The patient had slight pain on forward flexion of the neck. She was unable to put her chin down onto her chest because of the pain. There was, however, no local tenderness on palpation over the spinous processes of the vertebrae.

LABORATORY DATA:

1. Cerebrospinal fluid examination indicated an increased number of white blood cells, 9 lymphocytes, and 6 polys per cubic mm. Cerebrospinal protein was elevated to 85 mg./100 ml.; spinal fluid sugar was normal at 60. When this test was repeated on June 10, 1968, 26 lymphocytes per cubic mm. were present.

2. The serum serological test for syphilis was negative.

HOSPITAL COURSE:

The patient was transferred to the Infectious Disease Service of the New England Center Hospital on June 14, 1968 where polio virus type 1 was isolated from the stool. A rise in antibody titer to polio virus was apparent when samples of acute and convalescent serum were compared.

The severe muscle cramps of which the patient complained at the time of admission were relieved by warm wet packs. Over a period of several days following admission, the right triceps deep tendon reflex returned, and within several days, strength in the right upper extremity had returned to normal. After several additional weeks some return of strength occurred in the left leg, in terms of knee flexion. The right lower extremity remained virtually unchanged despite intensive physiotherapy, at the time of hospital discharge on September 27, 1968. Because no additional improvement was occurring in the function of the lower extremity the patient was fitted with long leg braces and crutches with which, at the time of discharge, she was able to ambulate and to accomplish the activities of daily living.

COMMENT:

Acute anterior poliomyelitis was formerly a disease primarily of children and young adults, since this was the population with the lowest previous exposure and therefore the lowest level of immunity. Occasional cases did occur in middle-aged or older adults (one of the most notable being that of Franklin D. Roosevelt). With the development of immunization to the common strains of the virus, there has been a marked decrease in frequency of the disease. The few cases that occur are primarily in nonimmunized individuals, often older adults.

From the neurological standpoint, the neurological findings were restricted to a lower motor neuron syndrome, manifested by flaccid weakness, a loss of deep tendon reflexes, and fasciculations. Fasciculations represent apparent spontaneous contractions of motor units, the group of muscle fibers supplied by a single anterior horn cell. Although occasional fasciculations may occur in many normal individuals, the frequent occurrence of fasciculations usually represents the dysfunction of a diseased anterior horn cell. At times the basic pathological process is actually present in the anterior root or the proximal peripheral nerve. Although actual atrophy was not noted in the immediate protocol of the present case, it is not unusual to find, when these patients are examined in later years, a significant degree of atrophy in the muscles affected by a flaccid paralysis.

The spinal fluid findings in this case were typical of a mild aseptic meningitis (i.e., a nonbacterial meningitis.) This variety of spinal fluid abnormality is often found in a viral infection of the central nervous system.

There is uncertainty as to the reason for the painful muscle cramps and muscle tenderness often seen early in the course of the paralysis. These symptoms have been explained in terms of involvement of the posterior horn interneurons; such involvement of the posterior horn neurons is noted in acute cases which come to autopsy. Involvement of gamma motor neurons might as easily be implicated in the etiology of this symptom. In closing this section, we should again emphasize that the major impact of this disease is, however, on large motor neurons.

Amyotrophic Lateral Sclerosis (Motor System Disease), Progressive Muscular Atrophy Variety: Amyotrophic lateral sclerosis is a degenerative disease of unknown etiology which occurs predominantly in the age group 40 to 60. From an anatomical standpoint there are essentially three aspects of the disease process: (1) degeneration and loss of the motor neurons in the anterior horn cells of spinal cord, (2) degeneration and loss of the motor neurons of the cranial nerves in the brain stem, and (3) degeneration of the corticospinal and corticobulbar tracts, in large part secondary to degeneration and loss of their large and giant pyramidal cells of origin in the motor cortex (Figs. 8–20 and 8–21). It is possible then to distinguish relatively pure examples or combinations of three clinical syndromes. Almost all cases will demonstrate some involvement in all three areas as the disease progresses. A predominance of anterior horn cell disease is perhaps the most common syndrome. This is termed progressive muscular atrophy because the predominant symptoms are widespread muscular atrophy, flaccid weakness, fasciculations, and loss of deep tendon reflexes. The following case history illustrates the visual findings and course of this syndrome.

Case History 11. Date of consultation: 6/19/68.

This 66-year-old, white, married merchant

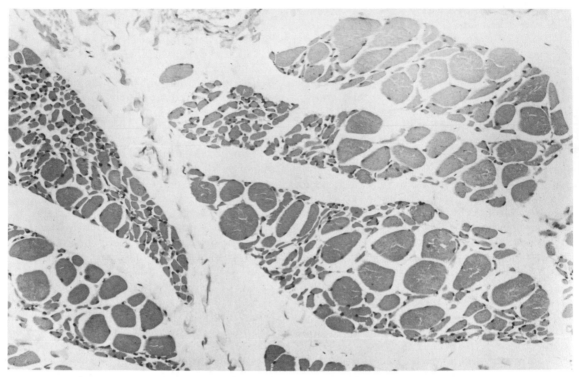

Figure 8–20 Amyotrophic Lateral Sclerosis. Loss of alpha motor neurons in the anterior horn has resulted in a grouped atrophy of muscle fibers within the supply of a motor unit (the clusters of small shrunken fibers). The clusters of large muscle fibers are motor units which are still relatively unaffected by the disease (H & E ×10). (Courtesy of Dr. Emanuel R. Ross.)

(Mr. J.R.) was referred for evaluation of progressive weakness and atrophy of both lower extremities. This had begun in an insidious manner 9 months previously. The upper extremities were shortly involved by atrophy and weakness to a lesser degree. Three months prior to admission the patient had an onset of thickness of speech, a difficulty in swallowing solids, and a less marked difficulty in swallowing liquids. No actual nasal regurgitation had resulted. During this 3-month period, a stiffness in both legs had been noted. There had been no sensory symptoms and no alteration in mental status.

A weight loss of 30 pounds had occurred during this period. There had, however, been no relevant pulmonary or gastrointestinal symptoms.

NEUROLOGICAL EXAMINATION:

1. *Mental status:* No definite deficits were present.

2. *Cranial nerves:*
   a. The jaw jerk was hyperactive (deep tendon reflex involving the fifth cranial nerve).
   b. There was a paucity of facial expression with a suggestion of a bilateral peripheral (or nuclear) paralysis of cranial nerve VII.
   c. Although a gag reflex was present, elevation of the uvula was poor.
   d. The voice was hoarse and speech was of low volume.
   e. Ridges of atrophy and fasciculations were present along the lateral borders of the tongue.

3. *Motor system:*
   a. Widespread muscular atrophy was present about the shoulders and in the intrinsic hand muscles and proximal leg muscles. The left leg showed greater atrophy than the right.
   b. Widespread fasciculations were noted, at rest, in all four extremities.
   c. A significant degree of weakness was present in all four extremities. Lower extremities were affected to a greater degree than upper, particularly the distal muscle groups. Strength was as follows: shoulder abductors, 60

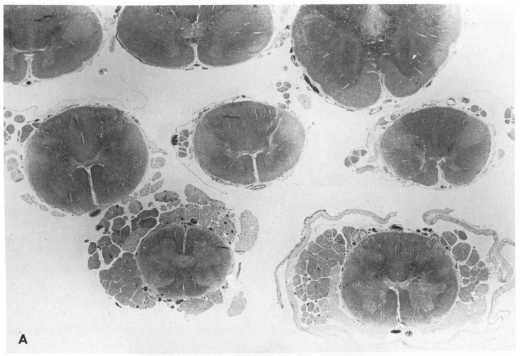

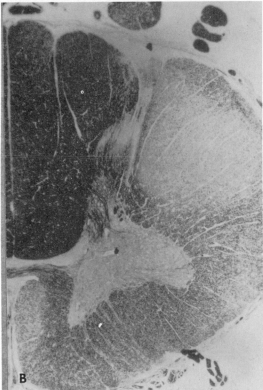

Figure 8–21 Amyotrophic Lateral Sclerosis. *A,* Degeneration of the corticospinal tracts is demonstrated in this myelin stain. Loss of myelin has occurred in medullary pyramids and in lateral columns as shown at various spinal cord levels. (Courtesy of Dr. Jose Segarra.)

B, Enlargement from another advanced case demonstrating marked involvement of lateral and anterior corticospinal pathways. (Courtesy of Dr. Emanuel R. Ross.)

per cent of normal; elbow flexors and extensors, 50 per cent of normal; wrist extensors, 70 per cent of normal; hand grip, 70 per cent of normal; finger abductors, 60 per cent of normal; long-thumb abductor 40 to 50 per cent of normal; opponens, 70 per cent of normal; hip flexors and extensors, 50 per cent of normal; knee flexors and extensors, 40 to 50 per cent of normal; ankle dorsiflexors and toe extensors, 30 per cent of normal on the right, 10 to 20 per cent of normal on the left.

d. The patient was able to arise from a chair and to walk a short distance without assistance.

e. Cerebellar tests were normal.

4. *Reflexes:*

a. The deep tendon reflexes of the biceps, triceps, and quadriceps were hyperactive at 3+. The right Achilles reflex was 2+, the left was decreased at 0–1+.

b. The plantar responses were both extensor (bilateral Babinski signs).

5. *Sensory system:* All modalities were intact.

LABORATORY DATA:

A complete evaluation had been undertaken by the patient's referring physician with the following findings:

a. Complete blood count and sedimentation rate were normal.

b. Chest x-rays had revealed cardiac enlargement to a minor degree which was unrelated to his neurological problem. The lungs were normal.

c. The pneumoencephalogram indicated a mild degree of enlargement of the lateral ventricles of the cerebral hemispheres.

d. Cerebrospinal fluid was normal as regards cells, protein (20 mg./100 ml.), sugar, and serological reaction.

e. Muscle biopsy (right quadriceps) revealed the changes seen in the various stages of denervation atrophy. The distribution of atrophy and fatty replacement was clearly in a motor unit pattern; that is, where a particular stage of degeneration occurred, all of the fibers of a motor unit showed that particular change.

SUBSEQUENT COURSE:

The patient experienced additional difficulty in swallowing. Information was subsequently received that the patient had expired approximately 3 months after the above evaluation.

COMMENT:

The history in this case suggested combined involvement of the anterior horn cells at the spinal cord level, brain stem motor function, and possible involvement of the corticospinal pathways (stiffness in legs). The examination confirmed the marked involvement of anterior horn cells (atrophy, weakness, and fasciculations). The loss of the left Achilles tendon reflex is consistent with the marked weakness and atrophy involving this extremity. (A certain degree of asymmetry may often be found as regards the involvement of the extremities.) In addition, there was definite evidence of involvement of the motor neurons of the brain stem (atrophy and fasciculations involving the tongue plus hoarseness and low volume of the voice, plus poor elevation of the uvula). The apparent bilateral facial weakness may have indicated bilateral involvement of the motor neurons supplying the facial musculature, or in view of the lack of atrophy and fasciculations involving these muscles, it may have indicated bilateral corticobulbar involvement. Such corticobulbar disease certainly was present in view of the hyperactive jaw jerk. The jaw jerk is a stretch reflex; hyperreflexia indicates a release of reflex function resulting from an upper motor neuron lesion.

The increased deep tendon reflexes and the bilateral extensor plantar responses indicated involvement of the corticospinal pathways in an upper motor neuron lesion. As we have noted, the decreased left Achilles tendon reflex indicated a greater prominence of anterior horn involvement affecting this extremity. The actual state of the deep tendon reflexes, then, will depend on the relative degree of involvement of the lower motor neuron and upper motor neuron. In cases where anterior horn cell involvement is marked, the patient may manifest relatively quiet deep tendon reflexes in the presence of a bilateral sign of Babinski.

As regards prognosis, the majority of patients die from the complications involving the bulbar motor neurons. The progressive difficulty in swallowing leads to a progressive weight loss and an inability to maintain oral nutrition. The involvement of pharyngeal musculature leads to aspiration of material into the trachea and bronchi with the subsequent development of pneumonia. In some patients respiratory failure is the result of progressive destruction of the anterior horn cells supplying the muscles involved in respiration: the diaphragm and intercostal and accessory muscles of respiration.

In general the prognosis for life is poorest for those patients whose illness begins with involvement of the bulbar motor neurons. In the series reported by Mackay (1963), the average duration of life for these patients after onset of symptoms is 17 months. Those cases beginning with involvement of the anterior horn cells of the spinal cord had an average duration of life of 33 months after onset of symptoms. The longest duration of life occurred in patients whose disease began with lateral column involvement (average of over 36 months after onset of symptoms).

Other Diseases Affecting Primarily the Anterior Horn Cells. *Werdnig-Hoffmann disease* (infantile muscular atrophy) is a relatively rare familial disease which begins in the first year of life and is characterized by progressive weakness and atrophy. The primary pathology involves degeneration of anterior horn cells.

Kugelberg-Welander disease (hereditary proximal neurogenic muscular atrophy) is a rare familial disease beginning in childhood or early adult life. The pathology is assumed to involve a very slowly progressive degeneration of anterior horn cells. The proximal limb muscles are primarily involved. The brain stem and lateral columns are not affected.

DISEASE OF THE POSTERIOR ROOT
WITH SUBSEQUENT ASCENDING
DEGENERATION OF POSTERIOR
COLUMNS (TABES DORSALIS)

Tabes dorsalis is a late complication of the venereal disease, syphilis. Syphilis involves a *primary* local infection (chancre) at the site of infection (skin or mucuous membrane). Within a matter of days to weeks, generalized dissemination of the infection occurs through invasion of the blood stream with a resultant generalized skin rash. At this stage or within an additional period of several weeks, invasion of the central nervous system may occur. Clinical evidence of this central nervous system invasion usually emerges only after many years. All of the later syndromes of syphilis are termed tertiary. The clinical syndromes of this central nervous system involvement (which occurs in approximately 30 per cent of all untreated cases of syphilis) are grouped together as neurosyphilis. Essentially four major clinical syndromes may be recognized: (1) asymptomatic (accounting for 31 per cent of cases) where examination of the cerebrospinal fluid indicates the presence of neurosyphilis but where clinical symptoms and signs are not yet evident; (2) meningeal and vascular involvement (accounting for 16 per cent of cases); (3) parenchymatous neurosyphilis involving the cerebral cortex (accounting for 12 per cent of cases), producing an alteration of psychological functions such as memory and personality in a process termed dementia paralytica or general paresis of the insane; and, (4) parenchymatous neurosyphilis involving the posterior root and posterior root ganglia, producing secondary degeneration of the posterior columns and a clinical syndrome termed *tabes dorsalis* (accounting for 30 per cent of all cases of neurosyphilis). Tabes dorsalis (prior to the penicillin-antibiotic era) occurred as a late complication of syphilis in 9 per cent of all cases. In general, males were predominantly affected. The latent period after infection was usually 10 to 25 years.

The symptoms and signs of tabes dorsalis relate to the primary involvement of the posterior root fibers.

1. The posterior roots are involved primarily at the level of the lumbar and sacral spinal cord. Degeneration of the long, heavily myelinated fibers entering the posterior columns occurs primarily in the fasciculus gracilis (Fig. 8–22) and results in a loss of conscious proprioception, such as joint position sense and of vibratory sensation in the lower extremities.

2. In addition, medium length fibers conveying nonconscious proprioceptive information, which will synapse in the nucleus dorsalis (Clarke's column) and which are eventually destined for the cerebellum, also degenerate in the posterior root. These fibers on their pathway to the cells of Clarke's column (or to the analogous lateral cuneate nucleus of the medulla) pass for a short distance upward in a portion of the fasciculus cuneatus adjacent to the posterior horn (Fig. 8–22). The loss of joint position sense

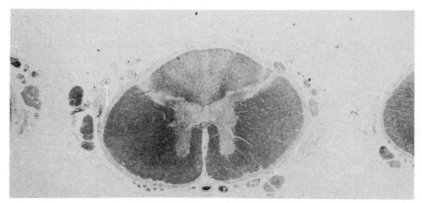

Figure 8-22 Tabes Dorsalis. Ascending degeneration of the posterior columns is demonstrated in this myelin stain of the spinal cord. This 67-year-old white male had multiple hospital admissions for tabes dorsalis, abdominal crises, luetic aortitis, and luetic optic neuritis. (Courtesy of Dr. Jose Segarra, Boston Veterans Administration Hospital.)

and of other proprioceptive information conveyed in the posterior columns, in addition to the loss of unconscious proprioceptive information destined for cerebellum, results in an *ataxia* (unsteadiness) of gait. (The name, locomotor ataxia, is sometimes applied to tabes dorsalis.)

There are several causes or types of ataxia. In this case, we may apply the term sensory ataxia because sensory information from the lower extremities fails to reach the cerebellum and cerebral cortex due to disease of the posterior roots. A similar ataxia would result from a peripheral neuropathy or from other disease processes involving the posterior columns. Other sensory cues (vision, for example) do reach the cerebellum and cerebral cortex.

Moreover, the cerebellum and cerebral cortex are intact. It is possible, then, to differentiate a sensory ataxia from other types of ataxia. Thus if a patient stands with feet together on a narrow base and is steady with his eyes open but is unsteady (sways or falls) when his eyes are closed (a positive *Romberg's sign*) we may conclude that a sensory ataxia is present. In contrast, a patient with disease of the cerebellum is as unsteady on a narrow base with eyes open as he is with eyes closed.

3. Loss of the heavily myelinated Ia fibers results in a third sign—*loss of stretch reflexes*. From a clinical standpoint, this is manifested by a loss of quadriceps and Achilles deep tendon reflexes.

4. Bladder dysfunction may also be present. Destruction of afferent fibers in the posterior root conveying information regarding stretch of the detrusor muscle of the bladder, secondary to distension, interferes with the reflex contraction of the detrusor muscle and subsequent emptying of the bladder. This reflex is integrated at the S2, S3, and S4 spinal cord segments. The result is an overdistended, flaccid bladder. This variety of bladder dysfunction is also referred to as *atonic neurogenic*. There are other possible causes of the atonic bladder: damage to the nerve roots of the cauda equina, which may interfere with the afferent or the efferent end of the reflex arc, or damage to the sacral segment of the spinal cord. When the afferent segments of the reflex arc are defective, as in tabes dorsalis, the patient may indicate a lack of desire to void despite the overdistension (500 to 2000 cc.) of the bladder. When the efferent segment of the reflex arc is defective, the patient may complain of a desire to void, but an inability to start the stream. In either case, overflow incontinence often occurs (the dribbling of urine from an overdistended bladder).

The atonic neurogenic bladder should be contrasted to the spastic neurogenic bladder. The spastic bladder reflects a release of spinal cord reflex activity from higher control; reflex emptying of the bladder will then occur in response to a minor degree of distension (50 to 100 ml. volume compared to a normal volume of 400 ml.). A spastic bladder usually indicates bilateral disease of the corticospinal pathways usually at a cervicothoracic spinal cord level.

5. Damage to the small diameter fibers

conveying pain sensation results in the characteristic *lightning pains,* i.e., fleeting sharp pains in the legs, and, occasionally, the back and face. At times, the viscera may be involved with the upper abdominal pain of the gastric crisis. On occasion, these latter episodes of pain may be accompanied by nausea and vomiting. With progression of pain fiber damage, actual zones of *decreased pain and touch sensation* may be found, e.g., over the cheeks, about the nipples, and on deep pressure over the Achilles tendon. The patient may also complain of paresthesias (numbness) of the extremities.

A small percentage of patients in the late stages of syphilis will develop changes in the joints (Charcot's joints), presumably as a result of defective sensation and subsequent trauma to the joints.

In addition to these clinical phenomena related to the posterior root, 90 per cent of patients with tabes dorsalis manifest abnormalities of the pupils. The classic findings in many cases is the Argyll Robertson pupil, usually bilateral but at times unilateral. In its fully developed form, an Argyll Robertson pupil is small (miotic) and irregular, fails to respond to light and fails to fully respond to sympathetic stimulation, but it does respond to accommodation-convergence. The basic site of pathology is not certain. The pretectal area or upper midbrain tegmentum has been suggested as a possible location, with the lesion so placed as to interrupt light reflex fibers passing to the third nerve nucleus and also interrupting sympathetic fibers passing down from the hypothalamus through the brain stem to the spinal cord.

As regards prognosis, tabes dorsalis may be prevented or its progression from an early stage avoided by treatment with adequate dosage of penicillin. Ataxia, lightning pain, and bladder disturbances, once present, are likely to continue despite treatment. The following case history illustrates the course of a case of tabes dorsalis.

Case History 12. NECH #110–666. Date of admission: February, 1957.

For 4 months prior to admission, this 49-year-old executive (Mr. L.J.B.) had noted lightning-like pains of the lower extremities with a girdle-like pain around the abdomen. He had also noted paresthesias of the soles of the feet and a tightening sensation of the entire body. In addition, there was a complaint of hypersensitivity of the skin of the abdomen and back.

PAST HISTORY: The patient had been treated 18 years previously (1939) with weekly buttock injections for 1 year because of "bad blood and loss of hair."

NEUROLOGICAL EXAMINATION:

1. *Mental status:* All areas were intact.

2. *Cranial nerves:* The right pupil was smaller than the left and failed to respond to light. Both pupils responded to accommodation.

3. *Motor system:* Strength was intact. There was no atrophy. Gait was intact.

4. *Reflexes:*
   a. Deep tendon reflexes were symmetrical and physiologic except for the Achilles tendon reflexes which were decreased bilaterally.
   b. Plantar responses were flexor.

5. *Sensory system:*
   a. Position sense was impaired in the toes bilaterally with a decrease in vibratory sensation.
   b. Deep pressure pain was absent on squeeze of Achilles tendon. Testicular pain was decreased on pressure.
   c. There was hyperesthesia to touch over the lower abdomen, the dorsal and lumbar spines, and the soles of the feet.

LABORATORY DATA:

1. Sixty lymphocytes and 2 polymorpholeukocytes were present in the spinal fluid.

2. Spinal fluid Hinton serological test for syphilis was positive. Blood serology for syphilis also was positive.

SUBSEQUENT COURSE:

The patient was treated with 15 million units of procaine penicillin. He improved except for hypersensitivity to tactile and thermal stimuli. The patient was readmitted in June 1957, for repeat spinal fluid examination: the Hinton serological reaction was still positive but the cell count was now normal. The patient was evaluated again in February 1958. He continued to complain of paresthesias about the trunk and about his ankles and the soles of his feet. Spinal fluid contained no significant cells but the serology of spinal fluid was positive. The patient continued to experience painful paresthesias of the abdominal wall and back when getting into the bath tub and rubbing himself with a towel. In addition, the patient continued to have short episodes (a few seconds duration) of dull, aching pain involving the heels or the thighs or the buttocks. Neurological examination in 1962 revealed that the right pupil failed to respond to light. The ankle jerks were still depressed as previously. Position and vibratory sensation of the toes was slightly impaired. There was still hyperalgesia to pin prick and touch over the soles of the feet, ankles, lower abdomen, and lower back. Serum Hinton continued to be positive. No significant cells were present in the spinal fluid, and spinal fluid protein was 15 mg./100 ml.

FOLLOW-UP EVALUATION IN MARCH 1969:

The patient continued to have lightning pain in the lower extremities with increasing frequency and intensity. He continued to complain of paresthesias, particularly when taking a bath. On neurological evaluation, pupillary findings were unchanged. Deep tendon reflexes were now symmetrical and physiologic. There was a decrease in vibratory sensation at the toes but position sense was intact. Serological examination was now normal.

COMMENT:

This patient presents a typical story for tabes dorsalis. Blood serology had been noted to be positive at least 18 years prior to the patient's onset of neurological symptoms ("bad blood"). The weekly injections at that time probably consisted of arsenicals and bismuth which were used with moderate effectiveness prior to the time of penicillin. His symptoms related primarily to paresthesias and lightning pains. Although evidence of posterior column disease was present, this had not yet progressed to any significant disability. A typical Argyll Robertson pupil was present on the right side. His spinal fluid findings were consistent with the diagnosis of tertiary lues. The cellular findings in the patient's spinal fluid improved with the use of penicillin although the serological reaction remained positive for some time after treatment, a not infrequent pattern. Posterior column findings improved and his subjective symptoms improved temporarily. It is not unusual for patients with tabes dorsalis to continue to experience shooting pains long after otherwise successful treatment. Thus, the alterations which occurred in the posterior root and posterior columns cannot be completely reversed. Of course, any progression of symptoms was clearly avoided in this patient. He never developed a significant degree of ataxia. We may also presume that any cardiovascular manifestation of tertiary lues also was prevented as a result of the treatment with penicillin. In addition to involvement of the central nervous system, patients in the tertiary stage of syphilis may have involvement of other organ systems. The wall of the thoracic aorta may develop a defect. This weakened wall may then balloon out in what is termed an aneurysm with the danger of subsequent rupture.

POSTERIOR LATERAL COLUMN SYNDROME

Subacute Combined Degeneration or Combined System Disease Due to Vitamin B12 Deficiency. The combination of posterior and lateral column degeneration may be seen in several disease states involving the spinal cord. Of these various causes, perhaps the most important characteristic syndrome is that of subacute combined degeneration secondary to vitamin B12 deficiency. The importance of this disease relates to the fact that a specific medical treatment exists which will prevent additional progression of the pathological process and which may reverse many of the early findings of the disease. If the disease is not recognized, progression is to be expected to a state of significant disability. This then is a nutritional, i.e., metabolic disease. The early symptoms may represent simply a dysfunction in nerve fibers; with persistence of the nutritional defect, permanent structural changes occur in nerve fiber.

The basic defect in most cases is a lack of intrinsic factor—an enzyme secreted by the parietal cells of the gastric mucosa and required for the absorption of vitamin B12 from the intestine. Usually atrophy of these cells results in the decreased secretion of intrinsic factor. In rare cases, the deficiency in absorption of vitamin B12 results from a gastrectomy or from an intestinal malabsorption syndrome. Vitamin B12 functions as a coenzyme with the formation of methionine and the nucleotide, thymidine. A deficiency of vitamin B12 results in a defect in synthesis of deoxyribonucleic acid (DNA) with a resultant failure of normal maturation of red blood cells. This is manifested in the megaloblastic anemia of pernicious anemia.

In approximately 30 to 70 per cent of patients with pernicious anemia, neurological symptoms occur related to posterior and lateral column disease. There is no one-to-one relationship between the severity of the anemia and the degree of neurological involvement. In actuality, a severe degree of neurological involvement may be present with little or no evidence of anemia. To some extent, then, the exact role of vitamin B12 in the nervous system remains unclear.

The basic pathological process involves a degeneration of white matter initially affecting myelin to a greater degree but eventually affecting axons as well. White matter in the spinal cord, cerebral hemispheres, and peripheral nerves are all affected in variable degree. In most cases, it is the spinal cord involvement which predominates.

The pathological process in its early stages is most prominent in the posterior columns; the patient complains of tingling paresthesias involving the toes and finger tips. An unsteadiness of gait is then noted. Examination at this time will show defects in joint position sense and vibratory sensation most severe in the lower extremities but also involving the finger tips. A positive Romberg sign will be

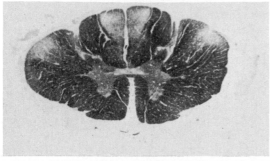

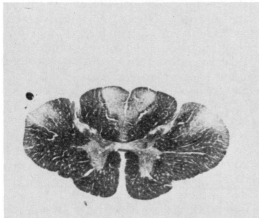

Figure 8–23 Combined Systems Disease. Degeneration of posterior and lateral columns is demonstrated in this myelin stain of cervical spinal cord. The degeneration in posterior columns is relatively restricted to fasciculus gracilis. (Courtesy of Dr. Emanuel R. Ross.)

See Filmstrip, Frame 14.

present and the gait slightly ataxic. If the disease is unrecognized and untreated, ataxia will become more severe and the signs of lateral column involvement will also appear: bilateral extensor plantar responses, a spastic weakness, and a spastic ataxic gait (Fig. 8–23). With additional progression in the disease, the basic pathological process may eventually affect other white matter systems of the spinal cord such as the spinothalamic and spinocerebellar pathways. The following case history provides an example of a patient evaluated and treated at an earlier point in the disease process.

Case History 13. NECH #76–89–66. Date of admission: 9/8/69.

This 65-year-old, white, married, male lathe operator (Mr. A.R.) was admitted to the hospital because of a 1-year history of difficulty in walking.

Following an uneventful cholecystectomy 1 year prior to admission, the patient first noticed a slowly progressive difficulty in walking, an unsteadiness rather than a weakness. There was an associated numbness (tingling pins and needles paresthesias) which began in the toes and gradually ascended to the level of the hips. Shortly after onset of the symptoms in the lower extremities, the patient also experienced tingling in all of the finger tips of the two hands. When driving an automobile, the patient had noted that he was unable to find the brake and gas pedal with his feet.

PAST HISTORY:

There was no history of diabetes and no evidence of excessive intake of alcohol. There had been no exposure to toxic substances. There was no family history of neurological disease.

GENERAL PHYSICAL EXAMINATION:

The patient was an alert, well-nourished although thin, white male.

NEUROLOGICAL EXAMINATION:

1. *Mental status:* Memory and orientation were intact. Serial 7 subtractions from 100 were poorly performed.

2. *Cranial nerves:* All areas were intact including pupillary responses.

3. *Motor system:*
    a. Strength was intact.
    b. Gait was broad-based and unsteady. The patient's degree of unsteadiness was markedly increased by eye closure. A positive Romberg test was present.

c. No spasticity was present.
4. *Reflexes:*
   a. Deep tendon reflexes were normal in the upper extremities (2+) but absent in the lower extremities at the quadriceps and Achilles tendon.
   b. Plantar responses were extensor bilaterally (bilateral Babinski signs).
5. *Sensory system:*
   a. Pain and temperature sensations were intact.
   b. Position sense decreased at the ankles and was absent at the toes.
   c. Vibration: There was a marked bilateral deficit in the lower extremities (absent from the hips down). There was a minor decrease at the fingertips as compared to the wrists.

LABORATORY DATA:

1. A minor degree of anemia was present. Hemoglobin was 12.6 grams, hematocrit was 38 per cent. The white blood count was normal at 8610 but many hypersegmented polymorphonuclears were present on blood smear, a finding often noted in pernicious anemia. Reticulocyte count was not increased (0.9 per cent).

2. Gastric analysis revealed no free acid even with histamine stimulation. The absence of free acid usually indicates that there is also a defect in the production of intrinsic factor, since both are produced by the parietal cells of the gastric mucosa.

3. The upper gastrointestinal series was normal. Cytology of the gastric aspirate was normal, revealing no malignant cells. (The incidence of carcinoma of the stomach is increased in pernicious anemia.)

4. Bone marrow showed megaloblastic changes consistent with a macrocytic type of anemia (e.g., pernicious anemia).

5. The Schilling test of radioactive B12 absorption indicated urinary excretion of 0.5 per cent of the oral dose. Normally 7 to 22 per cent of the oral dose should be excreted in the urine. The inability to absorb radioactive vitamin B12 reflects a defect in intrinsic factor. If B12 cannot be absorbed into the blood stream, it cannot be excreted in the urine.

6. The electroencephalogram was normal.

7. Cervical spine x-rays did not indicate significant pathology.

HOSPITAL COURSE:

Treatment with intramuscular injections of vitamin B12 was begun. The patient was instructed that it was necessary to continue to receive injections during the remainder of his life.

COMMENT:

This patient had definite symptoms suggesting a progressive and symmetrical involvement of the posterior columns, an ascending numbness beginning in the lower extremities and a sensory ataxia. Of course, an ascending numbness and sensory ataxia may also indicate progressive involvement of the peripheral nerve. In this case, however, examination clearly indicated selective involvement of those sensory modalities conveyed by the posterior columns. Moreover, the bilateral extensor plantar responses clearly indicated involvement of the lateral columns. The absence of deep tendon reflexes in the lower extremities is characteristic of combined systems disease. Several possible explanations may be considered: (1) a mild peripheral neuropathy is often present in vitamin B12 deficiency; (2) since the basic disease process begins in the posterior columns, essentially in Ia fiber, and since similar Ia fibers are passing through the posterior horn to the anterior horn as the afferent segment of the monosynaptic reflex arc, it would not be unusual for these fibers also to be involved by the basic metabolic lesion. Spasticity is usually absent in untreated cases, although the sign of Babinski is usually present. In severe terminal cases or in severe cases begun on treatment, a significant degree of spasticity may develop.

The essential metabolic lesion was documented in this case as a failure to absorb vitamin B12. In the present case, the involvement of the central nervous system was out of proportion to the involvement of the hematological system.

The purpose of parenteral treatment with vitamin B12 is to prevent additional neurological progression. A moderate improvement may also be noted. Thus in a metabolic disease some of the symptoms reflect functional alterations which have not yet progressed to structural alterations. Some reversal of these functional changes may be expected. In the present case, a severe degree of disability was not yet present. A significant improvement would be expected over the succeeding months.

Posterior Lateral Column Syndrome: Other Causes. Not all cases presenting with a syndrome of bilateral posterior-lateral column dysfunction will have a defect in vitamin B12 absorption. Other pathological processes may present a similar clinical pattern of involvement.

Compressive lesions anterior to the spinal cord, such as tumors, ruptured midline cervical discs, or midline osteophytes as in cervical spondylosis, may all result in this syndrome as discussed earlier in this chapter. Such cases are often asymmetrical in their involvement or may have evidence of nerve root involvement in addition to spinal cord involvement.

Multiple sclerosis may present, among other areas of myelin destruction, a large area involving the posterior and lateral columns at the level of the spinal cord. Such cases are often asymmetrical as regards the pattern of involvement. Multifocal lesions are often present elsewhere in the nervous system. Moreover, the history usually fails to follow the sequence noted for combined systems disease—progressive involvement of the posterior colums, followed by lateral column involvement. In addition, it is rare for deep tendon reflexes to be absent in multiple sclerosis, whereas it is usually the rule in combined systems disease.

Friedreich's ataxia is a progressive degenerative disease, often familial, involving the posterior columns, to a marked degree, with less marked involvement of the lateral corticospinal and spinocerebellar pathways. There are several important points of distinction. Friedreich's ataxia is a disease of childhood onset; combined systems disease, on the other hand, occurs in the adult during the middle and older years of age. Moreover, in Friedreich's ataxia there are signs such as nystagmus, tremor, ataxia of the trunk, muscle atrophy, and skeletal abnormalities which are almost never noted in combined systems disease. Aside from the clinical findings, the laboratory findings of combined systems disease are, of course, distinctive.

Finally, when all of these other disease entities have been excluded, there remains a group of cases of adult onset with relatively pure progressive involvement of the posterior and lateral columns with normal absorption and blood levels of vitamin B12. In these cases, the myelogram fails to reveal a compressive lesion of the spinal cord. Multifocal lesions are not present in the central nervous system and there is no familial history. These cases remain then as a degenerative disease of the posterior and lateral columns of unknown etiology. It is from this pool which was once much larger that the specific disease entities just considered were isolated and described in terms of particular pathological processes.

LATERAL COLUMN DISEASE

Relatively pure syndromes involving the corticospinal (pyramidal) pathways may reflect disease at various levels of the neural axis. Thus bilateral damage to the motor cortex (vascular disease or parasagittal meningioma) and bilateral damage to the internal capsule, midbrain, pons, medulla, or spinal cord may produce a spastic paraplegia with increased deep tendon reflexes and a bilateral sign of Babinski. The spinal cord disease may be intrinsic or extrinsic. From the standpoint of intrinsic cord disease, two relatively uncommon disease entities are usually considered: primary lateral sclerosis and familial spastic paraplegia.

A small proportion of cases of amyotrophic lateral sclerosis as previously discussed may begin as a syndrome of *primary lateral sclerosis,* presenting a picture of progressive spastic paraplegia for a number of years prior to the emergence of the signs of anterior horn cell and brain stem involvement.

Familial spastic paraplegia is a rare hereditary disease beginning in childhood or adolescence. The pathological changes of degeneration are usually limited to the corticospinal tracts in the thoracic and lumbar segments. As with most degenerative diseases involving the spinal cord and cerebellum, the basic etiology remains unknown.

SPINAL FORMS OF SPINOCEREBELLAR DEGENERATION

The spinocerebellar degenerations represent overlapping groups of degenerative diseases which are usually of unknown etiology, but are often familial. In some cases and families the predominant pathology involves peripheral nerve (peroneal muscular atrophy); in some, the cerebellum is involved; in others the cerebellum and brain stem are affected (olivopontocerebellar degeneration). Other cases involve the cerebellum and basal ganglia (dentatorubral degeneration). In others, the spinal cord is affected (Friedreich's ataxia and hereditary spastic paraplegia). In still other cases and families, there is a mixture of involvement, as for example, in a syndrome of hereditary ataxia with muscular atrophy which appears to be a mixture of Friedreich's ataxia and the muscular atrophy of the predominantly motor peripheral neuropathy found in peroneal muscular atrophy.

Friedreich's Ataxia. As we have previously indicated, this progressive disease begins in childhood or adolescence; the initial symptom is usually an ataxia of gait. The degeneration involves a loss of axons which is most severe in the posterior columns but which also involves the corticospinal and spinocerebellar pathways (Fig. 8–24). The involvement of the spinocerebellar pathways undoubtedly reflects the loss of cells in Clarke's dorsal cell column and in the posterior horn. There is a significant cell loss in the posterior root ganglia or atrophy of the posterior roots as well. This may in part account for the severe loss of axons in the posterior column since these axons have their nerve cells of origin in the posterior root ganglion. The ataxia of gait then reflects both posterior column degeneration and spinocerebellar degeneration. In addition, in some cases, minor loss of nerve cells in the cerebellum has been noted. The marked involvement of the posterior columns is reflected in the severe loss of joint position sense and of vibration sensation in the extremities. The loss of deep tendon reflexes reflects a loss of the afferent limb of the monosynaptic stretch reflex arc. As one might expect, there is a relative degree of hypotonia. Spasticity does not develop. Bilateral extensor plantar responses are present in most cases, signifying a degree of involvement of lateral corticospinal tracts. As the disease progresses, a

significant distal atrophy and sensory loss in the extremities may occur, suggesting a significant involvement of peripheral nerve.

Various skeletal deformities may be noted. The most frequent finding is that of pes cavus, a form of clubfoot (Fig. 8–25). A curvature of the spine (kyphoscoliosis) is also found in many cases. Pes cavus may occur as an isolated finding in family members unaffected by the neurological aspects of the disease. Abnormalities of cardiac function are frequently found as a result of disease of the myocardial muscle and conduction system (a chronic low-grade degeneration and inflammation). This aspect of the disease may contribute to the death of the majority of patients in the early adult years. In other patients, mortality is related to the eventual bedridden state during which intercurrent infection develops. The following case history illustrates a case of Friedreich's ataxia evaluated relatively late in the disease course.

Case History 14. Date of consultation: 3/3/68.

This 22-year-old, part-time college student (Mr. H.G.) was referred for evaluation of progressive ataxia. At 9 or 10 years of age, a slight change in handwriting had been noted. This became progressively worse with a loss of coordination of hand movement. When the patient was 12 or 13 years old, difficulty in walking and balancing was first noted.

Evaluation at the Children's Medical Center in 1963 when the patient was 15 years old indicated a wide-based gait. No weakness, spasticity, tremor, or dysdiadochokinesia (impairment in alternating hand movements) was present. Deep tendon reflexes were ab-

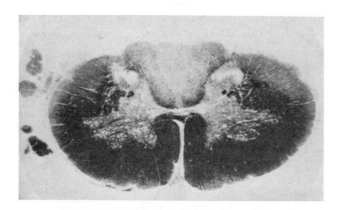

Figure 8–24 Friedreich's Ataxia. Degeneration of posterior columns and, to a lesser extent, of lateral columns is demonstrated in the myelin stain of cervical spinal cord. (From Wechsler, I.: *Clinical Neurology*, 9th Edition. Philadelphia, W. B. Saunders, 1963, p. 28.)

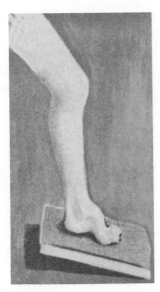

Figure 8–25 Friedreich's Ataxia: Pes Cavus. Note that a similar abnormality of the foot may occur in other disease states. (From Wechsler, I.: *Clinical Neurology,* 9th Edition. Philadelphia, W. B. Saunders, 1963, p. 123.)

sent bilaterally. A positive Romberg test was present and the patient was unable to walk with his eyes closed.

In the interim, ataxia had become progressively worse, particularly during the last year and especially during the last several months. The patient as recently as 1964 was able to walk holding onto walls. Then he needed the assistance of one person and during the last year he had required the assistance of two people. There had been a progressive change in voice after the last 3 to 4 years. At no time had the patient experienced numbness of his hands or legs. In addition to an ataxia of gait, the patient had noted, since 1964, weakness in the lower extremities with "collapsing at the knees." He had no bladder or bowel problems. He had had some change in vision with progressive changes of glasses. Despite these symptoms the patient continued to do relatively well in his studies at school. However, because of his significant disability in terms of traveling to his classes, he had to participate as a part-time student.

FAMILY HISTORY: The patient was adopted at an early age. No information concerning parents or siblings was noted.

GENERAL PHYSICAL EXAMINATION:

1. The patient was a thin, well-developed white male with a marked degree of ataxia of gait and marked truncal ataxia. He was unable to walk without the assistance of two individuals. He was unable to sit without back support.

2. No definite pes cavus or vertebral skeletal abnormalities were present.

3. There was no evidence of telangiectasia over the ears, the postauricular areas, posterior cervical areas, and conjunctiva (these dilated tangles of vessels are noted in these locations in one form of cerebellar disease: ataxia telangiectasia).

4. The heart was not enlarged to percussion. There was, however, an irregularity of the cardiac rhythm.

NEUROLOGICAL EXAMINATION:

1. *Mental status:*
   a. The patient was oriented for time, place, and person.
   b. His delayed recall within a 5-minute period and with assistance was 4-out-of-5.

2. *Cranial nerves:*
   a. Visual acuity and visual fields were intact. The optic fundi were normal.
   b. Extraocular movements were jerky but no definite nystagmus was noted.
   c. Frequent facial grimacing was noted. There was no clearly lateralized facial weakness present.
   d. There was no atrophy of the tongue.

3. *Motor system:*
   a. There was minor atrophy of the hand muscles. A greater degree of atrophy was evident in the muscles of the lower legs and feet. No definite fasciculations were present.
   b. There was mild weakness in the distal portions of the upper extremities and hands. There was a more significant weakness in the lower extremities, most marked distally but present to some extent at knee flexors as well.
   c. There was evidence of hypotonia with excessive rebound on passive motion and release.
   d. There was a marked intention tremor bilaterally. There was a marked impairment of alternating movements of the hands and fingers; an ataxia of the head was noted. (An intention tremor is an oscillating movement perpendicular to the line of movement and usually implies disease of a cerebellar hemisphere or of cerebellar pathways related to the lateral cerebellum.)
   e. There was a marked ataxia of the

trunk, previously noted; the patient was unable to stand except with the support of two individuals. Attempts to have him stand on a broad base indicated a marked truncal ataxia. (A truncal ataxia usually implies disease of the midline cerebellum or of fiber systems related to the midline cerebellum.)

4. *Reflexes:*
   a. There was absence of deep tendon reflexes everywhere.
   b. Plantar responses were equivocally extensor bilaterally.
5. *Sensory system:*
   a. There was a distal decrease in pain sensation in the lower extremities up to the ankles.
   b. Touch sensation was intact.
   c. There was a significant decrease in vibratory sensation with a total absence at the toes and ankles and a decrease at the knees. Vibratory sensation was practically absent at the fingers and markedly decreased at the wrists.
   d. Joint position sensation was markedly defective at the toes and defective to a lesser degree at the fingers.

LABORATORY DATA:

The electrocardiogram (EKG) demonstrated significant abnormalities with a marked sinus arrhythmia, occasional nodal beats, and premature atrial contractions. In addition, abnormal T wave inversions occurred.

COMMENT:

The early symptoms and findings in this case based upon neurological examination in 1963 when the patient was 15 clearly indicated predominant involvement of the posterior columns. His subsequent evaluation in 1968 indicated that significant progression of the posterior column findings had occurred. In addition, there was now evidence of significant disease of the cerebellum or cerebellar pathways: intention tremor, impairment of alternating movements, ataxia of the trunk, and a dysmetria of eye movements. Moreover, there was also evidence of a distal sensory-motor peripheral neuropathy whose motor components were somewhat more severe. Equivocal extensor plantar responses were present. The student should, of course, realize that a distal peripheral neuropathy will significantly interrupt the reflex pathway involved in the elicitation of the sign of Babinski.

In this case, as in many, mental status was relatively well preserved. Information received in September 1969 and September 1970 indicated that the patient was continuing his college studies although restricted to a wheel chair.

Other Predominantly Spinal Forms of Spinocerebellar Degeneration. Familial spastic paraplegia is often considered in this group and has already been briefly discussed.

Occasionally, one may encounter patients who have an onset in adult life of a progressive familial spinocerebellar degeneration which bears some resemblance to Friedreich's ataxia. Such cases, however, are less common than the other forms of cerebellar degeneration which occur in adults. (See chapter 25.)

MULTIFOCAL DISEASES OF THE SPINAL CORD

Essentially two categories of pathology produce multifocal symptoms and signs of central nervous system disease: demyelinating diseases and vascular diseases, particularly small vessel disease.

When the spinal cord is considered, the first category occurs relatively frequently; the second category has been encountered only rarely at the present time.

DEMYELINATING DISEASES

By demyelinating diseases we imply a pathological process in which there is a primary destruction of normally formed myelin. As we have indicated earlier, destruction of myelin may be a secondary aspect of other primary disease processes, in which the loss of myelin is but one step in the destruction of the axon, e.g., system diseases such as vitamin B12 deficiency. Similarly, destruction of myelin and axons may occur as a consequence of vascular infarction.

Moreover, there is another category of disease, the leukodystrophies, in which a diffuse loss of myelin occurs. The loss, however, involves the destruction of defectively formed myelin. The leukodystrophies are a rare group of diseases occurring primarily in infancy and childhood and need not concern us at this point.

Multiple Sclerosis. Among the primary demyelinating diseases, the most common variety is multiple sclerosis, also referred to as disseminated sclerosis. This is a disease of unknown etiology affecting primarily young adults. The disease is characterized by the dissemination of the pathological process in time and space. Thus a requirement for diagnosis is that the various lesions be acquired at different times. At any given moment, the various lesions will then be at a different pathological stage of development. It is, moreover, essential for diagnosis that multiple levels of the central neural axis be affected.

The basic pathological process of myelin destruction is followed by a stage in which destroyed myelin is removed by macrophages. There then follows a stage of astrocytic proliferation with the production of glial fibers. This gliosis results in the firm, (sclerotic) gray appearance noted in old lesions, thus the name multiple sclerosis. The areas of demyelination or sclerosis are referred to as plaques (Fig. 8–26). In the majority of cases, dissemination in time results in a characteristic picture of exacerbations and remissions. Other cases, however, follow a pattern of steady or stepwise progression.

There are in the early stages, predominant clinical syndromes which can be recognized, e.g., the spinal cord form, the brain stem-cerebellar form, the cerebral form, and the optic nerve form. In most patients encountered late in the course of the disease when they are bedridden, a mixture of clinical syndromes reflecting the multiple levels of involvement is seen. Not all cases seen in the early stages of the disease follow a progressive course to disability and incapacity. Some patients experience only one or two attacks or appear to recover completely after each of a series of attacks. Thus, in the series of 241 patients studied by McAlpine (1961) and followed for a minimum of 10 years, approximately one-third were dead, one-third were disabled, and one-third had no physical restrictions or disabilities as to work and home life. No specific therapy is available.

As regards the *spinal form*, the most common syndrome is that of posterior and lateral column involvement. When this symptom occurs early in the course, careful differentiation must be made from the other causes of this syndrome (see preceding discussion). In other cases, additional involvement of the lateral spinothalamic tract may indicate the apparent level of a spinal cord lesion with a compressive etiology to be ruled out. In both syndromes previously considered, a spastic

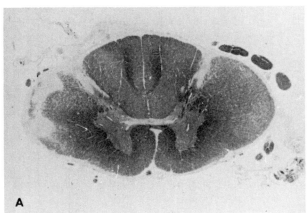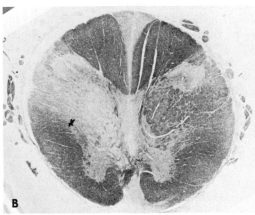

Figure 8–26 Multiple sclerosis affecting the spinal cord. *A,* This 58-year-old male expired after a long history of progressive multiple sclerosis. His later years were characterized by a bedridden state, severe flexion contractures, and decubitus ulcers. At postmortem examination multiple plaques of variable age were present in spinal cord, brain stem, and cerebral white matter. At cervical cord level, the major lesion involved the right lateral column; although evidence of ascending degeneration was also apparent in posterior columns. (Courtesy of Dr. Jose Segarra.)

B, This 44-year-old male 20 years previously had experienced an acute episode of multiple sclerosis involving spinal cord. He was asymptomatic in the interim until his acute death from an unrelated cause. In this section at the spinal medullary junction, demyelination is evident, lateral column, and contralateral medullary pyramid. The symmetrical demyelination in posterior columns probably represents ascending degeneration rather than primary demyelination. (Courtesy of Dr. Jose Segarra, Boston Veterans Administration Hospital.)

bladder is likely to be the result. Demyelination involving the sacral cord, however, may result in urinary retention. Such urinary retention, however, may also be the result of spinal shock stemming from a recent acute area of demyelination at a higher spinal cord level.

In the following case history, particular episodes related to spinal cord demyelination may be clearly distinguished.

Case History 15. NECH #155–379. Date of readmission: 3/2/67.

This 33-year-old, white, married real estate broker (Mr. B.W.) was re-evaluated on March 2, 1967 with a chief complaint of numbness of both lower extremities. The patient had awakened two days previously with a numbness and tingling paresthesias below the knees. This had gradually ascended to involve primarily the buttock area. Later that evening, the patient had begun to have difficulty in voiding and required catheterization by his local physician. The numbness had become more intense over the next day, particularly in the perianal area. In addition, a general sensation of weakness of the lower extremities had been noted.

The patient's neurological problem had begun in February 1963 when he awoke one morning with tingling, pins-and-needles paresthesias involving the left hand, which slowly spread to involve the left half of the body and left leg. There was then improvement followed by a recurrence of numbness on the left side and pain in the right arm. Shortly thereafter, incoordination of the left arm occurred. Neurological examination in April 1963 revealed mild weakness on the left side involving elbow flexion, wrist dorsiflexion, thumb abduction, and knee flexion. Touch, pain, and temperature sensation were decreased over the entire left arm, trunk, thigh, and left plantar surface. The cervical myelogram was normal. Cerebrospinal fluid protein was normal (35 mg./100 ml.), with a normal gamma globulin percentage. No significant cells were present and the serological test was negative. Blood sedimentation rate and other studies, including electroencephalogram, were normal.

The patient had subsequently, over several weeks, made a complete recovery and was well until November 1965, when, over a 7- to 10-day period, he had an insidious onset of weakness and tingling in the thumb and index and middle fingers of the left hand, accompanied by weakness of the left leg. The left arm weakness had progressed to a complete distal paralysis with a lesser involvement of the distal portion of the left leg. Eight days after onset of the left hand symptoms, numbness of the left side of the face developed. Neurological examination (November 15, 1965) had revealed a left central facial weakness and a left flaccid hemiparesis most marked distally. Deep tendon reflexes were increased on the left and a Babinski sign was present on the left. Laboratory studies were again all normal (including right carotid arteriogram, electroencephalogram, and brain scan). Within four days, a significant improvement had occurred. Examination on November 29, 1965, revealed only minimal weakness of finger and hand muscles (80 per cent of normal compared to 0 to 10 per cent on November 15, 1965). Deep tendon reflexes, however, were still hyperactive on the left and the sign of Babinski was still present on the left.

In April 1966, in relation to a minor viral infection and fever, the patient developed progressive weakness of right arm and leg. Within 10 days a disturbance of speech (dysarthria) had developed. Symptoms continued despite treatment with ACTH, and on May 28, 1966, a bilateral impairment of central vision was noted. On May 29, 1966, a weakness occurred on the left side. On May 30, 1966, the patient reported urinary retention with difficulty in beginning stream. Neurological examination at this time revealed a central and paracentral scotoma in the right eye (a defect in the field of vision suggesting a lesion of optic nerve). A scotoma was also present in the nasal field of the left eye. A mild distal right hemiparesis was present. Deep tendon reflexes were increased on the right side and a Babinski sign was present on the right. A mild cerebellar deficit was suggested by a mild ataxia on the heel to shin test. Within 2 days a significant degree of improvement was evident in all symptoms and signs.

The patient reported on June 13, 1966, that he had had burning pains for a short time on the right side of the face (eye, tongue, upper teeth). Re-evaluation in July 1966 revealed only a slight reflex asymmetry of deep tendon reflexes and the patient then was asymptomatic until there was an exacerbation of his condition in March 1967.

NEUROLOGICAL EXAMINATION:
1. *Mental status:* Intact.
2. *Cranial nerves:* Intact.

3. *Motor system:*
   a. Strength was intact except for a minor decrease bilaterally at hip flexors and ankle dorsiflexors.
   b. Gait was broad-based with an ataxia apparent on attempts to walk heel to toe tandem. Romberg test was positive.
4. *Reflexes:*
   a. Deep tendon reflexes were symmetrical.
   b. Plantar responses were flexor.
5. *Sensation:*
   a. A dense bilateral deficit in pain sensation was present over the lower sacral segments S3, S4, and S5 in a circular distribution about the anus. Temperature sensation was relatively well preserved.
   b. Touch sensation was intact.
   c. There was a marked bilateral decrease in vibratory sensation at the toes and ankles with a lesser decrease at the knees. Position sense was relatively well preserved.

LABORATORY DATA:

1. Cystometrogram indicated a defect in reflex voiding in response to distension of the bladder. The patient had no sensation of distension up to 450 cc. of saline. The patient, as distension of bladder was increased, had a progressive increase in discomfort, but no spontaneous voiding occurred even after a total of 750 cc. of saline had been instilled.

HOSPITAL AND SUBSEQUENT COURSE:

Significant improvement again occurred without specific therapy. By the second day in the hospital, the ability to void had returned. By the time of hospital discharge on March 7, 1967, neurological examination was normal except for the broad-based gait.

On March 14, 1967, the patient reported an exacerbation of symptoms. He was experiencing increasing difficulty in voiding, unable to start stream. A weakness and numbness of the right lower extremity had also developed the previous day. A significant degree of weakness in the right lower extremity was confirmed on neurological examination. His gait was more ataxic. Deep tendon reflexes in the lower extremities were now bilaterally hyperactive, but more marked on the right side. Bilateral extensor plantar responses were now present (sign of Babinski). Abdominal reflexes were absent bi-

laterally. Pain sensation was decreased below the level of the umbilicus (T10 dermatome). The deficit was marked on the left, moderate on the right. Touch sensation was intact. Vibratory sensation was markedly decreased in the lower extremities with a possible level at the T12 spinous process. The defect was greater on the right than on the left. Joint position sense was markedly defective at the toes on the right side (gross amplitude movements could not be distinguished). On the left, gross amplitude movements could be distinguished at the toes, but errors were made in the fine and medium amplitude movements.

After a one-week period of bed rest in the hospital, bladder function, strength, and pain sensation had returned to normal, and position sense had improved.

On April 1, 1967, symptoms again worsened. The patient experienced difficulty in voiding, and paresthesias were again noted, beginning in the feet and gradually spreading to the level of the umbilicus. After a 6-day period of bed rest at his local hospital, these symptoms gradually cleared.

In June 1967, the patient reported numbness (tingling paresthesias) of the left side of the face accompanied by a paralysis of all facial muscles on the left side. Shortly thereafter, a decrease in hearing in the left ear was noted. Examination two weeks after the onset of these symptoms, revealed a resolving peripheral type facial weakness on the left with defective perception of whisper and watch tick in the left ear.

Follow-up evaluation in October 1968, indicated no additional exacerbations. There was no actual disability on examination; the only neurological finding was a minor tremor of the hands. Periodic examinations over the next 2 years (the most recent in May 1970) indicated no significant exacerbations of the disease process. No significant disability was present. Only a minimal reflex asymmetry was present with deep tendon reflexes more active on the right. In the interim the patient had continued to pursue his usual business activities and had continued to pilot his own airplane.

COMMENT:

Unfortunately, the majority of patients afflicted with multiple sclerosis do not pursue the relatively benign course which, from a retrospective standpoint, was evident in this patient. From a diagnostic standpoint, it is evident that this patient presented symptoms and signs referable to pathological lesions disseminated in time and space. Dissemination in space was not evident at the time of the patient's initial episode in 1963. The combination of left hemiparesis and pain in the right arm with a negative myelogram suggested only the possibility of an intrinsic cervical cord lesion of unknown type. It should be noted that onset with a limited hemiparesis is somewhat atypical for multiple sclerosis. The second episode in November 1965, with symptoms in the left face, arm, and leg, suggested a lesion in the internal capsule or subcortical white matter of the right cerebral hemisphere. The third episode in April—May 1966 suggested multiple additional lesions: the scotomas in visual fields suggested multiple lesions of the optic nerves; the urinary retention suggested bilateral lesions of the sacral spinal cord. The episode in June 1966, of trigeminal neuralgia, suggested a lesion involving the trigeminal nerve or its descending spinal nucleus; that is, a pontine level of the brain stem. (It must be noted that trigeminal neuralgia has causes other than multiple sclerosis; most commonly, this occurs without any clearly established etiology.)

The episode of the present illness (March 2, 1967) with urinary retention and a perianal deficit in pain sensation over segments S3, S4, and S5 suggested a lesion affecting, in a bilateral manner, the white matter of the sacral spinal cord. The actual level of lateral spinothalamic tract involvement producing the deficit in pain sensation may have been as high as the S1 or S2 segment. Bilateral involvement of the posterior columns was also suggested by the deficits in position and vibratory sensation. The cystometrogram suggested that the urinary retention reflected involvement of both the afferent and efferent limbs of the reflex arc. (These axons would be involved as they pass within the substance of the spinal cord. The process of demyelination may affect axons within the gray matter as well as the white matter of the central nervous system.) Thus, the patient had no sensation of distension until 450 cc. Normally the sense of distension and desire to void begins to occur at 200 cc. Despite the sensation of distension, no spontaneous voiding occurred between 450 and 750 cc., suggesting that the defect in reflex activity involved more than a defect in the afferent limb of reflex arc. An apparent atonic bladder may

occur as one manifestation of spinal shock with a lesion at a higher level of the spinal cord. In such a case, one would expect a definite flaccid paraplegia with bilateral Babinski signs, signifying acute bilateral involvement of the pyramidal tracts, signs which were absent in this case during the present episode.

The subsequent exacerbation beginning on March 14, 1967 clearly suggested an additional lesion involving the lower thoracic spinal cord. The pattern of involvement suggested an atypical Brown-Séquard type lesion, primarily involving the right half of the spinal cord at approximately the T8 level. Thus, weakness involved the right lower extremity. Deep tendon reflexes were increased bilaterally but were more active on the right. There was a bilateral defect in position and vibration sense although this was clearly more marked on the right side. On the other hand, although a decrease in pain sensation was present below T10 bilaterally, this defect was clearly more marked on the left side. The difficulty in voiding at this time may well have reflected the additional "spinal shock" effects of an acute bilateral corticospinal tract lesion. The patient had a desire to void but was unable to start his stream. In this case, however, an exacerbation of the previous sacral cord lesion cannot be ruled out.

The last episode in June 1967 suggested an additional lesion involving the lateral tegmentum of the lower pontine brain stem on the left with involvement of the auditory division of the entering eighth (VIII) nerve, the facial (VII) nerve, and possibly the descending spinal tract of nerve V, with numbness of the face. (It should of course be noted that this syndrome taken in isolation might well suggest other types of pathology in the cerebellar pontine angle, e.g., an acoustic neuroma.)

The student might well raise the following question. "Granted that the patient had lesions disseminated in time and space, how can one be certain of the specific pathological nature of the lesion?" One of course cannot be absolutely certain until postmortem examination of the brain. At this time there are no specific diagnostic laboratory tests. An increased amount of gamma globulin is present in the spinal fluid of approximately 45 per cent of cases, with correlated changes in the colloidal gold tests (usually a first zone rise). The increased percentage of gamma globulin has suggested a possible autoimmune basis for the disease (as yet not proven). During acute exacerbations, an increased number of cells and an increase in protein may also be found in the spinal fluid. None of these changes are specific for multiple sclerosis.

Inflammation of blood vessels (vasculitis, periarteritis, or lupus erythematosus) may produce multifocal lesions within the central nervous system, in a sense disseminated in time and space. These diseases, however, are unlikely to involve the nervous system selectively. Moreover, when these diseases involve the central nervous system, they do not produce selective involvement of the myelin of axons, but rather involve both neurons and axons. In the present case, selective involvement of axons (white matter) was evident. Disease was limited to the central nervous system. Moreover, certain laboratory findings noted in a vasculitis or collagen disease were not noted in this case. Sedimentation rate, white blood count, and special preparations for lupus erythematosus were all negative.

We have indicated that the basic etiology remains unknown. In some cases, the initial episode or exacerbations may begin in relationship to trauma, fever, or nonspecific infections. Such a relationship to fever and infections was evident in several of the exacerbations experienced by this patient. In some cases, a familial or genetic factor may be suggested. In the present case, there was a clue to such a factor. The patient's brother had been hospitalized at age 33 in 1962 with a diagnosis of myelitis para infectious, manifested by a weakness of left arm and leg (accompanied by left-sided increased deep tendon reflexes and a left Babinski sign) and by a deficit in pain and temperature sensation below the C4 level. Symptoms developed over a 3-day period and cleared over a period of 3 weeks. Spinal fluid contained an increased number of cells (50 lymphocytes). Protein was increased to a minor degree (53 mg./100 ml.) but colloidal gold test suggested a significant increase in the percentage of gamma globulin. The patient had no residual disability and experienced no additional episodes during the succeeding 8 years. It would not be correct to label this second case as multiple sclerosis; the best diagnostic label would be acute postinfectious myelitis.

Acute Encephalomyelitis or Postinfectious Encephalomyelitis or Postvaccinal Encephalomyelitis. This is a less frequent demyelinating disease than multiple sclerosis with lesions disseminated in space but usually all occurring in one episode. The onset of symptoms is usually quite acute and severe. At times, the syndrome occurs 4 to 18 days after an acute system viral infection, e.g., measles, or after vaccination for smallpox or rabies. In contrast to multiple sclerosis, there is a significant perivascular inflammation reaction and a greater destruction of axons in addition to the more marked demyelination.

MULTIFOCAL VASCULAR DISEASE

As we have indicated, multifocal vascular disease is not presently a common problem with regard to the spinal cord. Occasional cases of *vasculitis* (an inflammation of blood vessel walls) may have spinal cord involvement. In the past, a somewhat more frequent cause was the spinal cord variety of meningo-vascular syphilis. The vascular components involved inflammation of the blood vessel walls and the perivascular space with subsequent thrombosis and infarction. The meningeal component involved a thickening and chronic inflammation of the meninges with subsequent compression of nerve roots, spinal cord, and spinal blood vessels.

In this regard, it should be mentioned that a multifocal spinal cord syndrome may also be noted in another circumstance in relation to chronic inflammation and thickening of the meninges—the *adhesive arachnoiditis* which follows the injection of foreign materials into the subarachnoid space, e.g., spinal anesthetic which has been contaminated by detergent agents employed in the cleaning of syringes.

References

Auld, A., and Buerman, A.: Metastatic spinal epidural tumors. Arch. Neurol., *15*:100–108, 1966.

Brain, Lord, and Wilkinson, M.: *Cervical Spondylosis.* Philadelphia, Lea and Febiger, 1967.

Brody, I. A., and Wilkins, R. H.: Neurological classics X: Brown-Séquard syndrome. Arch. Neurol., *19*: 347–348, 1968.

Elsberg, C. A.: *Surgical Diseases of the Spinal Cord Membranes and Nerve Roots.* New York, Paul B. Hoeber, 1941.

Garland, H., Greenberg, J., and Harriman, D. G.: Infarction of the spinal cord. Brain, 89:645–662, 1966.

Hogan, E. L., and Romanul, F. C.: Spinal cord infarction occurring during insertion of aortic graft. Neurol., 16:67–74, 1966.

Hughes, J. T.:*Pathology of the Spinal Cord.* Chicago, Year Book Medical Publishers, 1966.

Kurtzke, J. F., Beebe, G. W., Nagler, B., Nefzger, M. D., Acth, T. L., and Kurland, L. T.: Studies on the natural history of multiple sclerosis. V. Long term survival in young men. Arch Neurol., 22:215–225, 1970.

McAlpine, D.: The benign form of multiple sclerosis. Brain, 84:186, 1961.

McAlpine, D., Campston, N. D., and Lunsden, C. E.: *Multiple Sclerosis.* Edinburgh, E. & S. Livingstone, 1955.

Mackay, R. P.: Course and prognosis in amyotrophic lateral sclerosis. Arch. Neurol., 8:117–127, 1963.

Merritt, H. H.: *A Textbook of Neurology.* Philadelphia, Lea and Febiger, 1967.

Merritt, H. H., Adams, R. D., and Solomon, H. C.: *Neurosyphilis.* New York, Oxford University Press, 1946.

Slooff, J. L., Kernohan, J. W., and MacCarty, C. S.: *Primary Intermedullary Tumors of the Spinal Cord and Filum Terminale.* Philadelphia, W. B. Saunders, 1964.

Tarlov, I. M.: *Spinal Cord Compression: Mechanisms of Paralysis and Treatment.* Springfield, Ill., Charles C Thomas, 1957.

Wilkins, R. H., and Brody, I. A.: Neurological classics II: Babinski's sign. Arch. Neurol., 17:441–446, 1967.

Wilkins, R. H., and Brody, I. A.: Neurological classics VIII: Romberg's sign. Arch. Neurol., 19:123–126, 1968.

Wilkins, R. H., and Brody, I. A.: Neurological classics XI: Argyll Robertson pupil. Arch. Neurol., 19:443–447, 1968.

Williams, H. M., Diamond, H. D., Craver, L. F., and Parsons, H.: *Neurological Complications of Lymphomas and Leukemias.* Springfield, Ill., Charles C Thomas, 1959.

Wilson, C. B., Bertan, V., Norrell, H. A., and Hukuda, S.: Experimental cervical myelopathy: II Acute ischemic myelopathy. Arch. Neurol., 21:571–589, 1969.

Appendix to Chapter 8

ELLIOTT M. MARCUS

QUESTIONS FOR PROBLEM SOLVING

1. Assume that you have been given a single cross section slide of the spinal cord stained for cells and fibers. Indicate the distinctive features that will enable you to decide the approximate cord level of this cross section: (a) upper cervical, (b) midlower cervical, (c) middle thoracic, (d) lower lumbar, (e) lower sacral.

2. Indicate the pathways for the following sensory modalities:
   a. Position
   b. Vibration
   c. Pain
   d. Temperature
   e. Touch

3. a. Indicate the segmental lamination pattern within the lateral spinothalamic pathway at the upper cervical spinal cord level, by locating fibers from cervical, thoracic, lumbar, and sacral segments.

   b. What is meant by the term "sacral sparing" as used to distinguish intrinsic spinal cord disease (e.g., syringomyelia or glioma) from extrinsic, compressive spinal cord disease e.g., thoracic meningioma or neurofibroma or ruptured intervertebral disc at cervical or thoracic level)?

4. Indicate the segmental lamination pattern in the posterior columns (fasciculus gracilis and fasciculus cuneatus) at the upper cervical spinal cord level.

5. Indicate the segmental lamination pattern of the lateral corticospinal tract at the upper cervical spinal cord level.

6. Indicate at the level of the cervical enlargement the location within the anterior horn of the cell groups supplying distal hand muscles. Compare this to the location of cell groups supplying the proximal shoulder muscles. Which of these cell groups receives direct synaptic innervation from large corticospinal tract fibers, as opposed to indirect innervation (interneuron is interposed between corticospinal tract fibers and the anterior horn cells).

7. Indicate the pathways for conveying nonconscious sensory information from the periphery to the cerebellum.

8. The following diagrams indicate the location of lesions in various diseases affecting the spinal cord. For each diagram list the structures involved and the specific clinical effects which would be found on neurological examination. Be certain to lateralize the findings as to left or right. If possible indicate the spinal cord level involved. Be certain to consider the following, if applicable:

   a. upper motor neuron effects (due to involvement of descending motor pathways).

   b. lower motor neuron effects due to involvement of anterior horn cells, anterior roots, or peripheral nerves.

   c. ascending sensory tracts.

   d. local (segmental) sensory effects.

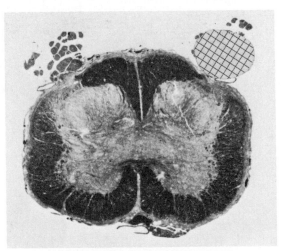

R   *Figure 8A–1.*   L

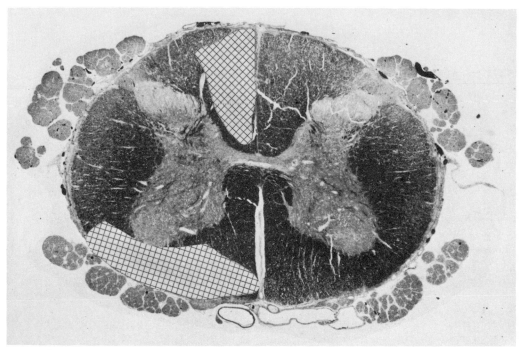

R   *Figure 8A–2.*   L

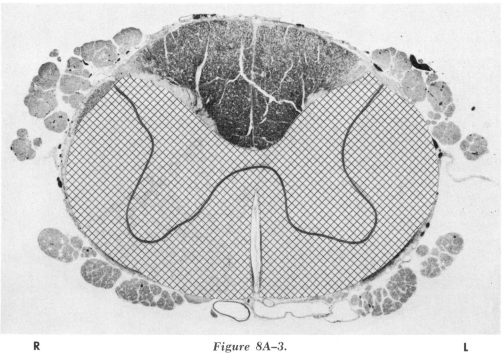

R   *Figure 8A–3.*   L

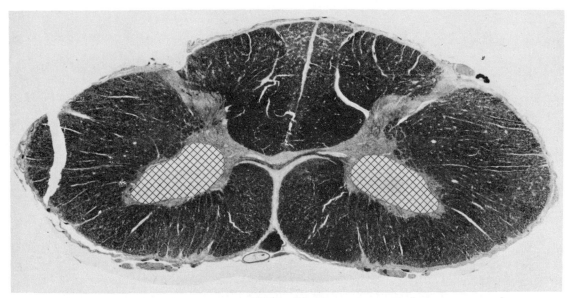

R   *Figure 8A–4.*   L

Figure 8A–5.

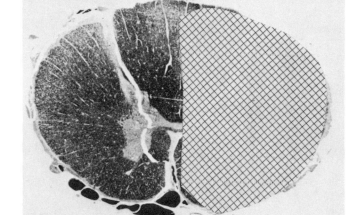

R   L

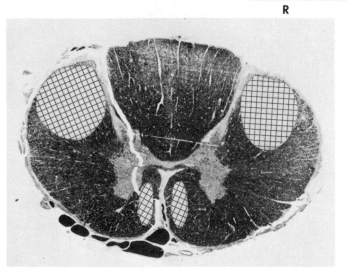

R   L

Figure 8A–6.

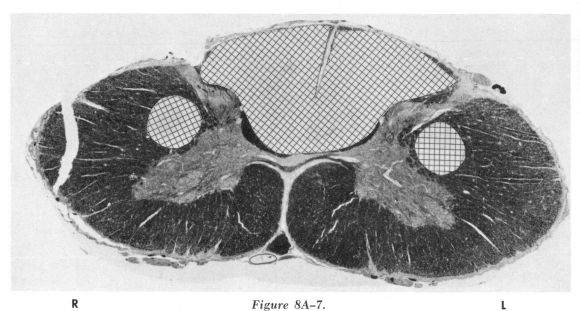

Figure 8A–7.

R   L

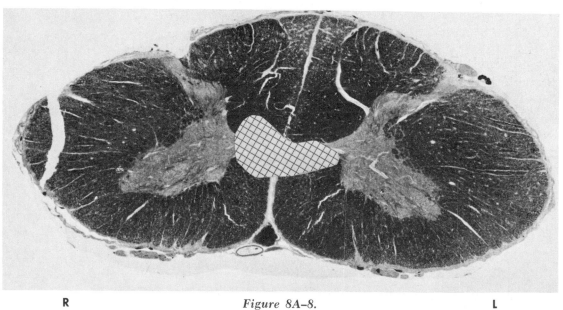

Figure 8A–8.

R   L

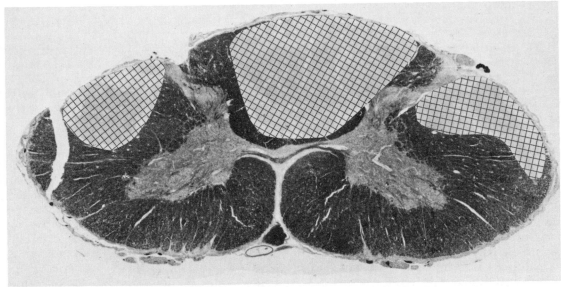

R   *Figure 8A–9.*   L

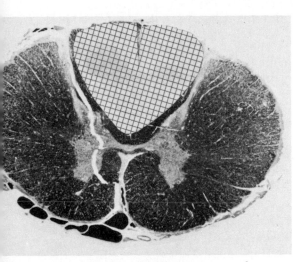

R   *Figure 8A–10.*   L

QUESTIONS AND PROBLEM SOLVING — CASE HISTORIES

Each of the following case histories deals with disease at the level of the spinal cord. In some of these cases the primary involvement may be that of anterior roots or of dorsal root ganglia rather than that of the spinal cord *per se.* For each case be prepared to draw a diagram of the lesion indicating as well the appropriate spinal cord level. Indicate the location of the lesion and the nature of the pathological process. If disease of the spinal cord is present, decide whether the process is intrinsic or extrinsic and whether it involves a single level lesion or is a system disease.

Case History 1A. NECH #170–087. Date of Admission: 10/68.

A 48-year-old, white male (Mr. W.T.) approximately 2 months prior to hospital admission, while lifting a heavy object, had the sudden onset of pain in the posterior cervical area radiating into the right shoulder, down the posterior aspect of the arm into the elbow. Coughing or straining at stool would result in a shooting burning electric shock type pain in the above distribution, also extending at times into the index finger and middle finger. In association with the pain, he experienced tingling "pins-and-needles" paresthesias in the right upper extremity in a distribution similar to that noted above. During this period the patient also noted minor weakness of the right hand. The lower extremities and bladder were not involved. When symptoms persisted, the patient was admitted to the hospital.

Neurological Examination:
1. *Mental status:* Intact.
2. *Cranial nerves:* II-XII intact.
3. *Motor system:*
   a. There was significant weakness of the right triceps (50 per cent of normal) with minimal weakness of the right wrist extensor and the finger abductors of the right hand. There was no weakness of the lower extremities.
   b. Gait was intact.
   c. No definite atrophy was present.

Rare fasciculations were noted in the right triceps muscles.

4. *Reflexes:*
   a. Deep tendon reflexes

Biceps:	right, 2+; left, 2+
Triceps:	right, 0; left, 2+
Radial:	right, 1–2+; left, 2+
Quadriceps:	right, 2+; left, 2+
Achilles:	right, 2+; left, 2+

5. *Sensation:* Minor decrease in pain sensation was present over the right middle finger. Pain, touch, position, and vibratory sensation were otherwise intact.

6. There was limitation of neck motion in all directions due to pain. Pressure over the lower cervical spinous processes produced a radiation of pain into the right upper extremity. There was also local tenderness on pressure over the right supraclavicular area.

HOSPITAL COURSE:

The patient had a reduction in pain and sensory symptoms following the use of cervical traction. Strength improved and the triceps deep tendon reflex returned.

QUESTIONS:

1. Is the spinal cord directly involved by this lesion? If so, indicate the level. If not, cite evidence against such involvement. Are the anterior roots involved? If so, indicate the level. If not, cite evidence against such involvement. Are the dorsal roots involved? If so, indicate the level. If not, cite evidence against such involvement.

2. What is the localizing significance of the relatively selective weakness of the right triceps muscle?

3. What is the explanation for the occasional fasciculations noted in the right triceps muscle?

4. What is the localizing significance of the selective depression of the triceps deep tendon reflex? Review also the segmental levels involved in the biceps, radial, quadriceps, and Achilles deep tendon reflexes.

5. What is the localizing significance of the distribution of pain and numbness experienced by the patient?

6. What is the localizing significance of the restricted pain deficit in the right hand?

7. Speculate concerning the pathology involved in this case.

8. Why did coughing and straining at stool produce an exacerbation of the pain?

Case History 2A. NECH #190–974. Date of Admission: 11/16/67.

This 51-year-old Negro male (Mr. H.B.) was in his usual state of health until October 6, 1967, when several boxes fell on his neck at work. He was knocked down but was not unconscious. He found that he was unable at this time to move either arms or legs. Shortly thereafter he noticed vague shooting pains down both arms and some tingling paresthesias of his right side involving both the arm and leg. The patient was hospitalized at his local community hospital.

Examination by the neurosurgical consultant shortly thereafter revealed a flaccid left leg, no voluntary movement in the left triceps or left hand. There was minimal movement in left elbow flexion. To a lesser degree there was weakness in the triceps on the right. A left extensor plantar response was present with an equivocal response on the right. Pain sensation was lost on the right side from the anterior chest downward to the sole of the foot. The pain loss extended into the axilla and in the right hand involved all of the fingers except the thumb.

The patient underwent an emergency laminectomy. After the laminectomy he regained the strength in his right arm and leg and left leg but his left arm continued to be weak.

NEUROLOGICAL EXAMINATION:

1. *Mental status:* Intact.
2. *Cranial nerves:* Intact.
3. *Motor system:*
   a. Fasciculations were present in the left deltoid muscle. Atrophy and fasciculations were present in the muscles of the left hand.
   b. There was marked weakness in the muscles of the left upper extremity. Finger flexion, thumb opposition, and triceps (elbow) extension were rated at 0 per cent of normal. Elbow flexion and the deltoid muscles were rated at 20 per cent of normal. In the left lower extremity, strength was intact except for weakness at the hip flexors (30 per cent of normal). Strength on the right side was intact except for minimal weakness at finger flexion, grip, and opposition.
   c. Moderate spasticity was present on passive motion at the left knee and ankle.
4. *Reflexes:*
   a. Deep tendon reflexes were increased on the left at the biceps, triceps,

quadriceps, and Achilles. Ankle clonus was present.

b. Plantar response was extensor on the left and equivocal on the right.

5. *Sensation:*

a. Position and vibration were intact.

b. Pain and temperature were absent on the right side of the body to the level of the clavicle, involving the entire arm, leg, and trunk.

QUESTIONS:

1. Indicate the level of involvement and the structures involved.

2. Diagram the lesion taking into account

a. the increased deep tendon reflexes on the left,

b. the spasticity of the left lower extremity,

c. the left Babinski response,

d. the defect in pain and temperature sensation on the right.

e. the atrophy and fasciculations involving the left deltoid and left hand.

3. This patient represents a partial example of a particular syndrome. Indicate the syndrome. What other components of the complete syndrome are missing in this case?

4. Indicate the nature of the pathological events which resulted in this syndrome.

Case History 3A. NECH #175–319.

Date of Admission: 11/9/65.

This 51-year-old, right-handed, white female (Mrs. E.S.) was transferred to Neurology Service for evaluation of pain present for 18 months in the left buttock and left posterior thigh. The pain had developed about 6 months after a fall. Initially, the pain was sharp and burning and localized to the left buttock area; it occurred in attacks lasting for a few seconds or minutes. Later the pain radiated as a shooting pain to the back and thigh. The pain was not increased by coughing or straining. Unrelated to the left buttock pain, the patient had also noted for several years sharp burning pains in both groin areas. The patient also reported that an unsteady gait had been present for many years (perhaps 20 years). A positive serological test had been noted in 1935 and the patient had received treatment for 3 months with a reversal of the serology. The patient's husband also in the past had a positive blood serology which under treatment had become negative.

NEUROLOGICAL EXAMINATION:

1. *Mental status:* The patient was a vague historian but all specific areas of mental status were intact.

2. *Cranial nerves:* The pupils were small (2 mm.) with little response to light. There was some pupillary reaction to accommodation.

3. *Motor system:*

a. Strength was intact.

b. The gait was broad-based. The patient was unable to walk a straight line. The Romberg test was positive.

c. Cerebellar test showed that no definite abnormality was present.

4. *Reflexes:*

a. Deep tendon reflexes were absent at biceps, triceps, radial, quadriceps, and Achilles.

b. Plantar responses were flexor.

5. *Sensation:*

a. Pain: There were multiple patchy areas of loss of pain sensation.

b. Vibration: There was a significant deficit in both lower extremities at the toes, ankles, and knees.

c. Joint position sense was intact.

QUESTIONS:

1. There was some question in this case whether we were dealing with one or with several disease entities. This was particularly the case as regards the leg pain. Indicate the diagnostic possibilities regarding this symptom and indicate what additional test you would perform to differentiate these possibilities.

2. What is the most likely explanation for the ataxia of gait, i.e., where is the pathology located and what is the nature of the pathology? How would you differentiate other remediable causes of the ataxia (i.e., what diagnostic procedures could be undertaken)?

3. How do the pupillary abnormalities aid in the establishment of a diagnosis?

Case History 4A. NECH #124–916.

Date of Admission: 3/16/59.

This 47-year-old, white, male, inspector of small parts (Mr. D.C.) entered the hospital complaining of weakness and numbness in both legs.

Five months prior to admission, the patient had noted a burning type pain extending over the right forearm. Soon thereafter, he became aware of a gradually increasing

numbness—"pins-and-needles" sensation—
involving his legs, first the right and then the
left. This was followed by a weakness of both
lower extremities which increased in severity. Urgency of urination, occasional bowel
incontinence, and increasing impotence were
also noted.

NEUROLOGICAL EXAMINATION:
1. *Mental status:* Intact.
2. *Cranial nerves:* Intact.
3. *Motor system:*
   a. Strength was intact in the upper extremities but decreased in the lower
   extremities to 50 per cent of normal.
   The involvement of the right leg was
   greater than that of the left leg.
   b. A mild degree of spasticity was present at the knees and ankles with a
   spastic gait.
   c. No atrophy or fasciculations were
   present.
4. *Reflexes:*
   a. Deep tendon: Triceps deep tendon
   reflexes were decreased bilaterally
   (0–1+) compared to biceps and radial
   periosteal which were active (2–3+).
   The quadriceps and Achilles deep
   tendon reflexes were markedly hyperactive (3–4+).
   b. Superficial reflexes: Bilateral extensor plantar responses were present (bilateral Babinski signs). Abdominal reflexes were decreased bilaterally.
5. *Sensation:*
   a. Position sense was defective for gross
   movements of the great toes bilaterally.
   b. Vibratory sensation was markedly
   decreased below the level of the T7
   spinous process.
   c. Pain and light touch were markedly
   decreased below the level of the umbilicus. Sacral segments were involved. There was also a poorly defined band of decreased pain sensation over the upper thorax. Pain
   sensation was somewhat greater on
   the left than on the right.

LABORATORY DATA:
1. *Glucose tolerance test* revealed a diabetic
type curve with a fasting blood sugar of 122,
30 minute sample of 205, 60 minute sample
of 218, and 150 minute sample of 142 mg./
100 ml.
2. *Lumbar puncture* revealed a partial dy-

namic block with the head in extension.
Cerebrospinal fluid protein was elevated to
80 mg./100 ml. (normal 45 mg./100 ml.).

HOSPITAL COURSE:
On February 17, 1959, surgery was performed by Dr. Samuel Brendler. Examination 2 weeks after surgery revealed some
return of pain sensation over the thorax,
abdomen, and lower extremities. Walking
had improved.

Evaluation 2 months after surgery indicated continued improvement as regards
gait. Position sense had returned to the
lower extremities, but vibration sense was
still absent.

QUESTIONS:
1. Indicate the level of the lesion in this
case and the structures involved by the
pathology.
2. Assuming that the pain in the upper extremities early in the course of the disease
had some localizing significance, why was
the sensory level for pain present only up
to the level of the umbilicus (T10) (i.e., pain
sensation absent or decreased below the umbilicus)?
3. Was the pathology in this case intrinsic
or extrinsic (compressive) to the spinal cord?
Cite the evidence for your conclusions.
4. What diagnostic procedures would you
undertake prior to surgery?
5. Granted that the patient had, among
other findings, posterior and lateral column
signs, why is the diagnosis of combined system disease unlikely in this case?

Case History 5A. NECH #79–39–63.
Date of Consultation: 8/25/70.
This 73-year-old retired executive (Mr.
S.G.) was referred for evaluation of paresthesias (pins-and-needles sensation and
numbness) involving all four extremities.
Approximately 8 months previously while
hospitalized for treatment of a febrile upper
respiratory illness, the patient had noted the
onset of a glove-and-stocking distribution of
paresthesias involving all four extremities in
a symmetrical manner. The symptoms over
the ensuing weeks and months gradually ascended; in the lower extremities it extended
as far as the perineum; in the upper extremities it ascended to the level of the elbows. The patient had also in the several
months prior to admission noted increasing
unsteadiness of gait, primarily when attempting to walk in the dark.

PAST HISTORY:

1. The patient at age 17 had developed a form of rheumatoid arthritis involving the spinal vertebrae: ankylosing spondylitis. This had produced a relatively rigid spine.

2. Family history revealed several relatives with pernicious anemia but no relatives with neurological disease.

NEUROLOGICAL EXAMINATION:

1. *Mental status:* Intact.
2. *Cranial nerves:* Intact.
3. *Motor system:*
   a. Strength was intact.
   b. Gait was broad-based, with unsteadiness on the turns. The degree of ataxia was increased by eye closure.
   c. The patient with eyes open and standing on a narrow base, was relatively steady. When his eyes were closed a significant swaying was apparent (Romberg test positive).
   d. Cerebellar tests, such as bringing the finger to the nose, when performed with eyes open were not remarkable.
4. *Reflexes:*
   a. Deep tendon reflexes were everywhere absent.
   b. Plantar responses were extensor bilaterally (bilateral Babinski signs).
5. *Sensation:*
   a. Vibratory sensation was absent at the toes and ankles and markedly decreased at the knees and iliac crests in a symmetrical manner. There was also a significant decrease at the fingers with a lesser decrease at the wrists and elbows.
   b. Joint position sense was defective for fine amplitude movements at the toes but elsewhere was intact.
   c. Pain and light touch sensation were intact.

QUESTIONS:

1. This patient presents a common neurological syndrome. Indicate the site of pathology. Present a differential diagnosis and indicate the most likely pathology. (You may disregard as nonrelevant the patient's other medical problem of ankylosing spondylitis.)

2. Does this patient have a single level lesion or a system disease?

3. Interpret the sensory symptoms and findings as to possible diagnosis.

4. Explain the absence of deep tendon reflexes.

5. What does the term "positive Romberg sign" mean?

6. Indicate the significance of the bilateral extensor plantar responses (sign of Babinski).

7. Outline what additional tests you would perform to confirm the diagnosis. What treatment would you undertake?

Case History 6A. NECH #79–15–65.
Date of Consultation: 8/17/70.
Date of Admission: 8/21/70.
This 65-year-old housewife (Mrs. C.T.) had complained for 5 months of a dull aching pain in the interscapular area radiating into the left axilla.

Four months prior to admission, the pain became sharp and burning radiating into an area on the inner aspect of the upper arm — essentially the T1 and T2 dermatomes.

Because the patient had long-standing epigastric pain and fatty food intolerance, a gallbladder series was performed, indicating a nonfunctioning gallbladder. When right upper quadrant pain developed, a cholecystectomy (removal of gallbladder) was performed on August 11, 1970. This revealed the presence of multiple gallstones (cholelithiasis) and of chronic inflammation (cholecystitis). Pathological examination of the specimen, however, subsequently revealed carcinoma of the gallbladder, extending through to the serosa and involving the cystic duct.

Despite the surgery, the patient continued to complain of pain over the T2, T3, and T4 vertebrae extending into the left axilla and accompanied at times by paresthesias in the same distribution.

NEUROLOGICAL EXAMINATION:

On August 17, 1970 examination had revealed that the patient's mental status, cranial nerves, motor system, reflexes, and sensations were intact. However, local tenderness was noted on palpation over the T3 and T4 spinous processes. There was also tenderness on palpation of the brachial plexus in the left axilla and in the left supraclavicular area. Possible enlarged lymph nodes were also noted in the axilla. Because of the elevated sedimentation rate, x-rays of the cervical and thoracic spine and more extensive evaluation were recommended.

On August 19, 1970, the patient noted minor weakness of the legs on climbing steps, with greater weakness in the right leg.

In addition she noted numbness and tingling of both legs. These symptoms were greater on the right than on the left.

On August 20, 1970 she found that she could not walk by herself and that she had no sensation in her lower trunk and legs. She fell and had a significant increase in weakness and numbness. Thereafter the patient was unable to void.

By 4:00 a.m. on August 21, 1970 she had progressed to a complete paralysis of both legs and an anesthesia below the midtrunk.

NEUROLOGICAL EXAMINATION:

1. *Mental status:* Intact.
2. *Cranial nerves:* Intact.
3. *Motor system:*
   a. No voluntary movement of the lower extremities was possible.
   b. Spasticity was present on passive motion at the knees and ankles.
4. *Reflexes:*
   a. Deep tendon reflexes were 2+ at biceps and triceps and 3+ at quadriceps and Achilles.
   b. Plantar responses were extensor bi-laterally. Abdominal reflexes were absent.
5. *Sensation:*
   a. There was complete anesthesia and complete analgesia below the nipples with no evidence of sacral sparing.
   b. Vibration sensation was absent below T3.
   c. Position sensation was absent in the lower extremities.
6. *Back:* Tenderness was present over the T2, T3 and T4 spinous processes.

HOSPITAL COURSE:

Examination one hour later indicated sensory level had extended upward to the sternal notch.

QUESTIONS:

1. Where is the lesion? Be specific. Indicate spinal cord level. Indicate whether lesion is epidural, intradural-extramedullary, or intramedullary.

2. What is the most likely nature of the pathology?

3. Indicate the diagnostic and therapeutic steps to be undertaken.

9

Brain Stem: Gross Anatomy

STANLEY JACOBSON

The constituent parts of the central nervous system (CNS) are the spinal cord, brain stem, cerebellum, and cerebrum. The brain stem is interposed between the spinal cord and cerebrum and has reciprocal connections with the spinal cord, cerebrum, and cerebellum.

The brain stem has four parts: medulla, pons, midbrain, and diencephalon (Fig. 9-1A, B, C). The cerebellum is attached to the pons but will be discussed as part of the motor system. In the central nervous system *in situ*, the spinal cord is continuous with the medulla; the medulla is continuous with the pons; the pons is continuous with the midbrain; and the midbrain is continuous with the diencephalon. The diencephalon is buried in the center of the cerebrum and is separated from and connected to it via the internal capsule. In the gross central nervous system only the anterior and lateral surfaces of the pons and midbrain are visible; the remainder of the pons and midbrain is covered by the cerebellum. Similarly, only the anterior surface of the diencephalon (hypothalamus) is visible (Fig. 9–2A: mammillary bodies median eminence): the bulk of the diencephalon being covered by the cerebrum (Fig. 9–2A). In Figure 9–2B the

medial surface of the hemisphere has been exposed and the diencephalon can be seen (hypothalamus, thalamus, epithalamus).

The spinal cord is divided into segments as evidenced by the spinal nerve roots, but the segmental arrangement of the spinal cord stops above the highest cervical level. The brain stem and cerebrum (cerebral cortex and striatum) are divided according to obvious gross sections.

DIVISIONS OF THE BRAIN STEM ACCORDING TO THE VENTRICULAR SYSTEM

The medulla, pons, and midbrain will be divided according to their relationship to the ventricular system which will herein become the central structure; all portions of the brain stem when superficially identified in terms of position will be described as being in front of, behind, or at the sides of the ventricular system (Fig. 9–3A). Structures lying anterior to the ventricular system form the tegmentum or floor, while structures lying posterior form the roof or tectum. The fiber tract connecting the cerebral cortex with the brain stem and spinal cord is the

217

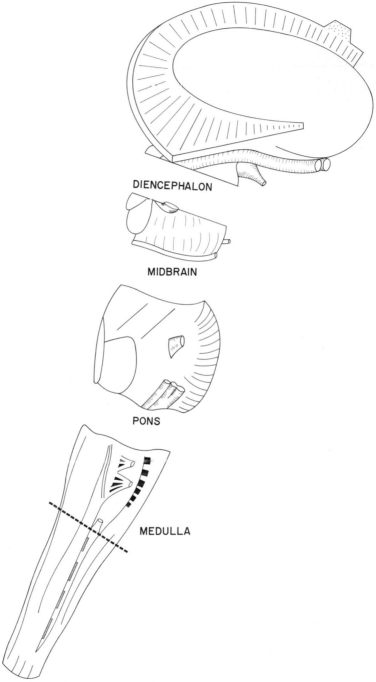

Figure 9–1A Lateral surface of brain stem identifying spinal cord, medulla, pons, midbrain, and diencephalon.

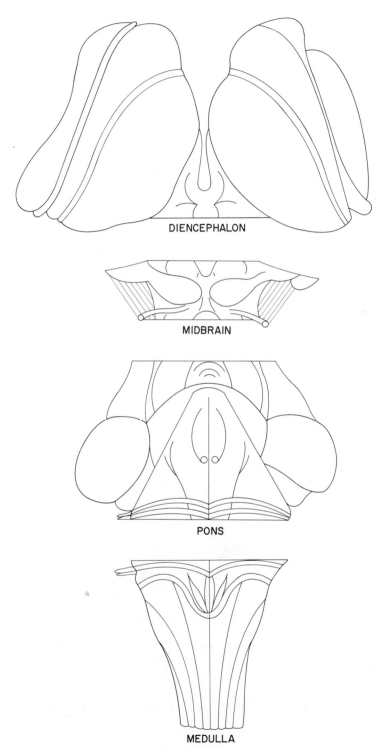

DIENCEPHALON

MIDBRAIN

PONS

MEDULLA

Figure 9–1 *Continued. B* Posterior surface of brain stem.

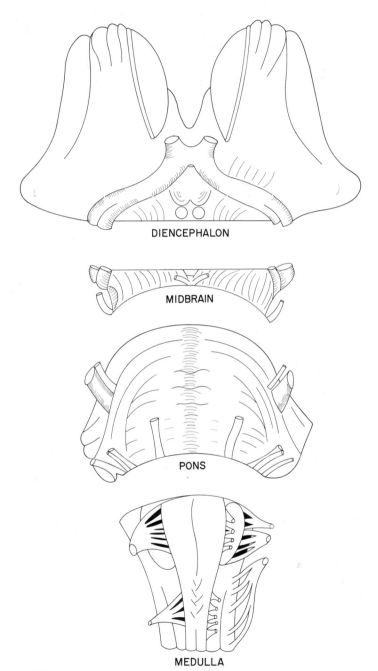

DIENCEPHALON

MIDBRAIN

PONS

MEDULLA

Figure 9–1 *Continued. C* Anterior surface of brain stem.

most recent addition to the brain; it forms the most anterior surface of the midbrain, pons, and medulla and is called the basis.

Structures lying lateral to the ventricle form the walls. The walls at the medullary and pontine levels are formed by cerebellar peduncles, while at the midbrain level the walls and roof are formed by the superior colliculi. At the diencephalic levels the corpus callosum and choroid plexus form the roof. The optic chiasm and mammillary bodies make up the floor, while the diencephalon proper forms the massive walls.

Throughout the medulla and pons, the undifferentiated gray (cellular) areas forming the walls or floor of the ventricular system will be called ventricular gray. In the midbrain the term used will be periaqueductal gray.

In *lower medullary regions,* the medulla looks like the spinal cord, with only a small canal present (Fig. 9-3A). The roof is formed by the fiber tract, conveying tactile and proprioceptive information from the body, and by the fasciculus gracilis and the fasciculus cuneatus. Internal to these fiber tracts are found the secondary nuclei (the nucleus gracilis and nucleus cuneatus) wherein the axons synapse. The floor of the medulla contains other fiber tracts and nuclei, with the corticospinal tract forming the basis at this level termed the medullary pyramids.

Progressing superiorly in the central nervous system, the ventricular system widens laterally as the medullary and pontine tegmentum expands due to the presence of nuclei which carry on special functions located in these segments of the brain stem.

The roof of the fourth ventricle in the lower medullary levels is nonnervous and is formed by the choroid plexus and the pia mater. In the upper medullary and pontine levels the cerebellum forms the tectum (Fig. 9-3A, B). Pontine levels of the brain stem (Fig. 9-3B) can be identified by the presence of the massive pontine basis which obscures the pontine tegmentum.

In *midbrain levels* (Fig. 9-3C. D), the ventricular cavity narrows to form the cerebral aqueduct which passes through the center of the midbrain. The superior and inferior colliculi form the tectum and walls of the midbrain. The midbrain tegmentum is continuous with the pontine tegmentum below and the hypothalamic zone of the diencephalon above. The basis of the midbrain is the massive paired cerebral peduncles which contain axons that connect the cerebral hemispheres to the brain stem and spinal cord.

In *diencephalic levels* (Fig. 9-3E), the ventricle (the third ventricle) is a slit separating the massive walls of the diencephalon. (Remember that the diencephalon and the third ventricle can only be visualized after the cerebral cortex and corpus callosum have been removed.) In diencephalic levels, the roof and floor of the ventricle are small, while the walls are massive and contain the nuclei and tracts that form the diencephalon.

CRANIAL NERVES

Scattered throughout the tegmentum of the brain stem are motor and sensory nuclei that innervate skin, muscles, and glands in the head and neck and the viscera in the thorax and abdomen; these are the cranial nerves (Fig. 9-4 A B). There are 12 pairs of cranial nerves, 11 of which are found in the brain stem. A detailed discussion of the cranial nerves will be found in Chapter 10. Here we will briefly identify them according to their location in the brain stem.

In the *medullary tegmentum* are five pairs of nerves innervating the tongue (nerve XII), the pharynx and larynx (nerves IX and X), the heart and lungs (nerve X), and the neck musculature (nerve XI). In the *medullary reticular formation* are several nuclei which control respiration and cardiovascular action and directly innervate the heart and lungs, thereby making the medulla and the adjacent pons the most vital portion of the central nervous system; complete destruction of this region produces death. The medulla also contains the motor neurons which control the vocal cords (ambiguous nucleus of nerve X), even though speech itself is a higher cortical function. Other nuclei within the medulla (ambiguous nuclei of nerves IX and X) innervate muscles in the pharynx and palate and permit food to be swallowed. The secondary neurons of the auditory and vestibular system (nerve VIII) are found in the medullary and pontine tegmentum.

The basis of the *pons* is the place where the cerebral cortex connects to the cerebellum, permitting integration of voluntary and reflex motor functions. In the pons tegmentum are located nerve VII, which innervates the

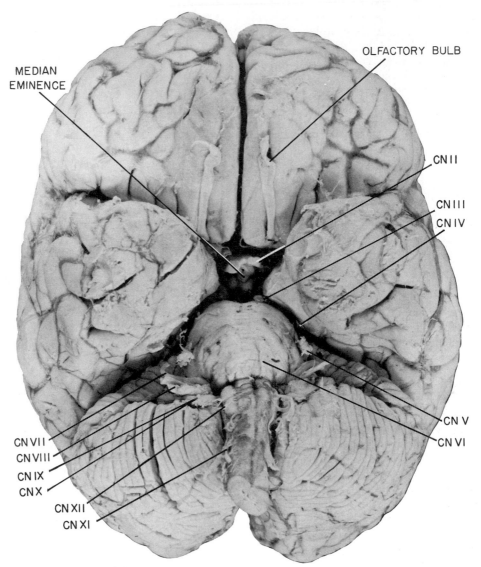

Figure 9–2A Ventral surface of gross brain.

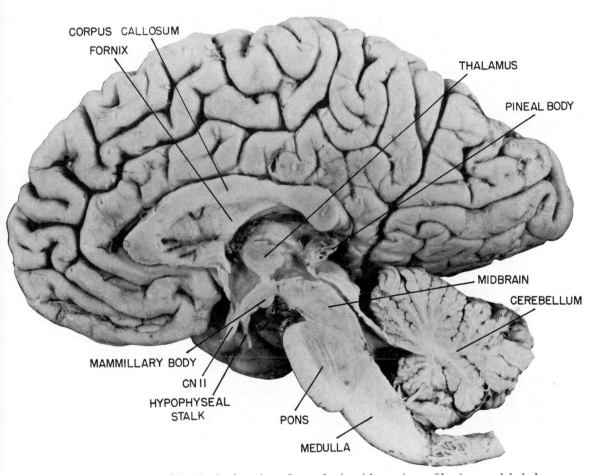

Figure 9–2 *Continued. B* Sagittal section of gross brain with portions of brain stem labeled.

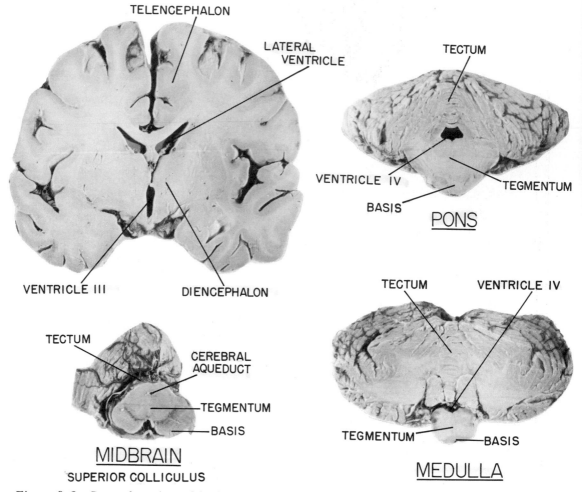

TELENCEPHALON

LATERAL VENTRICLE

TECTUM

VENTRICLE IV

TEGMENTUM

BASIS

PONS

VENTRICLE III

DIENCEPHALON

TECTUM

CEREBRAL AQUEDUCT

TEGMENTUM

BASIS

MIDBRAIN

SUPERIOR COLLICULUS

TECTUM

VENTRICLE IV

TEGMENTUM

BASIS

MEDULLA

Figure 9-3 Coronal section of brain stem: diencephalon, pons, superior colliculus, and medulla.

muscles of facial expression, and nerve V, which controls the muscles of mastication and mediates sensation from the skin, muscles, and joints in the head and neck. The nucleus of nerve VI, also located in the pons, controls the lateral rectus muscle which moves the eyeball laterally in the horizontal plane.

The inferior colliculus is actually two large paired nuclei which receive the ascending auditory pathway (Fig. 9-4 *A, B*). Cranial nerve IV is located in the tegmentum of the *midbrain* underlying the inferior colliculus; it controls the superior oblique muscle which pulls the eye down and out. The superior colliculus is laminated and receives input from the optic system as well as all the other sensory systems. It is important in coordinating eye movements to the position of the

head and body in space and is also an important center in relating pupil size to light levels. In the tegmentum underlying the superior colliculus is nerve III which provides the balance of innervation to the remaining extrinsic eye muscles and the intrinsic pupillary constrictor muscle.

The *thalamic* portion of the diencephalon is the last synaptic station before the cerebral cortex. All information going from subcortical regions in the brain and spinal cord must synapse in their respective thalamic nuclei before reaching the great analyzer, the cerebral cortex. Except for olfaction, all senses, including auditory, visual, somesthetic, gustatory, and visceral senses, have a thalamic relay nucleus.

The *hypothalamus*, located below the thalamus and adjacent to the third ventricle, controls the homeostatic mechanism, ionic balance, water, food intake, and endocrine levels) and plays an important role in behavior by controlling the autonomic nervous system. The thalamus interconnects with the cerebral cortex and basal ganglia via fiber tracts which run in the internal capsule. Fibers going from the cerebral cortex to the lower levels of the brain stem enter and run in the internal capsule. These fibers include the corticospinal, corticobulbar, and corticopontine tracts. The fibers connecting the thalamus to the cortex—the thalamocortical fibers—enter the internal capsule and continue up to the cortex.

DETAILED DESCRIPTION OF THE BRAIN STEM

As previously mentioned the segmental arrangement of the spinal cord stops superior to the first cervical spinal roots where the transition from spinal cord to medulla occurs. This transition is gradual and consists of a total reorganization of the pattern, seen in the spinal cord, of internal cell columns (gray matter) and external fiber columns (white matter). In the brain stem the columns of cells are organized into distinct nuclei, and individual tracts are recognizable in contrast to the nearly uniform pattern in the spinal cord. Finally, the tracts and nuclei are intermingled throughout the substance of the brain stem. The external sign of the segmental divisions of the spinal cord—the pairs of spinal nerves—stops at the spinomedullary junction. The rootlets attached to the brain stem represent the 11 pairs of cranial nerves, which are associated with the brain stem. The dorsal root ganglion of the spinal cord has an equivalent in the cranial nerve sensory ganglion associated with nerves V, VII, IX, and X.

The site of transition from the spinal cord to the medulla is found by passing a line from the superior border of the first cervical nerve root to the inferior border of the pyramidal decussation on the anterior surface (Figs. 9–5 and 9–6). Rostral to that line is the medulla. The separation of the medulla from the pons is made by passing a line from the superior border of the medullary stria on the floor of the fourth ventricle to the inferiormost margin of the massive pons itself; superior to this plane is the pons.

The boundary between pons and midbrain is found by passing a line from the inferior margin of the inferior colliculus to the superior margin of the pons; the midbrain is superior to this plane. The boundary between midbrain and diencephalon is formed by passing a line from the superior margin of the posterior commissure to the inferior margin of the mammillary bodies. The diencephalon is separated from the telencephalon laterally by the posterior limb of the internal capsule and superiorly by the lateral ventricles, corpus callosum, and fornix.

MEDULLA AND PONS: ANTERIOR SURFACE

In the midline on the anterior or ventral surface of the medulla and pons (Figs. 9–7 and 9–8) is found the *ventral median fissure* which continues from the spinal cord onto the medulla and stops at the basilar portion of the pons, the brachium pontis. The anterior spinal artery is found in the ventral median fissure. This fissure divides the two prominent pyramids which form the basilar portion of the medulla. These tracts provide voluntary control of all the skeletal muscles in the body. At the border between the spinal cord and medulla, the ventral median fissure may be obliterated by the decussation of the pyramids.

Lateral to the pyramids are the large inferior olives. In the medulla the rootlets of the hypoglossal nerve (cranial nerve XII) (Figs. 9–7 and 9–8) exit from the substance of the medulla between the olives and the pyramid. (The twelfth nerve innervates the intrinsic muscles of the tongue.) These rootlets identify the site of the usually inconspicuous ventral intermediate sulcus.

Exiting posterior to the olives are a nearly continuous series of nerve roots from cranial nerves IX X and XI. These rootlets identify the *ventral lateral sulcus* which is inconspicuous in the medulla. The rootlets for the spinal accessory nerve (nerve XI) originate from the upper cervical levels and the lowest portion of the medulla and usually stop at the inferior border of the olive. This motor nerve innervates the ipsilateral sternocleidomastoid and trapezoid muscles. The rootlets in a postolivary position come from the vagal (nerve X) and glossopharyngeal (nerve IX) nuclei. The inferior three-fourths of the rootlets originate from the nuclei of the

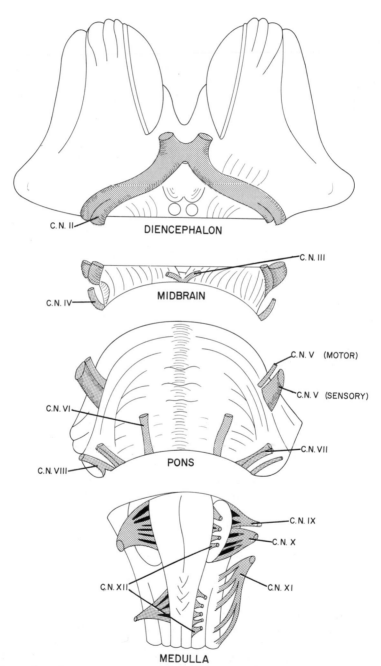

Figure 9-4A Ventral surface of brain stem showing the location of cranial nerves (C.N.) and nuclei.

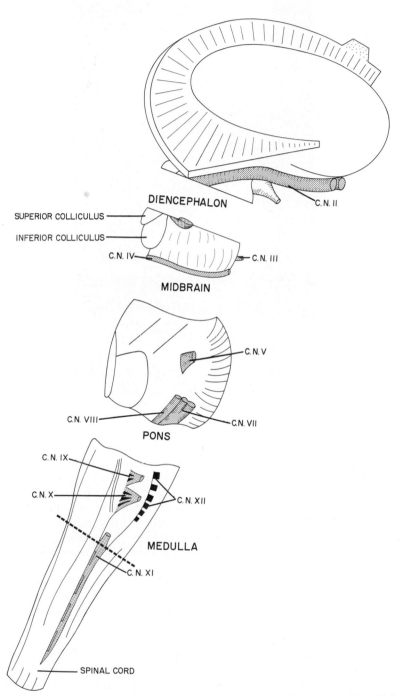

Figure 9-4 *Continued. B* Lateral surface of brain stem showing the location of cranial nerves (C.N.).

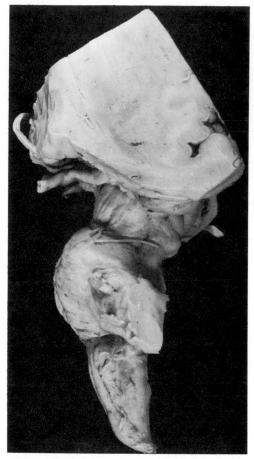

Figure 9–5 Lateral surface of brain stem.

vagus; the remaining one-fourth of the rootlets arise from the glossopharyngeal nuclei. The ninth cranial nerve carries sensations from the mucous membranes and taste buds in the posterior part of the mouth and pharynx and innervates the parotid gland and pharyngeal muscles. The vagus nerve (nerve X) provides motor innervation to the larynx and pharynx and preganglionic parasympathetic innervation to the viscera and conveys information from the gastrointestinal tract into the medulla.

The anterior surface of the massive pons consists of the *middle cerebellar peduncles*, or the *brachium pontis*, and contains nerve roots of cranial nerves V, VI, VII, and VIII. In addition to the middle cerebellar peduncles, there is also an inferior cerebellar peduncle, which interconnects the cerebellum and medulla, and a superior cerebellar peduncle, which connects the cerebellum to the mid-

brain; these tracts will be seen on the posterior surface of the medulla and pons.

The nerve rootlets of the abducens (VI) nerve emerge from the substance of the pons at the pontomedullary junctions, in a line with the hypoglossal rootlets. This nerve innervates the lateral rectus muscle of the eye.

The facial (VII) nerve and acoustovestibular (VIII) nerves emerge more laterally in the line with fibers of nerves IX, X, and XI; the fibers of nerve VIII are lateral to those of nerve VII. The rootlets of nerve VIII are more numerous than those of nerve VII and are divided into a smaller cochlear and a larger vestibular portion. Cranial nerve VIII is the receptor for hearing and balance. Cranial nerve VII has a smaller portion, the intermediate nerve, lying between the larger motor root of nerve VII and the vestibular portion of nerve VIII. These fibers are affer-

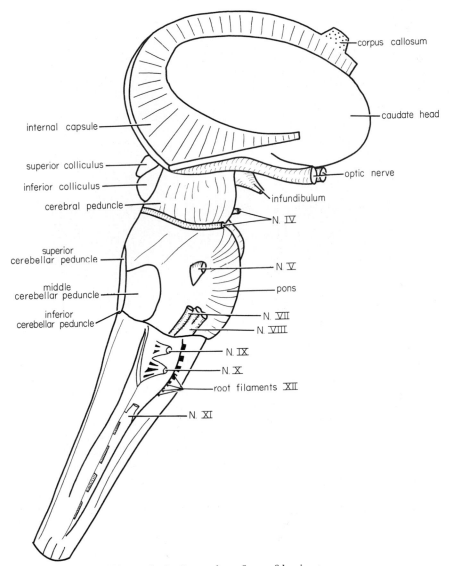

Figure 9-6 Lateral surface of brain stem.

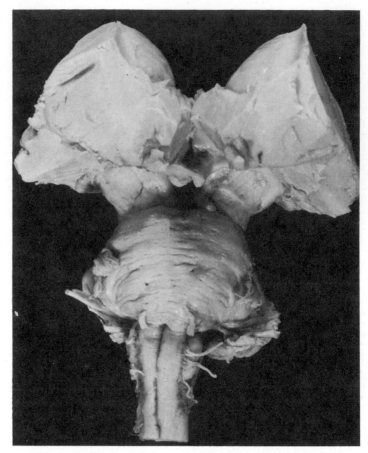

Figure 9-7 Anterior or ventral surface of brain stem.

ent and efferent visceral fibers, parasympathetic and special sensory; they carry sensations from mucous membranes and taste buds of the anterior two-thirds of the tongue and provide motor innervation to the facial muscles.

The trigeminal (V) nerve emerges from the substance of the pons laterally and usually consists of a small motor root and a large sensory root. Cranial nerve V carries sensory innervation for the head and innervates the muscles of mastication. The most anterior surface of the pontine basis contains a depression, the basilar sulcus, in which the basilar artery is found.

MEDULLA AND PONS: POSTERIOR SURFACE

In this view (Figs. 9–9 and 9–10), the cerebellar peduncles, which formed the medullary and pontine walls of the fourth ventricle, have been transected and the cere-

bellum removed, exposing the fourth ventricle. The posterior surface of the pons and medulla undergoes considerable change because of the presence of the fourth ventricle. The spinal canal is continuous with the most inferior portion of the fourth ventricle, which is a narrow channel in the lower medullary levels. In the lower medulla, the dorsal columns of the spinal cord (funiculus gracilis and funiculus cuneatus) migrate laterally, as the fourth ventricle enlarges from a narrow canal to a wide channel. The fiber tracts disappear as the tracts synapse on nuclei internal to the column, and the second order axons cross the midline and migrate to an anterior position behind the medullary pyramid, forming the medial lemniscus. The obex marks the place where the posterior neuronal roof of the spinal canal thins out and disappears, as the fourth ventricle opens and is covered only by pia mater and the choroid plexus, the tela choroidea.

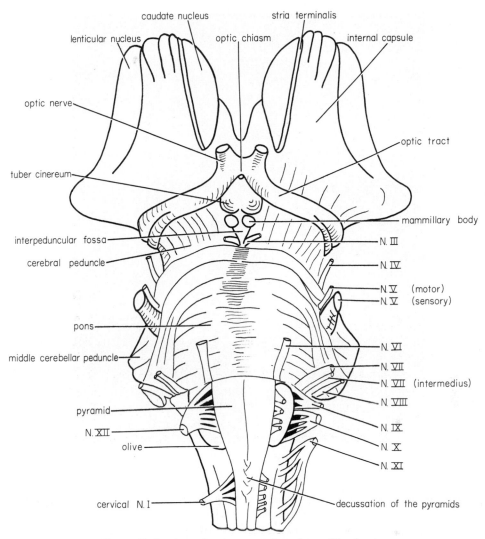

caudate nucleus
stria terminalis
lenticular nucleus
optic chiasm
internal capsule
optic nerve
optic tract
tuber cinereum
mammillary body
interpeduncular fossa
N. III
cerebral peduncle
N. IV
N. V (motor)
N. V (sensory)
pons
N. VI
middle cerebellar peduncle
N. VII
N. VII (intermedius)
N. VIII
pyramid
N. IX
N. XII
N. X
olive
N. XI
cervical N. I
decussation of the pyramids

Figure 9–8 Anterior or ventral surface of brain stem.

The dorsal median sulcus is seen at the midline on the spinal cord, medulla and pons. In lower medullary levels the funiculus gracilis is in a paramedian location. In the medulla, the tracts carrying primary somesthetic axons, the funiculus gracilis and the funiculus cuneatus, become more pronounced because of the presence of cell bodies which are internal to the fasciculus gracilis and the funiculus cuneatus and are called the gracile and cuneate nuclei. The enlargement of the funiculus gracilis is called the clava ("club-shaped"), while the enlargement of the cuneate funiculus is called the cuneate tubercle. The funiculus gracilis is separated from the funiculus cuneatus by the posterior intermediate sulcus which continues up from the spinal cord.

Lateral to the funiculus cuneatus is the trigeminal funiculus which is usually not prominent and continues down into the upper cervical level and contains the spinal tract and nucleus of the trigeminal nerve (nerve V). The primary axons of nerve V are so numerous that pontine, medullary, and upper cervical levels are required to provide enough secondary cell bodies for all the axons to terminate.

Lateral and anterior to the trigeminal funiculus is the lateral funiculus, which is also not usually prominent and is found posterior to the olivary eminence. On the sur-

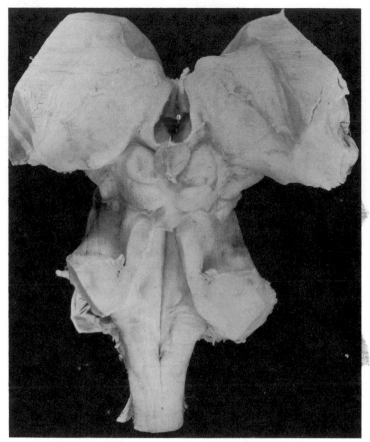

Figure 9–9 Posterior surface of brain stem.

face the lateral funiculus contains the dorsal and ventral spinocerebellar tracts; internally it contains the pain and temperature fibers, the lateral spinothalamic tract. At the upper medullary level the gracile and cuneate funiculi and nuclei have disappeared and the trigeminal funiculus is covered first by the dorsal spinocerebellar tract and then by the restiform eminence which contains the dorsal spinocerebellar tract and olivo-reticular fibers which unite and form the inferior cerebellar peduncle or restiform body.

In the medullary, pontine, and midbrain levels the floor of the fourth ventricle contains cranial nerve nuclei. Throughout the medulla, the paramedian hypoglossal trigone is separated by the dorsal median sulcus.

The hypoglossal trigone identifies the position of the nucleus of nerve XII, which innervates the intrinsic muscles of the tongue. Lateral to the hypoglossal trigone (nerve XII) lies the vagal trigone which marks the location of the dorsal motor nucleus of the vagus

nerve (nerve X). In lower medullary levels the nuclei of nerves X and XII are covered by the funiculus gracilis and the nucleus gracilis which disappear as the secondary axons form the medial lemniscus.

In pontine regions, the hypoglossal and vagal trigone are replaced by the median eminence which at inferior pontine levels has a prominent swelling, the facial colliculus. This marks the location of the nucleus of nerve VI and the genu of nerve VII.

Lateral to the vagal trigone and median eminence is a sulcus of variable constancy but of functional significance — the sulcus limitans. This sulcus marks the separation between the embryological alar and basal plates. Sensory nuclei develop in the alar plates while the basal plates form motor nuclei. This functional separation applies only to the nuclei in the floor of the fourth ventricle. In lower medullary levels the sensory area on the floor of the fourth ventricle receives both general and special sensations from the viscera via nerve X, while in upper

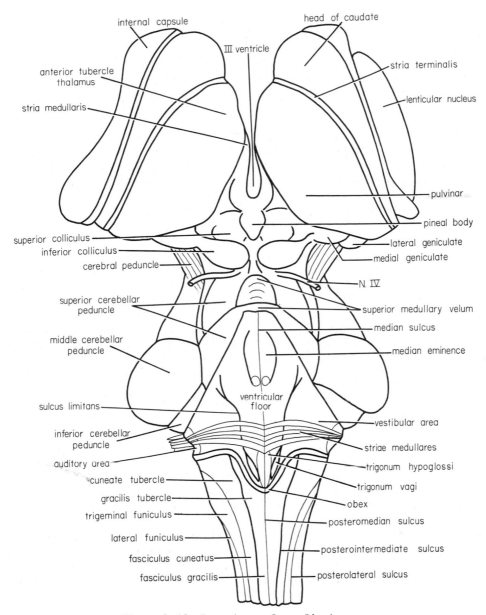

Figure 9-10 Posterior surface of brain stem.

medullary and lower pontine levels this region receives input from the inner ear via cranial nerve VIII.

The ventricular floor in this region also contains the second order auditory and vestibular nuclei. The vestibular fibers synapse in the medially placed vestibular area while the primary auditory fibers terminate in the more laterally placed acoustic tubercle (cochlear nuclei) which appears on the surface of the inferior cerebellar peduncle.

MIDBRAIN: POSTERIOR AND ANTERIOR SURFACES

The posterior surface (Figs. 9-9 and 9-10) of the midbrain has two pairs of conspicuous enlargements, the superior and inferior colliculi, which together form the tectum of the midbrain. The medial geniculate nucleus of the thalamus is attached to the lateral margin of the superior colliculus. A band of fibers, the brachium of the inferior colliculus, extends from each inferior colliculus along the border of the superior colliculus up to the medial geniculate nuclei of the diencephalon. Cranial nerve IV exits from the brain stem at the caudal margin of the inferior colliculus (Fig. 9–5). This is the only cranial nerve with rootlets on the posterior surface of the brain. Fibers of the optic tract may be traced past the lateral geniculate onto the superior colliculus.

The ventral or anterior surface of the midbrain is formed by the cerebral peduncles in which are found the corticospinal, corticobulbar, and corticopontine fibers. The cerebral peduncles are separated by the deep interpeduncular fossa where the arterial and venous supply enters the midbrain and where the rootlet of nerve III exits from the brain. Removal of these vessels leaves small perforations in the anterior surface of the midbrain forming the posterior perforated substance. The rootlets of nerve III exit from the tegmentum of the midbrain in the interpeduncular fossa on the most medial surface of the peduncle and innervate all extrinsic eye musculature except for the lateral rectus and superior oblique muscles.

DIENCEPHALON: VENTRAL AND POSTERIOR SURFACES

The only external features seen in the diencephalon are noted on the ventral surface of the brain (Figs. 9–7 and 9–8): the mamillary bodies, the hypophyseal stalk, and the optic chiasm and tract. Only after the cerebral hemispheres and corpus callosum are removed, as in Figures 9–9 and 9–10, can the entire diencephalon be seen. From the posterior surface the third ventricle is seen separating the diencephalon into two identical structures (Figs. 9–9 and 9–10). Commonly, a small mass, the massa intermedia, is seen in the third ventricle.

The diencephalon consists of four parts: (1) epithalamus, (2) thalamus and metathalamus, (3) hypothalamus, and (4) subthalamus (Fig. 9–11).

Epithalamus. On the superior surface, posteriorly, the epithalamus is visible at the midline; it consists of pineal gland, habenular trigone, and stria medullaris.

Thalamus and Metathalamus. The thalamus is seen only on the posterior surface (Figs. 9–9 and 9–10) and it forms the bulk of the diencephalon and appears to be continuous with the tegmentum of the midbrain. Anteriorly, it has a small prominence, the anterior tubercule, and posteriorly a larger swelling, the pulvinar. The detailed structure of the thalamus is best seen in coronal sections. In this coronal section (Fig. 9–11) the internal capsule, the tail of the caudate nucleus, and the stria terminalis mark the lateral boundary of the thalamus, while the lateral ventricle, the corpus callosum, and the fornix mark its superior and anterior borders. The thalamus is the primary relay center for all senses except smell. Crude awareness of pain, touch, temperature, and pressure are found here. All systems which connect with the cerebral hemispheres must synapse in the thalamus before they are projected onto the cerebral cortex.

The metathalamus (Figs. 9–9 and 9–10) consists of two nuclei located on the lateral surface of the midbrain: the medial and lateral geniculate nuclei. The medial geniculate nucleus receives the auditory fibers via the brachium of the inferior colliculus, and

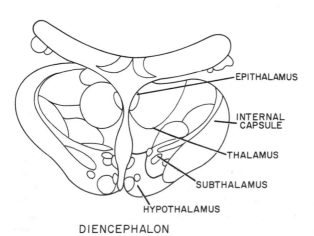

DIENCEPHALON

Figure 9–11 Coronal section of diencephalon.

the lateral geniculate nucleus receives fibers via the optic tract.

Hypothalamus. The hypothalamus is smaller than the thalamus and is functionally very important because of its relationship to behavior and emotions. The hypothalamus forms the walls and floor of the third ventricle below the hypothalamic sulcus. The following parts of the hypothalamus are seen on the anterior surface of the gross brain (Figs. 9–7 and 9–8): the infundibulum, the tuber cinereum, and the mammillary body. Other nuclear masses can be identified in brain sections stained with the Nissl method.

Subthalamus. The subthalamus cannot be seen in the gross brain or in a hemisected brain. In an appropriate coronal section (Fig. 9–11) it can be seen medial to the internal capsule below the thalamus and lateral to the hypothalamus. It consists of the zona incerta, the subthalamic nucleus, and the tegmental or prerubral field of Forel and small portions of substantia nigra and red nucleus. It is an important station in the extrapyramidal (involuntary) motor system.

BLOOD SUPPLY TO THE BRAIN STEM (Fig. 17–18)

The arterial blood supply to the medulla, pons, midbrain, and cerebellum originates from the posterior circulation (vertebral, basilar, and posterior cerebral arteries). The blood supply to the diencephalon originates from the anterior circulation (internal carotid, middle, and anterior cerebral arteries) and from the posterior circulation (posterior cerebral artery). The blood supply to the medulla, pons, and midbrain is derived from paramedian and circumferential branches of the posterior circulation.

Medulla. Paramedian branches of the vertebral artery supply the medullary pyramids, the inferior olive, the medial lemniscus, the tectospinal tract, the medial longitudinal fasciculus, and the hypoglossal nucleus and root. A circumferential branch of the vertebral artery (inferior cerebellar artery) irrigates the following structures in the tegmentum of the medulla: cranial nuclei of nerve X, ambiguous nucleus (of nerves X and XII), descending nucleus and root of nerve V, lateral spinothalamic tract, inferior cerebellar peduncles, the dorsal and ventral spinocerebellar tracts, descending and medial vestibular nuclei, and the descending sympathetic fibers.

Pons. Paramedian branches of the basilar artery supply the medial surface of the pontine basis and tegmentum, including the nucleus and rootlets of nerve VI. A circumferential branch of the basilar artery (anterior inferior cerebellar artery) supplies the lateral portion of the pontine basis and the lateral portion of the pontine tegmentum, including the rootlets and nuclei of nerves V and VII, the dorsal and ventral cochlear nuclei of nerve VIII, the superior, lateral, and rostral portions of the medial and descending vestibular nuclei, the lateral spinothalamic tract, and the middle and superior cerebellar peduncles.

Midbrain. Paramedian branches of the posterior cerebral artery supply the medial half of the cerebral peduncle, the nucleus and rootlet of nerve III, and much of the red nucleus. A circumferential branch of the basilar artery (superior cerebellar artery) supplies the superior cerebellar surface and a portion of the inferior colliculus, while a circumferential branch of the posterior cerebral artery (quadrigeminal artery) supplies the superior cerebellar peduncle, the remainder of the red nucleus, the lateral half of the cerebral peduncle, and the superior and inferior colliculus.

Diencephalon. The rostral part of the diencephalon is supplied by penetrating branches from the middle cerebral artery (striatal and thalamostriatal arteries), while the caudal part of the diencephalon, including the geniculate nuclei, subthalamus, pulvinar, ventral posterior medial, ventral posterior lateral, and ventral lateral nuclei of the thalamus, is supplied by penetrating branches from the posterior cerebral artery. The blood supply to the hypothalamus and hypophysis is discussed in Chapter 16.

Cerebellum. The posterior inferior surface of the cerebellum is supplied by the posterior inferior cerebellar artery (a circumferential branch of the vertebral artery). The anterior inferior surface of the cerebellum is supplied by the anterior inferior cerebellar artery (a circumferential branch of the basilar artery). The superior surface of the cerebellum is irrigated by the superior cerebellar artery (a circumferential branch of the basilar artery).

10

Cranial Nerves

STANLEY JACOBSON

COMPONENTS OF THE CRANIAL NERVES

In the spinal cord, the neurons are arranged in continuous columns of cells, each of which is connected to a structure with a specific function. This grouping of neurons with similar anatomical and physiological functions is called a *nerve component*. In the spinal cord, the neurons innervate general structures such as skin, skeletal muscles, blood vessels, glands, and viscera. They do not innervate the special sense organs: the eye, the ear, or the taste buds.

In the brain stem, cranial nerve nuclei that innervate structures of a similar embryonic origin are found in the same approximate position throughout the medulla, pons, and midbrain. These nuclei are arranged in discontinuous columns, usually in close proximity to the ventricular floor.

All the motor and sensory nuclei in the spinal cord are of a general nature and are designated as follows in the nerve component scheme of Herrick.

Motor (efferent)
Somatic (skeletal muscle)—GSE General somatic efferent
Visceral (smooth muscle)—GVE General visceral efferent
Sensory (afferent)

Somatic (cutaneous and proprioceptive)—GSA General somatic afferent
Visceral—GVA General visceral afferent

In the spinal nerves we recognize four types of neurons: GSE, GVE, GSA, and GVA. In the cranial nerves, in addition to these categories, we find neurons innervating more specialized sensory receptors (ear, eye, taste buds) or muscles in the face, pharynx, and larynx, which originated from pharyngeal arches. These special categories (abbreviated SVE for special visceral efferent, SVA for special visceral afferent, and SSA for special somatic afferent) are present only in cranial nerves. The components of the cranial nerves are designated as follows (See Fig. 10–1):

1. Motor innervation to muscles of presumed somite origin. The *general somatic efferent column* (GSE) consists of the motor nuclei of nerve III (superior colliculus), nerve IV (inferior colliculus), nerve VI (pons), and nerve XII (medulla). The column is adjacent to the midline underlying the ventricular gray.

2. Motor innervation from the cranial portion of the parasympathetic nervous system to smooth muscle (Fig. 10–13). The *general visceral efferent column* (GVE) contains the Edinger–Westphal nucleus of the superior colliculus, the superior salivatory nuclei of

236

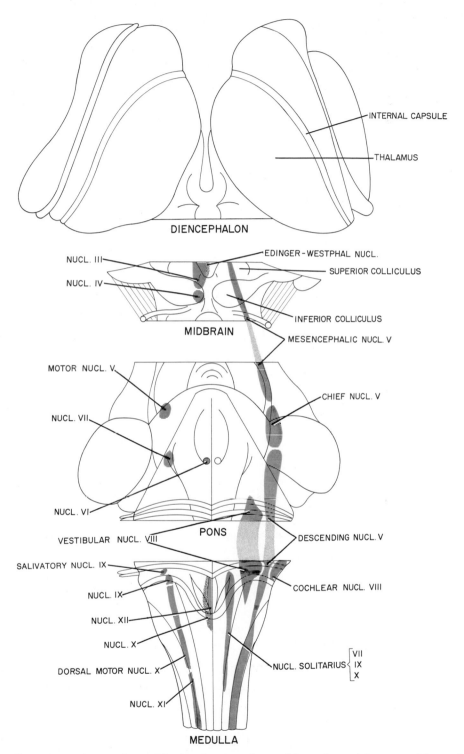

Figure 10–1 Posterior surface of brain showing the position of cranial nerves. Motor function is labeled on left side; sensory on right side.

cranial nerve VII (pons), the inferior salivatory nucleus of nerve IX (medulla), and the dorsal motor nuclei of nerve X (medulla). These nuclei are found lateral to the GSE column.

3. Motor innervation to muscles of visceral and pharyngeal origin. The *special visceral efferent column* (SVE) consists of the motor nucleus of nerves V, VII, IX and X (pons and medulla). These nuclei are not found near the ventricular system, but have migrated and are located in the ventral-lateral margin of the tegmentum.

4. Visceral and gustatory sensation. The *general and special visceral afferent column* (GVA and SVA) consists of the solitary nucleus in the medulla underlying the ventricular gray, lateral to the sulcus limitans. The

Table 10–1 *Cranial Nerve Components*

Cranial Nerve		Location of Cell Bodies	Functions
I Olfactory	SVA	Neuroepithelial cells in nasal cavity	Olfaction
II Optic	SSA	Ganglion cells in retinae	Vision
III Oculomotor	GSE	Oculomotor nucleus in tegmentum of upper midbrain	Eye movements, all eye muscles except the lateral rectus and superior oblique muscles
	GVE	Edinger-Westphal nucleus in tegmentum of upper midbrain—preganglionic to ciliary ganglion	Pupillary constriction and accommodation of lens for near vision
IV Trochlear	GSE	Trochlear nucleus in tegmentum of lower midbrain	Eye movements (contralateral), superior oblique muscle
V Trigeminal	GSA	Primary trigeminal ganglion, secondary mesencephalic (midbrain), sensory (pons), and descending nuclei (pons, medulla, upper cervical levels)	Cutaneous and proprioceptive sensations from skin and muscles in face, orbit, nose, mouth, forehead, teeth, and meninges, and anterior two-thirds of tongue
	SVE	Motor nucleus in pons	Innervation of muscles of mastication: masseter internal and external pterygoid, temporal, mylohyoid, and anterior belly of diagastric tensor velum palatini, and tensor tympani muscles
VI Abducens	GSE	Abducens nucleus in tegmentum of pons	Eye movements, ipsilateral, involving lateral rectus muscle
VII Facial	SVE	Motor nucleus in lateral margin of pons	Muscles of facial expression and platysma; extrinsic and intrinsic ear muscles; stapedius muscle
	GVE	Superior salivatory nucleus—preganglionic to ganglia associated with these glands	Secretions from glands of nose and palate and the lacrimal, submaxillary and sublingual glands
	SVA	Primary geniculate ganglion; Secondary Nucleus solitarius	Gustatory sensations from taste buds in anterior two-thirds of tongue

primary cell bodies are located in the sensory ganglia of nerves VII, IX, and X, and the axons of these cells enter the central nervous system, run in the fasciculus solitarius, and terminate in the solitary nucleus. General sensation fibers from the viscera as well as the taste fibers synapse in this column.

5. Cutaneous and proprioceptive sensations from the skin, and the muscle in the head and neck. The *general somatic afferent column* (GSA) is located throughout the brain stem and upper cervical levels and consists of the mesencephalic nucleus of nerve V (midbrain), the chief sensory nucleus of nerve V (midpontine), and the descending nucleus of nerve V (lower pons—upper cervical level). The mesencephalic nucleus is located in the lateral margins of the peri-

Table 10–1 *Continued.*

CRANIAL NERVE		LOCATION OF CELL BODIES	FUNCTIONS
VIII Vestibulo-acoustic	SSA	Primary spiral ganglion, temporal bone; Secondary cochlear nuclei in medulla	Audition
	SSA	Primary vestibular ganglion, temporal bone; Secondary vestibular nuclei in medulla and pons	Equilibrium, coordination, orientation in space
IX Glosso-pharyngeal	GVE	Inferior salivatory nucleus—preganglionic to optic ganglion	Secretions from parotid gland
	SVE	Nucleus ambiguus	Swallowing, stylopharyngeus muscle
	GVA	Primary inferior ganglion; Secondary Nucleus solitarius	Visceral sensations, introceptive palate and posterior one-third of tongue, carotid body
	SVA	Primary inferior ganglion; Secondary Nucleus solitarius	Gustatory sensations from taste buds in posterior one-third of tongue
X Vagus	GVE	Dorsal motor nucleus—preganglionic parasympathetic innervation	Smooth muscle in heart, blood vessels, trachea, bronchi, esophagus, stomach, intestine to lower half of large intestine
	SVE	Nucleus ambiguus	Phonation and glutination by innervators of larynx and pharynx
	GVA	Primary inferior ganglion; Secondary Nucleus solitarius	Visceral sensation from pharynx, larynx, aortic body and from thorax and abdomen.
	SVA	Primary inferior ganglion; Secondary Nucleus solitarius	Gustatory sensations from taste buds in epiglottis and pharynx
XI Spinal accessory	SVE	C1–C4	Motor innervation, trapezius and sternocleidomastoid muscles in neck
XII Hypoglossal	GSE	Hypoglossal nucleus in medulla	Motor innervation of intrinsic muscles of tongue

aqueductal gray of the cerebral aqueduct and the upper ends of the fourth ventricle. The main sensory and descending nucleus of nerve V is located in the lateral margin of the tegmentum of the pons and medulla and forms much of the substantia gelatinosa of the dorsal horn of the upper cervical levels. General sensations from structures innervated by cranial nerves III, IV, VI, VII, XI, and XII are conveyed by these nerves into the central nervous system (CNS) where they synapse in the descending nucleus of nerve V trigeminal nuclei.

6. Special sensory information from the olfactory mucosa, retinae, and inner ear. The *special somatic afferent column* (SSA) includes the four nuclei of the vestibular nerve, the two nuclei of the cochlear nerve, which together make up cranial nerve VIII, and cranial nerves I and II, which carry olfactory and visual sensations respectively. The vestibular and cochlear nuclei are located in the dorsal lateral tegmentum underlying the fourth ventricle in the lower pontine and medullary levels (vestibular area and acoustic tubercle). Cranial nerve I is found attached to the inferior surface of the frontal lobe, while nerve II ends in the lateral geniculate nucleus of the metathalamus.

Table 10–1 describes each of the cranial nerve components and its function:

GENERAL FUNCTION OF CRANIAL NERVES

I. Olfactory Nerve. The olfactory nerve originates from receptor cells in the nasal mucosa. The unmyelinated nerve fibers combine into about 20 bundles, pierce the cribriform plate, and end in the glomerular layer of the olfactory bulb. (See Chapter 18 where the visceral brain is discussed.) This is the only cranial nerve associated with the telencephalon.

II. Optic Nerve. The optic nerve (Fig. 10–2) is really a tract in the central nervous system, since it is invested with glia and not Schwann cells. The cells of origin of the optic nerve are tertiary neurons, the ganglion cells in the retinae. These axons form the optic nerve, chiasm, and tract, and they end in the optic thalamus (lateral geniculate nucleus) and superior colliculus (See Chapter 19 on Visual system).

III. Oculomotor Nerve. The oculomotor nucleus (Fig. 10–3) is a motor nucleus and is found in the tegmentum of the midbrain at the superior collicular levels and may be differentiated into a somatic and visceral portion. The somatic portion consists of the paired lateral nuclear complex and an unpaired central nucleus. The Edinger-Westphal nucleus forms the visceral portion and

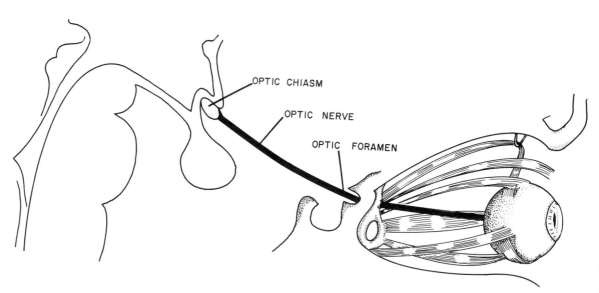

OPTIC CHIASM

OPTIC NERVE

OPTIC FORAMEN

Figure 10–2 Schematic view of the optic nerve and its central peripheral connections. (After House, E. L., and Pansky, B.: *A Functional Approach to Neuroanatomy.* New York, McGraw-Hill, 1967.)

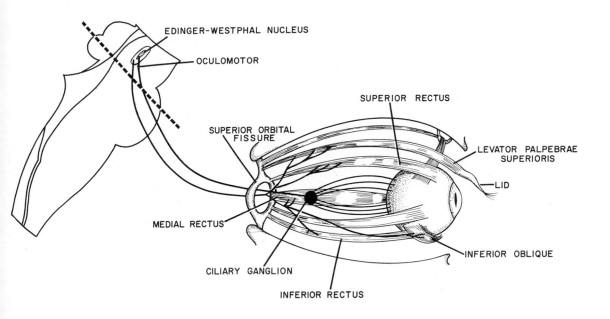

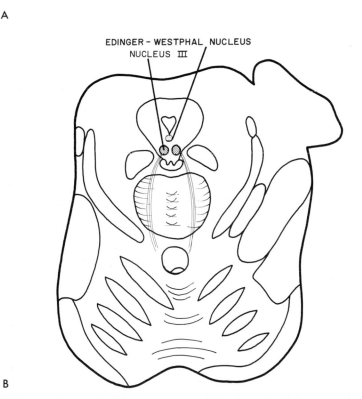

Figure 10–3   Schematic view of the oculomotor nerve, and its central and peripheral connections (*A*) as well as the location of the motor nuclei in midbrain (*B*). (After House, E. L., and Pansky, B.: *A Functional Approach to Neuroanatomy.* New York, McGraw-Hill, 1967.)

provides the preganglionic parasympathetic fibers to the ciliary ganglion from which postganglionic fibers pass to the muscles of accommodation and pupillary construction. There appears to be a representation of the individual muscles in the lateral nucleus but data is conflicting as to the exact location and extent of crossed and uncrossed innervation of the eye muscles.

The rootlet fibers from the nuclear complex of nerve III pass anteriorly through the tegmentum, some fibers running through the red nucleus and others going lateral or medial to it, finally entering the substance of the cerebral peduncle and uniting in the interpeduncular fossa to form nerve III. The fibers emerge superior to the pons between the superior cerebellar artery and the posterior cerebral artery, and the nerve penetrates the dura and enters the cavernous sinus where it is lateral to the internal carotid artery. The oculomotor nerve enters the orbit via the superior orbital fissure where it divides into superior and inferior divisions which then innervate the eye muscles.

The superior division innervates the levator palpebrae superioris and the superior rectus muscles, while the inferior division supplies the medial and inferior rectus and inferior oblique muscles and sends roots from the Edinger-Westphal nucleus to the ciliary ganglion.

In the physiological condition, normally the main axis of the eye is slightly adducted (slightly divergent) and the eyeballs and certain muscles work in tandem. The superior rectus muscle elevates the eyeball and turns it upward and inward. The medial rectus muscle adducts the eyeball. The inferior rectus muscle depresses the eyeball and adducts it to some degree, turning the eye downward and inward. The major action of the inferior oblique muscle occurs when the eyeball is adducted; contraction of the inferior oblique muscle will then elevate the eye. In the physiological position, contraction results in rotation. The levator muscle supplies the eyelid. The parasympathetic fibers from the Edinger-Westphal nucleus innervate the constrictor muscle of the pupil (via episcleral ganglia) and the ciliary muscle (via ciliary ganglia), permitting, respectively, dilation of the pupil and an increase in the thickness of the lens for accommodation (focus on objects within 6 inches of the eye).

Complete paralysis of nerve III produces ptosis of the lid, paralysis of medial and upward gaze, weakness in downward gaze, and dilation of the pupil. The eyeball deviates laterally and slightly downward; the dilated pupil does not react to light or accommodation. Paralysis of the intrinsic muscles (the ciliary, sphincter, or pupil) is called internal ophthalmoplegia, while paralysis of the extraocular muscles (recti and obliques) is called external ophthalmoplegia.

IV. Trochlear Nerve. The trochlear nucleus (Fig. 10–4) is purely motor and is located in the mediosuperior part of the tegmentum in the lower parts of the mesencephalon. It extends throughout the inferior collicular levels and is nearly continuous with the lateral nuclear complex of nerve III. The nucleus of nerve IV indents the medial longitudinal fasciculis (MLF).

Nerve IV is unique in that it is the only cranial nerve that has rootlets on the posterior surface of the brain stem. It originates on the floor of the cerebral aqueduct in the inferior collicular levels. The fibers proceed inferiorly and posteriorly in the periaqueductal gray, decussate in the anterior medullary velum, and exit from the substance of the brain at the caudal end of the inferior colliculus and run ventralward, lateral to the rootlets of nerve III. In the cavernous sinus the nerve is lateral to the rootlets of nerve III and enters the orbit through the superior orbit fissure where it terminates in the superior oblique muscle. The major action of the superior oblique muscle occurs with the eye adducted. With the eyeball in the physiological condition, contraction of this muscle will result in rotation of the eyeball. With paralysis of nerve IV these functions are lost. In a nuclear lesion of nerve IV the contralateral superior oblique muscle is paralyzed. A lesion in the nerve roots after decussation involves the ipsilateral muscle.

V. Trigeminal Nerve. The trigeminal nerve (Fig. 10–5) is the largest cranial nerve and provides sensory fibers to the face, including the posterior surface of the ear, the scalp up to the vertex, and the undersurface of the lower jaw, and motor fibers to the muscles of mastication. The sensory root is larger than the motor root. Associated with this nerve are one motor and three sensory nuclei in the brain stem and a large peripheral sensory ganglion, the semilunar

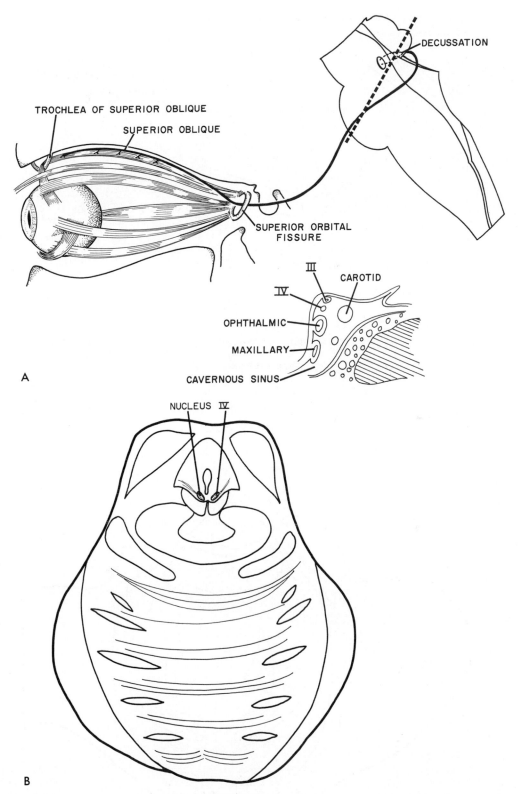

Figure 10-4 Schematic view of the trochlear nerve and its central and peripheral connections (*A*) as well as location of motor nuclei in the midbrain (*B*). (After House, E. L., and Pansky, B.: *A Functional Approach to Neuroanatomy.* New York, McGraw-Hill, 1967.)

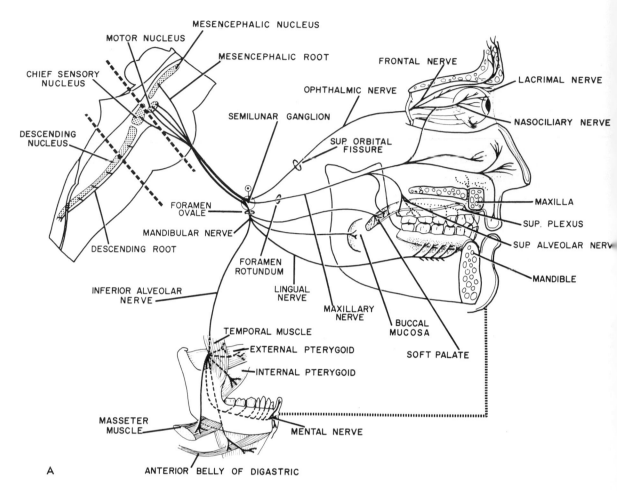

A

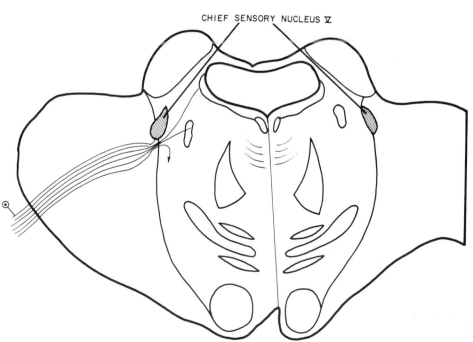

B

Figure 10-5 *See opposite page for legend.*

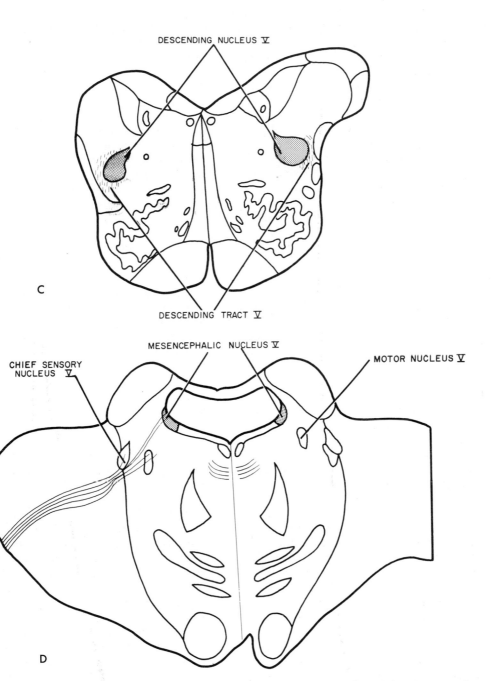

Figure 10–5 Schematic view of the trigeminal nerve and its central and peripheral connections (*A*) as well as the location of sensory nuclei in the pons (*B*) and medulla (*C*) and the location of motor and mesencephalic nuclei in pons (*D*). (After House, E. L., and Pansky, B.: *A Functional Approach to Neuroanatomy.* New York, McGraw-Hill, 1967.)

or gasserian ganglion. The motor nucleus of nerve V is located in midpontine levels medial to the trigeminal root at the lateral part of the reticular formation. The chief sensory nucleus of nerve V is found in the midpontine tegmentum, lateral to the root of nerve V. This nucleus is the equivalent of the gracile and cuneate nuclei. It receives cutaneous sensory information from the face and head and the nasal and oral cavities and transmits this information to the thalamus via fibers which travel with or adjacent to the medial lemniscus.

The descending or spinal nucleus of nerve V (Fig. 10–5C) is the equivalent of the dorsal horn of the spinal cord. Pain and temperature fibers synapse here. External to the cell bodies of the descending nucleus of nerve V is the descending tract of nerve V. Within this tract the fibers from the ophthalmic nerve descend to the third cervical level. The maxillary fibers descend to the first cervical level. Fibers from the mandibular and cranial nerves VII, IX, X, XI, and XII descend through the lower medullary levels. The secondary fibers are principally crossed as they ascend in the medial lemniscus to the ventral posterior medial nucleus in the thalamus.

The mesencephalic nucleus, located lateral to the fourth ventricle and the cerebral aqueduct in the upper pontine and midbrain levels, is proprioceptive from the facial muscles and the muscles of mastication. This is a unique nucleus since it is the only primary sensory nucleus (dorsal root ganglion equivalent) in the CNS. The mesencephalic nucleus and the motor nucleus provide a two-neuron reflex arc for the jaw jerk. There are three main branches of nerve V: ophthalmic, maxillary, and mandibular. The primary cell bodies for the sensory fibers are located, with one exception (mesencephalic nuclei), in the semilunar ganglion.

The *ophthalmic branch*, the smallest division of nerve V, innervates the skin of the forehead and scalp to the vertex, the upper eyelid, the skin of the anterior and lateral surfaces of the nose, the eyeballs, cornea, ciliary body, conjunctivum, and iris, the mucosa in the frontal and nasal sinuses, and the cerebellar tentorium. The nerve originates from the medial part of the ganglion, passes into the lateral wall of the cavernous sinus, and divides into its terminal branches in the superior orbital fissure.

The *maxillary division* of nerve V supplies the skin on the temples, the posterior half of the nose, the lower eyelid, the upper cheek and the upper lip, the dura in the middle cranial fossa (middle meningeal nerve), the gums and molar and premolar canine teeth (superior dental plexus), and the mucous membranes of the mouth, nose, and maxillary sinus. The nerve springs from the middle of the semilunar ganglion in the cavernous sinus. It leaves the middle cranial fossa via the foramen rotundum and enters the pterygopalatine fossa where it becomes the infraorbital nerve.

The *mandibular division* of nerve V is the largest of the three divisions and is formed by the union of the sensory and motor root at the inferior border of the ganglion. The motor root originates in the motor nucleus of nerve V in the pons, unites with the mesencephalic root, and exits from the middle cranial fossa in the foramen ovale where it then unites with the sensory root. The motor or masticator nerve innervates the muscles of mastication: the internal and external pterygoid, temporal, masseter, and mylohyoid muscles and the anterior belly of the digastric muscle.

These muscles function as follows: the *masseter muscle* elevates and slightly protrudes the mandible; the *temporal muscle* elevates and retracts the mandible; the external pterygoid muscle, working in unison with the other muscles, protrudes and depresses the mandible and singly causes the lateral motion of the jaw to the opposite side; the internal *pterygoid*, also working in unison with the other muscles, elevates and assists the external pterygoid muscle in protruding the mandible.

In mastication the jaws move up and down, forward and backward, and laterally. The masseter, temporal, and internal pterygoid muscles elevate the mandible; the external pterygoid muscle, in concert with the suprahyoid, mylohyoid, digastric, geniohyoid, and infrahyoid muscle and the depressors of the hyoid muscles (sternohyoid and amohyoid) along with gravity, depress the jaw. The internal and external pterygoid muscles assisted by the masseter muscle, protrude the jaw. The temporal and digastric muscles retract the jaw. The pterygoid muscles permit side-to-side movement.

The trigeminal nerve also innervates the tensor veli palatine and the tensor tympani muscles. The tensor veli palatine muscle tenses and draws the palate to one side which prevents food from entering into the nasal pharynx. The tensor tympani muscle pulls on the malleus which tenses the tympanic membrane and diminishes the amplitude of the vibration caused by a loud noise.

The sensory division of the mandibular branch of nerve V supplies the skin of the cheek, chin, lower jaws, and temporomandibular joint, and the dura in the middle and anterior cranial fossa, the lower teeth and gums (inferior dental plexus), the oral mucosa, and part of the ear.

Injury to the trigeminal nerve produces paralysis of the mastication muscles with the jaw deviating toward the side of the lesion. Injury also leads to loss of sensation of light touch, pain, and temperature in the face and to an absence of the corneal and sneeze reflexes.

Motor function of the trigeminal nerve is affected in various ways. Lesions in the pons may affect only the motor nuclei and produce a paresis or paralysis of the ipsilateral muscles. If the lesion is destructive, atrophy and fasciculations of the affected muscles result. The jaw jerk is also absent. As the cortical innervation of the muscles of mastication is bilateral, supranuclear lesions unilaterally may produce only a slight weakness with a minimal increase in the jaw jerk. A bilateral capsular or cortical lesion will produce marked paresis or even paralysis in the muscles of mastication with an exaggerated jaw jerk.

Pontine lesions usually produce injury to both the main sensory and motor nuclei causing paralysis of the muscles of mastication and diminished tactile sensation ipsilaterally. Tumors in the cerebellopontine angle or acoustic nerve may compress the trigeminal tubercle and cause an ipsilateral loss of the corneal reflex. Trigeminal neuralgia (tic douloureux) is a disorder of the sensory division of nerve V characterized by recurrent paroxysms of stabbing pains along the distribution of the involved branches. Trauma or infections in the area supplied by the nerve may account for the pathology, but in the majority of cases no known pathology is present. Medication may result in the remission of trigeminal neuralgia. In some cases a surgical approach is required to produce permanent relief.

VI. Abducent Nerve. The abducens nucleus (Fig. 10–6) is a purely motor nucleus and is located in the inferior pontine levels in the dorsal part of the pontine tegmentum posterior to the motor nucleus of nerve VII but surrounded by the looping fibers of nerve VII. Associated with the nucleus of nerve VI is the parabducens nucleus which relays impulses via the medial longitudinal fasciculus to coordinate contractions of the lateral rectus muscle of one eye with the medial rectus muscle of the other, producing conjugate horizontal deviations of the eyes. The nucleus of nerve VI and the fibers of nerve VII form a prominent structure in the floor of the pons, the facial colliculus. The fibers of nerve VI leave the nucleus medial to the rootlets of nerve VII. The fibers of nerve VI have the longest intracranial course of any cranial nerve which makes it most vulnerable to any disease process which affects the pons. The fibers pass inferiorly and emerge from the pons near the midline at the pontomedullary junction. The roots pierce the dura and enter the cavernous sinus below the medial to nerve III and lateral to the internal carotid artery. It enters the orbit via the superior orbital fissure and innervates the lateral rectus muscle which abducts or deviates the eye laterally. Injury to the nucleus or rootlets of nerve VI causes the eyeball to turn medially and makes it impossible to move the eye laterally on the side of the lesion.

VII. Facial Nerve. The facial nerve (Fig. 10–7) is primarily a motor nerve with a small sensory component. The motor root is larger than the sensory root. In the pons are one large motor nucleus and one sensory nucleus for nerve VII, while peripherally there is one sensory ganglion. The motor fibers supply the muscles associated with the second branchial arch (hyoid arch). The fibers originate from the motor nucleus of nerve VII in the lateral part of the reticular formation in the caudal pontine levels. The fibers leave the nucleus and pass medially and dorsally toward the fourth ventricle. Under the floor of the fourth ventricle, they pass over the dorsal surface of the nucleus of nerve VI and then turn anteriorly, forming the internal genu of the facial nerve. The fibers then pass laterally and anteriorly through the lateral portion of the pontine reticular formation and exit from the pons at its caudalmost border between the rootlets of nerves VI and VIII in the cerebellopontine angle. The nerve enters the posterior cran-

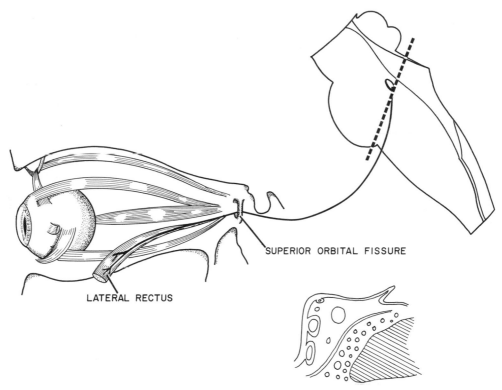

SUPERIOR ORBITAL FISSURE

LATERAL RECTUS

Figure 10–6 Schematic view of the abducens nerve and its central and peripheral connections. The location of the motor nucleus in the pons can be seen in Figure 10–7B. (After House, E. L., and Pansky, B.: *A Functional Approach to Neuroanatomy.* New York, McGraw-Hill, 1967.)

ial fossa and passes into the internal acoustic meatus where the motor and sensory divisions and nerve VIII lie separated from one another by only the arachnoid sheaths on the nerves.

In the meatus, the motor and sensory roots of nerve VII combine and enter the facial canal of the temporal bone. This nerve continues in the facial canal until it reaches the hiatus of the facial canal, where it bends around the anterior border of the vestibule of the inner ear forming the external genu of nerve VII. The geniculate ganglion is located at the external genu and provides the primary cell bodies of the intermediate or sensory root of nerve VII.

The sensory root fibers run through the facial canal into the internal acoustic meatus and then enter the pons, run through the lateral part of the reticular formation, and enter the tractus solitarius which is found just lateral to the sulcus limitans and is separated from the ventricular cavity by the aqueductal gray on the floor of the fourth ventricle. The

sensory root of nerve VII carries gustatory impulses from the taste buds in the anterior two-thirds of the tongue and cutaneous sensations from the anterior surface of the ear.

The motor and sensory roots continue in the facial canal between the inner and middle ear and turn and descend to the stylomastoid foramen where they emerge from the temporal bone. Just prior to leaving the stylomastoid foramen, the chorda tympani leaves nerve VII and enters its own small canal, then enters the tympanic cavity, and runs on the medial surface of the tympanic membrane, and onto the medial side of the manubrium. The nerve leaves the tympanic cavity and then emerges from the skull near the medial surface of the spine of the sphenoid and joins the lingual nerve at the medial surface of the lateral pterygoid muscle. It contains parasympathetic preganglionic fibers to the pterygopalatine ganglia and provides innervation to glands in the nasal cavity and palate and to the lacrimal gland, submandibular gland, and sublingual glands. It also carries taste sensation from the anterior two-thirds of the tongue.

The motor root innervates the stapedius muscle, the posterior belly of the digastric muscle, and the muscles of facial expression: frontal, orbicularis oculi, anterior auricular, corrugator supercilium, zygomatic, orbicularis oris, depressor labii, levator labii, levator anguli oris, nasalis, mentalis, platysma, buccinator, and risorius.

Injury to the facial nerve near its origin or in the facial canal produces paralysis of the motor, secretory, and facial muscles, a loss of taste in the anterior two-thirds of the tongue, and improper secretion in the lacrimal and salivary glands. The muscles in time will atrophy. Injury to nerve VII at the stylomastoid foramen produces ipsilateral paralysis of the facial muscles without affecting taste. Injury to the chorda tympani results in absence of taste in the anterior two-thirds of the tongue.

Injury to the facial nucleus in the pons produces ipsilateral paralysis of the facial muscles. Injury to just the nucleus or tractus solitarius is rare but it would produce a loss of taste on half of the tongue as the taste fibers from nerves VII and IX are found together in the tractus solitarius.

The cerebral innervation of the facial nucleus is unique in that the lower half of the facial muscles receive a crossed unilateral innervation, while the upper half of the facial muscles receive a bilateral innervation. A unilateral lesion in the appropriate part of the precentral gyrus will produce paralysis in the lower half on the opposite side, while a bilateral cortical involvement is necessary for paralysis of the upper facial musculature.

One of the more common involvements of the facial nerve is Bell's Palsy in which the entire nerve may be affected. This commonly results from swelling of the nerve somewhere in the facial canal, probably because of inflammation of the nerve. The patient will have sagging of the muscles in the lower half of the face and in the fold around the lips and nose, and widening of the palpebral fissure. There is an absence of voluntary control of facial and platysmal musculature. When the patient smiles the lower portion of the face is pulled to the unaffected side. Saliva and food tend to collect on the affected side. When the injury is distal to the ganglion there is excessive accumulation of tears as the eyelids do not move while the lacrimal gland continues to secrete.

VIII. Vestibulocochlear Nerve. The vestibulocochlear nerve (Fig. 10–8) has two divisions: the vestibular and cochlear nerves. The vestibular and cochlear nerves are attached to the medulla at its border with the pons lateral to the root of nerve VII. The cochlear nerve is smaller than the vestibular nerve and is lateral to it.

The vestibular nerve is concerned with equilibrium. Its primary bodies are bipolar and are located in the vestibular ganglia in the internal acoustic meatus. The fibers terminate in the vestibular nuclei located in the ventricular floor of the medulla. The vestibular nerve has five branches which originate from the hair cells in maculae of the saccule and utricle and from the cristae of the ampullae of the three semicircular canals.

The cochlear division of cranial nerve VIII originates from the spiral ganglion and terminates in the dorsal and ventral cochlear nuclei located on the external surface of the inferior cerebellar peduncle. The primary auditory fibers enter the cochlear nuclei and bifurcate, ending in the dorsal and ventral cochlear nuclei. Throughout the auditory system there is a tonotopic arrangement (see Chapter 14).

The secondary auditory fibers arise from the dorsal and ventral cochlear nuclei and form the three acoustic striae. The ventral acoustic stria originates from the ventral cochlear nucleus and courses through the ventral boundary of the pontine tegmentum, forming the trapezoid body. These fibers pass through the medial lemniscus, reach the superior olive, and migrate laterally to form the lateral lemniscus. The dorsal and intermediate striae arise from the dorsal cochlear nucleus and the dorsal one-half of the ventral cochlear nucleus. The dorsal stria crosses the midline ventral to the medial longitudinal fasciculus and joins the contralateral lateral lemniscus. The intermediate stria runs through the center of the reticular formation, crosses the midline, and enters the contralateral lateral lemniscus.

Some secondary auditory fibers end in the superior olivary nuclei, trapezoid nucleus, nucleus of the lateral lemniscus, and reticular formation. The superior olivary nucleus, the trapezoid nucleus, and the nucleus of the lateral lemniscus give origin to tertiary axons which ascend, primarily crossed, to the in-

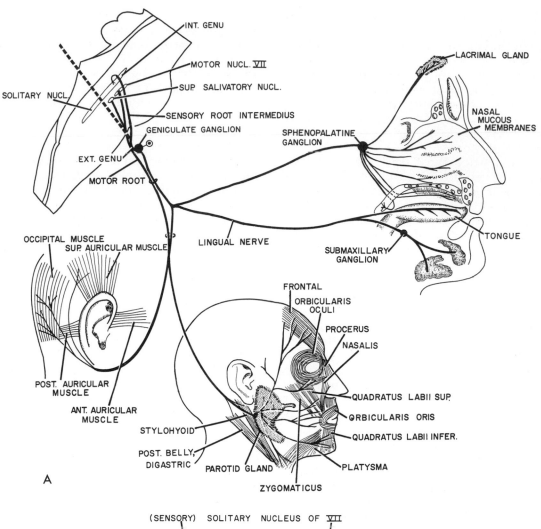

INT. GENU

MOTOR NUCL. VII

SOLITARY NUCL.

SUP. SALIVATORY NUCL.

SENSORY ROOT INTERMEDIUS

GENICULATE GANGLION

EXT. GENU

MOTOR ROOT

LACRIMAL GLAND

NASAL MUCOUS MEMBRANES

SPHENOPALATINE GANGLION

OCCIPITAL MUSCLE

SUP. AURICULAR MUSCLE

LINGUAL NERVE

TONGUE

SUBMAXILLARY GANGLION

POST. AURICULAR MUSCLE

ANT. AURICULAR MUSCLE

FRONTAL

ORBICULARIS OCULI

PROCERUS

NASALIS

QUADRATUS LABII SUP.

ORBICULARIS ORIS

QUADRATUS LABII INFER.

STYLOHYOID

POST. BELLY, DIGASTRIC

PAROTID GLAND

ZYGOMATICUS

PLATYSMA

A

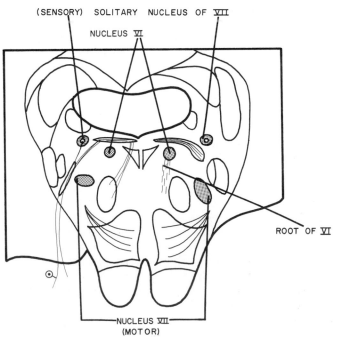

(SENSORY) SOLITARY NUCLEUS OF VII

NUCLEUS VI

ROOT OF VI

NUCLEUS VII (MOTOR)

B

Figure 10–7 *See opposite page for legend.*

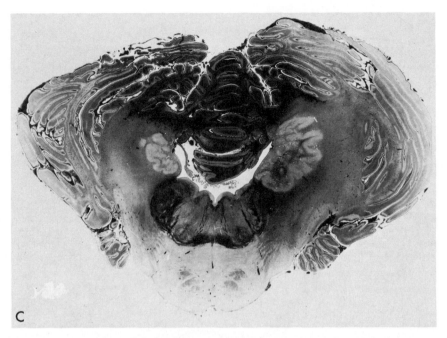

Figure 10-7 Schematic view of the facial nerve and its central and peripheral connections (*A*) as well as the location of the motor nuclei in the pons and the relation of the nucleus of nerve VI to the nucleus and rootlets of nerve VII (*B*). *C* is from term infant, myelin stains. (After House, E. L., and Pansky, B.: *A Functional Approach to Neuroanatomy.* New York, McGraw-Hill, 1967.)

ferior colliculus where many of the axons terminate or send collaterals into the inferior collicular nuclei. Fibers from the inferior colliculus and fibers from the lateral lemniscus form the brachium of the inferior colliculus which ends in the medial geniculate nucleus of the thalamus. All auditory fibers synapse in the medial geniculate and are projected from there into the auditory cortex, the transverse temporal gyri of Heschel.

Throughout the auditory system there are crossed and uncrossed fibers, so that a bilateral representation is found throughout the auditory system.

The cochlear nerve is concerned with hearing and originates from the spiral ganglion of Corti in the petrous portion of the temporal bone. The peripheral process originates from the hair cells in the spinal ganglion and the central process terminates on the cochlear nuclei or other nuclei in the auditory pathway.

The vestibular nerve originates from the vestibular ganglion. The primary fibers terminate mostly in the four secondary vestibular nuclei in the floor of the fourth ventricle. The secondary vestibular nuclei are the inferior (descending), lateral, medial, and superior nuclei (Fig. 10-8).

The inferior vestibular nucleus extends from the entrance of the vestibular nerve root, at the medullopontine junction, through the lower medullary levels. The medial vestibular nucleus is found medial to the inferior nucleus in these same levels. The medial and inferior vestibular nuclei form the prominent vestibular area on the floor of the fourth ventricle, lateral to the sulcus limitans. The inferior nucleus can be delimited by the presence of the myelinated bundles of the primary descending vestibular axons (Fig. 11-7). The lateral vestibular nucleus is found lateral to the roots of nerve VIII in the tegmentum. The superior vestibular nucleus lies in the angle formed by the floor and wall of the fourth ventricle and extends through the upper pontine levels in this same position. The superior cerebellar peduncle forms its dorsal border.

The primary vestibular fibers bifurcate into ascending and descending portions. The ascending axons end in the superior, lateral, and rostral portions of the medial nucleus, while the descending axons run in the in-

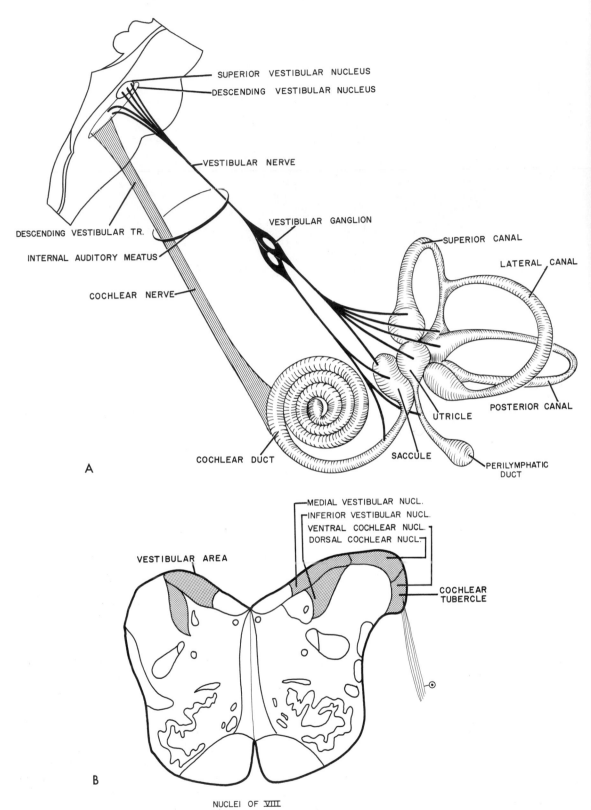

Figure 10-8 Schematic view of (*A*) the vestibulocochlear nerve and its central and peripheral connections and (*B*) the location of the vestibular and cochlear nuclei in the ventricular floor of the medulla. See Filmstrip frame 18. (After House, E. L., and Panksy, B.: *A Functional Approach to Neuroanatomy.* New York, McGraw-Hill, 1967.)

252

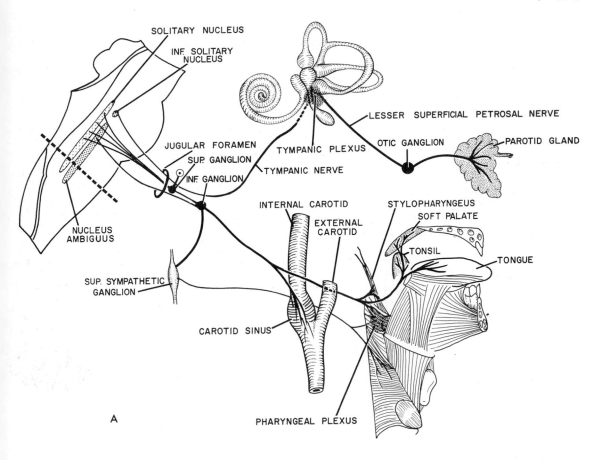

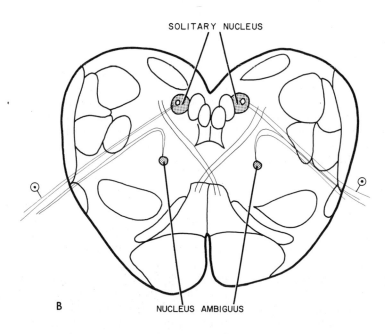

NUCLEI OF IX

Figure 10–9 Schematic view of the glossopharyngeal nerve and its central and peripheral connections (*A*) as well as the location of the motor nuclei in the medulla (*B*). (After House, E. L., and Pansky, B.: *A Functional Approach to Neuroanatomy.* New York, McGraw-Hill, 1967.)

ferior nuclei and provide collaterals to the medial nucleus. Primary vestibular fibers also run directly into the ipsilateral cerebellum, forming the juxtarestiform body (Fig. 29–9), projecting to the flocculus, nodulus, and uvula of the cerebellum. The secondary vestibular axons originate from the secondary vestibular nuclei and project to the cerebellum, reticular formation motor cranial nerve nuclei, and all levels of the spinal cord. Fibers from all the vestibular nuclei join the medial longitudinal fasciculus and are crossed and uncrossed with ascending and descending branches. Although there is no known vestibulothalamic pathway, vestibular impulses and responses have been noted in the temporal lobe of the cerebrum.

IX. Glossopharyngeal Nerve. The glossopharyngeal nerve (Fig. 10–9) is a mixed nerve and has sensory and motor nuclei in the medulla. The rootlets of nerve IX are found in the medulla in a postolivary position. The nerve trunk exits from the skull via the jugular foramen where it lies anterolateral to the vagus nerve. In the jugular foramen are found two swellings on the nerve trunk of nerve IX, the superior and inferior ganglia.

The sensory cell bodies are located in the superior and inferior ganglia and consist of SVA carrying gustatory sensations from the taste buds in the posterior third of the tongue and cutaneous sensations from the pharynx, auditory tube, middle ear, palatine tonsils, eustachian tube, and carotid sinus. The general and special visceral axons enter the medulla and run in the tractus solitarius in the middle and posterior medullary level, synapsing in the nucleus solitarius.

The secondary axons ascend bilaterally in the medial lemniscus up to the ventral posterior medial (VPM) nucleus in the thalamus.

The motor fibers of nerve IX originate from the most superior part of the nucleus ambiguus in the medulla. They pass posteriorly and laterally, exit from the medulla in a postolivary level, and distribute to the ipsilateral stylopharyngeus muscle in the pharynx. The preganglionic parasympathetic fibers originate from the inferior salivatory nucleus in the medulla and run via nerve IX to the otic ganglion, tympanic plexus, and smaller petrosal nerve below the foramen ovale. The postganglionic fibers pass via the auriculotemporal nerve to the parotid gland.

Lesions restricted to the nuclei or nerve roots of nerve IX are rare. Taste is lost on the posterior third of the tongue and the gag reflex is absent ipsilaterally. There is no response when the posterior pharyngeal wall and soft palate are stimulated. The functions of the parotid gland may also be impaired and can be evaluated by placing a highly seasoned food on the tongue and seeing if there is a copious flow from the duct.

X. Vagus Nerve. The vagus nerve (Fig. 10–10) has one sensory and two motor nuclei in the medulla and also has the most extensive distribution of any cranial nerve. Its roots are located in a postolivary position in the medulla in the posterolateral sulcus, in line with the fibers of nerve IX but inferior to them. They exit from the cranial cavity via the jugular foramen. In the jugular foramen is found the superior ganglion; the inferior ganglion is found just as the nerve leaves the jugular foramen of nerve X. In the neck the vagus nerve is found in the carotid sheath close to the common carotid artery and jugular vein.

The dorsal motor nucleus of the vagus nerve forms the vagal trigone on the floor of the fourth ventricle in the medullary levels. The dorsal motor nucleus of the vagus nerve provides preganglionic parasympathetic innervation to the ganglion in the walls of the pharynx, trachea, bronchi, esophagus, stomach, small and ascending portions of the large intestine, and the heart. The other motor division of the vagus nerve originates from the posterior two-thirds of the ambiguous nucleus in the medulla and connects to the striate muscles of the soft palate and pharynx, and the intrinsic muscles of the larynx and is thus important in swallowing and speech. The following muscles are innervated by the ambiguous portion of nerve X: the superior, middle, and inferior constrictors of the pharynx; the palatoglossus, palatopharyngeus, salpingopharyngeal, and levator palatine velum of the soft palate; the posterior cricoarytenoid, arytenoid, lateral cricoarytenoid, and thyroarytenoid of the larynx.

The primary cell bodies of the sensory fibers are located in the inferior ganglion and carry gustatory information from taste buds in the epiglottis and pharynx, cutaneous innervation from the base of the tongue and epiglottis, and general visceral sensation from all the structures receiving motor innervation – pharynx, larynx, heart,

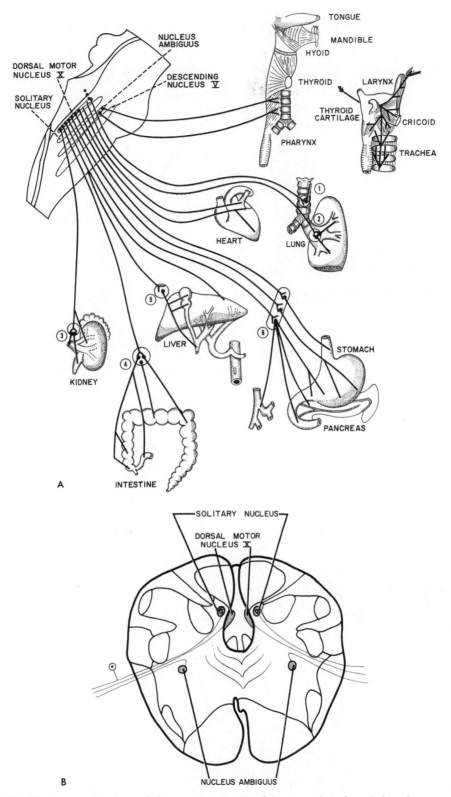

Figure 10-10 Schematic view of the vagus nerve and its central and peripheral connections (*A*) as well as the location of the motor and sensory nuclei in the medulla (*B*). (After House, E. L., and Pansky, B.: *A Functional Approach to Neuroanatomy.* New York, McGraw-Hill, 1967.)

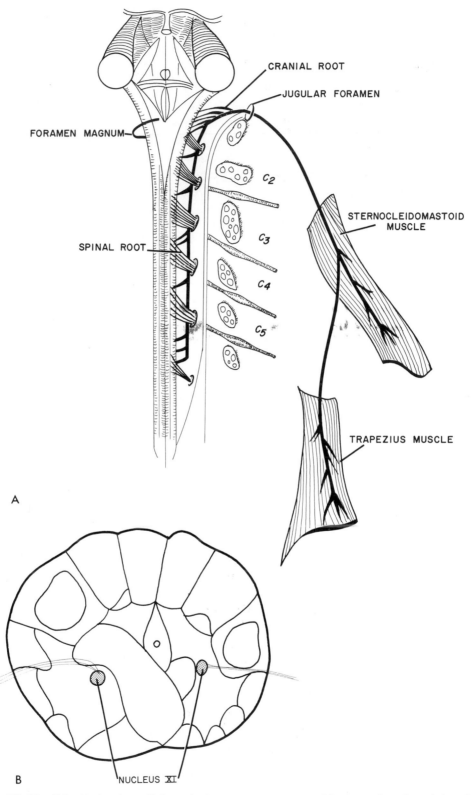

CRANIAL ROOT

JUGULAR FORAMEN

FORAMEN MAGNUM

C2

C3

C4

C5

STERNOCLEIDOMASTOID MUSCLE

SPINAL ROOT

TRAPEZIUS MUSCLE

A

B

NUCLEUS XI

Figure 10–11 Schematic view of the spinal accessory nerve and its central and peripheral connections (*A*) as well as the location of the motor nucleus in the medulla (*B*). (After House, E. L., and Pansky, B.: *A Functional Approach to Neuroanatomy.* New York, McGraw-Hill, 1967.)

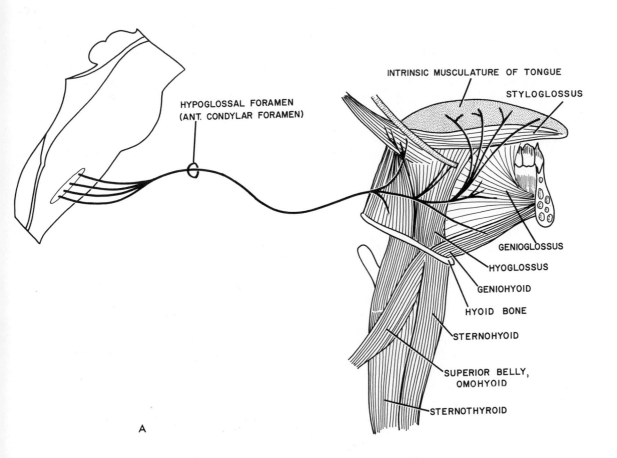

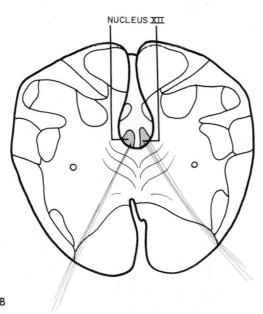

Figure 10-12 Schematic view of (A) the hypoglossal nerve and its central and peripheral connections and (B) the location of the motor nucleus in the medulla. (After House, E. L., and Pansky, B.: *A Functional Approach to Neuroanatomy.* New York, McGraw-Hill, 1967.)

tracheal bronchi, esophagus, small and large intestines, external ear, and dura of the sigmoid sinus. The fibers enter the medulla and synapse in the nucleus solitarius. The secondary axons ascend in the medial lemniscus to the ventroposterior thalamic nuclei.

Bilateral involvement of the vagal nuclear complex usually has a fatal result due to its proximity to the pneumotoxic, apneustic, and medullary respiratory centers. Unilateral lesions of the vagus nerve may or may not produce autonomic dysfunction. The heart rate, respiratory and gastronomic tract appear to function normally, but there may be minimal difficulty in swallowing. Injury to pharyngeal branches produces difficulty in swallowing. Lesions of the superior laryngeal nerve produce anesthesia of the upper part of the larynx and paralysis of the cricothyroid muscle. The voice is weak and the laryngeal muscles tire easily. Interruptions of the recurrent laryngeal

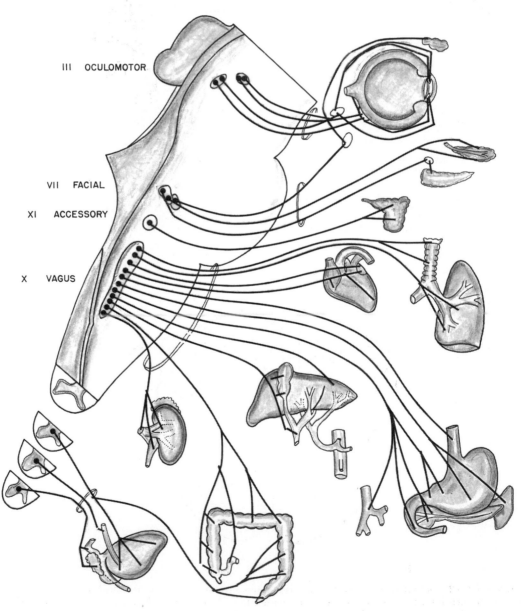

III OCULOMOTOR

VII FACIAL

XI ACCESSORY

X VAGUS

Figure 10–13 Schematic diagram of the parasympathetic preganglionic innervations from cranial nerves.

nerves produce paralysis of the vocal cords and hoarseness and dysphonia. Bilateral involvement of both recurrent laryngeal nerves produces aphonia and inspiratory stridor.

Lesions in the upper medulla produce dysphagia, while lesions in the lower medulla cause dysarthria. The palate on the affected side is paralyzed and the uvula deviates to the unaffected side with slurred or thickened speech. Speech is initiated from the cerebral cortex and will be discussed in the chapters on the cerebral hemisphere.

The dorsal motor nucleus of the vagus nerve inhibits and depresses heart rate and constricts the coronary circulation. Paralysis of the vagus nerve produces tachycardia. Stimulation of the vagus nerve produces contractions of smooth muscles in the trachea, bronchi, and bronchioli with resultant narrowing of the lumen. The dorsal motor nucleus of the vagus nerve generally stimulates alimentary functions by causing secretions of gastric and pancreatic juices important in peristalsis. It also stimulates the liver and spleen and inhibits the suprarenal glands. The vagus nerve is also important in many visceral reflexes: vomiting, swallowing, coughing, sneezing, sucking, hiccuping and yawning, and in the aortic sinus reflex. Any abnormalities in these responses usually involve structures in addition to the vagus nerve.

Supranuclear lesions involving the extrapyramidal pathways to the dorsal motor or ambiguous nuclei usually cause difficulty in swallowing but only become clinically significant when bilateral.

XI. Accessory Nerve. The accessory nerve (Fig. 10–11) is solely a motor nerve which originates from the medulla and spinal cord and is consequently divided into cranial (medullary) and spinal portions.

The cranial root arises from the most posterior part of the nucleus ambiguus, exits in a postolivary position, enters the jugular foramen, and then combines with the spinal root. The spinal portion arises from the ventrolateral part of the ventral horn in the upper four cervical segments, passes through the foramen magnum and combines with the cranial roots and distributes to the sternomastoid and trapezius muscles. General sensations from these muscles are carried by branches of the trigeminal nerve.

Injury to the ambiguous nucleus in the medulla causes paralysis and atrophy of the trapezius and sternomastoid muscles. There is weakness in movements of the head to the opposite side and weakness in shrugging. Supranuclear lesions produce only paresis due to the bilateral innervation.

XII. Hypoglossal Nerve. The hypoglossal nerve (Fig. 10–12) is solely a motor nerve and originates from the hypoglossal nucleus which forms the hypoglossal trigone in the medullary floor of the fourth ventricle. The fibers pass anteriorly, cutting inferiorly between the olive and pyramids. The fibers exit from the cranium via the hypoglossal canal and supply the intrinsic muscles of the tongue: the styloglossus, hypoglossus, and genioglossus. General sensations from the tongue musculature are carried by branches of the trigeminal nerve.

Unilateral injury to the nerve or nucleus produces atrophy and paralysis in the ipsilateral tongue with the tongue protruding toward the side of the lesion. Bilateral paralysis of the nucleus or nerve causes difficulty in eating and dysarthria. Supranuclear lesions rarely produce paralysis of the tongue.

Figure 10–13 summarizes the preganglionic parasympathetic innervation from the cranial nerves and spinal cord levels—S_2, S_3, and S_4.

11

Microscopic Anatomy of the Brain Stem

STANLEY JACOBSON

GENERAL DESCRIPTION

MEDULLA, PONS, AND MIDBRAIN

As previously indicated the medulla, pons, and midbrain are subdivided by their relationship to the ventricular system. One division, the tectum, forms the roof and walls or the posterior surface; the other division, the tegmentum, forms the floor or anterior surface. In the diencephalic levels the walls are massive and are formed by the nuclei of the thalamus, hypothalamus, and subthalamus. The floor and roof are greatly reduced. Many embryologists consider the thalamus to have been formed from the alar plate, and the hypothalamus from the basal plate. Others believe that the entire diencephalon originated from the alar plate. Irregardless of these arguments, the terms tectum and tegmentum are not usually applied to the diencephalon.

The *tectum* in medullary, pontine, and midbrain levels consists of regions which have highly specialized functions related to the special senses and movement. The tegmentum is less specialized and contains cranial nerve nuclei, the reticular formation, and tracts which interconnect higher and lower centers as well as tracts which inter-

connect the brain stem with other portions of the central nervous system (CNS).

Tectum. The tectum of the medulla and pons is formed by the cerebellum which is an important subcortical center for involuntary control of movement. The anatomy and functions of the cerebellum will be discussed in Chapter 25 on the motor system. The tectum of the midbrain is formed by the superior and inferior colliculi (corpora quadrigemini). The superior colliculus is an important reflex center in the visual system. It is laminated and receives fibers from the optic nerve and brain stem. The tectospinal tract originates in the deepest layers of the superior colliculus and connects that structure to motor nuclei in the brain stem and spinal cord.

The inferior colliculus is a large nucleus which receives fibers directly from the ascending auditory pathway, the lateral lemniscus. This region is an important subcortical reflex center in the auditory system.

Tegmentum. The tegmentum of the medulla, pons, and midbrain is continuous and for didactic purposes can be divided into five zones: dorsal, lateral, medial, ventral, and central.

The *dorsal zone* or ventricular floor in the upper medullary, pontine, and midbrain levels (Figs. 11–1, 11–2, and 11–3) contains

260

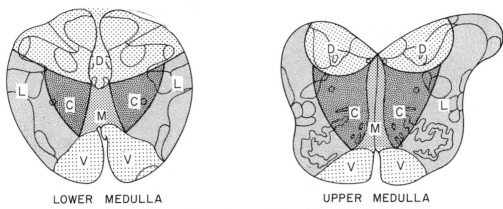

LOWER MEDULLA   UPPER MEDULLA

Figure 11–1 Cross section at a lower (*A*) and upper (*B*) medullary level of the brain stem tegmentum with dorsal, ventral, lateral, medial, and central zones identified.

the cranial nerves which innervate the skin (nerve V), the muscles and glands in the head and neck (nerves VII and IX), the viscera in the thorax and abdomen (nerve X), and the auditory and vestibular apparatus in the inner ear (nerve VIII). In midbrain levels the tectum is continuous with the ventricular floor, forming the dorsal region. In lower medullary regions the nuclei and fasciculus gracilis and the fasciculus cuneatus are found in the dorsal zone, which corresponds respectively to the funiculus gracilis and the funiculus cuneatus.

The *lateral zone* in the medulla (Fig. 11–1) contains the tracts that carry pain and temperature sensations from the body to the thalamus and connect the brain stem and spinal cord to the cerebellum (dorsal and ventral spinocerebellar tracts and inferior

cerebellar peduncle). It also contains a large nucleus, the inferior olive, that is also connected to the cerebellum. In medullary levels the dorsal and ventral spinocerebellar tracts are found on the surface, with the descending tract and the nucleus of nerve V and the spinothalamic and rubrospinal tracts being more internally placed. In pontine and medullary levels the first order axons conveying pain and temperature from the ipsilateral head and neck are found in the descending tract of nerve V, near the lateral surface of the brain stem internal to the dorsal spinocerebellar tract and inferior cerebellar peduncle. These fibers in the upper medullary levels are covered by the inferior cerebellar peduncle and in the pontine levels (Fig. 11–2) are covered by the middle cerebellar peduncle. Internal to the tract is found

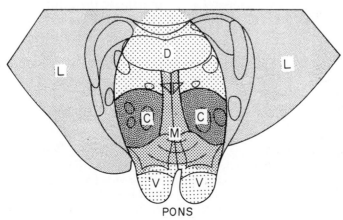

PONS

Figure 11–2 Cross section at a pontine level of the brain stem tegmentum with dorsal, ventral, lateral, medial, and central zones identified.

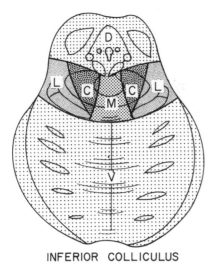

INFERIOR COLLICULUS

Figure 11-3 Cross section at a midbrain level of the brain stem tegmentum with dorsal, ventral, lateral, medial, and central zones identified.

the descending nucleus of nerve V (Fig. 11-3) where the primary axons synapse. In midbrain levels the lateral lemniscus (ascending auditory pathway) is found lateral to the medial lemniscus which has migrated from the midline to the lateral surface of the brain stem.

The *medial region* contains the paramedian long fiber tract which integrates eye movement, the medial longitudinal fasciculus. In medullary and pontine levels (Figs. 11-1 and 11-2) the second order neurons carrying somesthetic information, including proprioception and fine touch, run in the medial lemniscus to the thalamus and are found internal to the ventral zone.

The *central zone* throughout the medulla, pons, and midbrain (Figs. 11-1, 11-2, and 11-3) is the reticular formation which helps to maintain homeostatic mechanisms, including balance, and also determines our level of alertness. The ambiguous nucleus is found in the lateral margin of the reticular formation throughout the medullary levels (Fig. 11-1), and provides motor innervation to the muscles of the pharynx (nerves IX and X) larynx (nerve X), and neck (nerve XI). In the pons (Fig. 11-2) the motor nucleus of nerves V and VII are found in the lateral margin; these nuclei innervate, respectively, the muscles of mastication and facial expression. In the midbrain the red nucleus is found in this medial part of the reticular

formation; it is important in posture and orientation of the head in space.

Basis. The *ventral zone* corresponds to the basilar zone of the gross brain stem. In the midbrain regions (Fig. 11-3) it is formed by the cerebral peduncles which contain the corticopontine, corticospinal, and corticobulbar fibers. In pontine levels (Fig. 11-2) the pontine basis forms the ventral area. In medullary levels (Fig. 11-1) the pyramids form the ventral zone and contain corticospinal and corticobulbar fibers which innervate primarily the motor neurons in the spinal cord and brain stem.

Clinically Significant Tracts. Although all nuclei and tracts in the brain stem are important to the proper function of the CNS, lesions in certain tracts and nuclei produce abnormal responses which are detectable and important for diagnosis and treatment of disease. The tracts that produce clinically significant defects in function when affected are:

Lateral zone: Interruption of the lateral spinothalamic tract produces loss of pain and temperature from the contralateral body; interruption of the trigeminal root produces loss of pain, temperature, and touch from the ipsilateral head and neck.

Medial zone: Interruption of the medial lemniscus, depending on the level of the lesion, produces loss of touch, pain, and temperature from the head or body; the medial longitudinal fasciculus produces deficits in coordination of eye movements.

Ventral zone: Destruction of the corticospinal tract produces loss of volitional movement in the contralateral body muscles; interruption of the corticobulbar tract produces loss of volitional movement of the muscles in the contralateral head and neck.

Dorsal zone or central zone: Lesions here can produce abnormalities in the function of cranial nerve nuclei located in these regions. Involvement of any cranial nerve nucleus or root usually produces a clinically detectable abnormality in the function of that nerve. (See chapter on cranial nerves.)

DIENCEPHALON

The identified zones in the tegmentum of the medulla, pons, and midbrain are not visible in the diencephalon. The diencephalon is divided into three functionally distinct areas: thalamus, hypothalamus, and subthalamus (Fig. 11-4).

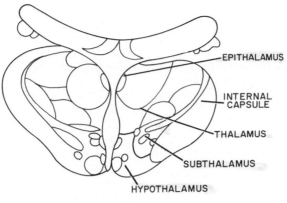

DIENCEPHALON

Figure 11–4 Cross section of the brain stem at the diencephalic level. The zones identified in the medulla (Fig. 11–1), the pons (Fig. 11–2), and the midbrain (Fig. 11–3) are not found in the diencephalon. Instead a functional division is used with the different functional regions identified as thalamus, hypothalamus, and subthalamus.

The *thalamic* portion of the diencephalon is the last synaptic stop before the cerebral cortex. All sensory systems, excluding olfaction, synapse here. Awareness of crude sensation associated with taste, temperature, pain, touch, and pressure is located here, but the actual ability to discriminate is located at the cerebral cortical levels. The *hypothalamus* is the most important subcortical center for emotions. It is also the regulator of homeostatic mechanisms (water balance, food intake, ionic levels, and endocrine levels). The *subthalamus* is part of the extrapyramidal system and is related to the involuntary control of movements. Its functions only become apparent when a disease process affects this region and causes involuntary, contralateral, and purposeless flinging of the limbs (hemiballismus).

MICROSCOPIC ANATOMY OF THE BRAIN STEM

Although the discussion in this chapter of each level is confined to the coronal section under examination, it should be noted that most nuclei and all tracts extend through more than just one level. Therefore, when reading this section the student should keep in mind the origin and destination of structures identified in isolated cross sections. It is especially important that the student understand the function and clinical importance of the anatomical structures he is studying. The cranial nerve nuclei and their relationships are all clinically important

since any abnormality in their functioning will help identify where the disease process is occurring in the CNS. Injury to the corticospinal, corticobulbar, and spinothalamic tracts and the cerebellar peduncles, medial lemniscus, and medial longitudinal fasciculus produces detectable clinical abnormalities.

The previous sections on the brain stem have discussed gross anatomy and cranial nerves. In this section, we will discuss the microscopic anatomy of the brain stem by examining cross sections. The analysis will start at the spinomedullary junction and continue superiorly through the medulla, pons, midbrain, and diencephalon.

LEVEL: MEDULLA–MOTOR DECUSSATION (FIG. 11–5)

Gross Features. The medulla at this level resembles the spinal cord; the dorsal columns and the funiculus gracilis and the funiculus cuneatus are conspicuous; the trigeminal funiculus is more laterally placed. In the gross brain, cord-like superficial structures are called *funiculi*, but in microscopic sections the axon bundles in these funiculi are called *fasciculi* or tracts. For example, the funiculus gracilis is equal to the fasciculus gracilis.

On the anterior surface of the cord, the medullary pyramids (corticospinal tracts) are evident. Note that the pyramid on the right side has shrunk as a result of the corticospinal tract shifting from the anterior surface of the medulla, crossing the midline, and entering what will be the lateral funiculus of the spinal cord. The narrow spinal canal is present in the gray matter above the pyramidal decussation.

Cranial Nerve Nuclei: Motor. Only the cranial portion of the nerve XI is present at the lateral margin of the reticular formation. It innervates the sternomastoid and trapezoid muscles which rotate the head and elevate the shoulders.

Cranial Nerve Nuclei: Sensory. The primary axons convey pain and temperature from the head and neck and are located in the spinal tract of the fifth cranial nerve. The second order axons originate from the underlying nucleus and then ascend contra-laterally to the ventral posterior medial nucleus of the thalamus. Tactile discrimination (fine touch, pressure, vibration sensation, and two-point discrimination) and proprioception from the extremities, thorax, abdomen, pelvis, and neck are carried via the dorsal columns. Nuclei can now be seen and

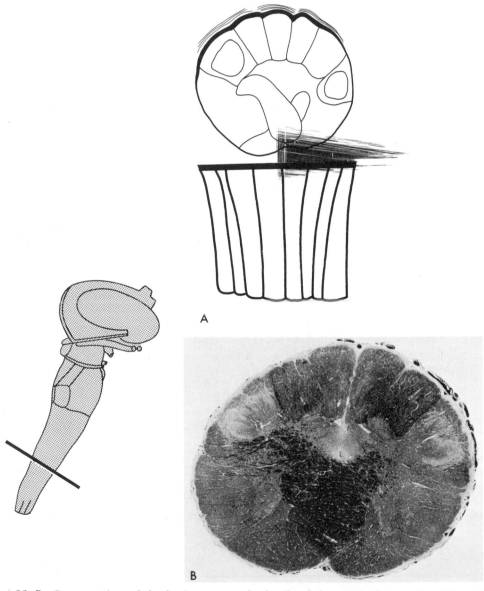

A

B

Figure 11–5 Cross section of the brain stem at the levels of the motor decussation (*A* and *B*). The nuclei are indicated in *C* and the tracts in *D*.

See Filmstrip, Frame 15.

will become the second order neurons in this pathway. The nucleus lateral to the pyramidal tract is the inferior reticular nucleus, a portion of the reticular formation.

White Matter. At this level the tracts are still in the same positions as in the spinal cord. The gracile and cuneate tracts (fasciculi) have reached their maximum bulk with the addition of the last of the fibers from the uppermost cervical levels. The segments of the spinal cord are represented so that the most medial fibers are sacral; then comes the lumbar, the thoracic, and finally, most laterally, the cervical fibers.

Pain and temperature from the extremities, abdomen, thorax, pelvis, and neck are carried by the lateral spinothalamic tract which is located at the lateral surface of the medulla. Light touch from the extremities, thorax, abdomen, pelvis, and neck is carried via the anterior spinothalamic tract which is seen on the surface of the medulla just posterior to the corticospinal tract.

The dorsal and ventral spinocerebellar tracts are found in the lateral funiculus. The rubrospinal and tectospinal tracts, which are important in supporting voluntary motor movements, are found respectively in the lateral funiculus and near the midline in the medullary and pontine levels.

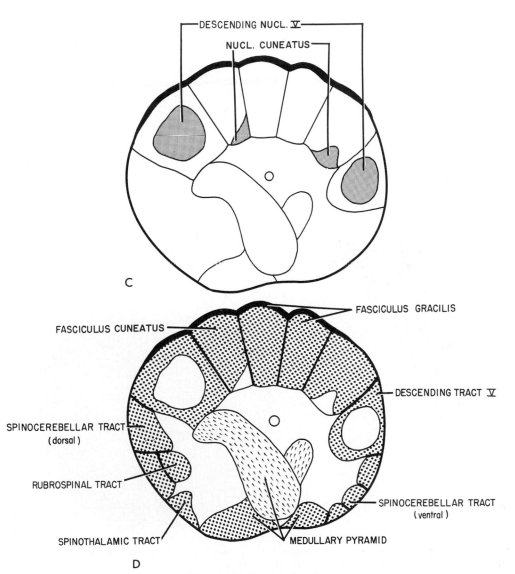

Figure 11–5 Continued.

LEVEL: MEDULLA — SENSORY
DECUSSATION (FIG. 11–6)

Gross Features. This level is representative of medullary levels below the appearance of the fourth ventricle. The funiculus gracilis and the funiculus cuneatus are conspicuous on the posterior surface of the spinal canal, while the medullary pyramids are prominent on the anterior surface.

Cranial Nerve Nuclei: Motor. This section contains the inferior extent of the hypoglossal nerve (XII) and the dorsal motor nucleus of the vagus nerve (X). The hypo-

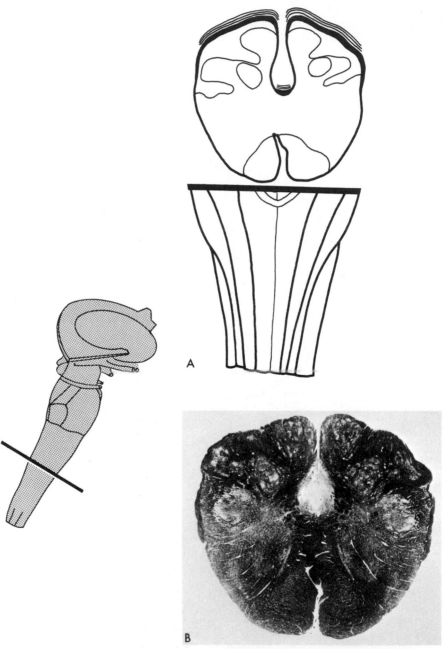

Figure 11–6 A cross section of the brain stem at the level of sensory decussation in the medulla (*A* and *B*). The nuclei are indicated in *C* and the tracts in *D*.

glossal nucleus innervates the intrinsic musculature of the tongue, while the dorsal motor nucleus of the vagus nerve provides parasympathetic preganglionic innervation of the viscera. This level marks the superior extent of the cranial portion of the eleventh cranial nerve in the ambiguous nucleus.

Cranial Nerve Nuclei: Sensory. Pain and temperature from the head are conveyed by the descending nucleus and tract of nerve V which is prominent anterior to the cuneate nucleus. It should be noted that myelinated second order axons are leaving the inner surface of the nucleus and passing toward

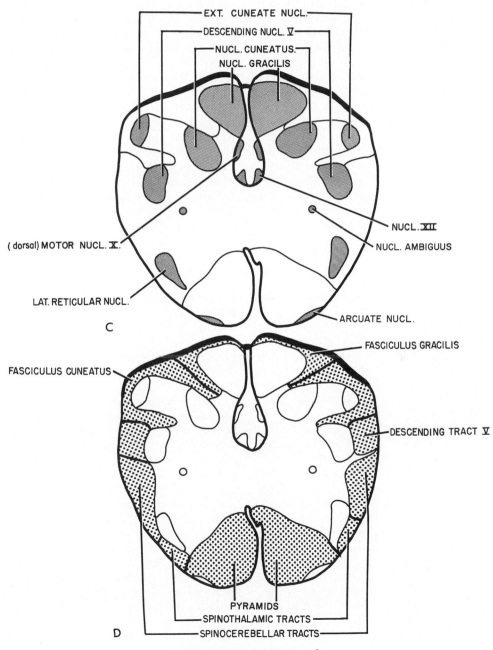

Figure 11-6 Continued.

the medial lemniscus, forming the trigeminothalamic (quintothalamic) tract.

White Matter. Tactile discrimination and proprioception are conveyed from the extremities, thorax, abdomen, pelvis, and neck by the axons in the fasciculus gracilis and cuneatus. The nucleus gracilis and the nucleus cuneatus form the second order neurons in this pathway and are conspicuous in this section. Internal arcuate fibers are seen leaving the inner surface of the gracile and cuneate nuclei, curving around the ventricular gray, crossing the midline (sensory decussation), and accumulating behind the pyramid as the medial lemniscus.

Unconscious proprioception is related to the external cuneate nucleus which corresponds to Clark's column in the spinal cord.

The central core of the medulla, pons, and midbrain consists of the reticular formation which is important for many vital reflex activities and for the level of attentiveness.

Pain and temperature from the extremities, thorax, abdomen, pelvis, and neck are carried via the lateral spinothalamic tract located in the lateral funiculus. The anterior spinothalamic tract is adjacent to the lateral spinothalamic tract.

The medial longitudinal fasciculus is located in the midline on the floor of the fourth ventricle below the hypoglossal nucleus. The vestibulospinal tract is found internal to the spinothalamic tracts.

The dorsal and ventral spinocerebellar tracts are seen on the surface of the medulla covering the spinal tract of nerve V and the spinothalamic tracts.

The rubrospinal tract is an important afferent relay to the alpha and gamma neurons in the spinal cord. It originates from the red nucleus in the tegmentum of the midbrain, crosses the midline, and descends. It is found in the *lateral funiculus* of the medulla internal to the spinocerebellar tract and anterior to spinal nerve V throughout the pons and medulla. It is important in postural reflexes. The tectospinal tract is phylogenetically an old tract, being the equivalent of the corticospinal tract in nonmammalian vertebrates. It originates from the deep layers of the superior colliculus and to some extent from the inferior colliculus. It is seen anterior to the medial longitudinal fasciculus throughout the medulla, pons, and midbrain and is important in coordinating eye movements and body position.

LEVEL: MEDULLA – INFERIOR OLIVE (FIG. 11–7)

Gross Features. At this level the medullary tegmentum expands laterally with the prominent inferior olive located behind the pyramids. The fourth ventricle contains the median eminence and the vestibular and cochlear tubercles. The median eminence consists of aqueductal gray, while the vestibular tubercle is formed by the medial vestibular nucleus and the descending root and nucleus of nerve VIII. The dorsal cochlear nucleus forms the cochlear tubercle. The ventricle at this level is at its widest extent. The sulcus limitans in the ventricular floor separates the medially placed motor cranial nuclei from the laterally placed sensory cranial nuclei.

Cranial Nerve Nuclei: Motor. This level marks the superior extent of nerve XII and the dorsal motor nucleus of nerve X. The ambiguous nucleus in the lateral margin of the reticular formation contains cell bodies innervating the pharynx and larynx (nerve X).

Cranial Nerve Nuclei: Sensory. Pain and temperature are conveyed from the face by nerve V. The descending nucleus and tract of nerve V are nearly obliterated by the olivocerebellar fibers.

Taste and visceral sensations are found in the solitary nucleus and tract in the tegmental gray below the medial vestibular nucleus. Fibers from nerves VII, IX, and X ascend and descend in this tract carrying general sensations from the viscera (nerve X) and gustatory sensations from the taste buds in the tongue (nerves VII and IX) and epiglottis (nerve X).

The medial and descending vestibular nuclei are present with first order axons found in the descending root of nerve VIII, interstitial to the descending nucleus. Fibers may be seen running from the vestibular nuclei into the medial longitudinal fasciculus.

The dorsal and ventral cochlear nuclei are second order nuclei in the auditory pathway and receive many terminals from the cochlear portion of nerve VIII seen within its borders.

The conspicuous inferior olivary nucleus in the anterior portion of the medullary tegmentum consists of the large main nucleus and the medial and dorsal accessory nuclei. This entire complex is important in supplying information to the cerebellum. Removal of the olive in animals produces contralateral increase in tone and rigidity in the extremities, with concomitant uncoordinated movements. The olive connects to the contralateral cerebellar hemispheres via the inferior cerebellar peduncle. The climbing fibers found on the dendrites of Purkinje's cells in the cerebellum originate in the olive. The olive also has strong connections with the red nucleus, the intralaminar nuclei in the thalamus, and the spinal cord. The inferior olivary nucleus receives input from the spinal cord, cerebellum, red nucleus, intralaminar nuclei, and basal ganglia. The central core of this section, as in other levels, consists of neurons of the reticular formation.

The position of the fiber tracts in this level corresponds to that in the previous levels.

LEVEL: MEDULLOPONTINE JUNCTION (FIG. 11–8)

Gross Features. The bulk of this section consists of the middle cerebellar peduncle (brachium pontis) and the cerebellum. In Figure 11–8 the bulk of the cerebellum has been removed. The fourth ventricle narrows as it nears the cerebral aqueduct. The medullary pyramids are present at the anterior surface. Note that the inferior olive is no longer present.

Cranial Nerve Nuclei: Motor. The nucleus of nerve VII is conspicuous at the lateral margin of the tegmentum. This nucleus innervates the muscles of facial expression. In the pons, in close proximity to the ventricular floor, the rootlet of this nucleus swings around the medial side of the nucleus of nerve VI forming the internal genu of nerve VII. These fibers then pass lateral to the nucleus of nerve VII and exit from the substance of the pons on the anterior surface in the cerebellopontine angle. The nucleus of nerve VI innervates the lateral rectus muscle of the eye. The rootlet leaves the anterior surface of the nucleus and has the longest intracerebral path of any nerve root. The fibers finally exit on the anterior surface of the brain stem near the midline at the pontomedullary junction. The close proximity of the nucleus of nerve VI to the rootlets of nerve VII demonstrates why any involvement of the nucleus of nerve VI usually produces a concomitant alteration in function of nerve VII. The nucleus of nerve VI and the internal genu of the rootlets of nerve VII form the prominent facial colliculus on the floor of the fourth ventricle.

Cranial Nerve Nuclei: Sensory. Pain and temperature are conveyed from the head. At pontine levels the descending nucleus of nerve V is small, while the tract is large. The superior vestibular nucleus is seen at the lateral margin of the ventricle with primary vestibular fibers present in its substance. Auditory sensation at this level is related to the superior olive which is seen inferior to the motor nucleus of nerve VII. The superior olive is one of the secondary nuclei in the auditory pathway. The auditory fibers are seen accumulating inferior to the superior olive and cutting through the medial lemniscus to form the lateral lemniscus.

White Matter. At this pontine level, some of the ascending tracts are starting to move more laterally. The medial lemniscus will shift laterally and the spinothalamic tracts will be found at its lateral margin. The corticospinal tract, which is actually descending, will be covered by the pons.

Tactile discrimination and proprioception from the limbs, thorax, pelvis, abdomen, and neck are conveyed by fibers in the medial lemniscus which is seen posterior to the corticospinal tract.

Pain and temperature from the head are conveyed by the secondary trigeminothalamic tracts which are found in the medial lemniscus and ascend to the nucleus ventralis posteromedialis in the thalamus.

Pain and temperature from the extremities, thorax, abdomen, pelvis, and neck are carried in the lateral spinothalamic tract which is near the anterior surface of the pons, close to the medial lemniscus.

Light touch is carried by the anterior spinothalamic tract which is mixed in with the lateral spinothalamic tract.

The gustatory fibers from the tongue are found in the solitary tract in the medullary tegmentum. These fibers will descend as the tract and the nucleus solitarius. The secondary fibers will ascend bilaterally in the medial lemniscus. Fibers carrying visceral sensations also synapse in the solitary nucleus. The medial lemniscus at this level will now contain secondary fibers from the dorsal columns and the spinothalamic, trigeminothalamic, and solitary tracts.

The medial longitudinal fasciculus and tectospinal tracts are still present near the midline in the floor of the fourth ventricle with the medial longitudinal fasciculus conspicuous under the floor and the tectospinal tract below it. In the center of the pontine tegmentum, the main efferent ascending

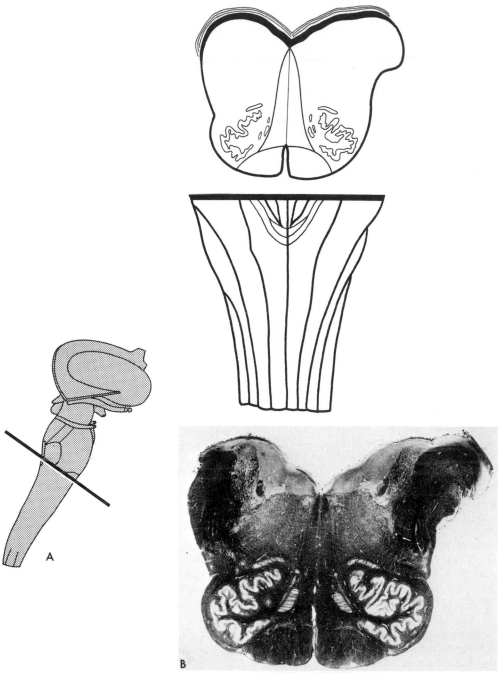

Figure 11–7 Cross section of the brain stem at the level of the inferior olive (*A* and *B*). The nuclei are indicated in *C* and the tracts in *D*.

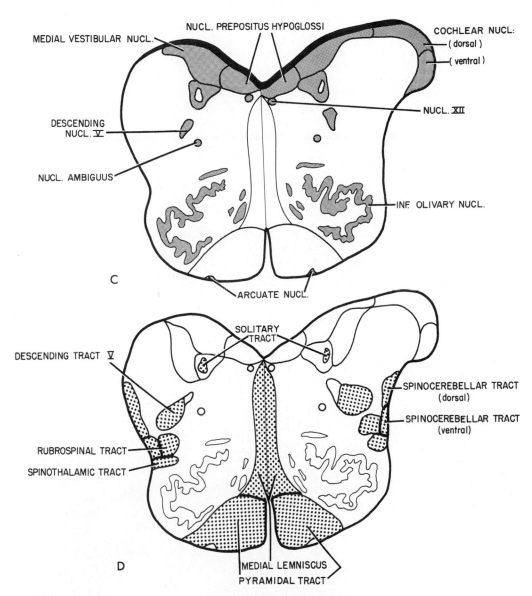

Figure 11-7 Continued.

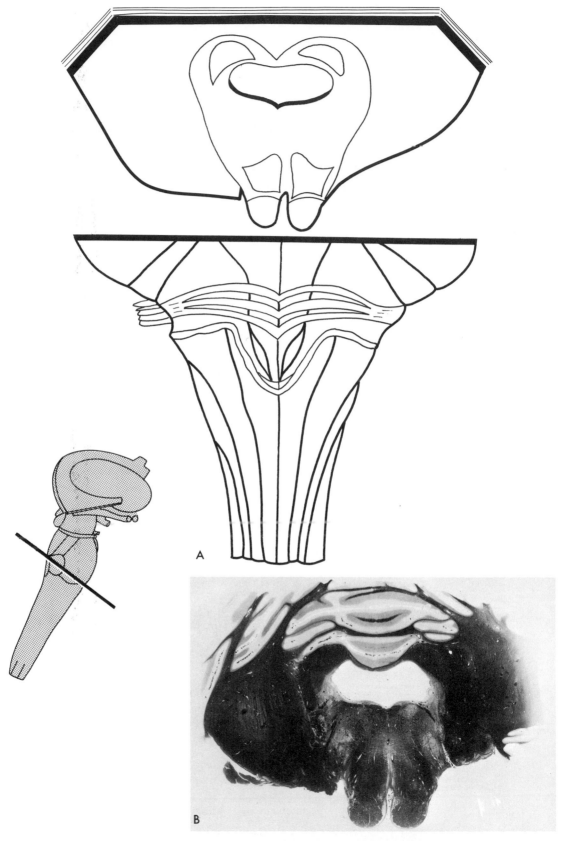

Figure 11-8 *See opposite page for legend.*

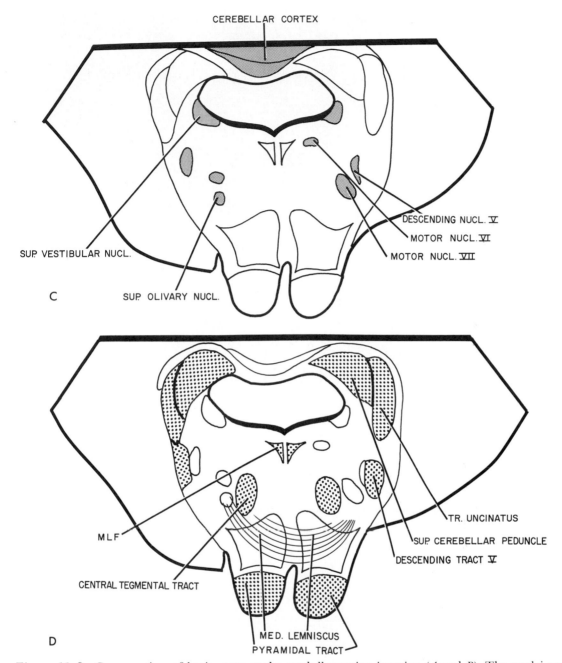

CEREBELLAR CORTEX

DESCENDING NUCL. V
MOTOR NUCL. VI
MOTOR NUCL. VII

SUP VESTIBULAR NUCL.

C

SUP OLIVARY NUCL.

MLF

TR. UNCINATUS
SUP CEREBELLAR PEDUNCLE
DESCENDING TRACT V

CENTRAL TEGMENTAL TRACT

D

MED. LEMNISCUS
PYRAMIDAL TRACT

Figure 11–8 Cross section of brain stem at the medullopontine junction (*A* and *B*). The nuclei are indicated in *C* and the tracts in *D*.

tract of the reticular system, the central tegmental tract, occupies the bulk of the reticular formation.

Cerebellum. The middle cerebellar peduncle forms the lateral walls of the ventricle as well as the bulk of the cerebellar medullary center. The ventral spinocerebellar tract is seen lateral to the superior cerebellar peduncle which it enters and then follows back into the cerebellum. The superior cerebellar peduncle consists primarily of axons carrying impulses from the dentate nucleus of the cerebellum to the red nucleus and the ventral lateral nucleus in the thalamus. This tract is also called the dentatorubrothalamic tract. The tractus uncinatus connects the deep cerebellar nuclei with the vestibular nuclei and reticular formation bilaterally.

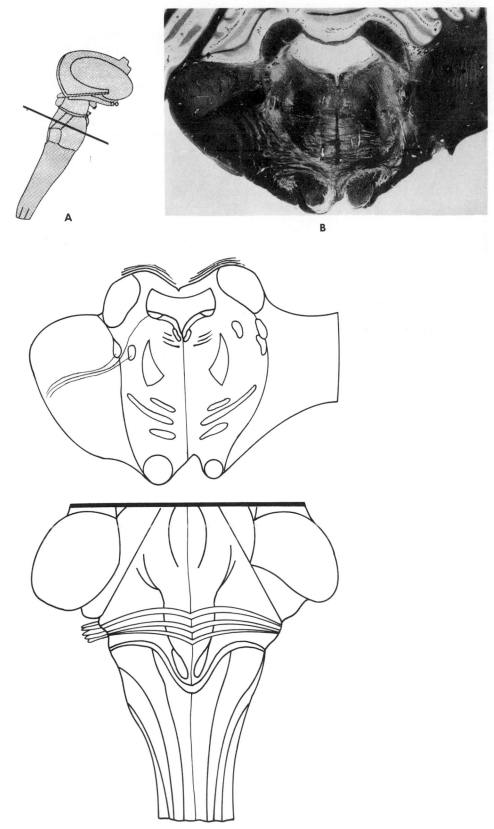

Figure 11-9 *See opposite page for legend.*

LEVEL: PONS—MOTOR AND MAIN SENSORY NUCLEI OF NERVE V (FIG. 11–9)

Gross Features. The bulk of this section consists of the middle cerebellar peduncle and cerebellar cortex. The fourth ventricle narrows as it nears the cerebral aqueduct.

Cranial Nerve Nuclei: Motor. The motor nucleus of nerve V is conspicuous bilaterally, medial to the entrance of the root of nerve V. Each of these nuclei provides innervation to the ipsilateral muscles of mastication.

Cranial Nerve Nuclei: Sensory. Tactile discrimination from the face is carried by the trigeminal root into the main sensory nucleus of nerve V, seen lateral to the intrapontine root of nerve V. The secondary fibers originate from this nucleus and ascend, crossed and uncrossed. The crossed fibers enter the medial lemniscus (ventral trigeminothalamic), while the uncrossed fibers run in the dorsal margin of the reticular formation (dorsal trigeminothalamic). Both fiber pathways terminate in the ventral posterior medial nucleus of the thalamus. Proprioception from the muscles in the head is carried in by the mesencephalic root and ends in the mesencephalic nucleus of nerve V which is located lateral to the walls of the fourth ventricle in the upper pontine and midbrain levels. These neurons are the only primary cell bodies (dorsal root ganglion equivalent) in the CNS. The jaw jerk is a monosynaptic stretch reflex. The receptor is the mesencephalic nucleus of nerve V and the effector is the motor nucleus of nerve V.

The superior olive is one of the nuclei in the auditory system. Auditory fibers are seen running through the superior olive or inferior to it cutting through the medial lemniscus and crossing the midline, forming the trapezoid body. The fibers are then found lateral to the medial lemniscus, and are known as the lateral lemniscus. The pontine nuclei are conspicuous in the basilar portion of the pons.

White Matter. At this level the medial lemniscus has moved from the midline to a more lateral position. The corticospinal tract is nearing the surface of the pons and is covered by pontine white matter. Either in the medial lemniscus or in close proximity to it at this level are found the following ascending sensory systems:

1. Tactile discrimination and proprioception from the limbs, thorax, pelvis, abdomen, and neck (dorsal columns).

2. Tactile discrimination and light touch from the head (dorsal and ventral trigeminothalamic).

3. Pain and temperature from the limbs, thorax, and pelvis (lateral spinothalamic).

4. Pain and temperature from the head (ventral trigeminothalamic).

5. Light touch from the limbs, abdomen, and neck (anterior spinothalamic).

6. Taste and visceral impulses from the tongue and viscera (viscerothalamic).

Cerebellum. The superior cerebellar peduncle (dentatorubrothalamic tract) forms the walls of the fourth ventricle. The medial longitudinal fasciculus is a conspicuous tract near the floor of the ventricle; it contains at this level many vestibular and cerebellar fibers which are necessary for accurate eye movements. The bulk of the reticular formation is taken up by the conspicuous central tegmental tract.

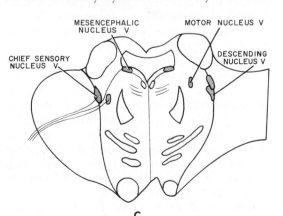

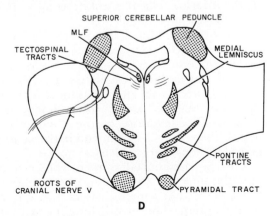

Figure 11–9 Continued. Cross section of the brain stem at the level of the motor and main sensory nuclei of nerve V in the pons (A and B). The nuclei are indicated in C and the tracts in D.

See Filmstrip, Frame 20.

LEVEL: INFERIOR COLLICULUS AND PONTINE BASIS (FIG. 11–10)

Gross Features. In this section the midbrain forms the roof and floor, while the pons makes up the basilar portion. The roof is the inferior colliculus, an important nucleus in the auditory pathway. The narrow ventricular lumen is the cerebral aqueduct.

Cranial Nerve Nuclei: Sensory. Proprioception is conveyed from the muscles in the head and neck. The mesencephalic nucleus of nerve V is located at the lateral margin of the periaqueductal gray. Remember these are the only primary sensory neurons in the CNS. These axons join the medial lemniscus and ascend to the ventral posterior medial nucleus in the thalamus. This nucleus controls the superior oblique muscle of the eye.

Cranial Nerve Nuclei: Motor. A small portion of cranial nerve IV (trochlear) is found in the ventricular floor adjacent to the medial longitudinal fasciculus.

Medial Lemniscus. At this level the medial lemniscus is near the lateral surface of the pontine tegmentum. It consists of second order fibers from the dorsal columns and the trigeminal, spinothalamic, and solitary tracts. Thus the following sensory modalities for the entire body are located there: tactile discrimination, proprioception, pain and temperature, and gustatory and visceral sensations.

Auditory Fibers. The lateral lemniscus is seen superior to the medial lemniscus. These secondary auditory fibers are now entering the inferior colliculus. Many of these fibers will synapse and then continue up into the medial geniculate as the brachium of the inferior colliculi and ultimately reach the auditory cortex. Other axons originating in the inferior colliculus will descend as part of the tectospinal tract.

Cerebellar Tracts. The superior cerebellar peduncle occupies most of the midbrain tegmentum. Some of these fibers have crossed the midline. Ultimately all these fibers will decussate and continue on up to the red nucleus where some fibers will synapse. The majority of these axons will bypass the red nucleus and end in the ventral lateral nucleus in the thalamus.

The periaqueductal gray is conspicuous in midbrain levels. Descending and ascending tracts associated with the visceral brain are found herein. The medial longitudinal fasciculus is again conspicuous in the floor of the ventricle; the fibers located within it are important in coordinating ocular movements.

Reticular Formation. In midbrain levels, the lower one-half of the periaqueductal gray and some other nuclei in the tegmentum, are part of the midbrain limbic area. This zone is important in our level of attentiveness. Bilateral lesions to the periaqueductal gray and midbrain tegmentum usually produce comatose patients.

LEVEL: SUPERIOR COLLICULUS AND PONTINE BASIS (FIG. 11–11)

Gross Features. In this section the roof and floor are formed by the midbrain, while the basilar portion is made up of peduncles and pons. The roof is the superior colliculus, an important station in the visual pathway. The cerebral aqueduct forms the narrow ventricular lumen. The superior colliculus is a laminated structure important in relating eye movements and body position. The tectospinal tract originates from its deepest layer and provides connections onto certain cranial and spinal neurons.

Cranial Nerve Nuclei: Sensory. Proprioception is conveyed from the muscles in the head and neck by the mesencephalic nucleus of nerve V, located at the lateral margin of the periaqueductal gray in the superior collicular levels as well as in the upper pontine and inferior collicular levels.

Cranial Nerve Nuclei: Motor. Cranial nerve III is visible in the floor of the cerebral aqueduct, adjacent to the medial longitudinal fasciculus. This nerve supplies the medial, inferior, and superior rectus muscles and the inferior oblique and superior levator muscles of the eyelid. The Edinger-Westphal nucleus of nerve III is also present; it provides preganglionic parasympathetic innervation to the constrictor muscle of the pupil via the ciliary ganglion.

Medial Lemniscus. This tract is stretched out over the inferior and lateral surface of the tegmentum, with the fibers that mediate pain and temperature from the extremities, thorax, abdomen, and pelvis located at its superior extent. The trigeminal fibers form its middle portion, and the fibers that mediate tactile, proprioceptive and visceral sensations are placed medially.

Auditory Fibers. The fibers from the inferior colliculus, which are called the brachium of the inferior colliculus, are seen at the inferior surface of the superior colliculus. On the left side they enter the medial geniculate nucleus of the metathalamus at which point they reach their final subcortical center.

Cerebellum. The superior cerebellar peduncle continues to cross in the tegmentum of the midbrain; just above this level many of these fibers will enter the red nucleus, while others will continue to the ventral lateral nucleus in the thalamus.

Cerebral Peduncles. At this level, the frontopontine fibers, which occupied the most medial part of the cerebral peduncles, enter the pons. The corticospinal fibers and many of the corticobulbar fibers are still in the peduncle.

The central tegmental tract is conspicuous in the midbrain tegmentum in the reticular formation. The medial longitudinal fasciculus in the floor of the cerebral aqueduct is conspicuous and is connected across the midline.

LEVEL: MIDBRAIN – DIENCEPHALIC JUNCTION (FIG. 11–12)

Gross Features. The diencephalon occupies the majority of this section, with the corpus callosum, fornix, and lateral ventricles forming its superior surface, and the third ventricle its medial surface. The lateral wall of the diencephalon is formed by the posterior limb of the internal capsule. The cerebral peduncles are prominent on the inferior surface; adjacent to them are the substantia nigra and more medially the red nucleus. The laminate lateral geniculate nucleus is prominent on the left side lateral to the cerebral peduncle.

Cranial Nerve Nuclei. Cranial nerves are found only in the medulla, pons, and midbrain. They are absent from diencephalic levels.

Epithalamus. This nuclear grouping with its associated tracts is functionally part of the visceral brain. The habenular nuclei and stria medullaris are present on the medial surface protruding in the third ventricle. The habenulopeduncular tract is seen on the left side connecting the medial habenular nucleus to the interpeduncular nucleus. At more posterior levels, the pineal gland is seen above the habenular nuclei and commissure.

Thalamus. The bulk of the thalamus at this level consists of the pulvinar nuclei which connect to the sensory associative cortex in the superior and inferior parietal lobule. A large ovoid nucleus is present about one-third of the way in from the third ventricle. This is the central median nucleus of the intralaminar group. The ascending tract of the reticular system ends here and makes this nucleus important in determining our level of consciousness. Lateral to this nucleus is the ventral posterior medial nucleus. It receives the second order gustatory and trigeminal fibers carried up to the thalamus in the medial lemniscus. This nucleus projects to the inferior one-third of the postcentral gyrus, areas 3, 1, 2 (See Chapter 20). Thus, we have reached the final subcortical center for gustatory and trigeminal impulses.

Optic Thalamus. On the left side, the laminate lateral geniculate nucleus is present. It receives the third order fibers which stem from the ganglionic cell layer of the retina via the optic nerve, chiasm, and tract. This thalamic nucleus projects to the striate cortex on the medial surface of the occipital lobe.

Red Nucleus. This nucleus is conspicuous near the wall of the third ventricle, and receives input from the cerebellum via the superior cerebellar peduncles. It connects to the ventral lateral nucleus of the thalamus and also to the alpha and gamma motor neurons in the spinal cord via the rubrospinal tract.

Substantia Nigra. This large pigmented nucleus is an important part of the extrapyramidal system. It connects with the globus pallidus, hypothalamus and midbrain tegmentum, and probably also the caudateputamen.

Deep Telencephalic Gray. Although the caudate nucleus is a part of the telencephalon its tail is found in diencephalic levels on the most lateral wall of the lateral ventricles separated from the thalamus by the external laminae of the thalamus. The stria terminalis is found on its medial surface; it is unrelated to the caudate nucleus and interconnects the amygdaloid nuclei. The caudate nucleus is an important part of the extrapyramidal system having to do with supporting volitional motor functions.

Fornix. This tract is an important part of the limbic or visceral brain. The fornix originates from the hippocampus located in the medial surface of the temporal lobe. It takes a circuitous pathway, following the inferior horn and body of the lateral ven-

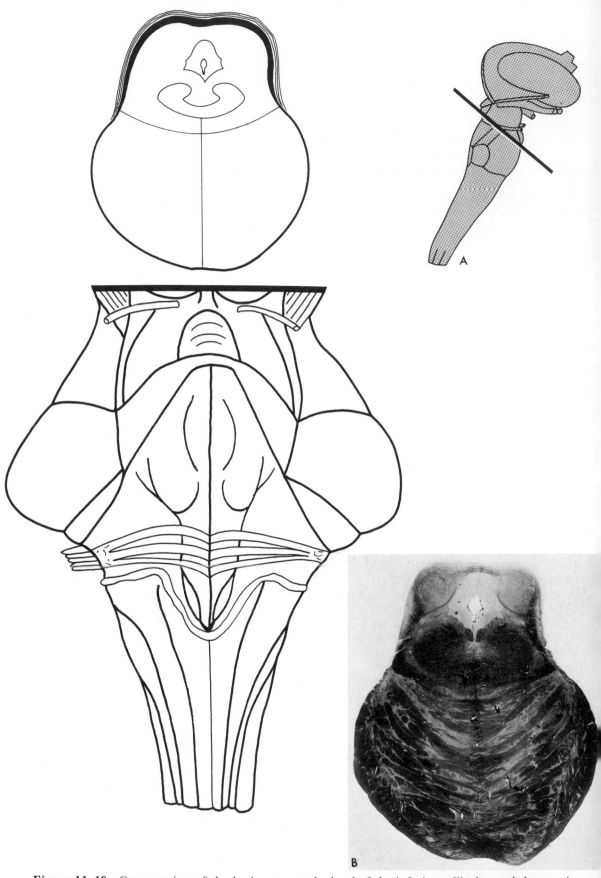

Figure 11-10 Cross section of the brain stem at the level of the inferior colliculus and the pontine basis (*A* and *B*). The nuclei are indicated in *C* and the tracts in *D*.

See Filmstrip, Frame 21.

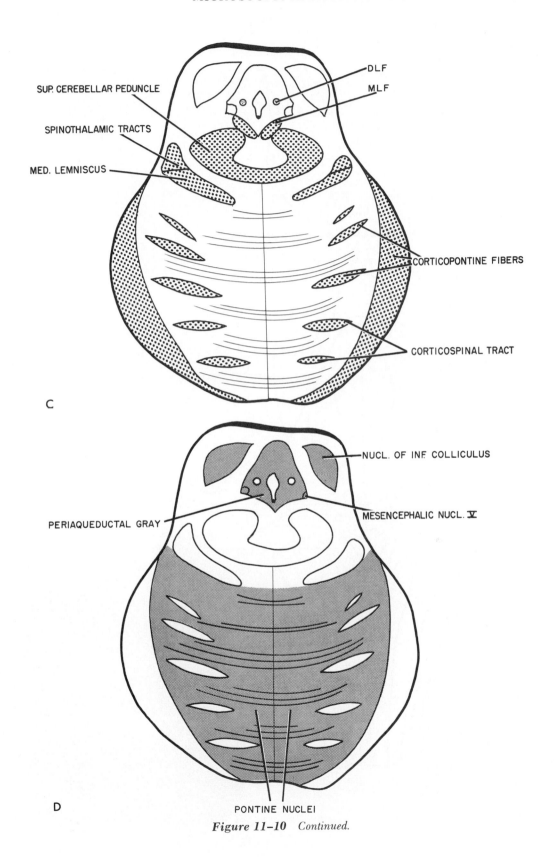

Figure 11–10 Continued.

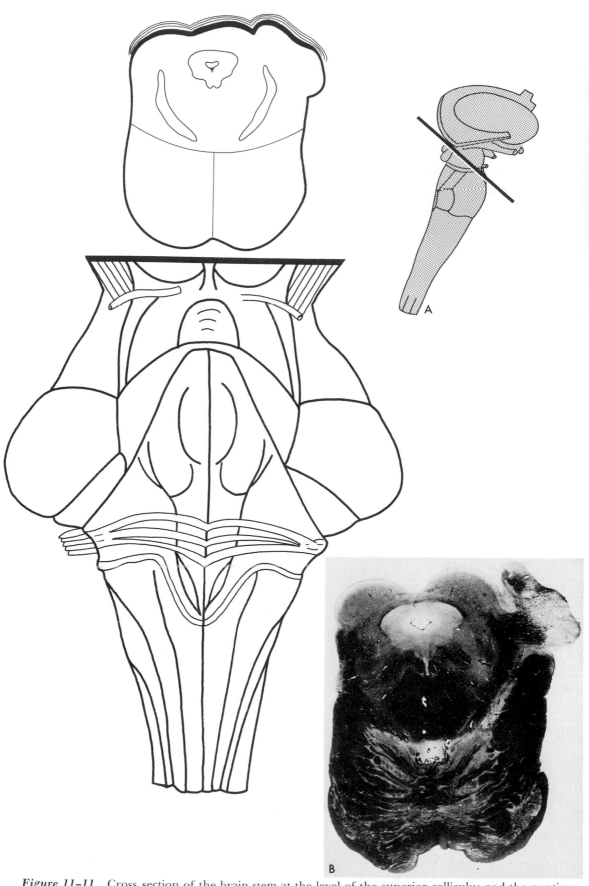

Figure 11–11 Cross section of the brain stem at the level of the superior colliculus and the pontine basis (*A* and *B*). The nuclei are indicated in *C* and the tracts in *D*.

See Filmstrip, Frame 22.

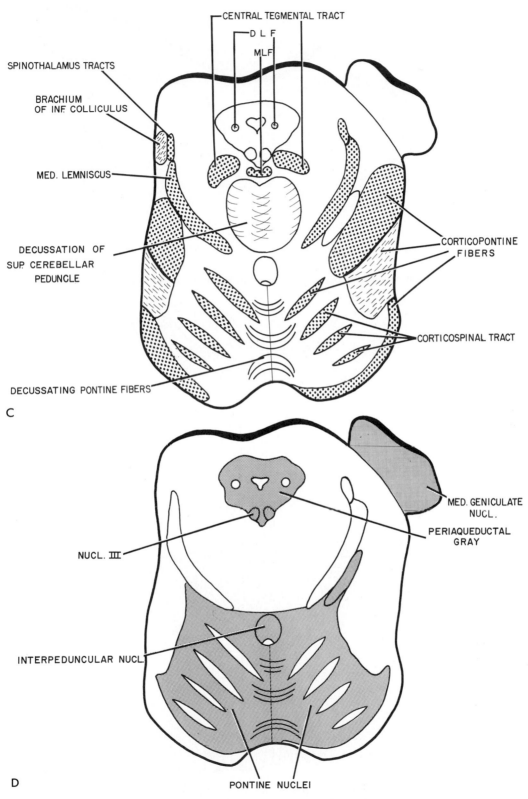

Figure 11–11 *Continued.*

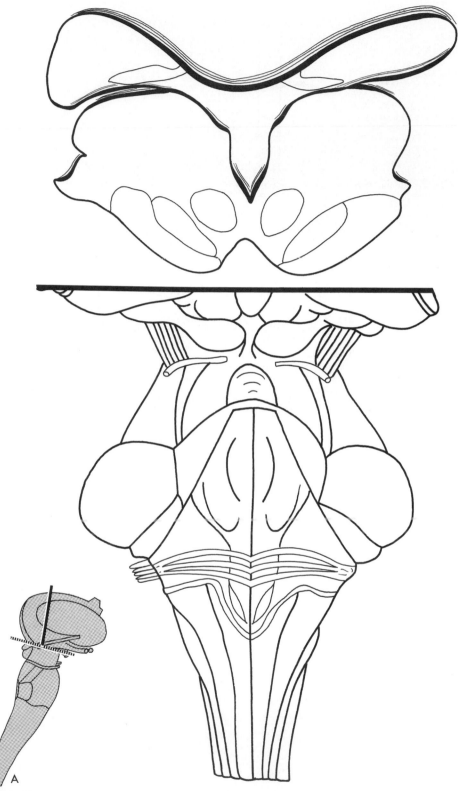

Figure 11-12 Cross section of the brain stem at the midbrain-diencephalic level (*A* and *B*). The tracts are indicated in *C*, and the nuclei in *D*. The thalamic nuclei are abbreviated as follows: CM = central median; LP = lateral posterior; M = medial dorsal; VPL = ventral posterior lateral; and VPM = ventral posterior medial.

See Filmstrip, Frame 36.

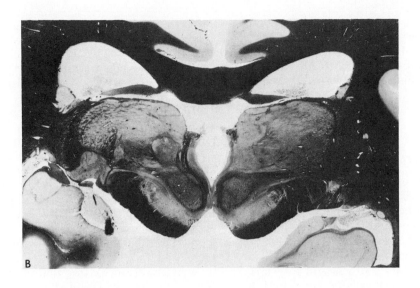

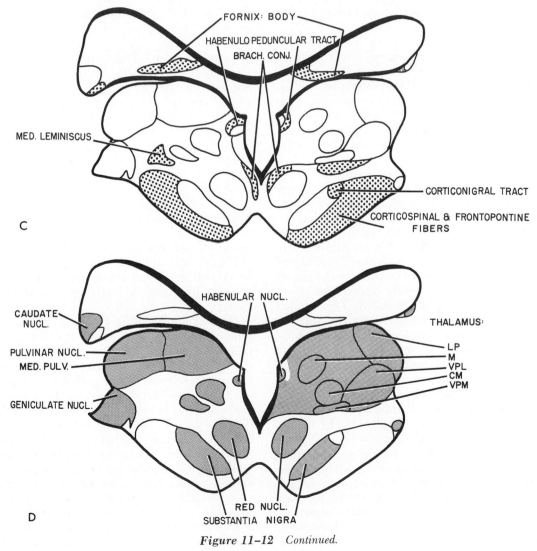

Figure 11–12 Continued.

tricle attached to the undersurface of the corpus callosum until it reaches the level of the interventricular foramen where it enters the hypothalamus and runs to the mammillary body. In this section we see the fornix under the corpus callosum; at other levels we will find it under the corpus callosum and in the substance of the hypothalamus.

LEVEL: MIDTHALAMUS (FIG. 11–13)

Gross Features. The diencephalon occupies the bulk of this section with the corpus callosum, fornix, and lateral ventricles forming its superior surface, the third ventricle, its medial surface, and the posterior limb of the internal capsule, its lateral surface. The optic tract is prominent inferiorly. Lateral to the internal capsule are found the deep telencephalic nuclei, the globus pallidus, and the putamen.

Epithalamus. The stria medullaris is seen on the superior margin of the third ventricle. This tract connects habenula with septum, amygdala, and hippocampus.

Thalamus. The thalamus at this level consists of two prominent divisions separated by the internal medullary laminar of the thalamus. The medial portion, the medial nucleus, connects to the prefrontal and orbital cortices and receives reciprocal innervation from these same regions as well as the hypothalamus. It is an important subcortical nucleus in the visceral brain. The lateral, more heavily myelinated portion consists of dorsal and ventral regions. Posteriorly the pulvinar is the continuation of this dorsal group. The ventral half consists of the nuclei which receive the specific ascending tracts from lower levels of the CNS. The ventral posterior medial nucleus receives the ascending gustatory and cutaneous and proprioceptive fibers from the head. Present also is the ventral posterior lateral nucleus, which receives the cutaneous (spinothalamic and dorsal columns), proprioceptive (dorsal columns), and visceral information via the medial lemniscus and projects to the upper two-thirds of the postcentral gyrus. The ventral lateral nucleus receives the superior cerebellar peduncle and projects to the motor and premotor cortices, areas four and six (see Chapter 20). Consequently in this section we have reached the final subcortical center for the dorsal columns, the spinothalamic and dentatorubrothalamic tracts.

Awareness of pain and temperature and crude touch are located in the ventral posterior lateral nucleus. More specialized sensory awareness is found in the postcentral gyrus, i.e., the position of digits in space and tactile discrimination.

Hypothalamus. The hypothalamic sulcus, at the midpoint of the third ventricle, marks the separation between the thalamus above and the hypothalamus below. At this level a cell stain would show several hypothalamic nuclei at or near the ventricular surface. On the right side, even in this fiber stain, the mammillary body is conspicuous with the mamillothalamic and mammillotegmental fibers forming a capsule on its medial surface. On the left side the fornix is seen anterior to the mammillary body. Near the ventricular surface a prominent pathway, the mammillothalamic tract, is present. This connects the mammillary body with the anterior thalamic nuclei.

Subthalamus. This zone lies medial to the cerebral peduncle, below the medullary laminae of the thalamus and lateral to the hypothalamus. It has three principal nuclei: (1) subthalamic, touching the cerebral peduncle, (2) zone incerta, below the external medullary lamina, and (3) the tegmental nucleus of Forel (or prerubral nucleus), lateral to the mammillothalamic tract. The lenticular fasciculus separates the zona incerta above from the subthalamic nucleus below. This region is an important region for relay in the extrapyramidal system because of its connections with the globus pallidus, thalamus, and hypothalamus. Fibers reach the subthalamic zone from the globus pallidus by going through the internal capsule.

Deep Telencephalic Gray. The caudate (tail) nucleus, the putamen, and the globus pallidus are present in this section. The caudate nucleus is seen near the superior surface of the thalamus. The globus pallidus and putamen are found lateral to the posterior limb of the internal capsule. The globus pallidus is the heavily myelinated nucleus just lateral to the internal capsule. It receives input from the caudate nucleus and putamen while it provides the only efferents from the basal ganglia to the subthalamus, the ventral anterior and the ventral lateral nuclei in the thalamus, hypothalamus, the substantia nigra, and the midbrain tegmentum. The fibers leave the globus pallidus and cut through or around the internal capsule to reach the aforementioned nuclei.

Fornix. This tract connects the hippocampus with the septum, habenula, lateral hypothalamic nucleus, and mammillary bodies. The fornix originates from the hippocampus in the medial portion of the temporal lobe. It is suspended from the undersurface of the corpus callosum up to the most anterior portion of the thalamus where it enters the hypothalamus and passes to the mammillary body. In this cross section, it is seen under the corpus callosum and in the substance of the hypothalamus. The hippocampus is an important part of the visceral brain and participates in recent memory.

LEVEL: ANTERIOR TUBERCLE OF THALAMUS (FIG. 11–14)

Gross Features. This section is near the anterior end of the thalamus and is at the superior end of the brain stem. The diencephalon is much smaller than in the previous levels, while the deep telencephalic nuclei, the globus pallidus and the putamen are much larger than in the previous section. The boundaries of the diencephalon are laterally the posterior limb of the internal capsule, medially the third ventricle, and superiorly the lateral ventricle and corpus callosum.

Epithalamus. The stria medullaris is conspicuous on the medial surface of the thalamus.

Thalamus. The thalamic nuclei at this level consist of two prominent divisions separated by the internal medullary laminae region containing anterior nuclei. The anterior nuclei are important subcortical nuclei in the visceral brain because of their connections to the cingulate cortex and the mammillary bodies. The internal medullary laminae which separate the anterior nucleus from the ventral anterior nucleus consist primarily of mammillothalamic fibers, while the external medullary lamina, which touches the superior surface of the anterior nucleus, contains fibers interconnecting the anterior nuclei and the cingulate cortex. The ventral anterior nucleus receives fibers from the intralaminar nuclei, the ventral anterior nucleus, and globus pallidus and projects to areas four and six (see Chapter 20), the motor and premotor cortices.

Hypothalamus. In this cross section the

fornix has just entered the hypothalamus. The optic chiasm forms the floor of the third ventricle. Note that a portion of the fornix is also seen under the corpus callosum.

Subthalamus. This is absent from this cross section. The subthalamus is seen in mid- and posterior thalamic sections (see preceding levels).

Deep Telencephalic Gray. The globus pallidus and putamen are conspicuous lateral to the posterior limb of the internal capsule. Fibers can be seen leaving the globus pallidus and sweeping around the internal capsule, as the ansa lenticularis, or cutting through the internal capsule, the pallidothalamic fibers.

Anterior Commissure. The anterior commissure is seen on the inferior border of the globus pallidus and putamen. This level is just caudal to the actual decussation of the anterior commissure. The anterior commissure interconnects portions of the temporal lobe, olfactory bulb, and olfactory cortex, as well as the amygdaloid nuclei (see Fig. 29–2).

Telencephalic Cortex. In this section the olfactory cortex forms the ventral surface of the hemisphere.

FUNCTIONAL LOCALIZATION IN BRAIN STEM

Now that the anatomical features of the brain stem have been discussed, it is appropriate to identify the important functions located in the brain stem. During this discussion, it will become evident that the cranial nerves are the pivotal point for many of these activities.

Reticular Formation. The central core of the medulla, pons, and midbrain tegmentum consists of the reticular formation. Upon microscopic examination this region is seen to consist of groupings of neurons separated by a meshwork of medullated fibers. With a Golgi neuronal stain the neurons are shown with their dendrites extending transversely and the axons bifurcating into ascending and descending branches which can run throughout the system, each neuron receiving input from at least 1000 neurons and each neuron possibly connecting to 10,000 neurons. It also appears that a majority of neurons in the reticular formation are Golgi Type I cells.

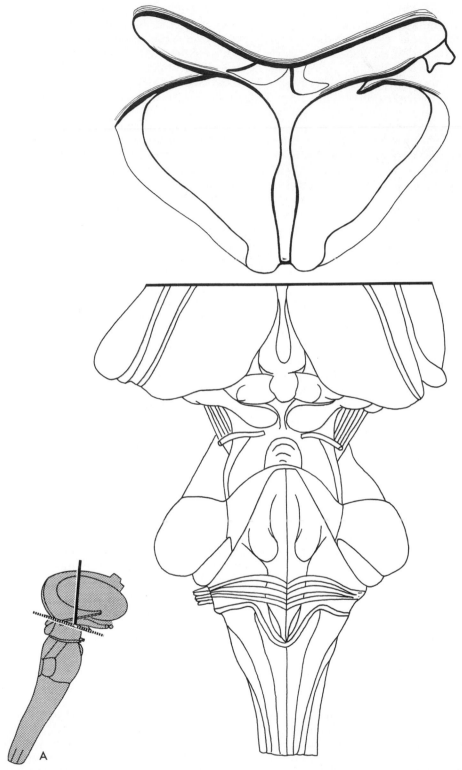

Figure 11–13 Cross section of the brain stem at the midthalamic level (*A* and *B*). The nuclei are indicated in *C* and the tracts in *D*. The thalamic nuclei are abbreviated as follows: LD = lateral dorsal, and VL = ventral lateral. The other abbreviations are explained in the legend for Figure 11–12.

See Filmstrip, Frame 37.

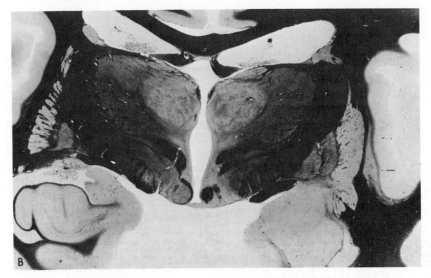

B

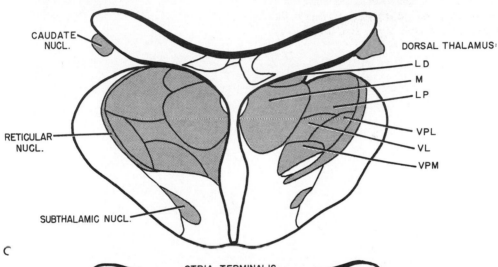

CAUDATE
NUCL.

DORSAL THALAMUS:

L D

M

L P

VPL

VL

VPM

RETICULAR
NUCL.

SUBTHALAMIC NUCL.

C

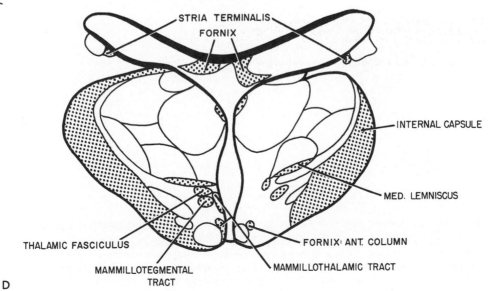

STRIA TERMINALIS

FORNIX

INTERNAL CAPSULE

MED. LEMNISCUS

THALAMIC FASCICULUS

FORNIX: ANT. COLUMN

MAMMILLOTEGMENTAL
TRACT

MAMMILLOTHALAMIC TRACT

D

Figure 11–13 Continued.

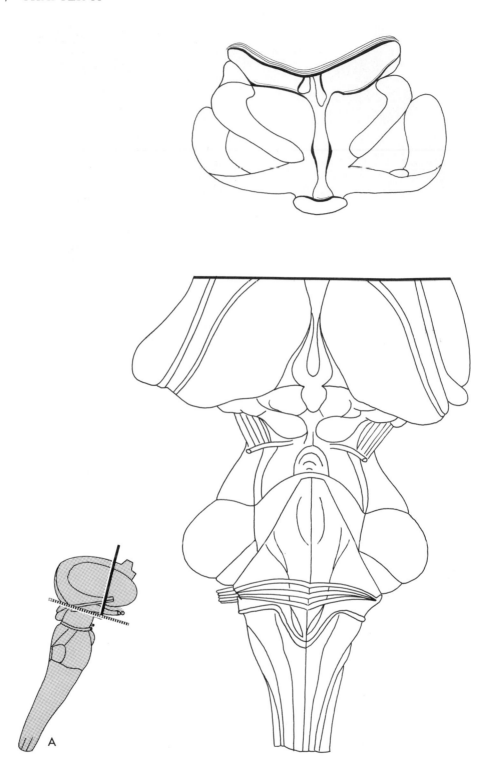

Figure 11–14 Cross section of the brain stem at the level of the anterior tubercle in the thalamus (*A* and *B*). The nuclei are indicated in *C* and the tracts in *D*.

See Filmstrip, Frame 39.

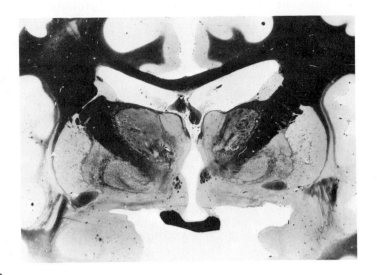

B

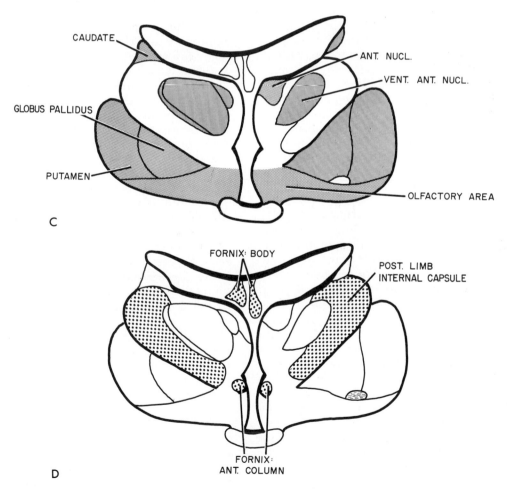

C

D

Figure 11–14 Continued.

Many nuclei have been identified in the reticular formation. In our discussion, however, only certain nuclei will be identified. The reticular formation in the medulla is especially important since it gives origin to the descending reticulospinal fibers and much of the ascending reticular system. The *nucleus reticularis gigantocellularis* is found at the rostral medullary levels, dorsal and medial to the inferior olive. This nucleus gives origin to much of the reticulospinal tract, which is primarily an ipsilateral tract, running in the lateral funiculus of the spinal cord in all levels and terminating on internuncial neurons. The axons from the *nucleus reticularis pontis oralis* and *caudalis* form much of the anterior reticulospinal tract which runs in the anterior funiculus in all levels and terminates on internuncial neurons. The lateral reticular nucleus is located in the lateral margin of the reticular formation dorsal to the inferior olive, while the ventral reticular nucleus is found in the caudal end of the medulla, dorsal to the inferior olive. These two nuclei, in conjunction with the nuclei in the pons and midbrain, form much of the ascending reticular fibers in the central tegmental tract distributing to neurons in the thalamus (intralaminar and reticular), hypothalamus, and corpus striatum. The paramedian reticular nucleus is found near the midline at mid-olivary levels, dorsal to the inferior olive, and provides direct input into the anterior lobe of the cerebellar vermis.

Input. The reticular formation receives information via the ascending spinal tracts (spinotectal, spinoreticular, spinothalamics, spinocerebellar), from the brain stem itself (olivoreticular, cerebellumreticular, vestibulospinal), and from the cerebral hemispheres (corticoreticular). The cranial nerves are another important source, especially nerves II, V, VII, VIII, and X. The visceral brain and striatum also project to the reticular system via the dorsal longitudinal fasciculus and the more diffuse descending fiber system.

Output. The medial lemniscus is a specific point-to-point relay system with few synapses (a closed system), while the fiber tracts of the reticular system are a multisynaptic nonspecific system (an open system). The central tegmental tract is the principal fiber tract of the reticular formation. Its descending portions are located in the medial tegmentum and its ascending portions are lo-cated in the lateral tegmentum. The ascending system projects to the thalamic intralaminar and reticular nuclei, the hypothalamus, basal ganglia, substantia nigra, and red nucleus. The descending system synapses via the reticulospinal tract onto interneurons which mediate their effects through alpha and gamma motor neurons in the spinal cord and via autonomic pathways and cranial nerves onto visceral neurons.

The ascending reticular system is the structural and functional substrate for determining the level of consciousness of the individual. The reticular system receives proprioceptive, tactile, thermal, visual, auditory, and nociceptive information via the spinal and cranial nerves. Many sensations including cutaneous, nociceptive, and erotic sensations activate the system. The reticular system is functionally important in controlling our "posture" by its reflex relationship to the position of our body in space and in controlling our internal milieu by maintaining the stability of our viscera. The sensory information ascends via the central tegmental tract into the limbic-midbrain area from which information can be more directly passed into the thalamus and hypothalamus; this midbrain to diencephalon and finally to telencephalon circuit seems especially important in determining our level of consciousness and motivation.

The reticular formation is also important in controlling posture and orientation in space. Stimulation of the caudal medulla inhibits the knee jerk. Laterally, stimulation facilitates the knee jerk.

The lateral part of the reticular formation is the receptor area, while the medial portion is the effector zone and the origin of centrotegmental and reticulospinal tracts. Many of the functions vital to the maintenance of the organisms are found in the medulla.

Respiration. Respiration is under the control of neurons in the *respiratory center* in the upper medulla and pons. Sensory fibers from the lungs ascend via nerve X and enter the solitary tract and proceed onto the neurons in the reticular formation in the medulla and pons. There are specific regions in the medulla which control either inspiration or expiration. The medullary respiratory center itself is responsive to the carbon dioxide content in the blood. Increased carbon dioxide produces increased respiration and decreased carbon dioxide produces decreased respiration.

In the pons the pneumotoxic centers are related to the frequency of the respiratory response. These centers play onto the medullary respiratory center to determine the respiratory output. The axons from cells in the medullary reticular center descend to the appropriate spinal cord levels to innervate the diaphragm and the intercostal and associated muscles of respiration. The vagus nerve itself provides preganglionic innervation of the trachea, bronchi, and lungs.

The respiratory response is also modified by cortical and hypothalamic control; i.e., emotionally stimulated individuals breathe more rapidly because of the hypothalamus influence of the brain stem and spinal cord. The actual respiration occurs with the intercostal muscles, the accessory muscles, and the lungs expanding and contracting in concert with associated vascular changes (autonomic nervous system).

Cardiovascular. The carotid body (innervated by sensory fiber of nerve IX) is found distal to the bifurcation of the common carotid artery, and the aortic body is found near the origin of the subclavian arteries. These carry information on blood pressure into the solitary tract and then into the medullary respiratory centers. These sites are sensitive to oxygen–carbon dioxide pressure; when oxygen is reduced, ventilation increases; when oxygen increases, ventilation decreases. Neural control over the tone of the arterioles is exercised through vasoconstrictor fibers; there may also be vasodilator fibers. There is a *vasomotor center* in the medulla which extends from the midpontine to the upper medullary levels. In the lateral reticular formation of the medulla, stimulation elicits an increase in vasoconstriction and an increase in heart rate—*pressor center*. In the lower medulla, stimulation of the *depressor center* produces a decrease in vasoconstriction and a decrease in heart rate. The carotid body of nerve IX and the aortic body of nerve X contain specialized receptors which are pressure receptors stimulated by an increase in the size of these blood vessels. This information runs via nerves IX and X to the medulla and depresses activity. Most sensory nerves, cranial and spinal, contain some nerve fibers which when stimulated cause a rise in arterial pressure by exciting the pressor region and inhibiting the depressor centers. Higher centers also influence respiratory and vascular centers in the medulla and other blood flow, depending on the psychic state; i.e., mental activity decreases peripheral blood (constricts vessels), while emotional states can produce increased blood flow, blocking vasodilation.

Deglutition. The act of swallowing starts volitionally but is completed by reflex activity. The food is first masticated (motor nucleus of nerve V) and reduced to smaller particles, called the bolus, which is lubricated by saliva. The bolus is propelled through the oral pharyngeal opening when the tongue is elevated (nerve XII) against the soft palate, and the facial pillars are relaxed. This opening is then closed and the superior and middle pharyngeal constrictor muscles (ambiguous nucleus of nerve X) force the bolus along into the laryngeal pharynx where the pharyngeal walls contract, closing this opening superiorly. At the same time, there is a closing of the trachea by the epiglottis and glottis, as the larynx, trachea, and pharynx move up. This movement is noted externally as the bobbing of the thyroid eminence. The inferior constrictor muscle contracts, pushing the bolus into the esophagus where peristaltic waves and gravity carry it through the esophagus.

Nerves V, IX, X, and XII perform the motor part of the activity, while nerves V, VII (taste), IX and X form the sensory function.

Vomiting. Vomiting is produced by many stimuli and is usually a reflex activity. The vomitus is composed of the gastric contents. Commonly, vomiting is caused by irritation of the oropharynx or gastrointestinal mucosa. Foci in the semicircular canals and genitourinary tract may also produce vomiting. The afferents travel via the vagus and glossopharyngeal tracts into the solitary tract. After synapsing on the dorsal motor nucleus of nerve X the information is conveyed via the vagus nerve to the stomach. Impulses are also passed down to the cervical and thoracic level onto the ventral horn cells which control the simultaneous contraction of the intercostal, diaphragmatic, and abdominal musculature.

Nausea and excessive salivation precede the deep inspiration associated with retching. The glottis is closed and the nasal passages are sealed off. The descent of the diaphragm and the contraction of the abdominal muscles exert the pressure that causes the stomach to contract in a direction contrary to normal peristalsis and forces vomitus through the relaxed cardia of the stomach and into the esophagus.

Coughing. Irritation of the lining of the larynx or trachea produces coughing. The stimulus is picked up by free nerve endings associated with nerve X which carries it up into the solitary tract, following the same pathway as in vomiting, except that the muscles contract alternately rather than simultaneously with the intercostal muscle contracting suddenly.

Coordination of Ocular Movements. The nuclei of nerves III, IV, and VI are located close to the medial longitudinal fasciculus and these nuclei are interconnected via the medial longitudinal fasciculus to permit conjugate movement. The medial longitudinal fasciculus also provides the ocular nuclei with information from the cerebellum, the red nucleus, the trigeminal and facial nerves, and the inner ear, as well as information from the neck and spinal cord. The medial longitudinal fasciculus permits head, body, and neck movements to be correlated with eye movements.

Lesions in the medial longitudinal fasciculus produce internuclear ophthalmoplegia with partial loss of conjugate movement and palsy of gaze. A lesion in the medial longitudinal fasciculus between the nuclei of nerves III and VI interrupts the connections between the parabducens nucleus of one side and nerve III on the other side, producing paralysis of the medial recti muscles on lateral gaze and nystagmus of the abducting eye. Bilateral involvement of the medial longitudinal fasciculus is usually indicative of multiple sclerosis.

The position of the eyes is influenced by information from the retinas, labyrinths, and cochleas, and by proprioceptive information from the facial and neck muscles. Any interruption of the normal balance of impulses between these systems can produce involuntary oscillations of the eyeballs, called nystagmus. The nystagmus usually represents the eyeball's attempt to compensate for these abnormal stimuli. Nystagmus is usually conjugate, but there may be unilateral nystagmus; it may occur in any direction, even rotatory, and at any rate. One can produce nystagmus in normal patients by rotating the person and stopping them suddenly or by stimulating one labyrinth. (See Chapter 14.)

A lesion in either the motor nucleus muscle or its rootlets or in the muscle itself produces a paralysis of one of the extraocular muscles and indicates a nuclear or infranuclear lesion. A lesion in the nucleus of nerve III can produce denervation of specific ocular muscles while infranuclear lesions usually produce complete paralysis of nerve III. In nerve IV, because of complete decussation of the rootlet, a nuclear lesion produces paralysis contralaterally while injury to the rootlets produces ipsilateral involvement. A nuclear involvement of nerve VI usually produces symptoms in nerve VII because the rootlets of nerve VII pass over the nucleus of nerve VI.

Ocular movements are examined by asking the patient to move his eyes in six directions—laterally, medially, upward and laterally, upward and medially, downward and laterally, and downward and medially. The coordination of eye movements through the medial longitudinal fasciculus prevents isolated movement of any one eye muscle and produces correlated (conjugate) movements of various eye muscles. In any eye movement, because of the intimate connection between the eye muscles, certain muscles contract and certain muscles relax. Therefore paresis or paralysis of any one muscle produces deviation of the eyeball from parallel action with the normal eyeball. This loss of conjugate or coordinated movements produces squint or strabismus. If the patient attempts to fix his vision on some object in the field of the affected muscle, the eyeball on the affected side will not move equally with that of the normal side. This produces an image on a different point of the retinae than that produced on the normal side and is called double vision or diplopia (Fig. 11–15). By tilting the head to compensate, the patient may see normally.

In addition to the movement of the eyeballs and lids, the pupil and lens are under the control of the parasympathetic (Edinger-Westphal nucleus of nerve III) and sympathetic nervous system (via descending sympathetic fibers to the thoracic cord).

Normally, the pupils are round, regular in outline, equal in size, and in the center of the iris. In light of average intensity, they are 3 to 4 mm. in diameter. In newborn children, the pupils react poorly to light. Pupils in young adults are normally larger than those of middle-aged or older individuals. Small pupils (miosis) are less than 2 mm. and may

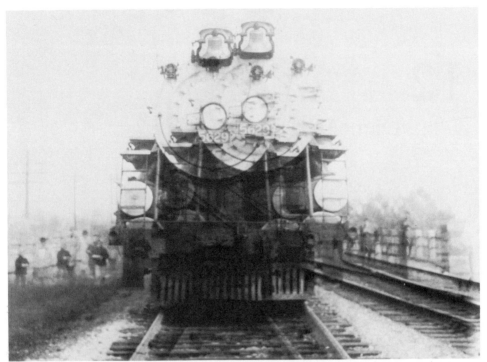

Figure 11–15   An example of double vision. This photograph demonstrates the most common double vision in which two separate images are seen in the horizontal plane.

be seen in bright light or in senility, arteriosclerosis, morphine or opium intoxication, sleep, deep coma, or with increased intracranial pressure and bilateral brain stem involvement. Unilateral miosis is caused by irritation or interruption of the sympathetic fibers in the brain stem or spinal cord. Dilated pupils more than 5 mm. in diameter (mydriasis) may be seen in decreased light or in anxious individuals (sympathetic activation) or may result from pain, deep anesthetic states, cardiac anesthesia, cerebral anoxia, and death. Unilateral mydriasis is seen with interruption of nerve III, which blocks the parasympathetic pathway.

The normal pupil contracts when light is focused on the ipsilateral retina and dilates when light is withdrawn — the *direct light reflex.* The contraction of the pupil occurs via the preganglionic fibers from the Edinger-Westphal nucleus and via the postganglionic fibers from the ciliary ganglion. Because of the partial decussation of the optic fibers in the optic chiasm, both pupils in the normal patient respond to light in one pupil. This is called the *consensual* or *crossed light reflex.* In a lesion of nerve III, the direct and crossed reflexes are absent on the affected

side and present on the intact side. Accommodation is seen when the eye shifts in focusing from a distant to a near object — the lens thickens, the eyes converge, and the pupils constrict. Accommodation is mediated by the parasympathetic fibers which innervate the sphincter of the iris causing constriction of the pupil and which stimulate the circular muscle fibers in the ciliary body, releasing the tension on the lens and increasing the convexity of the lens for near vision. The eye also reacts to painful stimuli (nerve V) or foreign bodies on the cornea with the pupil constricting (nerve III) and the eyelids closing (nerve VII).

The rotational control of conjugate eye movements is mediated from area eight in the posterior part of the middle and inferior frontal gyri. The fibers from this area course through the internal capsule, leave the peduncle, and, as the aberrant pyramidal fibers, innervate the nuclei of nerves III, IV, and VI. Unilateral destruction of area eight produces paralysis of the conjugate gaze with the eyes turning toward the affected side. Injury to the pretectal region may cause impairment of upward or downward gaze.

12

Diencephalon

STANLEY JACOBSON

The midbrain expands rostrally into the diencephalon. The diencephalon forms the superior end of the brain stem and consists of the following nuclear groupings: thalamus, epithalamus, metathalamus, hypothalamus, and subthalamus. As can be seen from the terminology associated with the diencephalon, all structures are described by their relationship to the thalamus, being either above, below, or behind it. Most of the diencephalon is covered by the telencephalon, so that in the gross brain only the ventral surface of the brain diencephalon is visible.

The border between the diencephalon and the midbrain is indistinct and may be arbitrarily assigned by passing a line from the inferior surface of the mammillary bodies to the posterior border of the habenula. A portion of the substantia nigra and red nucleus are also seen in the posterior portion of the diencephalon.

The lateral ventricle, corpus callosum, and fornix form the superior border of the diencephalon. The internal capsule and optic tract mark its lateral boundary, while the third ventricle denotes its medial border. Inferiorly the diencephalon is continuous with the tegmentum of the midbrain, while rostrally it ends at the lamina terminalis.

THALAMUS

The thalamus is the relay center interposed between the lower brain stem and the cerebral cortex. It is ovoid and is the largest portion of the diencephalon. It is bounded laterally by the posterior limb of the internal capsule and inferiorly by the subthalamus and hypothalamus. The boundary between thalamus and hypothalamus is determined by locating the hypothalamic sulcus on the medial wall of the diencephalon and labeling all nuclear structures superior to it as thalamus, and all nuclei below it, as hypothalamus.

NUCLEI OF THE THALAMUS

In gross material the nuclear groupings in the thalamus are indistinct, but in a coronal section (Fig. 12–1) one can identify the anterior tubercle at the rostral end of the diencephalon and the internal medullary lamina which divides the thalamus into lateral and medial and anterior cell masses (Fig. 12–2). Cell and fiber stains are needed to further subdivide the thalamus. With those stains the following nuclear masses are identifiable: anterior, medial, midline, intralaminar, lateral, reticular, and metathalamus. Each of

294

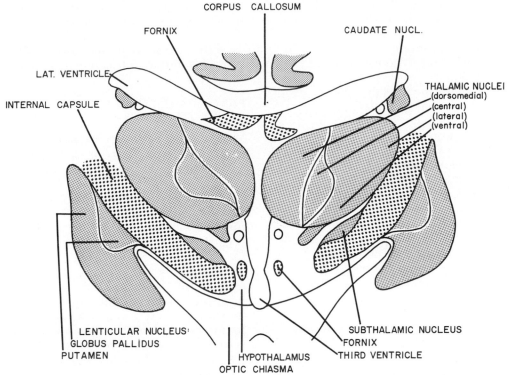

Figure 12-1 Coronal section through the diencephalon with thalamus, hypothalamus, subthalamus, basal nuclei, and related tracts identified.

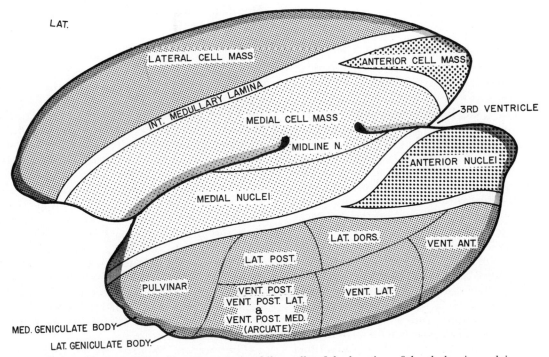

Figure 12-2 Schematic representation bilaterally of the location of the thalamic nuclei.

these nuclear groupings can be further sub-divided as follows (Fig. 12–2):

A. Anterior nuclei
   1. Nuclei anterior
   2. Nucleus anterodorsalis
B. Medial nuclei
   1. Nucleus medialis dorsalis
      a. Pars parvocellularis
      b. Pars magnocellularis
C. Midline nuclei
   1. Nucleus paratenialis
   2. Nucleus paraventricularis
   3. Nucleus reuniens
   4. Nucleus rhomboideus
D. Intralaminar nuclei
   1. Nucleus centrum medianum
   2. Nucleus parafascicularis
   3. Nucleus paracentralis
   4. Nucleus centralis lateralis
   5. Nucleus centralis medialis
E. Lateral nuclei
   1. Pars dorsalis
      a. Nucleus lateralis posterioralis
      b. Nucleus lateralis dorsalis
      c. Pulvinar
   2. Pars ventralis (ventrobasal complex)
      a. Ventralis anterior
      b. Ventralis lateralis
      c. Ventralis ventralis
      d. Ventralis posterior
         1) Posterolateral
         2) Posteromedial
F. Reticular nuclei
G. Metathalamic nuclei
   1. Lateral geniculate
   2. Medial geniculate

The thalamic nuclei may be grouped according to their subcortical and cortical major connections as follows (Fig. 12–3):

Specific Cortical Thalamic Nuclei. These nuclei receive their main input from the major ascending fiber systems from the spinal cord, brain stem, cerebellum, and visceral brain, and they project to specific cortical areas. They are the anterior, ventral lateral, ventral posterior, medial and ventral posterior lateral, lateral posterior nuclei and the geniculate nuclei.

Specific Associational Thalamic Nuclei. These nuclei receive the major portion of their input from other thalamic nuclei or ascending fiber systems and project primarily to associational areas of the the cortex. They are medial, midline, pulvinar, and reticular.

Nonspecific Thalamic Nuclei with Diffuse Cortical and Subcortical Connections. These nuclei receive input from many sub-cortical regions, including the reticular formation, visceral brain, and corpus striatum. They project to specific thalamic nuclei or associational areas in the cortex. They are ventral anterior, intralaminar, and midline.

FUNCTIONAL LOCALIZATION IN THE THALAMUS

The following nuclei are part of the *limbic* or *visceral brain:* anterior, medial, midline, and intralaminar nuclei (Figs. 12–3 and 12–4).

The *medial region* occupies most of the thalamus, and is found between the internal medullary laminae and the midline nuclei (Fig. 12–2). It consists of the anterior and medial nuclei.

The *anterior nucleus* (Fig. 12–2) is at the most rostral part of the thalamus and bulges in as the prominent anterior tubercle in the floor of the lateral ventricle. It consists of a large main nucleus (antroventral) and smaller accessory nuclei (anterodorsal). The internal medullary lamina splits and surrounds the anterior nucleus.

The anterior nuclei are important relay nuclei in the visceral brain and receive input from the mammillary body via the mammillo-thalamic tract. It projects to the cingulate gyrus (areas 23, 24, 32) and receives input from the hypothalamus, habenula, and cingulate cortex. Stimulation or ablation of this nucleus produces changes in blood pressure.

The *medial nuclear complex* consists of a large-celled and a small-celled division. The magnocellular portion of the medial nucleus is interconnected with the hypothalamus and midline nuclei and connects to the orbital cortex, while the large parvocellular division is interconnected with the orbito-frontal and prefrontal cortices (areas 9, 10, 11, 12). (See Chapter 20.) The medial nucleus is an important relay station between the hypothalamus and the prefrontal cortex and is concerned with interactions of visceral and somatic impulses which contribute to the emotional makeup of the individual. Destruction of this nucleus in cats results in a lower threshold for rage, so that the animal is easily aroused. In humans, ablation of the medial nucleus or a prefrontal lobotomy has been used as a therapeutic procedure to relieve emotional distress.

The *midline thalamic nuclei* (Fig. 12–2) are located in the periventricular gray above the hypothalamic sulcus. They are small and difficult to delimit in man, but these nuclei are intimately connected to the hypothalamus and the intralaminar nuclei and any functions must be considered in light of their relationship to these nuclei.

The *intralaminar nuclei* (Fig. 12–2) are found *interspersed* in the internal medullary lamina of the thalamus. The most prominent intralaminar nucleus is the centromedian, which is located in the midthalamic region between the medial and ventral posterior nuclei. The parafascicular nucleus is also easily delimited as it is at the dorsomedial portion of the habenular-peduncular tract. The intralaminar nuclei receive input from many regions throughout the central nervous system, ascending axons from the reticular nuclei and midbrain limbic nuclei, and subthalamus and hypothalamus as well as other thalamic nuclei. The intralaminar nuclei have no direct cortical projection but influence the cerebral cortex by their connections to the specific thalamic nuclei.

Electrical stimulation of the intralaminar nuclei activates neurons in both hemispheres throughout the cerebral cortex. More and more cortical neurons fire as the stimulation continues; this is called the recruiting response. The response finally reaches a maximum and then decreases and may increase again (waxes and wanes). The centromedian nucleus has a strong projection to ventral anterior and ventral lateral nuclei and has a direct projection to the caudate and putamen which permits interrelationship with the extrapyramidal motor system (Chapter 20).

The following nuclei are part of the *somatic brain* and receive direct input from the ascending lemniscal or sensory system, from the cerebellum, and from the optic tract: ventral lateral, ventral posterior lateral, ventral posterior medial, lateral geniculate, medial geniculate (Figs. 12–3 and 12–4).

The *lateral nucleus* is divided into three parts: lateral dorsal, lateral posterior, and pulvinar. It occupies the upper half of the lateral nuclear grouping throughout the thalamus. It is bounded medially by the internal medullary laminae of the thalamus and laterally by the external medullary laminae of the thalamus. In a stained preparation its ventral border with the ventral nuclear mass is distinct. The dorsal division of the lateral nucleus starts near the anterior end of the thalamus and runs the length of the thalamus with its posterior portion, the pulvinar, overhanging the geniculate bodies and midbrain. The lateral posterior projects to the parietal cortex and receives input from specific thalamic nuclei.

The *pulvinar* is the largest nucleus in the thalamus and is continuous with the posterior part of the lateral division. The pulvinar probably receives no direct sensory input but interconnects with many thalamic nuclei and is connected reciprocally with supramarginal, angular gyri, the superior parietal lobule, and occipital and posterior temporal regions.

The *ventral nuclear mass* consists of three distinct regions: ventral anterior, ventral lateral, and ventral posterior. The ventral anterior nucleus is the smallest and most rostral nucleus of this group. It can be identified by the presence of numerous myelinated bundles. This nucleus receives fibers from the globus pallidus, via the lenticular and thalamic fasciculi, and from the intralaminar nuclei and has some projections to areas four and six. Stimulation of this nucleus produces the same effects as stimulation of the intralaminar nuclei.

The *ventral lateral nucleus* occupies the middle portion of the ventral nuclear mass. It is a specific relay nucleus in that it receives fibers from the contralateral deep cerebellar nuclei (superior cerebellar peduncle or dentatorubrothalamic tract) and ipsilateral red nucleus. This nucleus receives fibers from the globus pallidus and from the intralaminar nuclei. This nucleus projects to area four and to a lesser degree to area six and has a topographical projection to the motor cortex. This nucleus is important in integrative somatic motor functions as a result of the interplay between the cerebellum basal ganglia and cerebrum in this nucleus.

The *ventral posterior nucleus* occupies the posterior half of the ventral nuclear mass and consists of two parts: the ventral posterior medial nucleus and the ventral posterior lateral nucleus. Both of these nuclei receive input from the specific ascending sensory systems. The ventroposterior medial nucleus (arcuate or semilunar nucleus) is located lateral to the centromedian nucleus and medial to the ventral posterior lateral nucleus. The secondary fibers of the trigeminal and gustatory pathways terminate in this nucleus; thus this nucleus is concerned primarily with taste and with general sensation

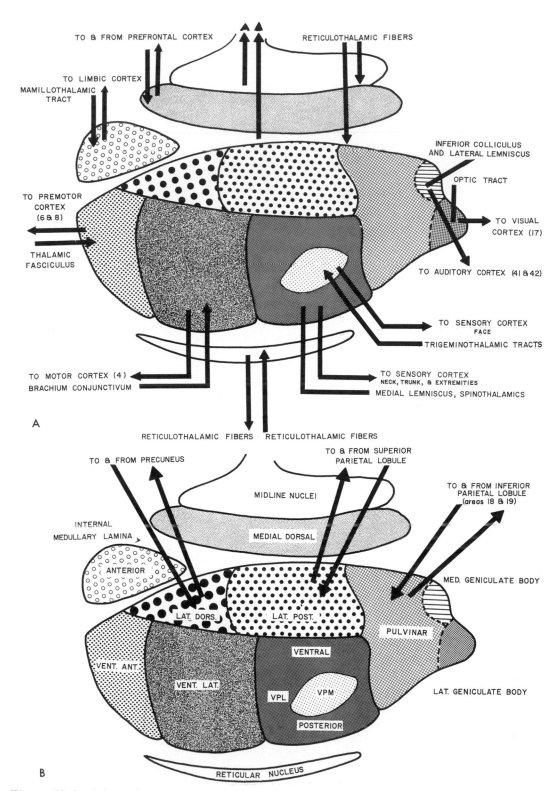

Figure 12–3 Schematic representation of the thalamic nuclei showing connections of lateral region of thalamus (*A*) and remainder of thalamic nuclei (*B*). (After Truex, R. C., and Carpenter, M. B.: *Human Neuroanatomy.* Baltimore, Williams and Wilkins, 1970.)

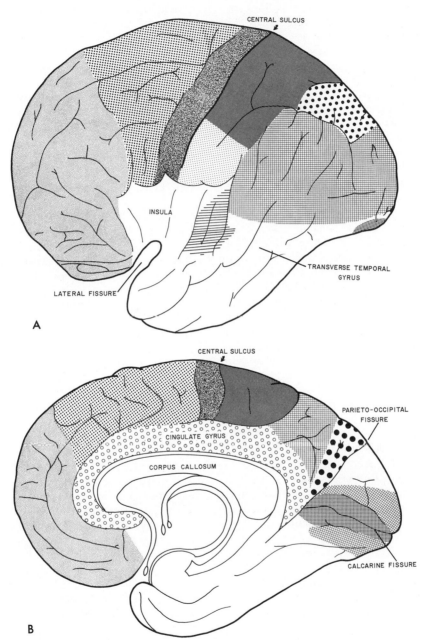

Figure 12-4   Schematic drawing of (*A*) the lateral surface of a cerebral hemisphere and (*B*) the medial surface, showing projections onto cerebral hemisphere of nuclei seen in Figure 12–3.

from the head and face. General sensations from the face, including pain, temperature, touch, and pressure, and proprioception, terminate in this nucleus. This nucleus projects to the face, ears, and head, and tongue regions on the inferior part of the postcentral gyrus, areas three, one, two. The *ventral posterolateral nucleus* receives fibers from the dorsal columns and spinothalamic tracts. The nucleus projects to the trunk and the upper and lower limb regions on the postcentral gyrus (areas 3, 1, 2).

The *medial geniculate nucleus* located on the most caudal portion of the thalamus receives the ascending auditory fibers originating from the following nuclei: cochlear, trapezoid, superior olivary, lateral lemniscal and inferior colliculus. The auditory fibers end on the medial geniculate pars parvocellularis. This nucleus projects to area 41, the transverse temporal gyrus of Heschl.

The *lateral geniculate nucleus* is a horseshoe-shaped laminate nucleus. It receives the optic tract and projects to area 17. Crossed fibers of the optic tract terminate in laminae 1, 4, and 6, while uncrossed fibers end in laminae 2, 3, and 5. This nucleus also connects with the pulvinar, ventral, and lateral thalamic nuclei. Some optic fibers precede to the pretectal area and the superior colliculus with or without synapsing in the lateral geniculate nucleus.

The thalamus is the final processing station for systems which project to the cerebral cortex. This makes the thalamus important to many integrative functions. Many sensations are first appreciated crudely at the thalamic levels. These sensations include pain, crude touch, crude taste, and vibration. The finite discriminative process associated with the aforementioned sensations as well as tactile discrimination, vision, audition, and taste, are elevated to consciousness in the cerebral hemisphere.

In man, lesions in the thalamus produce the "thalamic syndrome" in which there is diminished sensation on the contralateral half of the head and body (complete anesthesia results from injury to the ventral posterior lateral nucleus. Some pain and temperature from a contralateral side may be retained, and the face may be intact to all sensations. There is usually an upper motor neuron lesion of the contralateral limbs and trunk as a result of involvements of the internal capsule. The threshold for pain, temperature, touch, and pressure is usually elevated contralaterally. Mild sensory stimuli now produce exaggerated sensory responses on the affected side and may even lead to intractable pain. There may also be an emotional change. (See Chapter 22.)

SUBTHALAMUS (FIG. 12–1)

The subthalamus region is included in the diencephalon, but functionally it is part of the extrapyramidal system. The subthalamic nucleus, zona incerta, and prerubral field together form the subthalamus. This region is medial to the posterior limb of the internal capsule, lateral to the hypothalamus, and below the thalamus. The ansa lenticularis, subthalamic fasciculus, lenticular fasciculus and thalamic fasciculus provide input from the globus pallidus to the subthalamus. The zona incerta lies between the thalamus and lenticular fasciculus. The globus pallidus provides the principal input to the subthalamus via the subthalamic fasciculus which runs through the internal capsule. The motor and premotor cortex also project to this region. The subthalamus projects back to the globus pallidus via the subthalamic fasciculus and projects to the thalamus and contralateral subthalamus.

In man, a lesion in the subthalamus, usually vascular in origin, produces hemiballismus — purposeless, involuntary, violent, and forceful flinging movements of the contralateral extremity. These movements persist during wakefulness, but disappear with sleep. (See Chapter 24.)

13

Fiber Tracts
of the Brain Stem

STANLEY JACOBSON

INTRODUCTION

In this chapter the connections of the important fiber tracts of the spinal cord and brain stem will be discussed, including their location in the brain stem and their clinical importance. The student should refer to Chapter 11 for a discussion of the interrelationships between the tracts and the nuclei at each level.

The ascending tracts in the central nervous system function much as a railroad system. The information originates at a local station (a peripheral receptor) and is carried into the central nervous system by local tracts (nerve roots) which end at a station on the main line (a nucleus). From the station on the main line the information can be moved directly via the high speed line (the specific systems, i.e., the medial lemniscus), which constitutes the main line up to the union station in the big city (the diencephalon and cerebrum). Some nervous impulses must go through many local stations off the main line before reaching the main station. Consequently they reach the union station more slowly (the nonspecific systems, i.e., the reticular system).

The descending tracks, originating from the union station (corticospinal and cortico-

bulbar tracts), may operate at high speed and connect directly to the local stations (cranial nerve nuclei and other nuclei in the brain stem and spinal cord). There are also slow speed descending fiber systems (corticoreticulospinal, corticorubrospinal, and corticostriatal reticulospinal).

In essence then, the medial lemniscus is nothing more than a high speed ascending line so that information from all sensory systems can reach the diencephalon and ultimately the telencephalon as quickly as possible, while the corticospinal track is a main-line, high speed, descending system from the cortex so that voluntary movement can be provided with minimal delay.

The peripheral nervous system maintains two separate but identical systems to innervate the two body halves. In the central nervous system, even as neurons differentiate, axons cross the midline and form synapses with neurons on the other side of the sensory system. This integration of the body halves is necessary for the coordinate-integrative functions of the central nervous system.

Each sensory system has its first order neuron in a ganglia on one side of the peripheral nervous system or in a cranial nerve, but the axons of the second order neuron in the central nervous system usually ascend

301

in the opposite side of the central nervous system. *All ascending sensory systems follow this principle: primary cell body and axon are ipsilateral; a second order cell body is ipsilateral; second order axons are contralateral.* For example, pain and temperature fibers originate in free nerve endings in the skin, the primary cell body being located in an ipsilateral spinal ganglion. The axons of this primary neuron enter the spinal cord and synapse on ipsilateral neurons located in the dorsal horn of the spinal cord from which the second order axon crosses the midline and ascends as the lateral spinothalamic tract to the thalamus and subsequently to the sensory portion of the cerebral cortex. Thus, the right side of the body is represented in the left cerebral hemisphere not only as it regards motor function but also as it regards sensory function. It should also be noted that in the ascending sensory systems there are some axons which also ascend on the same side; thus there is some protective mechanism in the central nervous system. In case the fiber tracts of one side are interrupted some information from that region can still reach the cerebral cortex. However, this information does not have the same quality as that traveling in the major crossed pathway.

CORTICOSPINAL TRACTS (FIG. 13–1)

This tract innervates the motor neurons that control the skeletal muscles in the neck, thorax, abdomen, pelvis, and the extremities. It is essential for accurate voluntary movements and is the only direct tract from the cortex to the spinal motor neurons.

This system originates from the pyramidal cells and giant cells of Betz in the upper two-thirds of the precentral gyrus, area 4, and to a lesser degree from area 6 and parts of the frontal, parietal, temporal, and cingulate cortices. The fibers pass through the genu of the internal capsule into the middle one-third of the cerebral peduncles and enter the pons where they are broken into many fascicles and are covered by pontine gray and white matter. In the medulla, the fibers are again united and are found on the anterior medial surface of the brain stem in a pyramid-shaped region, the pyramids.

About 75 per cent to 90 per cent of the corticospinal tract fibers cross at the medullo-spinal junction and are thereafter found in the lateral funiculus of the spinal cord. The rest of the corticospinal fibers remain uncrossed in the anterior position but will slowly cross at lower levels. About 50 per cent of the corticospinal fibers end in the cervical levels with about 30 per cent going to the lumbosacral levels and the remainder to the thoracic levels.

Most of the corticospinal fibers end on internuncial neurons, but in regions in the spinal cord where the digits are represented (cervical and lumbosacral enlargement) the corticospinal fibers can end directly on the motor horn cells. The internuncial neurons are located in the base of the dorsal or ventral columns. Lesions in the corticospinal tract produce contralateral upper motor neuron symptoms, while lesions in the spinal motor neurons or rootlets cause lower motor neuron symptoms.

CORTICOBULBAR SYSTEM (FIG. 13–2)

This system distributes to the motor nuclei of the cranial nerves and provides voluntary and involuntary control of these structures. These fibers are found anterior to the corticospinal fibers in the genu of the internal capsule and medial to the corticospinal tract in the cerebral peduncle, pons, and medullary pyramids.

In upper midbrain levels, fibers to cranial nerves III and IV leave the cerebral peduncles and take a descending pathway through the tegmentum, usually in the medial lemniscus (corticomesencephalic tract).

The fibers supplying the muscles of facial expression (motor nerve VII), mastication (motor nerve V), and deglutination (ambiguous nuclei of nerves IX and X) originate from pyramidal cells in the inferior part of the precentral gyrus, area four. The fibers controlling eye movements originate from the frontal eye fields in the caudal part of the middle frontal gyrus and the adjacent inferior frontal gyrus, area eight. The fibers innervating the larynx originate from the inferior frontal gyrus and from the frontal operculum, the posterior part of the pars triangularis, area 44. It appears that many corticobulbar axons end on interneurons and not directly on the motor neuron of the cranial nerve.

The preganglionic parasympathetic inner-

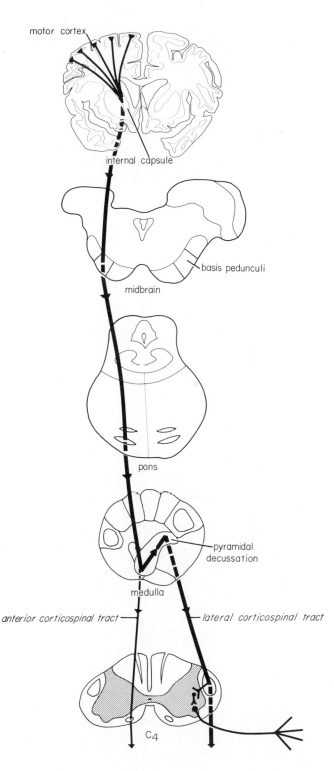

Figure 13–1 Corticospinal tract. This fiber bundle originates primarily from the motor cortex and descends in the basilar region of the brain stem until it reaches the spinal cord where a majority of the fibers cross.

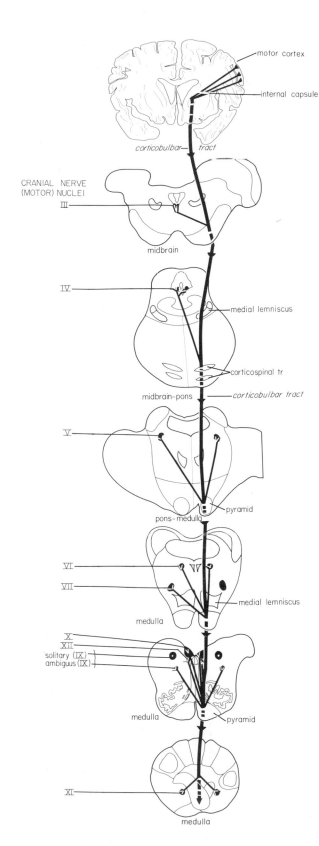

Figure 13-2 Corticobulbar tract. This fiber bundle originates primarily from the motor and premotor cortices and descends in the basilar region of the brain stem to supply bilaterally cranial nerves V to XII and contralaterally a portion of nerve VII, or it takes an aberrant pathway in the medial lemniscus to innervate cranial nerves III and IV.

vation of blood vessels, glands, and viscera is provided by motor nuclei of nerves VII (superior salivatory nucleus), IX (inferior salivatory nucleus) and X (dorsal motor nucleus). The motor, premotor, frontal associational orbital and cingulate cortices may also discharge directly onto the hypothalamus or midbrain-limbic nuclei and then, via a descending pathway, connect with cranial nerves VII, IX and X—the dorsal longitudinal fasciculus.

The cortical innervation of the cranial nerves is bilateral with the exception of the lower facial muscles which are innervated by the contralateral cortex; consequently unilateral lesions in the cortical bulbar system produce only weakness and not paralysis. Paralysis results only from bilateral lesions in the corticobulbar system. A lesion of the motor nucleus or rootlet produces a lower motor neuron syndrome, while supranuclear lesions produce upper motor neuron symptoms.

RUBROSPINAL AND TECTOSPINAL TRACTS

In lower animals not having corticospinal and corticobulbar tracts, fibers from the superior colliculus or optic tectum function similarly to the corticospinal and corticobulbar tracts. Fibers from the red nucleus also appear important in controlling the cranial and spinal nuclei. These tracts in man function normally as adjuncts to the direct corticospinal and corticobulbar tracts; only when disease affects the direct corticospinal pathway can the functions of these tracts be considered.

LATERAL SPINOTHALAMIC TRACT (FIG. 13–3)

This tract conducts pain and temperature from the neck, thorax, abdomen, pelvis, and extremities. The receptors for pain are the naked free nerve endings, while the corpuscles of Ruffini and of Krause detect warmth and cold. The primary cell bodies are located in the dorsal root ganglion; the axons enter the spinal cord and ascend or descend one segment ipsilaterally before ending on neurons in the dorsal horn. The axons of the secondary cells cross in the anterior commissure of the spinal cord and ascend in the ventrolateral part of the lateral funiculus in the spinal cord and medulla. In the pons they are found at the lateral margin of the medial lemniscus and continue up to the ventral posterior lateral nucleus of the thalamus. The axons in this tract convey information from the contralateral side.

The pain fibers in this tract are arranged segmentally with the most lateroposterior fibers representing the lowest part of the sacral levels of the body, and the more medioanterior fibers representing the upper extremities and neck. The temperature fibers have this same arrangement but are internal to the pain fibers. For surgical relief of pain this tract is located by identifying the denticulate ligament and then sectioning about 1 mm. below the ligament.

The sharp pain noted with most injuries is associated with the heavily myelinated direct or spinothalamic pathway to the ventral posterior lateral nucleus. In addition to the sharp pain, dull disagreeable throbbing pain is usually noted; it is carried up more slowly by a multisynaptic pathway, probably via the reticular system. Painful impulses set up in the viscera are transmitted with sympathetic nerves and referred to the periphery of the body—this is called referred pain. In this instance the organ in which the pain is felt is innervated by the same sensory dermatomes to which pain in these visceral structures would be referred: lungs, C8–T8; heart, C8–T8; bladder, T1–T9; testes, T10–T12; kidneys, T11–L1, and rectum, S2–S4.

A unilateral lesion of the spinothalamic tract in the spinal cord produces almost a complete absence of pain and temperature (analgesia and thermoanesthesia) contralateral to the site of the lesion. In the upper pontine levels, the lateral spinothalamic tract is usually closely associated with the medial lemniscus. Consequently, pain and temperature from the opposite side of the body, as well as touch, vibrational sensation, and proprioception, are diminished by a unilateral lesion.

Pain and temperature for the head are carried by the descending nucleus and root of nerve V. The primary cell bodies are found in the trigeminal ganglion with the secondary cell bodies originating in the descending nucleus of nerve V and the axons ascending contralaterally in the medial lemniscus up to the ventral posterior medial nucleus of the thalamus.

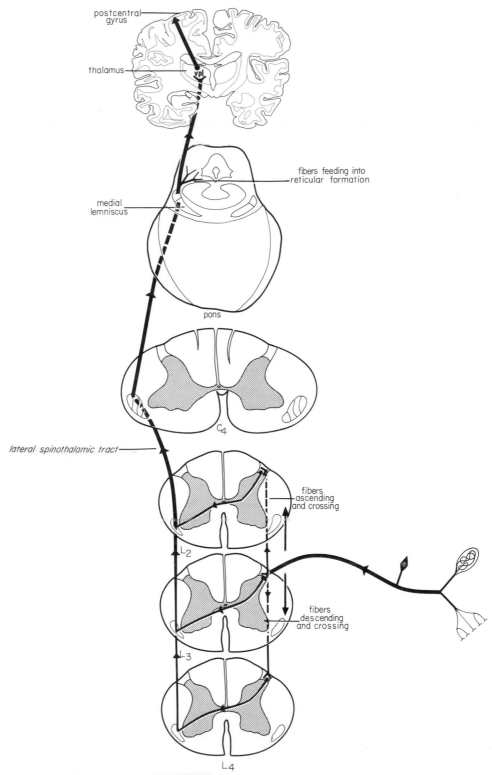

Figure 13–3 Lateral spinothalamic tract. This fiber bundle originates from temperature and pain receptors of the skin. The primary and secondary cell bodies are on the ipsilateral side of the spinal cord, while the secondary axons cross the midline and ascend in the lateral funiculus to the ventral posterior lateral nucleus (VPL) in the thalamus.

POSTERIOR COLUMNS (FASCICULI GRACILIS AND CUNEATUS)

The posterior columns—the fasciculus gracilis, and the fasciculus cuneatus (Fig. 13–4)—conduct proprioception (position sense), vibration sensation, tactile discrimination, object recognition, deep touch (pressure) awareness, and two-point discrimination from the neck, thorax, abdomen, pelvis, and extremities. The sensory receptors for the system are the Golgi tendon organs, the muscle spindles, the proprioceptors, and the tactile discs and Pacinian corpuscles (deep touch or pressure). The primary cell body is located in the dorsal root ganglion.

The well-myelinated fibers of this system enter the spinal cord as the medial division of the dorsal root and bifurcate into ascending and descending portions which enter the dorsal column.

The fasciculus gracilis contains fibers from the sacral, lumbar, and lower thoracic levels, while the fasciculus cuneatus contains fibers from the upper thoracic and cervical levels. Fibers from the sacral levels are the first to enter and lie most medial, followed by lumbar, thoracic, and, finally, cervical fibers. The primary axons ascend in the dorsal columns of the spinal cord to the secondary cell body of this system which is located in the nucleus gracilis and the nucleus cuneatus in the lower medullary levels.

From the secondary cell body the fibers cross the midline, form the medial lemniscus, and ascend to the ventral posterior lateral nucleus in the thalamus. From this nucleus these fibers are projected to the postcentral gyrus, areas 3, 1, 2. Fibers also descend in the dorsal columns, but their functional significance is unknown.

The fibers responsible for proprioception are crossed in the medial lemniscus. The fibers for vibration sensation and tactile discrimination primarily are bilateral in the medial lemniscus to the ventral posterior lateral nucleus. Consequently, proprioception can be abolished by a unilateral lesion, while tactile discrimination and vibrations will be impaired.

Lesions in the posterior column appear not to affect pressure, but vibration sense, two-point discrimination, and tactile discrimination are abolished or diminished, depending on the extent of the lesion. The ability to recognize differences in the shape and weight of objects placed in the hand is impaired. The extremities are more sensitive to these modalities than any other body regions; therefore, position sense is impaired again more severely in the extremities than elsewhere; the person has trouble identifying small passive movements of the limbs. Consequently, performance of voluntary acts is impaired and movements are clumsy (sensory ataxia).

ANTERIOR SPINOTHALAMIC TRACT

Light touch awareness from the neck, thorax, pelvis, and extremities is carried up the *anterior spinothalamic tract* (Fig. 13–5). The primary neuron is located in the dorsal root ganglion; the secondary neuron is located in the dorsal horn of the same side. The secondary fibers ascend contralaterally in the lateral funiculus, joining the medial lemniscus in the upper pontine levels. Light touch is evoked by stroking a hairless area of the skin with cotton. Lesions involving this tract produce no definite clinical deficiencies probably because a somewhat similar sensation is also carried in the uncrossed dorsal columns (fine touch, pressure).

TRACTS ORIGINATING FROM SECONDARY TRIGEMINAL NUCLEI (FIG. 13–6)

Proprioception from the Head. The primary cell body is located in the trigeminal ganglion and mesencephalic nucleus of nerve V. The primary axons project to the motor nucleus of nerve V and the reticular formation. Axons are also projected to the cerebellum and inferior olive.

The origin of the secondary neuron is unclear (probably the descending nucleus of nerve V). The secondary axons ascend in the medial lemniscus to the ventral posterior medial nucleus of the thalamus.

Pain and Temperature from the Head. The primary bodies are located in the trigeminal ganglion. The primary axons enter the pons, descend as the descending tract of nerve V, and terminate in the descending nucleus of nerve V. The ophthalmic fibers descend to C3, the maxillary to C1, and the mandibular to the lower medulla. The secon-

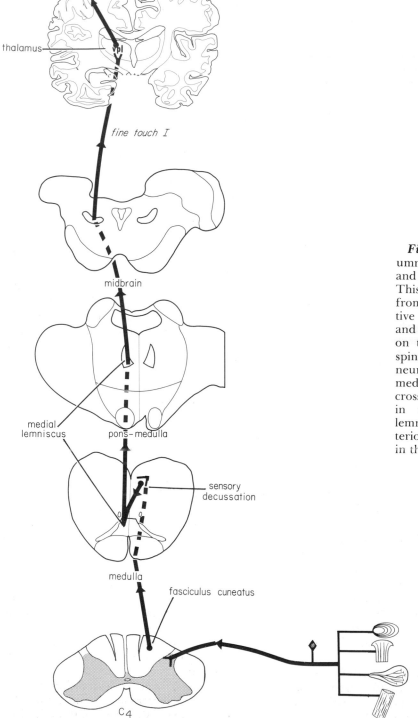

areas 3,1,2

thalamus

VPL

fine touch I

midbrain

medial lemniscus

pons-medulla

sensory decussation

medulla

fasciculus cuneatus

C4

Figure 13–4 Posterior columns or the funiculus gracilis and the funiculus cuneatus. This fiber bundle originates from tactile and proprioceptive receptors. The primary and secondary cell bodies are on the ipsilateral side of the spinal cord. The secondary neurons are found in the medulla. The secondary axons cross the midline and ascend in the contralateral medial lemniscus to the ventral posterior lateral nucleus (VPL) in the thalamus.

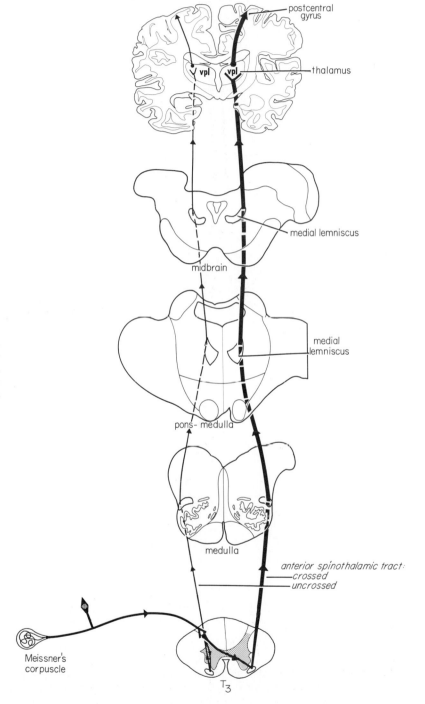

Figure 13–5 Anterior spinothalamic tract. This bundle originatcs from tactile receptors in the skin. The primary and secondary cell bodies are located on the ipsilateral side of the spinal cord while the secondary axons ascend bilaterally to the thalamus.

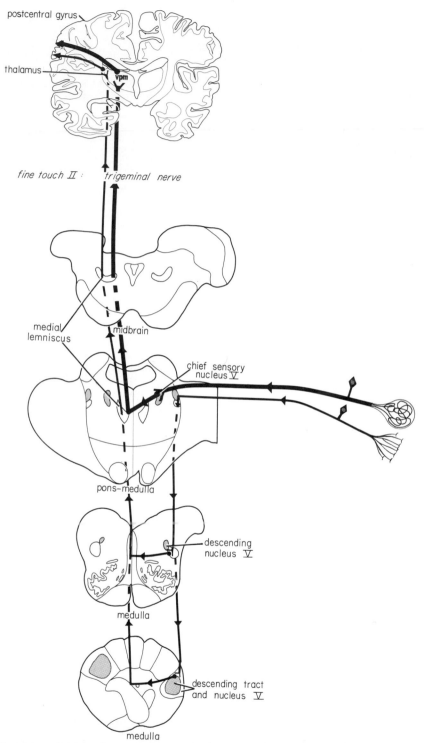

Figure 13-6 Trigeminal nuclei and tracts. All the cutaneous and proprioceptive impulses from the head and neck are carried into the CNS by nerve V. The pain and temperature fibers enter and descend ipsilaterally through pontine-medullary and upper cervical levels and synapse with the secondary cell bodies (descending nucleus of nerve V). The tactile fibers enter and synapse with the chief sensory nucleus in the pons. The proprioceptive fibers (not stains) enter and ascend in pontine and midbrain levels and synapse upon the mesencephalic nucleus of nerve V. The secondary axons ascend in the medial lemniscus to the ventral posterior medial nucleus (VPM) in the thalamus.

dary axons leave the descending nucleus of nerve V and ascend bilaterally in the medial lemniscus to the ventral posterior medial nucleus of the thalamus. The predominant component is crossed.

Tactile Discrimination, Vibration Sensation, and Pressure from the Head. The primary cell bodies are located in the trigeminal ganglion. The primary axons enter the pons and end on the main sensory nucleus of nerve V from which the secondary axons ascend contralaterally in the medial lemniscus or ipsilaterally in the dorsal trigeminothalamic tract to the ventral posterior medial nucleus, primarily on the contralateral side of the brain stem.

Lesions in the sensory nuclei cause an absence of sensation from the same side of the head, while lesions of the tracts produce diminished sensation.

CEREBELLAR TRACTS

The cerebellar cortex must have proprioceptive information to insure proper muscle tone and coordination. Fibers carrying this information run to the cerebellum in the following pathways:

Unconscious Proprioception from the Lower Extremity, Thorax, Abdomen, and Pelvis. This information is carried up to the cerebellum by the anterior and posterior spinocerebellar tracts. The receptors for both tracts are the neuromuscular spindles and Golgi tendon organs.

Posterior Spinocerebellar Tract (Fig. 13–7). The primary neuron is located in the dorsal root ganglion; the secondary neuron is located in Clarke's column in the dorsal horn in levels C8-L3 of the cord. The secondary axons ascend uncrossed in the lateral funiculus, enter the cerebellum via the inferior cerebellar peduncle, and terminate in the ipsilateral vermis (midline portion of the cerebellum).

The Anterior Spinocerebellar Tract (Fig. 13–7). The primary neuron is in the dorsal root ganglion, while the secondary neuron is in cells at the margin of the dorsal horn which are scattered throughout the spinal cord, especially in the lumbar levels. The secondary axon crosses the midline and ascends anterior to the posterior spinocerebellar tract in the lateral funiculus and medulla; it enters the cerebellum via the superior cerebellar peduncle and terminates in the same parts of the cerebellar vermis as the posterior spinocerebellar tract except it is located on the contralateral side.

Unconscious Proprioception from the Upper Extremity and Neck. The primary neurons are found in dorsal root ganglion at cervical levels; their axons ascend in the dorsal columns and end in the external cuneate nuclei in the lower medullary levels. The secondary axons ascend bilaterally with the posterior spinocerebellar tract and enter the cerebellum primarily uncrossed.

RETICULAR TRACTS

Fiber tracts interconnect all parts of the reticular formation as well as connecting the reticular formation with the vestibular nuclei, the inferior olive, the red nucleus, the thalamus, the basal ganglia, the spinal cord, and the cerebellum.

COORDINATION OF EYE MOVEMENTS — THE MEDIAL LONGITUDINAL FASCICULUS

This tract is present below the ventricular floor in the medulla, pons, and midbrain and in the anterior funiculus of the spinal cord. Fibers ascend and descend in this tract to coordinate eye movements with vestibular, visual, and postural information. The medial longitudinal fasciculus is ideally situated to coordinate eye movements because of its paramedian location in the ventricular floor adjacent to cranial nerves III, IV, and VI.

DESCENDING SYMPATHETIC AND PARASYMPATHETIC TRACTS

The visceral brain provides innervation for the preganglionic sympathetic neurons in the intermediolateral columns in the thoracic and lumbar levels as well as for the preganglionic parasympathetic neurons in the brain stem and sacral cord. The descending tracts are diffuse and are found in the lateral part of the reticular formation and in the anterior and lateral funiculi in the spinal cord. Lesions in these zones may produce sympathetic dysfunction; i.e., Horner's syndrome — paralysis of the sympathetic fibers to the dilator of the pupil, resulting in miosis (constricted

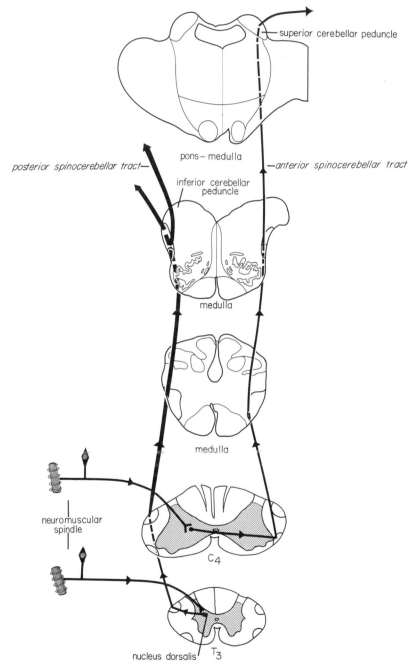

Figure 13–7 Anterior and posterior spinocerebellar tracts. These fiber bundles carry information from proprioceptive receptors in the body up to the cerebellum and also into the reticular formation.

pupil) and an absence of sweating (anhidrosis).

EXERCISE: IDENTIFY TRACTS AND NUCLEI IN FIGURES 13–8 TO 13–13

Figures 13–8 to 13–13 are taken from myelin-stained sections of a stillborn, term infant. In the developing central nervous system there is a sequence of myelination, so certain tracts are clearly seen in this stage. Fiber bundles which obscure these tracts in the adult will myelinate at some time in the future. Certain structures have been labeled; the student should identify the remaining unlabeled tracts and nuclei using the atlas chapter at the end of the book and Chapters 11 and 12 as references.

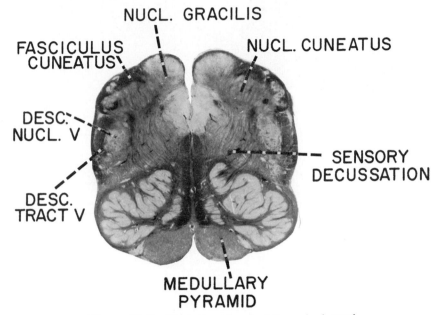

Figure 13–8   Medulla at level of the spinal canal.

See Filmstrip, Frame 16.

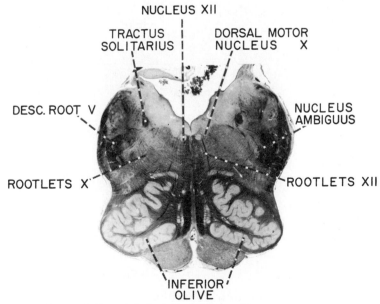

Figure 13–9   Medulla at level of the inferior olive.

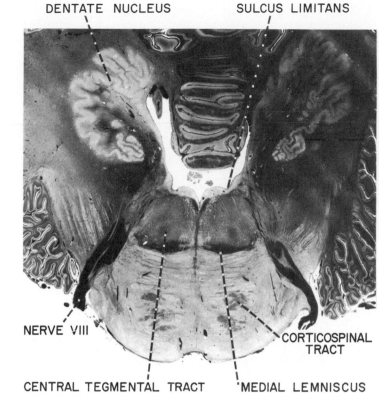

DENTATE NUCLEUS   SULCUS LIMITANS

NERVE VIII

CORTICOSPINAL
TRACT

CENTRAL TEGMENTAL TRACT   MEDIAL LEMNISCUS

Figure 13–10   Pons at level of root of nerve VIII.   See Filmstrip, Frame 18.

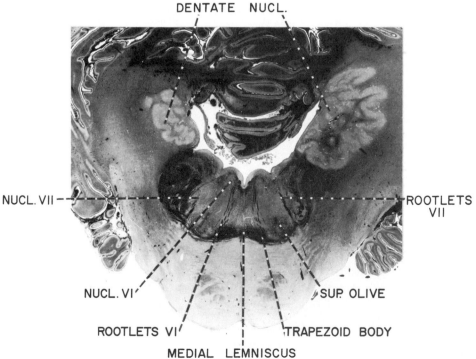

DENTATE NUCL.

NUCL. VII

ROOTLETS
VII

NUCL. VI

SUP. OLIVE

ROOTLETS VI   TRAPEZOID BODY

MEDIAL LEMNISCUS

Figure 13–11   Pons at level of roots of nerves VI and VII.   See Filmstrip, Frame 19.

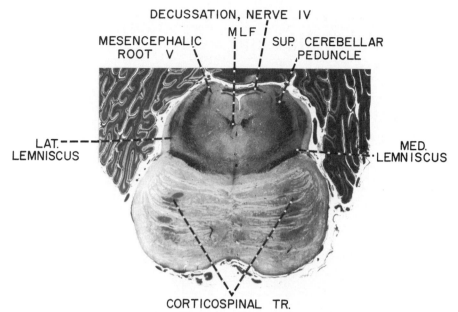

DECUSSATION, NERVE IV

MLF

MESENCEPHALIC
ROOT V

SUP. CEREBELLAR
PEDUNCLE

LAT.
LEMNISCUS

MED.
LEMNISCUS

CORTICOSPINAL TR.

Figure 13–12   Pons at level of root of nerve IV.

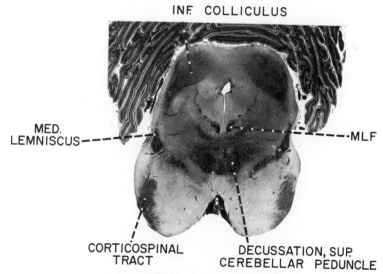

INF. COLLICULUS

MED.
LEMNISCUS

MLF

CORTICOSPINAL
TRACT

DECUSSATION, SUP.
CEREBELLAR PEDUNCLE

Figure 13–13   Inferior colliculus.

14

Vestibular and Auditory Systems

BRIAN CURTIS

THE VESTIBULAR SYSTEM

To maintain his upright, two-legged posture, man must have very precise information about his position in space. Visual clues provide probably the most important information. Next in importance are proprioceptive responses from the neck and leg muscles, and, lastly, the impulses from the vestibular system play a part in some righting responses. The integration of all of these types of input will be considered in Chapter 23, Motor Function.

The vestibular system is much more conspicuous in dysfunction than in function. However, you should be aware of the processes involved in its function.

The receptors of the vestibular system, the semicircular canals and the maculae, are located in the inner ear in close approximation to the organ of hearing, the cochlea. The primary nerve cells are in the inner ear; the axons enter the brain stem as cranial nerve VIII and end in the vestibular nuclei of the same side. Each set of semicircular canals consists of three canals in mutually perpendicular planes which interconnect at the utricle. The spatial location of each canal is shown in Figure 14–1. Tracing and cutting out part C of this figure should be of great

help in understanding the relationship of each canal. The sensory receptors in these canals respond to rotation in the plane of the canal and as such respond only to changes in position; they are acceleration receptors. For the rest of this discussion we will concentrate on the horizontal canals; the anterior and posterior canals function in the same manner.

Figure 14–2 shows a section through the right horizontal canal as well as the utricle and a third structure, the saccule. These structures are filled with an isotonic solution, *endolymph*, which is of high potassium and low sodium concentration.

The Sensory Receptors. The sensory receptor is in the ampulla and consists of the projections of many hair cells embedded in a gelatinous mass, the *crista* (Fig. 14–2). This mass almost fills the ampulla so that any movement of the fluid relative to the base of the crista will cause the crista to bend, deform the hairs, and fire the nerves. At the beginning of a rapid turning of the head, the base of the crista moves, but the endolymph does not because of its inertia. Consequently, the crista is bent (Fig. 14–4*A*). The nerve fibers from the crista are tonically active; they fire continuously even though there is no stimulus. When the crista is bent toward the utricle, the frequency of firing

316

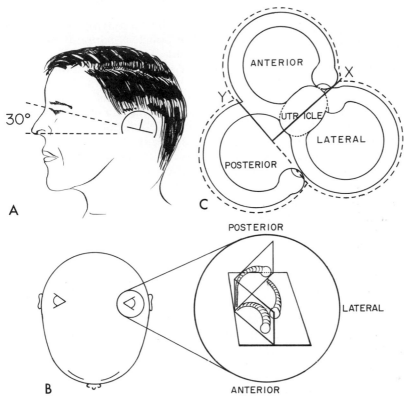

Figure 14-1 Parts *A* and *B* show the location of the semicircular canals in the head. Part *C* is a diagram to help in understanding the three-dimensional structure of the canals. Trace the lines on a sheet of paper and cut along the dotted lines; fold at X and Y. (Part *C* is based on Lithgaw, J. D.: J. Laryng., *35*:81, 1920.)

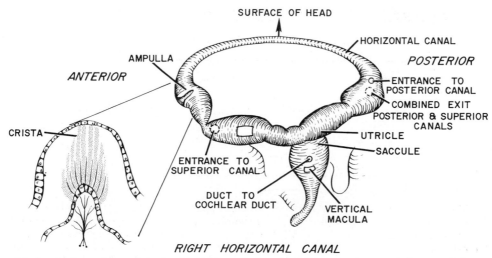

Figure 14-2 A view of the right horizontal canal, the ampulla and crista and the two right maculae.

is increased. When the crista is bent away from the utricle, the frequency decreases.

Records of firing, not of the vestibular nerve, but of a single unit in the vestibular nucleus in the cat are shown in Figure 14-3. As the cat is rotated to the right, the discharge is intense and lasts a short time on the swing back, but it dies out quickly as the cat is rotated to the left. The discharge from the other horizontal canal will show the reverse pattern. While not obvious in Figure 14-3, the receptor adapts fairly rapidly to rotation; the firing frequency returns to normal about 5 seconds after the rotation (as shown in Fig. 14-4) begins.

The lack of response to continued rotation is easy to understand; because of friction, the endolymph rapidly begins to rotate at the same speed as the head. Now there are no sheering forces on the crista (Fig. 14-4B), and the nerve discharge returns to normal.

When the body and the head stop rotating, the endolymph continues to rotate; a body in motion tends to remain in motion. The flow of endolymph past the crista bends the tip in the direction of motion (Fig. 14-4C) and causes a change in the nerve output. The crista bent toward the utricle is excited. The flow of endolymph rapidly ceases and the crista returns to normal.

A different set of terminology has been developed which is most useful when the head is stationary and endolymph is flowing. If the endolymph is flowing toward the ampulla, as happens on the left side at the end of a clockwise rotation (Fig. 14-4C), the crista is excited and the flow is called *ampullopetal*. In the same circumstances the flow in the right canal is away from the ampulla, *ampullofugal*, and the crista is inhibited.

The deflection of the crista in Figure 14-4C is identical to the pattern which would be seen at the beginning of a counter-clockwise rotation. The end organ has no mechanism for differentiating between the start of a counter-clockwise rotation and the end of a clockwise rotation. One method of showing this is to observe eye movement.

CONTROL OF EYE MOVEMENT

The output of the semicircular canals goes directly to the *vestibular nuclei*. Discrete portions of the nuclei respond to rotation in each plane. The vestibular nuclei influence a number of types of movement; one of the most important is eye movement.

Our heads are constantly in motion as we walk down the street, yet we have no impression of the world jiggling up and down in

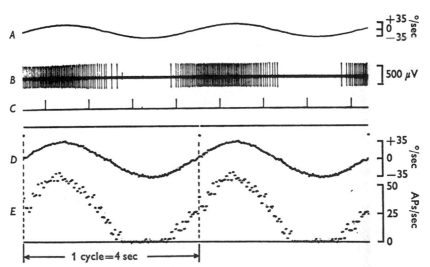

Figure 14-3 Response of a canal-dependent cell to *angular* oscillation in the plane of the lateral canals. The upper half of the figure is a sample of the photogalvanometer record and shows from above down: *A*, tachometer angular velocity signal; *B*, action potentials from microelectrode in the left medial vestibular nucleus, and *C*, time scale (sec.). The lower half of the figure shows the average stimulus (*D*) and concomitant average action potential frequency obtained over 10 cycles (*E*). The averaged data are written out twice to aid visual interpretation. (From Benson, A. J., Guedry, F. E., and Jones, M. J.: J. Physiol., *210*:475, 1970.)

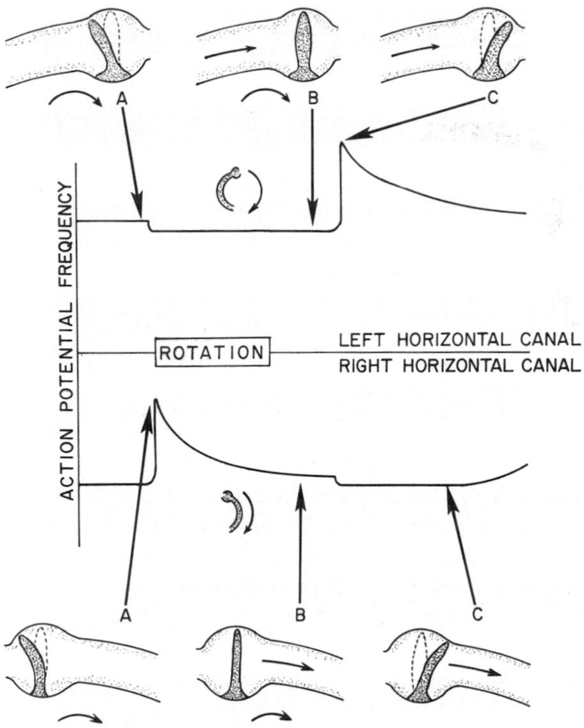

Figure 14-4 The response of the horizontal canals to the beginning, continuation, and cessation of rotation. Note that when one crista is stimulated the other is inhibited. (After Adrian, E. D.: J. Physiol., *101*:389, 1943.)

front of us. Persons without vestibular function often have just such a problem. They may fail to recognize their friends because faces are blurred. As we turn our heads, we can keep our eyes on an object. These and other eye movements show the influence of vestibular information.

This can easily be shown in the Bárány chair. Upon slow clockwise rotation, the eyes move counter-clockwise to keep objects in the visual field. The output from the vestibular nuclei to the medial longitudinal fasciculus (MLF) and the nuclei of nerves VI and III signals clockwise rotation; the response is anticlockwise eye movement.

Consider now the case of stopping suddenly after rotation; the output of the vestibular nuclei signals anticlockwise movement, so the response is clockwise eye movement. As the eyes move slowly clockwise, a stationary image moves out of the visual field and the eyes snap back to the center, find the image, and begin to move slowly again. This is the pattern of nystagmus. The direction of the nystagmus is named for the quick component. The physiologically meaningful component is the slow one.

Nystagmus. Nystagmus describes a rhythmic oscillation of the eyeballs, characterized by a slow drifting from a central gaze toward the periphery and then a sudden snap back to a central gaze position. Both eyes usually move together; it is a conjugate movement and is usually repeated many times. The easiest way to visualize this condition is to find a willing subject and have him look at Figure 14-5 held horizontally. It is important that the subject does not fixate on a single line, but gazes at your face. Move the book horizontally to your left. You should observe a slow movement of the subject's eyes to the right and then a quick snap back to the central position; this pattern will repeat several times as you move the book. You are observing *opticokinetic* nystagmus, but the eye movement pattern is the same for all types of nystagmus. A drum with vertical stripes is often used for testing. Opticokinetic nystagmus is mediated by the occipital lobe although the pathway to the lateral gaze center is not clear.

The nystagmus which originates from the vestibular apparatus has exactly the same form—slow movement followed by a quick jerk. The output of the vestibular nuclei enters the MLF, impinges on the lateral or vertical gaze center, and causes eye movement. Horizontal nystagmus is easily elicited,

Figure 14–5 A pattern to induce opticokinetic nystagmus. Hold the pattern horizontally at shoulder level about 2 feet from a willing subject. Instruct the subject to look at your face and not to fixate on the lines. Move the pattern back and forth horizontally; you should see your subject's eyes jerk — nystagmus.

as is vertical or rotatory nystagmus. Vestibular nystagmus occurs in a dark room or a blind person and involves pathways entirely within the brain stem.

Subjective Responses to Rotation. When a volunteer is placed in a special rotating chair (a Bárány chair), closes his eyes, and is spun slowly, he has no trouble identifying the direction of rotation. Even the direction of very slow rotation (½ degree per second, 12 minutes per revolution) will be correctly identified. After 20 seconds of a moderate spin, he is less certain about the direction and as he slows down the confusion increases. At some point, while still turning, he has a very strong impression that he is turning in the opposite direction. A student will often say, "I know this sounds funny, but I am sure I am turning the other way." At that point, the endolymph is rotating faster than the head and the crista is bent in the opposite direction as in Figure 14–4C. If the subject is stopped very quickly, the subjective impression of rotation in the opposite direction is very strong. Other outputs from the vestibular nuclei, such as to the MLF for eye movement and to the cerebellum for coordination, also show this disorientation upon the sudden cessation of rotation.

The cerebellum has rich connections with the vestibular nuclei, and the input from the vestibular nuclei is used to alter movement patterns in response to spatial movement. A simple example is the ability, when the eyes are closed, to raise the arm from a horizontal to a vertical position and return it to the same horizontal position. If the person rotates clockwise between the raising and lowering, the hand will have to move to the left to come down in its original position. After a long clockwise rotation, when the person has a strong impression of moving counterclockwise, the hand will come back down to the right of its initial position; this is termed past pointing. The output of the vestibular nucleus has convinced the cerebellum that the body is moving counterclockwise. The same problem occurs when the subject tries to walk straight toward a distant object after spinning. He thinks he is turning in the opposite direction and corrects accordingly.

Natural situations rarely cause this type of postrotatory confusion, and most of us have not adapted to it. Two types of performing arts have developed rapid turns: ballet and figure skating. These artists are trained to reduce postrotatory confusion. The ballet dancer rarely makes many rapid turns in succession, but employs a technique called spotting to help maintain balance after turning. At the beginning of a clockwise turn, the dancer will turn her head maximally over the right shoulder, in the direction of movement, will find a prominent object, and, as she turns, will move the head to keep the object in the visual field. When the head is finally turned over the left shoulder, she will snap it around and find the object again. She substitutes a strong visual image for misleading vestibular information.

Champion figure skaters spin much faster and are unable to spot on each turn. They develop, through much practice, the ability to completely disregard the vestibular output at the end of spinning. I had the opportunity to work with one of of our medical students, Lorraine Hanlan Comaner, who had been an Olympic figure skater. When she was rotated very rapidly in the direction she had been trained to spin, she showed no nystagmus after stopping even if her eyes were closed during rotation. She showed no past pointing and could walk straight toward a distant object. After the same rotation, an untrained person would be totally disoriented. When she was spun in the other direction, she showed minimal nystagmus or past pointing and deviated only slightly in walking. Her vestibular apparatus was perfectly normal by caloric testing.

The function of the individual semicircular canal can be determined through caloric testing, whereby the external auditory meatus is cooled by flushing ice water through it. When the subject lies supine with his head tilted back 60 degrees, the horizontal canal is vertical, and the part of it closely adjacent to the external auditory meatus can be cooled. This partial cooling sets up convection movements in the endolymph which bends the crista and causes stimulation of the vestibular nuclei. The function is usually evaluated by observing the resultant nystagmus. In the normal subject, the slow component of the nystagmus is toward the side where the cold water is infused. Both sides should be tested, but with a 10 to 15-minute pause between to allow the first to return to normal.

THE MACULAE

The semicircular canals are acceleration or dynamic receptors. The two maculae (Fig. 14–2) are static receptors; they continuously signal the position of the head. Their structure is shown in Figure 14–6. The hair cells are covered with a gelatinous mass, the otolithic membrane, in which are buried otoliths or crystals of calcium carbonate. Whenever the head tilts, the weight of the otoliths causes the gelatinous mass to shift and puts different stresses on the hair cells. Each hair cell is sensitive to movement in only one direction. When the hair cells bend toward the longest cilia, known as the *kinocilium*, the discharge rate increases; when the hair cells are bent away from the kinocilium, the discharge rate is inhibited. The kinocilia have different orientations in various parts of the macula so that tilt in various directions can be perceived. Recordings from the macular nerve show continuous nerve discharge after the head is tilted to a new position.

The macula is a static receptor; it continuously provides information on the location of the head, as well as on changes in position. In erect posture, the macula of the utricle is approximately horizontal and that of the saccule, vertical.

CONNECTIONS OF THE VESTIBULAR NERVE AND NUCLEI

The vestibular nerve is a portion of the cranial nerve VIII and enters the brain stem at the junction of the medulla and pons

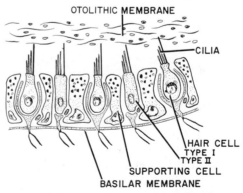

Figure 14–6 The structure of the macula. The cilia project into the gelatinous mass of the otolithic membrane in which are imbedded calcium carbonate granules. The longer, denser cilia apparently give the cell directional sensitivity since any one cell is sensitive to deflection in only one direction. (Based, in part, on Flock and Duvall: *J. Cell. Biol.*, 25:1, 1965.)

(Fig. 29–8). Most of the fibers end within the four vestibular nuclei, but a significant number end in the cerebellum, particularly the fastigial nucleus. The distribution of the endings within the four nuclei is well worked out (Brodal et al., 1962).

The secondary vestibular fibers run from the vestibular nuclei throughout the neuraxis. There are rich connections to and from the cerebellum via the inferior cerebellar peduncle. These cerebellar connections are particularly rich to the lateral vestibular nucleus which gives rise to the uncrossed vestibulospinal tract. This tract runs throughout the spinal cord in the anterior funiculus (Fig. 7–30). It is thought to be responsible for much of the influence the cerebellum and vestibular nuclei have on muscle tone and motor movement. The activity of the vestibular nuclei tends to facilitate motor neurons of the extensor muscles.

Secondary vestibular fibers enter the MLF; the descending ones project to the nuclei in the lower brain stem and account no doubt for the nausea and vomiting associated with extensive vestibular stimulation. The descending fibers project to nucleus XI and the upper cervical motor neurons to influence neck movement. The ascending fibers connect to all three nuclei (VI, IV, and III) controlling eye movement with both crossed and uncrossed fibers. Secondary vestibular fibers enter the reticular formation at many levels.

The vestibular nuclei project to the cortex of the temporal lobe by unknown pathways and are no doubt responsible for the conscious sensations of vertigo and dizziness.

DISTURBANCES OF THE VESTIBULAR SYSTEM

Motion Sickness. The most common affliction related to the vestibular system is motion sickness—air, car, or sea—which is characterized by vertigo, nausea, and vomiting. These symptoms are all caused by continual periodic motion; it seems likely that the repeated vertical movements are primarily responsible. Most people quickly adapt to the motion. In severe cases of sea sickness, however, the unfortunate person's major fear is that he *isn't* going to die. Motion sickness can usually be avoided by eating a light, fat-free meal and taking one of a number of antihistamine compounds, such as meclizine (Bonine) or dimenhydrinate (Dramamine), before traveling. These compounds do little good after the symptoms have appeared.

Vertigo. Intermittent attacks of vertigo, the false sensation that the person or his surroundings are whirling around, constitute a common problem associated with the vestibular system. These paroxysmal attacks can be very disabling since the patient is often thrown to the ground by his own reactions to these false clues of movement. Single attacks may occur in acute labyrinthitis.

Meniere's disease is one common cause of intermittent attacks of vertigo. Meniere's disease also attacks the organ of hearing and results in tinnitus, a constant ringing or humming in the ears; it is of unknown origin. There are a number of medical treatments for it. The surgical treatment is removal of the labyrinth or partial section of nerve VIII. Tumors of nerve VIII and prolonged treatment with streptomycin may also cause vertigo.

Labyrinth Destruction. Rapid destruction of one labyrinth causes only short-lived disturbances of equilibrium, some vertigo and nystagmus, and, occasionally, nausea and vomiting. The vestibular nuclei apparently work by comparing the signals from both labyrinths, a sort of differential amplifier. When one labyrinth is destroyed, the vestibular nuclei apparently overcompensate for the input from the other side.

Bilateral destruction of both labyrinths does not cause nystagmus or vertigo but a transient disturbance of equilibrium often lasting many months. Under water, patients with this disturbance are totally disoriented.

Vestibular deprivation in animals is usually much more severe than in man, probably because animals normally rely less heavily on visual input than man does.

THE AUDITORY SYSTEM

EXTERNAL AND MIDDLE EAR

The external ear consists of the cartilaginous pinna and the acoustic meatus. The *pinna* plays a role in collecting sound waves from the environment and channeling them into the other portion of the external ear. The external *acoustic meatus*, or ear canal, is about one-quarter of an inch (10 mm.) in diameter and 1 inch (25 mm.) long and ends blindly at the tympanic membrane (Fig. 14–

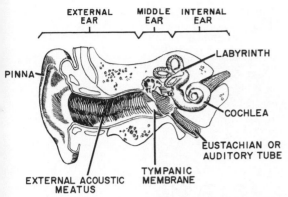

EXTERNAL EAR   MIDDLE EAR   INTERNAL EAR

PINNA

LABYRINTH

COCHLEA

EUSTACHIAN OR AUDITORY TUBE

EXTERNAL ACOUSTIC MEATUS

TYMPANIC MEMBRANE

Figure 14–7 The major structures of the auditory receptor.

7). It serves as a resonator for the average sounds of human speech (2500 to 5000 cps), and increases the sound pressure on the tympanic membrane two-fold for tones within this frequency range. In response to sound pressure, the *tympanic membrane* vibrates back and forth; compressions and rarefactions in the air are translated into movements of the membrane. In response to the sound pressure of a whisper, the membrane moves only a few angstroms.

The bones of the middle ear—the *malleus*, the *incus*, and the *stapes*—serve mainly as a lever to transform the large amplitude movements of a large diameter structure, the tympanic membrane, to low amplitude movements of a small area, the *oval window*. In the process, the force of movement is increased as much as 90 times. This increase in force can be described as a mechanical lever and serves as an impedance match between the low density of air and the high density of the fluid in the cochlea. The three bones are held in place by connections of the malleus to the tympanic membrane and of the stapes to the oval window and by five thin ligaments.

The process of transmission across the middle ear is influenced by two muscles: the tensor tympani and the stapedius. The *tensor tympani* is innervated by cranial nerve V. By tensing the tympanic membrane it dampens the vibration. The *stapedius* muscle is innervated by cranial nerve VII and, by pulling the stapes laterally and away from the oval window, tends to counteract force placed on the stapes from the tympanic membrane. When loud noises or tones are heard or anticipated, these muscles contract and reduce the percentage of the sound energy imping-

ing on the oval window. Since the stapedius is innervated by cranial nerve VII, it should not be surprising that persons with Bell's palsy (see Chapter 15) complain that ordinary sounds are excruciatingly loud.

While not shown on Figure 14–7, the *chorda tympani* nerve crosses the middle ear just behind the malleus. When the middle ear is infected, transmission of taste impulses from the anterior two-thirds of the tongue may be blocked here on their way to cranial nerve VII and the tractus solitarius.

INTERNAL EAR

The stapes transmits the vibration of the tympanic membrane to the oval window of the cochlea (Fig. 14–8). The *cochlea* is a spiral organ containing three cavities which spiral together. The function of the canals will be easier to understand if the spiral is unrolled (Fig. 14–9A). The cochlea is filled with fluid and embedded in bone. There are only two elastic points—the oval and round windows. Whenever the stapes compresses the oval window, the round window must bulge out since the rest of the structure and the fluid are incompressible. There are two routes by which a fluid wave can pass from the scala vestibuli to the scala tympani: through a hole (the helicotremia) at the extreme end of the spiral or through a deformation of the basilar membrane. Most of the energy is transmitted by deforming the basilar membrane. (Reissner's membrane seen in Figure 14–9 is too thin to warrant any consideration in this context.)

The *basilar membrane* is not uniform along its length; at the base it is very light and narrow while at the apex, it is thick and wide. Hydraulic pressure waves produce a rippling of the basilar membrane (Fig. 14–9B). The position of maximum movement depends upon the frequency of the sound (Fig. 14–10). The light, thin end moves when the sound is high pitched while the thicker, wider end at the apex vibrates in response to low pitched sounds. Any sound activates a considerable fraction of the total basilar membrane and the amplitude is proportional to the intensity of the sound. The beginning of frequency discrimination occurs on the basilar membrane yet is not completed there.

Movements of the basilar membrane are transformed by an unknown mechanism into action potentials at the organ of Corti,

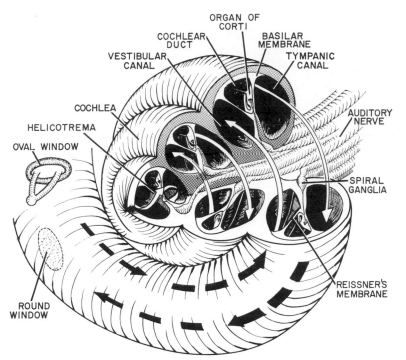

Figure 14–8   The cochlea.

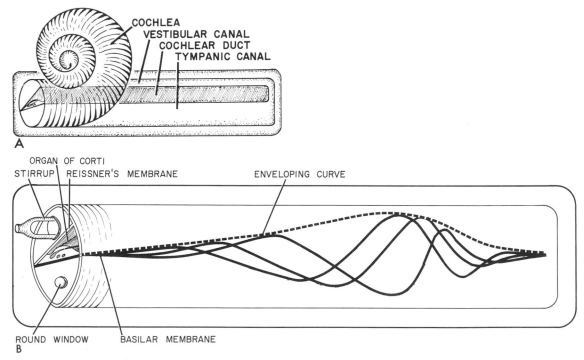

Figure 14–9   *A* shows how the cochlea can be unrolled to give a clearer idea of the function of the basilar membrane. When the stirrup vibrates, the basilar membrane vibrates also; the location of the peak of the enveloping curve varies as the pitch of the sound varies, as shown in *B*.

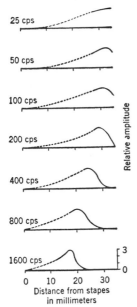

Figure 14–10 lists: 25 cps, 50 cps, 100 cps, 200 cps, 400 cps, 800 cps, 1600 cps, Relative amplitude, 3, 0, 0 10 20 30, Distance from stapes in millimeters

Figure 14–10 The amplitude of displacement of the basilar membrane for constant amplitude and different frequencies of stapes vibration. The solid lines were measured; the dotted lines were extrapolated from other observations. (From Békésy and Rosenblith: Chapter 27 *In* Stevens, S. S. (ed.): *Handbook of Experimental Psychology.* New York, John Wiley and Sons Inc., 1951.)

which lies on the basilar membrane (Fig. 14–11). The major sensory cells are three rows of outer hair cells and one row of inner hair cells. The hairs from the cells just touch the gelatinous *tectorial membrane.* Since the basilar membrane and the tectorial membrane are hinged at different points and are of different mass, it is thought that vibration of the whole complex gives rise to differential movement of the two structures and places a shearing force on the hair cells. If these cells respond in a similar manner to the hair cells in the macula, this bending is then translated into action potentials.

The nerves from the hair cells are bipolar and have their nuclei in the spiral ganglia close to their origins (Fig. 14–8). Their axons form the acoustic portion of nerve VIII. Recordings from a single auditory nerve fiber (Fig. 14–12) show it to respond to a wide range of frequencies; the greater the sound intensity, the greater the range. Other fibers have a different frequency response. This is consistent with the hair cell responding to movements of the basilar membrane since a greater length of the membrane will oscillate at greater sound intensities.

The first set of synapses in the auditory

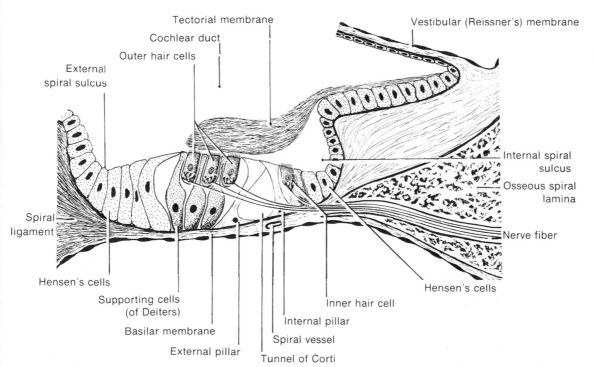

Figure 14–11 labels: Tectorial membrane, Cochlear duct, Outer hair cells, External spiral sulcus, Vestibular (Reissner's) membrane, Internal spiral sulcus, Osseous spiral lamina, Nerve fiber, Spiral ligament, Hensen's cells, Hensen's cells, Supporting cells (of Deiters), Basilar membrane, External pillar, Tunnel of Corti, Spiral vessel, Internal pillar, Inner hair cell

Figure 14–11 The organ of Corti. See Figure 14–8 for its location in the cochlea. The transduction between vibration and action potential firing occurs at the inner and outer hair cells. (From Bossy: *Atlas of Neuroanatomy.* Philadelphia, W. B. Saunders, 1970.)

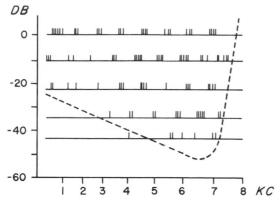

Figure 14-12 Responses of a single auditory nerve fiber to tones of differing frequency and amplitude. Each group of vertical bars represents a train of action potentials in response to a 10 msec. burst of tones at a given frequency and intensity. The responses on each line are to the same intensity but varying frequency. Note that the unit has a decreased range of frequency response as the intensity is reduced. The overall sensitivity is outlined by the dashed line. (After Tasaki, I.: J. Neurophysiol., *17*:97, 1954.)

pathway (Fig. 14–13) are in the dorsal and ventral cochlear nuclei of the pons (Fig. 29–8). Within the cochlear nucleus there is a very definite tonotopic organization. Each of these cells still responds to a range of frequencies, but the range is narrower than in the auditory nerve.

From the cochlear nucleus about one-half the fibers cross the midline and ascend on the opposite side. Consequently, only lesions in the cochlear nucleus, the auditory nerve, or the cochlea will produce deafness in one ear. Lesions of one entire auditory pathway above the pons, even though they destroy one-half of the fibers from each cochlear nucleus, have remarkably little effect on hearing.

The auditory fibers make several synapses before reaching the inferior colliculus, the medial geniculate of the thalamus and finally the transverse temporal gyrus (Fig. 14–13). These synapses occur anywhere along the pathway and there is no fixed number of synapses. At each locus the fibers retain a

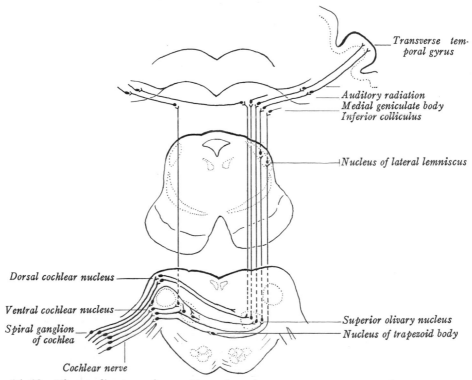

Figure 14-13 The auditory pathway. Note that there are many, nonsynchronous synapses. For clarity, the diagram shows most of the fibers crossing the neuroaxis; about half of the fibers do; the other half ascend on the same side. (From Ranson and Clark: Philadelphia, W. B. Saunders, 1954.)

tonotopic organization but with a gradually diminishing range of frequency sensitivity. On the transverse temporal gyrus the frequency sensitivity of any one cell is quite narrow. Further discussion of cortical function will be deferred to Chapter 21.

Branches of secondary and higher order auditory neurons go to the reticular activating system (p. 285) to mediate the very important auditory arousal mechanisms. Both the animal in the forest and the human can subconsciously discriminate between types of sounds and can awaken only to those of interest. A mother can awaken to the cry of her baby even though there are much louder sounds in the house. The reticular activating system is responsible for this function.

IMPAIRMENT OF HEARING

Hearing defects can be broadly classified as conduction deafness or sensory-neural deafness. *Conduction deafness* refers to disease which prevents the pressure waves from reaching the oval window; *sensory neural deafness* refers to disease of the cochlea and the auditory nerve. A simple test of air versus bone conduction will usually differentiate between these types and should be part of every physical exam.

A vibrating tuning fork is held against the mastoid bone and the patient is instructed to indicate when it is no longer felt. The tuning fork is immediately placed beside the pinna; a normal patient should hear the tuning fork. This is known as the Rinne test which is said to be positive when air conduction is greater than bone conduction. This should be tested in both ears. The vibration is conducted through the bones of the skull and activates the basilar membrane and the organ of Corti in the usual manner. If the patient hears neither, sensory-neural deafness is indicated.

A frequent form of sensory-neural deafness is a loss of hearing above 2 or 3000 cps; a high-tone loss, presbycusis. A Rinne test with a 128 cps tuning fork will not pick up this problem yet the loss is quite incapacitating since most of the consonant sounds are above 3000 cps. Since this form of neural deafness is quite common among older persons, it no doubt contributes to the isolation and depression so often seen in the elderly. Hearing aids are not often successful yet should be tried. Aside from acoustic neurinoma (p. 337), other types of neural deafness, such as that caused by loud noise or by neomycin intoxication, offer little hope of remediable action although consultation with an otolaryngologist should be sought.

An abnormal Rinne test, indicating that bone conduction is greater than air conduction, is a sign of a middle-ear defect or a blockage, such as a plug of wax, in the external auditory canal. These types of deafness are usually amenable to hearing aids or surgery.

Infections of the middle ear are common. The inflammation produces a redness of the ear drum and a fluid collects in the middle ear, temporarily interfering with hearing. If the tympanic membrane is red, middle-ear infection should be suspected.

There are many quantitative hearing tests which offer many diagnostic clues to the location, cause, and prognosis of the disease process. They are, however, beyond the scope of this test; one of the references should be consulted.

REFERENCES

Brodal, A., Pompeiano, O., and Walberg, F.: *The Vestibular Nuclei and Their Connections, Anatomy and Functional Correlations.* Edinburgh, Oliver and Boyd, 1962.

Burns, W.: *Noise and Man.* Philadelphia, J. B. Lippincott, 1969.

DeReuck, A. V. S., and Knight, J. (eds.): *Myotatic, Kinesthetic and Vestibular Mechanisms.* Boston, Little, Brown and Co., 1967.

DeReuck, A. V. S., and Knight, J. (eds.): *Hearing Mechanisms in Vertebrates.* Boston, Little, Brown and Co., 1968.

Pulec, J. L.: *Meniere's Disease.* Philadelphia, W. B. Saunders, 1968.

15

Clinical Considerations of the Brain Stem

ELLIOTT M. MARCUS

LOCALIZATION OF DISEASE PROCESSES IN THE BRAIN STEM

Pathological processes affecting the brain stem can usually be well localized from an anatomical standpoint. This is a direct consequence of the fact that these disease processes in general involve a particular combination of cranial nerves (as in acoustic neuroma at the cerebellar pontine angle) or produce a particular combination of ipsilateral cranial nerve dysfunction and contralateral long tract findings (as in the midbrain infarction of Weber's syndrome which results in a combination of ipsilateral third nerve dysfunction and contralateral pyramidal tract findings).

Moreover, when anatomical-pathological correlation is considered, the brain stem, of all sites in the central nervous system, provides the best example of how the anatomical pattern of involvement allows the prediction of actual pathological processes. The student has, of course, already encountered several examples of this phenomenon at the level of the spinal cord. Thus, the clinical finding of a selective dissociated loss of pain and temperature in a cape-like distribution over the shoulders and upper extremities implies an anatomical process in a pericentral location involving the anterior commissure. One could readily deduce that an intrinsic pathological process was present and, moreover, could assume that in most cases the pathological process was that of syringomyelia.

At the level of the brain stem such examples of close correlation occur frequently. Thus, the combined involvement of the ipsilateral cranial nerve VIII (auditory and vestibular), nerve VII (facial), and nerve V (trigeminal), manifested by deafness, tinnitus (a buzzing or ringing sound in the ear), dizziness, peripheral facial paralysis, and unilateral facial numbness, not only indicates the location of the pathology but also suggests the actual nature of the pathology: acoustic neurinoma (tumor arising from Schwann cells of the sheath of nerve VIII). While other pathological lesions may occur at this site, they are rare.

There are several possible approaches to the problem of localization of disease processes in the brain stem. We will first consider a number of guidelines for localization. We will then consider in greater detail the particular anatomical syndromes and the various types of pathology in terms of specific extrinsic and intrinsic syndromes.

When speaking of the anatomical syndromes of the brain stem in clinical neurology, we will limit our considerations to the medulla oblongata, pons, and midbrain. The neuroanatomist sometimes includes the diencephalon as a part of his consideration of the brain stem since the thalamus, hypothalamus, and subthalamus represent a natural rostral continuation of the midbrain. From a clinical standpoint, we have considered the syndromes involving the thalamus and hypothalamus as one aspect of diseases of the cerebral hemispheres. The subthalamus will be considered in relation to the motor system.

GUIDELINES FOR LOCALIZING BRAIN STEM DISEASE

In analyzing the clinical anatomy of the brain stem, the following major rules should be considered:

CORTICOSPINAL AND CORTICOBULBAR PATHWAYS

1. *The pyramidal (corticospinal) tracts* decussate low in the medulla. Damage to the pyramidal tract above this decussation will produce upper motor neuron signs on the contralateral side of the body. Within the brain stem, the left and right pyramidal tracts are situated closest together at the level of the pyramidal decussation and are most widely separated at the level of the upper midbrain-internal capsule. Lesions in the medulla will often produce bilateral effects; in the midbrain, unilateral effects.

Throughout their extent in the brain stem, the corticospinal tracts are located in a ventral (or basilar) location. Lesions limited to the dorsal (tegmental or tectal) portions of the brain stem then are less likely to produce signs of pyramidal tract involvement.

2. In general, the *corticobulbar fibers* descend to the cranial nerve motor nuclei in close proximity to the corticospinal tracts. A lesion of the corticobulbar tract(s), then, will produce a supranuclear lesion, as regards motor control of the cranial nerves, below the lesion. Rather than decussating all at one point, the corticobulbar fibers for each cranial nerve motor nucleus (V, VII, XII, ambiguous) decussate, separately, somewhat above the level of that motor nucleus. Although in animals such as the cat there are very few direct corticobulbar fibers

(the fibers synapse instead on internuncial neurons in the reticular formation), in man direct corticobulbar fibers can be traced to the trigeminal, facial, hypoglossal, and spinal accessory motor neurons.

3. In general *corticobulbar control* of the cranial nerve motor nuclei is bilateral. Thus, stimulation of the motor cortex of one cerebral hemisphere produces bilateral contraction of the laryngeal, pharyngeal, palatal, and upper facial musculature. The motor neurons supplying the lower half of the face and the genioglossus muscle of the tongue receive predominantly unilateral corticobulbar fibers. The effects of a *unilateral* corticobulbar lesion then will be limited to an upper motor neuron type weakness of the contralateral lower facial muscles (termed supranuclear or central) and a minor weakness of the tongue (with slight deviation of the tongue on attempted midline protrusion to the side contralateral to the lesion). *Bilateral* damage to the corticobulbar fibers will produce an upper motor neuron type weakness of the muscles of the pharynx, larynx, tongue, face (upper and lower muscles), and jaw. The resulting syndrome, termed a *pseudobulbar palsy*, will have the qualities which the student has come to associate with an upper motor neuron lesion: impairment of voluntary control, weakness without atrophy, and a release of segmental brain stem reflex activity from higher control. Thus, the jaw jerk, a stretch reflex, will be hyperactive. Since the muscles and brain stem motor nuclei are also involved in emotional expression (consider laughing, crying, the facial expression of rage, and so forth), bilateral corticobulbar lesions will result in a loss of higher control and a release of these motor components of emotional expression.

MOTOR FUNCTION CRANIAL NERVES

1. The effects of a lesion involving the *motor nuclei* of a cranial nerve or of the motor fibers of a cranial nerve will be ipsilateral to the lesion. The effects will be those of a lower motor lesion: atrophy and weakness, and a loss of segmental reflex activity. With regard to the facial nerve, the effects are often referred to as peripheral.

In a local lesion of the brain stem, it is the segmental ipsilateral motor findings, in association with the contralateral corticospinal and corticobulbar findings below the level of the lesion, which allow for localization (termed hemiplegia alternans).

2. The nuclei of the *somatic motor cranial nerves* (III, IV, VI, and XII) are located close to the midline. These nuclei tend to be involved, then, by paramedian lesions rather than by lateral lesions. Intrinsic lesions in a paramedian location tend to produce, early in their course, a bilateral involvement of these nuclei. These nuclei are also all located in a relatively dorsal position. These nuclei would be involved early by a lesion in a dorsal or tegmental location.

LONG SENSORY SYSTEMS

1. Those fibers conveying *joint position sense and vibratory sensation* synapse in the nuclei gracilis and cuneatus and then decussate to form the *medial lemniscus*. This decussation occurs in the midportion of the medulla (below the full development of the olives and below the caudal extent of the fourth ventricle). Lesions above the point of decussation will then produce deficits in vibratory and position sensation in the contralateral arm and leg. (Note that the term medial lemniscus is used in a more limited anatomical sense than in the previous chapter.)

2. At its commencement in the medulla, the *medial lemniscus* is located in a paramedian location close to the midline and separate from the *lateral spinothalamic tract* which at this point is in a lateral retro-olivary location. As the fiber systems ascend toward the thalamus, the medial lemniscus shifts from its original paramedian position to a more lateral and ventral position, becoming contiguous to the spinothalamic pathways at the level of the upper pons and midbrain. These structural considerations have several clinical implications. At the level of the medulla, an intrinsic paramedian lesion is likely to produce bilateral involvement of the medial lemniscus. At the level of the midbrain, the left and right medial lemniscal pathways are now separated in space and such bilateral involvement is much less likely. At the level of the medulla, since the medial lemniscus is quite separate from the lateral spinothalamic pathway, selective involvement of contralateral position and vibratory sensation, as opposed to pain and temperature sensation, may occur. At the level of the midbrain and thalamus, such selective involvement is less likely.

SENSORY FUNCTION TRIGEMINAL NERVE

1. Sensory symptoms and findings relevant to the *fifth cranial nerve (trigeminal)* may provide significant clues as to localization. Thus, a lesion of the main sensory root of the trigeminal nerve, in its course within or external to the midpons, will produce ipsilateral deficits in pain, temperature, and touch over the face. On the other hand, a selective ipsilateral deficit in pain and temperature sensation over the face with sparing of facial touch sensation usually indicates selective involvement of the descending spinal tract of the trigeminal nerve or of its associated nucleus. In general, the lesion must be intrinsic. Because these structures are situated close to the lateral spinothalamic tract, the combination of contralateral pain and temperature deficit over the body and extremities with ipsilateral pain and temperature deficit over the face is frequently found as a consequence of lesions which involve the lateral portion of the medulla, e.g., occlusion of the posterior inferior cerebellar artery which supplies this sector.

2. The descending spinal tract of the trigeminal nerve is analogous to and, in a sense, the direct continuation of Lissauer's tract (dorsal fasciculus); the nucleus of this tract is the continuation of the substantia gelatinosa. The tract and nucleus descend into the upper cervical spinal cord. Although there is apparently considerable overlap, there is some tendency for the mandibular division fibers to synapse and then decussate at a lower pontine—upper medullary level; the maxillary division fibers do so at a medullary level, and the ophthalmic division fibers at a lower medullary and upper cervical cord level.

There is then the possibility of an overlap at the upper cervical cord level between the upper cervical segment pain fibers and the ophthalmic division pain fibers. It is not surprising, then, that pain originating in the C2 and C3 segments of the spinal cord may sometimes be referred to the ophthalmic division of the face (orbit and forehead).

3. The pain fibers, having decussated, join the ventral secondary trigeminal tract (also labeled trigeminothalamic or quintothalamic tract) which, at a medullary level, is located just lateral to the medial lemniscus. At a pontine and midbrain location, the secondary trigeminal tract is just lateral to and essentially continuous with the medial lemniscus and

adjacent to the lateral spinothalamic path. A lesion which involves this tract would then usually produce contralateral deficits in pain and temperature over a variable portion of the face in association with a contralateral deficit in pain and temperature or position and vibration on the affected arm, leg, and trunk.

CONTROL OF EYE MOVEMENT

1. The *medial longitudinal fasciculus* interconnects, through its ascending fibers, the vestibular nuclei, the abducens nucleus, and the oculomotor nuclei. A descending component of the medial longitudinal fasciculus interconnects these nuclei with upper cervical cord segments. Our major concern is with the ascending component of this fiber system. The functions of the medial longitudinal fasciculus and the effects of damage to this fiber system may be illustrated by considering the events and anatomical substrate for lateral conjugate eye movements.

Under normal circumstances, when a person is looking in a horizontal direction to right or left, the eyes move in a conjugate, coordinated manner as though yoked together. The movement is so smoothly coordinated that the single image always falls on corresponding retinal points, and the subject does not have the sensation of double images. This coordination requires a simultaneous, coordinated contraction of the lateral rectus muscle of one eye and the medial rectus muscle of the contralateral eye. The medial longitudinal fasciculus provides the system for this coordination, passing across the midline from one abducens nucleus and ascending to the contralateral medial rectus nucleus.

2. *Conjugate lateral gaze* may be triggered by impulses from several sources. Voluntary conjugate lateral movements presumably originate in the contralateral cerebral hemisphere in an area of the cortex known as the frontal eye field—area 8. Thus electrical stimulation of area 8 in the left hemisphere results in conjugate lateral eye movements to the right (contraversive or adversive movements). The fiber system from the frontal eye field descends in the anterior limb of the internal capsule. These fibers decussate at an upper pontine level and terminate in the pontine tegmentum close to the abducens nucleus in an area known as the lateral gaze center. Whether this "lateral gaze center" is a separate nuclei group (the para abducens nucleus) or the abducens nucleus itself or is simply composed of neurons within the adjacent pontine reticular formation is uncertain (refer to Goebel et al., 1971). It is clear that destruction of the abducens nucleus results in a long-lasting ipsilateral paralysis of conjugate lateral gaze in addition to an ipsilateral lateral rectus palsy; whereas, section of the abducens nerve results in only a lateral rectus palsy. Destruction of the cortical center for voluntary conjugate gaze results in a transient paralysis of conjugate gaze to the contralateral field of vision.

Conjugate lateral gaze may also originate from the cerebral cortex on a nonvoluntary basis as when the eyes follow a moving object. This is dependent on fibers originating in the occipital lobe and descending to the superior colliculi and other mesencephalic areas.

3. Of greater importance at this point is the consideration of *vestibular* influences on conjugate lateral gaze. Thus irrigation of the external auditory canal with cold water cools the endolymph in the horizontal semicircular canal resulting in a convection current. This current of fluid movements then stimulates the receptors at the crista, resulting in impulses in the vestibular nerve which are then conveyed to the vestibular nuclei. From the medial, lateral, and inferior vestibular nuclei, secondary ascending vestibular fibers arise, pass through or close to the ipsilateral abducens nucleus and enter the medial longitudinal fasciculus. The majority cross the midline at the level of the abducens nucleus to ascend in the contralateral medial longitudinal fasciculus to the contralateral medial rectus nucleus. Some of the fibers passing into the abducens nucleus (or collaterals of the fibers passing through) synapse in relation to neurons of the ipsilateral abducens nucleus.

The resulting effect of the caloric stimulation is a slow conjugate movement to the side of stimulation. The slow movement is regularly interrupted by a rapid return movement to the opposite side, presumably for the purpose of recentering the eyes. These alternate movements are termed *nystagmus.* It might be logical to indicate the direction of the nystagmus from the slow component, since this would also correspond to the side of vestibular nucleus stimulation and the side of abducens nucleus stimulation. However, the direction of the rapid component is used for the notation. It is important to note that the movements of nystagmus are conjugate and synchronous, the normal subject does not usually experience diplopia. This synchrony is again dependent on the coordination provided by fibers passing from the vestibular nucleus to the ipsilateral abducens nucleus and then on to the contralateral medial rectus. In the comatose patient, the production of nystagmus on caloric stmulation provides valuable information concerning the intactness of the brain stem fiber systems interconnecting the vestibular and extraocular motor nuclei.

4. The effects of a lesion involving the medial longitudinal fasciculus should then be quite predictable. Assuming a unilateral lesion on the left side at a pontine level above the abducens nucleus, when right lateral gaze is attempted, the right eye will fully abduct but the left eye will fail to adduct fully. The left medial rectus, however, will be otherwise intact for adduction in other movements, such as convergence. A similar defect, lack of coordination, will be noted in vestibular induced movements. Thus, horizontal nystagmus, whether occurring spontaneously or induced by caloric stimulation, will be most prominent in the abducting eye. Thus, the specific example of cold water stimulation of the right ear would result in nystagmus most prominent in the abducting right eye, with lesser and dysconjugate movements of the left eye.

Usually the *syndrome of the medial longitudinal fasciculus (sometimes referred to as internuclear ophthalmoplegia)* is a bilateral syndrome since the fasciculus maintains throughout the brain stem a paramedian location in the dorsal tegmentum with the fiber systems of the two sides relatively close one to the other. The cause of the syndrome is almost always intrinsic disease: multiple sclerosis, vascular disease with infarction, or an infiltrating glioma. These intrinsic lesions also usually produce a vertical nystagmus on upward gaze.

5. We have already indicated that there is an inferior division of the medial longitudinal fasciculus which descends into the upper cervical spinal cord level. This then provides a pathway by which proprioceptive information originating in the muscles, tendons, and joints about the cervical vertebrae may influence extraocular movements. This pathway can be utilized in the comatose patient (but not in the conscious patient) to elicit eye movements and in a sense to test the integrity of the medial longitudinal fasciculus. The movements induced by head turning (the *oculocephalic reflex*) are commonly referred to as the *dolls' head eye phenomenon.* Side to side rotation results in contraversive conjugate eye deviation. Flexion of the neck leads to upward deviation of the eyes; extension of the neck to downward deviation of the eyes. This reflex is not dependent on the presence of the cerebral cortex. Although some have postulated a vestibular basis for the reflex, it is clear that the reflex may be obtained in patients in whom the ocular response to caloric vestibular stimulation can no longer be obtained (Plum and Posner, 1966).

6. *Conjugate gaze in the vertical plane* is disturbed in lesions which involve the pretectal area, that portion of diencephalic-mesencephalic junction just rostral to the superior colliculus. Fibers controlling conjugate upward gaze are believed to reach the oculomotor nuclei from the frontal area of the two hemispheres (bilateral) passing through the pretectal-posterior commissure area. The older view held that paralysis of the conjugate upward gaze followed damage to the superior colliculus; however, limited lesions of this area do not affect ocular movements. Most actual lesions are found to involve pretectal area as well as the superior colliculus. This paralysis of upward gaze is often accompanied by a paralysis of downward gaze and by a paralysis of pupillary response to light. The paralysis of pupillary response may relate to damage to the pretectal area, the Edinger-Westphal nucleus (which is located in a relatively rostral position in the oculomotor complex) or to the fibers running between these two areas. In general, paralysis of vertical gaze (Parinaud's syndrome) is found in lesions which are extrinsic to and compressing the pretectal area and the superior colliculus: pinealoma and hemorrhage into the posterior thalamus. Some impairment of upward gaze is, however, found in a significant proportion of the elderly population without specific localizing significance.

7. A role as a *center for convergence* has been postulated as the function of the nucleus

of Perlia, a midline component of the third nerve nuclear complex. From a theoretical standpoint, selective damage to this nucleus could occur without involvement of the nuclei supplying the medial rectus muscles. Such a selective lesion, however, would not be common in view of the fact that the entire oculomotor complex occupies a relatively small area. An intrinsic lesion would be implied. A relative defect in convergence may be commonly encountered in any circumstance in which consciousness has been impaired.

8. It is perhaps useful to point out at this time that *third cranial nerve symptoms and signs* may be frequently noted in mass lesions which involve the cerebral hemisphere. Thus, space-occupying lesions such as collections of blood in the epidural or subdural space, brain tumor, or abscess in the temporal lobe may all displace the temporal lobe medially and downward. The medial aspect of the temporal lobe (uncus and hippocampal gyrus) is then forced through the tentorial opening compressing the third cranial nerve. Compression of the third nerve produces, as its initial sign, paralysis of the pupillary constriction, resulting in a fixed dilated pupil, apparently because these pupillary constrictor fibers are most peripheral among the third nerve fibers. As compression continues, the fibers to the levator palpebrae and then to the other extraocular muscles are involved, resulting eventually in a complete third nerve paralysis.

On the other hand, small intrinsic lesions tend to produce selective involvement of particular extraocular nuclei. Such intrinsic paramedian lesions are also likely to produce partial bilateral involvement rather than complete unilateral involvement, since the third nerve nuclei on the left and right side are located close, one to the other. The student should recall at this time that myasthenia gravis often produces incomplete involvement of the extraocular muscles supplying one or both eyes. The superior rectus and medial rectus muscles, particularly, are most likely to be involved. There are, of course, in myasthenia gravis, no sensory findings and no long tract findings since the basic pathology is at the neuromuscular junction.

9. Symptoms and signs referable to the *sixth cranial nerve* may provide clues to localization. Thus, a small paramedian infarction in the tegmentum of the lower pons may produce the combination of ipsilateral peripheral facial palsy and ipsilateral lateral rectus palsy, due to involvement of the abducens nucleus and of the facial nerve fibers in the genu about the abducens nucleus. As we have already indicated, such a lesion would also produce a paralysis of conjugate lateral gaze, due to involvement of the "lateral gaze center." This combination of cranial nerve findings may be associated with a contralateral hemiplegia due to a more extensive paramedian infarction (the Millard-Gubler syndrome).

The sixth cranial nerve may be involved in its extramedullary course, producing an extraocular palsy limited to the lateral rectus muscle. A bilateral involvement is frequently seen in any situation where an increase in intracranial pressure has occurred. This susceptibility of the sixth nerve is due to its long course along the floor of the skull. At times, the problem may begin as a unilateral paralysis and then become bilateral.

A unilateral paralysis is also frequently found in locally invasive disease involving the base of the skull (nasopharyngeal carcinoma). Such a lesion would progress to involve other cranial nerves at the base of the skull.

An isolated neuropathy of the sixth cranial nerve may occasionally occur in a diabetic patient. Such an isolated neuropathy of the sixth nerve is less frequent than the isolated neuropathy of the seventh cranial nerve: peripheral facial palsy of Bell.

10. *Combined unilateral involvement of all extraocular muscles* indicates disease extrinsic to the brain stem. Growths within the orbit may involve all three nerves (or the muscles supplied) in addition to the optic nerve. Compression at the superior orbital fissure or within the cavernous sinus may involve all three nerves (III, IV, and VI) in addition to the ophthalmic division of the trigeminal nerve. At times, the adjacent maxillary division is involved as well. The types of pathology to be considered within the cavernous sinus are thrombosis of the sinus due to spread of infection from the face or orbits, or an aneurysmal dilatation of the internal carotid artery. *Bilateral involvement of the extraocular muscles* may occur in myasthenia gravis or in a familial degenerative disease involving the extraocular muscles in the process of muscular dystrophy (progressive ophthalmoplegia). More recently, studies

have suggested an intrinsic loss of extra-ocular motor neurons on a degenerative basis in this rare disease. In these diseases the extraocular muscles are selectively involved; the pupillary reactions remain intact.

11. *Selective involvement of the pupillary reactions,* on the other hand, may also occur. As we have indicated, compressive lesions involving the third nerve may, in their early stage, produce a unilateral paralysis of pupillary constriction to both light and accommodation. Selective impairment of the response to light, with preservation of the response to accommodation, occurs in *tabes dorsalis* (discussed earlier in Chapter 8 dealing with diseases of the spinal cord). The pupillary response to light is dependent on fibers from the retinal ganglion cells. These fibers pass through the optic nerve and tract. Rather than terminating in the lateral geniculate, these fibers diverge from the optic tract just rostral to the lateral geniculate and enter the pretectile region at the level of the posterior commissure. Fibers then pass to the Edinger-Westphal nucleus of the same side (for the direct pupillary response).

On the other hand, the pathways for pupillary constriction in response to accommodation (the shift in gaze from a distant to near object) and to convergence depend on fibers in the optic tract reaching the occipital-calcarine cortex via the lateral geniculate. Fibers from the occipital association cortex then reach the superior colliculus and the nucleus of Edinger-Westphal. The lesion in the pretectal area which has been postulated for tabes dorsalis then would affect pupillary response to light but not to accommodation. Involvement of descending sympathetic fibers in this area could be postulated to explain the fact that in tabes dorsalis the pupil is relatively small and constricted in the resting state. A *pseudotabetic pupil* may occur in other diseases, e.g., diabetic peripheral neuropathy. A *tonic pupil* (once dilated is slow to respond to light, once constricted is slow to dilate in the dark) may be noted as one aspect of the benign *Adie's syndrome* in which there is variable association with absence of deep tendon reflexes in the lower extremities.

CEREBELLAR DYSFUNCTION

1. *Cerebellar symptomatology* may be noted frequently in diseases affecting the brain stem and may provide information as to localization. On the other hand, expanding lesions of the cerebellum may secondarily compress the brain stem. Diseases affecting the cerebellum will be considered later in greater detail (Chapter 25). We will simply indicate certain general rules at this point.

In general, diseases affecting the *midline* cerebellum (vermis) or its fiber systems result in a disturbance of equilibrium (sense of balance) and *an ataxia (unsteadiness) of the trunk.* This may be evident on sitting, standing, or walking. If an ataxia in walking occurs, we speak of an *ataxia of gait.* Diseases affecting the *lateral* aspects of the cerebellum (the cerebellar hemispheres) or of the fiber systems related to the lateral cerebellum produce lateralized symptoms affecting the limbs. Thus, an unsteadiness (ataxia) of arm and leg will be noted. In addition, a characteristic tremor will be present—*intention tremor,* in which oscillations of movement perpendicular to the line of movement occur. The lateralized unsteadiness of the lower extremity will result in an impairment of gait. The ataxia of gait will have, however, a lateralized quality in the sense that the patient will tend to fall or deviate to a particular side.

2. In general, pathology affecting the cerebellar hemisphere produces symptoms ipsilateral to the side of involvement. This reflects the fact that the dorsal spinocerebellar and cuneocerebellar pathways are essentially uncrossed. Moreover, the major outflow from the cerebellar hemisphere, the dentatorubrothalamic pathway of the superior cerebellar peduncle, decussates in the upper pons before reaching the rubral and ventral lateral thalamic areas. Data from the cerebellum-ventral lateral thalamus is then projected on to the motor cortex. The major efferent pathways from the motor cortex cross again in the pyramidal decussation. Because of this double decussation, data then from the right cerebellar hemisphere will eventually influence the anterior horn cells of the right arm and leg.

It should be evident then that lesions of the restiform body and the adjacent spinocerebellar and cuneocerebellar pathways in the lateral medulla will produce ipsilateral symptoms. Lesions of the superior cerebellar peduncle below its decussation will produce ipsilateral symptoms; above the decussation, contralateral symptoms.

3. Whether lateralized cerebellar symptoms reflect intrinsic disease of the brain stem

or disease of the cerebellum will depend on the associated signs and symptoms. Thus, the ipsilateral intention tremor and ataxia seen in the lateral medullary infarction and due to damage of the restiform body and the adjacent spinocerebellar and cuneocerebellar pathways is clearly associated with the signs and symptoms referrable to the involvement of the adjacent intrinsic structures: the ipsilateral descending spinal tract of the fifth nerve; the lateral spinothalamic pathway (producing contralateral deficit in pain and temperature), the ipsilateral Horner's syndrome, and the ipsilateral nucleus ambiguus or vagal dysfunction producing hoarseness, defective gag reflex, and dysarthria. On the other hand, the ipsilateral intention tremor and ataxia due to an abscess or tumor (e.g., cystic astrocytoma) of the lateral cerebellum will not have this association but rather will be associated with the signs and symptoms of increased intracranial pressure. Common midline lesions of the cerebellum secondarily compressing the brain stem are tumors such as medulloblastomas and hemangioblastomas. The ependymoma, although arising from the floor of the fourth ventricle, is sometimes included in the midline cerebellar syndrome category.

DECEREBRATE RIGIDITY

We should introduce at this time another effect of brain stem transection: *decerebrate rigidity,* a state characterized by a marked increase in extensor tone due to a marked increase in stretch reflexes. This subject will be discussed in greater detail later (Chapter 23). The essential anatomical points, however, may be outlined at this time. The essential level of transection for the occurrence of decerebrate rigidity is at some point between the vestibular nuclei and the red nuclei; in general, damage has occurred at a midbrain or upper pontine level. The pyramidal tracts and lesions of the pyramidal tracts are not involved in the phenomena. Instead, the decerebrate state relates to the release of an extensor facilitory area in the reticular formation in the tegmentum of the pons and midbrain. Stimulation of this area results in a facilitation of muscle spindle discharge through effects exerted on the gamma motor neuron by the reticulospinal pathway. Normally, the action of this facilitory system is opposed to (or in balance with) another area within the medullary tegmentum reticular formation: the bulbar inhibitory area, stimulation of which decreases muscle spindle discharge. The inhibitory area must be driven from higher centers: the cerebral cortex and caudate nucleus. Transection removes this drive from the inhibitory center, leaving unopposed the action of the facilitory center. The facilitory center has little dependence on higher centers: its main impetus is derived from afferent inputs from below.

EFFECTS OF BRAIN STEM PATHOLOGY ON MENTAL STATUS

1. *Diseases involving the brain stem do not directly affect most aspects of mental status* such as memory, abstract reasoning, comprehension, and the ability to perform calculations—functions usually associated with the cerebral cortex. Brain stem lesions may interfere with the ability to test these functions in the sense that a patient with a transection of the upper pons or midbrain will usually be unable to convey information from the cerebral cortex to the cranial nerve and spinal cord motor neurons so that expression of the cortical functions cannot occur. The patient is akinetic and mute. Lesions involving the reticular formation at the diencephalic and mesencephalic junction will interfere with mental status in the sense that the alertness and arousal aspects of consciousness are defective. The patient then remains in a comatose state, either failing to arouse from this state when stimulated, or arousing only for brief periods.

2. Pathological processes which involve the brain stem may have effects moreover which are not simply limited to the brain stem. Thus, occlusion of the basilar artery may not only produce infarction (ischemic damage) of the brain stem but also may produce infarction of the territory supplied by the posterior cerebral arteries. This includes the calcarine cortex, the medial and inferior aspects of the temporal lobe, and the diencephalon. The medial aspects of the temporal lobe (the hippocampus) and the medial thalamic areas apparently provide the anatomical substrate for recent memory (the learning of new information). In this instance, the patients with brain stem symptoms may also manifest a selective disturbance of this aspect of mental status.

3. Space-occupying lesions of the brain

stem or posterior fossa may also secondarily interfere with mental status through a blockade of the ventricular system. With blockade of the fourth ventricle or aqueduct (or for that matter the third ventricle), cerebrospinal fluid pressure increases and is transmitted to the lateral ventricle. The lateral ventricles dilate and since the skull is a rigid container (after closure of the sutures), the white matter and gray matter of the cerebral hemisphere are subjected to compression with an alteration in mental status. The patient frequently presents a drowsy appearance and when roused he often manifests a diffuse defect in memory, comprehension, and abstract reasoning. With relief of the obstruction to the flow of cerebrospinal fluid, a rapid reversal in this state should occur.*

SPECIFIC SYNDROMES AND DISEASE ENTITIES

Specific syndromes and disease entities will now be considered. Our emphasis will be on various classic syndromes, each of which implies a single level lesion. The reason for this emphasis in the teaching of clinical anatomical correlation is obvious. *However, the student should realize that, in actuality, a number of the diseases involving the brain stem are not simply limited to a single level but rather affect multiple levels; that is, they are multifocal.* Thus, although we will consider in detail patients with limited focal infarcts, it is more frequent to have infarction at several levels of the brain stem in occlusive disease of the basilar-vertebral system (perhaps the most common disease involving the brain stem). Another rather common disease of the brain stem, multiple sclerosis, almost always follows a multifocal pattern.

Although several approaches are possible, we will employ the same categories of disease already familiar to the student from his study of the spinal cord: extrinsic and intrinsic. We found that at the level of the spinal cord, extrinsic diseases were much more common. At the level of the brain stem, the intrinsic diseases occur much more frequently. (We will also find this to be the case at the level of the cerebral hemisphere.)

Nevertheless, extrinsic diseases have an importance outside of their actual frequency of occurrence. As we have already noted, at the level of the spinal cord, extrinsic diseases represent progressive compression type problems. In general, these are tumors. Early diagnosis and surgical relief of the compression will prevent the development of disability and will preserve life. All lesions compressing the brain stem have a life-threatening potential as they progress to the vital respiratory centers of the medulla.

In distinguishing extrinsic and intrinsic diseases, several differential points have already been mentioned. The following patterns of disease suggest *extrinsic lesions:*

1. Multiple involvement of cranial nerves occurring in succession early in the course of the disease, with fiber systems involved later in the disease.

2. Increased intracranial pressure tends to occur early in the course of the disease and the symptoms are usually prominent: headache, nausea, and vomiting. Occasionally, as in midline cerebellar lesions, the symptoms of increased intracranial pressure (plus or minus truncal ataxia) may be the only symptom.

3. A syndrome in which symptoms are limited to the midline cerebellum: loss of equilibrium and truncal ataxia.

4. Early involvement of the eighth cranial nerve (as in acoustic neuroma).

The following points are in favor of *intrinsic lesions:*

1. There is segmental involvement simultaneously of the nuclei or cranial nerves and the long tracts, as in a lateral medullary infarction.

2. There is bilateral involvement of cranial nerves and long tracts, as in infiltrating glioma.

3. There is involvement of the descending spinal tract of the fifth cranial nerve with selective involvement of pain sensation over the face.

4. There is involvement of the medial longitudinal fasciculus, as in multiple sclerosis, glioma, or infarction with the occurrence of internuclear ophthalmoplegia and vertical nystagmus.

5. When the intrinsic disease is an infiltrating tumor, the symptoms of increased intracranial pressure tend to occur late in the disease.

---

*An increase in intracranial pressure, particularly when sudden, is often associated with headache, nausea, and vomiting.

EXTRINSIC DISEASES OF THE BRAIN STEM

The following outline gives a summary view of extrinsic diseases of the brain stem.

A. Tumors
   1. Cerebellopontine angle syndrome
      a. Acoustic neuroma
      b. Meningioma
      c. Cholesteatoma
   2. Midline cerebellar—fourth ventricle syndrome
      a. Medulloblastoma
      b. Ependymoma
      c. Hemangioblastoma
      d. Metastatic tumors
   3. Cerebellar hemisphere
      a. Cystic astrocytoma
      b. Hemangioblastoma
      c. Metastatic tumors
      d. Abscess
      e. Tuberculoma
      f. Hemorrhage
   4. Superior colliculus (pretectal) syndrome
      a. Pinealoma
      b. Posterior thalamic hemorrhage
   5. Tentorial notch syndrome
      a. Meningioma
      b. Supratentorial herniation
   6. Foramen magnum syndrome
      a. Meningioma
      b. Cerebellar pressure cone
B. Developmental-bony degenerative diseases
   1. Platybasia
   2. Basilar impression
C. Vascular diseases
   1. Cerebellar hemorrhage
   2. Aneurysm

EXTRINSIC TUMORS

As we have indicated, almost all of the problems within the extrinsic category are tumors. When we use the term "extrinsic" in the present context, we mean extrinsic to the actual substance of the brain stem. Some of the tumors to be considered are actually invasive intrinsic tumors of the cerebellum which are secondarily compressing the brain stem. Some of these tumors are actually derived from cells of the glial series, e.g., cystic astrocytomas of the cerebellum, medulloblastomas, and ependymomas. Some are locally invasive malignant tumors, e.g., nasopharyngeal carcinoma infiltrating the bone of the skull or carcinoma of the lung or breast, metastatic to the cerebellum. (In general, carcinomas do not spread in a metastatic manner to the brain stem *per se*.)

The Cerebellopontine Angle Syndrome

Acoustic Neuroma (Fig. 15–1). Most tumors encountered at the cerebellar pontine angle are acoustic neuromas arising from the Schwann cells about cranial nerve VIII. This is a disease of the middle-aged or older adult. The early symptoms and findings relate to a progressive involvement of nerve VIII (progressive loss of hearing of a neural type and a dead labyrinth on caloric stimulation). As the tumor enlarges, symptoms referrable to nerves VII and V and to the cerebellum develop. The following case history illustrates the clinical problem.

Case History 1. NECH #191–003. Date of admission: 11/17/67.

This 64-year-old, white, right-handed housewife (Mrs. M.B.) was admitted to the hospital for evaluation of progressive loss of hearing in the right ear, right facial weakness, and increasing headaches.

A progressive decrease in hearing had been present in the right ear for at least 10 to 15 years. Recently, the patient had noted total deafness in the right ear. A minor change in hearing on the left had also been noted.

For two years prior to admission the patient had noted the gradual development of an unsteadiness in walking (ataxia of gait). This had recently worsened, leading to several falls.

For 1 to 2 years prior to admission the patient had noted a progressive numbness on the right side of the face. Recently a weakness of the right side of the face had also been noted.

During recent months, a bifrontal or right-sided frontal and vertex headache had been present. The patient had no nausea or vomiting but reported occasional recent diplopia.

GENERAL PHYSICAL EXAMINATION: Was not remarkable.

NEUROLOGICAL EXAMINATION:

1. *Mental status :* Orientation, memory, and fund of knowledge were intact.
2. *Cranial nerves:*
   a. Fundi—There was evidence of an increase in intracranial pressure with bilateral papilledema (elevation of the discs with old and new retinal hemorrhages).

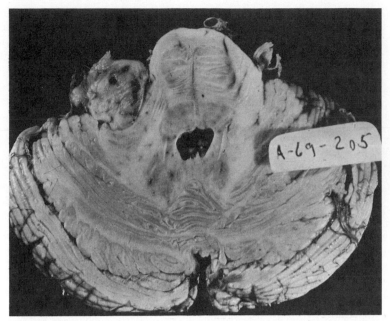

Figure 15–1 Acoustic neuroma at the cerebellar pontine angle. This elderly male had been hospitalized for treatment of carcinoma of the thyroid metastatic to the lung and kidney. When 4 days prior to death he suddenly became unresponsive with a left peripheral facial weakness and a right Babinski response, the actual pathological process was assumed to be metastatic disease. At postmortem examination, the only pathology found in the central nervous system was this well-encapsulated mass in the left cerebellar pontine angle arising from the eighth nerve and compressing the pons. Histological examination confirmed the diagnosis of acoustic neuroma. (Courtesy of Dr. Jose Segarra and Dr. Remedios Rosales, Boston Veterans Administration Hospital.)

See Filmstrip, Frame 23.

b. There was a decrease in pain and light touch over the maxillary and mandibular divisions of the right trigeminal nerve. The right corneal reflex was absent and the patient did not feel touch over the cornea.

c. A moderate right peripheral facial weakness was present with a droop to the right corner of the mouth, a widened right palpebral fissure, and an absence of blinking with the right eye.

d. Hearing was markedly decreased in the right ear (both air and bone) compared to the left.

e. Ice water caloric labyrinthine stimulation indicated no response of the right ear; there was normal response of the left ear.

f. There was a fine nystagmus on gaze to the left and to the right.

3. *Motor system:*
a. Strength was intact.
b. Gait was slightly broad-based with some weaving to the right or left. She was unable to walk a tandem gait.

c. No ataxia was present in the upper extremities.

4. *Reflexes:*
a. Deep tendon reflexes were symmetrical.
b. Plantar responses were flexor.

5. Sensation: All modalities were intact.

LABORATORY DATA:

1. Brain scan was negative.

2. Bilateral brachial arteriograms were negative.

3. A ventriculogram (a needle was placed in the frontal horn of the right lateral ventricle through a burr hole and contrast media was instilled) revealed a mass lesion displacing the aqueduct and fourth ventricle posteriorly, slightly upwards and to the left. This type of shift suggested a lesion at the right cerebellopontine angle, e.g., an acoustic neuroma.

HOSPITAL COURSE:

On December 15, 1967 a right suboccipital craniotomy was performed by Dr. Samuel Brendler. When the right cerebellar hemisphere was retracted and the right lateral third of the cerebellum amputated, a large acoustic neuroma was exposed, enveloping cranial nerves VII and VIII as they extended into the internal auditory meatus. At its lower end, the capsule of the tumor was also loosely attached to nerves IX, X and XI. At its superior end, the tumor was adherent to nerve V. A portion of the tumor extended superiorly through the hiatus of the tentorium. At several points, the tumor capsule was adherent to the brain stem. In the removal of the tumor, neither cranial nerves VII or VIII could be spared. A small portion of nerve V was also removed with the tumor capsule. As the tumor was being freed from the tentorium and brain stem, there were several episodes of hypotension and cessation of spontaneous respiration. It was therefore necessary to terminate the procedure after 60 per cent of the tumor had been removed. Subsequent histological examination of the tumor confirmed the operative impression of schwannoma (neuroma).

The patient's postoperative course was complicated by the development of congestive heart failure and pulmonary edema. At the time of hospital discharge 10 weeks after surgery, neurological examination revealed the following:

1. Mental status was intact.

2. There was no evidence of papilledema.

3. Pain and touch were decreased on the right side of the face and the right masseter was weak.

4. A complete right peripheral facial palsy was present. (The right eyelids had been sutured closed to avoid injury to the right cornea — tarsorrhaphy.)

5. Hearing was completely absent in the right ear and decreased on the left.

6. There was difficulty in swallowing; the gag reflex was depressed and speech was indistinct.

7. The patient was able to walk with assistance. Her gait was unsteady. A slight appendicular ataxia was evident bilaterally on finger-to-nose and heel-to-shin tests.

8. Strength, sensation, and reflexes were otherwise intact.

A follow up summary 9 months after surgery from the chronic disease hospital to which the patient had been transferred, indicated that no additional improvement had occurred.

COMMENT:

The symptoms and findings presented by this patient were those to be expected with a large tumor in the right cerebellar pontine angle. There was a combination of cranial nerve findings involving cranial nerves VIII, VII, and V, in addition to cerebellar findings. The tumor, moreover, had displaced brain stem structures, distorting the aqueduct and fourth ventricle. A significant increase in intracranial pressure had been produced. The occasional diplopia reported by the patient may well have suggested some of the bilateral cranial nerve VI dysfunction to be expected when a significant increase in intracranial pressure occurs.

The student may logically inquire as to how one may attribute the origin of the tumor to the Schwann cells of cranial nerve VIII, in view of the operative findings. Thus at surgery, the tumor was also adherent to nerves VII, V, IX, and X, in addition to cranial nerve VIII, and the origin was not clear cut. Certainly in occasional cases, neurofibromas (schwannomas) may arise from cranial nerves VII, V, IX; the most common site, however, remains nerve VIII. Moreover, the clinical history alone in this case would suggest such a nerve VIII origin. Thus the hearing deficit in the right ear was clearly the initial symptom beginning 10 to 15 years prior to admission, whereas those symptoms attributed to cranial nerves V and VII had been present for a shorter period of 1 to 2 years.

The patient had been seen relatively late in her disease course. The tumor at operation was certainly very large and presented a formidable problem for the neurosurgeon. The complications of the surgical procedure were not unusual when one considers that nerve VII was completely surrounded by the tumor and that cranial nerve V was also attached to the tumor. In some of these cases, the best result involves a subtotal removal of the tumor, attempting to preserve the continuity of the involved cranial nerves. It should of course be noted that prime indications for neurosurgical intervention were present: increased intracranial pressure and distortion of brain stem structures.

Because of the obvious papilledema, indicating an increase in intracranial pressure, a lumbar puncture was not performed in this case. Lumbar puncture performed in cases without papilledema almost always indicate protein values increased to over 100 mg./100 ml. (normal 45 mg./100 ml).

Other Tumors in the Cerebellopontine Angle. Rarely, other types of pathology are found in this location: meningiomas arising from arachnoidal cell nests and cholesteatomas (epidermoids). In general, the initial symptoms in these cases are not referrable to nerve VIII, and the vestibular response to caloric stimulation may be present.

Midline Cerebellum (Fourth Ventricle) Syndrome. The midline cerebellar syndrome is frequently encountered in neurology, presenting a disturbance of balance with ataxia of the trunk and gait but no clearly lateralized symptoms. In general, the etiology is neoplastic. The type of tumor varies as a function of age. The most common cause in an infant or child is a *medulloblastoma* (Fig. 15–2A). This tumor arises from nests of external granular cells in the nodulus, an older portion of the cerebellum relating to the vestibular system. Since this portion of the cerebellum projects as a roof into the fourth ventricle, early obstruction is to be expected. A typical case is presented in Chapter 25, p. 702, and the student should review this example at this time.

In older children and young adults, the most common cause is the *ependymoma* which arises from ependymal cells in the floor or roof of the fourth ventricle. The mass of tumor grows into the ventricle, obstructing this cavity but also exerting upward pressure on the midline nodulus (and other aspects of the cerebellar vermis). At times however, the ependymoma may extensively invade the tegmentum of the medulla and pons. Taken together, the medulloblastoma and the ependymoma constitute the most common central nervous system tumors of the pediatric age group.

In the middle-aged adult, the most common cause of the syndrome is a midline *hemangioblastoma*. These are tumors derived from embryonic vascular elements. In contrast to the medulloblastoma and the ependymoma, the hemangioblastoma is a surgically curable lesion. It is often found that a nodule of tumor exists within a nonneoplastic cystic cavity, allowing for removal of the tumor without sacrifice of a large amount of the cerebellum.

The following case history illustrates the course of such a midline tumor.

Case History 2.   NECH #189–434.
Dates of admission: 9/6/67–9/15/67; 12/8/67–11/7/68.

This 50-year-old, white, male accountant

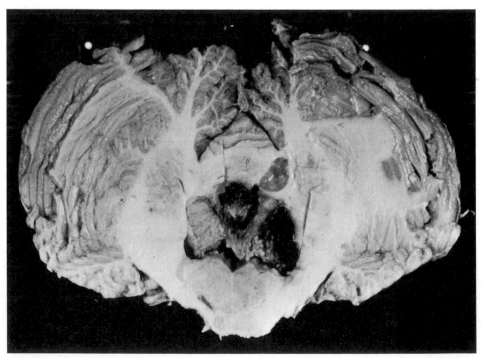

Figure 15–2A Medulloblastoma arising from vermis of cerebellum and obstructing the fourth ventricle. The clinical summary of this 27-month-old child is presented in Chapter 25, p. 702. (Courtesy of Dr. John Hills, New England Center Hospitals.)

See Filmstrip, Frame 24.

(Mr. F.H.) first noted the onset of a minor degree of unsteadiness of gait in March 1966. This unsteadiness did not become a prominent symptom until May 1967. Over the next 4 months, symptoms progressed so that the patient felt as though he were staggering constantly. He did not actually fall and had no rotational vertigo. The sense of staggering was no worse in the dark than in good light. On two occasions when the patient went directly from a sitting to a supine position, he had episodes of light-headedness with confusion and nausea. During the 5 to 6 months prior to initial admission, the patient had also noted frequent headaches, at times bifrontal, at times bioccipital. The bioccipital headaches were sharp and knife-like and would occur with straining and when the patient assumed sitting position from the supine. They were relieved by lying down on the right side. The patient's wife reported that he had experienced some gradual change in personality over a 5-year period.

NEUROLOGICAL EXAMINATION: (9/6/67)

1. *Mental status:* All aspects were intact except for considerable anxiety.

2. *Cranial nerves:* Intact.

3. *Motor system:* Intact except for gait. The patient had a variable and intermittent ataxia in walking. He swayed when standing on a narrow base. The ataxia could be corrected on command.

4. *Reflexes:* Deep tendon reflexes and plantar responses were normal.

5. *Sensation:* All modalities were intact.

LABORATORY DATA:

1. Complete blood count was normal.

2. Skull x-rays were normal.

3. Electroencephalogram was normal.

4. Brain scan was normal.

5. Cerebrospinal fluid pressure was normal but protein was elevated to 112 mg./100 ml.

On repeat exams, protein was elevated to 98 and 64 mg./100 ml.

HOSPITAL AND SUBSEQUENT COURSE:

The patient's ataxia, headaches, and anxiety increased during hospitalization despite treatment with tranquilizers (chlorpromazine). Psychiatric consultation suggested a mild schizoid personality disorder with conversion reaction (component of conversion hysteria).

Following discharge from the hospital, the patient's gait became more ataxic, so that he was described as staggering constantly rather than intermittently. In addition he had been noted to be ataxic in sitting as well. Headache had apparently also progressed. The patient was therefore readmitted to the hospital.

NEUROLOGICAL EXAMINATION: (12/8/67)

1. *Mental status:* Minimal deficits were present in all areas: delayed recall, digit span, and calculations. ("He did not perform as one would expect for an accountant.")

2. *Cranial nerves:*
   a. All were intact except for a left central facial weakness.
   b. Hearing was again normal.

3. *Motor system:*
   a. Strength was intact.
   b. Hand coordination was intact. Heel-to-shin and finger-to-nose tests were normal.
   c. When attempting to walk, gait was wide-based and reeling. Walking was virtually impossible without support. The patient tended to fall in all directions. When sitting the patient fell slowly backwards, being unable to maintain his balance.

4. *Reflexes:*
   a. Deep tendon reflexes were slightly brisker on the left than on the right.
   b. Plantar response on the left was extensor; the right was flexor.
   c. An excessive grasp reflex was present in both hands. A right foot grasp was present.

LABORATORY DATA:

1. The *electroencephalogram* now revealed bilateral bursts of slow waves, most prominent in the frontal areas and somewhat more prominent over the right hemisphere than left. (These findings *per se* did not have localizing significance.)

2. *Right brachial arteriogram* indicated a downward and forward displacement of the posterior inferior cerebellar artery. A downward displacement of this vessel usually indicates a herniation of cerebellar tonsils. In addition, a well-defined vascular tumor was present in the superior lobule of the midline cerebellum.

3. A *ventriculogram* indicated a mass lesion in the superior vermis of the cerebellum with anterior displacement of the aqueduct of Sylvius and the fourth ventricle.

HOSPITAL COURSE:

A suboccipital craniotomy was performed

by Dr. Samuel Brendler on December 20, 1967 (removal of a portion of occipital bone about the posterior rim of the foramen magnum). The dura covering the posterior fossa was tight, indicating increased intracranial pressure. A needle was passed through the mid vermis. At a depth of 2 cm., a cyst was encountered which contained 40 cc. of clear yellow fluid. The cerebellar vermis was then opened along its entire length and several cysts were encountered. Upon opening the largest cyst, a cherry red mural nodule was found anteriorly at the superior pole of the vermis. This large cyst was removed completely with the mural nodule. An additional cyst containing 15 cc. of fluid was then found anterior to the mural nodule, compressing the roof of the fourth ventricle. All of these cysts were then removed and the posterior fossa closed. Histological examination of the tumor confirmed the operative impression of hemangioblastoma.

Except for pneumonia involving the lower lobe of the right lung and treated with antibiotics, the patient's postoperative course was uneventful. The patient's ataxia gradually subsided and he began to ambulate without assistance. By the time of hospital discharge on January 7, 1968 only a minimal degree of ataxia was still present.

Follow-up evaluation in February 1968, 2 months after surgery, revealed no ataxia on routine gait, but a slight ataxia on tandem gait (narrow-based heel-to-toe walking). All changes in mental status had cleared; the patient was already preparing income tax returns for his clients.

A note from the patient's wife in September 1968 indicated that the personality changes noted in the several years prior to surgery had cleared to a significant degree.

Follow-up evaluation in January 1970, 2 years after surgery, indicated the same minor degree of ataxia which was apparent only on tandem gait.

COMMENT:

In the analysis of this case history, it is important to focus our attention on the patient's actual major complaints. It is also important from the standpoint of localization that we deal with those major symptoms and findings which were apparent early in the course of the disease. It is then evident that his major neurological complaints were related to a loss of equilibrium and a progressive ataxia of gait and trunk. These symptoms clearly suggested a midline cerebellar location of lesion. There was an accompanying headache which had several ominous features: the headache would occur with straining (which increased the intracranial and intraventricular pressure) and could be precipitated by a change in posture (supine to sitting). A headache with such mechanical qualities often indicates a space-occupying lesion in relation to the ventricular system.

It is important to realize that as such a mass lesion increases in size, several secondary effects occur with associated signs and symptoms. (1) Blockage of the ventricular system occurs. The resultant increase in intraventricular pressure will alter cortical function. In this case, mental status and personality were altered in a nonselective manner. Frontal lobe function was altered resulting in the release of a grasp reflex. Nonspecific changes also occurred in the electroencephalogram. (2) There is compression of brain stem structures, perhaps explaining the reflex asymmetry noted at the time of the second hospital admission. (3) There are indirect vascular effects because some vessels are compressed by the tumor mass.

It is also important to note that a significant increase in intracranial pressure may be present without papilledema being present on funduscopic examination.

At the time of the patient's initial hospitalization, a significant variability in the degree of gait ataxia was apparent. Moreover, worsening or improvement in the gait appeared to follow suggestions from the examiner. A primary diagnosis of psychiatric disease was therefore entertained. The student should keep in mind that conversion hysteria in general does not develop at age 48 in a patient who has never previously manifested this problem. In a similar vein, one should be suspicious in making a primary diagnosis of depression in a 60-year-old patient who has not previously presented this problem. Such a patient may have underlying medical or neurological disease. Gait disturbances and ataxia of trunk in particular often appear to be strongly influenced by anxiety and suggestion. This is more so the case because there often appears to the examiner to be a marked contradiction between the abilities of the patient when recumbent (no ataxia, able to do heel-to-shin test, and so forth) and the patient's severe ataxia when upright. The alterations in personality function which occur reflect both the anxiety and depression to be seen in any patient with chronic symptoms (neurological or non-neurological) and the effects on cortical function of an increase in intracranial pressure to be seen in a posterior fossa mass lesion.

The specific diagnosis as to the type of midline cerebellar mass depends, of course, on the age of the patient and the laboratory and operative findings. An almost identical picture of somewhat briefer course could be seen in a 15- or 20-year-old with an ependymoma or a child of 2 or 3 years of age with a medulloblastoma. When the patient is 50 years old, hemangioblastomas and metastatic lesions constitute the major midline entities. Metastatic carcinomas in general, however, are more often found in a non-midline cerebellar hemisphere location.

Lateral Cerebellar Hemisphere Syndrome. The syndrome of the cerebellar hemisphere with its lateralized symptoms affecting the ipsilateral arm and leg has

already been mentioned. The syndrome is discussed in greater detail with an illustrative case history in Chapter 25, p. 707. The student should refer to this section at this time.

As regards the specific mass lesions, this in large part depends on the patient's age. In the child and young adult, the most common lesion is probably the *cystic astrocytoma.* These are essentially low-grade gliomas, often composed of a cyst with a nodule of tumor projecting from the inner wall of the cyst. Such lesions offer the possibility of surgical cure. (Refer to Chapter 22, p. 603 for discussion of histological grading of gliomas.)

In the middle-aged and older age groups, the most common lesions are *metastatic carcinoma* and the *hemangioblastoma.* The metastatic carcinoma may represent a solitary metastasis from a primary lesion in lung, breast, ovary, or kidney or may be only one of multiple lesions (Fig. 15–2B). The cerebellar lesion in any case is often surgically removed since it does represent a relatively

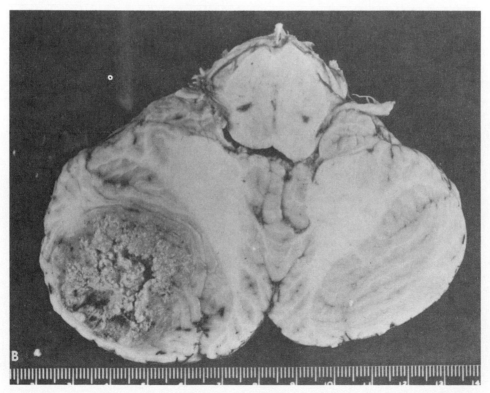

Figure 15–2B Lateral cerebellar syndrome. This patient with bronchiogenic carcinoma had multiple metastatic lesions in the cerebral hemisphere in addition to the lateral cerebellum. His symptoms included nystagmus and appendicular ataxia. (Courtesy of Dr. John Hills, New England Center Hospitals; and Dr. Jose Segarra, Boston Veterans Administration Hospital.)

See Filmstrip, Frame 25.

acute life-threatening lesion. The hemangioblastoma has already been discussed and is illustrated as noted.

Other types of lesion involving the cerebellar hemisphere are less common today, although in former years they occurred more frequently. Thus, the cerebellar hemisphere was often the site of a *tuberculoma* or of a *brain abscess*. The source of infection in brain abscesses was usually the adjacent middle ear and mastoid.

Hypertensive *hemorrhages* may occur into the cerebellar hemisphere presenting as an acute mass lesion. The cerebellum is an uncommon site when compared to the much more frequent locations: putamen and thalamus of the cerebral hemisphere. (See Fig. 15–8.)

Syndrome of Compression of the Pretectal Area and Superior Colliculus. There are essentially two causes of this syndrome: *tumors of the pineal* (Fig. 15–3) and *posterior thalamus hemorrhages* compressing this area in the form of mass lesions.

Tumors of the pineal are of two types: (1) *pinealomas* arising from the cells of the pineal and occurring most commonly in males in the age groups 15 to 25 years, and (2) *teratomas,* arising from congenital cell nests of a mixed type and occurring most commonly in the age group under 10 years. Both types of tumor are relatively rare. Hemorrhages of the posterior thalamus occur most commonly in middle-age or older patients with hypertension.

The following case history illustrates the clinical finding and course of a pinealoma.

Case History 3. NECH #144–613.
Date of admission: 10/2/61.

This 16-year-old, white male (Mr. J.M.) in November 1960 was first noted to be lethargic. Gradually from November 1960 to March 1961 there was progressively poor performance in school with apathy and somnolence. In December 1960 the patient had an onset of diplopia with difficulty in reading. In March 1961 he began to sleep

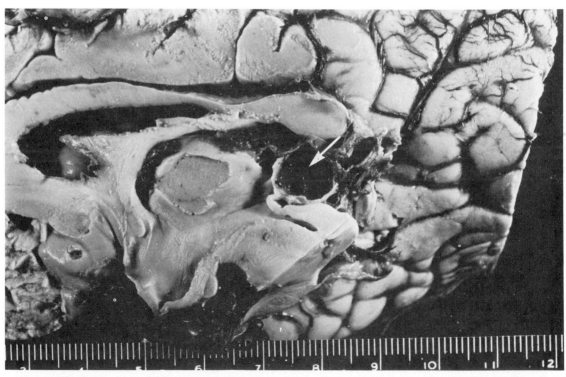

Figure 15–3 Tumor of the pineal. This is an enlarged nonmalignant cyst arising from the pineal gland (arrow). The relation of this tumor to the pretectal area, superior colliculus, aqueduct of Sylvius, and the posterior portion of the third ventricle clearly demonstrates the effects that a pinealoma would produce. (Courtesy of Dr. John Hills, New England Center Hospitals; and Dr. Jose Segarra, Boston Veterans Administration Hospital.)

See Filmstrip, Frame 26.

throughout the day and could be awakened only with difficulty. Headaches on arising, with nausea and vomiting, had been noted. In April 1961 evaluation at the Buffalo General Hospital had revealed that the pupils failed to respond to light but did respond to accommodation. Upward gaze was intermittently defective, and conjugate lateral gaze was intact. Findings improved to some degree over a 3-day period.

In August 1961, 2 months prior to admission, he had an onset of a progressive defect in coordination of gait as well as a defect in hearing, predominantly in the right ear with tinnitus. To a lesser degree the left ear was also affected.

In September 1961 there was a 1-day period of hiccoughs. At the same time, there was an onset of a slow, slightly slurred speech.

On the day of admission, an episode of urinary incontinence occurred.

NEUROLOGICAL EXAMINATION:

1. *Mental status:* All areas were relatively intact except for a slowness of response, emotional lability, and immaturity of behavior and questions.

2. *Cranial nerves:*
   a. The fundi were normal. Visual fields were intact on confrontation.
   b. The right eye was deviated outward; the patient was unable to converge. There was a paralysis of upward and downward gaze. Bilateral lid ptosis was present. However, spasm of the eyelids was easily stimulated. Pupils were sluggish in response to light. The right pupil was slightly larger than the left. Horizontal nystagmus was present.
   c. The jaw jerk was hyperactive.
   d. Guttural and lingual sounds were slurred in a pattern that was consistent with pseudobulbar palsy.
   e. Hearing was decreased bilaterally.

3. *Motor system:*
   a. Strength was intact.
   b. Spasticity was present on passive motion in the lower extremities and possibly in the upper extremities.
   c. There was slowness in alternating hand movements. A fixed facies was present.
   d. A bilateral intention tremor was present on finger-to-nose testing.
   e. Gait was broad-based with truncal ataxia.

4. *Reflexes:*
   a. Deep tendon reflexes were hyperactive bilaterally with ankle clonus.
   b. Plantar responses were extensor bilaterally (bilateral sign of Babinski).

5. *Sensory system:* Intact.

LABORATORY DATA:

1. Cerebrospinal fluid showed normal pressure; normal cells, and protein elevated to 100 mg./100 ml. Gamma globulin percentage was not increased.

2. Skull and chest x-rays were normal.

SUBSEQUENT COURSE:

(We are grateful to Dr. Walter Olszewski and Dr. Walter Stafford of the Buffalo General Hospital for information concerning the subsequent course of this case.)

The patient was readmitted shortly thereafter to the Buffalo General Hospital where a pneumoencephalogram revealed a mass displacing the aqueduct of Sylvius posteriorly. On October 25, 1961, radiation therapy was begun (a total of 4500 rads over 30 days). Within 10 days improvement in hearing occurred. Tremor of the arms and legs decreased; speech became less slurred, and a few degrees of upward gaze of the eyes returned. Ataxia of gait subsequently decreased so that the patient was able to walk rapidly although on a wide base. His pupils remained fixed to light but responded to accommodation. The eyes were divergent and askewed. Downward gaze never returned and only vertical nystagmus was present on attempted upward gaze. Bilateral Babinski signs remained. This condition remained relatively static until January 1967, when over a two-week period, the patient had a decrease in initiative, gait became more ataxic, headaches returned, and a marked ptosis of the left eyelid developed. Neurological examination on February 7, 1967 now revealed a bilateral ptosis. The pupils were irregular and constricted; the right measured 2.5 mm. in diameter, the left 1.5 mm. Neither reacted to light. The patient could not elevate, depress, or converge the eyes. The patient could look to either side. Nystagmus developed in the left eye on gaze to the right. As previously, intention tremor and bilateral Babinski signs were present. Shortly thereafter, a terminal coma developed with a marked elevation of temperature (104 to 106°) and blood pressure (200/80).

Postmortem examination revealed a significant degree of ventricular dilatation from infiltration and obstruction of the aqueduct. There was an area of apparent necrotic tissue sharply localized to the midbrain tectum and tegmentum, extending from the pretectal area down into the superior and inferior colliculi. The cerebellum and pons were not involved but there was slight bilateral invasion of the thalamus. A small necrotic nodule was also present at the presumed site of the pineal. While some of the necrosis may have been due to radiation, microscopic sections of the necrotic areas of midbrain tegmentum revealed the typical appearance of a pinealoma (a lobulated sinusoidal tumor containing large vesicular cells and a focal cluster of small cells resembling lymphocytes). A more complete discussion of the pathological features of pinealomas is presented in Chapter 22.

COMMENT:

The clinical findings in this case clearly suggested a lesion involving the pretectal area (pupillary response to light was defective, but response to accommodation was intact) and the pretectum-superior colliculus (defect in upward and downward gaze). The lethargy, apathy, and somnolence early in the course may have related in part to increased intracranial pressure. Increased intracranial pressure often occurs in these lesions because of the early compression of the aqueduct of Sylvius. However, in view of the early prominence of the somnolence prior to headache and vomiting, we may presume that there was compromise of tegmental structures including the reticular activating system at the diencephalic-mesencephalic junction. The bilateral impairment of hearing undoubtedly related to the bilateral involvement of the inferior colliculi. Bilateral involvement of the brachium of the inferior colliculus would also explain this symptom. The bilateral Babinski signs, the signs of pseudobulbar palsy (hyperactive jaw jerk, and slurring of speech sounds) indicated that compression of the corticospinal and corticobulbar pathways had occurred. The bilateral intention tremor and the marked ataxia of gait and trunk may have related to downward pressure on the cerebellum or to involvement of the superior cerebellar peduncles (brachium conjunctivum) and their rostral continuation within the tegmentum. As progression occurred

additional involvement of the oculomotor nuclei occurred.

Precocious puberty occasionally develops in preadolescent males with pinealomas. This usually indicates invasion or compromise of the hypothalamus. Cells of the teratoma of the pineal may seed into the structures about the third ventricle.

The usual treatment of pinealomas is based on shunting procedures to bypass the blockage at the aqueduct or radiation therapy. This patient had a relatively long survival, particularly long in view of the fact that a shunting procedure was not performed. His eventual demise apparently related to the obstruction at the aqueduct of Sylvius and brain stem compression.

Tentorial Notch Syndrome. *Meningiomas* may occur in the posterior fossa but are rare in this location compared to their various supratentorial sites. There are three usual sites for the origin of these tumors in the posterior fossa: (1) the cerebellopontine angle previously discussed, (2) the basilar groove—foramen magnum, and (3) the tentorium of the cerebellum.

Those arising from the *tentorium* may produce variable syndromes: (a) midline obstructing mass with increased intracranial pressure but without definite localizing features, (b) mass lesion extending above the tentorium to involve the temporal and occipital lobes, (c) mass lesion extending below the tentorium, displacing or invaginating the cerebellum and compressing the brain stem and cranial nerves.

Tentorial meningiomas are rare. A much more common syndrome in relation to the tentorial notch is *herniation of the medial aspects of the temporal lobe (uncus and parahippocampal gyrus) secondary to supratentorial mass lesions.* We will encounter several examples of this complication when we consider specific diseases affecting the cerebral hemisphere. We have already indicated that the earliest sign of this herniation is the development of an ipsilateral dilated fixed pupil and an ipsilateral paralysis of the levator palpebrae muscle, due to incomplete compression of the third cranial nerve. As the degree of compression increases, a complete ipsilateral third nerve palsy develops. Moreover, the herniating temporal lobe shifts the brain stem to the contralateral side. The tentorium is a relatively rigid structure; the tentorial opening, relatively small. The contralateral cerebral peduncle is soon compressed against the rigid free margin of the tentorium resulting in a hemiparesis which (considering the subsequent pyramidal decussation) is ipsilateral to the side of the herniation (Fig. 15–4). (The compression of the contralateral cerebral peduncle is referred to by neuropathologists as Kernohan's notch.) As compression of the brain stem continues, multiple small (Duret) hemorrhages develop within the tegmentum and, to a lesser degree, within the basal portions of the midbrain and pons, resulting in coma and bilateral fixed pupils with ensuing decerebrate state (Fig. 15–5). Once this stage has been reached survival and recovery is unlikely. The etiology of the hemorrhages probably relates to the obstruction of veins, within and without the substance of the midbrain and pons. Although we have indicated that the entire process resulting from temporal lobe herniation is a stepwise process, in actuality, the rate of progression is often so rapid that each separate stage may not appear as a discrete event to the examiner. This entire syndrome obviously represents an event to be avoided. Steps must be taken to remove or to decrease the size of the supratentorial lesion before these complications occur.

Foramen Magnum Syndromes. *Meningiomas* arising in relation to the foramen magnum produce a variable picture. Their growth may be primarily in the posterior fossa with compression of the lower cranial nerves, brain stem, and cerebellum. On the other hand, the tumor may extend down through the foramen magnum, compressing the upper and middle cervical roots and then the long tracts on one or both sides of the spinal cord. In some cases, a mixture of posterior fossa and cervical cord findings will be present.

Foramen magnum meningiomas are not common. On the other hand, *cerebellar tonsillar herniation* (sometimes referred to as cerebellar pressure cone) is a frequent complication of untreated posterior fossa mass lesions (Fig. 15–6). When gradually acquired, head tilt and stiff neck and pain in the neck may be early symptoms. When acutely acquired, a rapid and fatal arrest of respiratory and circulatory function is likely to occur. Such an acute event may be precipitated by the performance of a lumbar puncture in a patient with a posterior fossa mass lesion. At times in subacute cases, this final stage of arrest of respiration and fall in blood pressure is preceded by a period of irregular respiration, slow pulse, and rising blood pressure.

The student should note that once tentorial herniation has occurred in a supratentorial mass lesion, one has a situation of increased mass in the posterior fossa. In addition, hemorrhage into the brain stem and edema of the brain stem act to increase the mass in the posterior fossa. Tonsillar

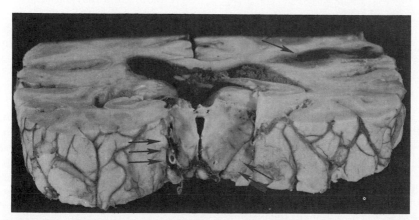

Figure 15–4 Tentorial herniation with brain stem compression. A large intracerebral hematoma and hemorrhagic infarction (single arrow) in right cerebral hemisphere has produced herniation of the medial aspect of temporal lobe (double arrow). Shift of the brain stem has occurred with compression of the left cerebral peduncle against the tentorium (tentorium no longer present in this photograph). Infarction of the left cerebral peduncle has resulted (triple arrow). (Courtesy of Pathology Department, Tufts New England Medical Center.)

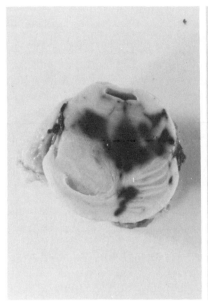
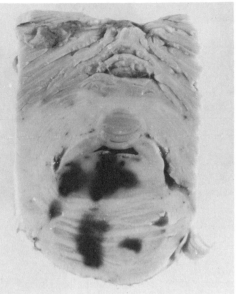

Figure 15–5 Duret hemorrhage. Multiple small hemorrhages are present in the pontine tegmentum and to a lesser extent in the basilar pons. This patient had a massive infarction of cerebral hemisphere with temporal lobe herniation and brain stem compression. (Courtesy of Dr. John Hills, New England Center Hospitals.)

See Filmstrip, Frame 27.

herniation with medullary compression would then in this situation also be the expected terminal event. (For a more complete discussion of the clinical pathophysiology of the tentorial and tonsillar herniation syndromes, the student is referred to the monograph by Plum and Posner, 1966.)

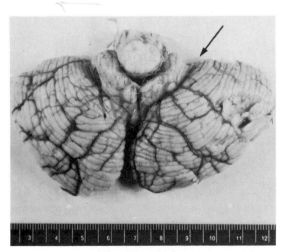

Figure 15–6 Herniation of the cerebellar tonsils. The cerebellar tonsils have been compressed downward through the foramen magnum, producing the notching of the inferior surface (arrow). In the process, the lower end of the medulla has been compressed. (The pathological process in this case was teratoma arising from the pineal.) (Courtesy of Dr. John Hills, New England Center Hospitals; and Dr. Jose Segarra, Boston Veterans Administration Hospital.)

See Filmstrip, Frame 28.

FORAMEN MAGNUM SYNDROMES DUE TO DEVELOPMENTAL AND BONY MALFORMATION

Deformation of the bones at the base of the skull occurs in a platybasia, a flattening of the sphenoid and occipital bones (sometimes referred to as basilar impression because the bones about the foramen magnum are pushed into the posterior fossa). There are essentially two causes for this deformation: Paget's disease, and various developmental malformations.

Paget's disease is a chronic metabolic disease of bone occurring in the adult, the cause of which is unknown. There is both excessive bone destruction and excessive and disorganized bone formation. Bony overgrowth may result in pressure on nerve roots, on cranial nerve VIII and on the facial nerve. Involvement of the vertebrae may result in spinal cord compression. Involvement of the skull is common. When the disease process affects occipital and sphenoid bones at the base of the skull, a softening, flattening, and distortion occurs. As a result, the odontoid process projects up into the posterior fossa. The posterior fossa in its normal state is a relatively small cavity. The end result is a compression of the contents of the posterior fossa—medulla, cerebellum, and lower cranial nerves—in addition to the upper cervical spinal cord. The following case history illustrates this problem.

Case History 4. NECH #89–782. Date of admission: 9/14/54.

This 57-year-old, white insurance salesman (Mr. A.DeA.) in 1949 first noticed difficulty in obtaining a standard-size hat. In 1952, the patient first noted the gradual onset of a steadily progressive difficulty in walking, characterized by a loss of balance. He had experienced increasing difficulty in standing erect and had fallen on several occasions. Beginning also in 1952, the patient had noted increasing discomfort at the occipital area of the head. In 1954, over a period of several months, the patient had noted a hoarseness of his voice, a weakness or tremor of the tongue, a difficulty in articulating words, and a difficulty in swallowing. More recently (1954) the patient had noted numbness of all fingers, the right more than the left, and a correlated clumsiness in the manipulation of small objects. In the several weeks prior to admission, the patient had noted difficulty in focusing his eyes. He had also noted diplopia particularly when gazing to the right.

NEUROLOGICAL EXAMINATION:

1. *Mental status:* Intact.
2. *Cranial nerves:*
   a. A right lateral rectus weakness was present with a resultant diplopia. Horizontal nystagmus on lateral gaze to either side was present.
   b. Pain sensation was significantly decreased in the ophthalmic and maxillary divisions of the left fifth nerve. Corneal reflex was decreased on the left. To a lesser degree touch sensation was decreased in the same distribution over the left face.
   c. Hearing was decreased bilaterally. Both bone and air conduction were affected.
   d. Gag defect was decreased and pharyngeal tactile sensation was decreased on the left more than the right. The uvula pulled to the right.
   e. Lingual movements and lingual

sounds were slowly performed although no definite weakness or atrophy of the tongue was present.
3. *Motor system:*
   a. Strength was intact
   b. Gait was grossly reeling and ataxic
   c. Ataxia was present on finger-to-nose and heel-to-shin tests of cerebellar function
4. *Reflexes:*
   a. Deep tendon reflexes were symmetrical and physiologic
   b. Plantar responses were flexor
5. *Sensory system:* All modalities were intact
6. *Head and neck:* The head was large. The neck was short. There was limitation of movement on turning the head laterally

LABORATORY DATA:

1. Skull x-rays showed marked thickening of the diploe with the changes characteristic of Paget's disease. Well advanced platybasia was present with the tip of the odontoid of the axis found to be 25 mm. above McGregor's line. (This is a line drawn from the posterior margin of the hard palate to the inferior surface of the basal occipital bone; normally the odontoid should not extend above this line by more than 4 to 5 mm.)

2. Alkaline phosphatase was elevated to 7.5 units, compared to a normal of 1 to 4 units.

SUBSEQUENT COURSE:

A suboccipital decompression was performed by Dr. Bertram Selverstone on October 5, 1954. The bone of the cranium was very thick. There was marked compression of the lower medulla and upper cervical cord by the anterior rim of occipital bone forming the posterior margin of the foramen magnum. The posterior arch of the first cervical vertebra was also compressing the underlying cervical spinal cord. Postoperatively, there was a significant improvement in symptoms and signs. Follow-up in November 1954 indicated that the patient had regained fine-movement skills in the hand. His gait was markedly improved, although still slightly wide-based. Lower cranial nerve findings were no longer present. The sixth and eighth cranial nerve findings were unchanged. Follow-up evaluation in September 1955 indicated continued improvement in gait. Nystagmus was present but the weakness of nerve VI had been resolved. Evaluation in 1957 indicated bilateral medial rectus weakness with gait still mildly ataxic.

Re-evaluation in 1963 indicated that beginning in 1961, the patient had increasing ataxia of gait and increasing diplopia. In addition, decreasing vision in the left eye had been noted. Gait was now moderately ataxic. Bilateral medial rectus weakness was present and there was decreased sensation as previously in right trigeminal distribution. Re-evaluation in 1967 indicated progression of ataxia. Skull x-rays indicated a progression of the degree of basilar invagination. The problem was now more complex in the sense that the patient now also had symptoms relevant to other disease processes: (a) cervical spondylosis with root and possibly cord compression, (b) insufficiency in the basilar vertebral circulation with dizziness on assumption of upright posture, and (c) a bilateral internuclear ophthalmoplegia. Any additional surgical procedures were refused by the patient.

COMMENT:

The findings in this case indicated involvement of the cerebellum and lower cranial nerves, particularly the vagus and glossopharyngeal nerves: hoarseness of voice, defect in elevation of the uvula and defective sensation in the posterior pharynx. In addition, there was involvement of the sixth and trigeminal nerves. Whether the fifth nerve involvement related directly to platybasia or whether this reflected occlusion of the ostia of the skull by Paget's disease would not be certain. Involvement of nerve VIII usually reflects narrowing of the internal auditory foramen with compression of the nerve.

Basilar impression occurs in conditions other than Paget's disease. In the majority of cases, the defect reflects a congenital malformation of the basal occipital bone. There are often associated malformations of bone: a fusion of the occipital bone with the atlas, a dislocation of the odontoid, a fusion of the vertebrae (Klippel-Feil abnormality), cervical spina bifida, or a small foramen magnum. There may also be associated malformations of the central nervous system, e.g., the Arnold-Chiari malformations — elongation of the inferior portion of the cerebellum through the foramen magnum into the cervical canal or persistence of the embryonal cervical flexure with apparent downward displacement of the medulla and cervical cord (Fig. 15–7). Malformations of the meninges (arachnoid cysts) or of the roof of the fourth ventricle, with absence of the foramina

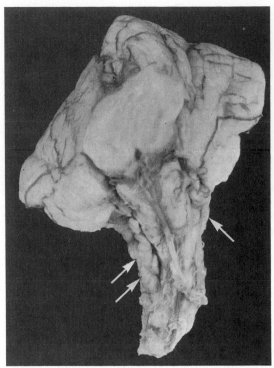

Figure 15–7 Arnold-Chiari malformation. The medulla, cerebellar tonsils (arrows), and a portion of the pons have been elongated downward through the foramen magnum. An abnormal flexure is present, resulting in a distortion of the medulla. The upper level of brain stem section is actually through the cerebral peduncles in this specimen. In this case, a meningomyelocele, hydrocephalus, and other malformations were also present. (Courtesy of Dr. John Hills, New England Center Hospitals.)

of Luschka and Magendie (Dandy-Walker syndrome) may be present. In occasional cases, syringomyelia or hydrocephalus also will be found. Although many of these malformations will produce their effects in infancy or childhood, not infrequently the first neurological manifestation may be delayed until adult life.

VASCULAR SYNDROMES AFFECTING THE BRAIN AS EXTRINSIC LESIONS

Aneurysms. At points of congenital weakness in the wall of an artery (usually points of bifurcation) a dilated thin-walled sac may form, termed an aneurysm. Intracranial aneurysms produce symptoms in several ways: (1) the dilated sac may act as a space-occupying lesion compressing adjacent structures such as cranial nerves, (2) rupture of the aneurysm may occur with leakage of blood into the subarachnoid space, and (3) circulation of blood in the artery beyond the point of the aneurysm may be impaired, producing ischemia and destruction of tissue supplied by the artery.

The majority (85 to 90 per cent) of aneurysms arise from what is termed anterior circulation at essentially three locations: (1) the anterior cerebral-anterior communicating junction, (2) the middle cerebral artery bifurcation, and (3) the junction of the posterior communicating and internal carotid arteries. At this last location, an enlarging saccular aneurysm may compress cranial nerve III. The finding of a fixed, dilated pupil and ptosis of the lid in a patient with subarachnoid hemorrhage may provide a valuable clue for localization. Such a case is presented in Chapter 22 p. 563, where a more detailed discussion of aneurysms and subarachnoid hemorrhage is presented.

Approximately 10 to 15 per cent of saccular aneurysms are found in relation to the basilar vertebral system. Common sites include the bifurcation of the basilar artery. In addition to saccular aneurysms, fusiform dilatations of the basilar artery may occur in atherosclerosis resulting in an enlarged tortuous vessel which may compress adjacent structures.

Intracerebellar Hemorrhage. Occurring in hypertensive patients, intracerebellar hemorrhage may secondarily compress the fourth ventricle and brain stem (Fig. 15–8). The early symptoms of dizziness, vomiting, and ataxia are often followed by coma and evolving extraocular muscle findings.

INTRINSIC DISEASES OF THE BRAIN STEM

Our discussion of intrinsic diseases of the brain stem will proceed according to the following outline.

A. Ischemic-occlusive vascular disease of the basilar vertebral arteries
  1. Vertebral arteries
  2. Medullary syndromes
    a. Lateral medullary (syndrome of the posterior inferior cerebellar artery)
    b. Medial medullary (paramedian medullary syndrome)
  3. Basilar artery and its branches including posterior cerebral arteries

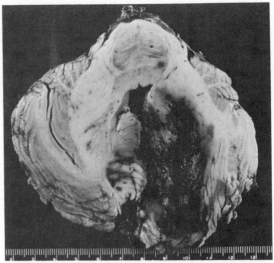

Figure 15–8 Intracerebellar hemorrhage. This 61-year-old patient with elevated blood pressure (240/110) had sudden onset of headache, vomiting, dizziness, marked ataxia of gait and trunk, nystagmus on left lateral gaze, and minor incoordination of left hand. The intracerebellar hemorrhage had extended into fourth ventricle and into subarachnoid space. Blood was present in the cerebrospinal fluid on lumbar puncture (16,500 red blood cells/cu. mm.). (Courtesy of Dr. John Hills, New England Center Hospitals; and Dr. Jose Segarra, Boston Veterans Administration Hospital.)

See Filmstrip, Frame 29.

  4. Inferior pontine syndromes
    a. Lateral inferior pontine (syndrome of the anterior inferior cerebellar artery)
    b. Medial (paramedian) inferior pontine
  5. Superior pontine syndromes
    a. Lateral superior pontine (syndrome of the superior cerebellar artery)
    b. Medial (paramedian) superior pontine
  6. Midbrain syndromes
    a. Paramedian (peduncular) syndrome
    b. Tegmental syndrome
  7. Combined syndrome: thrombosis of the basilar artery
B. Hemorrhage (Refer to Chapter 22.)
  1. Intrapontine
  2. Intracerebellar
C. Subarachnoid hemorrhage
    (Refer to forementioned extrinsic disease)

(Refer to diseases of cerebral hemispheres, Chapter 22)

D. Intrinsic tumors: pontine gliomas
E. Demyelinating diseases
   1. Multiple sclerosis
   2. Acute postinfectious encephalomyelitis
F. Degenerative diseases
   1. Focal disease: syringobulbia
   2. System diseases
      a. Amyotrophic lateral sclerosis: bulbar palsy
      b. Poliomyelitis
      c. Variants of cerebellar degenerations also involving brain stem: olivopontocerebellar degeneration, dentatorubral degeneration.

The disease entity affecting the brain stem which is most frequently encountered in clinical practice is vascular disease, predominantly of the ischemic-occlusive type. Ischemic-occlusive cerebrovascular disease usually produces its initial clinical manifestations in patients over the age of 50. The basic pathological process of atherosclerosis which underlies occlusive vascular disease (the deposition of lipids such as cholesterol in the walls of vessels) certainly may begin in an asymptomatic manner earlier in life. On the other hand, multiple sclerosis, which is the second most frequent brain stem disease entity encountered, usually produces its initial manifestations in the age group 20 to 40. Of the other intrinsic diseases affecting the brain stem, the next most frequently encountered are brain stem gliomas (occurring predominantly in the pediatric age group under 20 years) and the bulbar variety of amyotrophic lateral sclerosis (occurring predominantly in the age group over 40 years).

ISCHEMIC-OCCLUSIVE DISEASE OF THE BASILAR VERTEBRAL ARTERIES

Stenosis (narrowing) or occlusion of the vertebral and basilar arteries may occur at a number of sites. In general, maximum areas of atherosclerosis disease occur at the points of origin, bifurcation, or angulation of the extracranial and intracranial portions of the large and medium size cerebral arteries. There is no one-to-one relationship of a particular site of stenosis or occlusion to a specific pattern of clinical symptoms. Thus, occlusion of a vertebral artery may

occur with no resultant clinical symptoms in evidence. In other instances, such an occlusion may result in transient symptoms indicating ischemia (a temporary decrease in blood flow below a critical level) within the distribution of a particular vessel or combination of vessels arising from the vertebral or basilar arteries. In still other instances, such an occlusion may result in actual tissue destruction, infarction (encephalomalacia) within the distribution of one or more vessels taking origin from the vertebral or basilar arteries; e.g., the posterior inferior cerebellar artery arising from the vertebral artery or the posterior cerebral artery from the basilar artery.

In still other instances, one may find that infarction within the distribution of a particular vessel has occurred without actual occlusion of that particular vessel or even of the parent vessel. Instead, stenosis with a decrease in blood flow has occurred.

As we will discuss in greater detail in relation to vascular diseases affecting the cerebral hemispheres, several factors account for this lack of correspondence between the state of a particular vessel and the vascular status of the region supplied by that vessel.

1. There are significant congenital variations with regard to the normal patency of the two vertebral arteries. Thus, in a particular individual one vertebral artery may be vestigial or may terminate as the posterior inferior cerebellar artery. Thus, the basilar artery may be dependent entirely or predominantly on a single vertebral artery.

2. There are significant congenital variations in the circle of Willis. Thus, in a particular individual one or both of the posterior cerebral arteries may originate from the internal carotid artery as a continuation of a large posterior communicating artery, with only a thin proximal portion originating from the basilar artery. This may have several possible consequences. In occlusion of the basilar artery, the territory of the particular posterior cerebral artery will not be infarcted since this area is essentially supplied by the carotid system. In such a case, moreover, the posterior communicating artery could not be expected to supply blood from the carotid system in a retrograde manner to the basilar system. On the other hand, in this situation, infarction of the territory supplied by the posterior cerebral artery could occur on the basis of carotid artery disease without significant occlusive disease

of the usual source of supply—the basilar vertebral system.

3. There are significant leptomeningeal anastomoses over the surface of the cerebral hemisphere between the anterior, middle, and posterior cerebral arteries. Such anastomoses could in part contribute to blood flow in the area supplied by the posterior cerebral artery. Similar leptomeningeal anastomoses occur over the surface of the cerebellum between the posterior inferior, the anterior inferior, and the superior cerebellar arteries providing for an overlap in supply.

4. To a variable degree anastomoses may occur providing blood flow from extracranial noncerebral blood vessels. Such anastomoses will allow bypass of a block in the innominate, subclavian, or lower (extracranial portion) vertebral artery. For example, anastomotic flow may occur from the external carotid system via the deep descending branch of the occipital artery to the muscular branches of the vertebral artery. These muscular branches of the vertebral artery in the neck may also receive anastomotic flow from other branches of the subclavian artery: the ascending cervical artery arising from the thyrocervical trunk and branches of the transverse cervical artery.

5. Variations may also reflect the fact that often atherosclerosis affects more than one major artery. Thus, while total occlusion of one vertebral artery may have little effect, in the presence of intact carotid arteries, stenosis without occlusion of one vertebral artery and of both internal carotid arteries may have very significant effects.

6. Considerable variability may also occur because of certain general systemic and metabolic factors. Thus, a narrowed vessel may still deliver sufficient blood when the systemic blood pressure is 190/170, but then fails to do so when the head of pressure falls to 120/70. Such falls in blood pressure occur during sleep, on sudden standing after a long period of recumbency and in response to overtreatment with various agents which are designed to lower blood pressure.

7. Finally, certain mechanical factors may introduce a degree of variability. Thus, a patient may have stenosis of a vertebral artery without clinical symptoms when the head is in a neutral position. When the head is rotated or extended, a decrease in blood flow in the vertebral system normally occurs. In a borderline situation, this fall in blood flow may be sufficient to produce symptoms. The student should recall that the vertebral arteries pass through the foramina of the transverse processes of the cervical vertebrae and thus would be easily compressed by maneuvers such as rotation and extension.

We will now consider syndromes involving the territories of particular arteries. In addition to the large vessels, the vertebrals and basilar, we will deal with the major branches of these vessels. There is a general plan of brain stem vascular architecture. The basilar artery and vertebral arteries are placed on the basal (ventral) surface of the brain stem. One can visualize a midline or paramedian wedge-shaped area extending into the brain stem with a base on this ventral area. This paramedian wedge is supplied by penetrating vessels, termed *paramedian*. The lateral tegmental portions of the brain stem are supplied by branches, *long circumferential arteries*, named for their areas of supply over the surface of the cerebellum: posterior inferior, anterior inferior, and superior cerebellar arteries. In addition, at the upper midbrain level, quadrigeminal arteries from the posterior cerebral arteries function as long circumferential arteries. Ventral lateral portions of the pons and midbrain are supplied by variable transverse arteries, termed *short circumferential*, arising from the basilar artery. At each level of the brain stem, we will be dealing primarily with paramedian as opposed to lateral tegmental syndromes.

The Vertebral Artery. The vertebral artery usually arises from the subclavian artery (the left vertebral artery may arise directly from the aorta in 6 per cent of cases). The artery ascends to enter the foramen of the transverse process of the sixth cervical vertebra, then passes upward through the foramina of the successive cervical vertebrae; then, after passing behind the superior articular process of the atlas, it enters the foramen magnum. After passing upward and medially, the artery unites with its opposite number at the lower border of the pons to form the basilar artery. During its course in the neck, the vertebral artery gives rise to radicular branches (which anastomose with the anterior and posterior spinal arteries) and to muscular branches whose anastomoses have already been considered. The intracranial branches are the posterior inferior cerebellar, the anterior spinal, the posterior spinal, and the paramedian arteries (Fig. 17–16).

The syndromes associated with occlusive disease of the vertebral artery are variable. Occlusion or absence of *one* vertebral artery, particularly at a proximal point in an otherwise intact individual, is usually well tolerated (as we have indicated, it is not unusual to find one vertebral artery hypoplastic).

Stenosis or occlusion of the *proximal portions* of both vertebral arteries in the series of patients reported by Fisher (1970) was associated with transient symptoms: faintness, blurred vision, dizziness, loss of balance, diplopia, numbness of an arm or of the face. The symptoms are essentially those of transient insufficiency of circulation in the more distal distribution of vertebral and basilar arteries.

Stenosis or occlusion of the intracranial segment of the vertebral artery or arteries may result in infarction over a variable area: the distribution of the basilar artery, the distribution of the paramedian branches of the vertebral artery, or the distribution of the posterior inferior cerebellar artery. Actually, occlusive disease of the intracranial segment of the vertebral artery is a much more frequent cause of the lateral medullary syndrome than is limited occlusion of the posterior inferior cerebellar artery.

Medullary Syndromes (Fig. 15–9)

Lateral Medullary Syndrome: Syndrome of the Posterior Inferior Cerebellar Artery (Wallenberg's Syndrome) (Figs. 15–9, 15–10). Of all the various classic vascular syndromes of the brain stem, this syndrome, either alone in a relatively pure form or in a modified form, is the one most frequently encountered.* The brain stem territory of the posterior inferior cerebellar artery includes the following structures (Fig. 15–9A): (a) the restiform body (the inferior cerebellar peduncle) and the adjacent dorsal and ventral spinocerebellar pathway, (b) the descending spinal tract and nucleus of the trigeminal nerve, (c) the lateral spinothalamic tract, (d) the descending sympathetic pathway, (e) the nucleus ambiguus and the fibers of cranial nerve X, and (f) the vestibular nuclei (primarily spinal and medial at this level). The resultant clinical findings are illustrated in the following case history.

---

*The student should, of course, realize that nonclassic vascular syndromes of the brain stem are more commonly encountered than the classic syndromes involving isolated vascular territories.

Case History 5. NECH #155–057. Date of admission: 5/15/66.

This 60-year-old, white male (Mr. W.McM.) was admitted to the hospital in May 1966 with a chief complaint of left occipital headaches of three weeks duration. Two weeks prior to admission, the patient noted a sudden onset of diplopia on forward gaze and a sensation of dizziness (? vertigo). One day prior to admission the patient noted a relatively sudden onset of ptosis of the right eyelid.

PAST HISTORY: The patient had been under treatment for hypertension for 2 years with blood pressure in the range of 180/110.

GENERAL PHYSICAL EXAMINATION: Blood pressure was elevated to 192/96.

NEUROLOGICAL EXAMINATION:
1. *Mental status:* Intact.
2. *Cranial nerves:*
   a. The findings of a Horner's syndrome were present. The right pupil measured 3 mm.; the left was 5 mm., but both responded to light and accommodation. Ptosis (drooping) of the right eyelid, a slight degree of enophthalmos (recession of the eye), and decreased sweating on the right side of the face were also present.
   b. Nystagmus was present on left lateral gaze.
   c. The patient reported inconsistent diplopia, but extraocular movements were full.
   d. Pain sensation but not touch was decreased on the right side of the face. The right corneal reflex was diminished.
   e. A minor right central facial weakness was present.
   f. The uvula deviated to the left and there was deficient elevation of the right side of the palate. There was also a suggestion of hoarseness.
3. *Motor system:*
   a. Strength was intact.
   b. No spasticity was present.
   c. Cerebellar testing: An ataxia was evident in the right upper extremity on finger-tapping, hand-patting, and finger-to-nose tests. A side-to-side intention tremor was present. Ataxia was also present in the right lower extremity on heel-to-shin and tibial tapping tests.
4. *Reflexes:*
   a. Deep tendon reflexes:

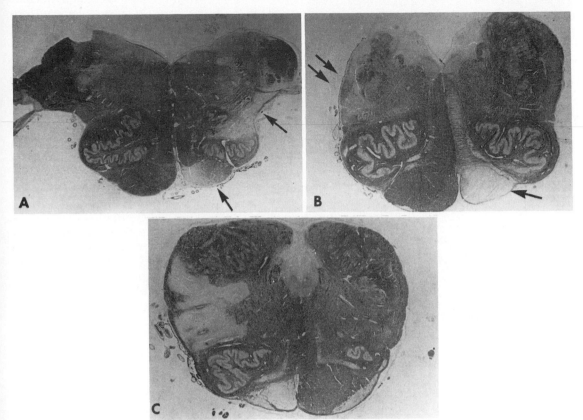

Figure 15–9 Medullary syndromes. *A*, This 65-year-old hypertensive male expired in 1964 following an acute occlusion of the basilar artery with acute infarction of the midbrain. The old infarct noted on the left side of the medulla (arrows) correlated with his hospital admission in 1959 when the patient had complaints of difficulty swallowing, "dizziness," ataxia, and numbness of the left side of the face and the right side of the body. Examination had revealed, in addition, a left-sided Horner's syndrome, a decrease in pain sensation on the left side of the face, deviation of the tongue to the left but increased deep tendon reflexes on the right side. These findings were associated with old occlusions of the left vertebral and left posterior inferior cerebellar arteries.

B, This 50-year-old male had extensive atherosclerosis, expiring in 1965 following surgery for occlusion of the femoral artery. Old infarcts were present in the medulla — one corresponding to a right-sided lateral medullary syndrome in 1959 (double arrows) and the other to repeated episodes of a basilar-vertebral insufficiency accompanied by a right hemiparesis in 1962–1963, correlated with the left-sided paramedian infarct (arrow). Stenosis of vertebral arteries and occlusion of right posterior inferior cerebellar artery were present at autopsy. **See Filmstrip, Frame 30.**

C, This patient presented a lateral medullary syndrome. The medullary pyramidal lesion in this case reflected a degeneration of axons from a pyramidal tract lesion at a higher level (independent capsular infarct). (Courtesy of Dr. Jose Segarra, Boston Veterans Administration Hospital.)

NOTE: In each case, the territory of the posterior inferior cerebellar artery is indicated by the retro-olivary lesion; the territory of the vertebral paramedian branches by the medullary pyramid lesion.

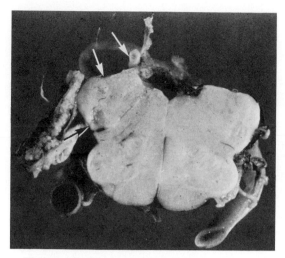

Figure 15–10 Lateral medullary infarct. This 72-year-old white male diabetic, 2 months prior to death, had the acute onset of nystagmus on left lateral gaze, decreased pain sensation on the left side of face and right side of body, with difficulty swallowing, slurring of speech, and deviation of the uvula to the right. The occluded left posterior inferior cerebellar artery (arrow) can be visualized just above the area of infarction (arrows) and adjacent to the choroid plexus of the fourth ventricle. Atherosclerosis of the right vertebral artery is also apparent. The tissue adherent to the lateral medullary infarct probably consists of infarcted adjacent cerebellum. (Courtesy of Dr. Jose Segarra, Boston Veterans Administration Hospital.)

See Filmstrip, Frame 31.

Biceps: right, 2+; left, 3+
Quadriceps: right, 2+; left, 3+
Achilles: right, 2+; left, 2+
 b. Plantar responses: The right was flexor; the left, equivocal.
5. *Sensation:*
 a. There was decreased pain on the left side of the body, the left arm, and the left leg.
   The patient was unable to distinguish between hot and cold on the left side.
 b. Position, vibration, and touch modalities were intact.
LABORATORY DATA:
1. A mild degree of anemia was present (hematocrit 39 per cent). White blood count was increased to 16,350. The differential revealed an increased number of polymorphonuclears (80 per cent). Sedimentation rate was increased to 89 mm. per hour. These findings were consistent with his subsequent course.

2. Chest and skull x-rays were normal.
3. Cerebrospinal fluid was clear and under normal pressure. Protein was normal.
HOSPITAL COURSE:
Two days after admission, the patient complained of severe right lower quadrant abdominal pain and began to vomit. Surgical exploration indicated an infarction of small bowel due to an inflammatory disease of blood vessels: *periarteritis.*

A limited small bowel resection was performed. The patient received treatment with steroids because of the inflammatory nature of his disease, and there was considerable improvement in symptoms.

On May 29, 1966, the patient developed a weakness of the left arm and leg over a 3-day period. Examination now revealed the additional findings of difficulty in conjugate lateral gaze to the right with diplopia on right lateral gaze and a mild weakness of the left arm and leg. As previously, deep tendon reflexes were increased on the left and there was an equivocal plantar response on the left. The cerebellar findings in the right arm and leg were no longer present. The Horner's syndrome and deficit in pain and temperature sensation on the left side of the body were still present. Improvement in the hemiparesis occurred over the next 3 weeks.
COMMENT:
The initial history of the present illness in this case does not allow for a clear-cut localization at a given level of the brain stem. A much more typical history in a lateral medullary infarction would have indicated the sudden onset of dizziness or vertigo, vomiting, numbness of the right side of the face and of the left side of the body, in addition to an ataxia of the right arm and leg and symptomatic difficulty in swallowing and speech.

Although the clinical history provided by the patient was relatively vague, the findings on neurological examination were clear-cut and allowed for a relatively precise localization.

The ptosis of the right eyelid might have suggested a third nerve lesion. However, the associated findings of a small pupil on the right (miosis), recession of the right eye (enophthalmos), and decreased sweating on the right side of the face provided the combination of findings known as Horner's syndrome. A lesion of the sympathetic pathways was indicated. The exact level of this lesion was unclear. A Horner's syndrome may be found with a lesion at almost any point in the sympathetic pathway in the brain stem, cervical spinal cord, sympathetic ganglion, and postganglionic fibers.

The associated findings, however, clearly indicate a lesion in the brain stem. The combination of decreased pain and temperature over all three divisions on the right side of the face with sparing of touch indicates that the lesion had involved the descending spinal tract and nucleus of the trigeminal nerve in the brain stem (upper medulla or lower pons). This finding provided a reasonable degree of certainty, moreover, that the lesion involved the lateral tegmentum of the brain stem.

This conclusion is reinforced by finding that pain and temperature were decreased in a selective manner over the left side of the body, arm, and leg, indicating involvement of the adjacent lateral spinothalamic pathway.

Additional confirmation of the lateral tegmental localization and more specific identification of the rostral-caudal level of involvement of the brain stem is provided by the additional findings relevant to the nucleus ambiguus: hoarseness and defects in movements of the uvula and soft palate. (In other cases, such damage to the nucleus ambiguus also produces difficulty in swallowing.) Thus, the lesion can now be localized to the lateral portion of the upper medulla.

Confirmation of this lateral medullary location is provided by the finding of ipsilateral ataxia of the right arm and leg (ipsilateral also to the descending spinal tract of nerve V, and the nucleus ambiguus) indicating involvement of the restiform body or the adjacent spinocerebellar pathways.

The student should note that in classic cases of this syndrome, no reflex asymmetry is present and the plantar responses are flexor. The finding of a reflex asymmetry should then indicate some slight involvement of the corticospinal tracts in the medullary pyramids or at a pontine or midbrain location. Such involvement should provide one small clue that the basic arterial lesion is localized not in the posterior inferior cerebellar artery but rather in the vertebral artery itself. Confirmation is provided by the patient's subsequent course: the development of the left hemiparesis. Since the face was not involved, the level of involvement of pyramidal pathway was presumably below the level of the nucleus of the facial nerve (pontomedullary junction).

As we have indicated, since it is usually the occlusion of the vertebral artery which is responsible for the syndrome, it is more common to encounter variations of the syndrome rather than the pure syndrome.

Keeping this in mind, the student should be able to explain the initial symptom of diplopia. This could indicate involvement of the sixth cranial nerve or of its nucleus or of the third nerve fibers or its nucleus. In view of the subsequent finding of a defect in conjugate lateral gaze to the right, we may assume that the localization was probably at the level of the right abducens nucleus.

Paramedian Medullary Syndrome (Fig. 15–9B). Occlusion of the paramedian penetrating branches from the vertebral artery may result in a syndrome characterized by ipsilateral paralysis and atrophy of one-half of the tongue (hypoglossal fibers or nucleus) in addition to a contralateral hemiparesis (medullary pyramid). There may be involvement of the adjacent medial lemniscus as well, producing a contralateral deficit in position and vibratory sensation and a relative decrease in tactile sensation. This syndrome, which bears the name of Hughlings Jackson's syndrome, is rarely encountered in its pure form.

Syndromes of the Basilar Artery. The basilar artery is formed by the union of the two vertebral arteries. As with the vertebral artery, it is customary to distinguish paramedian and circumferential branches. (Refer to Fig. 17–16 and Fig. 17–18B.)

The initial circumferential branch is the anterior inferior cerebellar artery which supplies the lateral tegmentum of the lower pons (Fig. 15–11A): the facial nerve, the cochlear nucleus and eighth nerve, the descending spinal tract and nucleus of the fifth nerve, the lateral spinothalamic tract, the sympathetic pathway, the middle and inferior cerebellar peduncles, and the anterior inferior portion of the cerebellum. The area of supply may also include the main sensory nucleus of the fifth nerve at a midpontine level. The internal auditory artery which supplies the inner ear may arise from this vessel or independently from the basilar artery.

The next circumferential branch is the superior cerebellar artery which supplies the tegmentum of the upper pons and caudal midbrain (Fig. 15–11B), including the brachium conjunctivum, the medial longitudinal

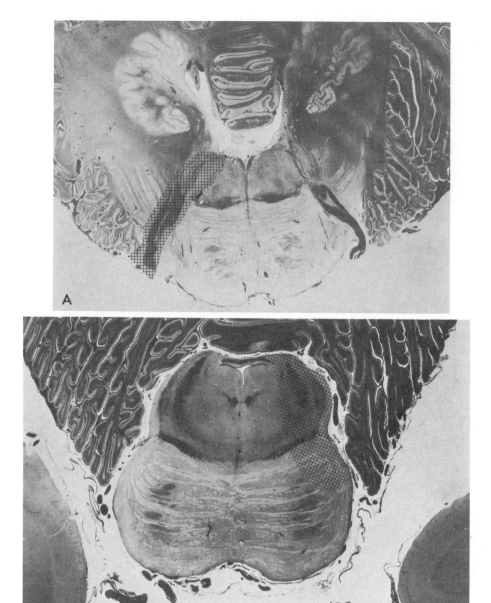

Figure 15–11 Syndromes of the basilar artery. Circumferential branches. *A*, The cross-hatched portion of lateral inferior pons represents the pontine area supplied by the anterior inferior cerebellar artery. *B*, The cross-hatched portion of lateral superior pons represents the pontine area supplied by the superior cerebellar artery. At times, the paramedian tegmental area is included within the supply of the artery.

fasciculus, the motor and main sensory nucleus of the trigeminal nerve, the medial lemniscus, the lateral spinothalamic tract, and the central tegmental tract, and then proceeds to supply the superior cerebellum. The basilar artery then terminates at the pontine-midbrain border into two posterior cerebral arteries. Each posterior cerebral artery in its proximal segment provides a series of vessels to supply the midbrain: penetrating paramedian branches from this vessel supply the medial one-half of the cerebral peduncle, the third nerve fibers, the third nerve nucleus, and the medial one-half of the red nucleus. Short circumferential vessels from the posterior cerebral artery supply the remainder (lateral one-half) of the cerebral peduncle and red nucleus. The lateral tegmentum and tectum of the midbrain is supplied by somewhat longer circumferential branches also called quadrigeminal arteries. Other penetrating branches (thalamoperforating and thalamogeniculate) of the posterior cerebral artery in this location supply the subthalamus and much of the thalamus: pulvinar, ventral lateral, ventral posterior, medial geniculate, lateral geniculate, centromedian, and the dorsal median nuclei.

The main posterior cerebral artery then passes around the cerebral peduncle and midbrain close to the tentorial opening, supplying branches to the medial aspect of the temporal lobe and then dividing into the parieto-occipital and calcarine branches to supply the occipital lobe.

The syndromes of the posterior cerebral arteries relevant to the thalamus, subthalamus, and the temporal and occipital lobes are discussed in the chapters on the cerebral hemispheres and motor system.

As atherosclerosis involves the basilar and vertebral arteries, there may be transient symptoms suggesting ischemia in the distribution of the various vessels originating from these major arteries. In some cases, infarction may occur within the distribution of these branches. Thus, the patient may experience episodes of vertigo or dizziness and diplopia, a bilateral blurring of vision, or a weakness or numbness of one side of the body or face, and then in a later attack, of the contralateral side of the face or body. In some cases, the transient symptoms are precipitated by extension or rotation of the head which reduces blood flow in the vertebral arteries. Sudden *drop attacks* without loss of consciousness are not unusual, due to ischemia of paramedian branches supplying the motor pathways: corticospinal tracts and the pontine-medullary reticular formation. Episodes of bilateral blindness may occur due to ischemia of the territory supplied by the posterior cerebral arteries.

With total occlusion of the basilar artery, various combinations of cranial nerve findings, coma, decerebrate rigidity, and quadriplegia will be found. Before we examine the situation of total basilar artery occlusion, we will consider the various syndromes of the branch territories. In general, these partial segmental syndromes are relatively uncommon compared to the syndrome of the lateral medulla. The student, moreover, will recognize that histories do not really provide pure examples. There will be some signs or symptoms in each case suggesting involvement at several segmental levels of the brain stem. As with the vertebral artery we will distinguish between paramedian (penetrating branch) and lateral tegmental (circumferential branch) syndromes.

Inferior Pontine Syndrome

Lateral Tegmentum (Syndrome of the Anterior Inferior Cerebellar Artery) (Fig. 15–11*A*). Infarction of the lateral tegmentum at a caudal pontine level results in a sudden unilateral deafness in association with an ipsilateral peripheral facial weakness, ipsilateral Horner's syndrome, vertigo (due to involvement of the vestibular nucleus), and ipsilateral cerebellar symptoms. There may be involvement of the descending spinal tract and nucleus of the trigeminal nerve resulting in an ipsilateral loss of pain and temperature over the face, or the main sensory nucleus may be involved resulting in involvement of facial tactile sensation as well. If the lateral spinothalamic tract is involved, a contralateral loss of pain and temperature will be evident over the arm, leg, and trunk.

Case History 6.   NECH #197–702–2. Date of admission: 10/15/68.

This 55-year-old, white, married, machinery salesman (Mr. C.K.), while driving, on October 14, 1968, had the sudden onset of pain on the left side of the head, accompanied by dizziness (counter-clockwise vertigo). The headache soon became generalized and within a short time nausea, projectile vomiting, and anorexia developed. At the same time, the patient noticed that he could not hear sounds in the left ear. Diplopia was present on left lateral gaze.

The patient was able to continue driving slowly to his home. When he walked from the car and as he was sitting on the edge of his bed, he noted that he tended to fall to the left.

The symptoms were unrelieved by a night of rest; the patient was brought to the hospital emergency room and subsequently admitted to the hospital.

PAST HISTORY:

In July 1966 the patient had had a "dizzy spell" and headache requiring bed rest for 10 days. Elevated blood pressure had required treatment from that time with antihypertensive medication. Obesity of a marked degree had been present for 20 years.

GENERAL PHYSICAL EXAMINATION:

1. The patient was an obese male who was alert and cooperative.
2. Blood pressure was elevated to 220/110.
3. Skin color was florid.

NEUROLOGICAL EXAMINATION:

1. *Mental status:*
   a. Orientation and recent and distant memory were all intact.
   b. Although speech was dysarthric, there was no impairment of higher language functions.
2. *Cranial nerves:*
   a. Fundi and visual fields were intact.
   b. Pupillary responses were intact.
   c. A marked coarse horizontal nystagmus was present at rest on forward gaze and in all directions of gaze but was most marked on left lateral gaze. On upward and downward gaze, vertical nystagmus was also noted. Eye movements were described as "unstable and rolling over" with lack of sustained fixation. One examiner felt that a bilateral weakness of the lateral rectus muscle was present. Convergence and upward gaze were noted to be intact.
   d. Pain sensation was selectively decreased over the left trigeminal distribution, most significantly over the mandibular division. The left corneal reflex was absent and left corneal sensation was reduced. There was a marked weakness of the left masseter muscle.
   e. An incomplete left peripheral facial palsy was present with greater involvement of the lower half of the face.
   f. Taste sensation was absent on the anterior two-thirds of the left side of the tongue.
   g. The left ear was totally deaf.
   h. The gag reflex was absent on the left. The left half of the uvula and soft palate failed to move on elevation.
   i. On protrusion, the tongue deviated to the left.
3. *Motor system:*
   a. Strength was intact except for very minimal weakness in extending the left wrist and elbow.
   b. Tone was normal.
   c. Alternating movements of the left

hand and foot were impaired. There was an ataxia and side-to-side intention tremor apparent in the left upper extremity on finger-to-nose test and in the left lower extremity on heel-to-shin test.
   d. On attempting to sit or stand, the patient fell to the left.
4. *Reflexes:*
   a. Deep tendon reflexes were ques tionably more active on the left at the biceps, triceps, and quadriceps. The asymmetry was of minimal degree.
   b. Plantar response on the right was extensor, on the left equivocal.
5. *Sensation:* All modalities were intact.
6. *Vessels:* The carotid pulses in the neck were strong. The blood pressure in the two arms was equal.

LABORATORY DATA:

1. Skull x-rays were negative.
2. Electroencephalogram was normal.
3. Electrocardiogram was abnormal and suggested left ventricular hypertrophy (presumed secondary to the patient's hypertension).
4. Brain scan was negative.
5. Lumbar puncture demonstrated an elevated cerebrospinal fluid pressure of 275 mm. of water. No cells were present and the protein was normal at 35 mg./100 ml.
6. Brachial arteriogram demonstrated an area of relative avascularity in the inferior one-half of the cerebellum. There was a marked tortuosity of the basilar artery secondary to atherosclerosis with an aneurysmal dilatation present at the apex of the basilar artery.

HOSPITAL COURSE:

Because of the severe headache and elevated cerebrospinal fluid pressure, arteriograms were performed to rule out an atypical but treatable space-occupying lesion in the posterior fossa (such as an intracerebellar hematoma) with the results as indicated. By October 20, 1968 eye movements were described as more stable and a left lateral rectus weakness could now be more clearly defined. The slight reflex asymmetry was no longer present, plantar responses were flexor, and strength was intact. The persistent findings at this time related to nystagmus, left cranial nerves V, VI, VII, and VIII, and to cerebellar findings involving the left arm and leg. By October 30, 1968 the patient was able to walk with assistance, although he still tended to fall to the left. The patient had continued improvement and was transferred to the rehabilitation division. By the time of his eventual hospital discharge, on December 6, 1968 the patient was able to walk with a cane. He was described as independent in dressing and shaving. A variable but improving diplopia was still present on lateral gaze to the left or right and at times on superior gaze. On upward gaze, the separation of images was vertical, suggesting an involvement of the superior rectus muscle.

COMMENT:

The combination of vertigo, left-sided deafness, vomiting, left peripheral facial palsy, and left-sided ataxia, suggests a disease process involving the lateral tegmentum of the caudal pons or the cerebellar-pontine angle. Thus, this particular combination of symptoms, accompanied by headache, might also be found in a tumor (an acoustic neuroma) at the cerebellar-pontine angle. The suddenness of onset of symptoms, however, is more in favor of a vascular accident, in this case ischemia and infarction within the territory of the anterior inferior cerebellar artery. The vertigo and vomiting may be related to the acute involvement of the vestibular nuclei or nerve. The deafness is due to involvement of the entering auditory division of nerve VIII or of the cochlear nuclei. The left-sided ataxia suggests a lesion involving the inferior or middle cerebellar peduncle or the left half of the cerebellum. The facial palsy suggested damage to the left facial nerve or to the motor nucleus of this nerve. The partial nature of the palsy with greater involvement of the lower face but with some involvement of the upper face is usually more in favor of nuclear rather than peripheral nerve involvement.

The decrease in taste on the anterior two-thirds of the tongue in all likelihood indicates involvement of fibers which have entered the brain stem from the geniculate ganglion in company with the facial nerve to join the tractus solitarius (or involvement of the tractus solitarius per se). These fibers whose bipolar neurons are located in the geniculate ganglion have traversed in turn the lingual nerve, the chorda tympani, and then the facial nerve to the geniculate ganglion. The taste fibers as they pass from the geniculate ganglion to the brain stem often appear to be grouped in a separate bundle of fibers, the nervus intermedius. Taste sensation from the posterior one-third of the tongue is con-

veyed by the glossopharyngeal (superior petrosal ganglion); from the epiglottis, by the vagus nerve (nodosa ganglion). These fibers then enter the brain stem to join the tractus solitarius at the medullary level.

It was of course evident at once, from the time of onset, that additional structures outside the distribution of the anterior inferior cerebellar artery were involved by the disease process. It is this more widespread involvement of brain stem structures which makes a vascular process even more likely. Thus, the basic process of stenosis is not in the anterior inferior cerebellar artery per se (although its point of origin may be narrowed or occluded by the process of atherosclerosis) but in the parent basilar artery.

Thus, the patient had diplopia as a prominent symptom. At times early in his hospital course, a bilateral palsy of nerve VI was evident. At times, a palsy of left nerve VI was evident with failure of movement of the left lateral rectus muscle. Such findings suggested some involvement of the paramedian areas in the lower pons (abducens nucleus or more likely abducens nerve fibers), areas usually within the territory of the paramedian branches of the basilar artery in this region. The extraocular findings later in the hospital course suggested a definite vertical separation of images due to dysfunction of the left superior rectus and left inferior oblique muscles. Such findings then would implicate the paramedian branches to the midbrain.

The involvement of pain sensation over the left side of the face, most prominent in the mandibular division, is certainly consistent with involvement of a portion of the descending spinal tract and nucleus of the trigeminal nerve in the lateral tegmentum of the caudal pons. The involvement of the masseter muscle, and the motor nucleus of nerve V, suggests involvement of the lateral tegmentum at a midupper pontine level. This area is on the border between supplies of the anterior-inferior and the superior cerebellar arteries.

The deviation of the tongue to the left was of uncertain explanation and might have suggested that the hypoglossal nucleus (perhaps its rostral portion) was involved by the lesion. The deviation, however, was not accompanied by any actual atrophy. Thus a significant lesion of the hypoglossal nucleus was unlikely. Some apparent deviation of the tongue is almost always seen where a significant degree of facial paralysis is present, be this central or peripheral. The patient may also have had involvement of the cortico-bulbar fibers to the hypoglossal nucleus before or after the decussation of these fibers.

The slight and transient reflex asymmetry with greater activity on the left, accompanied by an equivocal plantar response, suggested a transient involvement of the corticospinal tracts at a pontine location.

The decreased gag reflex on the left with defect in movement of the uvula and soft palate on the left, indicating involvement of the nucleus ambiguus, suggests some extension of the area of ischemia and infarction into the adjacent lateral tegmentum of the rostral medulla.

As regards treatment of the cerebrovascular disease in this particular case, there was little specific or definitive therapy that could be undertaken.

We may indicate at the onset that the basic disease process was atherosclerosis with ischemia and infarction. The aneurysmal dilatation at the apex of the basilar artery was secondary to the atherosclerosis. This aneurysm in any case was essentially above the level of the infarction and could not be implicated in the disease process from the standpoint of subarachnoid bleeding or brain stem compression. Surgical treatment of this aneurysm, even if feasible from a technical standpoint (it is not), would have little effect on the basic disease process.

In cases where recurrent episodes of transient basilar vertebral ischemia occur, anticoagulation therapy may be instituted with a reduction in frequency of the attacks. Occasionally patients with an occlusion or infarction in evolution may benefit from this therapy. Such therapy has little or no value in a completed infarction. Although the patient had "dizzy spells" 2 years previously, this probably related in a nonspecific manner to hypertension and does not necessarily indicate an earlier ischemic episode. Hypertension (present in this case) and a past history of gastrointestinal bleeding are contraindications for anticoagulation therapy. The combination of hypertension and anticoagulation may result in a secondary hemorrhagic infarction. Therapy in the present case was not specific: gait training, reasonable reduction of blood pressure, weight reduction, and dietary control.

Paramedian Lower Pontine (Fig. 15–12). Infarction within the territory supplied by the paramedian vessels of the basilar artery supplying the lower half of the pons results in the combination of an ipsilateral lateral rectus weakness and a contralateral hemiplegia due to involvement of the emergent fibers of nerve VI and the corticospinal tract in the basilar portion of the pons (syndrome of Millard-Gubler). If the area of infarction extends into the tegmentum, there would be evidence of involvement of the nucleus of nerve VI (with an ipsilateral paralysis of lateral gaze) and of the genu of nerve VII

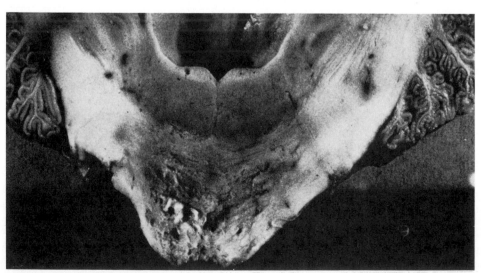

Figure 15–12 Infarct of basilar pontis at a midlower pontine level. This 74-year-old female was found motionless and speechless in bed. She could, however, open and close her eyes on command. Death occurred two weeks later. (Courtesy of Dr. John Hills, New England Center Hospitals.)

about the nucleus of nerve VI (with an ipsilateral peripheral palsy of cranial nerve VII), (syndrome of Foville). The medial longitudinal fasciculus would often be involved, with a unilateral (or bilateral) internuclear ophthalmoplegia. Involvement of the medial lemniscus would produce a contralateral hemianesthesia with deficits in position and vibratory sensation. Damage to the central tegmental tract in the pontine tegmentum may result in rhythmical contractions of the palate (palatal myoclonus). A paramedian midpontine infarct is shown in Figure 15–12.

Superior Pontine Syndromes (Caudal Midbrain)

Lateral Superior Pontine Syndrome of the Superior Cerebellar Artery (Fig. 15–11*B*). Ischemia or infarction of the tegmentum of the rostral pons involves the medial lemniscus and the lateral spinothalamic pathways, producing a contralateral hemianesthesia and hemianalgesia. Since the secondary trigeminothalamic (quintothalamic) fibers have already crossed the midline below the level and have essentially merged with the medial lemniscus, the sensory deficits involve the contralateral side of the face as well as the contralateral arm, leg, and trunk. There is, in addition, damage to the superior cerebellar peduncle (the brachium conjunctivum). The cerebellar symptoms are ipsilateral to the lesion when the damage to the brachium conjunctivum occurs below the level of decussation. However, since the superior cerebellar artery also supplies the lateral tegmentum of the midbrain at a caudal level, the brachium conjunctivum may be involved above its decussation. If so, the cerebellar symptoms will be contralateral to the lesion. Moreover, the disturbance of movement is likely to be more variable. Thus, a coarse tremor at rest or instability of sustained posture may be seen in addition to the expected intention tremor. As at lower levels of the pons, the central tegmental tract may also be involved. The lesion (and the territory of the superior cerebellar artery) may extend into the paramedian tegmentum. If so, damage to the medial longitudinal fasciculus may occur.

Paramedian Upper Pons (Fig. 15–13) When infarction of the corticospinal and corticobulbar tracts of the basilar pons occurs, the clinical effect is a contralateral, upper motor neuron paralysis of the face, arm, and leg. This produces a relatively pure motor syn-

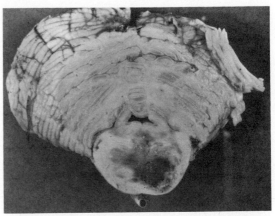

Figure 15–13 Paramedian syndromes of the upper pontine. This 64-year-old patient had repeated transient ischemic attacks within the distribution of the basilar artery involving predominantly left- or right-sided hemiplegia. Eventually thrombosis of the basilar artery occurred with hemorrhagic infarction involving the basilar pons (left half greater than right). The details of this patient's course are presented in Case History 8, p. 365. (Courtesy of Dr. John Hills, New England Center Hospitals; and Dr. Jose Segarra, Boston Veterans Administration Hospital.)

See Filmstrip, Frame 32.

drome. If one considers all cases of a pure motor vascular syndrome involving the face, arm, and leg contralaterally, it is found that such pontine infarcts are not the most frequent cause (Fisher and Curry, 1965). The most frequent site of infarction is the posterior limb of the internal capsule.

It is, moreover, important to realize, as demonstrated in Figures 15–12 and 15–13, that disease of the basilar artery often produces a bilateral paramedian syndrome with a bilateral infarction of the basilar pons.

Midbrain Syndromes

Paramedian Syndrome (Weber's Syndrome) (Fig. 15–14). Infarction in the territory supplied by paramedian-penetrating branches from the posterior cerebral artery involves the cerebral peduncle, the ipsilateral third nerve fibers, and, to a variable degree, the substantia nigra. The resultant clinical syndrome is that associated with the name of Weber: contralateral upper motor neuron paralysis of the face, arm, and leg, in association with an ipsilateral paralysis of third nerve function (Fig. 15–14). The clinical effects of the damage to the substantia nigra are usually not apparent. (Refer to Chapter 24.)

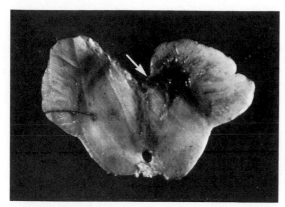

Figure 15-14 Weber's syndrome. An area of infarction is noted in the right cerebral peduncle (arrow), so located as to involve the fibers of the right third cranial nerve. This 61-year-old patient with rheumatic heart disease, endocarditis, and auricular fibrillation had the sudden onset of a paralysis of the left face, arm, and leg, plus a partial right third nerve palsy (among other neurological findings). (Courtesy of Dr. John Hills, New England Center Hospitals; and Dr. Jose Segarra, Boston Veterans Administration Hospital.)

See Filmstrip, Frame 33.

Case History 7. NECH #75-47-35-2. Date of admission: 3/5/70.

This 57-year-old white housewife (Mrs. S.L.) on the day prior to admission suddenly developed double vision and drooping of the right eyelid. In addition, the patient had difficulty walking. Examination of the patient in the emergency room revealed weakness of adduction of the right eye, ptosis of the right eyelid, and a left extensor plantar response. The patient was admitted to the neurology service.

PAST HISTORY:

1. Moderate hypertension had been present for many years.

2. The patient had had previous episodes suggesting cerebral vascular ischemia since 1966. These consisted initially of sudden 30-minute episodes of right-handed weakness and dysarthria. In January 1968, she had a 15- to 20-minute episode of bilateral blurred vision, unsteadiness of gait, and tingling paresthesias of the right hand and face. In May 1968, she had episodes of paresthesias, at times involving the left leg and arm; the following day the right arm and leg were at times affected. On examination in 1968, deep tendon reflexes were noted to have increased on the right side and

plantar responses were flexor. In September 1968 10-minute episodes of numbness of the left hand and face occurred as well as renewed numbness of the right hand. Examination again revealed minor right-sided findings. The patient was then free of episodes until she again experienced an episode of right-handed weakness 3 days prior to admission.

3. The patient had been receiving anticoagulant therapy (Coumadin) for phlebitis for several months prior to admission.

PHYSICAL EXAMINATION:

1. Blood pressure was 160/100.

2. The patient was obese and anxious.

NEUROLOGICAL EXAMINATION:

1. *Mental status:*
   a. The patient was alert and oriented.
   b. Recent memory was poor and delayed recall was limited to 2-out-of-4 objects. Similar findings were noted in September 1968.

2. *Cranial nerves:*
   a. Ptosis of the right eyelid was present.
   b. At rest, the right eye was deviated out to the right and down. There was no medial or upward movement of the right eye. (Note change from September 1968.)
   c. Pupillary responses were intact.
   d. A minor left central supranuclear facial weakness was present. (Note change from September 1968.)

3. *Motor system:* Strength was intact.

4. *Reflexes:*
   a. Deep tendon reflexes were now increased in the left lower extremity compared to the right. (Note change from September 1968.)
   b. There was now a left Babinski response and the abdominal reflex was absent on the left. (Note change from September 1968.)

5. *Sensation:* All modalities were intact.

6. *Carotid pulses:* Were strong bilaterally.

LABORATORY DATA:

1. Skull x-rays revealed calcifications in the cavernous portions of the carotid arteries.

2. The electroencephalogram revealed multifocal slow waves, right frontal central and temporal, left central and temporal, suggesting a mild multifocal damage.

3. Electrocardiogram was normal.

4. Blood counts, serology, and blood sugars and cholesterol were normal.

5. Lumbar puncture and arteriography were refused by the patient.

6. Prothrombin time was 68 per cent of normal, not actually within the therapeutic range for anticoagulation.

HOSPITAL COURSE:

The patient had a gradual clearing of the third nerve findings. At the time of discharge, 8 days following admission, she could move her eye fully in all directions with minimal diplopia on extremes of left lateral gaze.

COMMENT:

This patient had experienced multiple transient ischemic attacks. Many of these, including the present episode, were within the basilar vertebral distribution. Several episodes in which symptoms were limited to the hand and face suggested carotid disease as well. The actual state of the large vessels of the cerebral circulation could not be ascertained in this case.

As regards the episode of the present illness, the major symptoms involving the levator palpebrae and the medial and superior rectus muscles related to the partial involvement of the right third nerve. One of course could argue that the partial involvement reflected ischemia of the nucleus of the third nerve rather than the third nerve fibers. The third nerve fibers in passing through the brain stem fan out so that a small lesion could produce partial involvement. This patient, moreover, did not present the picture of a complete Weber's syndrome with a contralateral hemiplegia involving the face, arm, and leg. She did, however, present a contralateral supranuclear-type of facial weakness and a left Babinski response which were not present at the time of the evaluation in 1968. The fact that there was facial weakness without weakness of the arm and leg may relate to the relatively more medial location of direct corticobulbar fibers in the cerebral peduncle, compared to the adjacent corticospinal tracts.

The uncertainties in the evaluation of therapy for cerebrovascular disease could be well illustrated by this case. Thus, despite multiple transient ischemic attacks involving the basilar vertebral circulation the patient had little residual deficits 4 years after onset of symptoms. The basic difficulty may well have been in the extracranial portion of the vertebral artery, as in the cases described by Fisher (1970) rather than in the basilar artery *per se*. Moreover, despite frequent attacks in 1968, the patient then experienced a 2-year period free of attacks. Had anticoagulation been employed in 1966, the improvement might well have been attributed to this therapy. The eventual outcome of transient ischemic attacks is, of course, not always so benign. In particular, when these attacks involve the carotid artery distribution, infarction with residual neurological disability is a frequent eventual outcome.

Associated Tegmental Involvement (Benedikt's Syndrome). Involvement of the adjacent midbrain tegmentum (red nucleus, dentatorubralthalamic fibers) will produce a contralateral tremor and movement disorders in association with an ipsilateral third nerve lesion. There may be involvement of the cerebral peduncle as well, producing a contralateral hemiparesis.

Paramedian Periventricular Mesencephalicdiencephalic Junction. This involves the periaqueductal, pretectal, posterior-medial thalamic, and subthalamic areas. Infarction of this territory supplied by the penetrating branches of the proximal posterior cerebral arteries results in a drowsy, relatively immobile state (apathetic akinetic mutism) from which the patient can be roused with strong stimulation. The lesion interrupts the ascending reticular system fibers to the thalamus and subthalamus. Third cranial nerve findings are often present as associated findings, due to involvement of the third nerve nuclei. This syndrome has been recently considered in greater detail by Segarra (1970). (Refer to Chapter 26.)

Combined Syndrome: Thrombosis of the Basilar Artery. The following case history illustrates a case of thrombosis of the basilar artery in which several midbrain and pontine syndromes previously discussed were combined.

Case History 8. BVAH 069317, A64–416, (NECH NP 65–16).
Date of admission: 11/27/64.

This 64-year-old, white, right-handed, male house painter (Mr. W.A.) had been admitted on November 20, 1964, to his local community hospital with paralysis and numbness of the left arm and leg of several hours duration. Onset of symptoms had been relatively acute. The patient was noted to be slightly confused and unable to speak clearly (dysarthric). These symptoms apparently improved; but approximately 7 days later, the patient had an onset of weakness of the right arm and leg accompanied by increased difficulty in speech, necessitating his transfer to the neurological service of the hospital.

His past history was significant. Beginning in May 1964 the patient had experienced a series of 15 to 20 attacks of unsteadiness of gait, attributed to transient weakness of the right or left side of the body (predominantly the left side) and associated with vertigo and occasional tinnitus ("motor sounds") of the left ear. Initially, the vertigo was precipitated by head turning. Six months prior to admission, because of a sensation of dizziness when climbing his ladder, the patient had been forced to stop his work.

High blood pressure had been present for at least 6 months. Weakness and cramps in the legs on walking, relieved by rest, had been present for 1 year (suggesting the intermittent claudication of peripheral vascular disease).

GENERAL PHYSICAL EXAMINATION:
1. Blood pressure was elevated to 200/90.
2. Pulses in the lower extremities were decreased or absent.

NEUROLOGICAL EXAMINATION:
1. *Mental Status:* Although speech was severely dysarthric (speech was hardly intelligible to observers), the patient was alert and cooperative. He was able to follow commands, and to identify objects. There was no evidence of left-right confusion.
2. *Cranial Nerves:*
   a. The left pupil was slightly longer than the right.
   b. A right lateral rectus weakness was present.
   c. Nystagmus was present on gaze to the left or right.
   d. Pain sensation was decreased about the right corner of the mouth. The right corneal response was decreased. Jaw jerk was hyperactive.
   e. There was a paralysis of the lower half of the face on the right side.
   f. Gag reflex was decreased; the patient was unable to swallow on command. The uvula did elevate on phonation.
   g. The tongue was midline, but lateral tongue movements were weak.
3. *Motor:*
   a. Strength was uniformly decreased in the right arm and leg, but intact on the left.
   b. Truncal ataxia was apparent in the sitting position.
   c. Ataxia was evident on the right in finger-to-nose and heel-to-shin tests. Interpretation of these findings was clouded by the presence of right-sided weakness.
4. *Reflexes:*
   a. Deep tendon reflexes were hyperactive throughout with clonus apparent at the quadriceps. As noted above, the jaw jerk was 3–4+.
   b. Plantar responses were extensor bilaterally (bilateral Babinski signs).
5. *Sensation:*
   a. Pain sensation was decreased in the left leg.
   b. Vibratory sensation was decreased in both lower extremities.
   c. Position sense was defective in the left toes.

LABORATORY DATA:
1. Blood and spinal fluid serology were normal.
2. Cerebrospinal fluid was under normal pressure, with no cells. The protein content, however, was increased to 120 mg./100 ml. (explanation never certain).
3. Skull x-rays were negative except for calcifications in the internal carotids adjacent to the sella.

HOSPITAL COURSE:
The patient's inability to swallow progressed so that by the third day in the hospital, it was necessary to make use of a nasogastric feeding tube. On the fifth day, a temperature elevation occurred, related to aspiration pneumonitis. Death occurred on December 4, 1964.

Postmortem examination of the brain revealed that the major supply of the basilar artery was derived from the left vertebral artery. The right vertebral artery was rudimentary. In the lower portion of the basilar artery, significant atherosclerosis and calcification was present with narrowing of the lumen. The lower midportion of the vessel was occluded by thrombus. The proximal (caudal) portion of the thrombus was older, fibrous, and well organized; the distal portion was more recent. This suggested distal propagation from the more proximal thrombus.

The pons was soft to palpation. Serial sections revealed a recent area of infarction (with swelling and some hemorrhagic component) involving the entire left cerebral peduncle at the level of the midbrain, extending in a massive manner into the basilar pontis on the left. The areas of softening extended into the left and right paramedian areas of the pontine tegmentum (Fig. 15–13). A similar but possibly older lesion was present involving the right cerebral peduncle and right basilar pons. On the right the infarct extended up to the capsule of the red nucleus, to the subthalamus nucleus, and into the posterior and lateral portions of the thalamus.

Old infarcts were also noted in the right lenticular nucleus and the head of the left caudate nucleus. In addition, the right occipital cortex demonstrated old infarction.

COMMENT:

The symptoms and signs in this case would appear to be well correlated with the findings at postmortem examination. Thus, the appearance of the basilar artery and of the brain stem suggests several events from a chronological standpoint.

The recent massive lesion in the left cerebral peduncle and basilar pons corresponded to the right hemiparesis and right central facial weakness. The previous episodes of primarily left-sided involvement of the arm and leg would correlate with the older infarcts on the right side of the brain stem. The bilateral involvement of the basilar pons and cerebral peduncles must have resulted in a pseudobulbar syndrome, as regards the hyperactive jaw jerk and the movements of the tongue and the pharynx (reflecting bilateral corticobulbar involvement). The bilateral hyperactivity of deep tendon reflexes and the bilateral extensor plantar responses reflected bilateral corticospinal tract damage. The infarction of the right paramedian area of the pontine tegmentum must presumably correlate with the right lateral rectus muscle weakness and with deficit in position sense in the left toes. At some point, the infarction must have extended sufficiently lateral in the right pontine tegmentum to have involved the descending portion of the spinal tract and nucleus of the right fifth cranial nerve in addition to the lateral spinothalamic tract (decreased pain sensation in the left foot).

HEMORRHAGE

Intrapontine Hemorrhage (Fig. 15–15). (Refer to Chapter 22 for a more complete discussion of this disease process.)

The most common location of hypertensive hemorrhages is intracerebral (putamen predominantly, thalamus and cerebral white matter somewhat less commonly). In a small percentage of cases, the pons is the primary location of the hemorrhage. A large hemorrhage in the relatively small space of the pons produces rapid effects: coma and bilateral involvement of the long tracts within seconds or minutes, death within minutes or hours. Rupture into the ventricular system is common.

Primary Intracerebellar Hemorrhages. These uncommon hemorrhages may involve the pons secondarily by compression or rupture into the ventricular system (p. 351).

SUBARACHNOID HEMORRHAGE

(Refer to extrinsic diseases of the brain stem and to diseases of the cerebral hemispheres.)

Figure 15–15 Pontine hemorrhage. This 58-year-old hypertensive (200/100) patient had had a presumed brain-stem infarct 4 weeks previously. Anticoagulant therapy was then complicated by this massive pontine hemorrhage. (Courtesy of Dr. John Hills, New England Center Hospitals.)
See Filmstrip, Frame 34.

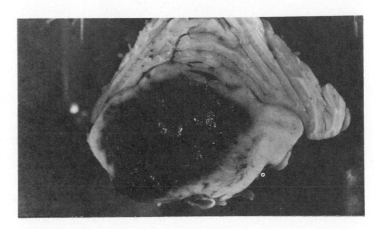

INTRINSIC TUMORS

The substance of the brain stem is a very uncommon site for metastatic tumors. Almost all tumors found within the substance of the brain stem are intrinsic, arising from glial elements, generally the astrocyte. Various histological grades of malignancy may be encountered. In contrast to gliomas of the cerebral hemisphere, the majority of which are of a very malignant variety (the glioblastomas), the majority of those involving the brain stem are astrocytomas with a lower grade of malignancy and with a longer course. The tumor slowly infiltrates the pons and medulla, producing a gross external enlargement of these structures (Fig. 15–16). On section, the distinctions between gray and white matter are obliterated. Areas of necrosis may be found within the tumor. The essential clinical syndrome is characterized by the progressive development of bilateral long tract and bilateral cranial nerve findings. The cranial nerve findings suggest involvement over adjacent segments of the brain stem, rather than a single segmental level. This tumor occurs primarily in children, adolescents, and young adults. A typical example is provided by the following case history.

Case History 9. NECH #139–821.
Date of admission: 7/2/62.

This 24-year-old white housewife and secretary (Mrs. J.W.) was referred for evaluation of progressive headache, diplopia, and left-sided weakness.

In March 1960 approximately 2 weeks after the delivery of her second child, the patient had an onset of diplopia with an apparent horizontal separation of images. Her family noted that the right eye was "turned in." The symptom was intermittent for a week, then persistent and static for approximately one year. In June 1961 one year prior to admission, the double vision worsened. Moreover, a weakness of the left leg, an unsteadiness of gait, and clumsiness of the left hand were now noted. These symptoms steadily progressed so that the patient fell in November 1961, sustaining a fracture of the left ankle. Skull x-rays and lumbar puncture at that time were normal and the diagnosis of multiple sclerosis was entertained. As the previous symptoms worsened, the patient in the 3 months prior to admission noted a progressive numbness of both sides of her face and of the oral cavity. She had lost all of her ability to taste food or even to tell where food was located in the mouth. She had experienced increasing difficulty in attempting to swallow food. Liquids such as coffee were frequently regurgitated into the nasopharynx on swallowing. Her speech had developed a nasal quality and hoarseness had been noted. A bilateral occipital headache had developed, at times precipitated by flexion of the neck. In recent days, the headache had been accompanied by vomiting.

GENERAL PHYSICAL EXAMINATION:
No remarkable features were present.
NEUROLOGICAL EXAMINATION:
1. *Mental status:*
    a. The patient was alert with intact memory and orientation.
    b. Although speech was slurred and the voice was low and hoarse, lan-

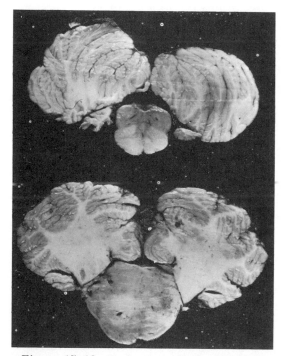

Figure 15–16 Brain stem glioma. Marked enlargement of the pons and medulla have occurred with obscuration of the usual anatomical landmarks. Note the size of pons and medulla relevant to cerebellum. This 8½-year-old patient had a month course of diplopia, ataxia, and dysarthria. Death occurred despite radiation therapy. (Courtesy of Dr. John Hills, New England Center Hospitals.)

See Filmstrip, Frame 35.

guage function *per se* was intact with no evidence of aphasia.

2. *Cranial nerves:*
   a. Bilateral papilledema was evident on examination of the fundus with marked blurring of disc margins, elevation of the discs, and retinal hemorrhages. Visual acuity was intact.
   b. Bilateral lateral rectus weakness was present, more marked on the right than on the left. Vertical nystagmus was present on upward gaze.
   c. Pain and touch sensation were decreased over all three divisions of the trigeminal nerve, more marked on the right than the left. Corneal reflexes were absent bilaterally.
   d. A mild right central (supranuclear) facial weakness was present.
   e. The uvula deviated to the left on attempted elevation. The gag reflex was decreased bilaterally. Speech was of low tone and slurred.
   f. A bilateral weakness of the sternocleidomastoid muscles was present. The upper half of the left trapezius was weak.
   g. The tongue deviated to the right on protrusion.

3. *Motor system:*
   a. Marked weakness accompanied by spasticity was noted in the left arm and leg.
   b. Gait was unsteady with a spastic quality evident in the movements of the left leg.
   c. Coordination was poor on the left side. Whether this reflected cerebellar deficits in addition to weakness was not certain.

4. *Reflexes:*
   a. Deep tendon reflexes were symmetrical and physiologic.
   b. Plantar responses were extensor on the left, flexor on the right.

5. *Sensation:*
   Except for the findings over the face, no deficits were present.

LABORATORY DATA:
1. Skull and chest x-rays were negative.
2. Electroencephalogram was normal.
3. Left brachial arteriogram indicated a probable low position of the posterior inferior cerebellar artery, suggesting the possibility of cerebellar tonsillar herniation. Basilar and vertebral arteries were in a normal position.
4. A pantopaque ventriculogram revealed an intrinsic pontine and medullary tumor. The fourth ventricle and aqueduct were midline but were displaced posteriorly. This study was performed by instilling a radio-opaque dye (pantopaque) into the ventricular system by means of a needle placed in the frontal horn.

HOSPITAL AND SUBSEQUENT COURSE:
A suboccipital craniotomy with removal of the lamina of C1 and C2 was performed by Dr. Samuel Brendler on July 3, 1962, with the aim of decompressing the cerebellum, brain stem, and cervical cord. The cerebellar hemispheres were found to be under marked tension. The medulla oblongata was markedly enlarged to twice the normal size, displacing the cerebellar hemispheres laterally. The upper cervical cord was also markedly enlarged. Although a firm yellow discolored mass could be visualized within the medulla, no definite delineation from the surrounding normal tissue could be made. No cyst was present within the tumor mass. The upward extent of the tumor could not be visualized because the suboccipital approach does not allow inspection of the pons.

Surgical decompression was followed by x-ray therapy (total of 4846 roentgens). An improvement in neurological status was subsequently noted. At the time of hospital discharge, 10 weeks after surgery, papilledema had disappeared. Corneal reflexes had returned. Gag reflex was now present and swallowing was intact. Sternocleidomastoid muscles and tongue were intact. Bilateral lateral rectus weakness and bilateral facial weakness were still present. There was still a slight bilateral decrease in pain sensation over the face. The patient was able to ambulate using a walker. Strength in the left upper extremity had improved.

Improvement continued to such an extent that the patient returned to her job as a secretary in April 1964 and walked to work each day. Her only residual symptoms were a minor degree of diplopia and a minor ataxia of gait.

Follow-up in October 1965 indicated an increased degree of diplopia and vertigo. Nystagmus of a rotary type was now present in all directions of gaze. Moderate weakness was present in the sternocleidomastoid muscles and fasciculations were noted bilaterally in the tongue.

In November 1965, the patient was readmitted to the hospital because of increasing ataxia, slurred speech, numbness of the right side of the face (pain and touch were now decreased over all three divisions of the trigeminal nerve), loss of taste, and decreased hearing in the right ear. In addition the gag reflex was decreased on the right. A greater degree of hoarseness was now evident and laryngoscopy demonstrated no movement of the right vocal cord. The sternocleidomastoid muscles were weak. Atrophy and fasciculation involving the right half of tongue was now evident. Intention tremor was now present. Pneumoencephalogram demonstrated an enlargement of the substance of the brain stem with posterior displacement of the fourth ventricle and narrowing of the pontine cistern. High voltage radiotherapy was started but had to be discontinued when symptoms progressed.

Follow-up evaluation in March 1966 demonstrated continued progression with additional neurological findings. Adduction and convergence of the right eye was now defective. A right peripheral facial weakness was now present. Marked intention tremor was present in the right upper extremity with a marked heel-to-shin ataxia in the right lower extremity.

Re-evaluation in May 1966 now indicated additional progression. A bilateral peripheral facial weakness was now present. Bilateral Babinski signs were present. In addition to the marked right-sided cerebellar findings previously noted, a significant involvement of the trunk and, to a lesser degree, of the left arm and leg was now apparent.

The patient was treated with steroid therapy (Decadron) and with an experimental chemotherapeutic drug, 8-azaguanine. The latter agent was administered by continuous irrigation from the lateral ventricle to the lumbar subarachnoid space. This therapy was discontinued when infection of the meninges developed (meningitis). Although this complication responded promptly to antibiotic therapy, progression of the basic disease process continued at the time of hospital discharge in July 1966. There were now additional findings of atrophy of the muscles of the left upper extremity particularly in the deltoid. In addition, the hypalgesia on the right side of the face was now accompanied by a loss of pain sensation on the left side from the clavicle to the toes. The patient was unable to stand and unable to arise from bed. The patient was transferred to a chronic disease hospital where death occurred on September 3, 1966.

COMMENT:

The course of events in this case over a 6-year period clearly indicates the progressive involvement of cranial nerves and long fiber systems over a wide extent of the brain stem. In the later stages, the cervical spinal cord was involved as well. The initial diplopia was related to involvement of the right sixth nerve. The long duration of this finding, its unilateral nature, the fact that headache and other symptoms and signs of increased intracranial pressure were absent (despite examinations by competent ophthalmologists and neurologists) all suggested that this was not the nonspecific effect of increased intracranial pressure. (Thus a patient with the symptoms and signs of increased intracranial pressure may present a bilateral sixth nerve palsy.)

With the subsequent development one year later of left-sided cerebellar findings, involvement of both sides of the brain stem was suggested, a somewhat unusual combination for a focal extrinsic compressive lesion. The subsequent development 3 months prior to admission of bilateral fifth nerve symptoms more clearly suggested a bilateral intrinsic lesion involving the pons. The difficulties in swallowing and the hoarseness in speech suggested involvement of the nucleus ambiguus or the vagus nerve at a medullary level. The loss of all sense of taste may have indicated bilateral involvement of the tractus solitarius or, less likely, of the various entering fibers passing via the facial and glossopharyngeal nerves. At later stages, the motor neurons or associated fibers at a medullary level supplying the tongue and sternocleidomastoid muscles were involved as indicated by the significant atrophy and fasciculations present in these muscles.

In very late stages, defects in adduction and convergence of the right eye suggested spread to a midbrain level. The atrophy of muscles in the left upper extremity suggested spread to a spinal cord level.

Increased intracranial pressure (with headache, vomiting, papilledema) was certainly present at the time of hospital admission in 1962; but this was certainly not an early finding. Thus diplopia was present for 2 years without evidence of an increase in pressure. This is the usual situation in intrinsic tumors of the brain stem—increased intracranial pressure is absent in early stages. In contrast, extrinsic tumors involving the brain stem usually manifest increased intracranial pressure early in their course.

Having concluded that an intrinsic lesion is present, the identification of the type of pathology as glioma should be evident when one considers the differential diagnoses. Thus, vascular disease, multiple sclerosis, amyotrophic lateral sclerosis and syringobulbia represent other intrinsic diseases of the brain stem.

Vascular disease would be unlikely in view of the gradual but progressive nature of the problem and the age of the patient. Multiple sclerosis would be unlikely since both neurons and long tracts were involved. Moreover, the symptoms were limited to the brain stem (although certainly involving several rostral-caudal segments of the brain stem). The progressive nature of the problem without definite remissions is also to some extent against the diagnosis of multiple sclerosis. The diagnosis of a bulbar form of amyotrophic lateral sclerosis would be unlikely in view of the early age of onset of symptoms, the presence of sensory signs and symptoms, the presence of cerebellar symptomatology, and to some extent the asymmetrical nature of the motor neuron and long motor tract involvement. Syringobulbia is also unlikely. This is a relatively rare disease. The brain stem involvement is often associated with a relatively typical syndrome of syringomyelia. The involvement of the brain tends to be localized to several wedge or slit type areas extending in from the fourth ventricle at a medullary level.

As regards treatment of brain stem gliomas, the general principles are similar to those considered for intrinsic tumors of the spinal cord. There is no surgical cure. Surgery often confirms the diagnosis and eliminates the possibility of extrinsic tumor. In addition, surgical decompression provides greater room for expansion of the brain stem. At times, when the tumor has produced obstruction of the fourth ventricle or aqueduct, the use of a bypass shunt will produce a considerable reduction in those symptoms related to an increase in intracranial pressure. The tumor often has a significant response to radiation with the production of a temporary remission as in the present case.

DEMYELINATING DISEASES

A general discussion of demyelinating diseases will be found in Chapter 8, Clinical Consideration of the Spinal Cord. The student should also refer to the specific illustrative case history. (Spinal cord case history 15; p. 202). That case of multiple sclerosis presented, in addition to lesions involving the spinal cord, several episodes suggesting discrete lesions at various levels of the brain stem.

Multiple sclerosis, the most common type of demyelinating disease, frequently involves the brain stem and cerebellum (Figs. 15-17 and 15-18). The classic triad of Charcot includes: nystagmus, intention tremor, and scanning speech—symptoms which are often present in the later stages, but which may be absent early in the disease course.

The following example illustrates a case of multiple sclerosis with predominant involvement of brain stem.

Case History 10. NECH #148–402. Date of admission: 4/29/62.

This 25-year-old, white, married, male mechanic (Mr. J.De.) was admitted with a chief complaint of diplopia of three weeks duration. Four weeks prior to admission the patient had noted the gradual onset of persistent tingling paresthesias of all fingers of the left hand. Three weeks prior to admission he had the gradual onset of a diplopia with a diagonal separation of images. Four days prior to admission paresthesias of the upper and lower lip on the left side were noted; these gradually spread within one day to the left half of the face and tongue.

During the three weeks prior to admission, occasional episodes of weakness of both legs had been noted.

NEUROLOGICAL EXAMINATION:
1. *Mental status:* All areas were intact.
2. *Cranial nerves:*
   a. A scotoma was present in the superior field of the left eye.
   b. Weakness of the left medial rectus was present both on conjugate lateral gaze to the right and on convergence. A coarse horizontal nystagmus was

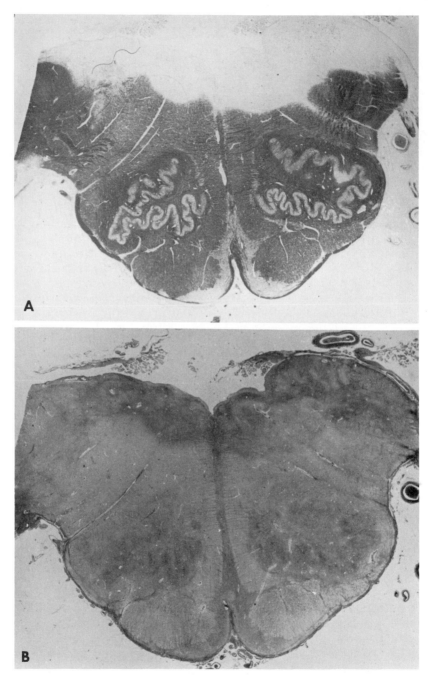

Figure 15–17 Multiple sclerosis affecting the brain stem.

A, Multiple irregular areas of myelin loss are evident in this myelin stain of the medulla from a 58-year-old male who expired after a long history of progressive multiple sclerosis. A spinal cord lesion from this same case is demonstrated in Figure 8–26*A*, p. 201.

B, Holzer stain for glial fibers of the same section demonstrates darkly staining areas of gliosis corresponding to the areas of old demyelination. (Courtesy of Dr. Jose Segarra, Boston Veterans Administration Hospital.)

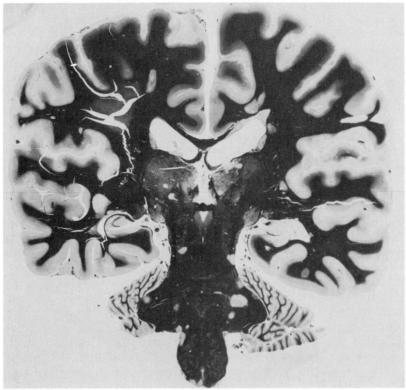

Figure 15–18 Multiple sclerosis. Multiple areas of demyelination in the white matter of brain stem and cerebral hemispheres are demonstrated in this myelin stain. (Courtesy of Dr. Harry Zimmerman, Montifiore Hospital.)

present on lateral gaze to the right or left (more marked on gaze to the right). The nystagmus was, however, dissociated in that there was a greater degree present in the abducting eye. Vertical nystagmus was present on upward gaze.

   c. A mild left central type facial weakness was present.

3. *Motor system:*

   a. No weakness, atrophy, or abnormal movements were present.

   b. Resistance to passive motion was normal.

   c. Gait was normal.

   d. Cerebellar tests were negative.

4. *Reflexes*

   a. There was a slight increase in deep tendon reflexes on the left compared to the right.

   b. Plantar response was possibly extensor on the right and definitely extensor on the left.

5. *Sensation:* All modalities were intact.

LABORATORY DATA:

1. X-rays of skull and cervical spine were normal.

2. Cerebrospinal fluid was normal with protein of 47 mg./100 ml. and 2 lymphocytes per cu. mm.

3. Complete blood count and sedimentation rate were normal.

SUBSEQUENT COURSE:

Patient was discharged on May 3, 1962. The diplopia became more marked. Two weeks later on May 17, 1962 he noted difficulty in walking. No actual weakness was noted but he felt unsteady as if the floor were moving. On May 21, 1962 a thickness of speech was noted. The patient was then readmitted to the hospital on May 25, 1962. Neurological examination now demonstrated, in addition to the previously noted findings, a wide-based, slow, mildly ataxic gait and a minor slurring of speech. A bilateral side-to-side tremor was present on finger-to-nose test, being slightly greater on the left than on the right. Rapid alternating movements were disorganized bilaterally, to a greater extent on the left than on the right. The crossed diplopia was now more marked and present on either right or left lateral gaze. Nystagmus was still greater in the abducting eye on horizontal gaze to the right or left. Vertical nystagmus was also present. Cerebrospinal fluid examination now revealed a total protein of 56 mg./100 ml. but the gamma globulin of 3.0 mg./100 ml. constituted only 5.2 per cent of the total. The colloidal gold curve was now slightly elevated at 1122211000.

The patient was begun on high dosage steroid treatment (80 mg. of prednisone per day). Over a two-and-a-half-week hospital course, the patient had a significant improvement as regards diplopia, ataxia of gait, and intention tremor. This improvement may have related to the steroid therapy.

COMMENT:

The diagnosis of multiple sclerosis is based on evidence in the history and in the examination of lesions disseminated in time and space. There was then little question of the diagnosis in this case. At the time of initial hospital admission, the patient had evidence of a left optic nerve lesion (scotoma) and of one or more brain stem lesions. The dissociated nystagmus, greater in the abducting eye, on right or left lateral gaze, suggested a bilateral lesion of the medial longitudinal fasciculus. Multiple sclerosis is the most common cause of such a bilateral lesion. (Vascular disease with infarction may produce either a unilateral or bilateral type of internuclear ophthalmoplegia. A pontine glioma may also produce this syndrome.) The defect in medial rectus movement, which was present also on convergence, may have reflected a minor involvement of the third nerve fibers in their passage through the substance of the midbrain.

At the time of the patient's second hospital admission, ataxia, intention tremor, and dysarthria were present in addition to the previously noted symptoms.

There is no specific therapy for multiple sclerosis. In some acute cases, particularly with involvement of the optic nerve or optic chiasm, a significant improvement may follow the use of high doses of adrenocortical steroids (or their synthetic analogues). Before concluding that the remission which occurred was directly related to therapy, the student should review the previously presented spinal cord case (p. 202) in which similar remission occurred without benefit of such therapy.

DEGENERATIVE DISEASES

Focal Disease: Syringobulbia. We have already studied the effects produced by the paracentral canal cavity of a syrinx at a spinal cord level. A similar defect may appear in the medulla as an irregular wedge or cavity. When one considers that the fourth ventricle represents an opening up of the central canal, then the usual location of the cavity as a wedge extending anteriorly and laterally between the motor and sensory nuclei in the floor of this ventricle is quite understandable. In this location, the nucleus ambiguus, nucleus and tractus solitarius, vestibular nuclei, and the descending tract and nucleus of the trigeminal nerve are likely to be involved. At a midmedullary level, the internal arcuate fibers from the nuclei gracilis and cuneatus are likely to be damaged. At a low medullary level, the decussating pyramidal fibers may be damaged as they shift from a ventral medullary to a lateral column location. The cavity is, however, often irregular; at times extending across the midline, at times extending into the spinal cord. At times an independent cavity may be present, between the medullary pyramid and inferior olive, producing damage to the pyramidal tract and hypoglossal nerve fibers.

In addition to the clinical manifestations previously discussed for syringomyelia, the patient would demonstrate loss of pain and temperature sensation over one side of the face, nystagmus, vertigo, hoarseness, and dysarthria. Damage to the nucleus ambiguus may interfere with the coordinated movements of the larynx and epiglottis during respiration so that respiration is noisy and difficult (respiratory or laryngeal stridor). Atrophy of the tongue and of muscles supplied by the accessory nerve may also be noted in addition to pyramidal tract findings.

System Diseases. These diseases are discussed and illustrated in other chapters.

Amyotrophic Lateral Sclerosis. (Refer to p. 187). This disease produces symptoms and signs referrable to the brain stem in two ways: degeneration of brain stem motor neurons (bulbar palsy), and degeneration of corticobulbar fibers—in part secondary to a loss of giant pyramidal cells in the motor cortex. Brain stem symptoms may be the early and predominant manifestations or may appear as a late manifestation in cases characterized in their early stages by predominant involvement of the anterior horn cells of the spinal cord or involvement of the lateral column.

The duration of the disease is essentially determined by the degree of involvement of the bulbar motor neurons.

The illustrative case history provided in

the spinal cord chapter (Case History 11, p. 187) indicates also the nature of the brain stem involvement. There were clearly lower motor neuron findings relevant to the cranial nerves: bilateral peripheral facial weakness, poor elevation of the uvula, hoarseness of speech, and atrophy of the tongue. There was also evidence of bilateral corticobulbar involvement with a hyperactive jaw jerk. In some cases, the pseudobulbar syndrome resulting from bilateral involvement of the corticobulbar tracts may be more prominent.

Poliomyelitis: (Refer to pp. 185 and 589). This virus produces its major effects by invasion of motor neurons. The bulbar motor neurons may be selectively implicated, but more often they are involved in addition to the anterior horn cells of the spinal cord. As already indicated, the bulbar involvement with paralysis of the pharyngeal muscles and impairment of the respiratory centers leads to many of the complications of the disease.

Spinocerebellar Degenerations. Several of the relatively rare variants of cerebellar degeneration also involve pontine or midbrain nuclei or fiber systems: olivopontocerebellar or dentatorubral degeneration. (Refer to Chapter 22 p. 632.)

References

Adams, R. D., and Sidmar, R. L.: *Introduction to Neuropathology.* New York, McGraw Hill, 1968.

Carpenter, M. B., McMasters, R. E., and Hanna, O. R.: Disturbances of conjugate horizontal eye movement in the monkey: I. Physiological effects and anatomical degeneration resulting from lesion of the abducens nucleus and nerve. Arch. Neurol., 8:231–247, 1963.

Cogan, D. G.: *Neurology of the Ocular Muscles,* 2nd Edition. Springfield, Ill., Charles C Thomas, 1956.

Cogan, D. G., and Wray, S. H.: Internuclear ophthalmoplegia as an early sign of brain stem tumors. Neurology, 20:629–633, 1970.

Fazekas, J. F., Alman, R. W., and Sullivan, J. F.: Vertebral basilar insufficiency. Arch. Neurol., 8:215–220, 1963.

Fisher, C. M.: Occlusion of the vertebral arteries causing transient basilar symptoms. Arch. Neurol., 22:13–19, 1970.

Fisher, C. M., and Curry, H. B.: Pure motor hemiplegia of vascular origin. Arch. Neurol., 13:30–44, 1965.

Fisher, C. M., Gore, I., Okabe, N., and White, P. D.: Atherosclerosis of the carotid and vertebral arteries— extracranial and intracranial. J. Neuropath. exp. Neurol., 24:455–476, 1965.

Fisher, C. M., Karnes, W. E., and Kubik, C. S.: Lateral medullary infarction—The pattern of vascular occlusion. J. Neuropath. exp. Neurol., 20:323–379, 1961.

Ford, F. R.: *Diseases of the Nervous System in Infancy, Childhood and Adolescence,* 5th Edition. Springfield, Ill., Charles C Thomas, 1966. Chapter VI, Neoplasms and Related Conditions Involving the Nervous System, pp. 890–1028.

Goebel, H. H., Komatsuzaki, A., Bender, M. B., and Cohen, B.: Lesions of the pontine tegmentum and conjugate gaze paralysis. Arch. Neurol., 24:431–440, 1971.

Harrington, R. B., Hollenhorst, R. W., and Sayre, G. P.: Unilateral internuclear ophthalmoplegia. Arch. Neurol., 15:29–34, 1966.

Hatcher, M. A., and Klintworth, G. K.: The sylvian aqueduct syndrome. Arch. Neurol., 15:215–224, 1966.

Haymaker, W.: *Bing's Local Diagnosis in Neurological Disease,* 15th Edition. St. Louis, C. V. Mosby, 1969.

Ingraham, F., and Matson, D.: *Neurosurgery of Infancy and Childhood.* Springfield, Ill., Charles C Thomas, 1954. Part IV, Intracranial Tumors, pp. 221–340.

Ingvar, D. H., and Sourander, P.: Destruction of the reticular core of the brain stem. Arch. Neurol., 23: 1–8, 1970.

Kemper, T. L., and Romanul, F. C. A.: State resembling akinetic mutism in basilar artery thrombosis. Neurology, 17:74–80, 1967.

Kubik, C. S., and Adams, R. D.: Occlusion of the basilar artery—clinical and pathological study. Brain, 69:6–121, 1946.

Merritt, H. H.: *A Textbook of Neurology,* 4th Edition. Philadelphia, Lea and Febiger, 1967.

Olszewski, J., and Baxter, D.: *Cytoarchitecture of the Human Brain Stem.* Basel, Karger, 1954.

Pasik P., Pasik, T., and Bender, M. B.: The pretectal syndrome in monkeys. I: Disturbances of gaze and body posture. Brain, 92:521–534, 1969.

Pasik, T., Pasik, P., and Bender, M. B.: The pretectal syndrome in monkeys. II: Spontaneous and induced nystagmus and lightning eye movements. Brain, 92:871–884, 1969.

Plum, F., and Posner, T. B.: *The Diagnosis of Stupor and Coma.* Philadelphia, F. A. Davis, 1966.

Pool, J. L., and Pava, A.: *Early Diagnosis and Treatment of Acoustic Nerve Tumors.* Springfield, Ill., Charles C Thomas, 1957.

Ross, A. T., and DeMyer, W. E.: Isolated syndrome of the medial longitudinal fasciculus in man. Arch. Neurol., 15:203–205, 1966.

Segarra, J. M.: Cerebral vascular disease and behavior: I. The syndrome of the mesencephalic artery (basilar artery bifurcation). Arch. Neurol., 22:408–419, 1970.

Truex, R. C., and Carpenter, M. B.: *Human Neuroanatomy,* 5th Edition. Baltimore, Williams and Wilkins, 1964.

Wilkins, R. H., and Brody, I. A.: Neurological classics XII: Horner's syndrome. Arch. Neurol., 19:540–542, 1968.

Wilkins, R. H., and Brody, I. A.: Neurological classics XXX: Wallenberg's syndrome. Arch. Neurol., 22: 379–382, 1970.

Williams, D., and Wilson, J. G.: The diagnosis of the major and minor syndromes of basilar insufficiency. Brain, 85:741, 1962.

Appendix to Chapter 15

ELLIOTT M. MARCUS

QUESTIONS AND CASE HISTORIES FOR PROBLEM SOLVING

For each of the following diagrams indicate the structures involved by the cross-hatched lesion(s). For each structure involved indicate the expected clinical effects. Be certain to indicate the appropriate lateralization, i.e., left or right (ipsilateral or contralateral). Where appropriate, indicate the vascular territory involved.

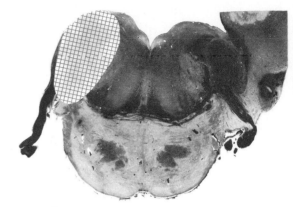

R *Figure 15A–1.* L

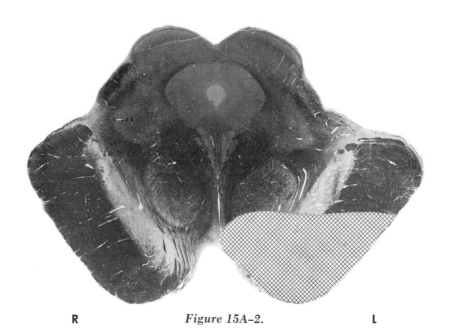

R *Figure 15A–2.* L

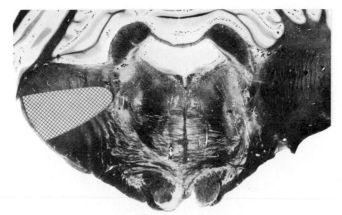

R   *Figure 15A–3.*   L

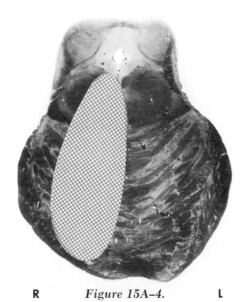

R   *Figure 15A–4.*   L

R   *Figure 15A–5*   L

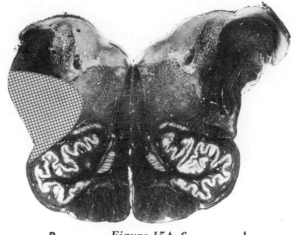

R   *Figure 15A–6*   L

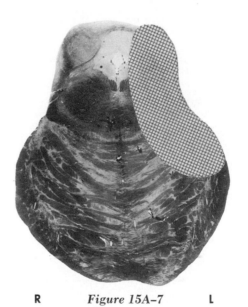

R   *Figure 15A–7*   L

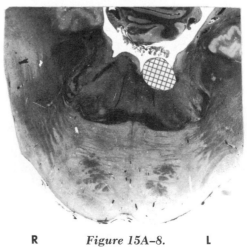

R   *Figure 15A–8.*   L

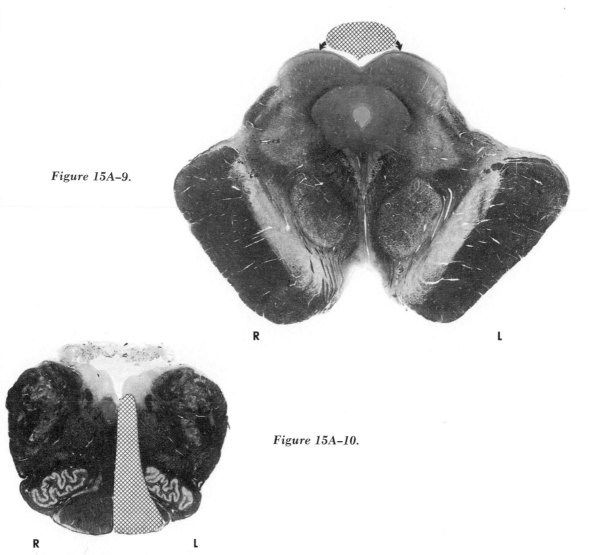

Figure 15A–9.

R   L

Figure 15A–10.

R   L

PROBLEM SOLVING: CASE HISTORIES

Each of the following case histories deals with disease at the level of the brain stem. In some cases, it will be evident that the disease process involves the spinal cord as well as the brain stem. Some of the cases deal with intrinsic disease, some with extrinsic disease. For each case indicate and diagram the location of the lesion and indicate the nature of the pathological process.

Case History 1A.   NECH #176–136. Date of admission: 7/3/66.

This 57-year-old, white, male sales manager (Mr. S.J.) had an onset of difficulty in walking and progressive weakness in the legs in January 1965. He had fallen in the snow and had difficulty standing up. Shortly there-

after, he noted weakness of the right arm and leg and, some time thereafter, weakness of the left arm and leg. In November 1965, he had to stop work because of progressive weakness involving the arms and legs. In addition, he had difficulty in chewing and swallowing food. Increased difficulty in swallowing was noted as was hoarseness in talking. The patient had noted no numbness or pain during the course of the disease.

Neurological Examination:
1. *Mental status:* Intact
2. *Cranial nerves:*
   a. Extraocular movements were intact.
   b. Masseter and pterygoid muscles were weak with significant atrophy.
   c. Sensation over the face was intact. Bilateral facial weakness of central type was present.
   d. Sensation in pharynx was intact but

only a minimal gag occurred on stimulation.

   e. Tongue movement was weak to left or right. Fasciculations were present.

   f. Severe weakness and atrophy of the sternocleidomastoid and trapezius muscles were present.

3. *Motor system:*

   a. There was marked weakness and atrophy in all muscle groups of the extremities and trunk—left leg greater than right leg, proximal greater than distal.

   b. Widespread fasciculations were present at rest, e.g., deltoids, biceps, small hand muscles, quadriceps.

   c. Gait: The patient was bedridden and unable to sit up or to stand.

   d. Tone: No definite resistance was present on passive motion.

   e. Coordination: No tremor.

4. *Reflexes:*

   a. Deep tendon reflexes:
     Biceps: right, 2+; left, 1+
     Triceps: right, 2+; left, 2+
     Quadriceps: right, 3+; left, 2+
     Achilles: right, 0-1+; left, 0

   b. Superficial reflexes:
     Plantar response: right, ↑; left, ?
     Abdominal: right, 0; left, 0
     Cremasteric: right, 0; left, 0

5. *Sensation:* Pain, position, touch, and vibration were all intact.

QUESTIONS:

1. Can this disease be localized to a particular level of the nervous system, or is the basic problem that of a system pathology? Indicate level or system.

2. Why are the bilateral Babinski signs present?

3. What is the localizing significance of the weakness and atrophy involving the masseter and pterygoid muscles? What is the significance of the atrophy in the trapezius and sternocleidomastoid muscles?

4. What is the localizing significance of the diffuse atrophy and fasciculations at rest involving the upper and lower extremities?

5. What is the significance of the fasciculations in the tongue?

6. Pharyngeal sensation was intact but the gag reflex was weak. Explain.

7. What would you expect a muscle biopsy to reveal?

Case History 2A. NECH #142–349.
Dates of admission: 7/3/61 and 9/19/61.
This 56-year-old white housewife (Mrs.

H.B.) was admitted for evaluation of episodes of stupor and cyanosis associated with severe laryngeal stridor (high pitched and harsh respiratory sounds) and stertorous breathing. Laryngeal stridor had been present for 20 years and had grown worse during the last 5 to 6 years. An episode of anoxia during a cesarean section 18 years prior to admission may have been a complication of this problem.

Sixteen years prior to admission numbness and weakness of the right leg had been noted. Progression had occurred in the last 2 years and episodic unsteadiness of gait had been noted. During this same period, weakness of the right hand had developed. During the one year prior to admission the patient had three hospital admissions related to episodes of coma and cyanosis. Each had followed a several-week period in which there was increased stridor and increased accumulation of tracheobronchial secretions with frequent periods of daytime sleepiness.

NEUROLOGICAL EXAMINATION:

1. *Mental status:* Intact.

2. *Cranial nerves:*

   a. Pain sensation was decreased over all three divisions of the right side of the face with decreased right corneal reflex.

   b. Laryngoscopy revealed paralysis with atrophy of the left vocal cord. The right cord moved but was inhibited on abduction, indicating partial paresis.

3. *Motor system:*

   a. Atrophy of the right upper extremity was present including the shoulder, arm, and hand.

   b. Weakness was present in the right upper extremity—approximately 50 per cent of normal strength at shoulder, elbow, wrist, and fingers. Weakness *without* atrophy was present in the right lower extremity and to a lesser degree in the left lower extremity.

   c. Spasticity was present on passive movement at the right knee and ankle and to a lesser degree at the left knee.

   d. Gait: There was circumduction of the right leg with unsteadiness on rapid turns.

   e. Cerebellar tests were otherwise negative except for horizontal nystagmus on lateral gaze and minimal vertical nystagmus on upward gaze.

4. *Reflexes:*
   a. Deep tendon:
      Biceps: right, 0; left, 0
      Triceps: right, 0; left, 0
      Radial: right, 0; left, 0
      Quadriceps: right, 4+; left, 3+
      Achilles: right, 4+; left, 3+
   b. Superficial reflexes:
      Plantar: extensor on the right and possibly extensor on the left
      Abdominal: right, 0; left, 0
5. *Sensation:*
   a. Position, vibration, and touch were intact.
   b. Pain and temperature were decreased in a cape-like distribution over the shoulders.

LABORATORY DATA:

1. Cerebrospinal fluid: normal (pressure 150, cell count 0, protein 45 mg./100 ml.)
2. Skull x-rays were negative.
3. Cervical spine x-rays revealed minor nonsignificant degenerative changes at C5–C7.

SUBSEQUENT COURSE:

The patient was readmitted to the hospital 10 weeks later in a semicomatose and cyanotic condition. She required a tracheostomy and 48 hours of respiratory assistance. Subsequent neurological examination was unchanged from that recorded earlier.

QUESTIONS:

1. Where is the lesion? Does this lesion involve a single localized segment or are several segments involved?
2. Is the pathology limited to the brain stem? To the spinal cord?
3. Indicate what structures are involved to produce:
   a. laryngeal paralysis,
   b. cape-like deficit in pain and temperature but sparing touch and vibration,
   c. atrophy of all muscle groups in right upper extremity,
   d. absence of deep tendon reflexes in both upper extremities, and
   e. defective pain sensation on the right side of the face.
4. Indicate the most likely pathology and the probable prognosis.
5. What diagnostic tests should be undertaken to establish the diagnosis?

Case History 3A. NECH #193–771. Date of admission: 4/68.
This right-handed, 43-year-old white housewife (Mrs. B.W.) had the onset of deafness in the right ear in June 1967. Rapid progression of deafness was noted; some tinnitus (sensation of ringing) was also noted. Caloric testing of labyrinthine function at that time indicated no response to cold or hot water on the right side. In July 1967, the onset of a minor unsteadiness of gait was noted. In December 1967 the patient noted defects in coordination of the right hand, particularly in typing, with a progression of unsteadiness of gait. At the same time a "numbness" sensation of pins-and-needles — "like novocaine given by a dentist" — was noted over the entire right side of the face. Relatively continuous pain was noted extending from the right side of the neck to the suboccipital area and right postauricular area. In January 1968 difficulty in swallowing solids and liquids was noted.

PAST HISTORY: Episodes of vertigo 5 to 6 years prior to admission. Right frontal headache since age 33.

NEUROLOGICAL EXAMINATION:

1. *Mental status:* Intact.
2. *Cranial nerves:*
   a. Pain and touch sensation were decreased over all 3 divisions of the trigeminal nerve on the right side, including the face, cornea, and the right side of the tongue.
   b. There was minimal flattening of the right nasolabial fold and a poorer degree of eye closure on the right side than the left (orbicularis oculi).
   c. There was no perception of voice in the right ear.
   d. No vestibular response was present to ice water caloric testing in the right ear.
   e. Minimal rotatory nystagmus was present on horizontal gaze with a minor degree of vertical nystagmus on upward gaze.
   f. A minimal degree of dysarthria was apparent as regards guttural sounds.
3. *Motor system:*
   a. Strength and tone were intact.
   b. Cerebellar tests revealed a slight clumsiness in fine finger movements of the right hand.
   c. Gait was slightly ataxic when performed on a narrow base with eyes open.
4. *Reflexes:*
   a. Deep tendon reflexes were symmetrical and physiologic.
   b. Plantar responses were flexor.
5. *Sensation:* All modalities were intact.

LABORATORY DATA:
Cerebrospinal fluid protein was slightly elevated to 50 mg./100 ml. Skull x-rays were negative.

HOSPITAL COURSE:
Following a diagnostic contrast study of the posterior fossa, a suboccipital craniotomy was performed.

QUESTIONS:
1. This patient presents a typical example of a classic neurological syndrome. Locate the lesion.
2. What is the most likely pathology to be found by the neurosurgeon in this location?
3. The initial involvement of the functions of cranial nerve VIII prior to involvement of other cranial nerves should provide a clue as to the structure from which this lesion arises.
4. Does the pattern of sensory disturbance over the right side of the face indicate primary involvement of the trigeminal nerve extrinsic to the brain stem or of the descending spinal tract and associated nucleus of the trigeminal nerve within the brain stem?
5. Were long sensory and motor tracts within the brain stem involved by this lesion?
6. Predict the clinical picture that would have occurred if the lesion had progressed.
7. During the course of surgery, aimed at total resection in these cases, the facial nerve must often be sacrificed or damaged. Based on your understanding of the anatomical considerations in these cases, indicate why this occurs.

Case History 4A. NECH #75–58–95.
Date of admission: 3/25/69.

This 66-year-old, retired, white male (Mr. E.T.), 10 days prior to admission, noted at his evening bath that he was unable to detect the temperature of water with his left foot and ankle. Several hours later he awoke from sleep to void and found that his balance was defective; he tended to fall over to the right side. He also had a strange sensation over his right ear and face.

The following morning, the patient noted numbness of the right side of the face, dysarthria, headache, nausea, and vomiting.

The patient was admitted to his local community hospital where skull x-rays and lumbar puncture were essentially normal. His symptoms had begun to clear at the time of his referral.

PAST HISTORY: Approximately 6 weeks prior to his admission the patient had developed mild symptoms of congestive heart failure and had begun appropriate treatment.

NEUROLOGICAL EXAMINATION:
1. *Mental status:* The patient was alert, well oriented with memory intact. Language functions and ability to do calculations were intact.
2. *Cranial nerves:*
   a. A partial Horner's syndrome was present on the right with ptosis of the eyelid and a slightly smaller pupil. Extraocular movements were intact.
   b. Nystagmus was present on lateral gaze and at times on forward gaze.
   c. Pain sensation was decreased over the entire right half of the face, and the corneal reflex was absent on the right half of the face.
   d. The uvula deviated to the left. The gag reflex was slower on the right. The voice was hoarse.
3. *Motor system:*
   a. Strength was intact.
   b. The patient was ataxic on a narrow base, tending to fall to the right.
   c. An intention tremor was present in the right upper extremity on finger-to-nose testing. A side-to-side tremor was apparent in the right lower extremity in heel-to-shin testing.
4. *Reflexes:*
   a. Deep tendon reflexes were physiological (2–3+) and symmetrical.
   b. Plantar responses were flexor.
5. *Sensation:*
   a. Pain sensation was decreased over the left lower extremity. (Examination shortly after onset of symptoms at his local hospital had demonstrated a decrease in pain sensation involving all of the left side of the body — below C2.)
   b. Position, vibration, and light touch were intact.

HOSPITAL COURSE:
By the time of hospital discharge on April 9, 1969 neurological symptoms and findings had almost completely disappeared.

QUESTIONS:
1. The findings in this case, when taken in combination, constitute a classic syndrome: (decreased pain sensation on the right side of the face and the left side of the body plus right-sided cerebellar findings plus right-

sided Horner's syndrome plus hoarseness plus nystagmus). Indicate the location of the lesion and the name of the syndrome.

2. Indicate the most likely etiology. If vascular, indicate the appropriate vessel.

Case History 5A. BFH #38797.
Date of admission: 7/60.

This 7-year-old white male (R.F.), in June 1960, was noted to turn his head to look at objects rather than looking directly at them. Over the next month, the patient, who was right-handed, began to use his left hand for activities. His gait became clumsy and ataxic. In addition he tended to walk with a "stiff" right leg. The patient had begun to complain of headaches mainly in the morning on awakening. He was first examined in July 1960.

EXAMINATION:

1. *Mental status:* Intact.
2. *Cranial nerves:*
   a. Occasional coarse nystagmus was present on left lateral gaze.
   b. Left corneal reflex was decreased on the left.
3. *Motor system:*
   a. Mild weakness of the right arm and leg.
   b. Tests of cerebellar function demonstrated impairment of fine movements and of alternating movements of the right arm (dysdiadochokinesis). Ataxia was present on heel-to-shin test on the right.
4. *Reflexes:*
   a. Deep tendon reflexes were increased on the right in the arm and leg with unsustained clonus at the right ankle.
   b. Plantar responses were bilaterally extensor (sign of Babinski).
5. *Sensation:* Intact.

SUBSEQUENT COURSE:

In August 1960 difficulty in swallowing was noted with nasal regurgitation. Diplopia was reported.

NEUROLOGICAL EXAMINATION:

1. *Cranial nerves:*
   a. Decreased pain sensation involving all three divisions of the left side of the face.
   b. Weakness of the left lateral rectus.
   c. On the left there was weakness in wrinkling the forehead with wider palpebral fissure and flattening of the nasolabial fold. On the right there was flattening of the right nasolabial fold. All other findings were as noted

above. Some improvement occurred following radiation therapy.

Re-evaluation in January 1961, however, indicated progression with decreased pain sensation over the right ophthalmic and maxillary divisions. A sagging of the right soft palate was also present. The right hemiparesis was present, as previously, with right hyperreflexia, right ankle clonus, and bilateral extensor plantar responses.

In February 1961, in addition to the forementioned signs, a left lateral rectus palsy was present. Nystagmus was now present on lateral gaze to the right or left. Weakness of the right sternocleidomastoid muscle was now noted. Ataxia had now returned in the right upper extremity.

Re-evaluation in March 1961 indicated additional progression. A bilateral deficit in corneal sensation was present and the left lateral rectus weakness was more marked with coarse nystagmus on lateral gaze bilaterally. A bilateral facial weakness was present. The gag reflex was absent bilaterally. A bilateral weakness of the sternocleidomastoid muscles was present; the patient was unable to shrug the right shoulder and was unable to support the head. The tongue deviated slightly to the left with atrophy of the left half. Speech was slurred. No voluntary movement was present in the right arm and leg (which were spastic on passive motion). Deep tendon reflexes were now hyperactive bilaterally with bilateral Babinski signs. Improvement again occurred with radiation therapy.

However, re-evaluation in June 1961 indicated paralysis of conjugate gaze to the left. Vertical nystagmus was also present on upward gaze as well as horizontal nystagmus on lateral gaze to the right. A symmetrical weakness of jaw movement was also noted. Ataxia was now present in the left upper extremity. The tongue now deviated to the right. Minimal papilledema was noted.

Examination in July 1961 indicated that extraocular movements were limited to upward and downward gaze with no lateral gaze to either side possible. Weakness of facial muscles on the left progressed so that the patient was unable to close the left eye.

Death occurred on July 15, 1961 when the patient had increasing difficulty breathing.

QUESTIONS:

1. It is evident that this patient had a progressive disease affecting the brain stem. In view of the insidious onset, the age of the

patient, and the progressive course over a 1-year period, is the diagnosis of vascular disease of an occlusive or hemorrhagic variety likely?

2. Those diseases which affect primarily white matter in a selective manner, producing foci of myelin loss, are also unlikely for the same reasons, and, in view of another fact, does this disease selectively involve white matter or have neurons as well as long fiber systems been involved?

3. What is the most likely diagnosis in this case?

4. Are we dealing with a level disease or are the findings distributed over several levels in a rostral caudal extent? If over several levels, indicate the upper limit and lower limit.

5. At a given horizontal level is this lesion localized in the sense that a lateral medullary infarction is limited?

6. List the cranial nerves involved on the left, those involved on the right. List the long motor tracts, cerebellar and sensory fiber system involved on the left and right. For each listed, indicate the clinical effects.

7. Diagram the lesion.

8. Having answered these questions you should be able to decide whether this tumor was intrinsic to (infiltrating) or extrinsic to (compressing) the brain stem. The absence of papilledema until very late in the disease course should also be consistent with your answer.

9. What is suggested by the fact that early in the course of the disease the patient had to turn his head to look at objects?

10. The patient eventually had marked impairment of lateral eye movements. Moreover, conjugate lateral gaze to the left was paralyzed. Late in the course, there may well have been paralysis of conjugate lateral gaze to the right as well. Yet, even late in the course upward and downward gaze were preserved. Convergence was not recorded in the record but it would probably have been intact. Indicate why these findings are consistent from an anatomical standpoint.

Case History 6A. Boston V. A. H. A64–284. NECH NP #64–85.
Date of admission: 5/13/64.
This 61-year-old white male, manager of an apartment house, (Mr. W.E.R.) was admitted to the Boston Veterans Administration Hospital shortly after being found on the floor of his home with a left hemiplegia and difficulty with speech.

PAST HISTORY:
There was no previous history of neurological disease. There was a significant past history, however, of peripheral vascular disease with involvement of the left lower extremity. Amputation of the left fourth toe had been performed in April 1962 for this reason. The patient was also known to have had arteriosclerotic heart disease and had been taking digitalis since 1961 for congestive failure. There had been a chronic problem with excessive alcohol intake.

PHYSICAL EXAMINATION:
1. The patient, acutely ill, was confused, frothing at the mouth, and having difficulty in handling secretions. He had an obvious hemiplegia.

2. The heart rate was irregular at 76. There was evidence of atrial fibrillation.

3. No pulses could be felt at the posterior tibial or dorsal pedal points bilaterally, suggesting significant bilateral peripheral vascular disease.

NEUROLOGICAL EXAMINATION:
1. *Mental status:* Speech and evaluation of mental status were hampered by a severe dysarthria. Spoken words were barely intelligible and barely audible. The patient did appear confused and only seemed able to understand and respond to simple questions.

2. *Cranial nerves:*
   a. There was a question of a right homonymous hemianopsia.
   b. There was significant ptosis of the right eyelid. The right pupil appeared larger than the left. The right pupil measured 3 mm., the left 1.5 mm. There were full eye movements to the left. The left eye, however, could not adduct past the midline to the right. Cold water irrigation of the auditory canals failed to produce any significant movement of the eyes. Extraocular movements were often described as dysconjugate.
   c. Left corneal reflex was absent and sensation was diminished over the left face.
   d. There was a left supranuclear type of facial weakness.
   e. Gag reflex was diminished and there was difficulty swallowing.
   f. Tongue moved towards the left.

3. *Motor system:* There was a moderately severe left hemiparesis with increased tone

(spastic quality) of the left arm and leg. Spasticity was also present in the right upper extremity.

4. *Reflexes:*

   a. Deep tendon reflexes were hyperactive on the left.

   b. The left toe was clearly extensor on plantar stimulation (left Babinski response).

5. *Sensory system:* Pain sensation was diminished over the left leg and body. Position sense was absent in the left lower extremity.

LABORATORY DATA:

1. EKG revealed atrial fibrillation.

2. Spinal fluid was clear; pressure was normal. Protein was increased to 76 mg./100 ml.

HOSPITAL COURSE:

Several hours following admission, the patient was noted to be less alert although arousable. The right pupil was noted to be more dilated. Eye movements were roving and at times skewed. Bilateral extensor plantar responses were now present, with a hyperactive jaw jerk. The patient rallied from his initially grave, semicomatose condition and stabilized over the next 1 to 2 weeks. Because of his inability to swallow and to handle secretions, he required constant suction as well as nasogastric feeding. After recovery from the initial crisis the patient was noted to be fully alert with good cooperation and comprehension. The marked dysarthria and inability to swallow persisted.

On transfer to the neurology service on April 28, 1964 the patient was, however, found to be disoriented for time and place. His visual fields were full. On examination of cranial nerves, his right pupil was larger than his left. On forward gaze, a skew was noted with the right eye elevated and abducted. There was diminished conjugate lateral gaze to the left. On right lateral gaze there was full abduction of the right eye but poor adduction of the left eye. On right lateral gaze there was sustained horizontal nystagmus of the right eye, greater in the abducting eye, diminished in the left. Upward gaze was limited bilaterally, more so as regards the left eye. A dense left hemiplegia was still present with increased reflexes on the left, a left Babinski response, and an associated left central facial weakness. There were no findings on sensory examination.

Following recurrent episodes of aspiration pneumonia due to the patient's difficulties in handling secretions, he expired on August 5, 1964.

QUESTIONS:

1. At the time of the patient's initial evaluation, there was a combination of ptosis of the right eyelid and a dilated sluggish pupil on the right in addition to a supranuclear (upper motor neuron type) paralysis of the left face, arm, and leg. Locate the responsible lesion. Assign a name to this combination of symptoms and indicate the responsible vessel.

2. The patient's eye movements were later (April 28, 1964) described as dysconjugate with a skew deviation on forward gaze. On right lateral gaze, there was full abduction of the right eye but poor adduction of the left eye. On right lateral gaze there was sustained horizontal nystagmus in the right abducting eye but very little nystagmus in the left eye. Consider for the moment this combination of extraocular findings taken in isolation. Assign a name to the syndrome and localize the lesion. Indicate the responsible branch vessels.

3. In considering the localization of question 2 (as regards the left or right side of the brain stem) you may also wish to note that there was diminished conjugate lateral gaze to the left. Discuss the localizing significance of this finding. (Several explanations are possible.)

4. Upward gaze was diminished bilaterally more so as regards the left eye. Discuss the localizing significance of these findings if taken in isolation.

5. There was no response to caloric stimulation. Indicate the significance of this finding.

6. The jaw jerk was hyperactive. There was a severe dysarthria. The patient was unable to swallow and had difficulty in handling secretions. Assign a name to this syndrome and discuss its localizing significance.

7. At various times the patient was reported as confused and disoriented for time and place. In addition there was at the time of admission a possible right homonymous hemianopsia. Discuss these findings if taken in isolation from the standpoint of relevant arterial supply.

8. Now considering the case as a whole, indicate the location of pathological process as regards the arteries involved.

9. Indicate the nature of the pathological process.

16

Hypothalamus and Autonomic Nervous System

STANLEY JACOBSON

HYPOTHALAMUS

The hypothalamus forms the medial part of the floor of the diencephalon and is located on the wall of the third ventricle from the anterior margin of the optic chiasm to the posterior margin of the mammillary bodies. It is bounded dorsally by the thalamus and laterally by the subthalamus and internal capsule and it is connected to the hypophysis by the hypothalamic-hypophyseal tract. The hypothalamus consists of nuclei with their associated fiber systems.

For didactic reasons the hypothalamus can be divided into three zones (Fig. 16–1): (1) the anterior zone, including preoptic and supraoptic nuclei; (2) the middle zone, including the dorsal medial, ventral medial, lateral nuclei, and tuberal nuclei; and (3) the posterior area, including posterior hypothalamic nuclei and mammillary nuclei. In addition, there are periventricular nuclei adjacent to the third ventricle in all zones.

ANATOMICAL ORGANIZATION

Although the hypothalamus weighs only four grams, this small area controls our in-

ternal hemostasis and establishes behavior patterns.

Source of Input. The major subcortical input into the hypothalamus includes: (1) ascending reticular input from the multisynaptic ascending pathways in the mesencephalic reticular nuclei via the medial forebrain bundle, dorsal longitudinal fasciculus, and mammillary peduncle; (2) the globus pallidus; (3) the dorsal medial nucleus and intralaminar nuclei; and (4) the optic nerve-retinohypothalamic fibers. The major cortical input into the hypothalamus comes from the hippocampus (fornix), amygdala (stria terminalis), cingulate cortex, and frontal associational cortex (corticohypothalamic fibers). Thus we see that the hypothalamus is so located that it serves as an important integrating center between the brain stem-reticular system and the limbic forebrain structures.

Source of Output. The output of the hypothalamus is mediated via fiber tracts and the neurosecretory system.

The efferent pathways from the hypothalamus are: (1) the mammillothalamic tract which links the medial mammillary nucleus with the anterior thalamic nucleus and,

386

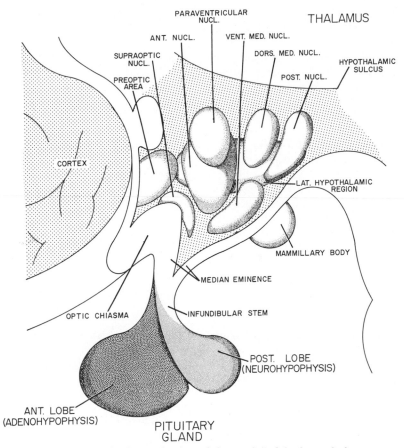

Figure 16–1 The hypophysis and the nuclei of the hypothalamus.

ultimately, with the cingulate cortex; (2) the paraventricular system which arises in the supraoptic, tuberal, and posterior nuclei in the hypothalamus to supply the medial thalamic nucleus and join the medial forebrain bundle; (3) the mammillotegmental tract which connects the medial mammillary nuclei with the midbrain reticular nuclei; (4) medial forebrain bundle and dorsal longitudinal fasciculus which receive fibers from the lateral hypothalamic nucleus and paraventricular nuclei and connect to the midbrain tegmentum and autonomic neurons in the brain stem and spinal cord; and (5) the hypothalamic-hypophyseal tract which connects supraoptic, paraventricular, and other hypothalamic nuclei via the hypophyseal stalk with the neural hypophysis, that is, the neurosecretory system.

FUNCTIONAL LOCALIZATION

The hypothalamus through its relationship to the autonomic nervous system and hypophysis maintains a more or less stable, controlled, internal environment which permits the individual to exist almost in spite of the external environment. It affects body temperature, water balance and neurosecretion, food intake, sleep, and the parasympathetic and sympathetic nervous system.

Body Temperature. Maintenance of a constant body temperature is vital to a warmblooded animal. The hypothalamus acts as an automatic thermostat, establishing a balance between vasodilation, vasoconstriction, sweating, and shivering. It does this by means of two opposing thermoregulatory centers: one to regulate heat-loss and one to regulate heat production. Lesions in either of these centers will interfere with the regulation of body temperature.

Control Center for Regulating Heat Loss. A destructive lesion in the anterior hypothalamus at the level of the optic chiasm or in the tuberal region renders an animal incapable of controlling its body heat in a warm environment; a tumor in the third ventricle may produce a similar picture. The human can no longer control the heat-loss mechanism which consists of cutaneous vasodilation and sweating. Without this mechanism the body temperature rises (hyperthermia), the patient becomes comatose, and may even die.

Control Center for Regulating Heat Production and Conservation. Lesions in the posterior hypothalamus above and lateral to the mammillary bodies interrupt an animal's ability to maintain normal body temperature in a warm or cold environment. In normal animals, exposure to cold produces vasoconstriction, shivering, piloerection, and secretion of epinephrine, all of which tend to increase body temperature. Following a lesion in the posterior hypothalamus the body temperature tends to match that of the environment, whether warm or cold, relative to 37° C. (poikilothermy). This probably results from damage to the fibers descending from the heat-loss center as well as from direct injury to the heat production and conservation center.

The thermoreceptors are located in the skin (end bulbs of Krause and end bulbs of Golgi-Mazzoni; Fig. 3–22) or in the hypothalamus itself monitoring the temperature of the cranial blood. Thus, some receptors respond to cold and others to warmth. Cold receptors excite the caudal heat production and conservation center and inhibit the rostral heat-loss center. Warm receptors reverse this pattern.

Water Balance and Neurosecretion (Fig. 16–2). Water balance is regulated by the hypothalamic-hypophyseal tract, which originates in the supraoptic and paraventricular nuclei and runs through the median eminence and hypophyseal stalk to terminate in close proximity to blood vessels in the neural hypophysis. A lesion in the region of the supraoptic nucleus or in the hypothalamic-hypophyseal system causes diabetes insipidus with polyuria (excessive formation of urine). The patient drinks copious amounts of water (polydipsia) and may excrete 20 liters of urine a day. The symptoms of diabetes insipidus may be relieved by the administration of pitressin (ADH) or extract from the neural hypophysis.

The hypothalamic-hypophyseal tract controls the formation and release of the antidiuretic hormone (vasopressin, ADH), which causes water to be reabsorbed from the distal

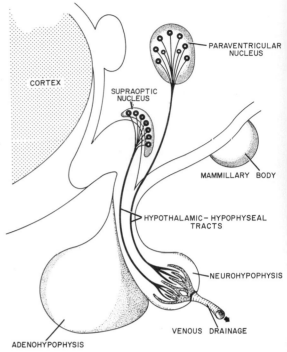

Figure 16–2 The hypothalamic-hypophyseal tract (neurosecretion). This tract provides a direct connection between the hypothalamus and the neurohypophysis. The neurosecretory granules pass down the axons of this tract and are stored in the neural lobe until they are released into the blood stream.

convoluted tubule and collecting duct of the kidneys into the bloodstream, thereby limiting the amount of water lost in the urine. Ingestion of large amounts of water causes a drop in ADH level and a reduction of tubular reabsorption with resultant diuresis. Water deprivation increases the ADH level and causes increased reabsorption and a very concentrated urine.

Current evidence suggests that the cells in the supraoptic nuclei form ADH or its precursors. The ADH is formed in the cell body, travels down the axons of the hypothalamic-hypophyseal tract, and is stored in the posterior lobe of the hypophysis as neurosecretory granules. The osmoreceptors in the aortic and carotid body and in the hypothalamus itself detect the concentration of water in the blood. This information is passed on to the hypothalamic nuclei which will then control the release of ADH into the circulation.

Water intake is probably also controlled

by hypothalamic neurons, but the exact site of these cells is yet unknown.

Food Intake. Bilateral lesions restricted to the *ventromedial* hypothalamic nuclei produce hyperphagia with resultant obesity. Stimulation of this center inhibits eating. Further experimentation has shown that these animals are not motivated to eat more, they just do not know when to stop eating; thus the *satiety center* is located here.

Bilateral lesions in the *lateral* hypothalamic region produce anorexia, whereby the animal refuses to eat and eventually dies. If this same region is stimulated and not destroyed, the animal eats more than normally. Appetite, the stimulus for eating, is dependent on many factors, including glucose concentration in the blood, stomach distension, smell, sight, taste, and the mood of the individual. Lesions in other portions of the limbic system also may affect appetite. However, most cases of obesity in man are not related to a neurological lesion; yet in some rare cases obesity has been traced to lesions in the ventromedial nuclei.

Sleep Cycle. The hypothalamus is important in our level of alertness due to the input from the reticular system and cerebral cortex. The posterior portion including the mammillary body is important in controlling the normal sleep cycle. Lesions in this region may produce an inversion in the sleep cycle, hypersomnia. Lesions in the anterior hypothalamus may produce insomnia (see Chapter 26, p. 750).

Parasympathetic and Sympathetic Nervous Systems. Stimulation of the *anterior* hypothalamus (anterolateral region) excites the parasympathetic nervous system and inhibits the sympathetic nervous system. The heart beat and blood pressure decrease (vagal response), the visceral vessels dilate, peristalsis and secretion of digestive juices increase, the pupil constricts, salivation increases.

Stimulation of the *posterior* hypothalamus (posteromedial region) excites the sympathetic nervous system and inhibits the parasympathetic nervous system. The heart beat and blood pressure increase, the visceral vessels constrict, peristalsis and secretion of gastric juices decrease, the pupil dilates, and piloerection occurs.

A lesion in the anterior or parasympathetic zone produces a sympathetic response, while destruction of the posterior or sympathetic zone may produce a parasympathetic response. The effects on blood vessels are produced by stimulation of the smooth muscles in the tunica media, and the effects on the sweat glands result from the stimulation of the glands through the cranial or peripheral nerves.

NEUROENDOCRINE RELATIONS OF THE HYPOTHALAMUS

HYPOTHALAMIC RELEASING FACTORS

The adenohypophysis receives no direct innervation from the hypothalamus, but the hypothalamus triggers the release of substances from the adenohypophysis. Experimental results have shown that releasing factors are produced in the hypothalamus and that these substances travel down the hypothalamic-hypophyseal portal system to stimulate formation of certain hormones in the adenohypophysis. The region in which these releasing factors are produced is called the *hypophysiotrophic* area since it is necessary for hormone production in the adenohypophysis.

Hypothalamic-Hypophyseal Portal System. The hypothalamus and adenohypophysis are connected by the hypothalamic-venous hypophyseal portal system (Fig. 16–3) which is the means by which humoral agents travel from the hypothalamus to the adenohypophysis.

The hypophysis receives its blood supply from two pairs of arteries: the superior hypophyseal artery and the inferior hypophyseal artery. The *superior hypophyseal arteries* leave the internal carotid and posterior communicating arteries and supply the median eminence, infundibular stalk, and adenohypophysis; in the infundibular stalk and median eminence the artery terminates as a capillary network which empties into veins that run down the infundibular stalk. In the anterior lobe these veins form another capillary network or sinusoid. The *inferior hypophyseal arteries* leave the internal carotid and distribute to the posterior lobe where they form a capillary network which flows into the sinus in the adenohypophysis. The hypophyseal veins finally drain into the cavernous sinus. The releasing factors enter the venous drainage of the hypothalamus which drains into the median eminence and hypophyseal stalk. These factors are then car-

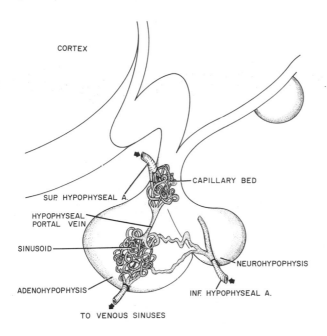

CORTEX

CAPILLARY BED

SUP. HYPOPHYSEAL A.

HYPOPHYSEAL
PORTAL VEIN

SINUSOID

NEUROHYPOPHYSIS

ADENOHYPOPHYSIS

INF. HYPOPHYSEAL A.

TO VENOUS SINUSES

Figure 16–3 The hypothalamic-hypophyseal venous portal system. These venous channels provide a vascular continuity between the hypothalamus and the adenohypophysis. The releasing factors from the hypophysiotrophic area of the hypothalamus drain into the veins of the hypothalamus which connect to the capillary bed in the infundibular stalk and median eminence. The factors are then carried to the adenohypophysis.

ried via the hypophyseal portal system to the adenohypophysis.

The capillary loops in the infundibular stalk and neural hypophysis drain in close proximity to the neurosecretory axons of the hypothalamic-hypophyseal tract.

Hypophysiotrophic Area. The hypophysiotrophic area is a paramedian zone which extends rostrally at the level of the optic chiasm dorsally from the ventral surface to the paraventricular nuclei. Caudally this area narrows down to include only the ventral surface of the hypothalamus at the level of the mammillary recess of the third ventricle. The hypophysiotrophic center includes neurons in the following hypothalamic nuclei: paraventricular, arcuate, and tuberal.

Releasing Factors Produced by Hypothalamus. Releasing factors are produced in the hypophysiotrophic area and stimulate the adenohypophysis to produce the following hormones: adrenocorticotrophin, lactogenic hormone, gonadotropins (which are luteinizing and follicle-stimulating), somatotropin, and thyrotropin. These factors traverse the hypothalamic-hypophyseal portal system and trigger the formation and eventual release of hormones from the adenohypophysis. These adenohypophyseal hormones are released into the blood stream and transported to a target organ on which their effect is produced.

Adenohypophyseal Hormones. Somatotropin and the lactogenic hormone are produced in acidophilic cells in the adenohypophysis. The gonadotropin and thyrotropic hormones are produced by basophilic cells in the adenohypophysis. The exact origin of the adrenocorticotrophic hormone is uncertain.

Adrenocorticotrophic Hormone (corticotrophic hormone, ACTH). This hormone is produced by basophilic cells and stimulates the formation of adrenal glucocorticoids (hydrocortisone) and, to a lesser degree, mineral corticoids (aldosterone). In conditions of stress (cold, heat, pain, fright, flight, inflammation, or infection) ACTH is produced.

Lactogenic Hormone (prolactin). This substance promotes development of the mammary glands and lactation.

Gonadotropins (luteinizing hormone, LH; or interstitial cell-stimulating hormone, ICSH): In females gonadotropin is necessary for ovulation as it causes luteinization of follicles after they are ripened by FSH (follicle-stimulating hormone); in males it activates the interstitial cells of the testis to produce testosterone.

Follicle-Stimulating Hormone (FSH). This substance stimulates growth of the ovarian follicle in the female and stimulates spermatogenesis in males.

Growth Hormone (somatotropin, STH). This hormone is important in the normal growth of the body after birth. It specifically affects the growth of the epiphyseal cartilage. The growth hormone is also important in the metabolism of fat, protein, and carbohydrates. Cessation of growth follows hypophysectomy, while gigantism is produced by an excessive dose of somatotropin prior to closure of the epiphyseal plate. *Acromegaly* is produced by adenohypophyseal tumors after the closure of the epiphyseal plate.

Thyrotropic Hormone (TH). This substance stimulates the thyroid gland.

HORMONES PRODUCED BY HYPOTHALAMUS

Two hormones, vasopressin and oxytocin, are manufactured in the hypothalamus, are carried down the hypothalamic-hypophyseal tract, and are stored in the neurohypophysis before being released into the blood stream.

Vasopressin (ADH) is an antidiuretic hormone, formed in the supraoptic nucleus and carried down the hypothalamic-hypophyseal tract. This substance acts on the distal convoluted tubules and collecting ducts in the kidney causing resorption of water.

Oxytocin is formed in the paraventricular nucleus and is carried down the hypothalamic-hypophyseal tract. This substance stimulates the mammary gland, causing them to contract and expel milk concomitant with suction upon the nipple. Oxytocin also contracts the smooth muscle in the pregnant uterus and dilates the uterus, cervix, and vagina.

LIGHT LEVELS AND THE HYPOTHALAMUS

Light appears to produce effects which are mediated through the hypothalamus via the retinohypothalamic tract. In many animals abnormal variations in the light levels may alter the sexual cycle and prevent estrus. Light levels may also affect the formation of melanin.

EMOTIONS AND THE HYPOTHALAMUS

As noted in Chapter 18 on the emotional brain, the hypothalamus sets the foundation for emotional responses and controls the functions in the viscera. It exerts these powerful influences through the multisynaptic descending autonomic pathways in the lateral margins of the reticular formation as well as by controlling the release of the catecholamines—epinephrine and norepinephrine—from the adrenal medulla.

Norepinephrine causes vasoconstriction of the peripheral vessels with resultant increased blood flow in the large vessels. The blood pressure and pulse rate rise and the flow of blood in the coronary muscles increases.

Epinephrine increases the heart rate and the force, amplitude, and frequency of contractions.

Epinephrine has other effects. It dilates the pupils and the sphincters of the gastrointestinal system and the urinary bladder causing voiding and defecation. It inhibits the motility of the gut and causes the bronchial musculature to relax, thereby dilating the bronchial passages. Epinephrine increases oxygen metabolism and the basic metabolic rate. It causes hyperglycemia by triggering an increasing phosphorylase activity which accelerates glycogenesis in the muscles and liver. And it increases the rate of resynthesis of lactic acid to glycogen, thereby prolonging the contraction of the skeletal muscles.

AUTONOMIC NERVOUS SYSTEM

Much of the effectiveness of the hypothalamus is produced by its innervation of the nuclei in the central nervous system which form the autonomic nervous system. In this section we will identify these neurons in the central and peripheral nervous systems and list the responses produced by the autonomic nervous system in each organ. It should be noted that there is normally a balance between the functions of the parasympathetic and sympathetic systems. However, this equilibrium may be modified by environmental stresses as well as disease processes.

The somatic nervous system has its own receptors and effectors which provide cutaneous and motor innervation to the skin and muscles in the head, neck, and body. The visceral or autonomic nervous system also has its own receptors and effectors which provide visceral motor and sensory innervation to the glands, smooth muscles, cardiac muscles, viscera, and blood vessels. These axons run part of the way with somatic fibers, but they also have separate pathways.

In the somatic nervous system the efferent neuron is the ventral horn cell. Its axon leaves the central nervous system to innervate a skeletal muscle.

In the visceral nervous system two efferent neurons are found: the preganglionic neuron and the postganglionic neuron.

The preganglionic neuron is found in the intermediate horn in the thoracic and lumbar levels of the spinal cord. The axon of this cell leaves the central nervous system via the ventral root and ends in an autonomic ganglion which parallels the spinal cord or is found near the target organ.

The postganglionic neuron, or the motor ganglion cell, is located outside the central nervous system and ends in the appropriate gland, smooth muscle, or cardiac muscle.

PARASYMPATHETIC AND SYMPATHETIC SYSTEMS

The autonomic nervous system is divided into parasympathetic and sympathetic systems. The preganglionic cell bodies are found in the CNS at the following sites:

a. Cranial parasympathetic (cranial nerves III, VII, IX, and X

b. Thoracolumbar sympathetic (all thoracic segments and lumbar segments 1 and 2)

c. Sacral parasympathetic (sacral segments 2 to 4)

The cranial and sacral portions are parasympathetic, while the thoracolumbar cells are sympathetic.

The nerve fibers are further classified as being adrenergic or cholinergic, depending on which nerve transmitter is involved—epinephrine or acetylcholine. Injections of epinephrine into the blood stream produces an effect similar to that which results when the thoracolumbar or sympathetic nervous system is stimulated. Most postganglionic sympathetic fibers release a substance similar to epinephrine; these are called *adrenergic* fibers. Small doses of acetylcholine injected into the blood stream produce the same effect as stimulation of the craniosacral column—*cholinergic* endings. Most postganglionic parasympathetic fibers release acetylcholine at their terminals.

The axons ending on sweat glands, though receiving innervation from the thoracolumbar system, are cholinergic. Pilomotor axons, which also receive thoracolumbar innervation, are adrenergic.

The two systems provide dual innervation to glands and viscera and act to produce optimal balances for maintaining the internal milieu under any environmental condition.

PARASYMPATHETIC SYSTEM

Cranial Fibers

Cranial Nerve III. The fibers originate in the Edinger-Westphal nucleus in the midbrain and innervate the constrictors of the pupil.

Cranial Nerve VII. The axons originate in the superior salivatory nuclei of the pons and innervate glands in the nasal cavity and palate and the lacrimal, submandibular, and sublingual glands.

Cranial Nerve IX. The fibers originate in the inferior salivatory nucleus in the medulla. The axons exit with nerve IX and end in the otic ganglion which innervates the parotid gland.

Cranial Nerve X. The dorsal motor nucleus of the vagus nerve provides preganglionic parasympathetic innervation to the pharynx, larynx, esophagus, lungs, heart, stomach, and small intestine and large intestine up to the transverse colon. The postganglionic fibers originate from ganglia in the respective organs and in the nodes of the submucosal plexus of Meissner and in the myenteric plexus of Auerbach in the alimentary tract.

Sacral Plexus. The parasympathetic sacral plexus originates from sacral segments S2 and S4 and supplies the genitalia, sigmoid colon, rectum, bladder, and ureter. The ganglia are located in the organ and are named for the organ.

SYMPATHETIC TRUNK

The preganglionic fibers originate in the intermediolateral column of grey matter in the spinal cord from T1 to L2; they exit in the white rami and enter the paravertebral sympathetic ganglionic chain. The ganglia form a continuous paravertebral trunk in the cervical, thoracic, lumbar, and sacral segments.

The postganglionic fibers originate in the ganglia and exit via the grey communicating rami. The postganglionic fibers reach their destinations by plexuses enwrapping the arteries or via cranial and spinal nerves.

Cervical Ganglia. The cervical ganglia extend posterior to the great vessels from the level of the subclavian artery to the base of the skull. There are usually three ganglia in the cervical region: superior, middle, and inferior.

The *superior cervical ganglion* is the largest, being flat and 25 to 35 mm. long. The internal carotid nerves leave the superior border of the superior cervical ganglia and pass into the cranial cavity with the carotid artery in the carotid canal. These fibers form the plexus around the carotid artery and in the cavernous sinus. This ganglion provides postganglionic innervation to the eye, lacrimal gland, parotid gland (otic ganglia), submaxillary and sublingual glands (sublingual ganglia), and some branches to the heart.

The *middle cervical ganglion* is small and variable and is found at the level of the cricoid cartilage. It gives postganglionic fibers to the heart.

The *inferior cervical ganglion* is usually fused with the first thoracic ganglion and forms the stellate ganglion. It is also small and irregular in shape and lies posterior to the vertebral artery. The postganglionic fibers innervate the heart.

Thoracic Ganglia. The thoracic portion of the sympathetic trunk extends anterior to the heads of the first through tenth rib and then passes along the sides of the lower two thoracic vertebrae. The number of thoracic ganglia varies from 10 to 12.

The ganglia of T1 to T4 provide postganglionic fibers to the heart and lungs. The postganglionic fibers from T5 to T12 form the splanchnic nerves. The greater splanchnic nerve is formed by preganglionic rootlets from T5 to T10; the axons pass through the thoracic ganglia and end in the celiac ganglion, from where postganglionic axons run above the aorta, esophagus, thoracic duct, and azygos vein to reach the stomach, small intestine, and adrenal glands. The lesser and least splanchnic nerves arise from spinal cord segment T11 and T12 and run through the paravertebral ganglion to the celiac and superior mesenteric ganglion from where the postganglionic axons run to the small intestine, the ascending portion of the colon, and the kidneys.

Lumbar Ganglia. The lumbar sympathetic trunk consists of small ganglia which lie along the anterior border of the psoas muscle. The preganglionic fibers originate from the intermediate column of spinal cord segments L1 and L2, pass through the lumbar ganglia, and end in the inferior mesenteric ganglion where they innervate the descending colon, rectum, urinary bladder, ureter, and external genitalia.

INNERVATION OF SPECIFIC STRUCTURES

Eye

Parasympathetic: The preganglionic cell bodies are found in the Edinger-Westphal nucleus associated with cranial nerve III. These axons end in the ciliary ganglion. The postganglionic fibers run in the short ciliary nerve, providing innervation to the ciliary muscle and the constrictor of the iris, and permit accommodation for near vision.

Sympathetic: Preganglionic axons originate from the intermediolateral nucleus in cord levels C8 to T2. The fibers ascend in the sympathetic chain to reach postganglionic neurons in the superior cervical ganglion. The postganglionic axons join the carotid plexus and the ophthalmic branch of nerve V to innervate the dilator muscle of the iris and the levator palpebrae and radial ciliary muscles, producing eye opening (lifting of the lid) and dilation of the pupil for distant vision.

Lacrimal Glands

Parasympathetic: Preganglionic fibers originate in the superior salivatory nucleus of nerve VII and run to the sphenopalatine ganglion. The postganglionic fibers join the maxillary division of nerve V, resulting in vasodilation and secretion.

Sympathetic: The preganglionic fibers originate from T1 to T2, exit from the central nervous system, and ascend in the sympathetic trunk to the superior cervical ganglion, from whence they join the carotid plexus. The resulting action is vasoconstriction and reduced secretion.

Salivary Glands

Parasympathetic: The preganglionic axons to the submaxillary and sublingual glands orginate in the superior salivary nucleus of nerve VII. The preganglionic axons to the parotid originate from the inferior salivatory nucleus of nerve IX. The resulting action in this case is vasodilation and secretion.

Sympathetic: These fibers originate from the intermediolateral column in the upper thoracic level, exit from the central nervous system, run up to the superior cervical ganglion, and then proceed to the glands. Vasoconstriction and reduced secretion result.

Heart

Parasympathetic: The preganglionic fibers originate in the dorsal motor nucleus of nerve X, exit from the central nervous system, and run in the vagus nerve to the postganglionic ganglia in the cardiac plexus and atria. These axons reach coronary vessels and atrial musculature, causing cardiac deceleration.

Sympathetic: The preganglionic fibers originate in the T1 to T4 segments, exit from the central nervous system, and reach the postganglionic neurons in the upper thoracic ganglion and all three cervical ganglia. The fibers form the cardiac nerves and enter the cardiac plexus. The resulting effect is cardiac acceleration.

Lungs

Parasympathetic: The preganglionic fibers originate in the dorsal motor nucleus of nerve X and run in the vagus to the pulmonary plexus in the bronchi and blood vessels, causing constriction of the bronchi and decreased respiration.

Sympathetic: The preganglionic fibers originate in T1 to T4. The postganglionic originate in the upper thoracic and lowest cervical ganglia. The result in this case is dilation of the bronchi and increased respiration.

Abdominal Viscera

Parasympathetic: These fibers originate from the dorsal motor nucleus of nerve X and S2 to S4, and end in the intrinsic plexus in the organ. They stimulate peristalsis and gastrointestinal secretions.

Sympathetic: The sympathetic fibers originate from the lower thoracic and lumbar segments, pass through the paravertebral ganglia and form the splanchnic nerves which end in the celiac and superior and inferior mesenteric ganglia. Postganglionic fibers from these ganglia end on smooth muscle or glands. The resulting action is to inhibit peristalsis and gastrointestinal secretion, stimulate secretion from the adrenal medulla and cause vasoconstriction of the visceral vessels.

Pelvis

Parasympathetic: These fibers originate from segments S2 to S4 and end in ganglia in the organs. Postganglionic fibers supply the uterus, vagina, testes, erectile tissue (penis and clitoris), sigmoid colon, rectum, and bladder. They cause contraction and emptying of the bladder and erection of the clitoris or penis.

Sympathetic: These fibers originate from the lowest thoracic segments and segments L1 to L3 and run in the hypogastric nerves to the target viscera where the ganglia are found. They cause vasoconstriction and ejaculation of semen and inhibit peristalsis in the sigmoid colon and rectum.

Cutaneous and Deep Vessels, Glands, and Hair

Blood vessels receive only sympathetic postganglionic innervation from the appropriate paravertebral ganglion. Activation of this system produces vasoconstriction (cooling of the skin), sweating, and piloerection.

The innervation of the peripheral blood vessels and glands is summarized in Table 16–1.

DISORDERS OF THE AUTONOMIC NERVOUS SYSTEM

Disorders of the autonomic nervous system can affect any of the organs innervated by the autonomic nervous system. Only a few will be discussed here. The student is referred to any standard neurology text for further details.

Eye. A lesion in the nucleus or nerve root of cranial nerve III produces Horner's syndrome, drooping of the eyelid, and pupillary dilatation. The Argyll Robertson pupil does not react to light but will accommodate

Table 16–1 Sympathetic Innervation of Peripheral Blood Vessels and Glands

	LOCATION OF PREGANGLIONIC NEURONAL CELL BODY	LOCATION OF POSTGANGLIONIC NEURONAL CELL BODY
Head and neck	T1–T2	Superior cervical ganglion
Forelimb	T5–T9	Middle and inferior ganglion, T1 and T2 of paravertebral chain
Hindlimb	T10–L2	Lumbar and sacral ganglion
Thorax	T1–T5	Thoracic ganglion, T1–T5
Abdomen	T6–L2	Abdominal ganglion, T6–T12

and is commonly seen in neurosyphilis in the central nervous system. (Refer to discussion, Tabes Dorsalis, p. 191.)

Blood Vessels. Raynaud's disease (vasomotor disease), most common in young women, causes the patient to be abnormally sensitive to cold. The extremities upon exposure to cold become cyanotic and then red and very painful. It seems that the sympathetic innervation does not dilate the vessels. Vasodilators will help, but section of the preganglionic sympathetic innervation to the limb brings relief by vasodilation.

Heart and Gastrointestinal Tract. These organs respond to any change in our emotional behavior. Consequently they are affected by psychosomatic diseases, i.e., hypertension and ulcers.

Bladder. The bladder is a reflex organ and contracts in response to stretch. The afferents are carried into the sacral spinal cord. The efferents are supplied by the parasympathetic (S2–S4) and sympathetic (L1–L2) ganglia. The parasympathetic axons initiates the reflex contraction to empty the bladder or urine (micturition). This action is voluntarily exerted through the nerve to the external sphincter. Sympathetic axons do not act on micturition but control blood vessels and closure of the internal sphincter during sexual intercourse.

Micturition. Under normal conditions, the bladder fills and expands, stretching the receptors in the bladder walls. The pressure build-up is carried into the CNS by the sensory nerves. Following the voluntary contraction of the external sphincter the bladder contracts reflexly; the internal and external sphincters open and the muscles in the pelvic floor relax (control from cerebral cortex). The urine passing through the urethra continues the stimulation until the bladder is empty. The external sphincter then closes. We can also initiate this voluntarily with the assistance of the abdominal muscles.

Any interruption of the autonomic, sensory, or voluntary pathways produces abnormality in this function. Interruption of the cortical pathways (bilateral involvement of the cerebral hemispheres) produces the *uninhibited bladder,* in which sensation is normal, but the patient no longer has control over voiding. Thus, as the bladder fills and becomes distended it voids suddenly without cortical control.

Destruction of the parasympathetic supply via injury to the motor roots produces the *autonomic bladder,* in which there is no sensation and no longer any reflex or voluntary control. The need to void occurs from abdominal discomfort produced by increasing intra-abdominal pressure.

Injury to the sensory roots or ganglia or dorsal column produces the *sensory paralytic bladder,* in which there is no sensation and no reflex ability to void. The bladder visually enlarges and then dribbles. Voiding is also difficult without sensory feedback.

Isolation of the bladder from the upper motor neurons either by transsection of the spinal cord above the sacral level or by extensive brain disease produces the *reflex bladder.* In this condition the descending autonomic fibers are interrupted as well as the corticospinal fibers, but the spinal reflex circuit remains intact. Micturition is involuntary and results from just the stretch reflex which will produce sudden and uncontrollable voiding.

REFERENCES

Bodian, D.: Cytological aspects of neurosecretion in opossum neurohypophysis. Bull. Johns Hopk. Hosp., *113*:57, 1963.

Bodian, D.: Herring bodies and neuroapocrine secretion in the monkey: An electron microscopic study of the fate of the neurosecretory product. Bull. Johns Hopk. Hosp., *118*:282, 1966.

Green, J. D.: The comparative anatomy of the portal vascular system and of the innervation of the hypophysis. *In* Harris, G. W., and Donovan, B. T. (eds.): *The Pituitary Gland.* Berkeley, University of California Press, 1966, Vol. I, p. 127.

Haymaker, W., Anderson, E., and Nauta, W. J. H.: *The Hypothalamus.* Springfield, Illinois, Charles C Thomas, 1969.

Palay, S. L.: The fine structure of the neurohypophysis. *In* Waelsch, H. (ed.): *Progress in Neurobiology: II. Ultrastructure and Cellular Chemistry of Neural Tissue.* New York, Paul B. Hoeber, 1957, p. 31.

Scharrer, E.: *Endocrines and the Central Nervous System.* Baltimore, Williams and Wilkins, 1966.

Szentagothai, J., Flerko, B., Mess, B., and Halasy, B.: *Hypothalamic Control of the Anterior Pituitary.* Budapest, Akademiai Kiado, 1968.

Wislocki, G. B.: The vascular supply of the hypophysis cerebri of the rhesus monkey and man. Proc. Assoc. Res. nerv. Dis., *17*:48, 1938.

17

Telencephalon

STANLEY JACOBSON

GROSS ANATOMY OF THE TELENCEPHALON

The telencephalon or cerebrum consists of an external or cortical portion and an internal or subcortical division separated by a core of white matter. The cerebral cortex forms the external part, while the basal ganglia forms the internal portion. Gross inspection of the cerebral hemispheres shows that the surface consists of irregularly shaped folds called convolutions or gyri. The gyri are separated from each other by depressions of varying depth. The deepest depressions are called fissures, while shallower ones are labeled sulci. It should be noted that about 30 per cent of the neurons in the cerebral hemispheres are found on the surface; the remaining 70 per cent are located in the walls of the sulci and fissures.

LATERAL SURFACE

The lateral surface of the brain (Fig. 17–1) has four divisions named after the bones of the cranium overlying these regions: frontal, parietal, occipital, and temporal. Only the frontal, occipital, and temporal regions or lobes have poles.

The four lobes can be delineated by locating certain sulci and fissures (Fig. 17–2). The

anteroposterior lateral running fissure separates the superiorly placed frontal and parietal lobes from the inferiorly placed temporal lobe. The central fissure separates the frontal lobe from the parietal lobe. On the medial surface of the hemisphere, near the occipital pole, is found a deep fissure, the parieto-occipital fissure. A line drawn from this fissure to an indentation on the inferior border of the brain (the preoccipital notch) will delimit the occipital lobe. If a line is drawn which follows the curvature of the lateral fissure to intersect the line which delimits the occipital lobe, all cortex behind the central sulcus above this line forms the parietal lobe, while all cortex below the line forms the temporal lobe.

The lateral surface of the cerebrum may be divided into two roughly equivalent halves separated by the central fissure. The frontal lobe forms the anterior half; the parietal and occipital lobes form the posterior half.

Frontal Lobe (Figs. 17–3 and 17–4). Parallel to the central fissure is the precentral sulcus which varies in extent, being either continuous or divided into an upper portion (superior precentral) and a lower portion (inferior precentral). The precentral gyrus or motor strip lies between the central fissure and the precentral sulcus. Arising from the upper part of the precentral sulcus is the

396

superior frontal sulcus, which is continuous and runs anteriorly toward the frontal pole. The inferior frontal sulcus originates from the lower part of the precentral sulcus and runs toward the frontal pole. In some brains a middle frontal sulcus separates the middle frontal gyrus into two portions. The superior frontal gyrus lies above the superior frontal sulcus; the middle frontal gyrus lies between the superior and inferior frontal sulci, while the inferior frontal gyrus lies below it.

The inferior frontal gyrus is divided into an opercular, triangular, and orbital portion. The pars opercularis is continuous with the precentral gyrus. The pars triangularis is separated from the pars opercularis by the anterior ascending limb of the lateral fissure.

Parietal Lobe (Figs. 17–3 and 17–4). Posterior to the central sulcus and paralleling it is the postcentral sulcus which is either continuous or divided into superior and inferior portions similar to the precentral sulcus. The postcentral or *sensory cortex* lies between the central and postcentral sulci. About half way up the postcentral sulcus, the intraparietal sulcus extends posteriorly, dividing the parietal lobe into superior and inferior parietal lobules. The inferior parietal lobule consists of the supramarginal and angular gyri. The supramarginal gyrus surrounds the posterior ascending limb of the lateral fissure. The angular gyrus is behind the supramarginal gyrus and surrounds the posterior end of the superior temporal sulcus.

Occipital Lobe. The lateral occipital gyrus consists of visual associative cortex. The visual receptive cortex is found on the medial surface of the hemisphere.

Temporal Lobe (Fig. 17–4). The temporal lobe lies below the lateral fissure and has three anteroposterior-running gyri on the lateral surface of the brain: the superior, middle, and inferior temporal gyri. The inferior temporal gyrus extends onto the ventral surface of the cerebrum. The superior temporal gyrus forms the temporal operculum. Near its posterior end two gyri are seen running into the lateral fissure (Fig. 17–5). These gyri are the transverse temporal gyri, consisting of the primary receptive auditory cortex. If the lateral fissure is enlarged by opening the frontal, parietal, and temporal operculum, the insula is seen (Fig. 17–5). This cortical region, consisting of short and long gyri, is functionally part of the emotional brain.

MEDIAL SURFACE

The medial surface (Fig. 17–6) is revealed after separation of the cerebral hemispheres by a section through the corpus callosum in the midline.

Corpus Callosum. The great cerebral commissure, the corpus callosum, dominates the medial surface of the hemisphere. It consists of a ventral part, the rostrum (1 in Fig. 17–7); a large genu (2 in Fig. 17–7) which is continuous with the rostrum; a body (3 in Fig. 17–7), and posteriorly a very thick splenium (4 in Fig. 17–7). The corpus callosum permits the transfer of learning and memory from one hemisphere to the other and it connects portions of the frontal, parietal, occipital, and cingulate cortex in one hemisphere with the same regions in the other hemisphere. The anterior commissure (Fig. 17–7), located at the posterior end of the septum, has a function somewhat similar to the corpus callosum, and interconnects parts of the temporal lobe and olfactory bulb.

Cingulate Cortex. The callosal sulcus (Fig. 17–8) separates the corpus callosum from the overlying cingulate gyrus or lobe (Fig. 17–9) which is a portion of the emotional brain (see Chapter 18). The cingulate gyrus is separated from the overlying superior frontal gyri by the cingulate sulcus. The superior frontal gyrus (Fig. 17–7) stops inferiorly at the parolfactory sulcus while the cingulate gyrus is continuous inferiorly with the subcallosal gyrus. The septal region lies posterior to the parolfactory gyrus and is functionally connected with it. The cingulate gyrus continues around the splenium of the corpus callosum and connects to the hippocampal gyrus. This narrow zone is called the *isthmus* of the cingulate gyrus.

Other Landmarks of Medial Surface. The superior frontal gyrus (Fig. 17–9) stops at the precentral sulcus. The portions of the pre- and postcentral gyri on the medial hemispheric wall form the *paracentral lobule* and are related respectively to motor and sensory functions. The region of the superior parietal lobe, extending on the medial surface from the postcentral sulcus to the parieto-occipital fissure, is called the *precuneus* (Fig. 17–7) and is sensory association cortex.

The caudalmost portion of the medial surface is formed by the occipital lobe (Fig. 17–9) which is bounded anteriorly by the parieto-occipital fissure and inferiorly by the

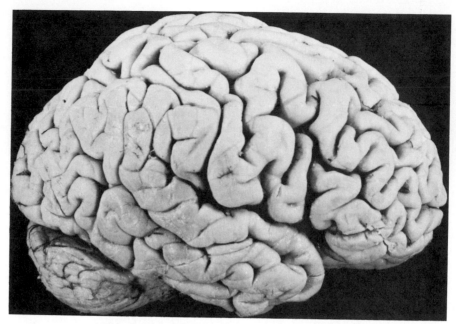

Figure 17-1 Lateral surface of the cerebrum.

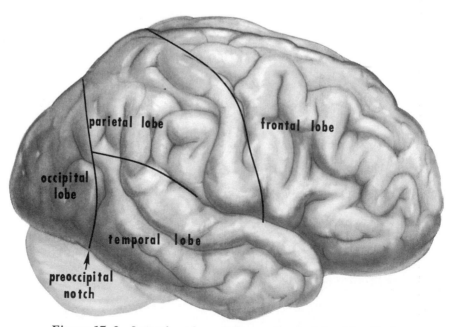

Figure 17-2 Lateral surface of the cerebrum; lobes identified.

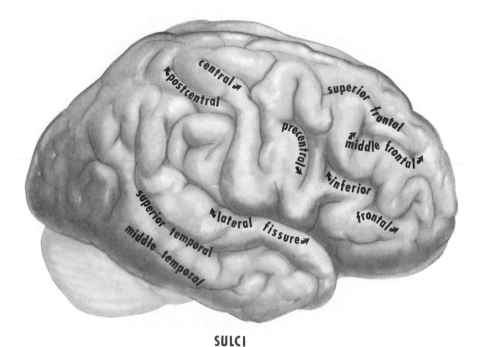

SULCI

Figure 17–3   Lateral surface of the cerebrum; sulci and fissures identified.

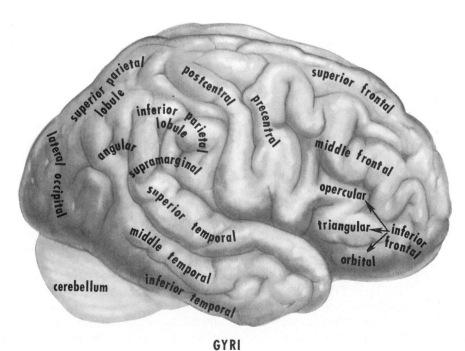

GYRI

Figure 17–4   Lateral surface of the cerebrum; gyri identified.

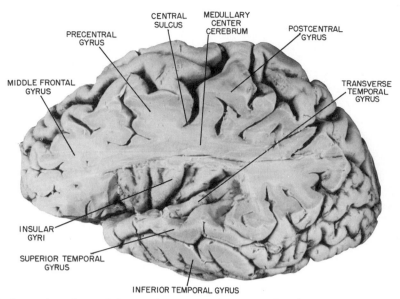

CENTRAL
SULCUS

MEDULLARY
CENTER
CEREBRUM

PRECENTRAL
GYRUS

POSTCENTRAL
GYRUS

MIDDLE FRONTAL
GYRUS

TRANSVERSE
TEMPORAL
GYRUS

INSULAR
GYRI

SUPERIOR TEMPORAL
GYRUS

INFERIOR TEMPORAL GYRUS

Figure 17-5   Lateral surface of the cerebrum with frontal and parietal operculum removed demonstrating insula and transverse temporal gyri.

collateral sulcus (Fig. 17–8). The *calcarine fissure* (Fig. 17–8) originates near the occipital pole and runs anteriorly to intersect the parieto-occipital fissure. The visual radiation ends in the cortex surrounding the calcarine fissure which is the primary visual cortex.

The area lying between the calcarine and parieto-occipital fissure (Fig. 17–8) is wedge-shaped and thus is called the *cuneus* (Fig. 17–7). The lingual gyrus (*lingula*) is found below the calcarine fissure and is continuous rostrally with the occipitotemporal gyrus (Fig. 17–7).

VENTRAL SURFACE

Olfactory Bulb and Tract.   The olfactory bulb and tract are seen on the ventral surface of the brain. The olfactory bulb rests on the cribriform plate of the ethmoid bone and is connected to the base of the hemisphere by the olfactory tract (see Fig. 18–2). The olfactory tract lies in the olfactory sulcus and fuses with the hemisphere dividing into a medial and lateral striae. The medial stria enters into the anterior commissure and interconnects the two olfactory bulbs, while the lateral striae continue posteriorly into the olfactory cortex.

Frontal Lobe.   The ventral surface of the frontal lobe consists of orbital cortex. The most ventromedial portion of the frontal lobe is called the *gyrus rectus*. The orbital and most anterior portions of the frontal lobe form the frontal associative region which is important in controlling our behavior patterns.

Temporal Lobe.   The bulk of the ventral surface is formed by the temporal lobe (Fig. 17–9) which is divided into anteroposterior-running gyri. The most medial gyrus (Fig. 17–7) is the *parahippocampal gyrus* which is separated from the adjacent occipitotemporal gyrus by the collateral sulcus. The inferior temporal gyrus is the most lateral gyrus on the anteroventral surface of the hemisphere and is separated from the occipitotemporal gyrus by the inferior temporal sulcus.

Medial to the parahippocampal gyrus is the *hippocampus* which is more easily seen after the diencephalon is removed (Fig. 18–6). The cerebral peduncle and optic tract are adjacent to the hippocampus. The *fornix* exits from the substance of the hippocampus and connects it to the septum and hypothalamus. The *uncus* (Fig. 17–7) is found anterior to the hippocampus and consists of the olfactory cortex and amygdaloid nuclei. The amygdala, hippocampus, parahippocampal gyrus, and cingulate gyrus collectively are called the *fornicate gyrus.* They form the bulk of the visceral or "emotional" brain. The hippocampus is also involved in short-term memory.

BASAL GANGLIA AND WHITE MATTER OF CEREBRAL HEMISPHERES

BASAL GANGLIA

The deep telencephalic nuclei, the basal ganglia, are separated from the cerebral cortex by the medullary center and are formed by the caudate, putamen, globus pallidus, and claustrum. The globus pallidus and putamen are lens-shaped in profile and are called the *lenticular nuclei*. Collectively the lenticular nuclei and caudate are called the *corpus striatum*. All these structures are deep to the insula.

A coronal section at this level (Fig. 17–10) shows in sequence from lateral to medial surface the following cellular regions: insular cortex, claustrum, putamen, globus pallidus, caudate, and lateral ventricle. The cells in the caudate and putamen are either small or large multipolar neurons. The small cells are very numerous and provide the connections within the nuclei. The myelinated axons of the large multipolar cells project to both portions of the globus pallidus.

Caudate (Fig. 17–11). The large anterior portion or head of the caudate bulges into the lateral wall of the anterior horn of the lateral ventricle. Its narrow tail begins at the interventricular foramen of Monro and continues along the dorsolateral border of the thalamus at the lateral margin of the body of the lateral ventricle to the posterior end of the thalamus, where it runs within the roof of the inferior horn of the lateral ventricle, finally fusing with the corticomedial portion of the amygdaloid nuclei.

The *stria terminalis* accompanies the tail of the caudate lying medial to it and connects the amygdala with the hypothalamus. At its most anterior end, the head of the caudate and the putamen are continuous (Fig. 17–26), and in levels rostral to the thalamus the caudate and putamen are connected by cellular bridges. The terminal vein lies medial to the stria terminalis. This vessel drains the corpus striatum, septum, and choroid plexus in the lateral ventricle.

Putamen. The putamen (Fig. 17–11) is the largest and most lateral portion of the basal ganglia; it is separated from the more medially placed globus pallidus by the external medullary stria. The putamen extends from the most anterior end of the lateral ventricle to about the level of the mammillary bodies.

Globus Pallidus. The globus pallidus (Fig. 17–11) is found medial to the putamen adjacent to the anterior and posterior limbs of the internal capsule. This nucleus is divided into two portions by the internal medullary stria. Many myelinated axon bundles run in the globus pallidus; consequently in gross material it appears paler than the caudate and putamen. The caudate and putamen connect to the globus pallidus which provides the efferent connections for the basal ganglia.

Fiber Tracts of the Globus Pallidus. The following fiber tracts leave the globus pallidus: subthalamic fasciculus, ansa lenticularis, and lenticular fasciculus. These tracts either cut directly through the posterior limb of the internal capsule or swing around it.

The *subthalamic fasciculus* passes through the posterior limb of the internal capsule and interconnects the globus pallidus and the subthalamic nucleus (Figs. 17–12, 17–13, and 17–14).

The *ansa lenticularis* swings around the posterior limb of the internal capsule and connects to the thalamus and prerubral field (tegmental field).

The *lenticular fasciculus* passes through the posterior limb of the internal capsule and runs between the zona incerta and subthalamic nucleus and reaches the prerubral field (Figs. 17–12, 17–13, and 17–14). Many of the fibers from the lenticular fasciculus and ansa lenticularis enter the thalamic fasciculus which is found at the inferior medial border of the thalamus.

The fibers in the *thalamic fasciculus* enter the following thalamic nuclei: ventral anterior, ventral lateral, and central medial. Some axons in these tracts also connect to the hypothalamus, zona incerta, midbrain tegmentum, and substantia nigra. The caudate, putamen, globus pallidus, claustrum, subthalamus, and substantia nigra form part of the extrapyramidal or old motor system.

Extrapyramidal System. Volitional, skilled movements are initiated in the cerebral cortex and executed by the pyramidal system. The reflex maintenance of the motor response and the integrative functions associated with the volitional movements are controlled through the extrapyramidal system. The extrapyramidal system thus pro-

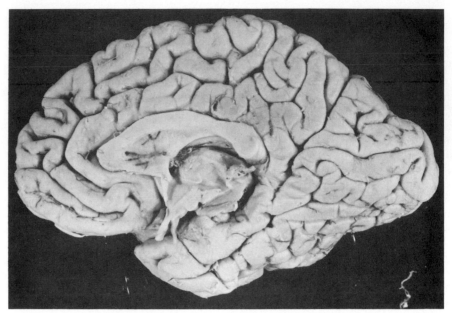

Figure 17–6　Medial surface of the cerebrum.

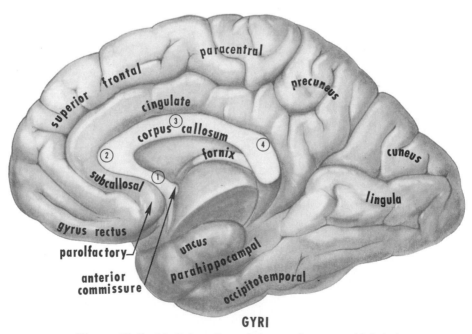

GYRI

Figure 17–7　Medial surface of the cerebrum; gyri labeled.

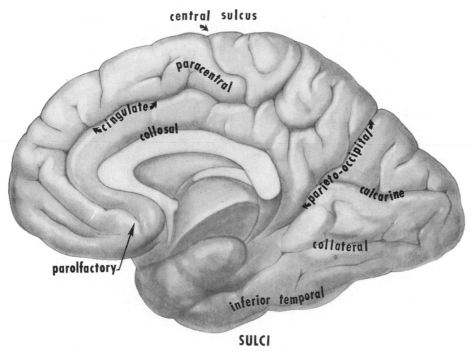

SULCI

Figure 17–8   Medial surface of the cerebrum; sulci and fissures identified.

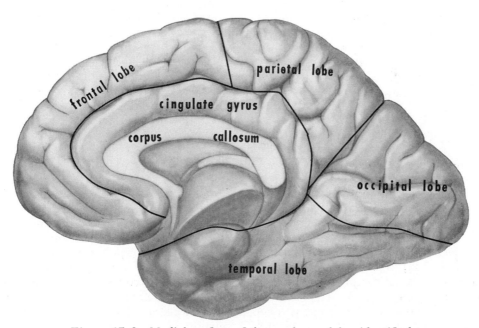

Figure 17–9   Medial surface of the cerebrum; lobes identified.

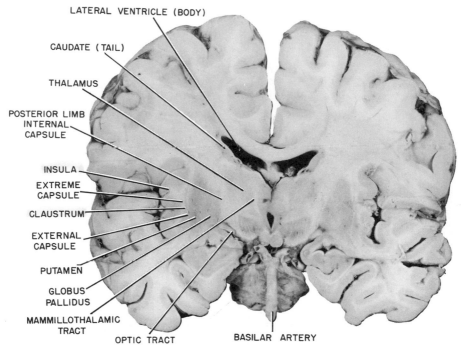

LATERAL VENTRICLE (BODY)

CAUDATE (TAIL)

THALAMUS

POSTERIOR LIMB
INTERNAL
CAPSULE

INSULA

EXTREME
CAPSULE

CLAUSTRUM

EXTERNAL
CAPSULE

PUTAMEN

GLOBUS
PALLIDUS

MAMMILLOTHALAMIC
TRACT

OPTIC TRACT

BASILAR ARTERY

Figure 17–10   Coronal slice of the cerebrum at level of lenticular nuclei.

vides the postural support which permits execution of voluntary movements; however, the extrapyramidal system is incapable of initiating movements. Lesions in the basal nuclei produce purposeless involuntary movements and loss of automatic movements, i.e., Parkinson's disease, choreiform movement, athetosis, and hemiballismus.

MEDULLARY CENTER OF THE CEREBRUM

The white matter of the cerebral hemisphere separates the cortex from the subcortical nuclei. Three different classes of fibers run in the medullary centers: projectional, commissural, and associational.

PROJECTION FIBERS

The projection fibers either arise in the cortex and end in the subcortical nuclei, brain stem, and spinal cord or terminate in the cortex (thalamocortical). The corticobulbar, corticospinal, corticothalamic, corticostriatal, fornix, external capsule, internal capsule, and thalamocortical fibers comprise the bulk of the projection fibers.

The *corona radiata* consists of bundles of corticoprojectional and thalamocortical fibers subjacent to the cortex. The axons tend to form bundles due to the intermingling with the callosal fibers.

Internal Capsule. The corona is continuous with the internal capsule which is a mass of medullated axon bordered medially from anterior to posterior by the head of the caudate, the thalamus, and the tail of the caudate and laterally by the lenticular nuclei (Fig. 17–11).

In horizontal sections (Fig. 17–32) the entire internal capsule is visualized and seen to consist of three parts: the anterior limb, genu, and posterior limb.

The *anterior limb* is found between the putamen and head of the caudate. The *genu* is bounded anteriorly by the head of caudate, posteromedially by the thalamus, and laterally by the lenticular nuclei.

The *posterior limb* lies medial to the lenticular nuclei and lateral to the thalamus. The posterior limb consists of the following portions: thalamolenticular, retrolenticular, and sublenticular. The *thalamolenticular* portion lies between the thalamus and lenticular nuclei and contains the corticospinal and sensory radiations. The *retrolenticular* portion of the posterior limb projects to the

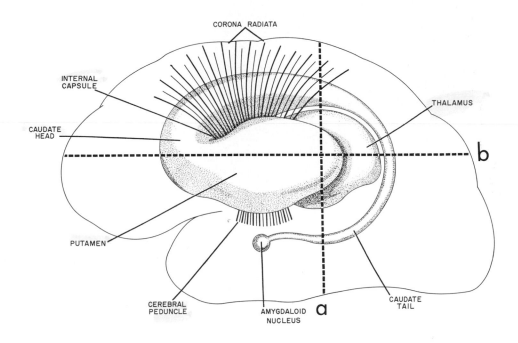

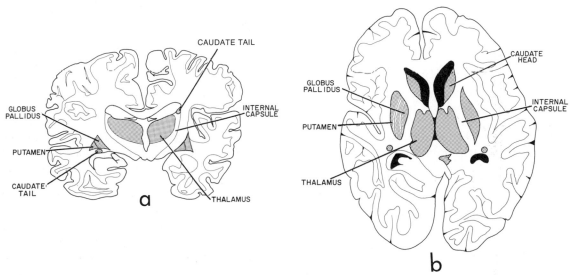

Figure 17–11 Diagrammatic representation showing relationship between basal ganglia, thalamus, and cerebral cortex in sagittal section (*top*) and coronal (a) and horizontal (b) sections. Figure 17–10 is a photograph at the same level as Figure 17–11a.

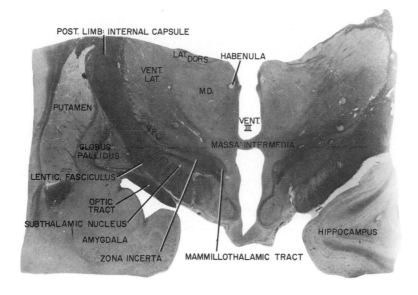

POST. LIMB: INTERNAL CAPSULE

LAT. DORS.   HABENULA

VENT. LAT.

M.D.

PUTAMEN

VENT. III

GLOBUS PALLIDUS

V.P.L.

MASSA INTERMEDIA

LENTIC. FASCICULUS

OPTIC TRACT

SUBTHALAMIC NUCLEUS

AMYGDALA

HIPPOCAMPUS

ZONA INCERTA   MAMMILLOTHALAMIC TRACT

Figure 17–12 Coronal section, level of massa intermedia, demonstrating relationship between basal nuclei, internal capsule, and diencephalon.

visual cortex, while the *sublenticular* portions connect to the auditory, parietal, and occipital cortex.

Many clinically significant fiber bundles run in the internal capsule. In the genu are found corticobulbar fibers which provide voluntary control of muscles in the head and neck. In the posterior limb are found: (a) corticospinal fibers which exert voluntary control over muscles in the extremities; (b) thalamocortical sensory radiations from the entire body, head, and neck; (c) visual radiations; and (d) auditory radiations.

A lesion in the internal capsule commonly due to the occlusion of the lenticular branches of the middle cerebral arteries will produce a hemiparesis resulting in loss of voluntary control of muscles of the contralateral face, arm, and leg. Impairment in contralateral sensation and the contralateral visual field may also occur.

External Capsule. The external capsule forms the lateral border of the putamen. Fibers from all cortical lobes enter the external capsule and connect to the putamen and globus pallidus.

The fornix will be discussed in detail in the visceral brain; it connects the hippocampus to the hypothalamus.

COMMISSURAL FIBERS

This category of axons connects the two hemispheres. The hippocampal commissure, the anterior commissure, and the corpus callosum are the cerebral commissures.

The *hippocampal commissure* connects the hippocampus, fornix, and portions of the parahippocampal cortex of one hemisphere to the other.

The *anterior commissure* interconnects the olfactory bulbs, olfactory cortex, basilar amygdaloid nuclei, and neocortex in the middle and inferior temporal gyri and occipitotemporal gyri. The fibers from the temporal gyri form the bulk of the anterior commissure.

The *corpus callosum* or great cerebral commissure is the largest telencephalic commissure and consists primarily of myelinated axons. It is divided into a rostrum, genu, body, and splenium. It forms the roof of the anterior horn and the roof of the body of the lateral ventricles. Its anterior radiations toward the frontal pole are called anterior forceps, while its posterior radiations toward the occipital pole are called the posterior forceps. The corpus callosum permits learning and memory in one hemisphere to be shared with the other hemisphere. All cortical regions are not interconnected via the corpus callosum, i.e., digital regions of the sensory and motor cortex and most of the visual cortex.

ASSOCIATION FIBERS

Association fibers interconnect cortical areas in the same hemisphere. They may be any length, connecting distant areas and frontal and occipital regions, or as close by as the adjacent gyrus. The external capsule

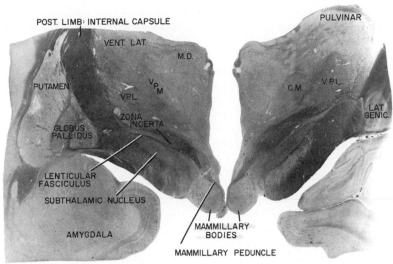

Figure 17–13 Coronal section, level of mammillary bodies I, demonstrating relationship between basal nuclei, internal capsule, and diencephalon.

is included in the association category. Lesions in the associational fibers may produce deficits in memory, speech, and other higher cortical functions. These fiber systems will be discussed in greater detail in Chapters 20 and 21.

ARTERIAL SUPPLY

Two arterial trunks supply the brain: the internal carotids and the vertebrals. The internal carotids provide the circulation to the anterior part of the brain, while the vertebrals provide the blood supply to the posterior and inferior part of the brain.

Internal Carotids. The internal carotids pass through the carotid canal in the petrous portion of the temporal bone and enter the middle cranial fossa. In the cavernous sinus the ophthalmic artery arises to supply the orbital contents. The terminal branches of the internal carotid are the anterior cerebral, middle cerebral, posterior communicating, and choroid arteries.

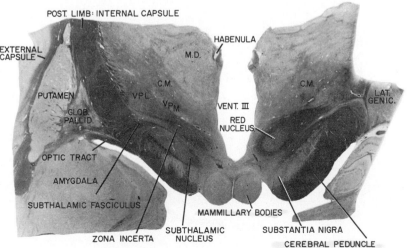

Figure 17–14 Coronal section, level of mammillary bodies II, demonstrating relationship between basal nuclei, internal capsule, and diencephalon.

Choroid Artery. The choroid artery supplies the optic tract, the choroid plexus in the lateral ventricles, and the posterior limb of the internal capsule and globus pallidus.

Anterior Cerebral Artery. The anterior cerebral (Fig. 17–15) irrigates the optic chiasm, the anterior limb of the internal capsule, the head of the caudate, the rostrum, genu, and body of the corpus callosum, and the medial surface of the hemisphere up to the parietooccipital fissure.

Middle Cerebral Artery. The middle cerebral artery passes laterally around the anterior perforated substance into the lateral fissure (Fig. 17–16). This vessel irrigates anterior and medial parts of the thalamus, the genu of the internal capsule, all of the putamen, and portions of the globus pallidus and caudate (lenticulostriate arteries), as well as most of the lateral surface of the hemisphere (Fig. 17–17).

Communicating Arteries. The anterior and middle cerebral arteries are connected with the posterior cerebral by the posterior communicating artery which completes the cerebral arterial circle of Willis (Fig. 17–16 *A, B*).

The anterior cerebrals (Fig. 17–16) are interconnected by the anterior communicating artery. The anterior cerebral connects directly with the middle cerebral, while the posterior communicating artery connects the middle and posterior cerebral arteries.

Normally the communicating vessels are small, and the flow is such that the middle and anterior cerebrals are supplied directly by the internal carotid, and the posterior cerebrals by the vertebral arteries. Occasionally one of the posterior cerebral arteries is connected to the internal carotid which then provides a direct channel between the anterior and posterior circulation. Small vessels originate from the circle of Willis and irrigate the hypothalamus, median eminence, and hypophyseal stalk.

Vertebrals. The *posterior circulation* (Fig. 17–16) consists of the vertebral arteries which arise from the subclavian artery and enter the cranial cavity via the foramen magnum and provide irrigation to the dura mater (posterior meningeal artery), the spinal cord (anterior and posterior spinal arteries), the medulla (paramedian branches), and the cerebellum (posterior inferior cerebellar artery). Each vertebral artery terminates by fusing with the other vertebral artery to form the basilar artery at the inferior border of the pons. The anterior spinal artery is a paramedian branch of the vertebral arteries.

Basilar Artery. The basilar artery irrigates the anterior part of the inferior cerebellar surface (anterior inferior cerebellar artery), the internal ear (labyrinthine artery), the pons (paramedian, short circumferential and long and circumferential pontine arteries), and the superior surface of the cerebellum (superior cerebellar artery). It terminates as

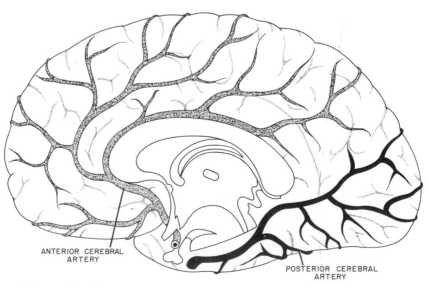

ANTERIOR CEREBRAL
ARTERY

POSTERIOR CEREBRAL
ARTERY

Figure 17–15 Distribution of posterior and anterior cerebral arteries.

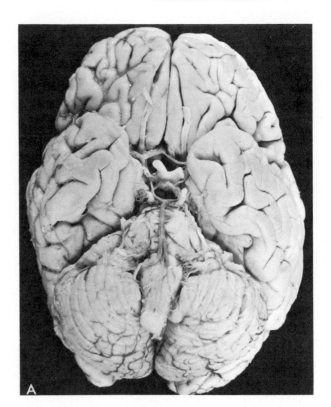

Figure 17-16 Arterial supply to the brain, circle of Willis. *A*, Base of brain with blood vessels. *B*, Arterial circle of Willis dissected out and labeled.

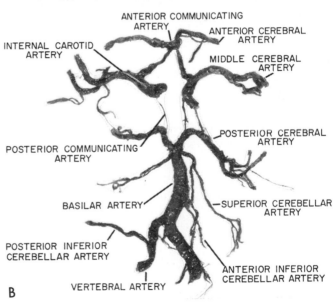

ANTERIOR COMMUNICATING ARTERY

ANTERIOR CEREBRAL ARTERY

INTERNAL CAROTID ARTERY

MIDDLE CEREBRAL ARTERY

POSTERIOR CEREBRAL ARTERY

POSTERIOR COMMUNICATING ARTERY

BASILAR ARTERY

SUPERIOR CEREBELLAR ARTERY

POSTERIOR INFERIOR CEREBELLAR ARTERY

ANTERIOR INFERIOR CEREBELLAR ARTERY

VERTEBRAL ARTERY

B

the posterior cerebral artery which unites with the posterior communicating artery to form the posterior part of the circle of Willis.

The supply to the medulla, pons, and cerebellum arises from the vertebral and basilar vessels and is divided into paramedian, short circumferential, and long circumferential vessels (Fig. 17–18). The paramedian branches originate from the main trunk and pass directly into the anterior surface of the pons or medulla. The short circumferential vessels go to the lateral surface, the long circumferential finally reach as far as to the ventricular lumen on the posterior surface.

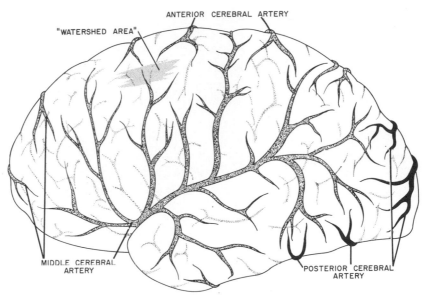

"WATERSHED AREA"

ANTERIOR CEREBRAL ARTERY

MIDDLE CEREBRAL ARTERY

POSTERIOR CEREBRAL ARTERY

Figure 17–17 Distribution of middle cerebral artery.

Posterior Cerebral Artery. The posterior cerebral artery (Fig. 17–15) passes laterally and posteriorly around the peduncles and continues onto the inferior surface of the hemisphere and irrigates the cerebral peduncles, midbrain, posterior thalamus, geniculate nuclei (thalamogeniculate artery), medial surface of the temporal lobe, and cuneus; it terminates by supplying the visual cortex.

Communicating Links. There are some anastomotic channels between the various cortical arteries but usually they are inadequate, explaining why a blockage of blood supply usually produces some neuronal death with resultant neurological deficit. A common interruption of arterial circulation results from insufficiency of the carotid artery, with a resultant ischemia to the hand region on the pre- and postcentral gyrus. This region is called the "water shed" or border zone and receives its blood supply from the middle cerebral artery with little collateral circulation from the anterior cerebral artery (Fig. 17–17). If the anterior cerebral artery on one side has decreased flow, the arterial blood from the opposite anterial cerebral artery will supply the affected side via the anterior communicating artery.

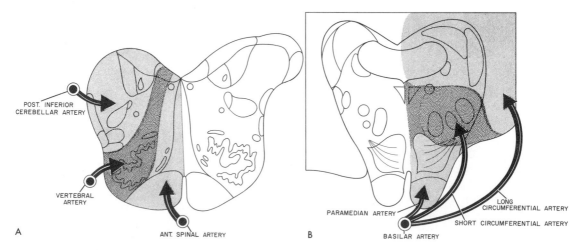

POST. INFERIOR CEREBELLAR ARTERY

VERTEBRAL ARTERY

ANT. SPINAL ARTERY

A

PARAMEDIAN ARTERY

BASILAR ARTERY

LONG CIRCUMFERENTIAL ARTERY

SHORT CIRCUMFERENTIAL ARTERY

B

Figure 17–18 Arterial supply to medulla (*A*) and pons (*B*). The anterior spinal artery is a paramedian branch of the vertebrals.

VENOUS DRAINAGE FROM CEREBRAL HEMISPHERES (Fig. 17–19)

The cerebral veins have very thin walls, no muscular layer, and no valves. They are found on the surface of the brain or in the substance of the central nervous system.

Superficial Cerebral Veins. The superficial cerebral veins lie in the sulci and are thinner and usually more external than the arteries. They consist of the superior, middle, and inferior cerebral veins. A variable number of *superior cerebral veins* drain the superior surface of the cerebral cortex and empty into the superior sagittal sinus. The *middle cerebral veins* drain the bulk of the lateral and inferior surface; these vessels are found in the lateral fissure and empty into the cavernous sinus. The *inferior cerebral veins* drain the lateral occipital gyrus and the temporal lobe; this vessel opens directly into the transverse sinus.

Internal Cerebral Veins. The internal cerebral veins and the basal vein are the principal cerebral veins. These vessels conduct blood from the center of the cerebrum and converge upon the single great *cerebral vein* (of Galen) which empties into the straight sinus. The vein of Galen collects venous blood from the medullary center, diencephalon, basal ganglia, and midbrain.

Each of the internal cerebral veins is formed near the foramen of Monro by the union of veins from the lenticular nuclei, caudate, septum, and choroid plexus. The internal cerebral veins run backward in the velum interpositum in the roof of the third ventricle.

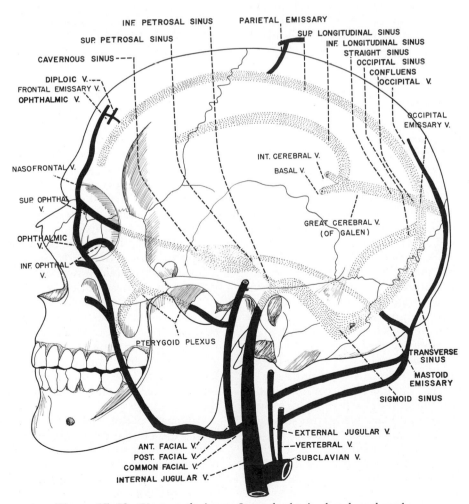

Figure 17–19 Venous drainage from the brain, head, and neck.

Basal Vein. The paired *basal vein* (of Rosenthal) originates near the anterior perforated substance by the union of vessels from the corpus callosum, thalamus, insula, and anterior temporal lobe. Each vein passes posteriorly around the cerebral peduncle and unites with the internal cerebral veins behind the splenium of the corpus callosum to form the cerebral vein (of Galen).

Superior Cerebellar Veins. The superior cerebellar veins ramify on the superior surface of the cerebellum. Some branches join the straight sinus and great cerebral vein, while other branches run into the transverse and superior petrosal sinus.

Inferior Cerebellar Veins. The inferior cerebellar veins drain the inferior surface of the cerebellum. Some vessels go superiorly into the inferior petrosal sinus and transverse sinuses, while other branches pass posteriorly into the occipital sinus. The veins which drain the medulla and pons terminate in the superior and inferior petrosal sinuses.

Sinuses. The sinuses in the dura mater consist of blood vessels lined with endothelium enwrapped between the periosteal and meningeal layers of the dura mater. These channels convey blood from the superficial and deep cerebral veins and the veins in the orbit, meninges, and diploe into veins in the neck and ultimately back to the superior vena cava. The sinuses can be divided into median unpaired channels and lateral paired channels. The unpaired median sinuses are the superior sagittal, inferior sagittal, straight, occipital confluens, circular, and basilar sinuses. The paired lateral sinuses are the transverse, sigmoid, superior and inferior petrosal, and cavernous sinuses.

The *superior sagittal sinus* is found in the attached margin of the falx cerebri in the inner surface of the cranium from the sagittal groove on the foramen cecum to the internal occipital protuberance. It is small anteriorly and enlarges as it proceeds posteriorly. At the internal occipital protuberance the superior sagittal sinus curves downward and joins the transverse sinus at the confluens.

The superior sagittal sinus communicates with the superficial temporal veins by means of the parietal emisssary veins; the superior cerebral veins empty directly into it.

The arachnoid granulations (Fig. 17–22), which are located in the margins of the sinus, provide a means for the cerebrospinal fluid in the subarachnoid space to pass into the venous circulation.

The *inferior sagittal sinus* is found in the free margin of the falx cerebri at the junction of the falx and the cerebelli tentorum. It joins the great cerebral vein to form the straight sinus.

The *straight sinus* continues into the confluens and then onto the *transverse sinus* which lies horizontally in a groove along the squamous portion of the occipital bone, the mastoid angle of the parietal bone, and the petrous portion of the temporal bone. It also lies in the attached margin of the cerebellar tentorum.

The *sigmoid sinus* is the continuation of the transverse sinus to the jugular fossa where it becomes continuous with the internal jugular vein. The sigmoid sinus lies in the temporal and occipital bones.

The *cavernous sinus* consists of numerous venous channels which are found in the dura mater on either side of the sella turcica. It continues from the medial portion of the superior orbital fissure to the apex of the petrous bone. The rootlets of nerves III and IV and the ophthalmic and maxillary divisions of nerve V (carotid siphon) are within its lateral walls. The internal carotid, with the rootlet of nerve VI on its lateral surface, is also found within the sinus, separated from it by the endothelial lining. The cavernous sinus anteriorly receives the ophthalmic vein, middle cerebral veins, and veins from the hypophyseal plexus.

Posteriorly the *superior* and *inferior petrosal sinuses* drain the cavernous sinus and connect it respectively with the transverse sinus and the internal jugular vein. The superior and inferior petrosal sinuses lie in grooves with the same name in the petrous portion of the temporal bone. Anteriorly the superior and inferior ophthalmic veins connect the cavernous sinus to the anterior facial vein.

The *circular sinus* surrounds the hypophysis and connects to the cavernous sinus. The basilar plexus connects the cavernous sinus with the vertebral plexus.

It has been demonstrated that venous blood leaves the brain principally via the internal jugular and vertebral veins and plexus.

Alternate pathways by which venous blood leaves the cranial cavity are provided by the following emissary veins: frontal, parietal, occipital, and mastoid (Fig. 17–19). In addition the superior and inferior ophthalmic veins provide another channel by which blood leaves the cavernous sinus and enters the anterior facial vein. The venous plexus of the internal carotid connects the cavernous sinus and the internal jugular vein.

MENINGES

The brain and spinal cord are enclosed by three membranes: (1) an inner more delicate membrane, the pia, in which the blood vessels are found; (2) an intermediate two-layer membrane filled with cerebrospinal fluid, the arachnoid; and (3) an outer tough protective membrane, the dura.

Pia Mater. The pia mater appears to be part of the brain and spinal cord (Fig. 17–20). It is actually attached to the central nervous system by the network of blood vessels which run in the pia and then penetrate the central nervous system with a portion of pia extending onto the blood vessels. The pia fuses with the dura and is continuous with the perineurium of the cranial and peripheral nerves.

The cranial pia mater invests the entire external surface of the brain, running into the sulci and fissures of the cerebrum and cerebellum. It also forms the non-nervous roof of the third, lateral, and fourth ventricles in combination with the choroid plexus and ependyma, the tela choroidea.

The pia is perforated at the midline of the roof and at the lateral recess of the fourth ventricle respectively by the foramina of Magendie and Luschka which permits cerebrospinal fluid to pass into the subarachnoid space from which it can escape into the venous sinuses.

The denticulate ligaments of the pia anchor the spinal cord to the dura. This fibrous band extends from the lateral surface of the spinal cord to the inner surface of the dura between the dorsal and ventral roots. The lateral margin of this ligament has a denticulate appearance because it is attached to the dura at regular intervals at 21 points. The most superior attachment is at the foramen magnum, and the most inferior at the conus medullaris.

Arachnoid. The arachnoid is a delicate membrane between the dura and pia (Fig. 17–20). The space between the arachnoid and pia is maintained by trabeculae consisting of fibrous and elastic connective tissue connecting the inner arachnoid surface to the outer pia surface. This space (subarachnoid) is filled with cerebrospinal fluid. The arachnoid membrane bridges over the sulci in the cerebrum and extends from the posterior surface of the medulla to the cerebellum (cisterna magna) and below the neural end of the spinal cord (lumbar cistern), forming large cisterns which contain pools of cerebrospinal fluid. These cisterns are clinically important since a needle can be inserted into the cistern and the cerebrospinal fluid drawn out and tested to determine if the patient has had any disease or trauma.

Other cisterns are also formed by the arachnoid membranes (callosal, pontine, postchiasmaticus, prechiasmaticus, interpeduncular lamina terminalis, and postcollicular), but only the lumbar cistern or occasionally the cisterna magna is tapped.

The arachnoid membrane is usually separated from the dura by the subdural space, but in some places it may push into the dura and form arachnoidal villi (Figs. 17–20 and 17–21) which may also be found in the highly organized arachnoid granulation

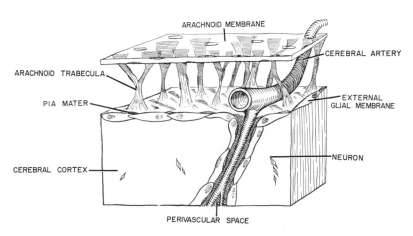

Figure 17–20 Diagrammatic representation showing the relationship between the meninges and blood vessels and brain.

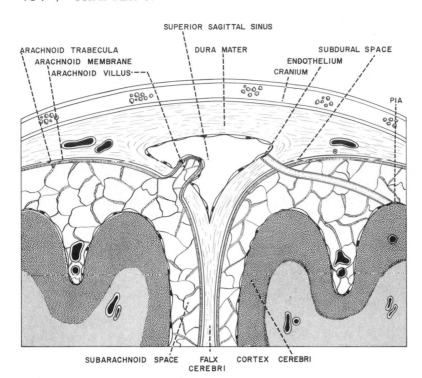

SUPERIOR SAGITTAL SINUS

ARACHNOID TRABECULA
ARACHNOID MEMBRANE
ARACHNOID VILLUS

DURA MATER

SUBDURAL SPACE

ENDOTHELIUM
CRANIUM

PIA

SUBARACHNOID SPACE   FALX   CORTEX CEREBRI
CEREBRI

Figure 17–21 Diagrammatic representation showing the relationship between subarachnoid space, arachnoid granulations, and venous sinuses.

(Fig. 17–22). This is most common in the cerebral venous sinuses and permits the cerebrospinal fluid to pass into the venous drainage.

Dura Mater. The dura (Fig. 17–21), the external and thickest membrane enclosing the brain and spinal cord, consists of fibrous connective tissue. In the cranium the dura consists of a periosteal and meningeal portion; in the spinal cord the dura has only a meningeal portion.

SPINAL DURA. The spinal dura forms a sac surrounding the spinal cord from the foramen magnum to the second sacral vertebrae. The vertebrae have their own periosteal membrane. The spinal dural sac is attached at the margins of the foramen magnum and to the second and third cervical vertebrae and is continuous with the perineurial sheaths of the spinal nerves. It is also loosely attached to the inner surface of the second or third sacral vertebrae. It forms a covering for the filium terminale and becomes continuous with the periosteum on the dorsal surface of the coccyx as the coccygeal ligament. The extensive epidural space intervenes between the dura and the periosteum on the vertebrae. It contains loose areolar tissue and a venous plexus.

The sheath is much larger than the spinal cord and most of the interval between the cord and dura is filled by the fluid in the subarachnoid space.

In the adult the spinal cord stops at L1 while the dural tube continues to the level of the second sacral vertebrae from where the dura invests the filium terminale and the nerve roots. The subarachnoid space below the end of the actual spinal cord, the lumbar cistern, is filled with fluid which can be withdrawn and examined serologically, cytologically, and chemically to determine if any disease process is occurring.

CRANIAL DURA. In the cranial cavity the dura forms the periosteal membrane on the inner surface of the cranial bones. The inner or meningeal layer forms partitions between the cerebral hemispheres (falx cerebri), between the cerebellum and cerebrum (tentorum cerebelli), and between the cerebellar hemispheres (falx cerebelli). In the adult the periosteal and meningeal portions of the cranial dura may be fused.

The *falx cerebri* extends into the interhemispheric fissure and is attached to the inner surface of the cranial cavity from the crista Galli to the internal occipital protuberance where it is continuous with the tentorum

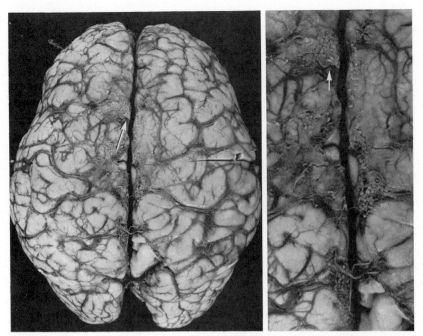

Figure 17–22 Dorsal surface of the brain demonstrating arachnoid granulation.

cerebelli. It contains at its attached margin the superior sagittal sinus while at its free margin it contains the inferior sagittal sinus.

The *tentorium cerebelli* separates the occipital lobes from the cerebellum. It is attached laterally and posteriorly to the transverse sinuses and anteriorly to the superior margin of the petrous portion of the temporal bone and to the posterior choroid process, leaving a space for the superior petrosal sinus. In the midline it is continuous with the falx cerebri and forms the straight sinus. Its free border, from the junction with the free edge of the falx cerebri to the anterior clinoid process, leaves an oval opening, the tentorial notch, for the passage of the brain stem.

The *falx cerebelli* is triangular and is attached to the occipital crest and the tentorum. Its free edge projects between the two cerebellar hemispheres.

The *diaphragma sellae* is a small fold which extends between the two clinoid processes and forms a roof over the hypophysis lying in the sellae turcicae. The infundibulum passes through a circular opening in the center of the diaphragm sellae. The circular sinus is found in the margin of the circular opening.

The *cavum trigeminal* (Meckel's cave) is a narrow cleft between the dural layers, on each side, at the trigeminal impression which is found on the apex of the petrous portion of the temporal bone. The ganglion of cranial nerve V is encased in this membrane.

VENTRICULAR SYSTEM

The lumen of the central nervous system initially is a hollow tube, which becomes greatly modified in appearance as the central nervous system develops. Within the first trimester, the simple tube is changed into the definitive structures: the paired lateral ventricles, third ventricle, cerebral aqueduct, fourth ventricle, and spinal canal.

Lateral Ventricle. The lateral ventricles are found within the cerebral hemispheres and are divided into an anterior horn, body, posterior horn, and inferior horn.

The relationships between the lateral ventricles and the cerebrum is best shown in a horizontal section through the cerebrum (Fig. 17–23). This slice demonstrates that the anterior horn lies in the frontal lobe and is continuous with the third ventricle at the level of the interventricular foramen (Fig. 17–23, arrows). The posterior horn is short and extends into the occipital lobe beginning at the junction of the body and inferior horn at the level of the splenium of the corpus callosum. The inferior horn curves downward into the temporal lobe.

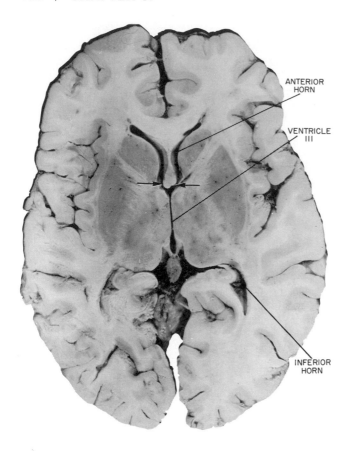

ANTERIOR
HORN

VENTRICLE
III

INFERIOR
HORN

Figure 17–23   Horizontal section showing ventricular system. Arrows identify the interventricular foramen.

Coronal sections will be used to demonstrate the structures which form the walls, floors, and roof of the lateral ventricles. The roof of the anterior horn and the inferior horn (see Fig. 17–26) is formed by the corpus callosum. The medial wall of the anterior horn is formed by the septum and genu of the corpus callosum. The walls and floor of the anterior horn are formed by the head of the caudate nucleus. The body is bounded medially by the septum and fornix and posteriorly by the splenium of the corpus callosum. The lateral walls of the body (see Fig. 17–29) are formed by the tail of the caudate and the stria terminalis and the medullary center of the cerebrum, while the floor is formed by the thalamus.

The inferior horn curves into the temporal lobe (see Fig. 17–29). The hippocampus and amygdala form its floor and medial walls while the medullary center of the temporal lobe forms the lateral wall. The lateral wall of the posterior horn is formed by the visual radiation, with the medullary center of the occipital lobe forming the remainder of the walls, floor, and roof. The choroid plexus is seen in the roof of the body and inferior horn.

Third Ventricle.   In the coronal sections (see Fig. 17–28) the third ventricle is seen as a narrow slit between the paired diencephalic masses.

In a sagittal section (Fig. 17–24) only one wall is shown. Rostrally the interventricular foramen is evident, while posteriorly the ventricular system narrows, becoming the cerebral aqueduct in midbrain levels. The *cerebral aqueduct* is bounded by the tegmentum (floor) and tectum (roof) of the midbrain and is inferiorly continuous with the rhomboid-shaped fourth ventricle which is found in pontine and medullary levels.

Fourth Ventricle.   The tegmentum of the pons and medulla forms the floor of the fourth ventricle. In pontine and upper medullary levels, the cerebellum and its fiber tracts form the roof of the fourth ventricle, while in lower pontine levels, the pia and choroid plexus (tela chorioid) form the roof. The fourth ventricle extends laterally and is continuous with the subarachnoid space at the foramen of Luschka. In the midline,

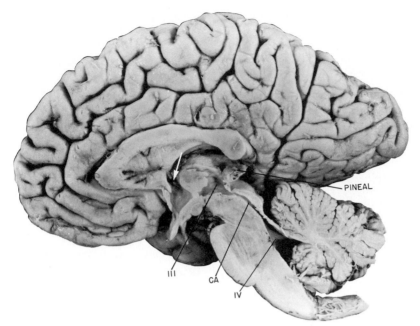

Figure 17–24 Sagittal section showing ventricular system. (CA = cerebral aqueduct; III = third ventricle; IV = fourth ventricle; arrow identifies interventricular foramen.)

where the roof of the fourth ventricle consists of the tela chorioid, the ventricle is also continuous with the subarachnoid space through the foramen of Magendie. Both the foramen of Luschka and the foramen of Magendie are usually not demonstrable in the gross brain, but they can be seen under experimental conditions. These foramina permit circulation of the cerebrospinal fluid from the ventricular system into the subarachnoid space and then into the venous circulation via the arachnoid villi in the venous sinuses.

The fourth ventricle is continuous with the narrow spinal canal which is completely surrounded by the gray matter of the spinal cord.

The ependymal cells form the lining of the ventricular system. These cells are cuboidal and ciliated (Fig. 3–29). The choroid plexus consists of modified ependymal cells placed external to the endothelial cells of the capillary network in the roof of the lateral ventricles and fourth ventricle. Current data suggests that the choroid plexus produces much of the cerebral spinal fluid which fills the ventricular system and subarachnoid space.

Subarachnoid Space. The subarachnoid space is maintained by fibrous trabeculae which extend from the inner surface of the arachnoid membrane onto the outer surface of the pia mater. The pia invests the central nervous system and dips into the sulci and fissures, while the arachnoid bridges the sulci and fissures. Consequently, the subarachnoid space varies and is very extensive in the sulci and fissures of the cerebrum, at the base of the brain between the optic chiasm and rostrum of the corpus callosum (cisternae chiasmaticus), and in the cerebral peduncles (cisterna interpeduncularis basalis), the cerebellum and the posterior surface of medulla (cisterna magna).

The blood vessels enter the nervous system through the subarachnoid space and are invested with a sleeve of the arachnoid which follows the blood vessels a short distance into the nervous system. The perivascular spaces provide another extensive area for accumulations of the cerebrospinal fluid.

CEREBROSPINAL FLUID

The cerebrospinal fluid (CSF) in the ventricles and subarachnoid space in concert with the meninges encases the brain in a fluid medium which provides a protective suspension for the brain. All parts of the ventricular system and subarachnoid space are in communication.

The normal CSF (lumbar puncture) in the adult consists of (a) 100 to 140 ml. of clear, colorless fluid with a specific gravity of 1.003 to 1.009, (b) a pH of 7.35 to 7.4 (c) 50 to 75 mg. of glucose/100 ml. of CSF, (d) 15 to 40 mg. of protein, (e) 3 to 5 mononuclear cells/cu mm., and (f) 120 to 130 mEq/L. of chloride. The pressure of the CSF when the adult patient lies on one side is 70 to 200 mm. of water.

The cerebrospinal fluid is formed primarily in the choroid plexus and absorbed principally through the arachnoid villi in the dural sinuses, with some absorption also occurring in the capillaries of the choroid plexus. The arachnoid villi form only a thin two-cell barrier (arachnoid and endothelium) between the cerebrospinal fluid and the venous supply and appear to be the preferred channel of absorption.

Blockage of the ventricular-subarachnoid-arachnoid villi circulation produces increased intracranial pressure due to the continued production of cerebrospinal fluid and the decreased absorption. In these circumstances, the ventricular system dilates, but since there

is very little extra space in the cranial cavity, the swelling of the ventricular system produces compression of the nervous system with concomitant neurological symptoms. This condition is termed *hydrocephalus* (Fig. 2–16). Blockage of the subarachnoid space, i.e., by meningeal adhesions, is called communicating hydrocephalus. Any blockage of the ventricular system produces a noncommunicating hydrocephalus. Congenital abnormalities in the formation of the ventricular system (stenosis or atresia) can also produce a noncommunicating hydrocephalus.

CORONAL AND HORIZONTAL BRAIN SECTIONS

The previous section has detailed the gross anatomy of the brain, blood vessels, and meninges. This section will identify many of these structures in coronal and horizontal slices of the brain.

Coronal Slice I (Fig. 17–25). Level: genu of the corpus callosum. In this slice only the

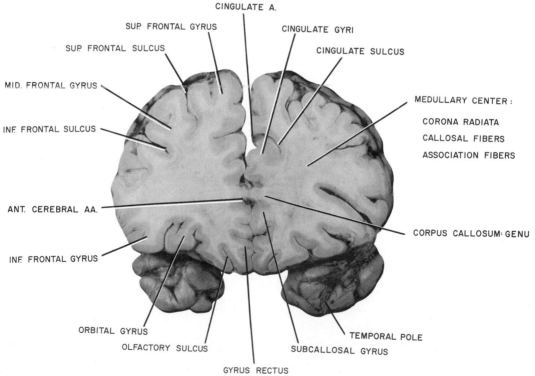

Figure 17–25 Coronal slice: level – genu of the corpus callosum.

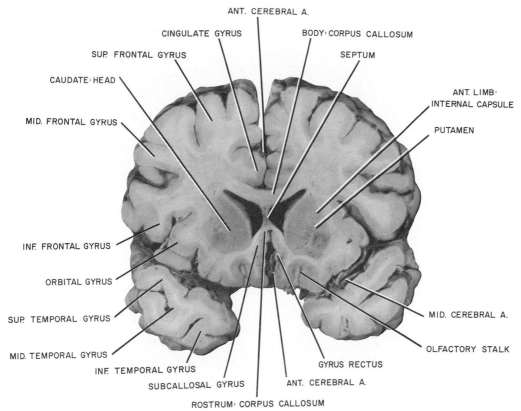

ANT. CEREBRAL A.

CINGULATE GYRUS

SUP. FRONTAL GYRUS

CAUDATE: HEAD

MID. FRONTAL GYRUS

INF. FRONTAL GYRUS

ORBITAL GYRUS

SUP. TEMPORAL GYRUS

MID. TEMPORAL GYRUS

INF. TEMPORAL GYRUS

SUBCALLOSAL GYRUS

ROSTRUM: CORPUS CALLOSUM

BODY: CORPUS CALLOSUM

SEPTUM

ANT. LIMB: INTERNAL CAPSULE

PUTAMEN

MID. CEREBRAL A.

OLFACTORY STALK

GYRUS RECTUS

ANT. CEREBRAL A.

Figure 17–26   Coronal slice: level—rostrum of the corpus callosum.

cerebral cortex and medullary center of the telencephalon are present.

Gyri.   Portions of the frontal and cingulate lobes are present on this slice. The temporal pole is present beneath the inferior surface of the brain.

Arteries.   Note that the anterior cerebral arteries are curving around the genu of the corpus callosum. This vessel supplies the medial surface of the hemisphere up to the parieto-occipital fissure.

Coronal Slice II (Fig. 17–26).   Level: rostrum of corpus callosum. In this section a portion of the deep telencephalic gray is now seen (caudate and putamen). The temporal lobe is still separated from the remainder of the cerebrum. The corpus callosum is now a thick band of fibers forming the roof of the anterior horn of the lateral ventricle. The olfactory stalk in the olfactory sulcus on the base of the frontal lobe is attached to the inferior surface of the frontal lobe.

Frontal Lobe.   The following gyri are present: superior, middle, inferior, orbital, and

rectus. These are the frontal associational areas.

Temporal Lobe.   The most anterior tip of the superior, and middle, inferior gyri are present.

Cingulate Lobe.   This cortex is found above the corpus callosum in all levels from the genu through the splenium.

White Matter.   The anterior limb of the internal capsule separates caudate from putamen.

Arteries.   Note that the anterior cerebral arteries are seen in the interhemispheric sulcus above and below the corpus callosum. The middle cerebral arteries are seen entering the lateral fissure.

Coronal Slice III (Fig. 17–27).   Level: anterior commissure. The temporal lobe is now connected to the remainder of the cerebral hemisphere.

Frontal Lobe.   The same gyri are present as in slice II.

Temporal Lobe.   The superior, middle, inferior, occipital-temporal, and parahippo-

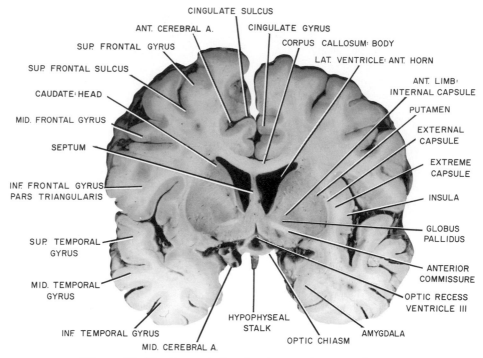

Figure 17-27 Coronal slice: level—anterior commissure.

campal gyri are present from the lateral to the medial surface.

Note the location of the insular and cingulate cortex: respectively internal to the lateral fissure and above the corpus callosum. The anterior commissure is seen below the lenticular nuclei (globus pallidus and putamen) and above the olfactory area.

White Matter. The optic chiasm is seen attached to the base of the brain. The optic recess of the third ventricle is the lumen above the optic chiasm. The septum forms the medial wall separating the body of the lateral ventricles. The anterior limb of the internal capsule is seen between the caudate and putamen.

Arteries. The middle cerebral artery is seen at its point of origin from the internal carotid and in the lateral fissure. Identify the anterior cerebrals in the interhemispheric fissure.

Hypophyseal Stalk. This structure is seen medially on the inferior surface of the brain.

Coronal Slice IV (Fig. 17-28). Level: anterior nucleus of the thalamus. This is the first level to include part of the diencephalon.

Frontal Lobe. The superior, middle, inferior, and precentral gyri are present.

Parietal Lobe. This is the first slice to in-

clude parietal cortex. The postcentral (sensory) gyrus is seen forming the roof of the lateral fissure.

Temporal Lobe. The superior, middle, inferior, occipitotemporal, and parahippocampal gyri are present. A portion of the transverse temporal gyri (auditory cortex) is found internal to the superior temporal gyri in the depths of the lateral fissure. The hippocampal formation, with the inferior horn of the lateral ventricle at its medial surface, is the most medial portion of the temporal lobe.

Thalamus. The anterior nucleus protrudes into the floor of the lateral ventricle (body). The mammillothalamic tract is seen entering the inferior surface of the anterior nucleus.

Hypothalamus. The mammillary bodies are prominent on the base of the diencephalon. The fornix is seen suspended from the body of the corpus callosum, and the column of the fornix is seen in the hypothalamus. This tract connects the hippocampus to the hypothalamus.

White Matter. The posterior limb of the internal capsule is seen lateral to the thalamus. Many of the fibers of the internal capsule continue to the inferior surface of the brain where they form the cerebral ped-

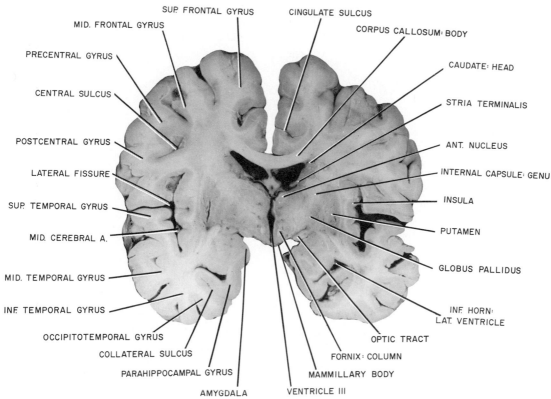

SUP. FRONTAL GYRUS

MID. FRONTAL GYRUS

PRECENTRAL GYRUS

CENTRAL SULCUS

POSTCENTRAL GYRUS

LATERAL FISSURE

SUP. TEMPORAL GYRUS

MID. CEREBRAL A.

MID. TEMPORAL GYRUS

INF. TEMPORAL GYRUS

OCCIPITOTEMPORAL GYRUS

COLLATERAL SULCUS

PARAHIPPOCAMPAL GYRUS

AMYGDALA

CINGULATE SULCUS

CORPUS CALLOSUM: BODY

CAUDATE: HEAD

STRIA TERMINALIS

ANT. NUCLEUS

INTERNAL CAPSULE: GENU

INSULA

PUTAMEN

GLOBUS PALLIDUS

INF. HORN:
LAT. VENTRICLE

OPTIC TRACT

FORNIX: COLUMN

MAMMILLARY BODY

VENTRICLE III

Figure 17-28   Coronal slice: level—anterior nucleus of the thalamus.

uncles. The base of the pons is seen behind the basilar artery.

Arteries. (Fig. 17–10). The basilar artery is seen blending into the posterior cerebral arteries which irrigate the medial and inferior surface of the hemisphere behind the parieto-occipital fissure. A portion of the posterior cerebral artery is also seen medial to the hippocampal formation. The middle and anterior cerebral arteries should be identified respectively in the lateral and interhemispheric fissure.

Coronal Slice V (Fig. 17–29). Level: habenular nucleus. In this section only a small portion of the caudate and putamen remains.

Frontal Lobe. Only the most medial portion of the precentral gyrus (motor cortex) remains.

Parietal Lobe. The postcentral and inferior parietal lobule are present.

Temporal Lobe. The transverse temporal (auditory cortex), superior, middle, inferior, occipitotemporal, and parahippocampal gyrus and hippocampus are found in this level. Cingulate and insular cortex are also evident.

Brain Stem. The bulk of the thalamus at this level consists of the pulvinar nuclei. The laminated lateral geniculate nucleus is found at the inferior, lateral margin of the telencephalon. The fibers of the optic tract synapse in this nucleus. The habenular nucleus of the epithalamus protrudes into the third ventricle. The red nucleus and the pigmented substantia nigra are prominent in the tegmentum of the midbrain. The visual radiation is seen leaving the lateral surface of the geniculate nucleus.

White Matter. The body of the fornix is suspended from the undersurface of the corpus callosum. The visual radiation is seen leaving the lateral surface of the lateral geniculate. The massive brachium pontis forms the base of the brain. The posterior commissure is seen crossing below the habenular nuclei; this fiber bundle interconnects the pretectal, tectal, and posterior portion of the thalamus.

Coronal Slice VI (Fig. 17–30). Level: splenium of the corpus callosum. This level is posterior to the thalamus. Frontal and insular cortex are absent from this level.

Parietal Lobe. The bulk of the cerebrum

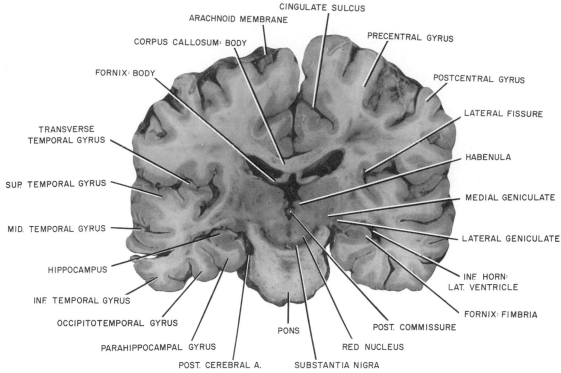

Figure 17–29 Coronal slice: level—habenular nuclei.

consists of the parietal lobe: the paracentral, superior, and inferior, parietal lobules are present.

Temporal Lobe. The superior, middle, inferior, occipitotemporal, parahippocampal, and hippocampus are present.

Midbrain. The tectum and tegmentum of the inferior colliculus are present.

Pons and Medulla. The pontine basis (middle cerebellar peduncle) and the medullary basis (medullary pyramid) are evident.

Cerebellum. The cerebellar hemispheres are noted below the temporal lobe.

Arteries. The posterior cerebral artery is found on the medial surface of the parahippocampal gyrus.

Ventricular System. In this section the inferior horn of the lateral ventricles is continuous with the body of the lateral ventricles. The cerebral aqueduct is seen in the midbrain.

White Matter. The bulk of this section consists of the medullary center of the cerebrum and the splenium of the corpus callosum. The visual radiations form much of the lateral wall of the ventricle.

Arteries. The posterior cerebral artery is seen on the lateral surface of the cerebral peduncle. The choroid plexus is prominent in the body of the lateral ventricles and third ventricle.

Meninges. On the superior surface of the cortex the arachnoid is seen bridging the sulci, showing how a large subarachnoid space is formed in these regions.

Coronal Slice VII (Fig. 17–31). Level: calcarine fissure. In this section, parietal, occipital, and temporal gyri are present.

Parietal Lobe. The superior parietal lobule and angular gyrus can be seen.

Occipital Lobe. The lateral occipital gyrus, lingula, and cuneus are present.

Temporal Lobe. The superior, middle, inferior, and occipitotemporal gyri form the main portion of the temporal lobe seen at this level.

Brain Stem. The cerebellar hemispheres and vermis cover the medulla.

Arteries. The posterior cerebral artery is seen adjacent to the calcarine fissure.

Ventricular System. The posterior horn of the lateral ventricles and the fourth ventricle are present. Note the choroid plexus in the fourth ventricle.

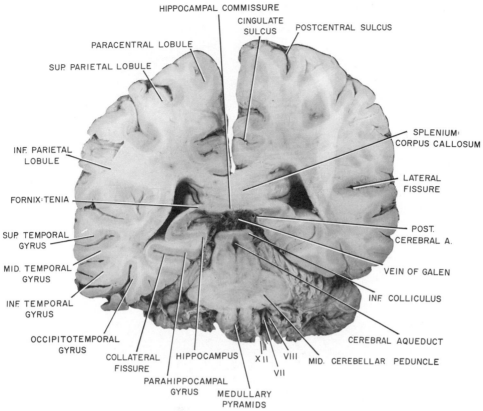

HIPPOCAMPAL COMMISSURE

CINGULATE SULCUS

POSTCENTRAL SULCUS

PARACENTRAL LOBULE

SUP. PARIETAL LOBULE

SPLENIUM: CORPUS CALLOSUM

INF. PARIETAL LOBULE

LATERAL FISSURE

FORNIX: TENIA

POST. CEREBRAL A.

SUP TEMPORAL GYRUS

VEIN OF GALEN

MID. TEMPORAL GYRUS

INF COLLICULUS

INF. TEMPORAL GYRUS

OCCIPITOTEMPORAL GYRUS

CEREBRAL AQUEDUCT

COLLATERAL FISSURE

HIPPOCAMPUS

X II

VIII

MID. CEREBELLAR PEDUNCLE

VII

PARAHIPPOCAMPAL GYRUS

MEDULLARY PYRAMIDS

Figure 17–30   Coronal slice: level—splenium of the corpus callosum.

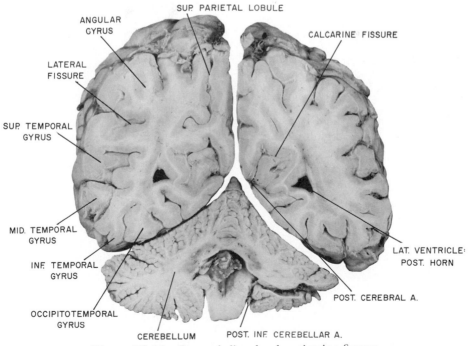

SUP. PARIETAL LOBULE

ANGULAR GYRUS

CALCARINE FISSURE

LATERAL FISSURE

SUP. TEMPORAL GYRUS

MID. TEMPORAL GYRUS

INF. TEMPORAL GYRUS

LAT. VENTRICLE: POST. HORN

OCCIPITOTEMPORAL GYRUS

POST. CEREBRAL A.

CEREBELLUM

POST. INF. CEREBELLAR A.

Figure 17–31   Coronal slice: level—calcarine fissure.

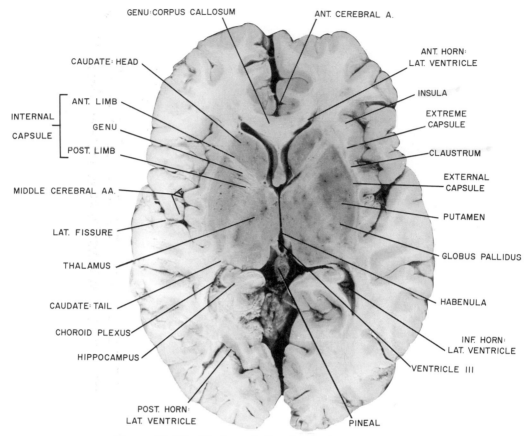

Figure 17–32 Horizontal slice: level — internal capsule.

Horizontal Slice (Fig. 17–32). Level: internal capsule. In this slice both hemispheres are present and connected by the corpus callosum.

Gyri. Identify the lateral fissure and the location of the frontal and occipital poles. Note that the interhemispheric fissure is wider occipitally.

White Matter. Identify the anterior limb, genu, and posterior limb of the internal cap-sule. Note the relationship between the anterior limb, head of the caudate and puta-men, posterior limb, thalamus, and globus pallidus. Locate the fornix.

Blood Vessels. Identify the anterior, mid-dle, and posterior cerebrals.

Ventricular System. Locate the third ven-tricle, anterior horn, body, and inferior horn of the lateral ventricle and note their re-lationship to the caudate and thalamus.

18

Taste, Olfaction, and the Emotional Brain

STANLEY JACOBSON

TASTE

The receptors for taste are the taste buds or gustatory cells located on the tongue, soft palate, palatoglossal arch, posterior wall of the pharynx, and posterior wall of the larynx.

Lingual Taste Buds. Three types of papillae are found on the dorsal surface of the tongue: filiform, fungiform, and circumvallate. Taste buds are associated only with the fungiform and circumvallate papillae. The fungiform and filiform papillae are scattered throughout the tongue, while the circumvallate papillae are arranged in a V-shaped region in the terminal sulcus (gustatory zone) where the free body of the anterior two-thirds of the tongue becomes continuous with the root of the tongue.

The taste buds (Fig. 18–1) are ovoid and consist of supporting cells and neuroepithelial cells with a pore opening onto the lingual surface. The neuroepithelial cells, numbering 6–20 per taste bud, are scattered between the supporting cells and have microvilli which project into the pore.

There are four distinct gustatory modalities: sweet, salt, bitter, and sour (acid). Certain regions of the tongue are most sensitive to one of these modalities. Although the tip of the tongue is sensitive to all modali-

ties, it is especially sensitive to sweet and salt. The sides of the tongue are most sensitive to sour or acid while the base is most sensitive to bitter.

Taste Sensation. Taste sensation is a mixture of gustatory sensation and olfactory impulses (Zotterman, 1963). The neuroepithelial cells in the taste buds have a brief life cycle, but their gustatory response continues unabated. The application of a substance to the tongue produces a generator potential in the neuroepithelium which is somehow transmitted across the basal laminae to the sensory axons where the all-or-none response originates. It appears that each neuroepithelial cell responds to all stimuli but it is usually most sensitive to only one modality.

Innervation of Taste Buds. The taste buds on the anterior two-thirds of the tongue are innervated by nerve VII (chorda tympani), while those on the posterior one-third of the tongue, including the circumvallate papillae, are innervated by nerve IX. The taste buds in the palatoglossal arch, pharynx, and larynx are innervated by nerve X. The course of nerve VII to the tongue should be reviewed in the chapter on cranial nerves (Chapter 10).

The primary axons of nerves VII, IX, and X enter the medulla, form the tractus solita-

425

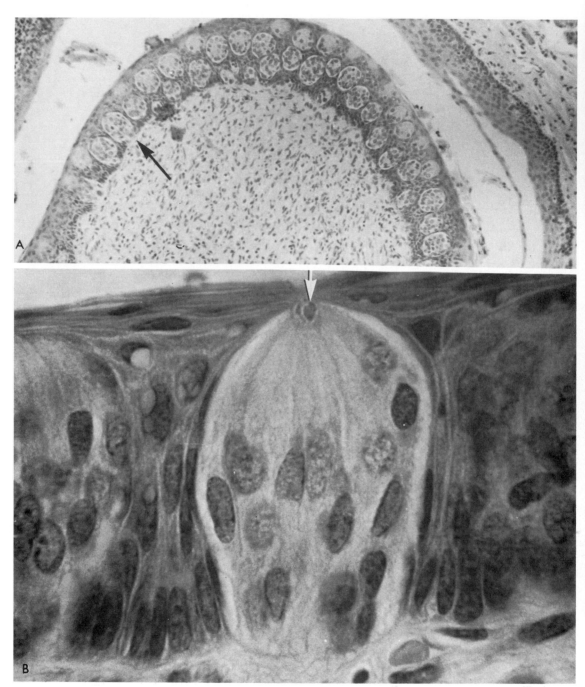

Figure 18–1 Taste buds. *A*, Circumvallate papillae of a rhesus monkey showing numerous taste buds. *B*, Taste bud; arrows identify gustatory pore into which the neuroepithelial cilia project. H & E stain.

rius, and terminate in the adjacent nucleus solitarius. The secondary gustatory fibers originate from the nucleus solitarius and ascend bilaterally in the medial lemniscus to the ventral posterior medial nucleus in the thalamus. The gustatory portion of the cortex is buried in the Sylvian fissure in the post-central gyrus. Crude awareness of taste occurs in the thalamus, but discrimination between different foodstuffs occurs at cortical levels.

Taste and Food Selection. Recent evidence has shown that taste plays a critical role in determining what an infant eats. In most animals, gustatory sensations from each foodstuff exercise great influence over the animal's intake, but in man this is not necessarily the case. We are affected by environmental pressure which produces bizarre eating habits that may even lead to obesity.

OLFACTION

OLFACTORY CORTEX

The olfactory portion of the brain (rhinencephalon-archipallium) comprises much of the telencephalon in fish, amphibians, and most mammals. In the higher primates, including man, the olfactory portion of the brain is found in the base of the frontal lobe on the inferior surfaces of the telencephalon and is greatly overshadowed by the great overgrowth of the neocortex (Fig. 18–2).

The term "rhinencephalon" initially denoted those areas which appeared to receive olfactory information, including the olfactory bulb, olfactory tract, pyriform cortex, hippocampus, isthmus cinguli, hippocampal gyrus, amygdala, septum, and cingulate cortex. In recent years it has been shown that only the olfactory bulb, olfactory tract, olfactory tubercle, pyriform cortex, and corticoamygdaloid nuclei receive olfactory impulses; the other portions of the telencephalon are now known to form the cortical regions of the emotional brain.

OLFACTORY SYSTEM (Fig. 18–3)

Olfactory Nerve. The olfactory nerve (cranial nerve I) originates from the uppermost portion of both nasal fossae which occupy the mucous membrane covering the superior nasal conchae and adjacent septum. The mucous membrane is attached to the walls of the nasal septum which in this region is formed by the ethmoid bone.

The 100 million or more bipolar receptor

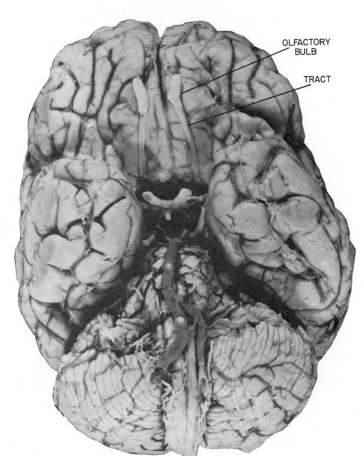

Figure 18–2 Gross view of ventral surface of brain demonstrating olfactory bulb and olfactory tract.

OLFACTORY BULB

TRACT

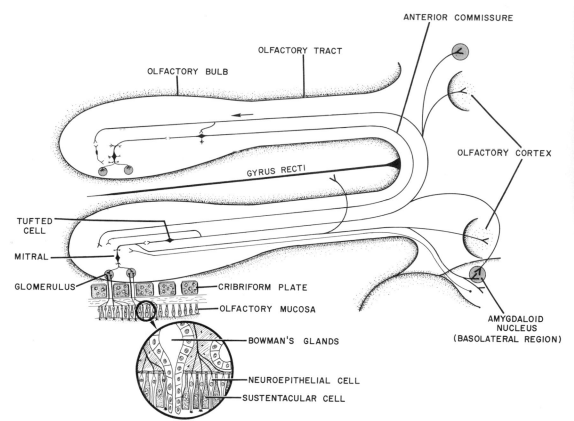

ANTERIOR COMMISSURE

OLFACTORY TRACT

OLFACTORY BULB

OLFACTORY CORTEX

GYRUS RECTI

TUFTED
CELL

MITRAL

GLOMERULUS

CRIBRIFORM PLATE

OLFACTORY MUCOSA

AMYGDALOID
NUCLEUS
(BASOLATERAL REGION)

BOWMAN'S GLANDS

NEUROEPITHELIAL CELL

SUSTENTACULAR CELL

Figure 18–3 Diagrammatic representation of the olfactory system. A portion of the olfactory mucosa is shown with the olfactory nerve. Cranial nerve I is seen ending in the glomeruli of the olfactory bulb. The axons of the mitral cells form most of the projections from the olfactory bulb to the septum, opposite the olfactory bulb via the anterior commissure or to the olfactory cortex.

cells are embedded in sustentacular, supporting cells. The dendrites of the receptor cells are short and ciliated. The cilia are embedded in the odor absorbing secretion which covers the mucosa and is secreted by the Bowman glands in the mucous membrane. All the axons from the olfactory neuroreceptor cells are unmyelinated and gather together into about 20 bundles (fila olfactoria) which then pass through openings in the cribriform plate of the ethmoid bone.

Olfactory Bulb. The olfactory bulb lies on the cribriform plates and upon microscopic inspection is seen to be laminated. The unmyelinated olfactory axons form the external layer of the bulb. They synapse with dendrites of mitral cells and tufted cells in the subjacent glomerular layer. The axons of about 20–30,000 bipolar olfactory cells terminate in one glomerulus. In addition, the axons of mitral cells and tufted cells also converge upon one single glomerulus. This

summation of olfactory information permits a high sensitivity to odoriferous substances.

There is probably no point-to-point relationship between the olfactory mucosa and olfactory bulb; instead there is wide overlap throughout the bulb due to the axon collaterals from the mitral and tufted cells diverging throughout the bulb. It has also been noted (Adrian, 1950) that each mitral cell is more sensitive to one class of odoriferous substances. Evidence points to discrimination between two odors in the bulb itself, with more complex discrimination and recognition found in the olfactory cortex (pyriform cortex).

Olfactory Stria. As previously noted the primary axons in the olfactory system originate from the olfactory receptor cells in the nasal fossae. The secondary axons originate from mitral and tufted cells and pass posteriorly as the olfactory stalk, enter the base of the hemisphere, and divide into a lateral, medial, and intermedial olfactory stria. The place where the olfactory tract enters the ventral surface of the telencephalon and divides is called the *olfactory trigone;* posterior to the trigone is the anterior perforated substance (olfactory tubercle) which is characterized in the gross brain by small perforations resulting from removal of small penetrating blood vessels.

The intermediate stria terminates in the olfactory tubercle. The medial olfactory stria terminates primarily in the septal region or continues into the anterior commissure and connects with the opposite olfactory bulb, while the lateral olfactory stria terminates in the olfactory cortex of the uncus and in the corticomedial amygdaloid nuclei.

Olfactory Discrimination. Vertebrates with a well-developed sense of smell are called "macrosomatic," while those with a poorly developed sense of smell are called "microsomatic." Dogs and cats are macrosomatic animals, while man and all of the great apes are microsomatic. Nevertheless man can still distinguish many different substances; in fact many people have built careers on their olfactory acuity: wine and coffee sniffers and perfumers. There is also the example of humans, without vision or hearing (blind or deaf), who can detect differences in their environment because of their acute sense of smell.

In all other sensory systems, such as vision and audition, it is possible to speak in terms of a basic measuring system, but in the olfactory system, degree of smell is a subjective matter. So only general rules for smell can be listed. In order for man to detect an odor, it must have some degree of volatility and water and lipid solubility. These qualities are necessary for the odor to reach the superior portion of the nasal conchae and penetrate the aqueous mucous membrane.

The loss of smell in man commonly occurs during a cold and causes food to have a bland taste due to the absence of any odor. The loss of smell can also result from injury to or compression of the olfactory nerves. This may occur from trauma or from tumors in the floor of the anterior and middle cranial fossa or from tumors involving any portion of the frontal lobe overlying the olfactory system. Disease of either uncus produces uncinate fits in which the patient has an olfactory aura of a disagreeable odor with associated visual and emotional aura (for more details see Chapter 21).

In these days of air pollution one wishes we were free of olfactory senses. However, the olfactory system is necessary for our survival as individuals and as a species: the aroma of food stimulates salivation, the musky scent of a female stimulates a male, unpleasant aromas produce nausea, vomiting, and tearing, and the strong odor of smoke produces fear.

EMOTIONAL BRAIN

Since the initial observations of Kluver and Bucy and Papez, which localized emotions in the telencephalon, many other investigators have added information concerning the localization of behavior so that now we know that many cortical and subcortical regions are incorporated into the "emotional brain."

Different investigators have coined different terms to succinctly describe this region: visceral brain, vital brain, emotional brain, and limbic system. The term visceral brain would seem appropriate since much of our emotional response is characterized by specific responses in the viscera. On the other hand, the importance of the emotional responses to the self-preservation of the individual and the perpetuation of the species has led other investigators to call this region the "vital brain" (MacLean, 1955). The term which has been used most commonly by investigators is limbic lobe (limbus = margin) because the region involved is located on the medial margin of the cerebrum.

The current author, however, chooses to use the term "emotional brain" because it best sums up, for didactic purposes, the functions of this region. By describing a large region of the brain as being devoted to the emotions, we can separate the entire central nervous system into a "somatic brain," which controls the external environment through the skeletal muscles, and an "emotional brain," which controls the internal environment through the smooth muscles and glands.

GROSS ANATOMY OF THE EMOTIONAL BRAIN

The structures related to the emotional brain are divided into cortical and subcortical regions. With the exception of the frontal association cortex (areas 9, 10, 11, and 12), the cortical structures are found on the medial and ventral surface of the hemisphere.

The medial surface of a hemisphere and brain stem, as shown in Figure 18-4, demonstrates the following structures: the cingulate cortex at the cortical level and the thalamus and hypothalamus (unlabeled) in the subcortical region.

In Figure 18-5 the brain stem has been sectioned at the mesencephalic-diencephalic junction and the midbrain, pons, medulla, and cerebellum removed. Now the ventral and medial surface of the cerebrum are visible and the following cortical structures are seen: uncus, amygdaloid nuclei and olfactory cortex, parahippocampal gyrus, isthmus cinguli, cingulate cortex and subcallosal gyrus, subcortical-thalamus, septum, and the mammillary body of the hypothalamus.

In the final figure of this series (Fig. 18-6), the entire diencephalon has been removed so that the relationship between the uncus, hippocampus, and fornix can be seen.

It should be noted that the *fornix* is the efferent pathway from the hippocampus and is connected to the hypothalamus, septum, and thalamus. This tract takes a rather circuitous pathway to reach the hypothalamus.

The fornix originates from the hippocampus in the medial surface of the temporal lobe and runs in the medial wall of the inferior horn of the lateral ventricle, and in the medial wall of the body of the lateral ventricle suspended from the corpus callosum, finally entering the substance of the hypothalamus at the level of the interventricular foramen. Different portions of the fornix have specific names. Thus the portio-fimbria of the fornix may be found in the dorsal surface of the hippocampus, the portio-tenia connects from the hippocampus to the corpus callosum, the portio-corpus is located underneath the corpus callosum, entering the hypothalamus, and the portio-columnis is found in the substance of the hypothalamus. These relationships should be traced out in Figures 17-21 to 17-31 and in the atlas section (Figs. 29-21 to 29-24).

The pathway of the *stria terminalis* (the efferent fiber tract of the amygdala) parallels the fornix but it is found in relationship to the body and tail of the caudate nucleus on its medial surface (Figs. 29-16 and 29-17). The stria terminalis interconnects the amygdaloid nuclei as well as connecting the amygdala to the hypothalamus and septum.

The *septum* consists of two parts: (a) the rostral septum and septum pellucidum and

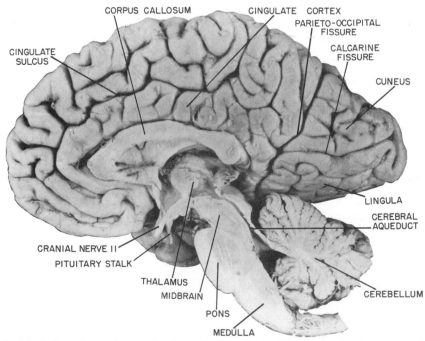

Figure 18-4 Medial surface of a cerebral hemisphere including entire brain stem and cerebellum.

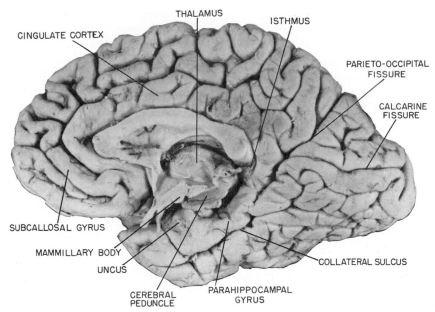

Figure 18-5 Medial surface of a cerebral hemisphere with medulla, pons, and cerebellum removed.

(b) the caudal velum interpositum. The septum pellucidum is rostral to the interventricular foramen. It consists primarily of a glial membrane with a few neurons which separates the anterior horn of the lateral ventricles. The lower part of the septum pellucidum consists of many neurons and glia, the septal area. Caudal to the interventricular foramen, the medial wall of the ventricle consists of glial membrane and some pia arachnoid (velum interpositum) with the bulk consisting of the fornix. This paired glial membrane, along with the fornix, separates the body of each lateral ventricle.

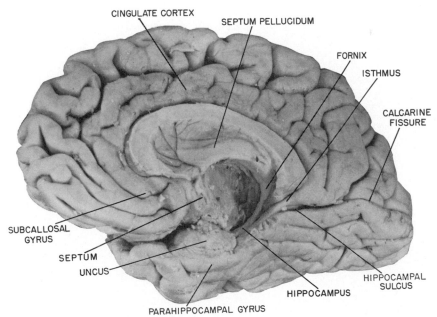

Figure 18-6 Medial surface of a cerebral hemisphere with thalamus removed, demonstrating relationship between fornix and hippocampus.

NUCLEI AND CIRCUITRY IN THE EMOTIONAL BRAIN

The structures of the visceral brain may be divided into subcortical neurons and cortical neurons and their associated fiber tracts.

SUBCORTICAL STRUCTURES

The subcortical nuclei in the emotional brain are the hypothalamus (preoptic, lateral, lateral mammillary nuclei), thalamus (midline, intralaminar, anterior, and dorsal medial nuclei), epithalamus, midbrain limbic nuclei (interpeduncular nucleus, paramedian nucleus, ventral tegmentum area, ventral half of the periaqueductal gray), septum, and the reticular formation of the brain stem and spinal cord.

Reticular Formation of Brain Stem and Spinal Cord.

The spinal and cranial nerve roots are the first order neurons for the somatic and visceral brain (Fig. 18–7). These peripheral nerves send axon collaterals into the reticular formation of the spinal cord, medulla, pons, and midbrain. The reticular formation is organized longitudinally, with the lateral zone being the receptor and the medial zone being the effector. In the medial zone are the ascending and descending multisynaptic fiber tracts of the reticular formation—the central tegmental tract. The mesencephalic portion of the reticular formation seems to be especially important since this zone provides a direct reciprocal pathway to the hypothalamus, thalamus, and septum.

Hypothalamus.

The hypothalamus is the highest subcortical center of the emotional brain; it receives input from all portions of the emotional brain as well as from the reticular formation, basal ganglia, and frontal associational cortex. The hypothalamus connects to the thalamus, midbrain, pons, and medulla via the medial forebrain bundle and the dorsal longitudinal fasciculus. Autonomic fibers from the hypothalamus run in the lateral portion of the reticular formation and descend to the thoracolumbar (sympathetic) and sacral levels (parasympathetic). The most potent effects result from the hypothalamic control of the adrenal medulla. The adrenal medulla releases epinephrine and norepinephrine which produce a decrease in peripheral blood flow, an increase in central blood flow, and an increase in heart rate and force. These agents also stimulate release of glycogen stores from the liver, providing energy for muscular contractions which accompany the response.

The *mammillary nuclei* of the hypothalamus connect to the anterior thalamic nuclei and habenula, via the mammillothalamic tract, and to nuclei in the brain stem tegmentum via the mammillotegmental tract. The lateral

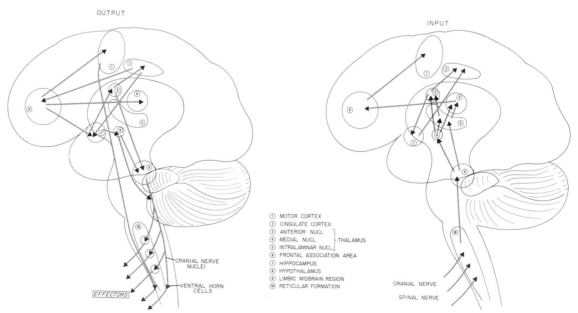

① MOTOR CORTEX
② CINGULATE CORTEX
③ ANTERIOR NUCL.
④ MEDIAL NUCL. ⎤ THALAMUS
⑤ INTRALAMINAR NUCL. ⎦
⑥ FRONTAL ASSOCIATION AREA
⑦ HIPPOCAMPUS
⑧ HYPOTHALAMUS
⑨ LIMBIC MIDBRAIN REGION
⑩ RETICULAR FORMATION

Figure 18–7 Circuitry in emotional brain. *A*, Input; *B*, output.

mammillary nucleus receives axons via the fornix from the hippocampus and also receives axons from other portions of the hypothalamus and septum through the medial forebrain bundle. Input from the midbrain tegmentum and substantia nigra via the mammillary peduncle is also received by the lateral mammillary nucleus.

Thalamus. The anterior, medial, midline, and intralaminar thalamic nuclei receive input from the hypothalamus, reticular system, and especially the midbrain reticular formation and cingulate and frontal associational cortex. The intralaminar and midline nuclei connect to the medial and other specific thalamic nuclei which then project to the cerebral cortex.

Interpeduncular Nucleus. The interpeduncular nucleus (posterior perforated substance) is found on the anterior surface of the midbrain in the interpeduncular fossa extending from the posterior end of the mammillary body to the anterior end of the pons. It receives fibers from the habenular nuclei (habenular peduncular tract) and has reciprocal connections with the hypothalamus and the midbrain limbic region.

Epithalamus. The habenular nucleus (epithalamus) gives origin to the habenulopeduncular tract which projects to the midbrain tegmentum and interpeduncular nuclei. The habenular nuclei receive afferents from the septum and preoptic region via the stria medullaris and connect to the intralaminar nuclei.

Septum. The septum connects with (1) the hypothalamus, interpeduncular nucleus, and the midbrain tegmentum via the medial forebrain bundle; (2) the habenula via the stria medullaris; and (3) the basolateral amygdaloid nuclei through the diagonal band.

CORTICAL STRUCTURES

The cortical structures of the emotional brain are as follows: hippocampal formation, perihippocampal cortex, cingulate cortex, portions of the temporal lobe, cingulate isthmus, supracallosal gyrus and longitudinal stria, subcallosal gyrus, and amygdaloid nuclei (uncus), and frontal associational areas.

Limbic Structures. The central cortical structures in the emotional brain are the limbic structures: amygdalae, hippocampal formation, and cingulate cortex.

The *amygdala* consists of two main groupings of nuclei: corticomedial and basolateral. The corticomedial group receives olfactory information from the lateral olfactory stria and interconnects with the contralateral-corticomedial and ipsilateral-basolateral nuclei. The primary efferent pathway of the corticomedial nucleus is the stria terminalis which projects to the septum and preoptic nucleus of the hypothalamus, and to the corticomedial nucleus in the opposite hemisphere.

The basolateral nuclear grouping is associated with the visceral brain, exchanges connections with the perihippocampal cortex, and receives projections from the temporal pole, frontal lobe, orbital gyrus, and cingulate lobe. The efferent pathways project to the septum, the preoptic, lateral, and ventral hypothalamus, and the dorsomedial, intralaminar, and midline thalamus. The uncus consists of the amygdaloid nuclei and the olfactory cortex.

The *hippocampal formation* (hippocampus, dentate gyrus, and subiculum) receives afferents from (1) the adjacent perihippocampal cortex which in turn receives its input from many parts of the frontal, orbital, temporal (amygdalae), and cingulate cortex; (2) the septum; and (3) the contralateral hippocampus, via the hippocampal commissure.

The efferents from the hippocampal formation only leave via the fornix (axons of hippocampal pyramidal neurons) and connect to (1) the septum, preoptic region, and parolfactory and cingulate cortex via the precommissural fornix and supracallosal fornix; (2), via a column of the fornix, to the lateral mammillary nuclei, habenular nuclei, anterior midline and intralaminar thalamic nuclei, lateral hypothalamic nuclei, midbrain tegmentum, and periaqueductal grey.

The *cingulate cortex* receives reciprocal innervation from the anterior thalamic nuclei, contralateral and ipsilateral cingulate cortex and temporal lobe, as well as projecting to the corpus striatum and most of the subcortical limbic nuclei.

Frontal Associational Areas. The frontal associational areas (areas 9, 10, 11, 12) receive their input from cingulate regions and cortical associational areas (i.e., somesthetic, auditory, visual). They also have a strong thalamic connection from the dorsal medial thalamic nucleus via the anterior thalamic radiation. The dorsal medial thalamic nucleus in turn receives most of its input from the hypothalamus and the midbrain limbic nuclei. The frontal associational region has strong projections onto the hypothalamus and thalamus.

Temporal Gyri. The inferior and middle temporal *gyri* are also important cortical centers. They have connections with the cingulate cortex, the perihippocampal gyrus, and the frontal associational cortex (via the uncinate fasciculus).

FUNCTIONAL LOCALIZATION IN THE EMOTIONAL BRAIN

Temporal Lobe. The work of Kluver and Bucy initially localized emotions in the limbic lobe. These findings were based on experiments with animals with bilateral ablation of temporal pole, amygdaloid nuclei, and hippocampus. In these experiments, the monkeys became hypersexual and copulated excessively and indiscriminately. They showed lack of response to adversive stimuli and showed no recollection or judgment. The animals could see and find objects but they could not identify objects (visual agnosia). They also had very strong oral tendencies and compulsively placed objects in their mouths, which, if not edible, were dropped. These animals also had lost their fear (release phenomenon) and, in the case of wild monkeys, became tame and docile creatures. They had a marked absence of response to anger or fear. They also had lost fears of unknown objects or objects that previously had frightened them. They also ate food not normally a part of their diet.

The human with bilateral amygdaloid-hippocampal lesions is unable to remember recent events but will remember events prior to the operation (see Chapter 27, Memory). The human will also have visual agnosia, will become docile, and may become hypersexual.

In later experiments, Kluver and Bucy found that the animals became placid and emotionally unresponsive after removal of only the amygdaloid-pyriform cortex and portions of the adjacent hippocampus. These behavioral effects are of limited duration and usually disappear within weeks.

Amygdala. Stimulation of the amygdaloid region in monkeys, cats, and rats produces a variation in behavior; with stimulus the animal becomes aggressive; without stimulus they are peaceful. The stimulated

cats have a sympathetic response of dilated pupils, increased heartbeat, extension of claws, piloerection, and attack behavior. Upon removal of stimuli, they become friendly. Animals will even fight when the amygdala is stimulated and stop fighting when the stimulus is off. Stimulation here may also stimulate eating, sniffing, licking, biting, chewing, and gagging. Stimulations of the amygdala in man produce feelings of fear or anger.

Hippocampus. The hippocampus has a low threshold for seizure discharge; consequently stimulation of any region which supplies hippocampal afferents or stimulation of the hippocampus itself may produce seizures. Stimulation of the hippocampus produces respiration and cardiovascular changes, as well as face, limb, and trunk movements.

Cingulate Cortex. Stimulation of cingulate cortex also produces respiratory, vascular, and visceral changes, but these changes are of less magnitude than those produced by hypothalamic stimulation.

Septum. Destruction of the septum in cats causes docile animals to become fearful and aggressive. These effects usually wear off. Complete destruction of the septum may produce coma, probably as a result of the strong connections between the septum and hypothalamus.

Hypothalamus. The basic function of this region is to maintain internal homeostasis (body temperature, appetite, water balance, pituitary functions) and establish some control of our emotional state. It is a most potent subcortical center due to its control of the autonomic nervous system.

Stimulation in the anterior hypothalamus produces parasympathetic responses: a decrease in heart rate, respiration, and blood pressure, an increase in peristalsis and in gastric and duodenal secretions, constriction of the pupils, increased salivation, and, depending on the internal milieu, even evacuation of bowels and bladder. Concomitant with the parasympathetic excitation there is sympathetic inhibition.

Stimulation in the posterior hypothalamus produces a sympathetic or anxiety response: increased heart rate and blood pressure, decreased peristalsis and secretions, sweating, dilation of pupils, and piloerection. Concomitant with sympathetic excitation there is parasympathetic inhibition.

Stimulation in the hypothalamus can produce flight (fear) and fight (rage). Stimulation can also produce visceral responses: sweating, salivation, defecation, and retching. The aforementioned responses can be produced in regions adjacent to one another or by moving the electrode site or changing stimulation parameters (varying current). Another interesting result has been noted in cats made docile with amygdaloid lesions; these same animals become savage when a lesion is placed in the ventromedial hypothalamic nuclei.

Frontal Associational Cortex. The highest expression of behavioral control and inhibition is found in the prefrontal or frontal associational areas 9, 10, 11, and 12; they are connected with many sensory cortical areas including the cingulate cortex, and they have strong projections to the hypothalamus and the medial thalamic nucleus.

For over a century it has been recognized that disease in the anterior part of frontal lobes in man produced changes in intelligence and personality. In 1936, Moniz produced changes in severely disturbed patients by separating the prefrontal lobes, resulting in a less excitable, less creative, less anxious, more passive individual who was no longer bothered by events which previously were disturbing. Frontal lobotomy has also been performed on patients with intractable pain from carcinoma; the patient still perceives the pain but he can ignore it and is no longer anxious or fearful about it.

The surgical procedure to produce personality change (prefrontal lobotomy or leukotomy) has since fallen into disuse. This personality change results from the isolation of the prefrontal lobe from input from the limbic subcortical structures.

A somewhat similar but less drastic change in personality is produced by bilateral severance of the anterior thalamic radiation from the medial nucleus or by direct destruction of the medial nuclei or orbital cortex. This latter, less massive resection of cortex produces loss of anxiety with less marked personality changes. Bilateral ablation of the anterior cingulate regions will also produce this less drastic change.

The results of partial or complete prefrontal lobotomy have shown that this region is important in motivation, intellect, judgment, abstract reasoning, and emotional control. Disease in this region produces deterioration in intellect and changes in personality which are somewhat similar to temporal lobe extirpations, except that they are permanent. Many of the emotional changes associated with disease or lesions in the frontal association cortex can be found to a lesser degree with disease processes in the temporal lobe. (Additional discussion of frontal lobe functions will be found in Chapter 21.)

Pleasure-Punishment Areas. Throughout the visceral brain are located "pleasure centers" or "punishment centers" (Olds, 1958). Experimentally, electrodes are implanted at various subcortical sites in an animal and the animal is trained to press a bar which connects the electrode to an electrical current. In certain regions of the visceral brain the animal will self-stimulate until exhausted — a pleasure center! In fact the animal would rather press the lever than eat. The pleasure centers are located throughout the visceral system, but especially in the septum and preoptic region of the hypothalamus. There are also centers in the brain which when stimulated produce fear responses — a punishment center: dilation of pupils, piloerection, sweating. In these regions the animal quickly stops pressing the bar. These zones are located in the amygdala, hypothalamus, thalamus, and midbrain tegmentum.

THE EMOTIONAL BRAIN AS A SYSTEM

The emotional brain is organized into a hierarchy of function proceeding from the reticular formation including mesencephalic midbrain nuclei to the hypothalamus and thalamus to the limbic and neocortical regions.

Reticular Formation. The reticular formation is the site where information is received from the peripheral nerves. This system is so organized that only certain stimuli will trigger the reticular activating system which will then alert the brain. If it were possible for any response to trigger this system, then the individual's survival would be endangered. The responses, however, become selective because throughout our years of development, and in fact throughout our life, we have evolved an emotional set of responses which determine whether we will respond to a situation calmly or with rage or fear. What happens is that the reticular system, based on the sensory information with probably some cortical subconscious assistance, focuses the attention of the central nervous system by sorting out the relevant information, thus enabling the central nervous system to continue to function efficiently throughout a crisis.

Hypothalamus. By the time the data reaches the hypothalamus there are already clearly well-organized emotional responses. The hypothalamus, with some assistance from the thalamus, will set the basic level of energy needed for the emotional state and will organize and mobilize the cortical and subcortical centers (especially the autonomic nervous system).

If the situation is nonthreatening, the normal operations of the viscera continue. In a mildly stressful condition, such as that involving anger or heavy work, some of the digestive processes slow down and the heart rate and blood flow increase. If the situation is threatening, triggering any of the following reactions—fear, pain, great hunger or thirst, and sexual drive—most of the digestive processes slow down and heart rate, blood flow, and respiration increase. Once the threatening situation passes conditions will return rapidly to a normal balance between the sympathetic and parasympathetic nervous system.

Limbic Cortical Regions. The limbic cortical regions are strongly influenced by the emotional patterns which are set in the hypothalamus and are transmitted with only a very few synapses into the limbic cortex where the emotional pattern is elaborated and organized efficiently. The neocortex (frontal associational cortex and, to a lesser degree, the temporal lobe), based on past experience, examines the situation, sorts out the emotional responses from the intellectual, and inhibits or controls the situation based on what past experience has proven to be expedient for the survival of the individual.

Consider the following examples: a mother responds to her baby's crying, while the father sleeps on; in the middle of the night a jet airplane thundering overhead causes no response, while a whiff of smoke or breaking glass quickly arouses the central nervous system and keeps it focused.

References

Adrian, E. D.: Sensory discrimination with some recent evidence from the olfactory organ. Brit. med. Bull., 6:330, 1950.

Fulton, J. F.: The limbic system: A study of the visceral brain in primates and man. Yale J. Biol., 26:107, 1953.

Green, J. D.: The rhinencephalon: Aspects of its relation to behavior and the reticular activating system. In Jasper, H. H. (ed.): Reticular Formation of the Brain. Boston, Little, Brown and Company, 1958, p. 607.

Jasper, H. H., and Proctor, L. O. (eds.): Reticular Formation of the Brain. Henry Ford Hospital Symposium, Boston, Little, Brown and Company, 1958.

Kluver, H.: Brain mechanisms and behavior with special reference to the rhinencephalon. J. Lancet (Minneapolis), 72:567, 1952.

Kluver, H.: The "temporal lobe syndrome" produced by bilateral ablations. In Wolstenholme, E. E., and O'Connor, C. M. (eds.): Neurological Bases of Behaviour. Foundation Symposium, London, J. A. Churchill, 1958, p. 175.

Kluver, H., and Bucy, P. C.: Psychic blindness and other symptoms following bilateral temporal lobectomy in Rhesus monkeys. Amer. J. Physiol., 119:352, 1937.

MacLean, P. D.: The limbic system (visceral brain) and emotional behavior. Arch. Neurol. Psychiat. (Chicago), 73:130, 1955.

Nauta, W. J. H.: Central nervous organization and the endocrine motor system. In Nalbandov, A. V. (ed.): Advances in Neuroendocrinology. Urbana, University of Illinois Press, 1963, p. 5.

Olds, J.: Self-stimulation experiments and differentiated reward systems, In Jasper, H. H. (ed.): Reticular Formation of the Brain. Boston, Little, Brown and Company, 1958, p. 671.

Papez, J. W.: A proposed mechanism of emotion. Arch. Neurol Psychiat. (Chicago), 38:725, 1937.

Papez, J. W.: The visceral brain, its components and connections, In Jasper, H. H. (ed.): Reticular Formation of the Brain. Boston, Little, Brown and Company, 1958, p. 591.

Sheer, D. E. (ed.): Electrical Stimulation of the Brain. Austin, University of Texas Press, 1961.

Zotterman, Y. (ed.): Olfaction and Taste. New York, MacMillan, 1963, p. 309.

19

Visual System

BRIAN CURTIS

Of all of man's senses, vision is by far the most important; most of our perception of the world comes to us through our eyes. Even though the light intensity changes 10 million times between the brightest snowy day and a bright starlit night, our eyes and visual system adapt to these intensity changes so that we see clearly. Furthermore, we can discriminate colors, something that only a very few primates can do. Lastly, our eyes are set in our heads in such a way that each eye sees almost the same visual field, making depth perception possible.

THE STRUCTURE OF THE EYE

The anatomy of the receptor organ, the eye, is shown in Figure 19–1. It is made up of three major layers or tunics: the outer tunic, the choroid, and the retina. The outer tunic consists of two parts; the clear cornea and the tough, white sclera. The *cornea*, the window to the world, allows light rays to enter the eye. Most of the focusing or refraction of light rays on the retina occurs at the air-cornea junction. The *sclera* forms the white of the eye and the rest of the outer covering. The middle tunic, the *choroid*, is richly vascular and provides oxygen and nutrients to the inner, photoreceptor layer, the *retina*.

The *lens* delineates the anterior chamber from the vitreous body and completes the refraction of the entering light. The ciliary muscle (Fig. 19–2) can alter the shape of the lens by an undefined mechanism; contraction of the muscle allows close objects to be brought into focus. A normal consequence of aging is a decreased ability to focus on close objects.

The *iris* is a circular structure which acts as a diaphragm to control the amount of light falling on the retina. It is analogous to the f-stop setting of a camera. The eye has a range of f2 to f22. The ability of the iris to change the size of the pupil (the opening) will be discussed later (p. 444).

THE RETINA: VISUAL PIGMENTS

The inner tunic, the retina, contains the photopigments and the nerve cells. They are organized so that the cells containing the photopigments are closest to the sclera with the nerve cells above them. These nerve cells send fibers to the optic nerve through a pigment-free area, the *optic disk*.

The first principle of vision is that we cannot hope to see light which cannot be absorbed by a photopigment.

There are four types of photoreceptor cells. Three are cone-shaped, each *cone cell* containing one of the three pigments of color vision. Color vision requires light levels greater than bright moonlight and has high resolution so that fine detail can be seen.

The fourth type of cell, the *rod*, also con-

437

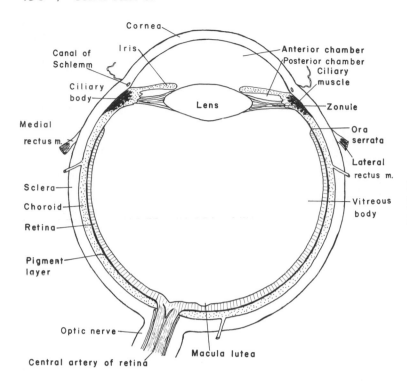

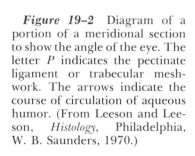

Figure 19–1 Diagram of a horizontal meridional section of the eye. (From Leeson and Leeson, *Histology,* Philadelphia, W. B. Saunders, 1970.)

Figure 19–2 Diagram of a portion of a meridional section to show the angle of the eye. The letter *P* indicates the pectinate ligament or trabecular meshwork. The arrows indicate the course of circulation of aqueous humor. (From Leeson and Leeson, *Histology,* Philadelphia, W. B. Saunders, 1970.)

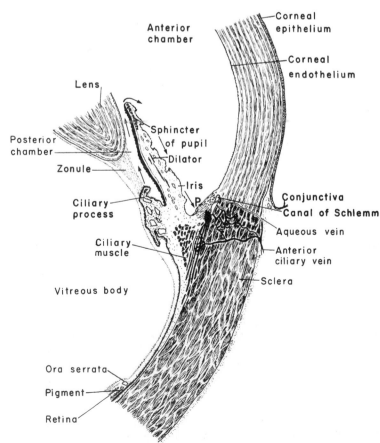

tains a single pigment, rhodopsin, and is responsible for night vision. This system has very poor resolution; newspaper headlines are the smallest letters which can be recognized.

The rods and cones are not uniformly distributed on the retina. Most of the 6 million cone cells are all located in an area 2 mm. in diameter, the *macula lutea* (Fig. 19–1), which can be seen through the ophthalmoscope. In the center of the macula lutea lies a zone of pure cones, the *fovea* (Fig. 19–3). The rest of the macula lutea is composed of both rods and cones, while most of the peripheral retina contains only rods. There are about 120 million rods.

Scotopic Vision. The rods contain a single pigment, *rhodopsin*, which is related to vitamin A1. The spectral sensitivity of night or scotopic vision is identical to the absorption spectra of rhodopsin (Fig. 19–4). Light which can be absorbed by rhodopsin is seen; light which cannot be absorbed, such as infrared light, is not seen at these low light intensities. Scotopic vision has quite poor definition; two light sources must be quite far apart to be distinguished as two sources rather than one. The definition gets progressively worse as the vision becomes more peripheral—"out of the corner of the eye."

The modern human uses this system very little since we have bright portable light sources.

The biochemistry of rhodopsin has been elegantly worked out by Wald (1968) and his colleagues and will not be discussed further here.

In daylight all of the rhodopsin is largely inactivated and inoperative. After 5 minutes in the dark, scotopic vision begins to return and is maximally sensitive after 15 to 20 minutes. Since the rhodopsin does not absorb red light, it is not inactivated by red light; night vision can be conditioned or preserved by using red goggles.

Color Vision. Color vision requires much higher light intensities and occurs primarily when the image is focused upon the macula. Each cone contains one of the three color pigments whose absorption spectra is shown in Figure 19–5. To distinguish the color orange, 600 nm (nanometers), the visual system compares the relative absorption by two visual pigments, in this case the red and green cones. Any wavelength which does not excite two pigments, such as deep purple, 400 nm, and deep red, 650 m, will be hard to discriminate from a close wavelength; these color discriminations are apparently made on the basis of the intensity of absorp-

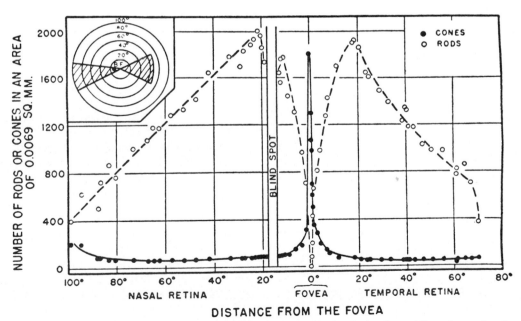

Figure 19–3 The density of cones and rods on or near the horizontal meridian through a human retina. The inset is a schematic map of the retina showing the fovea (*F*) and the blind spot (*B*). The striped area represents the regions of the retina which were sampled in obtaining the counts plotted here. (From Chapanis after Østerberg, Acta ophth., 1935, Suppl. 6.)

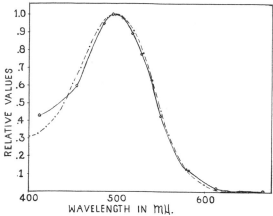

Figure 19–4 Comparison of the absorption curve of pure visual purple (interrupted line) with the scotopic luminosity curve (continuous line) as obtained with an equal quantum spectrum. (From Ludvigh, Arch. Ophthal., *20*:713, 1938.)

tion relative to the brightness of other colors in the field of view. For example, a color of 660 nm could, in bright intensity, mimic (in the percentage absorption) a color of 640 nm in weaker intensity. Only when two types of cones are excited can color and brightness be determined independently.

THE RETINA: ELECTROPHYSIOLOGY

We have jumped from the absorption of light by a pigment to "seeing." What are the intermediate steps? The cells of the retina

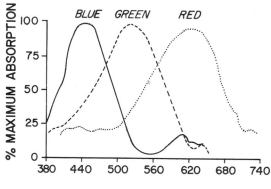

Figure 19–5 The absorption spectrum of the three types of cones. (Drawn from records *In* Marks, Dobelle, and MacNichol, Jr., Science, *143*: 1181, 1964; and Brown and Wald, Science, *144*: 45, 1964.

are shown in Figure 19–6; remember that the rods and cones are innermost and that the light shines through the nerve plexus before reaching them.

The rods and cones make synaptic contact with bipolar cells. The number of cells in contact with one bipolar cell varies enormously. In the peripheral portion of the retina, 60 degrees from the center, as many as 600 rods may innervate a single bipolar cell, while in the fovea, one or two cones may do so. In the macula lutea both rods and cones may innervate a single bipolar cell. The dendrite of the bipolar cell synapses with a ganglion cell. Once again the degree of convergence on the ganglion cell depends upon the region of the retina. There are ganglion cells in the fovea which connect with only one bipolar cell. The axons of the ganglion cells form the optic nerve. There are about 1 million optic nerve fibers. It is clear that a great deal of data reduction has occurred between the 126 million rods and cones and the one million optic nerve fibers.

There are two other types of neurons in the retina: horizontal cells and amacrine cells. *Horizontal cells* are found in the outer plexiform layer; their dendrites make contact with numerous rods and cones over a 2 to 400 μ field. The axon runs transversely along the retina and branches to make contact with many other rods or cones at the bipolar cell junction. The horizontal cells connect groups of visual receptors in one area with groups in another area. The processes of the *amacrine cells* lie in the inner plexiform layer. The dendrites make contact with numerous ganglion cells; no axon has been described.

Electrical recording from these cells gives many clues to their function: the retina of the mudpuppy is most informative, due, in part, to the large size of the cells. Recordings from the receptor cells (Fig. 19–7) show a resting potential of −30 mv and a hyperpolarization in response to light (column A). When the receptor is dark and the area 250 μ away is light (column B), there is a very slight response due to scattered light. Both rods and cones show this hyperpolarizing response. The horizontal cell also hyperpolarizes in response to light (columnA), but has a large receptive field. Even when the light is shining on receptor cells 250 μ away, there is a strong hyperpolarizing response (column B).

Both of these inputs impinge on the bipolar

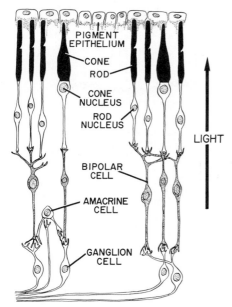

Figure 19-6 The principal cells of the retina.

cell: direct receptor potential and horizontal cell output. When only a few, near-by, receptors are illuminated, the bipolar cell hyperpolarizes (column A, Fig. 19–7), but when the area 250 μ away is *also* illuminated, the bipolar cell depolarizes. Here we see the first type of data reduction carried out in the retina—*contrast enhancement.* The bipolar cell has one type of output, hyperpolarization, for a bright spot on a dark field and another, depolarization, for a continuous bright field.

Recordings from the amacrine cell show it to respond primarily to sudden changes in light intensity. Note that the major activity is at the onset or cessation of the light. This is the second type of processing or data reduction, *dynamic detection*, which takes place in the retina.

Two types of ganglion-cell responses are seen. One reflects the amacrine cell response, primarily a dynamic response to turning the light on or off. Some cells will react more strongly to on than off or vice versa. These cells are inhibited by illumination of both a spot and the surrounding area.

The second type of response reflects the bipolar cell activity. When only a spot is illuminated the ganglion cell responds with an intense train of action potentials during the illumination and abruptly stops as the light ceases. The frequency of the action potentials during the illumination is proportional to the logarithm of the brightness of the light. When both the spot and the surrounding area are illuminated, the background level of firing is inhibited.

THE OPTIC PATHWAY

Electrical recording from optic nerve fibers also shows the types of data reduction occurring in the retina. First, there is convergence which involves many receptors firing to activate one bipolar cell, except in the fovea. Consequently the "grain" of the visual image will vary depending on the location on the retina. Second, brightness can be detected. Third, there is a center-surround contrast enhancement. Lastly there is dynamic or motion detection.

A bar of light on the retina will be "seen" in terms of its brightness and its edges. As it is turned on and off, the dynamic receptors will fire to alert higher centers. The bar of light will receive much more attention in the optic nerve if it is moved around since each tiny movement will set off a new set of dynamic or movement receptors which make up about half the total optic nerve fibers.

The fibers from the ganglion cells run along the inner surface of the retina to the optic disk where they turn and continue on toward the brain stem. The artery and vein to and from the retina also run through the optic nerve and spread out on the retinal surface; they are readily observed with the ophthalmoscope. Since the retinal vein runs through the subarachnoid space, increased intracranial pressure will result in venous congestion and engorgement as well as a protrusion of the normally depressed optic disk. This combination is called papilledema and should be considered a danger sign whenever found.

The pathway of fibers from the retina to the occipital lobe is shown in Figure 19–8. The patient's visual field is divided in two by a vertical line running through his nose. Figure 19–8 shows visual fields for each eye; these, however, are really one, but are shown this way for convenience. The visual fields are named for the patient's right and left hands. The left visual field projects onto the nasal retina of the left eye and the temporal retina of the right eye. At the chiasm, the fibers from the left nasal retina cross the midline and run, with the fibers from the right temporal retina, to the lateral geniculate body of the thalamus (see Fig. 29–14).

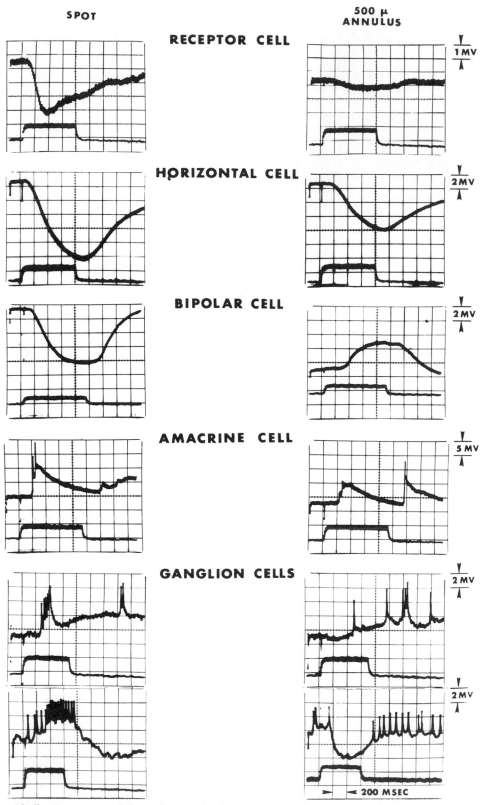

Figure 19-7 Responses of the cell types in the Necturus retina. (From F. S. Werblin and J. Dowling, J. Neurophysiol., *32*:339, 1969.)

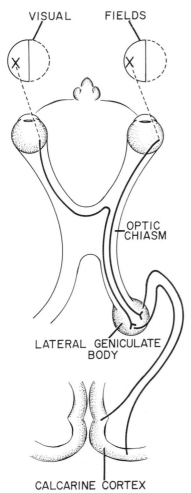

VISUAL FIELDS

OPTIC CHIASM

LATERAL GENICULATE BODY

CALCARINE CORTEX

Figure 19-8 The optic tract. The (X) in the right and left fields should be much further away and in reality represents the same point.

By this crossing, all the information from the left visual field is brought together in the right lateral geniculate body and subsequently on the right calcarine cortex. The fibers of the right nasal retina also cross in the chiasm, Thus, the visual pathway repeats the usual pattern of sensory systems; the right side is represented on the left cerebrum.

THE CALCARINE CORTEX

The cellular physiology of the calcarine cortes will be discussed here while the structure and gross function will be discussed later (pp. 508–512). Of the cells in the calcarine cortex, the ones with the simplest response are those that react very much as

retinal ganglion cells respond—an excitatory region surrounded by an inhibitory region. The opposite contrast—the surrounding area is excited; the center inhibited—is also seen in higher mammals; they are excited by an annulus of light.

Three types of higher order, more sophisticated cells have been described in the visual cortex by Hubel and Wiesel (1968). The first is termed a simple cell and responds best to a bar of light in a critical orientation and location. The receptive fields of several simple cells are shown in Figure 19–9. The excitatory field of each simple cell is bordered on one or both sides by an inhibitory field as shown for simple cell *a*. The small portion of the visual field outlined in Figure 19–9 will drive thousands of simple cells, each with a discrete location and orientation. It would appear that each simple cell receives input from a number of ganglion cells which have their excitatory and inhibitory fields in a straight line.

Every simple cell can be driven through either eye, but they usually show a preference for one eye or the other. For example, a simple cell may be strongly excited by looking at a bar through the right eye and only weakly stimulated by the same bar seen through the left eye. This differential sensitivity may form the basis of binocular vision.

A number of simple cells having the same orientation activate a complex cell. An example of this is shown as complex cell α in Figure 19–9. The complex cell has a definite orientational preference, but a very much larger receptive field. Complex cell α will be excited by any horizontal line of any length within the visual field outlined. Lines with different orientations in the same visual field will drive other complex cells.

The final cell type described is a *hypercomplex cell*. It has characteristics very similar to the complex cell except it discriminates on the length of the line. The bottom light bar in Figure 19–9 will inhibit hypercomplex cell 2. If its left-hand border were moved into the visual field, it would strongly excite cell 2. Once again it is excited by lines of a critical orientation anywhere within a large portion of a visual field, but they must not be too long.

About one-half million fibers of the optic tract enter the occipital lobe. It should be clear that there is enormous increase in the number of cells processing this information, and indeed the banks of the calcarine cor-

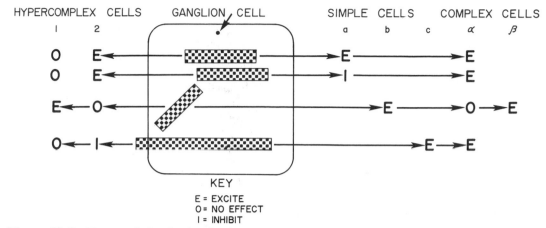

Figure 19–9 Types of visual stimuli which excite each of the four types of cells found in the calcarine cortex. The square represents a box ½″ by ½″, 5 feet away from the monkey's eye. The actual stimuli are bright bars of light on a dark field. (Data from Hubel and Wiesel, J. Physiol., *195*:215, 1968.)

tex contain many millions of cells. How the image is processed beyond this region is still unknown and we must jump to what a person consciously perceives as we will do in Chapter 21.

CLINICAL CONSIDERATIONS

Lesions of the Optic Pathway. There are a number of common lesions of the visual tract with which all students should be familiar. Visual fields are tested by asking the patient to cover one eye and look directly at the examiner's nose while the examiner stands about 4 feet away. A white-headed pin is slowly brought into the visual field until the patient sees it. The pin should be brought in from the top, the bottom, and the two horizontal and the four midpoints. The visual field can be tested quantitatively with a perimeter, an instrument which does the forementioned maneuvers and marks them on a card. The records in Figure 19–10 were obtained with a perimeter. The normal visual field is not symmetrical because the nose blocks vision toward the center.

If the retina or the optic nerve is destroyed (2 in Fig. 19–10) there is no sight in that eye — *monocular blindness.* When the lesion is in the chiasm, the fibers from both nasal retina, temporal visual fields, are cut; the result is *bitemporal hemianopia* (3 in Figure 19–10). A frequent cause of this lesion is a pituitary tumor expanding upward. The lowermost

fibers are interrupted first so that the superior temporal fields are impaired first. The physician who performs careful visual field tests during a physical examination will have the greatest chance to save the vision of the majority of his patients.

Complete cuts in the optic tract, the lateral geniculate body, or the geniculocalcarine radiation will result in blindness in one visual field — *homonymous hemianopia* (4 in Fig. 19–10). Partial lesions of the geniculocalcarine radiations are quite common and produce a *quadrantanopia* (5 in Fig. 19–10). Lesions close to the occipital pole will often spare the macular region since it is represented on the anterior end of the calcarine cortex. This lesion is referred to as *macular sparing* (6 in Fig. 19–10) and helps to differentiate lesions of the optic tract and geniculocalcarine radiation from occipital cortical lesions. Further examples of lesions to this pathway are to be found in Chapter 20.

Pupillary Reflexes. There are two sets of muscles in the iris which control the size of the pupil. When the circular muscles (the sphincter pupillae) (Fig. 19–2), contract, the iris is drawn together and the pupil constricts much as purse strings close the mouth of the purse. The second set of muscles, (the dilator pupillae), are radial and draw the iris back toward the sclera.

The sphincter pupillae is supplied by the parasympathetic nervous system via the ciliary nerves, the fibers of which run together with nerve III. The transmission is cholinergic. The dilator pupillae is supplied by

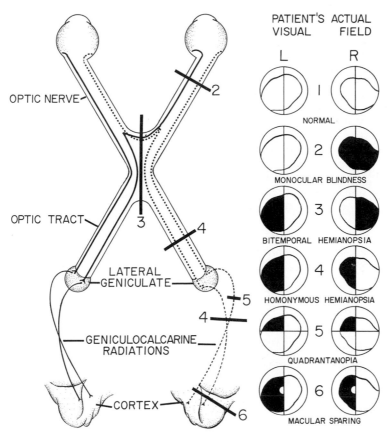

Figure 19-10 Common lesions of the optic tract.

the sympathetic system via the cervical ganglion.

The pupil constricts when light is directed into either eye (the light reflex) and when the eye focuses on close objects (accommodation). The light reflex involves fibers which arise in the retina and travel with the optic nerve and tract, but continue past the lateral geniculate body to the pretectal region of the midbrain and then to the Edinger-Westphal nucleus. Fibers from each eye reach the Edinger-Westphal nucleus. The constrictor response when light is shone in the same eye is called the *direct light reflex*; when shone in the opposite eye, the *indirect light reflex*. From the Edinger-Westphal nucleus preganglionic parasympathetic fibers run together with the third cranial nerve to the ciliary ganglion, and the past ganglionic fibers run to the constrictor fibers. The pathway which subserves accommodation is more complex but apparently arises in the occipital lobe and reaches fibers running together with nerve III.

Fixed dilated pupil or pupils are often a

sign of pressure on the third cranial nerve, usually from supratentorial structures, and should always be treated with concern and the reason for them determined.

A dissociation of the light and accommodation reflexes occurs, with a syndrome called the Argyll Robertson pupils. This describes a pupil which does not react to light but does react by constriction upon viewing near objects; it accommodates but does not react to light. This disorder is usually bilateral. The pupils are small and the retinas are sensitive to light. Argyll Robertson pupils almost always indicate central nervous system syphilis.

An interruption of the sympathetic supply leads to an imbalance in the pupillary muscles and very constricted pupils. This is usually accompanied by ptosis (drooping) of the upper eyelid. These two signs are part of Horner's syndrome and may be either unilateral or bilateral. Horner's syndrome is accompanied by a red flush due to vasodilation of surface blood vessels and a lack of sweating.

Drugs are often introduced into the conjunctival sac to cause mydriasis (enlargement of the pupil) as an aid in examination of the retina. A 2 to 5 per cent solution of homatropine hydrobromide or hydrochloride will cause wide dilation of the pupil and will also paralyze the ciliary muscles so that focusing is not possible. Recovery is usually complete in 24 hours. A 5 to 10 per cent solution of eucatropine hydrochloride is useful only as a mydriatic agent, causes little disturbance of accommodation, and has a rapid onset and a duration of a few hours. These and other belladonna alkaloids act by blocking the postganglionic parasympathetic synapses.

Ephedrine (3 to 5 per cent) and phenylephrine (1 to 2 per cent) also cause mydriasis by stimulating the postganglionic sym-pathetic fibers and consequently the radial muscles of the iris. The effect lasts only an hour or so, with no effect upon focusing.

References

Alpern, M., Rushton, W. A. H., and Torii, S.: Signals from cones. J. Physiol., *207*:463, 1970.

Cambell, F. W., and Rushton, W. A. H.: Measurement of the scotopic pigment in the living human eye. J. Physiol., *130*:131, 1955.

Dowling, J.: Organization of the vertebrate retinas. Invest. Ophthal., *9*:655, 1970.

Hubel, D., and Wiesel, T. N.: The functional architecture of the striate cortex *In* Carlson, F. D. (ed.): *Physiological and Biochemical Aspects of Nervous Integration.* Englewood Cliffs, New Jersey, Prentice-Hall, 1968.

Wald, G.: Molecular basis of visual excitation. Science, *162*:230, 1968.

20

Cerebral Cortex: Cytoarchitecture and Electrophysiology

ELLIOTT M. MARCUS

ANATOMICAL CONSIDERATIONS

A firm knowledge of the structure and function of the cerebral cortex and the relationship of the cerebral cortex to the subcortical centers is of crucial importance for all who wish to understand the behavior and accomplishments of man as opposed to other animal forms. The use of the thumb and fingers for fine manipulations with tools, the use of linguistic and mathematical symbols for communication in the auditory and visual spheres, and the capacity for postponement of gratification all reflect the evolution of the cerebral cortex. This development of the cerebral cortex has led to a laminar arrangement of 16 billion nerve cells with an almost infinite number of synapses. The almost infinite number and variety of circuits present not only has provided the anatomical substrate for the recording of an infinite number of past experiences but has also allowed for a plasticity of future function projected both in time and in space.

The attempt to relate functional differences to the differences in structure of the various areas of the cerebral cortex was a scientific outgrowth of the earlier philosophical arguments concerning the relationship of mind and body. We may indicate at the onset that to a certain degree cytoarchitectural differences do reflect functional differences. This is never, however, a one-to-one relationship. Moreover, at times, architectural differences are not sharp; strict borders may not be present.

The various areas of cerebral cortex differ as regards several parameters:

1. Thickness, evident on simple visual inspection (average thickness is 2.5 mm., motor cortex: 4.5 mm., visual cortex 1.45 to 2.0 mm.). In addition to differences in overall thickness, some areas differ in the thickness of the various layers that constitute the laminar pattern.

2. Relative density of the various cell types, as evident in Nissl stain or other cellular stains, e.g., the presence of giant pyramidal cells or the relative numbers of large pyramidal cells as opposed to stellate (granule) cells. It must also be noted that within a given area of cortex, the various layers of cortex differ as regards the relative distribution of these various types of cells (Fig. 20–1).

3. Density of horizontal fiber plexuses (stripes) (evident on myelin and silver stains) and density of axodendritic and other synapses (evident on Golgi stain and Fink-Heiner stains).

4. Degree of myelination of intracortical

447

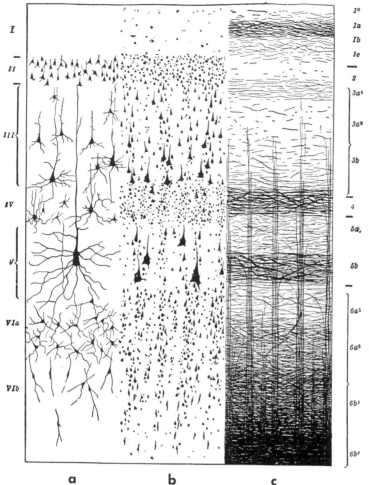

a   b   c

Figure 20-1 Diagram of the structure of the cerebral cortex. The results obtained with (*a*) a Golgi stain, (*b*) a Nissl stain or other cellular stain, and (*c*) a myelin stain are contrasted. I = molecular layer; II = external granular layer; III = external pyramidal layer; IV = internal granular layer; V = large or giant pyramidal layer (ganglionic layer); VI = fusiform layer. The following features should be noted in the myelin stain: 1a = molecular layer; 3a[1] = band of Kaes Bechterew; 4 = outer band of Baillarger; 5b = inner band of Baillarger. (After Brodmann, from Ranson, S. W., and Clark, S. L.: *The Anatomy of the Nervous System*, Philadelphia, W. B. Saunders, 1959, p. 350.)

fiber systems (evident on myelin stain). To some extent the various myelinated bands may be seen with the naked eye in freshly cut sections of the cerebral cortex. For example, a white line in the cortex near the calcarine fissure had been noted independently by Gennari in 1782 and Vicq d'Azyr in 1786. The various features to be noted in the several types of stains are demonstrated in Figure 20–1.

CYTOLOGY

There have been extensive studies of the architecture of the cerebral cortex as seen in myelin and silver preparations. However, most of our concepts of laminar pattern and of regional differences are based on cytology as seen in the Nissl stain or other cellular stains. Two main cell types may be distinguished: pyramidal cells and stellate cells (Fig. 20–2). Pyramidal neurons have cell bodies of variable height—small 10 to 12 μ;

medium 20 to 25 μ; large 45 to 50 μ, and giant 70 to 100 μ. The giant pyramidal cells are characteristic of the motor cortex. The upper end of the pyramidal cell continues on toward the surface as the apical dendrite. Numerous spines are found on the dendrite providing sites for synaptic contact. In general, the larger the cell body, the larger the apical dendrite and the wider the spread in terms of ramifications of the terminal horizontal branches. The wider the spread of the apical dendrite, the greater the number of possible axodendritic synapses. The larger the cell body, the greater the number of possible axosomatic synapses. In addition to the apical dendrite, shorter basal dendrites arise from the base of the cell body and arborize in the vicinity of the cell body. The axon emerges from the base of the cell body and descends toward the deeper white matter. In general the axons of small- and medium-sized pyramidal cells terminate as association fascicles within the cortex. The axons of

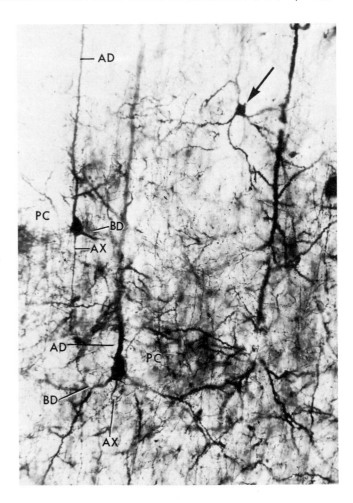

Figure 20-2 Pyramidal and stellate cells as demonstrated in Golgi stain of cat cerebral cortex. PC = pyramidal cells; arrow = stellate cell; AD = apical dendrite of pyramidal cell; BD = basal dendrite of pyramidal cells; AX = axons of pyramidal cell. (Courtesy of Dr. Stanley Jacobson.)

large and giant pyramidal cells enter the deeper white matter as (a) association fibers to other cortical areas, (b) commissural fibers to the contralateral hemisphere, or (c) projection (efferent) fibers to subcortical, brain stem, and spinal cord areas. In addition recurrent collateral association fibers may branch off from these axons within the cortex.

The stellate cells (or granular or star-shaped cells) have oval or circular bodies and are Golgi type II cells—with a short axon which branches near the cell body and usually ramifies near the cell body. The axons of some stellate cells descend into the white matter or ascend into the outermost cortical layers. The stellate cells lack a major apical dendrite; their thin dendrites have few, if any, spines. These cells function primarily as interneurons (Fig. 20–3). Several additional specialized types of stellate cells have been described. The double bush-cells (cellule à double bouquet dendritique of Cajal) possess an extremely ramified vertically oriented

arborization of the axon which forms a column, making multiple synaptic contacts with apical dendrites or bodies of pyramidal cells. The horizontal cell of Cajal, noted in the immature cortex, is oriented in a horizontal manner in the superficial layer. The cell of Martinotti has a long ascending axon which ramifies in one or more cortical layers. Spindle-shaped cells are found in the deepest cortical layers.

MAJOR CYTOARCHITECTURAL SUBDIVISIONS

Meynert in 1867 described a fundamental five layer horizontal distribution of neurons within the cerebral cortex. Betz in 1874 described the presence of the giant pyramidal cell in the fifth layer of Meynert in the human precentral gyrus. Cajal between 1899 and 1902 described the differences between human precentral and postcentral gyri. Cytoarchitecture as a major area of study began in

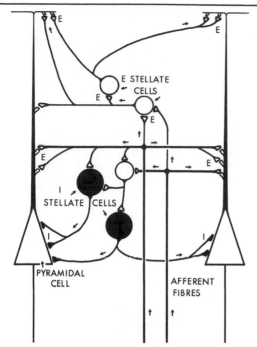

Figure 20-3 Diagram showing the possible function of stellate cells as interneurons. E represents excitatory (axodendritic) and I inhibitory (axosomatic) synapses. Note that the specific afferent fibers are postulated to synapse not only directly with the proximal apical dendrite of the pyramidal cell but also indirectly by a longer pathway involving stellate cell interneurons with the superficial axodendritic synapses. (From Eccles, J. C. (ed.): *Brain and Conscious Experience.* New York, Springer Verlag, 1966, p. 45.)

1903 with the independent work of Campbell, Vogt, and Brodmann who advocated a basic architectural plan of six layers (actually based on an earlier diagram of Bevan Lewis in 1878) and who demonstrated how various cortical areas differed from this fundamental plan. Brodmann then indicated that two fundamental types of cerebral cortex could be distinguished: *homogenetic* and *heterogenetic.* The homogenetic cortex has a six-layered pattern present at some time during development (recognizable by the end of the third fetal month). The six-layered pattern may or may not be apparent during the adult stage. This type of cortex is also called *isocortex, neocortex, neopallium,* or *supralimbic.*

The *heterogenetic* cortex in contrast does not show six layers at any time during development or during adult life. This type of cortex is also called *allocortex.* Two types of heterogenetic cortex may be recognized: *archipal-*

lium (hippocampus, dentate gyrus, and subiculum) and *paleopallium* (pyriform area) portions of the parahippocampal gyrus medial to the rhinal sulcus and the anterior perforated substance. Since there must be an area where heterogenetic cortex borders homogenetic cortex (cingulate gyrus of limbic lobe), a transitional type of cortex has been designated as *mesocortex.* The fundamental difference between heterogenetic and homogenetic cortex is demonstrated in Figure 20-4.

FUNDAMENTAL SIX-LAYERED SCHEME OF NEOCORTEX (HOMOGENETIC)

Our concern in the remainder of this chapter is with the neocortex (refer to Fig. 20-1 and Fig. 20-5). The following features can usually be distinguished in cellular stains of those areas of cerebral cortex showing the classic six-layered pattern in adult life (beginning from the pial surfaces).

Layer I: Molecular or plexiform layer. This layer contains very few cells. The tangential plexus of fibers, composed of apical dendrites, ascending axons, and axon collaterals, occupies this layer and provides a dense collection of axodendritic synapses.

Layer II: External granular layer. This is a relatively densely packed layer of small pyramidal cells and granule cells. The apical dendrites of the pyramidal cells terminate in the molecular layer. The axons of these cells are sent as association fibers to the lower cortical layers.

Layer III: External pyramidal layer. This is a layer of medium and large pyramidal cells. Two or three sublayers are sometimes recognized with the larger pyramidal cells located in the lower portion of this layer. Apical dendrites of the pyramidal cells extend to layer I; the axons may enter the white matter as association or commissural fibers or may function as intracortical association fibers.

Layer IV: Internal granular layer. This layer is densely packed with (granule) stellate cells. This layer is also occupied by the dense horizontal plexus of myelinated fibers; the external band of Baillarger. These fibers are the terminal branches of the specific thalamocortical projection system. These fibers synapse in relation to the stellate cells of layer IV and the basilar dendrites of the pyramidal cells of layer III. Many of the

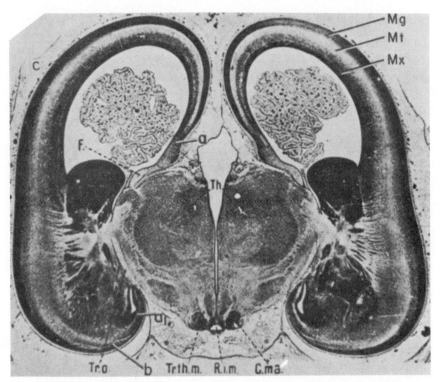

Figure 20-4 Frontal section through the diencephalic part of the prosencephalon of an 87 mm. (crown to rump), 3½-month embryo. a and al = anlage of the hippocampus (heterogenetic or rhinic allocortex); b = anlage of the parahippocampal cortex (limbic mesocortex); c = supralimbic isocortex (or homogenetic). Mg = marginal layer; Mt = mantle layer; Mx = matrix layer. (From Yakovlev, P. I.: Res. Publ. Assn. nerv. ment. Dis., *39*:3–46, 1962.)

stellate cells of layer IV function as interneurons interposed between the thalamocortical fibers (or collaterals of such fibers) and the pyramidal cells of other layers.

Layer V: Internal or large (and giant) pyramidal cell layer (also called ganglionic layer). The predominant cell type of this layer is the large or giant pyramidal cell. The apical dendrite of these cells ascends to the tangential plexus in the molecular layer. The axons of these cells enter the white matter as long projection fibers, association fibers, or commissural fibers. Collaterals from these axons may function as intracortical association fibers.

The internal band of Baillarger forms a dense horizontal plexus of fibers occupying the deeper portion of this layer.

Layer VI: Fusiform or spindle-cell or multiform layer. This layer contains a mixture of spindle-shaped cells and other stellate cells. The dendrites of the stellate cells ascend to various cortical layers. The axons enter the white matter as short association fibers or ascend to other cortical layers.

Layers I, II, and III are referred to as supragranular layers. Layer IV the internal granular layer is considered the major granular layer. Layers V and VI are referred to as infragranular layers. The supragranular layers are newer from a phylogenetic standpoint and are not found in the archipallium. In general these layers (supragranular) send out or receive predominantly association fibers. On the other hand, the infragranular layers are in general phylogenetically older and are related to more fundamental efferent activities.

FEATURES IN MYELIN OR SILVER STAINS

A series of horizontal fiber plexuses are present as indicated in the preceding section (refer to Fig. 20–1):

Layer I: Tangential fiber plexus; composed of apical dendrites and ascending axons.

Layers II−III (border): Stripe of Kaes-Bechterew − composed of collaterals given off from commissural, association, and nonspecific radiation fibers (? nonspecific thalamocortical).

Layer IV: External stripe or band of Baillarger composed of terminal ramifications of specific thalamocortical fibers which will synapse with stellate cells of layer IV and basilar dendrites of pyramidal cells of layer III.

Layers V and VI: Inner band of Baillarger composed of collaterals from ascending commissural, association, and nonspecific radiation fibers.

In addition to the horizontal plexuses of fibers, there are of course numerous vertically oriented fibers. Some of these enter the cortex (thalamocortical, commissural, association, and other projection fibers), some leave the cerebral cortex as long axons, and some originate and terminate in the cerebral cortex. One may include in the latter group the vertically oriented axonal arborization of the double bush stellate cell (described by Cajal) in the sensory cortex which makes multiple contacts with the dendrites and cell bodies of the pyramidal cells.

Although it has been clearly established that the specific thalamocortical projection fibers terminate in layer IV, the termination of nonspecific thalamic afferents remains uncertain. Nonspecific afferent fibers with diffuse connections were described by Lorente de No (1949), and this system has sometimes been identified with the diffuse thalamic system. As will be indicated, the major physiologic effects of this nonspecific thalamic system appear to occur mainly in the superficial layers of the cerebral cortex.

The callosal fibers originate from neurons in layers III and V. There is some uncertainty as to the termination. In the rat, these fibers terminate in layers I to VI with relatively dense termination in layers I, II, and III. In the monkey and chimpanzee, terminations appear to be mainly in layers III, IV, and V (Jacobson and Marcus, 1970).

CLASSIFICATION OF THE VARIOUS TYPES OF NEOCORTEX

It is evident that in the adult, all areas of the neocortex (the homogenetic cortex) do not have the same appearance. Brodmann termed those areas that show the typical six-layered pattern, as *homotypical*. Where such a typical six-layered pattern cannot be distinguished in the adult, the term *heterotypical*

is used. In a sense, two types of specialization are possible from the typical pattern. At one extreme is the agranular cortex of the motor area with many giant pyramidal cells present in layer V, but with a virtual absence of the entire internal granular layer (layer IV). Layers III and V are thick and continuous. At the other extreme is the granular sensory projection area; layers II, III, and IV appear as an almost continuous granular layer. Layers V and VI are thin and few large pyramidal cells are present.

Von Economo considered the various neocortical areas to fall into five basic categories (Figs. 20–5 and 20–6). Type 3 may be considered the midpoint of a continuum representing the stereotyped six-layered homotypical pattern. In man and the monkey, this type is best represented in nonsensory parietal cortex, e.g., inferior parietal lobule. Type I is the agranular extreme end of the continuum and as previously noted is represented in the motor cortex. Type 5 (granulous) is at the other (granular) end of the continuum and is represented in the primary sensory projection areas. Striate calcarine visual projection cortex is the best example. This type is also referred to as koniocortex (the densely granular cortex resembled a cloud of dust, konios). Type 2 is referred to as frontal homotypical (or frontal granular) and is represented in the superior frontal gyrus of the prefrontal area. Type 4 is referred to as polar and is represented in the nonstriate occipital cortex of area 18. Type 4 would then represent a point on the histological continuum between the parietal homotypical parietal (Type 3) and the granular koniocortex of the striate occipital cortex (Type 5).

CYTOARCHITECTURAL MAPS OF NEOCORTEX

Von Economo and Koskinas (Fig. 20–7) (more recently — 1951 — modified by Bailey and Von Bonin — (Fig. 20–8) have assigned cytoarchitectural designations to various neocortical areas based on a relatively logical letter scheme. Thus all frontal lobe areas receive the primary designation F followed by the secondary designation A, B, C, or D to indicate the various subtypes, e.g., FA, FB, FC, and FD. The letters A, B, C, D, and so forth represent definable histological gradations. Moreover, geographically FA, the agranular primary motor cortex, is adjacent

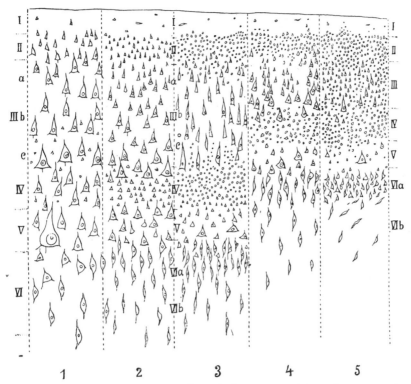

Figure 20–5 The five fundamental types of cortical structure: Type 1 = agranular motor cortex. Type 2 = frontal homotypical (frontal granular). Type 3 = parietal homotypical. Type 4 = polar, e.g., area 18. Type 5 = granular koniocortex. (From Von Economo, C.: *The Cytoarchitectonics of the Human Cerebral Cortex.* London, Oxford University Press, 1929, p. 16.)

to FB, the premotor cortex, which is adjacent to FC, the transitional premotor cortex, which in turn is adjacent to FD, the prefrontal granular cortex. In occipital areas the designations OA, OB, and OC are used. The letters A, B, and C again represent steps of a definable histological gradation. Moreover OC, the striate koniocortex, is surrounded by OB, which in turn is transitional to the outer surrounding cortex of OA (Fig. 20–9).

This scheme and terminology, however, have not come into widespread use. Instead, the older numbers scheme of Brodmann (Fig. 20–10) remains in common usage. Numbers were initially assigned, as histologically distinct areas were identified in successive horizontal slices, moving in anterior and posterior directions from the central sulcus. The crest of the postcentral gyrus, being the highest point, would then appear in the first horizontal section and would be assigned the number 1. Thus there is no logical reason why the numbers 6 and 8 are assigned to areas of the frontal lobe and 5 and 7 to areas in the parietal lobes. Nevertheless, some of

the numbers are used with sufficient frequency in everyday neurological language that the student should commit these to memory. The more commonly used numbers are listed in the following outline with a brief note as to function. The corresponding terminology of Von Economo and Koskinas is indicated in parentheses (Fig. 20–7):

FRONTAL LOBE

Area 4 (FA) corresponds in general to the precentral gyrus and functions as the primary motor cortex. It is continued onto the medial surface as the paracentral lobule (Fig. 20–10).

Area 6 (FB) located anterior to area 4 and thus referred to as premotor cortex, functions as a motor association or elaboration area (Fig. 20–10).

Area 8 (FC) located anterior to area 6 is often grouped with area 6 as premotor cortex. This area functions in relation to head and eye turning.

Areas 44 and 45 (FCB) correspond in general to the inferior frontal gyrus triangular and opercular portions. In the dominant

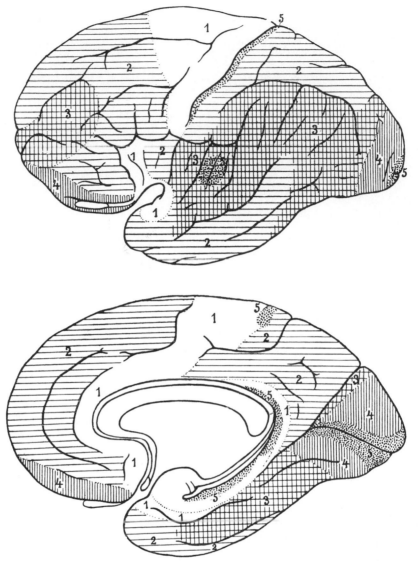

Figure 20-6   Distribution of the five cortical types of Figure 20–5 over the lateral and medial surfaces of the cerebral surface. The Sylvian fissure has been laid open. (From Von Economo, C.: *The Cytoarchitectonics of the Human Cerebral Cortex.* London, Oxford University Press, 1929, p. 18.)

hemisphere this constitutes Broca's motor speech center.

Areas 9, 10, 11 and 12 (FD), the prefrontal areas, are concerned with emotional control and other aspects of cognitive function (Fig. 20–10).

PARIETAL LOBE

Areas 3, 1, 2 (PB, PC, PD) correspond to the postcentral gyrus and function as the primary somatosensory projection areas (continue into paracentral lobule).

Areas 39, 40 (PG, PF) correspond to the inferior parietal lobule. These areas in the dominant hemisphere function in relation to reading and writing as higher integrative areas for language.

TEMPORAL LOBE

Areas 41, 42 (TC, TB) The transverse gyri of Heschl function as primary auditory projection areas.

Area 22 (TA) corresponds to the superior temporal gyrus and surrounds areas 41–42. This is an auditory higher association center. In the dominant hemisphere, this area represents an auditory association area concerned with the reception and interpretation

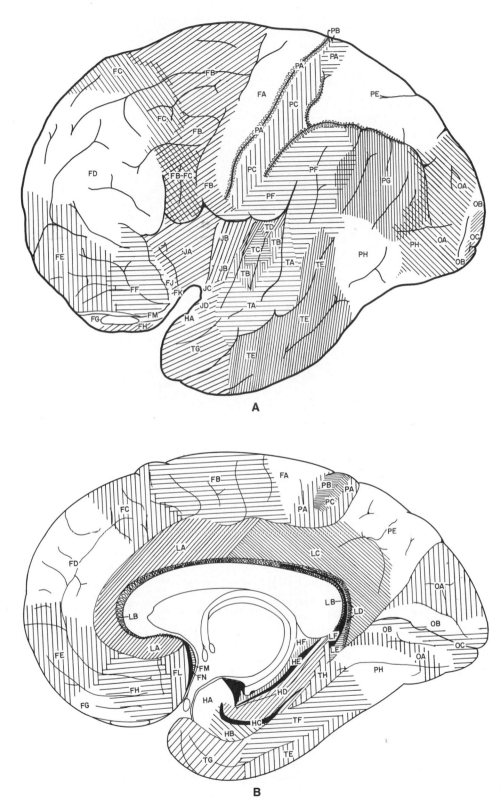

Figure 20-7 Cytoarchitectonic map of the cortex; scheme of Von Economo and Koskinas (1925). The original map has been considerably modified in this drawing with many subareas of the original map combined for the purpose of simplification. Note the logical sequence of cytoarchitectural designations in terms of FA, FB, FC, FD, OA, OB, OC, and so forth.

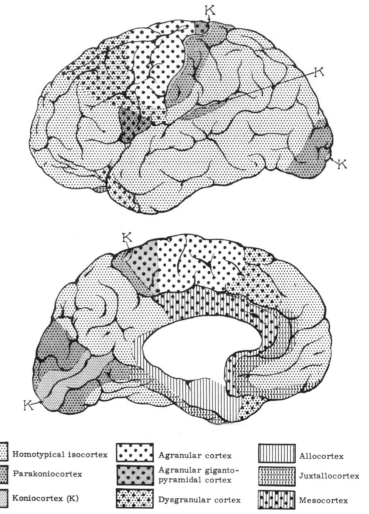

Figure 20-8 Map of human cerebral cortex based upon original color maps of Bailey and Von Bonin as modified by Chusid and McDonald (1964). In the original map, the transition from one cytoarchitectural area to the next is not sharp but rather gradually shades off. (From Chusid, J. G., and McDonald, J. J.: *Correlative Neuroanatomy and Functional Neurology,* 12th Edition. Los Altos, California, Lange Medical Publications, 1964, p. 9.)

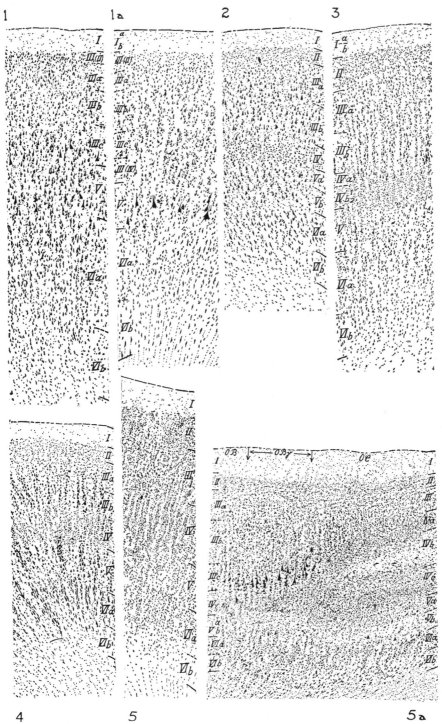

Figure 20-9 Sections of the cerebral cortex of man showing the arrangement of nerve cells in each of the five cortical types. Each section is enlarged to the same extent so that the thickness of the different types of cortex can be directly compared. 1, From the posterior part of the superior frontal gyrus (Type 1); 1*a*, from the anterior central gyrus, motor cortex (a variety of Type 1); 2, from the middle part of the middle frontal gyrus (Type 2); 3, from the supramarginal gyrus (Type 3); 4, from the lateral surface of the occipital lobe (Type 4); 5, from the anterior temporal gyrus, auditory cortex (Type 5); 5*a*, *oc*, the striate area, visual cortex (a variety of Type 5). Note the sharp transition from striate to peristriate cortex. (After von Economo from Ranson and Clark: *The Anatomy of the Nervous System.* Philadelphia. W. B. Saunders, 1959, p. 354.)

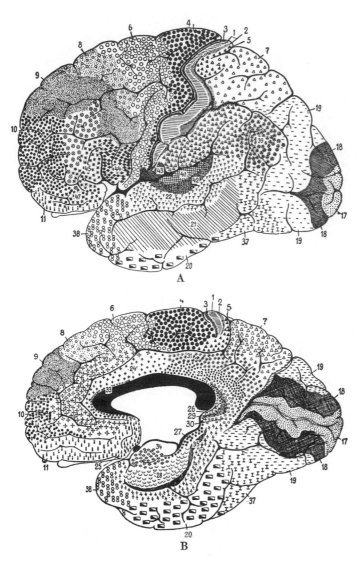

Figure 20-10 Cytoarchitectural areas of cerebral cortex as designated by Brodmann. (From Ranson and Clark: *The Anatomy of the Nervous System.* Philadelphia, W. B. Saunders, 1959, p. 356.)

See Filmstrip, Frames 61 and 62.

of spoken language. The area is often referred to as Wernicke's receptive aphasia center.

OCCIPITAL LOBE

Area 17 (OC) corresponds to the striate cortex bordering the calcarine fissure and functions as the primary visual projection area.

Areas 18, 19 (OB, OA) form surrounding strips around area 17. These areas function as visual association areas of varying complexity.

THALAMOCORTICAL RELATIONSHIPS *(Fig. 20-11)*

It has been indicated to you that certain of the thalamic nuclei have a specific rela-

tionship with certain cortical areas. Ablation of the specific cortical area then produces degeneration in a specific nucleus of the thalamus. Other nuclei of the thalamus are classed as nonspecific and do not have a relationship to a specific cortical area but rather relate to more general areas of cerebral cortex or relate via other thalamic nuclei. The following specific relationships may be indicated:

Lateral geniculate and area 17

Medial geniculate and area 41

Ventral posterior lateral ⎱
Ventral posterior medial ⎰ and areas 3, 2, 1

Ventral lateral ⎱
Ventral anterior ⎰ and areas 4, 6

Dorsomedial and prefrontal areas 9, 10, 11, 12

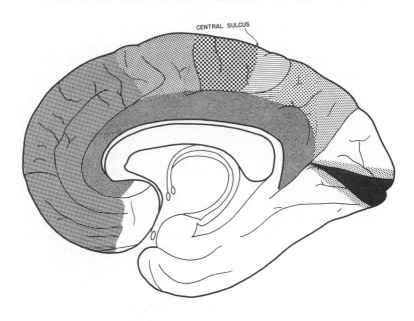

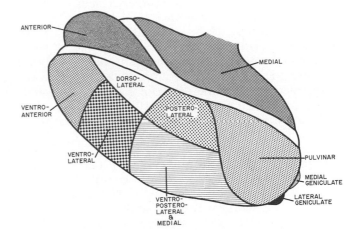

Figure 20–11 Thalamocortical relationships. The relationship of specific cortical areas to specific thalamic nuclei is demonstrated. (Based on Netter, 1953; Treux and Carpenter, 1964, and Akert, 1964.)

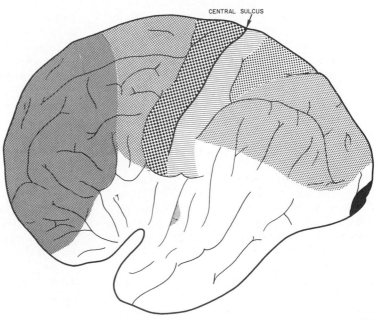

459

Anterior nuclei and cingulate gyrus

Lateral posterior and superior parietal lobule

Pulvinar and inferior parietal lobule and portions of 18, 19 visual association

CHANGES IN CORTICAL ARCHITECTURE AS A FUNCTION OF POSTNATAL AGE

During postnatal development the brain increases significantly in weight from an average of 375 to 400 grams at birth to 1000 grams at 1 year, to a maximum of 1350 to 1410 grams at age 15 years (males). This increased growth does not affect all areas of the brain to an equal extent. Thus this growth involves a rapid expansion of the convexities of the frontal, parietal, and temporal lobes. This results in a completion of the covering of the insular lobe by the surrounding operculum and a relative displacement of the parahippocampal gyrus and occipital lobe. In addition, the cortical surface area is in a sense being increased by the deepening of sulci, with increasing complexity of the primary and secondary fissures. This process continues after the second year with the development of tertiary fissures.

In addition to these grossly visible postnatal changes in the external appearance of the cerebral hemispheres, important changes are occurring as regards myelination. These changes parallel the successive stages of psychomotor development witnessed during these postnatal months. At birth most of the intrinsic fiber systems of the spinal cord and brain stem have myelinated. The long corticospinal tracts and corpus callosum begin to myelinate during the first postnatal months. The frontopontine, temporopontine, and thalamocortical projections myelinate during the second postnatal month.

Myelination is occurring not only as regards long fiber systems but also as regards the intrinsic fiber systems and plexuses seen at a microscopic level within the cerebral cortex. Flechsig pointed out that not all cortical areas myelinate at the same time and that the sequence of myelination followed a logical pattern (Fig. 20–12). The areas that showed stainable myelin before or at term, he designated as *primordial*. These areas correspond in general to the primary motor and sensory areas. The *intermediate fields*, corresponding to association areas around these primary zones, myelinate at approximately 6

to 12 weeks. The *terminal fields* which myelinate after the fourth postnatal month correspond to the higher order association or integration areas surrounding or lying as bridges between different modality sensory association areas—for example, the prefrontal and inferior parietal lobule. As regards the general relationship of these myelogenetic fields to the cytoarchitectural areas, it may be noted that the primordial fields correspond to the specialized heterotypical variants, and the terminal fields to the homotypical varieties of neocortex.

Although myelination of the cerebral cortex begins during the early postnatal months, it is evident that this process is not completed at this time (Fig. 20–13). Thus the initial myelination occurs in the vertically oriented fibers of the infragranular layers, then extends into the supragranular layers. The myelination of horizontal plexuses occurs at a later stage. Myelination continues to increase beyond 15 years of age, even until age 60, with a gradual increase in density of myelinated fibers particularly in the horizontal plexuses. It must of course be noted that even in the adult not all cortical areas will reach the same density of myelinated fibers, since the underlying cellular and fibrous structure will differ significantly among different cortical areas.

In addition to changes in the degree of myelination, more basic changes in the relationships between nerve cells are occurring. The cerebral cortex has received its full quota of neurons by the end of the sixth fetal month. During postnatal development, as shown in the silver stain, there is a progressive growth of the apical and basilar dendritic arborization, with a progressive increase in the number of synapses (Fig. 20–14). The studies of Conel have demonstrated that the more primitive allocortex (e.g., hippocampus) attains its final structural form at an earlier stage than the neocortex. The changes in structure may be correlated with changes in excitability patterns as shown by Purpura in studies of evoked potentials in the immature cortex of the cat. These studies have also shown that the adult pattern of evoked response and excitability is attained in the hippocampus at an earlier postnatal age than in the neocortex.

The possible role of environmental and other afferent stimuli in this progressive increase in synaptic contacts between nerve cells and between nerve cells and afferent

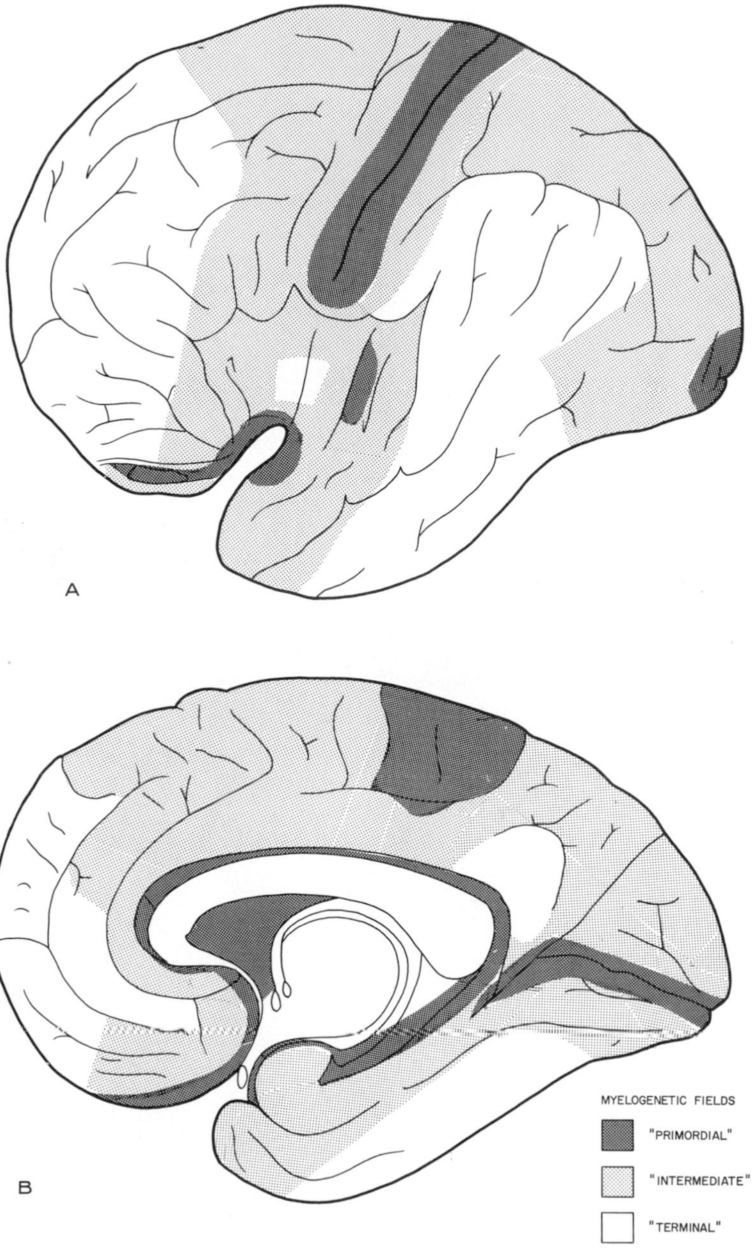

Figure 20–12 The myelogenetic fields of Flechsig, modified from Yakovlev (1962) to demonstrate "primordial fields" (fields 1–10 in the number sequence of Flechsig), "intermediate fields" (fields 11–30 in the number sequence of Flechsig), and "terminal fields" (fields 36–45 in the number sequence of Flechsig). Primordial fields show stainable myelin before or at term. Intermediate fields myelinate at 6–12 weeks. Terminal fields myelinate after the fourth postnatal month. *A* is lateral surface, *B* is medial surface.

MYELOGENETIC FIELDS

"PRIMORDIAL"

"INTERMEDIATE"

"TERMINAL"

fibers will be considered in a later chapter on learning.

SUBCORTICAL WHITE MATTER

Essentially three types of fiber systems occupy the subcortical white matter: (1) projection fibers, (2) commissural fibers, and (3) association fibers.

Projection fibers consist of the corticopetal afferent fibers, such as the thalamocortical radiations, and the corticofugal efferent fibers such as the corticospinal, corticoreticular, and corticorubral tracts (Fig. 20–15).

The major commissural systems are the corpus callosum, anterior commissure, and hippocampal commissure. The corpus callosum is the major commissure for the neocortical areas (except the middle and inferior temporal gyri) (Fig. 20–16). In general, homologous areas of the two hemispheres are interconnected. However, there are significant regional variations between homologous areas as regards fiber density (Fig. 20–17).

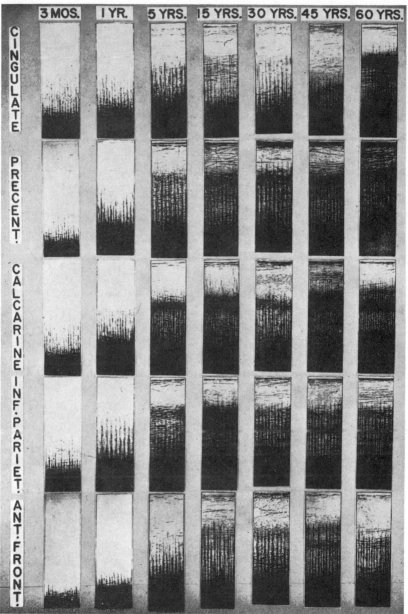

Figure 20–13 Progressive myelination of the vertical and horizontal or tangential plexus of cortical fibers in five sample areas of cerebral cortex from 3 months to 60 years. (After Kaes, from Yakovlev, P. I.: Res. Publ. Ass. nerv. ment. Dis., *39*:3–46, 1962, p. 28.)

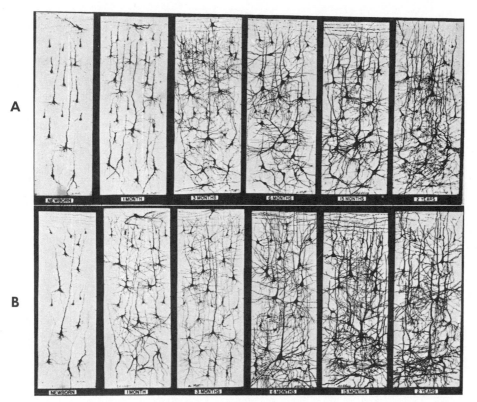

Figure 20–14 Progressive growth of the dendritic and axonal plexus in the supralimbic homotypical cortex. *A,* Frontal granular (FD). *B,* Parietal granular (PG) from birth to second postnatal year. (After Conel, from Yakovlev, P. I.: Res. Publ. Ass. nerv. ment. Dis., *39*:3–46, 1962, p. 44.)

Thus there is a high density of callosal fibers connecting the premotor areas of the two cerebral hemispheres. On the other hand, primary visual projection areas—area 17—has almost no direct callosal connection to the contralateral hemisphere. Area 17 transmits to the adjacent area 18 which has connections to contralateral area 18.

Cortical areas also differ as regards the spread of fibers to asymmetrical as well as to symmetrical points in the contralateral hemisphere. Thus area 6 has widespread connections in the contralateral hemisphere not only to area 6 but also to areas, 4, 5, 7, and 39, whereas area 4 has discrete contralateral connection only to the homotypic points.

The anterior commissure interconnects the middle and inferior temporal gyri, paleocortex, and amygdala. The hippocampal commissure interconnects the hippocampal formation and dentate gyri (archicortex). These fibers are conveyed via the fimbria of the fornix and cross at the point beneath the splenium of the corpus callosum, where the posterior pillars of the fornix converge.

Two types of subcortical association fibers may be distinguished (excluding from this discussion, the intracortical association fibers): (a) *short subcortical U or arcuate fibers* which interconnect adjacent gyri and (b) *long fiber bundles* which reciprocally interconnect distant cortical areas. The following long fiber bundles may be distinguished on blunt dissection of the cerebral hemisphere:

1. *The uncinate* fasciculus interconnects the orbital and medial prefrontal areas and the anterior temporal area (Fig. 20–18).

2. *The superior longitudinal fasciculus* interconnects the superior and lateral frontal, parietal and temporal, and occipital areas (Fig. 20–19). The extension of this fiber system into the temporal area, passing through the subcortical white matter of supramarginal and angular gyri, is often distinguished as the arcuate fasciculus. This fasciculus has considerable importance because of its role in connecting the receptive language centers of the temporal lobe with the expressive motor speech centers of the inferior frontal gyrus. Such a connection must be made if a sentence which has been heard is to be repeated.

3. *The cingulum* passes within the subcor-

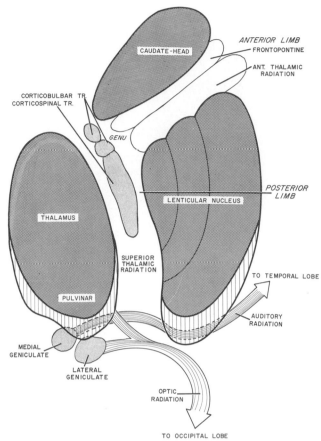

Figure 20-15 Projection fiber systems passing through the internal capsule. The superior thalamic radiation includes fibers projecting from ventral thalamus to sensory and motor cortex.

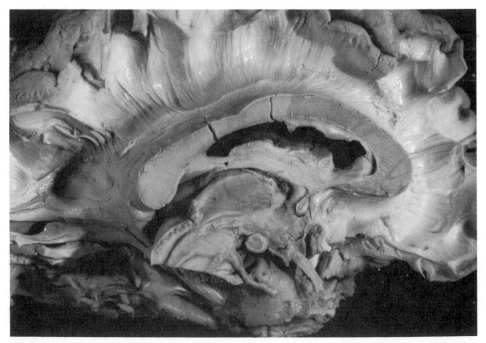

Figure 20-16 Radiation of fibers from corpus callosum as dissected in human brain.

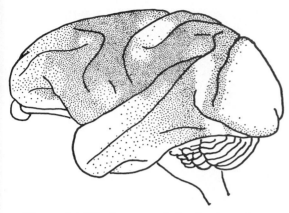

Figure 20–17 Pattern of distribution of commissural fibers over the cortical surface of the left hemisphere of the monkey (Macaca mulatta) as studied following section of major commissures. (From Myers, R. E.: *In* Ettlinger, E. G. (ed.): *Functions of the Corpus Callosum.* Boston, Little, Brown & Company, 1965, p. 142.)

tical white matter of the cingulate gyrus; it interconnects the subcallosal, medial-frontal, and orbital-frontal with the temporal lobe, occipital areas, and cingulate cortex.

4. The *inferior longitudinal fasciculus* interconnects the occipital and inferior temporal areas.

5. *The inferior frontal occipital fasciculus* interconnects the frontal and occipital areas. It is often difficult to clearly differentiate this fiber system from the uncinate fasciculus.

ELECTROPHYSIOLOGICAL CORRELATES OF CORTICAL CYTOARCHITECTURE

INTRODUCTION: METHODS OF ANALYSIS

The cerebral cortex of man and of other mammals is characterized by continuous rhythmic sinusoidal electrical activity of variable frequency. This electrical activity may be recorded through the scalp of man in the form of the electroencephalogram or directly from the cerebral cortex during surgery in the form of the electrocorticogram. In man, the basic resting electrical activity, as recorded from the posterior scalp areas, has an alternating voltage of 50 to 100 microvolts and an average frequency of 8 to 13 cps (called the alpha rhythm).

This basic continuous activity may be modified by various conditions of stimulation. The responses evoked in a group of cortical neurons by stimulation is referred to as the

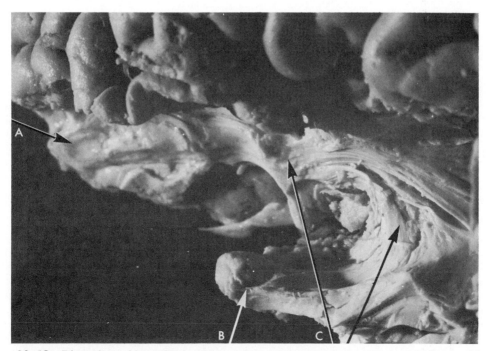

Figure 20–18 Dissection of long fiber systems; the uncinate fasciculus (C) passing from orbital frontal (A) to anterior temporal areas (B).

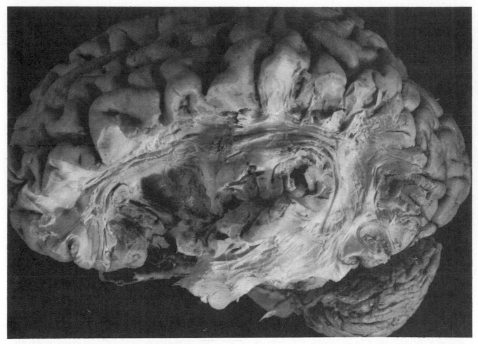

Figure 20–19 Dissection of long fiber systems: the superior longitudinal fasciculus demonstrating the arcuate fasciculus, passing beneath the cortex of inferior parietal, and posterior temporal areas. A small bundle of U fibers are also demonstrated incidentally at posterior, inferior margin of the temporal lobe interconnecting adjacent gyri.

evoked potential. We will be concerned in this chapter in attempting to relate these evoked cortical potentials to various features of cortical cytoarchitecture. We will also attempt to indicate how variations in cortical cytoarchitecture may be correlated with variations in cortical excitability. In Chapter 26 we will deal in greater detail with the underlying anatomical and physiological basis of the resting electroencephalogram. In addition we will consider the clinical use of the electroencephalogram in the diagnosis of diseases of the nervous system.

AXONAL ACTIVITY CONTRASTED TO SYNAPTIC ACTIVITY

Neurons of the cerebral cortex, when subjected to afferent stimulation, (via synaptic contacts on dendrites and cell body) are capable of two different types of electrical activity: (a) propagated axonal spike responses and (b) postsynaptic potentials. In this respect cortical neurons are similar to neurons elsewhere in the central nervous system. For example, the student has already encountered these two distinct types of activity in his earlier study of the conducted

axonal spike and of synaptic activity at the level of the spinal cord anterior horn cell.

Propagated axonal spike activity may be characterized as an all-or-nothing response triggered by a critical level of membrane depolarization. The spike is of high amplitude (i.e., intracellular recordings from Betz cells in the motor cortex after antidromic stimulation of the pyramidal tract have an amplitude of approximately +90 millivolts). Duration of the spike is short: 2 milliseconds at the cell body; 0.5 to 2.0 milliseconds at the level of the axon. There is an absolute refractory period of 2.0 to 2.5 milliseconds at the cell body and then a relative refractory period. There is, moreover, following the axon spike, a period of negative after potential of 12 to 20 milliseconds and then a more prolonged period of positive after potential (relative hyperpolarization) measuring 100 to 150 milliseconds at the level of the cell body.

In contrast, postsynaptic potentials are local graded (rather than all-or-nothing) responses of a much smaller amplitude. Spatial and temporal summation occurs. The summated potentials being considered are below the critical depolarization (10 millivolts) for the generation of the spike potential. Often voltages of less than 1 millivolt are under consideration (e.g., 50 or 200 microvolts). If the summated potential rises above the critical depolarization level then the all-or-nothing propagated axon spike is generated. The duration of the unitary postsynaptic potential is relatively long compared to the axon spike — 10 to 15 milliseconds (as recorded from cat alpha motor neuron). There is no refractory period. Therefore, spatial and temporal summation can occur over wide ranges of amplitude and duration. In contrast to the electrical propagation of the axon spike, the postsynaptic potential in the vertebrate nervous system is, in general, generated by the release of a chemical transmitter from the presynaptic membrane across the synapse.

The actual identity of the agents involved in synaptic transmission within the cerebral cortex is, in most instances, not completely established. Several agents must be involved since there is evidence of both excitatory and inhibitory synapses with corresponding excitatory and inhibitory postsynaptic potentials. As we have indicated previously, axodendritic synapses are generally related to excitatory postsynaptic potentials (EPSP's), and axosomatic synapses to inhibitory postsynaptic potentials (IPSP's). There are of course other differences between axonal propagation and synaptic impulse transmission. Axonal conduction is rapid and bidirectional. Synaptic conduction is slower (synaptic delay) and unidirectional.

Earlier attempts to explain the electrical activity of the cerebral cortex (as studied in the electroencephalogram or in evoked potentials) in terms of the axonal activity of the neurons were unsuccessful. This is understandable in view of the rapid short duration, all-or-nothing nature of the axon spike and the refractory period which follows this spike. There is, moreover, no one-to-one relationship between these spontaneous wave forms (recorded at the scalp or at the cortical surface or in closer relationship to a neuron) and the axon spike discharges of that neuron. On the other hand, the graded long duration and the nonrefractory nature of the postsynaptic potentials does provide a more reasonable basis for an understanding of the spontaneous and evoked cortical potentials. In particular the potentials recorded in the electroencephalogram have been linked to the summated postsynaptic potentials of the apical dendrites of many cortical neurons.

METHODS EMPLOYED IN ANATOMICAL CORRELATION STUDIES OF EVOKED CORTICAL POTENTIALS

Various sites of electrical stimulation have been employed: e.g., cortical surface, specific thalamic nuclei, nonspecific thalamic nuclei, basal ganglia, mesencephalic reticular formation, sciatic nerve, and optic nerve. It will be evident from the more detailed discussion that follows that the form of response and the cortical area from which the response is obtained will vary in part as a function of the site of stimulation. Evoked responses may be recorded from the cortical surface using macroelectrodes (usually a nonpolarized chlorided silverball electrode). Responses may also be recorded at various points below the cortical surface employing a microelectrode mounted on a micromanipulator. This laminar analysis allows a correlation of electrical events with particular cell layers or with a particular locus on the large neurons, e.g., apical dendrite, cell body, or basilar dendrites. Surface activity is usually recorded simultaneously with a macroelectrode on the surface to allow cross correlation with electrical events recorded by the microelectrode in the deeper layers of the cerebral cortex. Microelectrode recording may be made in an extracellular manner, or the microelectrode may be introduced into a large neuron to record intracellular events.

In general, when the electroencephalogram and evoked responses are recorded, the cortical electrical potentials are amplified with equipment (preamplifiers, cathode-ray oscilloscope, and ink-writing oscilloscopes) which record alternating currents. The electrical activity to be recorded consists of oscillating sinusoidal wave forms of alternating polarity. At times, however, particularly in intracellular recording, it is useful to evaluate shifts in membrane potential by means of direct current recordings. For this purpose special electrodes and amplifiers are employed.

At times in the analysis of evoked potentials, it is useful to modify the membrane potential of the neuron by passing current through an intracellular microelectrode to produce a relative depolarization or hyperpolarization.

Several pharmacological agents may also be employed in the analysis of evoked responses. Thus, active agents applied to the pial surface of the cerebral cortex will have their initial effects on superficial layers of the cerebral cortex. Those components of the evoked response which are due to the activation of synapses in the superficial layers of the cerebral cortex will be modified initially by these agents. Those components of the evoked response related to the neuronal structure in the deeper layers of the cortex will not be immediately modified by these agents. Certain agents such as procaine have a general depressing effect on all activities in the superficial layers of the cerebral cortex. Other agents, such as strychnine, gamma aminobutyric acid, and other amino acids, are considered to have more specific synaptic effects. For example, gamma aminobutyric acid acts primarily to block excitatory axo-dendritic synapses in the superficial layers. At times in order to localize various electrical events the superficial layers of the cortex may be destroyed by heating, while the deeper cortical layers are preserved.

In recordings, the potential voltage difference between two electrodes of a pair is displayed, after amplification, on a cathode-ray oscilloscope or on paper by means of an ink-writing oscillograph (as in the usual electroencephalogram). Recordings may be made in a bipolar manner (both electrodes of the pair over active brain tissue) or in a monopolar (or unipolar) manner (one electrode of the pair over active brain tissue, the other at a distant point which is relatively inactive electrically). By convention, when alternating currents are being recorded in electrophysiology, the connections from the electrodes to the differential input stage of the amplifying system are arranged so that when the electrode over active tissue becomes relatively negative to an electrode over inactive tissue an upward deflection is produced in the record. This arrangement involves the connection of the active electrode to grid I and the inactive monopolar reference (or the other active electrode of the bipolar pair) to grid II. When the electrode at grid I becomes negative to the electrode at grid II an upward deflection occurs. When a depolarization occurred, at the cortical surface immediately beneath an extracellular macroelectrode resting on the pial surface such an upward (negative) deflection would be recorded. On the other hand, hyperpolarization occurring at the surface close to the electrode would be recorded as a downward or positive deflection.

It is important to realize, however, that electrical events are occurring not only close to the cortical surface (in the superficial layers of the cortex) but also in the deeper layers of the cerebral cortex. These events in the deeper layers are not occurring as electrically isolated events: neuronal elements *in situ* within the brain (and for that matter also axons in peripheral nerve) exist embedded in tissue which is itself an electrical conducting medium (concept of volume conduction). The electrical activity at the surface will be influenced in a passive manner by events occurring in the deeper layers of the cortex.

At a point of excitation at the onset of depolarization there is a flow of current into the nerve. This area is spoken of as a "*sink*" of current and acts as a cathode. Cations are attracted to this area, and among these sodium enters the nerve. These cations must in a sense have originated from surrounding conducting tissue and neuronal elements relatively distant from the point of excitation. There is then an outflow of current and cations from this surrounding tissue. These surrounding areas are spoken of as "sources" of current. The sink and the sources are, relative to an indifferent electrode, undergoing electrical activities which are opposite in sign. An extracellular electrode at a sink, the point of excitation in the deeper layer (that is the point of depolarization), would record an upward or negative deflection. At this same time an electrode at the surface, "the source," (a point of relative hyperpolarization), would record a downward or positive deflection. One could speak of this as a passive surface hyperpolarization (as opposed to an active surface hyperpolarization due to events originating at the cortical surface in the superficial layers). Similarly, events occurring at the surface will influence the activity of deeper cortical layers (Fig. 20–20).

Using this same frame of reference, it should be evident that a significant active hyperpolarization occurring in the deeper layers of the cerebral cortex (for example, at the level of the nerve cell body) would be recorded as a downward or positive deflection by an extracellular electrode in the deeper layers close to this point. On the other hand, an electrode resting on the cortical surface at the same moment would record a passive relative depolarization—a negative or upward deflection.

In analyzing a negative wave recorded at the surface, the electrophysiologist must distinguish between active depolarization at superficial excitatory synapses and passive

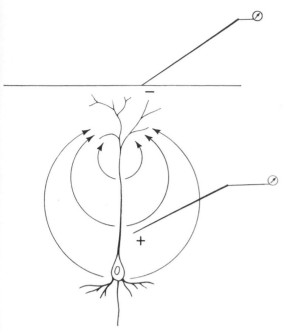

Figure 20-20 A diagrammatic illustration of volume conductor theory as applied to the pyramidal cell. A depolarization, (−) of the apical dendrites close to the surface has occurred, producing a "sink" (−) of activity. Current then flows into this area, the "sink," from the polarized deeper regions. The latter are referred to as "sources" (+). Electrodes recording at the superficial and deeper layers would record the voltage difference produced by this flow of current in the volume conductor. (From Ochs: *Elements of Neurophysiology.* New York, John Wiley, 1965, p. 376.)

depolarization (volume conductor effects) resulting from active hyperpolarization (inhibitory synapses postsynaptic potentials) in the deeper layers. This differentiation can be made by employing the methods previously described: laminar recordings, pharmacological blockage of the synapses in the superficial layers of the cortex, destruction limited to the superficial layers of the cortex, intracellular recording, and passive membrane polarization.

DEFINITION AND ANATOMICAL CORRELATION OF NEOCORTICAL EVOKED RESPONSES

We will now consider particular neocortical evoked responses. This will serve to introduce the student to the terminology employed by the cortical electrophysiologist and to briefly indicate current concepts of the anatomical correlates of these evoked responses. For a more detailed consideration of this subject the student should consult *The Electrical Activity of the Nervous System* by Brazier and the extensive review by Purpura.

SUPERFICIAL CORTICAL RESPONSE

Minimal electrical stimulation of the cortical surface produces a surface negative wave lasting from 15 to 20 milliseconds. The response is recorded close to the point of stimulation and results from the activation of excitatory (depolarizing) synapses on apical dendrites. The stimulus presumably produces local nonpropagated depolarization of the superficial presynaptic sites of axodendritic synapses. (This local depolarization never reaches the critical depolarization level that would generate propagated axon spikes in the presynaptic axons.) This leads to release of a transmitter substance and activation of excitatory postsynaptic sites on apical dendrites. Microelectrode studies indicate that the response is limited to the upper 0.5 mm. of the cerebral cortex, that is, the superficial layers (Fig. 20–21). Spread of activity along the surface to points distant from the point of stimulation does, however, occur as a result of conduction in the horizontally oriented fibers of the molecular layer.

The surface negative wave of the superficial cortical response may be considered a basic building block which will be encountered whenever synaptic activation of surface axodendritic synapses occurs.

DIRECT CORTICAL RESPONSE AND PROPAGATED AFTER-DISCHARGE

The term direct cortical response has at times been used interchangeably with the superficial cortical response. As used by Purpura, this term refers to the sequence of potentials obtained by stronger (supraliminal) stimulation of the cerebral cortex. Recordings are obtained close to the stimulating electrode. The stimulation produces an all-or-nothing axonal spike discharge in the presynaptic axons. Such a discharge must not only result in the release of considerable transmitter agent from presynaptic sites, but also must produce, in an antidromic manner, propagation of impulse to the nerve cell from which the axon originates and activation also of other axon branches. The transmitter agent released may produce sufficient

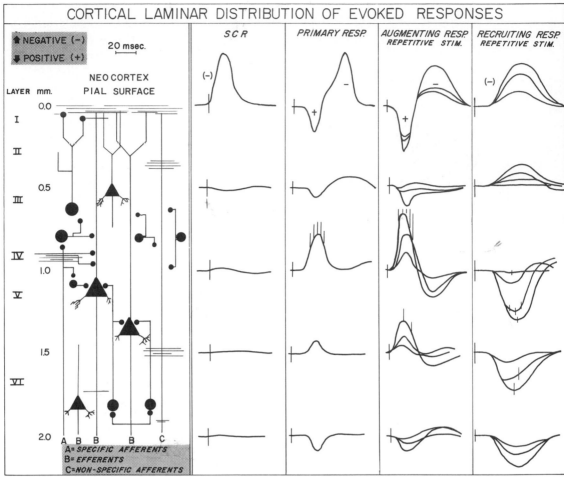

Figure 20–21 A laminar analysis of the various cortical evoked responses is indicated in terms of the type and magnitude of response recorded with an external microelectrode at various depths. The presumptive cortical layers are indicated and the cytoarchitectural pattern is diagrammed in a schematic manner. Specific afferent fibers terminate in layer IV and are shown making synaptic contact with both granule cell interneurons and adjacent pyramidal cells. Nonspecific afferent fibers are shown terminating in many layers including layer I. The efferent fibers of pyramidal cells (B) have axon collaterals which synapse with various types of interneurons. These interneurons may synapse in turn with the large pyramidal cells, e.g., axon collateral inhibition.

The *SCR* (superficial cortical response) is limited to the superficial layers of cerebral cortex. The initial surface positive component of the *primary evoked response* (specific stimulus, recording from specific cortical projection) originates in the deeper cortical layers (the vertical lines represent cell discharges). The subsequent surface negative wave originates in superficial cortical layers. The *augmenting response* is similar to the primary evoked response except that a specific thalamic nucleus is stimulated (e.g., VPL as compared to sciatic nerve for the primary evoked response). The origin of the *recruiting response* to stimulation of nonspecific thalamic nuclei is complex (see text). (Reproduced with modifications from an unpublished diagram by Purpura.)

summated postsynaptic depolarization to result in all-or-nothing propagated discharge of the synaptically activated neurons. With the development of propagated action potentials, there is the possibility of repetitive afterdischarge and of propagation to distant cortical, subcortical, and brain stem areas.

Propagation may of course also occur to the contralateral hemisphere.

TRANSCALLOSAL RESPONSE

With sufficient stimulation of the cortical surface as indicated, an all-or-nothing propagated discharge of neurons in the deeper cortical layers will occur with transmission of impulse via the corpus callosum to the contralateral hemisphere. Recordings from the homologous point in this contralateral hemisphere will reveal, after a latency period of 10 milliseconds, a surface positive response of 10 to 15 milliseconds followed by a surface negative wave of 10 to 20 milliseconds (Fig. 20–22). The surface positive wave is due to the generation of excitatory postsynaptic potentials in the deeper cortical layers (e.g., layers IV and V and deeper III). The surface negative wave indicates the sub-

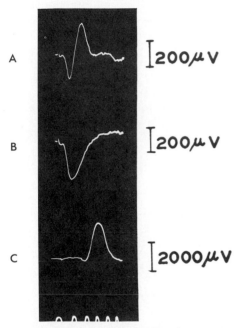

Figure 20–22 The transcallosal response. Potentials were recorded with a macroelectrode on surface of middle suprasylvian gyrus of cat, with the stimulus delivered to a symmetrical point in the contralateral hemisphere.

A, Typical normal wave (note the resemblance to the primary evoked response).

B, Same recording point after local application of 6.5% Nembutal (a barbiturate sedative and general anesthetic agent).

C, Same recording point after local application of 1.0% strychnine sulfate. Note that the amplification has been reduced (calibration signal reduced). Both of these agents modify the surface negative component (negativity is recorded as an upward deflection) without greatly modifying the initial surface positive wave. The surface negative wave must originate in superficial layers, the initial surface positive wave in deeper layers. The time signal is 60 cps. (From Curtis, H. J.: J. Neurophysiol., *3*:416, 1940.)

sequent generation of excitatory postsynaptic potentials at superficial axodendritic sites.

PRIMARY OR SPECIFIC EVOKED RESPONSE

These responses are obtained from specific sensory projection areas of the cerebral cortex following stimulation of specific sensory pathways. Thus stimulation of the sciatic nerve in the cat will produce, after a latency period of 10 to 20 milliseconds, a response in a limited locus (the leg representation) of the somatic sensory projection area of the contralateral hemisphere. This response is similar in form to the transcallosal response consisting of a surface positive wave of 10 to 15 milliseconds followed by a surface negative wave of 10 to 20 milliseconds (Fig. 20–23). The initial surface positive wave is associated with excitatory postsynaptic potentials generated in deeper cortical layers (layers III and IV) at a depth of approximately 1 mm. Electrodes at this depth often record, superimposed on this wave, brief spike discharges presumably originating in pyramidal cells at this level (Fig. 20–21). The subsequent surface negative wave again indicates the generation of excitatory postsynaptic potentials at superficial axodendritic sites. The surface negative wave is often followed by a series of waves of variable form which merge with the spontaneous background electrical activity.

With visual stimulation (a flash of light) a response is obtained from visual projection area which is, in general, similar in form to that described for somatosensory stimulation.

Following direct stimulation of the specific thalamic nucleus (ventral posterior lateral, lateral geniculate, or medial geniculate) a response may be obtained from the limited area of the cerebral cortex which is the appropriate sensory projection area for the specific thalamic nucleus. The form of response is similar to that obtained by stimulation of the sciatic nerve. The latency of the response is, of course, much shorter.

The primary evoked response has been mainly studied in the experimental animal. Occasionally recordings have been made directly from cerebral cortex in man during neurosurgical procedures. More recently the use of computers to average responses has allowed the recording with scalp electrodes in man of the response evoked by somato-

A

B

C

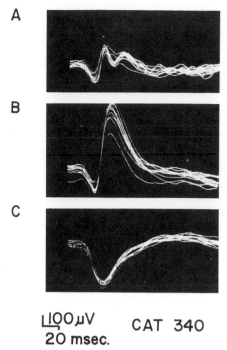

⌊100 μV
20 msec.   CAT 340

Figure 20-23 The primary evoked response. In lightly anesthetized cat stimulation of left sciatic nerve was performed at approximately 1 volt, 0.1 msec. duration and frequency of 1 cps. Recordings are from hind-limb projection area of right posterior sigmoid gyrus (10 superimposed responses).

A, Control response

B, Following topical application of 0.1% solution of strychnine sulfate (blocks IPSP's at surface). Effects were immediate. This recording was obtained 100 sec. after application.

C, Following topical application of 1.0% solution of gamma aminobutyric acid (GABA—blocks EPSP's at surface). Effects were immediate, this recording was obtained 5 minutes after application. Note that the primary effects of these agents is on the surface negative wave (negativity is recorded with upward deflection). The initial positive wave which originates in deeper cortical layers is relatively unchanged. (From unpublished experiments Marcus, E. M., and Bowker, R., 1966.)

sensory stimuli (ulnar nerve stimulation) or visual stimuli (short duration light flash). The recording electrodes must of course be arranged on the scalp so as to record from the specific sensory projection area.

SECONDARY DISCHARGE OR RESPONSE OF FORBES

Following sciatic stimulation, in addition to the primary evoked response described,

there is noted a second, relatively long (30 to 60 milliseconds) surface positive wave which occurs with a latency of 30 to 80 milliseconds. The surface positive wave is often followed by a surface negative wave. The secondary response was originally described by Forbes as occurring under conditions of relatively deep barbiturate anesthesia (sufficient to suppress the background electrical activity) (Fig. 20-24). However, this response may also be recorded in the unanesthetized animal.

In contrast to the limited cortical distribution of the primary evoked response, the secondary response is widespread in its distribution, appearing simultaneously over many cortical areas. The primary response to sciatic stimulation is conducted over specific pathways of the medial lemniscus to a specific thalamic nucleus and then projected to a specific cortical area. In contrast, the secondary response follows several (crossed and uncrossed) nonspecific pathways in the brain stem. It is uncertain whether these

↓ Stimulus

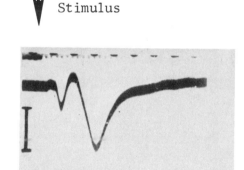

↑ Primary response   ↑ Secondary discharge

⊢⊣
40 msec.

Figure 20-24 The secondary response of Forbes. Cortical response ("sensorimotor cortex") to contralateral sciatic stimulation in the cat under deep pentobarbital anesthesia. The vertical calibration signal represents 200 uv. The peak of the secondary response occurs approximately 110–120 msec. after the stimulus. (Modified from Forbes, A., and Morrison, B. R.: J. Neurophysiol., 2:117, 1939.)

pathways are distinct from the ascending reticular formation. The pathway from the brain stem to the cortex apparently follows an extrathalamic pathway. Thalamic stimulation does not produce this response.

AUGMENTING RESPONSE

We have indicated that stimulation of a specific thalamic nucleus (e.g., ventral posterior lateral) will produce, in the appropriate cortical projection area, a localized response which is similar in form to the primary evoked response but is of much shorter latency (1 to 5 milliseconds). With repetitive stimulation at 6 to 12 cps the amplitude of each response progressively increases (or augments) (Fig. 20–25). There would appear little doubt that the basic cortical elements involved are the same as those involved in the primary evoked response. The initial surface positive wave is the result of excitatory postsynaptic potentials originating in the deeper cortical layers. Intracellular recordings from these areas indicate associated spike discharges of the neuron (Fig. 20–21). The subsequent surface negativity is related to subsequent synaptic activation of superficial excitatory axodendritic synapses.

RECRUITING RESPONSE

The augmenting response evoked in the cortex by stimulating a specific thalamic nucleus must be contrasted to the recruiting response which follows repetitive (6 to 12 cps) stimulation of nonspecific thalamic nuclei: the intralaminar group (centrum medianum, parafasciculus, limitans, paracentralis, and centralis lateralis) and the reticular nucleus within the external medullary lamina (Fig. 20–25). Responses are also obtained on stimulation of the ventral anterior and reuniens nuclei. The response obtained in the cortex consists of repetitive surface negative waves which wax (recruit) and then wane in amplitude (Fig. 20–26). The latency of the response (15 to 60 milliseconds) is long compared to the responses evoked by stimulating specific thalamic nuclei. The cortical distribution of the recruiting response is often considered to be diffuse with the implication that stimulation of a particular nonspecific thalamic nucleus produces a response throughout all areas of the cerebral cortex. The nonspecific thalamic

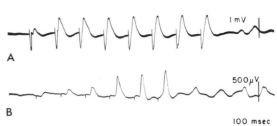

Figure 20–25 Comparison of augmenting and recruiting responses.

A, Augmenting responses recorded from anterior sigmoid gyrus of cat (motor cortex) following stimulation of the ipsilateral specific thalamic nucleus ventralis lateralis. The response in form is similar to the primary evoked response. The latency, however, is extremely short; the stimulus artefact merges with the initial surface positivity.

B, Recruiting responses recorded from the sensory motor cortex of the cat following stimulation of a nonspecific or diffuse system midline thalamic nucleus (nucleus reuniens). Note the long latency following the stimulus artefact for the appearance of the surface negative wave. (From Brookhart and Zanchetti: Electroenceph. Clin. Neurophysiol., *8*:431, 1956.)

nuclei and the related cortical elements involved in this response have been grouped together as the diffuse thalamocortical system. The original studies of Morrison and Dempsy (1942) indicated, however, that there were regional variations as regards those areas of the cortex from which the recruiting response could be obtained. Responses were more readily obtained from association cortex than from primary sensory projection areas. In the monkey, the response was obtained primarily from the frontal and parietal association areas (Starzl and Whitlock, 1952) (Fig. 20–27). Moreover the studies of Jasper (1949) indicated a significant degree of topographical organization within these nonspecific thalamic nuclei. In the cat, frontal recruiting responses were obtained predominantly by stimulating more rostral nuclei, and occipital responses, by stimulating more caudal thalamic areas. In addition the effects were predominantly ipsilateral, rather than bilaterally symmetrical.

The surface negative wave of the recruiting response is associated with excitatory postsynaptic potentials generated in the superficial layers at axodendritic synapses. Under particular conditions of light anesthesia and of stimulation, the initial surface negative wave may be followed by a second long duration surface negative wave of 100 to 200

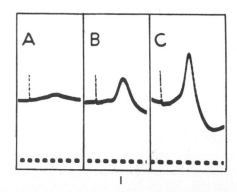

I

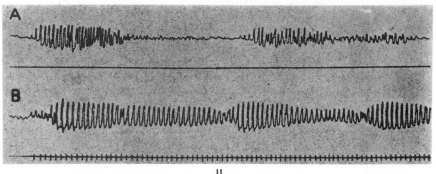

II

Figure 20–26 The recruiting response.

I. Cortical responses in anterior sigmoid gyrus of cat to successive stimulation (*A, B, C*) at 8 cps of intra-laminar nuclei of thalamus. Note the long latency and the progressive increase in amplitude of the surface negative response. The time marks indicate 10 msec. (From Morison, R. S., and Dempsey, E. W.: Amer. J. Physiol., *135*:288, 1942.)

II. The similarity of the recruiting response to the spontaneous 8–12 cps spindles which characterize sedation or anesthesia with Nembutal or other barbiturates. The waxing and waning amplitude of the recruiting response is also demonstrated. Recordings from middle suprasylvian gyrus of cat.

A, Spontaneous spindle burst.

B, Recruiting response to stimulation (stimulus marker) of intralaminar areas of thalamus. (From Dempsey, E. W., and Morison, R. S.: Amer. J. Physiol., *135*:297, 1942.)

milliseconds. This second wave is associated with a prolonged hyperpolarization of the neuron as recorded in the deeper cortical layers.

There remains considerable uncertainty as to the actual connections from nonspecific thalamic nuclei to the cerebral cortex. We have previously indicated in the section on cytoarchitecture that nonspecific afferent fibers enter the cerebral cortex and ascend giving off collaterals at many levels. The sub-cortical origin of these fibers, however, has never been clearly identified. No direct connections from these nonspecific nuclei to the cortex of the lateral convexity of the cerebral hemisphere have been demonstrated. More-over, the prolonged latency of the recruiting response would suggest that several synapses are involved.

The more recent studies in the cat by Velasco and Lindsley (1965), by Skinner and

Lindsley (1967), and by Clemente and Ster-man (1967) suggest that the nonspecific nuclei do not have diffuse connections to many cortical areas, but rather information from these nuclei is sent to the orbital frontal cortex via the preoptic region (basal fore-brain). From the orbital frontal cortex spread may then occur to other cortical areas via corticocortical association fiber systems. In these studies the recruiting response could be produced by direct stimulation of the basal forebrain or the orbital frontal areas.

Another possible pathway has also been implicated. Lesions of the ventral anterior nucleus of the thalamus also abolish or reduce the recruiting response. Connections of the centrum medianum nucleus to the caudate nucleus and putamen are known. The caudate nucleus and putamen project via the globus pallidus to the ventral anterior and ventral lateral nuclei of the thalamus. These

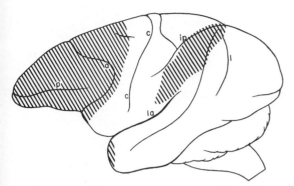

Figure 20–27 Cortical projection of the diffuse thalamic system (intralaminar and medial nuclei) in the monkey. On the dorsolateral surface of the hemisphere, the projections are primarily to the premotor prefrontal areas, inferior parietal lobule, and anterior temporal pole. The premotor area of response continues onto the medial surface of the hemisphere extending into the cingulate gyrus. The prefrontal and anterior temporal response areas continue onto their respective inferior surfaces. The system has been referred to as the frontal-parietal recruiting system since the response is primarily found in these areas. (From Starzl, T. E., and Whitlock, D. G.: J. of Neurophysiol., *15*:459, 1952.)

thalamic nuclei then project to the motor and premotor cortex.

AROUSAL OR ACTIVATION OR DESYNCHRONIZATION RESPONSE

High frequency (50 to 300 cps) stimulation of the ascending reticular formation in the tegmentum of the pons or mesencephalon (Fig. 20–28*I*) will convert the resting cortical activity from 3 to 12 cps waves of high relative amplitude (e.g., the activity present during drowsiness or sleep) to a high frequency (30 to 40 cps) activity of low relative amplitude (the activity present during alertness) (Fig. 20–28*II*). The response is widespread throughout all cortical areas. The response occurs with a latency of approximately 40 milliseconds and outlasts the period of stimulation. The long latency suggests a pathway involving several synapses as opposed to the classic short latency lemniscal sensory pathway.

A similar activation response follows stimulation in the periphery. Thus sciatic stimulation produces not only the short latency, localized, primary evoked response but also the long latency, generalized, arousal response. This reflects the fact that sensory

data enters the reticular formation via collaterals from the specific sensory pathways, particularly the spinothalamic system. However, multiple sensory modalities may synapse on the same neuron in the reticular formation. The system then is in a sense nonspecific as to the modality identity of the incoming stimulus. The ascending reticular formation follows several pathways involving the diencephalon. The intralaminar nuclei of the thalamus represent an upward continuation of the ascending reticular formation. Stimulation of these thalamic nuclei, e.g., centrum medianum, at high frequency (300 cps) produces the same effects on cortical electrical activity as stimulation of ascending reticular formation at a brain stem level. The pathways from this area to the cerebral cortex are uncertain but may be identical to those involved in the recruiting response which follows stimulation of these same intralaminar nuclei at a much lower frequency.*

However, at a mesencephalic level the arousal (desynchronization) effects of stimulation of the ascending reticular formation persist after destruction of the thalamus. The alternate pathway involves the subthalamus, dorsal hypothalamus, and septum. Stimulation of these areas at high frequency will produce the arousal effect. Fibers apparently pass from these areas into the internal capsule. The actual identity of the fibers at the level of the cerebral cortex remains uncertain. The "nonspecific afferents" (noted in the cortex) whose subcortical origin remains uncertain may be involved.

At the level of the cerebral cortex the discrete elements involved also remain uncertain. There is some evidence that there is a depression or blockage of axodendritic excitatory postsynaptic potentials, e.g., there is a depression of the surface negative wave, superficial cortical response during the arousal response (Fig. 20–29).

The use of the term desynchronization to describe the appearance of low voltage fast activity may be somewhat puzzling to the student. The term came into use in the early years of electroencephalography, when the high amplitude slow waves noted in sleep and other conditions were considered to represent the synchronized discharges of

---

*However, as indicated by Brodal (1969), some of these effects of high-frequency thalamic stimulation may be mediated by descending pathways from the thalamus to mesencephalic reticular formation.

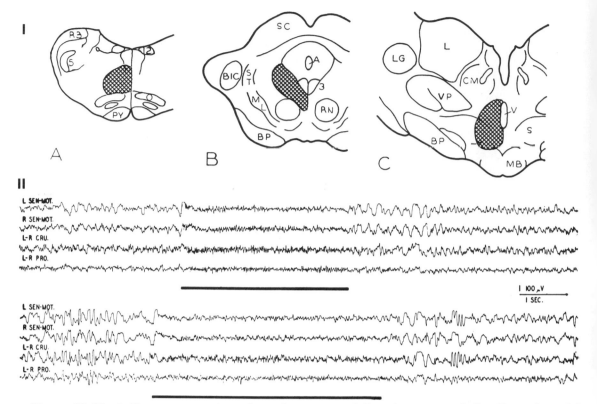

Figure 20–28 *I.* Transverse sections through upper medulla (*A*), mesencephalic (*B*), and caudal diencephalic (*C*) levels with cross hatching to indicate the areas from which the brain stem reticular activating system arousal responses were elicited with lowest voltage.

II. Effects of stimulation of the brain stem reticular formation upon electrocortical activity of cat under light chloralosone anesthesia. Note the replacement of high voltage slow waves by low voltage fast activity during stimulation (1.5 volts at 300 cps). SEN – MOT = sensory motor; CRU = cruciate gyrus; PRO = proreus gyrus (frontal). (From Moruzzi, G., and Magoun, H. W.: Electroenceph. clin. Neurophysiol., *1*:456, 458, 1949.)

many neurons. A change from this state to low voltage fast activity was considered as representing a loss of synchronization – a desynchronization.

The role of the reticular formation and other brain stem areas in sleep, consciousness, and attention will be considered in greater detail in a later chapter.

CLINICAL AND PHYSIOLOGICAL CORRELATES OF CYTOARCHITECTURAL VARIATIONS

In this section we will attempt to demonstrate that the significant cytoarchitectural differences between various neocortical areas have important physiological and clinical consequences.

THE RELATIONSHIP OF CYTOARCHITECTURAL VARIATION TO CAPACITY FOR SEIZURE DISCHARGE

Anatomical Observation. In the monkey as in man the motor cortex (area 4) of the precentral gyrus is characterized by the presence of giant and large pyramidal cells. These giant and large pyramidal cells are characterized by a long apical dendrite. Associated with these pyramidal cells, there is noted in the Golgi stain, the presence of a massive tangential plexus in the molecular layer with the presence of many axodendritic synapses. In contrast, the striate occipital cortex (area 17) has a dense external line of Baillarger in layer IV but only a thin tangential plexus in the molecular layer. Giant pyramidal cells are absent and large pyramidal cells are sparse.

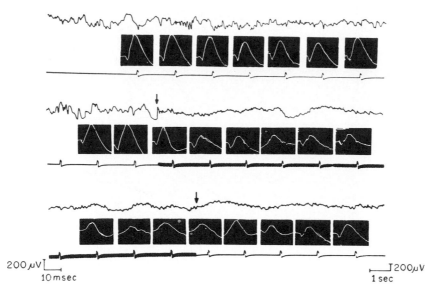

Figure 20-29 Effects of brain stem reticular stimulation on activity of superficial axodendritic synapses in cerebral cortex. Superficial cortical response (SCR) was evoked by stimulation of anterior suprasylvian gyrus and is shown during a control period. At the first arrow, stimulation of the brain stem reticular formation at 300 cps was begun (indicated also by the artefact superimposed on the signal marker for the SCR). During this period the surface negativity of the superficial cortical response was depressed. The background electrocortical activity (i.e., EEG activity) demonstrated the typical arousal (desynchronization) effect. These effects persisted beyond the cessation of stimulation (second arrow). Stimulation of the brain stem reticular formation then appears to inhibit the activity of the superficial axodendritic synapses. (From Purpura, D. P.: Science. *123*:804, 1955.)

Physiological Observations. The superficial cortical response represents the summated postsynaptic potentials generated at superficial axodendritic synapses. In the studies of Eidelberg et al. (1959) this response could be easily obtained at low threshold in the motor cortex. On the other hand, only a feeble response was produced in the striate occipital cortex (Fig. 20–30).

French et al. (1956) studied the threshold for generation of propagated seizure after discharge following electrical stimulation of monkey cerebral cortex. Low thresholds were found in the motor cortex with the ready development of generalized seizure discharge. On the other hand, high thresholds were present in the striate occipital cortex (Fig. 20–31).

Similar regional variations in capacity for generation of seizure discharge have been found by Walker (1964) as regards chemical convulsants.

Clinical Correlation. The capacity for a clinical seizure is directly related to the capacity for generation of repetitive discharge and of after-discharge. Thus whether a tumor involving the cerebral cortex announces its location with a seizure will be related to its location. There is, then, an extremely high incidence of focal or generalized seizures in patients with parasagittal meningiomas overlying the motor cortex. On the other hand, tumors in the prefrontal, posterior-temporal parietal, or occipital areas may grow to a large size without producing focal seizures. When focal seizures occur they may indicate a compromise of low threshold motor cortex with discharge originating at that area rather than at the primary site of involvement.

PHYSIOLOGICAL AND CLINICAL CORRELATIONS OF VARIATIONS IN CALLOSAL FIBER SYSTEM DENSITY

Anatomical Observation. Using the Nauta method to study degeneration of axons, Ebner and Myers (Myers, 1965) have evaluated the density of callosal projection approximately 10 days after section of the major interhemispheric commissures. A dense callosal projection was found in the frontal and parietal areas (particularly in premotor and precentral areas). Only a sparse callosal projection was present in

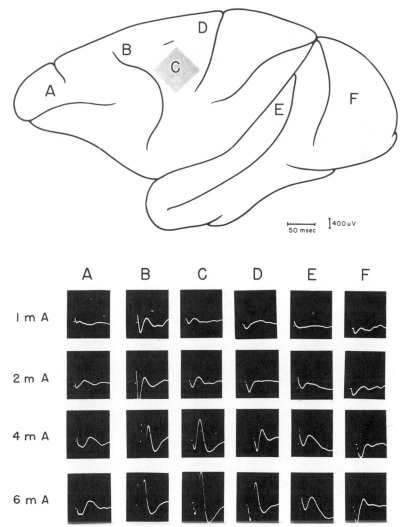

Figure 20–30 Variations in thresholds and amplitude of superficial cortical response (local cortical response) as a function of locus of stimulation in the monkey. Note the low threshold and relatively higher amplitude of the premotor and motor cortex responses (B, C, D) compared to those obtained in area 17 (F) posterior temporal (E) and prefrontal areas (A). The stimulation intensities were the same in all areas (0.10 msec. single shocks). (From Eidelberg, E., Konigsmark, B., and French, J. D.: Electroenceph. clin. Neurophysiol., *11*:123, 1959.)

Compare the cytoarchitectural patterns of these various areas as demonstrated in Figure 20–9 on page 457.

striate occipital and superior temporal areas (Fig. 20–17).

Physiological Observations. The original studies of Curtis (1940) on the transcallosal response in the monkey indicated significant regional differences in the capacity for generation of this response. The response was easily obtained on stimulation of the premotor, precentral, and parietal areas but could not be obtained on stimulation of the striate occipital cortex (Fig. 20–32). In general, similar differences were found in studies of McCulloch and his associates (1944) employing a local area of seizure discharge (strychnine neuronography) rather than direct electrical stimulation. Both series of studies also indicated that significant regional differences existed as regards the diffuseness of callosal projection. Thus, certain cortical areas (e.g., motor cortex) had limited projection only to the symmetrical area of the contralateral hemisphere. Other areas, such as the premotor area (area 6) had widespread projection to many points in the contralateral hemisphere (areas 6, 4, 1, 5, and 39 as regards area 6).

SUSCEPTIBILITY OF CORTEX
TO SEIZURE DISCHARGE

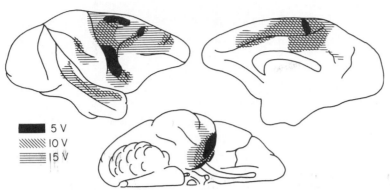

5 V
10 V
15 V

Figure 20–31 Regional Differences in Seizure Susceptibility in Monkey Cortex. The thresholds for electrical seizure after discharge in response to direct stimulation of cerebral cortex are shown. Note the low threshold of motor cortex of sectors in premotor cortex and of anterior medial temporal area as contrasted to striate occipital, (area 17) prefrontal posterior temporal, and parietal areas. Compare to Figure 20–30, note the similarity as regards pattern of regional variation. Note the cytoarchitectural differences of these areas summarized in Figure 20–9 on page 457. (From French, J. D., Gernandt, B. E., and Livingston, R. B.: Arch. Neurol. Psychiat., 75:270, 1956.)

A somewhat more complex experimental model has been employed by Marcus et al. (1968) in which bilateral foci of epileptic discharge are produced in symmetrical cortical areas of the two hemispheres. Although the spike discharges in the two hemispheres may be initially independent, an interaction soon occurs, resulting in the synchronization of the seizure discharges in the two hemis-

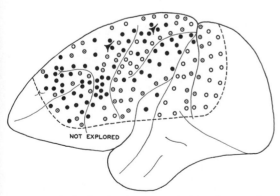

NOT EXPLORED

Figure 20–32 Regional variations in monkey cerebral cortex as regards the transcallosal response. Note that large potentials (black dots) are obtained from the precentral, premotor, and inferior parietal areas—corresponding to the heavy callosal degeneration in these areas demonstrated in Figure 20–17, whereas almost no potentials are obtained from area 17 (open dots). (From Curtis, H. J.: J. Neurophysiol., 3:408, 1940.)

pheres. In the monkey there are significant regional variations in the capacity for this interaction in a pattern which is consistent with the anatomical observations concerning the density of callosal projection. In the premotor and precentral areas a close and well-developed interhemispheric synchrony is evident (Fig. 20–33); in striate occipital and superior temporal areas, bilateral synchrony is poorly sustained (Fig. 20–34). Section of major commissures disrupts the fine synchrony (0 to 20 milliseconds interhemispheric differential) of discharge but a poorly sustained coarse type of synchrony (50 to 400 millisecond interhemispheric differential) remains in the precentral areas. This coarse synchrony is dependent on extra-callosal pathways (presumably multisynaptic with decussation at various brain stem levels). This latter pathway may well represent phylogenetically old pathways.

It is possible to modify the experimental procedure so that a metabolic disease of the cerebral cortex is studied from the standpoint of regional variations in the capacity for bilateral synchronous discharges. Intravenous injection of a threshold amount of pentylenetetrazol (metrazol) provides such an example of a diffuse toxic disease.

Following injection, bilateral synchronous discharges developed first in the premotor and precentral areas. Discharges in the tem-

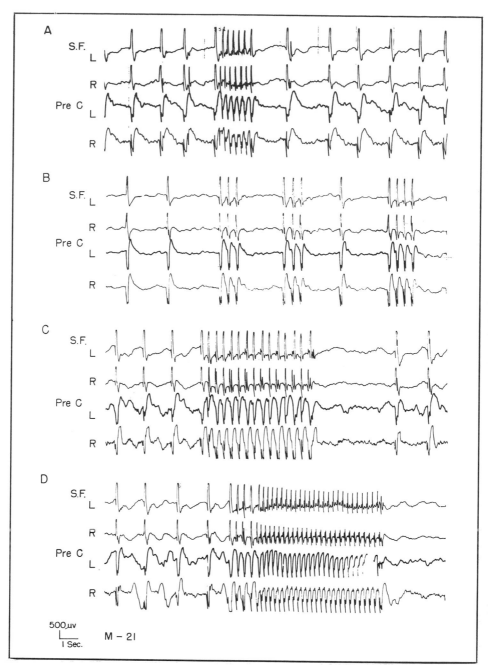

Figure 20–33 Capacity for bilateral synchrony in premotor area of monkey cerebral cortex. Experimental design of bilateral symmetrical discharging premotor foci. Foci were produced using a topical convulsant agent (1% conjugated estrogens). Recordings from superior frontal (S.F.) and precentral gyri (Pre C). Note the repetitive bilaterally synchronous discharges of spikes and spike slow wave complexes. Compare to Figure 20–34. Note also the density of callosal projections of premotor area as demonstrated in Figure 20–17. (From Marcus, E. M., and Watson, C. W.: Arch. Neurol., *19*:102, 1968.)

poral and striate occipital areas are independent and multifocal. Synchrony is lost following section of the corpus callosum.

Clinical Correlation. Seizure discharges, as recorded in the human electroencephalo-gram, may be focal, multifocal, or generalized with bilateral symmetry and synchrony of discharge. When the latter category of bilateral discharges is examined it is evident that the bilateral synchrony is usually best

Figure 20-34 Lack of capacity for bilateral synchrony in area 17 of monkey cerebral cortex. Experimental design of bilateral symmetrical discharging foci. Foci were produced employing a topical convulsant (1% solution of conjugated estrogens as in premotor cortex in Figure 20–34). Recordings from left and right occipital area. Note that the discharges in the two hemispheres were relatively independent, particularly when prolonged (A and C). Occasional bilateral discharges relatively synchronous at onset could occur (B). Synchronous discharges could be triggered by an extrinsic source, e.g., photic stimulation (PS) as in D. Compare to Figure 20–33. (From Marcus, E. M., and Watson, C. W.: Arch Neurol., *19*:107, 1968.)

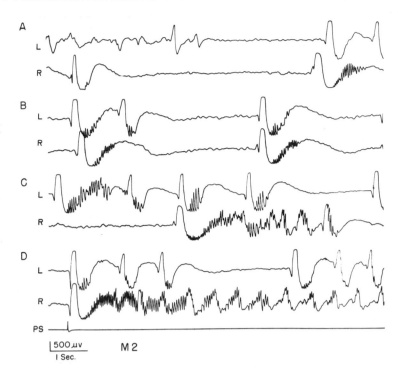

developed in the frontal and central areas. On the other hand, bilateral discharges in the temporal and occipital areas often appear to be independent, that is, multifocal. In view of the experimental studies previously summarized, the variation in density of the callosal fiber system may also explain the regional variations in patterns of bilateral discharge noted in the clinical laboratory.

It is also evident that when focal-seizure discharges are considered, the corpus callosum represents a preferential pathway for the spread of discharge to the contralateral hemisphere, although alternate pathways are also available. The tendency for secondary spread of discharge into the contralateral hemisphere does vary as a function of location of the discharging focus. Foci in the parasagittal frontal and medial frontal areas (essentially premotor areas), are often likely to present considerable secondary spread of discharge into the contralateral hemisphere. Section of the corpus callosum has been employed on rare occasions to limit spread of seizure discharge.

GENERAL CORRELATIONS OF CYTOARCHITECTURE AND FUNCTION

In general, regions that are specialized as regards cytoarchitecture have specialized physiological functions. Destruction of these areas will result in relatively specific defects which can be well localized.

Anatomical Observation. Both the motor cortex and granular koniocortex (of the postcentral gyrus or striate occipital area) have a specialized cytoarchitecture as previously discussed.

Physiological Observations. The short latency primary response evoked in the cerebral cortex by sciatic stimulation is limited to the projection area of the lower extremity in the postcentral gyrus of the contralateral hemisphere. The primary response evoked in the cerebral cortex by stimulation of the hand is likewise limited to a particular section of the contralateral somatosensory cortex.

In contrast a flash of light elicits a short latency, primary evoked response in the visual projection cortex but does not produce this response in the somatosensory cortex of the postcentral gyrus.

As regards motor activities, short latency, low threshold, discrete movements are elicited by stimulation of the motor cortex. Movements may be obtained by stimulating the adjacent cortical areas, e.g., premotor areas, but the thresholds are higher, movements are not discrete, and latency is often longer.

Clinical Correlation. Seizures resulting from epileptic foci located in these specific areas often have specific focal components of a motor or sensory variety. We should note the localizing significance of the "motor march of Jackson," the warning (aura) of localized paresthesias, or the warning prodromal symptom of flashing lights.

Stimulation of these areas at surgery in the unanesthetized patient at low threshold will identify the specific focal symptoms.

This specific focal symptom should be contrasted to the less specific symptoms which follow discharge originating in the nonspecialized homotypical cortex of the prefrontal area or posterior temporal lobe or posterior parietal area.

References

CEREBRAL CORTEX: CYTOARCHITECTURE

Bailey, P., and Von Bonin, G.: *The Isocortex of Man,* Urbana, Ill., University of Illinois Press, 1951.

Colonnier, M. L.: The Structural Design of the Neocortex *In* Eccles, J. C. (ed.): *Brain and Conscious Experience.* New York, Springer Verlag, 1966.

Colonnier, M. L.: The fine structural arrangement of the cortex. Arch. Neurol., *16*:651–657, 1967 (June).

Conel, J.: *The Postnatal Development of The Human Cerebral Cortex,* Vol. I-VI. Cambridge, Mass., Harvard University Press, 1939–1960.

Jacobson, S.: Intralaminar, interlaminar callosal and thalamocortical connections in frontal and parietal areas of the albino rat cerebral cortex. J. comp. Neurol., *124*: 131–146, 1965.

Jacobson, S., and Marcus, E. M.: The laminar distribution of fibers of the corpus callosum: a comparative study in rat, cat, monkey, and chimpanzee. Brain Res., *24*:517–520, 1970.

Lorente de Nó, R.: Cerebral Cortex: Architecture, Intracortical Connections, Motor Projections *In* Fulton, J. F. (ed.): *Physiology of the Nervous System,* 3rd Edition. New York, Oxford University Press 1949, pp. 288–330.

McCulloch, W. S.: Cortico-Cortical Connections *In* Bucy, P. (ed.): *The Precentral Motor Cortex.* Urbana, Ill., University of Illinois Press, 1944, p. 211–242.

Nauta, W. J. H., and Whitlock, D. G.: An Anatomical Analysis of the Nonspecific Thalamic Projection System *In* Delafresnaye, J. F. (ed.): *Brain Mechanisms and Consciousness.* Oxford, Blackwell Scientific Publications, 1954, pp. 81–116.

Purpura, D. P.: Relationship of Seizure Susceptibility to Morphologic and Physiologic Properities of Normal and Abnormal Immature Cortex *In* Kellaway, F., and Petersen, I. (eds.): *Neurological and Electroencephalographic Correlative Studies in Infancy,* New York, Grune and Stratton, 1964, pp. 117–157.

Yakovlev, P. I.: Morphological criteria of growth and maturation of the nervous system in man. Res. Publ. Ass. nerv. ment. Dis., *39*:3–46, 1962.

Von Economo, C.: *The Cytoarchitectonics of the Human Cerebral Cortex.* London, Oxford University Press, 1929.

CEREBRAL CORTEX: ELECTROPHYSIOLOGY

Brazier, M. A. B.: *The Electrical Activity of The Nervous System.* London, Pitman, 1968, 69–78, 92–114, 185–268, 183–261.

Brodal, A.: The Reticular Formation *In Neurological Anatomy in Relation to Clinical Medicine.* Chapter 6. New York, Oxford University Press, 1969, pp. 304–349.

Clemente, C. D., and Sterman, M. B.: Basal forebrain mechanisms for internal inhibition and sleep. Res. Publ. Ass. nerv. ment. Dis., *45*:127–147, 1967.

Curtis, H. H.: Intercortical connections of corpus callosum as indicated by evoked potentials. J. Neurophysiol., *3*:407–413, 1940.

Doty, R. W., and Smith, J. W.: Electrical Activity of the Brain *In* Freedman, A. M., and Kaplan, H. I. (eds.): *Comprehensive Textbook of Psychiatry.* Baltimore, Williams and Wilkins, 1967, pp. 112–125.

Eidelberg, E. Konigsmark, B., and French, J. D.: Electrocortical manifestations of epilepsy in monkey. Electroenceph. clin. Neurophysiol., *11*:121–128, 1959.

French, J. D., Gernandt, B. E., and Livingston, R. B.: Regional differences in seizure susceptibility in monkey cortex. Arch. Neurol. Psychiat., *72*:260–274, 1956.

Jasper, H.: Diffuse projection system: The integrative action of the thalamic reticular system. Electroenceph. clin. Neurophysiol., *1*:405–420, 1949.

Marcus, E. M., and Watson, C. W.: Symmetrical epileptogenic foci in monkey cerebral cortex: mechanisms of interaction and regional variations in capacity for synchronous discharges. Arch. Neurol., *19*:99–116, 1968.

Marcus, E. M., Watson, C. W., and Jacobson, S.: Role of the corpus callosum in bilateral synchronous discharges induced by intravenous pentylenetetrazol. Neurology, *19*:309, 1969.

McCulloch, W. S.: Cortico-cortical Connections *In* Bucy, P. C. (ed.): *The Precentral Motor Cortex.* Urbana, Ill., University of Illinois Press, 1944, pp. 211–242.

Morrison, R. S., and Dempsey, E. W.: A study of thalamocortical relations. Amer. J. Physiol., *135*:281–292, 1942.

Myers, R. E.: General Discussion: Phylogenetic Studies of Commissural Connections *In* Ettlinger, E. G. (ed.): *Functions of the Corpus Callosum.* Boston, Little, Brown & Company, 1965, pp. 138–142.

Purpura, D. P.: Nature of electrocortical potentials and synaptic organizations in cerebral and cerebellar cortex. Int. Rev. Neurobiol., *1*:47–163, 1959.

Scheibel, M. E., and Scheibel, A. B.: Structural organization of nonspecific thalamic nuclei and their projection toward the cortex. Brain Res., *6*:60–94, 1967.

Skinner, J. E., and Lindsley, D. B.: Electrophysiological and behavioral effects of blockade of the nonspecific thalamocortical system. Brain Res., *6*:95–118, 1967.

Starzl, T. E., and Whitlock, D. G.: Diffuse thalamic projection system in the monkey. J. Neurophysiol., *15*: 449–468, 1952.

Towe, A. L.: Electrophysiology of the Cerebral Cortex *In* Ruch, T. C., and Patton, H. D. (eds.): *Physiology and Biophysics* 19th Edition, Philadelphia, W. B. Saunders, 1965, pp. 455–464.

Velasco, M., and Lindsley, D. B.: Role of orbital cortex in regulation of the thalamocortical electrical activity. *Science, 149*:1375–1377, 1965.

Walker, A. E.: The Patterns of Propagation of Epileptic Discharge *In* Schaltenbrand, G., and Woolsey, C. W. (eds.): *Cerebral Localization and Organization.* Madison, University of Wisconsin Press, 1964, pp. 95–111.

21

Cerebral Cortex: Functional Localization

ELLIOTT M. MARCUS

INTRODUCTION

METHODS OF STUDY

A variety of methods have been employed to study the functions of the various areas of the cerebral cortex in man and animals. These methods fall into two general categories: stimulation and ablation.

Within the category of *stimulation* may be included the acute discharge produced by local application of electrical current or of chemical convulsants, such as strychnine or penicillin. The effects produced in part depend on the parameters of stimulation. For electrical stimulation, the frequency, duration, voltage, and wave form have significance. For chemical convulsants, the effects are in part dependent on the structural configuration of the agent and on the relationship of this configuration to the configuration of the pre- and postsynaptic sites on which they act. Some chemical convulsant agents may also be employed to provide a longer lasting seizure focus, e.g., cobalt or alumina gel. Such chronic areas of discharge may also be produced by local freezing of an area of the cerebral cortex. With the exception of local electrical stimulation (often a necessary procedure at the time of neurosurgery of the cerebral cortex), such methods cannot be employed to study cortical function in man. However, various disease processes in man involving the cerebral cortex may produce a local area of excessive discharge—in a sense, a local area of stimulation.

Actually our first understanding of cortical function was derived from the systematic study of such cases of focal discharge (focal seizures, focal convulsions, focal epilepsy, and epileptiform seizures) by Hughlings Jackson in 1863 and 1870. Jackson was able to predict that an area existed in the cerebral cortex which governed isolated movements of the contralateral extremities.

Initially, data as to the actual location of the disease process and its nature (old scar from traumatic injury, old area of tissue damage due to ischemia, infection, local compression, or invasive brain tumor) were dependent on final examination of the brain at autopsy. One may then speak of the method of clinical pathological correlation. With the development of neurosurgery and the specialized techniques of electroencephalography, arteriography, pneumoencephalography, and radioactive brain scan, it is possible to define and to confirm during life the anatomical boundaries of a disease process, often allowing for treatment or cure of the basic disease process.

The results obtained by the method of

stimulation are subject to several possible interpretations from the standpoint of functional localization:

1. The effect observed may be clearly related to the actual function of the area stimulated, e.g., stimulation of the motor cortex results in discrete movements.

2. The effect observed may be in part related to the spread of discharge to other cortical areas via corticocortical association pathways, e.g., orbital frontal area to anterior temporal area via the uncinate fasciculus.

3. The effects observed may in part reflect the spread of discharge to various subcortical and brain stem centers. The generalized convulsive seizure which may develop secondary to the focal seizure represents such a spread.

4. The effects observed may indicate that the remainder of the central nervous system is functioning without the participation of the area stimulated. Thus if all the neurons of a given cortical area are involved in a seizure discharge, they may be unable to participate in their usual activities, be they of an afferent, integrative, or efferent nature. Thus the effects of seizure discharges involving prefrontal or hippocampal areas may be in some aspects quite similar to the effect of ablation of these areas as regards intellectual functions, personality, and memory or learning. This concept also implies, in a sense, release of function in other areas (cortical and subcortical). Therefore, certain of the emotional responses of the patient with seizure discharges involving the prefrontal or temporal lobe areas are also similar to the effects obtained on ablation of these areas and suggest release of lower centers.

The method of *ablation* involves destruction of a specific area by operative resection, coagulation, or freezing to the point of tissue death. In man, the method of clinical pathological correlation has produced considerable information. The destructive lesions have been the result of a local area of tissue destruction due to blood vessel occlusion, hemorrhage, solitary metastatic tumor, or intrinsic tumor. Less frequently employed have been several methods that produce a temporary depression of function: controlled cooling and a process involving the spreading depression of cortical electrical activity.

The effects observed following ablation are subject to several interpretations:

1. The observed effects may indicate deficits directly related to a failure of a positive function normally subserved by the area destroyed. For example, after destruction of parietal somatosensory projection areas, deficits in stereognosis and position sense occur.

2. The effects may reflect the release of centers in other cortical areas or at other levels of the neural axis. This presumes that certain functions of these other centers are usually inhibited by the area ablated. The end result then is an enhancement of certain functions. Spasticity several weeks or months after ablation of the motor cortex is an example.

3. A temporary loss of function of a lower center may follow acute ablation of higher centers. For example, following acute unilateral ablation of all motor cortex in man, there will be observed a temporary loss or depression of deep tendon reflexes and of other stretch reflexes in the contralateral extremities. There will be initially a flaccid paralysis. This state (referred to as the "diaschisis of Von Monokow") is analogous to spinal shock or pyramidal shock. As recovery from this state occurs, deep tendon reflexes return and become progressively more active. The flaccid paralysis is replaced by a spastic paresis.

A third general method for the study of cortical function, the *evoked cortical response technique,* has also provided considerable information. This method has been employed predominantly as an experimental laboratory technique. The method involves the stimulation of an afferent pathway, while recording from the cortical receiving areas the short latency evoked response. For example, in the monkey stimulation of the sciatic nerve will evoke in the contralateral postcentral gyrus a short latency primary evoked response. The response is limited to that specific area of the postcentral gyrus devoted to the representation of the lower extremity. Stimulation of the upper extremity will elicit a similar response from a different portion of the contralateral postcentral gyrus—that devoted to representation of the upper extremity. Eventually it is possible to prepare a map of the somatosensory projection cortex of the postcentral gyrus. It is possible to refine this technique at the response end by using microelectrode recordings from within or just outside neurons at particular depths of the cortex. It is also possible to define more carefully the parameters of stimulation as Hubel and Wiesel have done in their analysis of responses in the visual cortex to specific types of visual stimuli.

By stimulating particular thalamic nuclei, one may map out specific thalamocortical relationships.

A modification of the technique is that of antidromic stimulation of an efferent pathway, such as the pyramidal tract, to map out the cortical nerve cells of origin of fibers in this tract.

CONCEPT OF REPRESENTATION AND REREPRESENTATION OF FUNCTION

In considering functional localization, one must keep in mind that a given function may be represented and rerepresented at the various levels of the neural axis. However, at a given level not all functions may be represented to the same degree.

ONTOGENETIC FACTOR

In considering the effects of ablation, one must also consider the ontogenetic factor. Thus bilateral ablation of the prefrontal cortex in the adult monkey produces impairment in the capacity to delay responses. Bilateral prefrontal ablation at one week of age in the infant monkey does not have this effect. Such a monkey when tested at 4 months, the usual age when delay response appears, is able to manifest this capacity. Similar observations may be made with regard to somatosensory and visual pattern discrimination in the infant cat as compared to adult cats following the appropriate resection of the somatosensory or visual projection cortex. Similar observations may be made in man. Thus, destruction in most adults of the inferior frontal convulution (areas 44 and 45) in the left hemisphere will result in a marked and lasting deficit in linguistic expression (so called Broca's expressive aphasia). Destruction of this same area in the infant or young child does not produce an enduring defect.

The functions of specific cortical areas will now be considered. Each area will be considered in terms of the effects of stimulation and then in terms of the effects of ablation. Our attention will be directed primarily to function as studied in man or in subhuman primates (Fig. 21–1A).

PRIMARY MOTOR CORTEX (Area 4)

Area 4 is distinguished by the presence of giant pyramidal cells in layer V. Occasionally giant pyramidal cells may also be found more anteriorly in area 6. In man, much of area 4, particularly as regards its lower half, is found on the anterior wall of the central sulcus. More superiorly, area 4 appears on the lateral precentral gyrus and continues onto the medial aspect of the hemisphere in the anterior half of the paracentral lobule.

It is important to note that the pyramidal tract is not named for its cells of origin but rather on the basis of its passage through the medullary pyramid. Of the approximately one million fibers in the pyramidal tract, 31 per cent arise from area 4; 29 per cent arise from area 6; and 40 per cent arise from areas 3, 1, 2, 5, and 7. Fibers with a large diameter (9 to 22 micra) number about 30,000 and correspond roughly to the number of giant pyramidal cells. Most of these large fibers then will originate from area 4. It is also important to note that the same cortical areas that give rise to the pyramidal tract also give rise to other descending motor pathways: corticoreticular, corticorubral, corticostriatal, and corticothalamic. From a phylogenetic standpoint this is a logical arrangement since this relatively new control center, the motor cortex, has available a relatively new fast conducting pathway to the anterior horn cells. At the same time the motor cortex also has available pathways to certain older brain stem centers which formerly exercised primary control, e.g., the reticular formation.

Area 4: Stimulation. Electrical stimulation of the motor cortex at threshold stimulus produces isolated movements of the contralateral portions of the body. The movements may be described as a twitch or small jerk. With increased strength or increased frequency of stimulation, repetitive jerks occur; the movements involve a larger part of the contralateral side of the body and an orderly sequence of spread may occur. The repetitive jerks are similar to the movements of a focal motor seizure. The orderly sequence of spread is duplicated in the "Jacksonian March" of a focal motor seizure.

In the conscious patient, these movements, which occur on stimulation of the motor cortex during surgery, are not clearly the same as consciously willed voluntary movements. According to Penfield, the patient recognizes that this is not a voluntary movement of his own. The patient will often attribute the causation to the neurosurgeon.

There has been considerable controversy as to whether muscles or movements are rep-

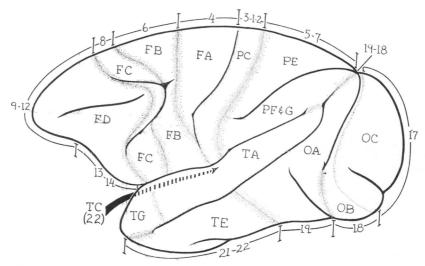

Figure 21–1A Reference diagrammatic cytoarchitectural map of monkey brain relating terminology of Brodmann (number system) to that of Von Bonin and Bailey (letter system). The borders are only approximate. (From Ruch, T. C., and Patton, H. D.: *Physiology and Biophysics*, 19th Edition. Philadelphia, W. B. Saunders, 1965, p. 256.)

resented in the motor cortex. Some single-unit recording studies have suggested a close topographic grouping of all the neurons for a given muscle. Occasionally stimulation will evoke the movement of a single muscle, usually a distal finger muscle, such as an interosseous. In general, however, stimulation produces contraction of a group of muscles concerned with a specific movement. Voluntary actions also occur in terms of the integrated movement of several muscles rather than the isolated contraction of a single muscle. It should then be apparent that the motor cortex "thinks" in terms of movements. This is, in a sense, inherent in the intracortical connections between the neurons

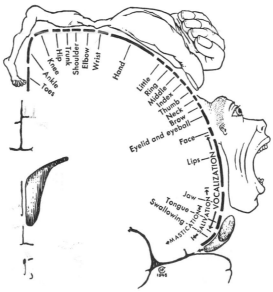

Figure 21–1B Motor representation as determined by stimulation studies on the human cerebral cortex at surgery. This motor homunculus is arranged over the surface of a coronal section of the cerebral hemisphere. Note the large area devoted to the thumb and fingers. (From Penfield, W., and Rasmussen, T.: *The Cerebral Cortex of Man*. New York, MacMillan, 1955, p. 215.)

representing the various muscles related to a given movement.

Although there is some overlap of the movements represented on the surface of the motor cortex, a certain sequence of arrangements is apparent (Fig. 21–1*B*). Thus movements of the pharynx and tongue are located close to the sylvian fissure. Unilateral stimulation of these areas results in bilateral movements. Next in upward sequence are movements of the lips, face, brow, and neck. In the middle third of the precentral gyrus, a large area is devoted to the representation of the contralateral thumb, fingers, and hand. In the upper third, the sequence of the contralateral wrist, elbow, shoulder, trunk, and hip is found. The remainder of the lower extremity in the sequence (knee, ankle, and toes) is represented on the medial surface of the hemisphere in the paracentral lobule. The centers for control of the anal and vesicle sphincters have been located lowest on the paracentral lobule. There is some evidence that this sequence in man differs somewhat from that found in subhuman primates. Thus, in the monkey, movements of the shoulder and elbow are located anterior to the wrist, hand, and finger representation on the precentral gyrus (Fig. 21–2).

It is important to note how large the areas devoted to the thumb, fingers, and face (particularly the lips and tongue) are in man, in view of the evolution in use of these structures as regards speech, writing, tool making and manipulation.

It is also important to note that not all areas of the motor cortex have the same threshold for discharge. As studied in the baboon (Phillips, 1966) the thumb and index finger are the region of lowest threshold. Slightly stronger shocks are required to produce a movement on stimulation of the great toe area; at slightly greater intensities of shock, movements of the face begin to occur on stimulation of the appropriate area. These findings may relate in part to the fact that those pyramidal fibers making direct connection to anterior horn cells are primarily those mediating cortical control of the distal finger and thumb muscles.

It must also be noted that at times on stimulation of the postcentral gyrus discrete movements will be produced similar to those elicited from the motor cortex. There is some evidence that such discrete movements

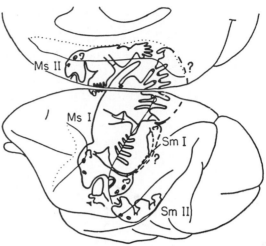

Figure 21–2 Diagram of monkey cerebral cortex demonstrating the pattern of representation within the precentral motor area (MSI) and the main postcentral sensory representation (SMI). The supplementary motor cortex (MSII) is also demonstrated on the medial surface of the cerebral hemisphere. A second sensory area is demonstrated buried in the sylvian fissure. Note the arrangement of body parts in the primary motor cortex (simunculus rather than homunculus) with the shoulder representation anterior to elbow, which is anterior to wrist and fingers. Note also that the proximal body parts extend into premotor cortex. (From Schaltenbrand, G., and Woolsey, C. N.: *Cerebral Localization and Organization.* Madison, University of Wisconsin Press, 1964, p. 18.)

are produced at a higher threshold than in the precentral cortex and that the ability to obtain such discrete movements is lost after ablation of the primary motor cortex. However, not all of this neurosurgical data on stimulation of postcentral gyrus in the human is consistent. There are also, of course, both pyramidal and nonpyramidal fibers originating from the postcentral sensory cortex.

Area 4: Ablation. The effects following ablation of the motor cortex must be distinguished from the more selective effects of limited section of the pyramidal tract in the cerebral peduncle or medullary pyramid. Damage to or ablation of the motor cortex affects not only the pyramidal tracts, but also the corticorubral, corticostriatal, and corticoreticular pathways.

The sequence of events in man following partial vascular lesions (infarcts) of the precentral cortex or of the motor pathways in the internal capsule have been studied by

Twitchell. There is initially a transient period of flaccid paralysis of the contralateral arm and leg and the lower half of the face, with a transient depression of stretch reflexes (decrease in resistance to passive motion at affected joints and depression of deep tendon reflexes). The duration of this paralysis is variable; it may be quite fleeting depending on the extent of the lesion (which is usually less than total). The sign of Babinski is present with an extensor plantar response on tactile or painful stimulation of the lateral border of the foot.

After a variable period of time, the deep tendon reflexes in the affected limbs return and become hyperactive. There is increased resistance on passive motion at the joints (when there are severe lesions even this stage may not be reached). This does not affect all movements equally but tends to have its greatest effect in the flexors of the upper extremity. The upper extremity is flexed at the elbow, wrist, and fingers and the leg is extended at the hip, knee, and ankle and externally rotated at the hip with circumduction in walking. The resultant posture is referred to as the hemiplegic posture and hemiplegic gait. Walking is possible with the hemiplegic limb as movement of the proximal limb begins to return. In general, recovery of function in the lower extremity is usually greater than in the upper extremity. Eventually, depending on the extent of the lesion, some return of distal hand movement may occur but such recovery is usually less than that which occurs for movements at more proximal joints, e.g., at the shoulder and hip.

The events may be quantitated to a greater degree in the monkey when a complete ablation of the precentral gyrus has been performed. There is an immediate flaccid hemiplegia of the contralateral lower face, arm, and leg with depression of stretch reflexes such as deep tendon reflexes. The weakness of hip muscles, however, is only partial. Within hours the monkey begins to use the proximal muscles of the lower limb. Within 2 to 3 days, the affected arm is used in climbing if the animal is frightened: hand and foot hook onto the cage wire. Deep tendon reflexes become more active. Within 7 to 10 days, spasticity is noted in the flexors of the upper limb and the extensors of the lower limb. There is then the appearance of a typical hemiplegic posture. After several additional weeks the wrist and fingers begin

to move independently of the proximal joints, but capacity to use the thumb and fingers in independent action never reaches the preoperative level. The actual details of recovery of motor function and an analysis of the reflex activity involved will be considered in greater detail in the chapter on the motor system.

The following case history illustrates the effects of focal disease involving the motor cortex.

Case History 1. NECH #186–869. Date of admission: 5/10/67.

This 37-year-old, right-handed, white male, steelmill employee (Mr. H.G.) in January 1967 had the onset of episodes characterized by repetitive jerks of the proximal portions of the left upper extremity, the episodes lasting a few seconds and occurring once every two days. These episodes occurred without warning and initially they did not involve the face, hand, or legs. At first no weakness was present after the episode. On January 23, 1967, the patient had two prolonged episodes of uncontrollable shaking of the left shoulder and arm, spreading down to the fingers of the left hand and progressing to unconsciousness with biting of the tongue. The patient was admitted to his local hospital where neurological examination, lumbar puncture, right carotid arteriogram, and pneumoencephalogram were all normal. The electroencephalogram was borderline with minor random focal slow wave activity in the right central and temporal areas. A second record was normal. Despite treatment with anticonvulsants (phenobarbital and Dilantin), the patient continued to have focal seizures involving the left arm with clenching and jerking of the left hand. Following several of these focal seizures, a transient weakness of the left arm was noted (referred to as a Todd's postictal palsy). Examination by Dr. John Sullivan in February 1967 demonstrated a mild degree of weakness of the left upper extremity and a slight increase in deep tendon reflexes in the left upper extremity. Re-evaluation in April 1967 indicated increasing weakness of the left upper extremity and the relatively rapid development of weakness in the left lower extremity with no voluntary movement below the knee. Deep tendon reflexes were now increased in the upper and lower left extremities. The left plantar response was extensor. The brain scan now indicated a slight uptake of radioisotope (Hg^{197}) high in the right hemisphere near the vertex. Hospital admission was advised.

NEUROLOGICAL EXAMINATION (May 11, 1967):

1. *Mental status:* Intact.
2. *Cranial nerves:* A minor left central facial weakness was present.
3. *Motor system:*
   a. A left hemiparesis was present involving the leg more than the arm which demonstrated only a mild degree of weakness. In the lower extremity there was marked involvement of the distal musculature at the ankle and toes with only minor involvement at the hip.
   b. Muscle tone was normal.
   c. The patient walked with a hemiplegic gait: decreased swing of the left arm and circumduction of the left leg.
   d. Cerebellar tests were negative.
4. *Reflexes:*
   a. Deep tendon: an increase was present on the left in the upper extremity.
   b. Superficial: The plantar response was extensor on the left (sign of Babinski).
5. *Sensation:* All modalities were intact.

LABORATORY DATA:

1. *Electroencephalogram:* Rare focal 5 to 7 cps slow waves were present in the right frontal area close to the midline, suggesting focal damage in this area.
2. *Brain scan:* There was a focal increased uptake of the isotope (Hg^{197}) in the right central area close to the midline; the appearance suggested an infiltrating tumor rather than a meningioma.

The brain scan employs a radiation detection device to measure the distribution within the cranial cavity of a gamma emitting radioisotope administered intravenously.*

---

*Normally radioactive isotopes when administered intravenously remain confined to the intravascular space and do not enter the brain substance per se. Radioisotopes, however, will accumulate within abnormal areas within or close to the brain. Such accumulation reflects a focal alteration in blood-brain barrier permeability or an increased vascularity of the lesion or a local alteration in metabolic activities. Significant focal dense uptake of radioisotopes will be noted when neoplasms such as metastatic tumors, meningiomas or glioblastomas are present. Other pathological processes, however, may also be localized due to abnormal accumulation of radioisotope. Examples include cerebral infarcts, hemorrhages, arteriovenous malformations and brain abscess. (Refer to Maynard and Janeway: Radioisotope Studies in Neurodiagnosis. *In* Toole, J. F. (ed.): Special Techniques for Neurologic Diagnosis. Philadelphia, F. A. Davis, 1969, pp. 71–91.)

3. *Right carotid arteriogram:* An avascular space-occupying lesion in the right, high posterior, frontal and anterior parietal area was suggested. The right anterior cerebral artery was displaced to the left with a branch of the pericallosal artery displaced down and laterally away from the falx. Stretching of the terminal branches of the anterior cerebral artery was also noted.

4. *Pneumoencephalogram:* The findings of the arteriogram were confirmed. Both ventricles were displaced downward. The roof of the right lateral ventricle was compressed. The septum pellucidum was displaced towards the left. Although air passed over the convexity of the left cerebral hemisphere, little air passed over the right.

SUBSEQUENT COURSE:

Because of increasing hemiparesis, subtotal removal of the tumor was performed on May 23, 1967 by Dr. Robert Yuan. In the right parasagittal posterior frontal area, a relatively superficial but intrinsic tumor of 4 to 5 cm. in diameter was found, containing areas of necrosis and a base of cystic cavities. It was possible to almost enucleate the tumor on the surface. Cortex, white matter, and tumor were resected until white matter of apparently normal appearance was encountered. Dissection of the medial aspect of the parasagittal area was also performed so that at the conclusion of the procedure the cerebral falx was totally exposed. Pathological examination of the tumor indicated a very malignant tumor of glial tissue: a glioblastoma (or spongioblastoma) multiforma with a marked variation in cell types and an abundance of mitotic figures.

Postoperatively there was no voluntary movement of the left upper extremity and only limited proximal movement of the left lower extremity. By the time of hospital discharge on June 9, 1967, two weeks after surgery, significant improvement in strength had occurred; a moderate weakness was present with the greatest deficit located at the left foot and ankle. Deep tendon reflexes were increased on the left with ankle clonus. A left extensor plantar response (sign of Babinski) was present. No sensory deficits were present. The patient then received supervoltage radiation therapy. He continued to have a left foot-drop and experienced occasional focal seizures, beginning in the left hand or leg. He otherwise did well until March 1968 when increasing spastic weakness in the left arm and leg developed. The patient had a progressive obtundation of consciousness with the development of increased intracranial pressure (papilledema) and fever. Death occurred on July 3, 1968.

COMMENT:

The location of disease in this case as found in laboratory studies and at operation correlates well with the clinical features. The initial focal seizures involving the left shoulder correspond to the representation of this area relatively high on the precentral gyrus, close to the area of involvement. The preoperative neurological status indicating marked weakness in the distal portion of the lower extremity corresponds closely to the parasagittal location of the lesion close to the midline.

It should be noted that, in general, focal seizures do not originate from areas of total destruction but rather from adjacent cortical areas of partial damage or of altered function. Thus although weakness was greatest in the distal portion of the lower extremity, seizures were originating from the shoulder or hand areas. The persistent left foot-drop following surgery corresponds to the area of greatest ablation.

The purpose of surgery in this case was to remove as much of the tumor mass as possible so as to reduce the effects which the tumor's pressure was having on the function of surviving relatively normal areas of the cortex within the closed cranial cavity. Glioblastomas are highly malignant tumors which usually lack clearly definable borders. Even though some "enucleation" may be performed, as in this case, cure is virtually impossible, since tumor cells have already invaded apparently normal appearing areas of white matter and cortex. The late effects reflect the regrowth of the tumor, the invasion of other areas, and the increased pressure effects of the tumor.

PREMOTOR CORTEX (Areas 6 and 8)

Area 6, area 8, and the supplementary motor cortex (the continuation of areas 6 and 8 onto the medial surface of the hemisphere) have been grouped by Penfield on clinical grounds as intermediate frontal areas. These areas may also be grouped as motor association areas. As we will see, there is considerable rationale for doing this from the standpoint of the results of stimulation studies. Moreover, there is also considerable

justification for such an approach from the cytoarchitectural standpoint. Histologically, area 6 is similar to area 4 but lacks, in general, giant pyramidal cells. Area 8 has some similarity to area 6 but is also transitional to the granular prefrontal areas. There are considerable variations when the several cytoarchitectural maps are compared as to the exact boundaries of area 8 in both man and monkey (compare, for example, the maps of Brodmann [Fig. 20–10] and the Vogts [Fig. 21–3]). Areas 44 and 45 in the inferior frontal convolution (Broca's motor speech or expressive aphasia centers) should also be included within this motor association or intermediate frontal grouping, from both the functional and cytoarchitectural standpoints. For simplicity of presentation, these areas will be considered later in relation to language function.

Area 6: Stimulation (Fig. 21–3). Stimulation of that portion of area 6 adjacent to area 4 (designated as area 6a alpha) has produced in man and monkey responses similar to those obtained by stimulation of area 4. The thresholds for production of these discrete contralateral movements are higher than those required when the stimulation is carried out in area 4. Moreover, these isolated movements as related to area 6 stimulation cannot be obtained after ablation of area 4, suggesting that transmission of impulse to area 4 is required to elicit the response.

Stimulation of the remainder of area 6 (designated as area 6a beta) produces the more characteristic responses associated with area 6; rotation of head, eyes, and trunk to the opposite side (termed adversive by Foerster) with associated movements of flexion or extension in the contralateral extremities; the contralateral arm is often abducted at the shoulder and raised with flexion at the elbow. These effects are tonic and more complex than the isolated movement elicited from area 4. A pattern of movement is produced. These movements occur independently of area 4 and continue to occur after ablation of area 4.

Area 6: Ablation. In man the ablation of area 6, not involving the precentral or supplementary motor cortex, produces no weakness and no definite change in tone. If the ablation of area 6 is combined with area 4 ablation, the degree of spasticity obtained is said to be greater than with area 4 lesions

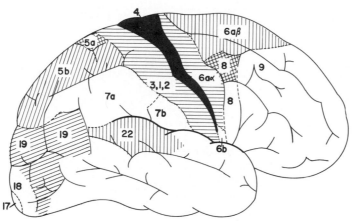

Figure 21-3 The motor cortical fields of man as determined by Foerster employing cortical stimulation. The results were then superimposed on a modified cytoarchitectural map which had been derived from the studies of the Vogts, and employed their terminology. Stimulation of the area indicated in black produced discrete movements at low threshold and was designated pyramidal. Other areas producing movements are indicated by lines or cross hatching. These movements were usually more complex synergistic and adversive movements. All these other motor areas were designated in a broad sense as extrapyramidal. Foerster included in this category the adversive responses obtained by stimulation of area 19. Each of the areas extending to the midline is continued on to the medial surface. (Modified from Foerster, O.: Brain, 59:137, 1936.)

alone. Again it must be noted that some of these studies have included ablation of the adjacent supplementary motor cortex with the area 6 ablation. These observations would however be consistent with the fact that both pyramidal and nonpyramidal motor fibers arise from area 6 as well as area 4.

Unilateral ablation of area 6 results in the transient release of contralateral instinctive tactile grasp reflex. A more permanent release of this reflex follows the combined ablation of areas 6 and 8 and the supplementary motor cortex. Such lesions also produce a significant gait apraxia—an impairment of ability to walk without actual weakness or sensory deficit. These problems will be discussed in greater detail in the chapter on motor system.

Area 8: Stimulation. As we have indicated there is disagreement regarding the exact boundaries of area 8. Some investigators (Vogts, Foerster, Penfield) (Fig. 21–3) have limited area 8 to those portions of middle frontal and inferior frontal gyri just anterior to the precentral gyrus. These authors have then designated all of the superior frontal gyrus between the prefrontal areas and the motor cortex as area 6. It is clear that conscious, adversive eye and head movements to the contralateral field occur most frequently in relation to stimulation of

that portion of the middle frontal gyrus just anterior to the precentral gyrus (Figs. 21–4 and 21–5). Adversive head and eye movements may also occur, of course, as part of a more complex movement on stimulation of area 6 or of the supplementary motor cortex. Moreover, adversive head and eye movements, as a seizure phenomenon following

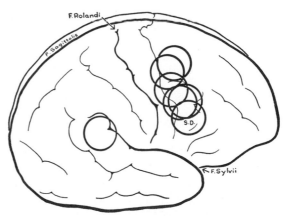

Figure 21-4 Simple (conscious) adversive seizures. Localization of the epileptogenic lesion at surgery in seven patients with this type of seizure. Note the concentration of cases about the middle frontal gyrus anterior to motor cortex. (From Penfield, W., and Kristiansen, K.: *Epileptic Seizure Patterns*, Springfield, Ill., Charles C Thomas, 1951, p. 30.)

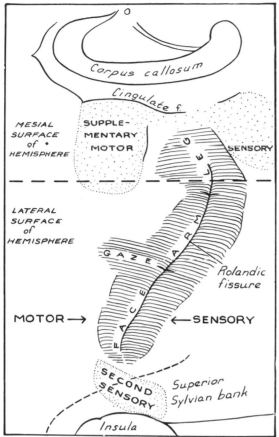

Figure 21–5 Map of somatic motor and sensory areas. Note that the primary motor and sensory areas extend into the depths of the Rolandic fissure. Note also the extension onto the medial surface of the hemisphere, which has been opened up to form a continuous map. Note the location of the adversive gaze field in relation to motor cortex. Compare to location of cross hatched portion of area 8 in map of Foerster (Figure 21–3). Note that the supplementary motor cortex represents the continuation of area 6 onto the medial surface of the hemisphere. (From Penfield, W., and Jasper, H.: *Epilepsy and the Functional Anatomy of the Human Brain.* Boston, Little, Brown, and Company, 1954, p. 103.)

loss of consciousness, may occur with foci of seizure discharge more anteriorly placed in the prefrontal areas (Fig. 21–6). In addition, stimulation in areas 18 and 19 will also produce eye turning. Thus the clinical neurologist must in each case weigh the localizing significance of seizures characterized by head and eye turning. Such seizure components do not have the more specific localizing significance of the focal motor seizure or of the olfactory hallucination.

In addition to head and eye turning, opening and closing of the eyelids may occur on area 8 stimulation. At times, eye movements, other than conjugate adversion, may occur, e.g., upward deviation of the eyes (Fig. 21–7).

Area 8: Ablation. Ablation of area 8, or (in man) infarction of this area following occlusion of the blood supply, results in a transient paralysis of voluntary conjugate gaze to the contralateral visual field. In general, in man, this paralysis of voluntary gaze does not occur in isolation but is associated with a sufficient degree of infarction to have produced a severe hemiparesis. The patient then lies in bed with the contralateral limbs in a hemiplegic posture and with the head and eyes deviated towards the intact arm and leg. This deviation may perhaps reflect the unbalanced effect of the adversive eye center of the intact hemisphere. The effect is usually transient, clearing in a matter of days or weeks.

These patients at times also appear to neglect objects introduced into the visual field contralateral to the lesion. The patients also neglect contralateral tactile and auditory stimuli. In the past, such a unilateral neglect has been attributed to associated involvement of the inferior parietal lobule. The studies of Kennard (1938) and of Welch and Stu-

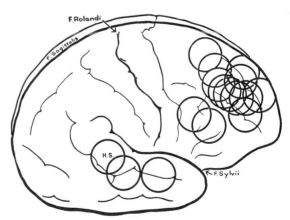

Figure 21–6 Unconscious adversive seizures. Localization of the lesion at surgery in 16 patients whose seizures began with unconscious adversion of head and eyes. Note that the majority of the lesions are located in the anterior portion of the frontal lobe and are certainly anterior to the lesions indicated in Figure 21–4 for conscious adversive movements. (From Penfield, W., and Kristiansen, K.: *Epileptic Seizure Patterns.* Springfield, Ill., Charles C Thomas, 1951, p. 22.)

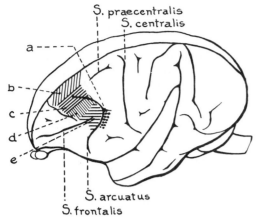

Figure 21-7 Functional subdivision of the frontal eye fields in the monkey. Under favorable conditions of relatively light anesthesia, it is possible to subdivide the frontal eye fields on the basis of eye movement obtained: *a,* closure of eyes; *b,* pupillary dilatation; *c,* eyelid opening ("awakening reaction"); *d,* conjugate deviation to the opposite side; and *e,* nystagmus to opposite side. (From Smith, W. K., *In* Bucy, P.: *The Precentral Motor Cortex,* Urbana, University of Illinois Press, 1944.) In the studies of Crosby, E. C., et al. (J. Neurol., 97:357–383, 1952) oblique and vertical movements were also obtained.

teville (1958), however, suggest that these unilateral neglect syndromes may occur as transient phenomena following ablation of area 8 in monkeys (area within the superior limb of the arcuate sulcus). These animals also had conjugate deviation of head and eyes to the side of the lesion and forced circling. Bilateral ablations within this area resulted in animals who, in a sense, had a bilateral neglect of the environment, remained apathetic, and neglected visual and auditory and tactile stimuli, although they could follow moving objects. Although some recovery occurred over a period of weeks to months, the animals continued to have a "wooden expression" and a fixed gaze. Some of these findings are seen in the human following bilateral frontal lobe damage. In addition, however, a similar state may occur in Parkinson's disease which will be discussed later.

SUPPLEMENTARY MOTOR CORTEX

Stimulation. The supplementary motor cortex is distinguished not on the basis of its cytoarchitecture (which is indistinct from that of areas 6 and 8) but on the basis of the effects produced on stimulation (Fig. 21–8). Even

these effects, moreover, overlap those of area 6. The threshold of this area is somewhat higher than that of the primary motor cortex. The effects produced consist of complex movements with the assumption of postures — raising of the contralateral arm with head and eye deviation towards this arm in the contralateral field. There are also associated bilateral movements of the trunk and lower extremities. The effects continue to occur after ablation of the primary motor cortex.

Ablation. Unilateral ablation of this area does not produce any significant weakness or significant alteration in tone. A transient release of the grasp reflex may occur. Bi-

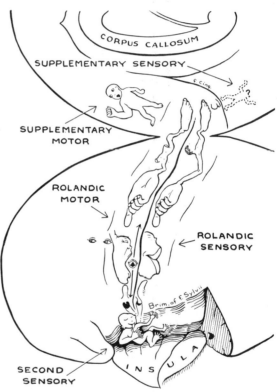

Figure 21-8 Somatic figurines. The primary motor and sensory (Rolandic) representation is demonstrated. In addition the effects usually produced by supplementary motor cortex stimulation are shown. Note that the latter effects are bilateral involving adversion and synergistic postural alteration. Note that similar effects were produced by Foerster by stimulation of area 6α β on the lateral convexity of the hemisphere (high parasagittal) as shown in Figure 21–3. Note the second sensory area buried in the parietal operculum of the Sylvian fissure. (From Penfield, W., and Jasper, H.: *Epilepsy and the Functional Anatomy of the Human Brain.* Boston, Little, Brown and Company, 1954, p. 105.)

lateral simultaneous ablation of this area produces no actual weakness, but increased tone (spasticity) develops, predominantly in the flexor muscles with an increase in deep tendon reflexes. A bilateral release of instinctive tactile grasp reflex also occurs.

SUPPRESSOR AREAS FOR MOTOR ACTIVITY

Dusser de Barenne and McCulloch found in the monkey that stimulation of that portion of area 4, adjacent to area 6 (designated area 4S), resulted in a suppression of the motor response elicited by stimulation of area 4. In addition, thresholds for obtaining responses from area 4 were raised, and after-discharge was aborted. Stretch reflexes and muscle tone were decreased. It was soon discovered that these effects could be obtained from a number of other cortical areas: area 8 (8S), 2S and 19S. On the medial aspect of the hemisphere, similar effects could be obtained from areas in relation to the cingulate gyrus: 24S and 32. These "suppressor" areas cannot be distinguished on cytoarchitectural grounds from adjacent cortical areas. Similar effects have been elicited from stimulation of the caudate nucleus and of the bulbar medullary inhibitory center. There has been some evidence that the cortical motor suppressor effects are mediated via cortical reticular and corticostriatal connections. In subsequent studies, Kaada (Fangel and Kaada, 1960) has indicated that arrest of movement may occur from stimulation of a number of distinct neocortical and rhinencephalic points. Note must of course be made that a nonspecific interference with voluntary movement may occur in relation to stimulation of the motor cortex. Thus, the patient who is experiencing a focal motor seizure involving the hand cannot use that hand in the performance of voluntary skilled movements. Similarly, arrest of speech is frequently produced by stimulation of the various speech areas of the dominant hemisphere; vocalization is only rarely produced.

PREFRONTAL CORTEX (Areas 9, 10, 11, and 12)

The term prefrontal refers to those portions of the frontal lobe anterior to the agranular motor and premotor areas. Most studies of stimulation or of ablation lesions involving the prefrontal areas have included, within the general meaning of the term prefrontal, not only areas 9, 10, 11, and 12 (sometimes grouped as orbital frontal) but also several adjacent areas. Thus the posterior orbital cortex (area 13) and the posteromedial orbital cortex (area 14) have been added to the orbital frontal group (Fig. 21–9). These areas all share a common relationship to the dorsomedial nucleus of the thalamus. Areas 46 and 47, located in man on the lateral surface of the hemisphere, are also often grouped with areas 9, 10, 11, and 12 as orbital frontal areas. Another area, the anterior cingulate gyrus (area 24), is also included in the prefrontal area, although it may be considered part of the limbic system and relates to the anterior thalamic nuclei.

Prefrontal Cortex: Stimulation. The threshold of the prefrontal areas is relatively high. In seizures beginning in this area, loss of consciousness may be the initial symptom with subsequent progression to adversive head and eye deviation and then to a generalized convulsive seizure. At times, in the experimental animal (the monkey), it has been possible to produce a prolonged, bilateral, electrical seizure discharge in the prefrontal areas (which remains limited to

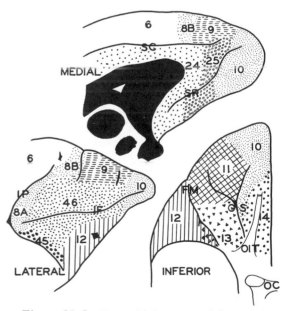

Figure 21–9 Frontal lobe areas of the monkey (Macaca Mulatta). Note location of orbital areas 13 and 14, anterior cingulate area 24, in addition to motoral prefrontal areas 9, 10, 11, 12. (From Walker, E. A.: J. Comp. Neurol., 73:81, 1940.)

these areas) (Marcus et al., 1968). Such animals do not show any gross impairment or alteration of behavior. They are able to reach for and grasp objects introduced into the visual field. They are able to respond appropriately to a beaker of water. More detailed testing of such animals as indicated by Weiskrantz et al., (1962) however, does reveal deficits in such tests as delayed response and delayed alternation. These deficits are similar to those noted following bilateral ablative lesions in the prefrontal areas.

Similarly, in a human patient with seizures, whom we have observed with electroencephalographic discharge in both prefrontal areas, a transient alteration in personality occurred during the seizures with changes similar to those described following prefrontal lobotomy. These personality changes with a compulsiveness of behavior and a release of inhibitions persisted for a period of several weeks into the postictal period. A similar interference effect of seizure discharge in this area has been described by Penfield and Jasper (1954).

Stimulation of the orbital frontal area (area 13) and the adjacent anterior cingulate gyrus (area 24) in the monkey and the human has produced various autonomic effects (both sympathetic and parasympathetic). In addition, arrest of respiration and alteration in blood pressure have occurred. In the understanding of these autonomic effects and of the effects on emotional behavior, the connections of these prefrontal and anterior cingulate orbital areas to the hypothalamic, anterior thalamic, and dorsomedial thalamic nuclei assume considerable importance.

Prefrontal Cortex: Ablation. In general, most studies of prefrontal function have dealt with bilateral ablation or with a unilateral lesion which, because of its parasagittal location in relation to the medial aspect of the prefrontal area, has produced essentially bilateral effects.

The first well authenticated case of the frontal lobe syndrome is the crowbar case of Mr. Phineas P. Gage reported by Harlow in 1868. In an explosion in 1848, a pointed tamping iron shot through the skull of the patient, an efficient, well-balanced, shrewd, and energetic railroad foreman. The bar 3.5 feet in length and 1.25 inches in greatest diameter entered below the left orbit and emerged in the midline vertex, anterior to the coronal suture, lacerating the superior

sagittal sinus in the process. Following the injury, a marked personality change was noted. The balance "between his intellectual faculties and animal propensities" had been destroyed. He was "impatient of restraint or advice when it conflicts with his desires; at times—obstinate yet capricious and vacillating devising many plans of future operations which are no sooner arranged than they are abandoned in turn for others appearing more feasible."

More discrete lesions in the monkey and chimpanzee have been correlated with more specific deficits. Thus lesions, restricted to the posterior orbital areas (area 13), have produced a syndrome of hyperactivity. Bilateral lesions involving the posterior and medial orbital areas, e.g., gyrus rectus (area 14), have also been associated with the release of a sham rage syndrome. Bilateral prefrontal lesions which did not necessarily involve posterior orbital areas produced a significant reduction in the emotional response to failure and stress. A similar decrease in fear and anxiety with the appearance of tameness in previously aggressive monkeys followed lesion of the anterior cingulate area (area 24). These effects on emotional response should be contrasted to the effects of restricted bilateral lesions involving the lateral prefrontal surface (particularly in the principal sulcus area) which produced deficits in the capacity for delaying response. In addition, deficits in the delayed alternation tests occurred with perseveration of response.

In man, there were a number of studies of prefrontal function in relation to the surgical procedure of bilateral prefrontal lobotomy or prefrontal leucotomy (disconnection of frontal lobe fiber connections to and from other cortical and subcortical areas). This procedure was introduced by Moniz in 1936 to modify the behavior and affect of psychotic patients, following the reports of Jacobsen and Fulton of the effects of these prefrontal lesions on the emotional responses of the chimpanzee. Subsequently, a number of lobotomies were performed to modify the emotional response of patients with chronic pain problems previously requiring large doses of narcotics. Such studies must be interpreted with a certain degree of caution. The lesions are produced in individuals with preoperative abnormalities of personality function. The effects are not necessarily those which the same lesion would produce in otherwise normal individuals. There is, however, a considerable resemblance to the effects produced by trauma (to the prefrontal areas) in relatively normal individuals.

It is clear that these procedures did produce an alteration in the emotional response with a reduction of anxiety generated in conflict and painful situations. Emotional response was often detached from the pain and conflicts.

These effects on emotion can now be produced by the use of the tranquilizing drugs. The development of these drugs, in addition to the prominence of certain postoperative personality alterations led to the discontinuation of the procedure.

These patients often were impulsive and distractable. Their emotional responses often were uninhibited with an apparent lack of concern over the consequences of their actions. A related finding was an inability to plan ahead for future goals; at times, the patients were unable to postpone gratification, responding to their motivations of the moment. (In a sense, a loss of the reality principle had occurred.) Although distractable, a certain perseveration of response was noted with an inability to shift responses to meet a change in environmental stimuli or cues. A rigidity and concreteness of response was apparent with deficits in abstract reasoning.

It must be noted that lesions (e.g., meningiomas) which were initially parasagittal or subfrontal in relation to the prefrontal areas may, as they progress, compromise the function of adjacent premotor areas (8 and 6 and the supplementary motor cortex). The resultant clinical picture may then include not only the changes in personality but also the release of an instinctive tactile grasp and of a sucking reflex. An incontinence of urine and feces may be present in addition to an apraxia of gait—an unsteadiness of gait which is apparent as the patient attempts to stand and as he begins to walk but clears up once the act has been initiated. The following case history illustrates many of these features of focal disease involving the prefrontal areas.

Case History 2. NECH #122–407.
Dates of admission: 10/1/58 and 9/30/65.

This white housewife and fashion designer (Mrs. B.C.) was first admitted to the hospital in 1958 at age 60 with a history of several years (? 2 to 5) of fatigue, loss of ambition, lack of enthusiasm, and a tendency to readily cry over minor problems. A depression of mood and a tendency to introspection had developed. The patient also reported a loss of her taste for food with a subsequent decrease in appetite and weight loss. These symptoms had progressed despite an adequate dosage of thyroid medication (60 mg. t.i.d.). Neurological examination was recorded as negative except for a slowness of speech and of thought processes. She was described by the psychiatric consultant as indecisive in her answers. Cerebrospinal fluid examination revealed no significant findings. Tests of thyroid function indicated hypothyroidism with protein bound iodine of 3.2 micrograms/100 ml. (normal; 4 to 8 micrograms/100 ml.) and a radioactive iodine uptake of 2.3 per cent in 24 hours (normal 20 to 50 per cent). Discharge diagnosis was chronic depression and hypothyroidism.

These symptoms continued to progress despite treatment with thyroid. The patient had increasing difficulty in walking. This was first noted in 1955 as a "phobia for heights." The patient would "freeze" at the top of a high flight of stairs. She then developed progressive difficulty in climbing stairs. Her husband reported that she would have marked difficulty in getting out of chairs. She would appear unsteady in gait after rising from a chair but would soon recover her equilibrium and would be able to walk in a relatively normal manner. Increasingly, the patient's motor and mental activities became slower. She "procrastinated in making decisions." Occasional urinary incontinence developed in 1964 and was attributed to her neurological disease (apparent senile dementia). Although her husband reported her memory as initially well preserved, other observers in 1964 reported a progressive deficit in memory. In September 1965 the patient began to complain of episodic fogging or blurring of vision:

Neurological examination on admission to the hospital in September 1965 at age 67 indicated: (a) slowness of speech and gait, (b) slight disorientation for date and year, (c) deep tendon reflexes 2+, plantar responses flexor, and (d) no significant sensory finding except a slight decrease in position sense at the toes. No details as to the patient's gait were recorded. The sense of smell was apparently not tested and no notes as to the presence or absence of a grasp reflex were recorded.

HOSPITAL COURSE:

On October 1, 1965 the patient developed headache and vomiting. She had difficulty walking unsupported and became increasingly more somnolent but could be roused by painful stimulation. Deep tendon reflexes were increased bilaterally with bilateral extensor plantar responses (bilateral Babinski signs). Grasp response was absent. Pupils responded to light but were sluggish.

Funduscopic examination was negative but lumbar puncture indicated a markedly increased pressure, greater than 400 mm. of H_2O. Cerebrospinal fluid protein was elevated to 125 mg/100 ml. The patient became unresponsive and emergency neurological and neurosurgical consultations were obtained.

NEUROLOGICAL EXAMINATION:

1. *Mental status:* The patient was semicomatose with periodic Cheyne-Stokes respirations.

2. *Cranial nerves:* Pupils were fixed, the left dilated, the right constricted.

3. *Motor system:*
   a. The patient moved all limbs in response to painful stimulation, right more than left.
   b. There was a spastic resistance in the upper and lower left extremities.

4. *Reflexes:*
   a. A generalized hyperreflexia was present with bilateral ankle clonus.
   b. Bilateral Babinski signs were present.
   c. A bilateral grasp reflex was present. Note, however, that in a semicomatose patient this has little localizing significance.

5. *Sensation:* Pain sensation was intact.

HOSPITAL COURSE:

Bilateral carotid arteriograms revealed that a large subfrontal butterfly-shaped mass (probable meningioma) was present in the anterior cranial fossa bilaterally. The intradural portions of both internal carotids were depressed. The anterior cerebral arteries as well as the frontal polar, pericallosal, and callosal marginal branches were displaced backwards. The anterior cerebral arteries were also displaced upwards. The middle cerebral arteries were displaced backwards. The tumor mass derived blood supply from the ophthalmic arteries.

A bifrontal craniotomy was immediately performed by Dr. Robert Yuan with total removal of a large bifrontal meningioma arising from the falx and olfactory groove. On the right side the tumor was estimated to occupy 75 per cent of the anterior cranial fossa, measuring $7 \times 5 \times 6$ cm. On the left the tumor was of approximately half this size, measuring 5 cm. in diameter. The thickness of the cerebral hemisphere covering the tumor in the right prefrontal area was reduced to 0.5 cm. Histological examination of the tumor indicated a benign meningioma (meningotheliomatous type).

The patient showed some immediate improvement at the conclusion of surgery, in the sense that both pupils were equal in size and reacted to light. By the time of discharge from the hospital, 2 months after surgery, considerable improvement had occurred. She could recognize the doctor by name but did not know the place, the season, or the month; she could, however, describe a picture she had just seen. A bilateral deficit in olfaction was present (anosmia). Assistance was required in walking. A bilateral grasp reflex was present.

Follow-up evaluation in July 1967 indicated continued improvement although the patient still had complaints relevant to impairment of recent memory and slight unsteadiness of gait. Deep tendon reflexes were symmetrical with plantar responses flexor. A bilateral grasp reflex was present and the patient was slow in walking and fell occasionally. Urinary incontinence occurred with wetting of the bed.

COMMENT:

In retrospect, the evolution of symptoms in this patient clearly indicates a tumor initially compressing both prefrontal areas and producing alterations in mood and personality. With continued growth of the tumor, compromise of the premotor areas with resultant apraxia of gait and release of grasp reflex began to occur, either as a result of direct compression or secondary to the distortion and compression of the anterior cerebral arteries. It is not unusual to witness the development of a dementia (deficits in recent memory) in large tumors in a subfrontal midline location. A similar dementia may occur in large aneurysms of the anterior communicating artery. The problem of dementia will be considered in greater detail in the section on memory.

The development of headache, vomiting,

and increasing somnolence indicated the development of increasing intracranial pressure. The sudden unresponsiveness following the lumbar puncture with the development of periodic Cheyne-Stokes respirations, pupillary changes, and bilateral corticospinal tract signs all indicated an additional acute exacerbation of the already compromised brain stem functions, a compromise which had already resulted from the backward displacement of the intracranial contents with distortion of the brain stem. In retrospect, one might hypothesize that the patient's complaint of a loss of taste for her food in 1958 might well have indicated some loss of olfactory sensation since much of our appreciation of food is dependent on olfaction. Specific tests for olfaction had apparently not been performed prior to surgery.

PARIETAL LOBE

POSTCENTRAL GYRUS: SOMATIC SENSORY CORTEX

The postcentral gyrus is not, from a histological standpoint, a single cytoarchitectural type. That portion at the base of the central sulcus, area 3, is typical granular koniocortex and receives the major projection from the ventral posterior nuclei of the thalamus. Area 1, on the crest of the postcentral gyrus, and area 2, on the posterior wall of the postcentral gyrus, are modified homotypical cortex and are more dependent on collaterals from area 3 for afferent input than on direct input from the ventral posterior thalamic nuclei.

Postcentral Gyrus: Stimulation. Stimulation of the postcentral gyrus produces a sensation on the contralateral side of the face, arm, hand, leg, or trunk described by the patient as a tingling or numbness and labeled paresthesias. Less often, a sense of movement is experienced. The patient does not describe the sensation as painful. These various phenomena, occurring at the onset of a seizure, may be described as a somatic sensory aura.

There is in the postcentral gyrus a sequence of sensory representation which, in general, is similar to that noted in the precentral gyrus for motor function (Fig. 21–10). The representation of the face occupies the lower 40 per cent; the representation of the hand, the middle-upper 40 per cent; and

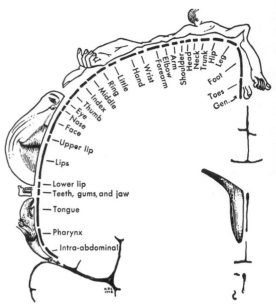

Figure 21–10 Sensory representation as determined by stimulation studies on the human cerebral cortex at surgery. Compare this sensory homunculus to the motor homunculus (Figure 21–1). Note the relatively large area devoted to lips, thumb, and fingers. (From Penfield, W., and Rasmussen, T.: *The Cerebral Cortex of Man.* New York, MacMillan, 1955, p. 214.)

the representation of the foot, the paracentral lobule. As in the precentral gyrus of man, certain areas of the body have a disproportionate area of representation, i.e., the thumb, fingers, lips, and tongue. In addition, at the lower end of the postcentral gyrus, extending into the sylvian fissure (the parietal operculum), there is found a representation of the alimentary tract, including taste.

Studies of cortical potentials evoked by tactile stimulation in the monkey have suggested that there is a secondary somatic sensory projection area in addition to the classic postcentral contralateral projection area. This second area has a bilateral representation and is found partially buried in the sylvian fissure at the lower end of the central sulcus (Fig. 21–2). A similar second area of representation has been reported by Penfield in seizure patients in whom an abdominal sensation (aura) was followed by a sensation of paresthesias in both sides of the mouth and in both hands (Fig. 21–8). Note also should be made that stimulation of the precentral gyrus of man by the neurosurgeon during surgery has at times produced contralateral tingling or numbness, in addition to the more frequent motor responses. (Penfield and Jasper, 1954).

Postcentral Gyrus: Ablation. Immediately following destruction of the postcentral gyrus, there will often be found an almost total loss of awareness of all sensory modalities on the contralateral side of the body. Within a short time there is usually a return of some appreciation of painful stimuli. The patient will, however, often continue to note that the quality of the painful stimulus differs from that on the intact side. An awareness of gross pressure, touch, and temperature also returns. Vibratory sensation may return to a certain degree. Certain modalities of sensation, however, never return or return only to a minor degree. (In partial lesions of the postcentral gyrus these various modalities may return to a variable degree.) These modalities are often referred to as the cortical modalities of sensation or as discriminative modalities of sensation. The following types of sensory awareness are usually included in the category:

1. Position sense: the perception of movement and the direction of movement when the finger or toe is moved passively at the interphalangeal joint.

2. Tactile localization: the ability to accurately localize the specific portion of the body or extremity stimulated.

3. Two-point discrimination: the ability to perceive that a double stimulus with a small separation in space has touched a given part of the body.

4. Stereognosis: the ability to distinguish the shape of object and thus to recognize objects based on their three-dimensional tactile form.

5. Graphesthesia: the ability to recognize numbers or letters which have been drawn on the finger, hand, face, or leg.

6. Weight discrimination: the ability to differentiate relative amounts of pressure.

7. Perception of simultaneous stimuli: the ability to perceive that both sides of the body have been simultaneously stimulated. When bilateral stimuli are presented but only a unilateral stimulus is perceived, "extinction" is said to have occurred.

8. Perception of texture: ability to perceive the pattern of surface stimuli encountered by the moving tactile receptors.

In contrast, the sensory modalities of pain, gross touch, pressure, temperature, and vibration are referred to as primary modalities of sensation. Perception of these modalities continues to occur after ablation of the postcentral gyrus, and it has been assumed that the anatomical substrate for such an awareness must exist at the thalamic level.

The following case history demonstrates the type of sensory deficits found in disease of the parietal lobe involving the postcentral gyrus.

Case History 3. NEMCH #184–743. Date of admission: 1/27/67.

This 62-year-old white, right-handed housewife (Mrs. L.B.) had undergone a left radical mastectomy in 1961 for carcinoma of the breast. In August 1966 a persistent cough had developed with left pleuritic pain and a collection of fluid in the left pleural space (pleural effusion). At this time, there was also noted the onset of daily headaches in the right orbit, occasionally awakening the patient from sleep.

In September 1966, the patient noted some weakness of both legs. It was soon evident that the problem mainly concerned the right lower extremity. Over a 3- to 4-week period, a progressive weakness and difficulty in control of this extremity developed. The patient's husband noted that the right leg was circumducted when the patient walked.

In September 1966, aching pain in the right index finger was also noted in addition to a progressive deficit in the use of the right hand which was more a "stiffness and incoordination" than any actual weakness.

In December 1966, episodes of pain in the toes of the right foot with numbness of right foot occurred, lasting 2 to 3 days at a time.

In January 1967, difficulty in memory and some minor language deficit, suggesting a nominal aphasia, was noted.

NEUROLOGICAL EXAMINATION:

1. *Mental status:*
   a. The patient was oriented for time, place, and person.
   b. Delayed recall was reduced to 3-out-of-five in 5 minutes.
   c. A slowness in naming objects was present—missed one item of 6.
   d. Calculations, reading, and attention were normal. There was no left-right confusion.

2. *Cranial nerves:*
   a. Nerve II: early papilledema was

noted: absence of venous pulsations, indistinctness of disc margins, minimal elevation of vessels as they pass over edge of disc.

b. Nerve VII: right central facial weakness was present.

3. *Motor system:*
a. A mild weakness of the right upper limb was present, more marked in the lower limb (most marked distally).

b. Spasticity was present at the right elbow and knee.

c. Gait: The right leg was circumducted; the right arm was held in a flexed posture.

4. *Reflexes:*
a. Deep tendon reflexes were increased on the right.

b. A right Babinski response was present.

5. *Sensation:*
a. Touch intact.

b. An ill-defined alteration in pain perception was present in the right arm and leg—more of a relative difference in quality of the pain than any actual deficit.

c. Repeated stimulation of the right lower extremity (pain or touch) produced dysesthesias (painful sensation).

d. Vibration sensation was decreased to a minor degree at the toes bilaterally but intact in the upper extremities.

e. Position sense was markedly defective in the right fingers with errors in perception of fine and medium amplitude movement in the right toes.

f. Simultaneous stimulation resulted in extinction in the right lower extremity.

g. Graphesthesia (identification of numbers, e.g., 8, 5, 4 drawn on cutaneous surface) was absent in the right hand and fingers and poor in the right leg.

h. Tactile localization and two-point discrimination were decreased on the right side.

LABORATORY DATA:

1. *Skull x-rays:* The pineal was shifted from left to right. Demineralization of the dorsum sellae also had occurred: consistent with the increase in intracranial pressure.

2. *Chest x-ray:* Several metastatic nodules were present in the left lung.

3. *Electroencephalogram:* A focal disturbance, having the quality of damage, was present in the left posterior frontal central and parietal areas (almost continuous focal 4 to 7 cps slow wave activity).

4. *Left carotid arteriogram:* A left posterior frontal parietal lobe lesion was suggested by a shift of the posterior portion of the anterior cerebral artery from the left to the right. The middle cerebral artery in the sylvian fissure was also depressed downwards.

5. *Brain scan:* The findings were consistent with a focal metastatic lesion with a focal uptake of radioisotope (Hg^{197}) in the left parietal area: high and close to the midline with uptake in the adjacent subcortical white matter (Fig. 21-11).

6. Erythrocyte sedimentation rate was elevated to 90 mm., consistent with metastatic disease.

SUBSEQUENT COURSE:

There was evidence in this case that the disease had spread to multiple organs: brain (findings as noted), lung (chest x-rays and biopsy), and liver (abnormal laboratory tests of liver function). Radiation and hormonal therapy were therefore administered rather than any attempt at surgical removal of the left parietal metastatic lesion. Follow-up examination one month later indicated that a significant improvement had occurred in motor function in the arm. Sensory deficits persisted. Speech was slow but relatively intact. The patient eventually expired in June 1967.

Autopsy was performed by Dr. Humphrey Lloyd of the Beverly Hospital and disclosed extensive metastatic disease present in lungs, liver, and lymph nodes. A single necrotic metastatic lesion was present in the brain. This was located in the upper postcentral gyrus of the left parietal area, 1.0 cm. below the pial surface and measuring $1.2 \times 1.0 \times 0.6$ cm.

COMMENT:

This patient had a progressive neurological deficit with headache and papilledema, a clinical course that clearly indicates the presence of a neoplasm. This diagnosis was supported by the ancillary laboratory studies.

In general, one should assume that a patient with a past history of carcinoma of the breast, carcinoma of the lung, malignant melanoma, or renal cell carcinoma, who de-

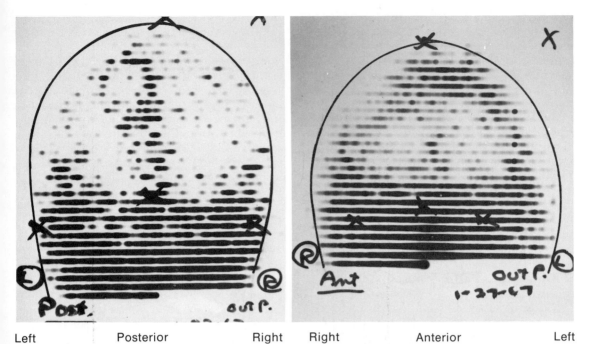

| Left | Posterior | Right | Right | Anterior | Left |

Figure 21–11 Brain Scan, Case History 3. The posterior scan demonstrates the posterior one-half of the hemispheres; the anterior scan, primarily the anterior one-half. A high uptake in the left parasagittal parietal central area is demonstrated. (Courtesy of Dr. Bertram Selverstone.)

velops symptoms of central nervous system disease, has metastatic disease until proven otherwise. Such symptoms at their onset may be minor and nonfocal and appear trivial: headache, subjective weakness, a change in personality. On the other hand more focal symptoms and signs may be present: focal weakness, focal seizure. The metastatic lesions may be single or multiple.

A diagnosis of metastatic disease does not imply that no treatment of central nervous system lesions is possible. Surgical resection of single lesions may be successfully performed. Often the apparent deficits are far out of proportion to the actual size of the tumor because of the surrounding swelling (edema) in the adjacent tissues.

The pattern of sensory involvement in this case clearly localized this lesion to the cortex (or white matter close to cortical surface) rather than to the thalamus. The relative intactness of pain, touch, and vibration sensation should be contrasted to the significant deficits in position sense, graphesthesia, tactile localization, and two-point discrimination with extinction on simultaneous stimulation. The occurrence of episodic pain in the involved arms and legs along with the production of an experienced painful sensation on repetitive tactile stimulation (dysesthesias) in patients with sensory pathway lesions is sometimes referred to as a "thal-

amic" or "pseudothalamic" syndrome. (Refer to discussion of Wilkins and Brody, 1969.) In this case, the anatomical locus for the pseudothalamic syndrome is apparent.

The effects of deficits in cortical sensation on the total sensory motor function of a limb are apparent in this case. The actual disability and disuse of the right arm and leg were far out of proportion to any actual weakness. Such an extremity is often referred to as a "useless limb." The actual weakness which was present undoubtedly reflected pressure effects on the precentral gyrus and the descending motor fibers in adjacent white matter.

Destructive lesions of the postcentral gyrus during infancy or early childhood often produce a retardation of skeletal growth on the contralateral side of the body. Such a patient examined as an adolescent or adult will be found to have not only cortical sensory deficits in the contralateral arm and leg but also a relative smallness of these extremities (shorter arm or leg, smaller hand and glove size, smaller shoe size).

SUPERIOR AND INFERIOR PARIETAL AREAS

The superior parietal lobule receives the numerical designations 5 and 7 in the cytoarchitectural map of Brodmann; the inferior parietal lobule receives the designations 39 and 40. From a practical standpoint we may consider both of these parietal areas as examples of homotypical cortex.

Stimulation. The threshold of the superior and inferior parietal lobules for discharge is relatively high. Although Foerster reported the occurrence of some contralateral paresthesias on stimulation in man, these results were not confirmed by Penfield. Stimulation in the inferior parietal areas of the dominant hemisphere did produce arrest of speech, but this is a nonspecific effect, occurring on stimulation of any of the speech areas of the dominant hemisphere. It must, of course, be noted that space-occupying lesions in the parietal lobules may produce sensory or motor seizures by virtue of their pressure effects on the lower threshold post- and precentral gyri.

Ablation. Earlier studies had suggested possible sensory deficits in relation to ablation of the inferior or superior parietal areas. The detailed studies of Corkin, Milner, and Rasmussen on patients subjected to limited cortical ablations of the inferior or superior parietal areas (in the treatment of focal epilepsy) have clearly indicated that no significant sensory deficits occurred. The postcentral gyrus rather than the parietal lobules is critical for somatic sensory discrimination. Again note must be made of the fact that large lesions in the parietal lobules may produce effects on the function of the post- and precentral gyri through pressure or invasion. Lesions involving the white matter deep to the inferior parietal lobule may damage the superior portion of the optic (geniculocalcarine) radiation, producing a defect in the inferior half of the contralateral visual field — a so-called inferior quadrantanopsia.

DOMINANT HEMISPHERE PARIETAL LOBULES

Destructive lesions of the parietal lobules produce effects on more complex cortical functions. Those lesions involving particularly the supramarginal and angular gyri of the dominant (usually the left hemisphere) inferior parietal lobule may produce one or more of a complex of symptoms known as *Gerstmann's syndrome.* These include (a) dysgraphia (a deficit in writing in the presence of intact motor and sensory function in the upper extremities), (b) dyscalculia (deficits in the performance of calcula-

tions), (c) left-right confusion, and (d) errors in finger recognition, for example, middle finger, index finger, ring finger, in the presence of intact sensation (finger agnosia). In addition disturbances in the capacity for reading may be present. Some patients may also manifest problems in performing skilled movements on command (an apraxia) at a time when strength, sensation, and coordination are intact. Usually only partial forms of the syndrome are present. Some patients with lesions in the parietal lobules will show a neglect of the visual space on the right side. To what extent this reflects actual parietal dysfunction is not certain. Such lesions might produce their effects by involvement of the adjacent occipital lobe or by involvement of the subcortical white matter of the optic radiation. The problem of the dominant parietal lobe in language function will be considered in greater detail and illustrated in the section on language and aphasia. The reader should refer to that section for an illustrative case history.

NONDOMINANT HEMISPHERE PARIETAL LOBULES

Patients with involvement of the nondominant parietal lobe, particularly the inferior parietal lobule, often demonstrate abnormalities in their concepts of body image, in their perception of external space, and in their capacity to construct drawings (Fig. 21–12).

The disturbance in concept of body image may include the following:

a. A lack of awareness of the left side of the body, with a neglect of the left side of the body in dressing, undressing, and washing. Despite relatively intact cortical and primary sensation, the patient may fail to recognize his arm or leg when this is passively brought into his field of vision.

b. A lack of awareness of a hemiparesis despite a relative preservation of cortical sensation (anosognosia).

c. A denial of illness. At times this may be carried to the point of attempting to leave the hospital since as far as the patient is concerned, there is no justification for hospitalization.

The disturbance in perception of external space may take several forms:

a. A neglect of the left visual field and of objects, writing, or pictures in the left visual field. At times this is associated with a dense defect in vision in the left visual field; at other

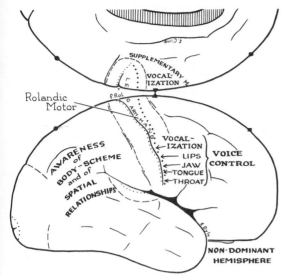

Figure 21–12 Functions of the nondominant inferior parietal lobule. A major lesion in the posterior temporal and inferior parietal region of the nondominant hemisphere in adult life would produce loss of awareness of body scheme and spatial relationship. The same destruction in the contralateral (dominant) hemisphere would result in a marked deficit in the understanding and use of language (aphasia). (From Penfield, W.: *In* Eccles, J. C. (ed.): *Brain and Conscious Experience.* New York, Springer-Verlag, 1966, p. 223.)

times there may be no definite defect for single objects in the left visual field, but an extinction occurs when objects are presented simultaneously in both visual fields. Again the problem of possible involvement of occipital cortex or of subcortical optic radiation should be considered as previously noted.

b. An inability to interpret drawings such as a map or to pick out objects from a complex figure. The patient is confused as to figure background relationship. He is disoriented in attempting to locate objects in a room. When asked to locate cities on an outline map of the United States, the patient manifests disorientation as to the west and east coasts and as to the relationship of one city to the next. Chicago and New Orleans may be placed on the Pacific Ocean; Boston on the Florida peninsula; and New York City somewhere west of the Great Lakes.

The disturbance in capacity for the construction of drawings has been termed a constructional apraxia or dyspraxia. An apraxia may be defined as an inability to perform a previously well performed act at a time when voluntary movement, sensation, coordination, and understanding are otherwise all intact. The following deficits may be present: the patient may be unable to draw a house or the face of a clock; he may be unable to copy a complex figure such as a three-dimensional cube, a locomotive, and so forth; in severe disturbances the patient may be unable to copy even a simple square, circle, or triangle.

Case History 4. NEMC #190–353.
Date of admission: 10/19/67.
Date of consultation in office of Dr. Marcus: 10/4/67.

This 70-year-old, single, white, female, right-handed, retired candy maker (Miss S.C.) underwent a left radical mastectomy for carcinoma of the breast in 1964, three years prior to admission. In June 1967, the patient became unsteady with a sensation of rocking as though on a boat. She no longer attended to her housekeeping and to dressing.

In October 1967, over a three-week period, a relatively rapid progression occurred with perseveration and deterioration of recent memory. The patient no longer was concerned with urinary and fecal continence.

For 2 weeks, right temporal headaches had been present. During this time, the patient was noted by her sister to be neglecting the left side of the body. She would fail to put on the left shoe when dressing. In undressing, the stocking on the left would be only half removed.

Family History: the patient's mother died of metastatic carcinoma of the breast.

NEUROLOGICAL EXAMINATION:
1. *Mental status:*
   a. The patient was oriented for time, place, and person.
   b. Delayed recall was 5-out-of-5 objects in 5 minutes.
   c. There was no evidence of an aphasia.
   d. The patient often wandered in her conversation.
   e. She often asked irrelevant questions and was often impersistent in motor activities.
   f. There was marked disorganization in the drawing of a house or a clock. A similar marked disorganization was noted in attempts at copying the picture of a railroad engine (Fig. 21–13). There was a marked neglect of the left side of space and of the

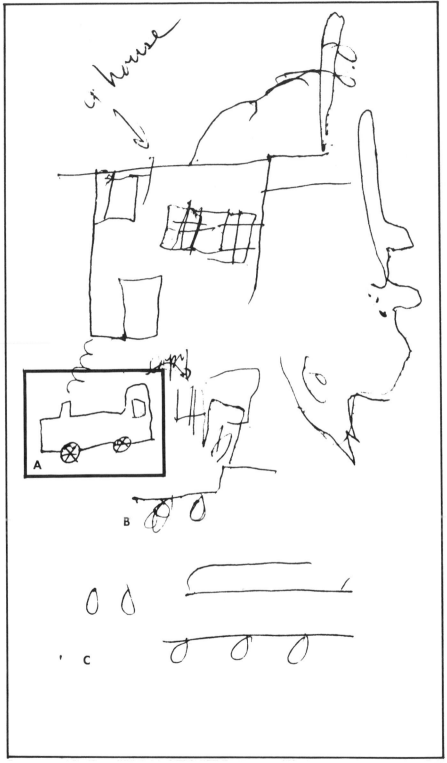

Figure 21-13 Nondominant hemisphere constructional apraxia: Case History 4. The patient's attempts to draw a house are shown on the upper half of the page. The patient was then asked to copy a drawing of a railroad engine. The examiner's (Dr. Leon Menzer) original (*A*) and the attempted copies of the patient are shown on the lower half of the page (*B* and *C*).

left side of the body. Patient failed to read the left half of a page. When she put her glasses on, she did not put the left bow over the ear. When getting into bed, she did not move the left leg into bed. She had slipped off her dress on the right side, but was lying in bed with the dress still covering the left side. The patient had been reluctant to come for neurological consultation. Although she complained of headache and nausea she denied any other deficits. Information concerning these problems was provided by her relatives. Much additional persuasion was required before the patient would agree to be hospitalized.

2. *Cranial nerves:*
   a. Nerve II: A dense left homonymous hemianopsia was present. When reading, the patient left off the left side of a page. She bisected a line markedly off center. Disc margins were blurred and venous pulsations were absent, indicating papilledema.
   b. Nerve III: The right pupil was slightly larger than the left.
   c. Nerve VII: A minimal left central facial weakness was present.

3. *Motor system:*
Strength was intact. There was, however, little spontaneous movement of the left arm and leg. Tone was normal.

4. *Reflexes:*
   a. Deep tendon reflexes were symmetrical and physiologic.
   b. Plantar responses were flexor.

5. *Gait:*
The patient was ataxic on a narrow base with eyes open with a tendency to fall to the left, and was unable to stand with eyes closed even on a broad base.

6. *Sensation:*
   a. Pain, touch, and vibration were intact. At times, however, there was a decreased awareness of stimuli on the left side.
   b. Errors were made in position sense at toes and fingers on the left.
   c. With double simultaneous stimulation, the patient neglected stimuli on the left face, arm, and leg.
   d. Tactile localization was poor over the left arm and leg.

LABORATORY DATA:
1. *Skull x-rays* were negative.

2. *Chest x-ray* indicated a possible metastatic lesion at the right hilum.

3. *Erythrocyte sedimentation rate* was elevated to 72 mm., suggesting metastatic disease.

4. *Electroencephalogram* (Fig. 21–14) was abnormal because of frequent focal 3 to 4 cps slow waves in the right temporal and parietal areas, suggesting focal damage in these areas.

5. *Brain scan* indicated that a large but well-defined area of increased uptake of isotope (Hg^{197}) was present in the right parietal area extending from the midline to the lateral surface, measuring $7 \times 5 \times 7$ cm. The most likely diagnosis was that of a solitary large metastatic lesion (Fig. 21–15).

6. *Right carotid arteriogram* showed that a large vascular tumor mass, probably metastatic, was present in the posterior section of the right temporal lobe. There was elevation of the middle cerebral artery and displacement of the anterior cerebral artery to the left side.

SUBSEQUENT COURSE:
Treatment with steroids (dexamethasone and estrogens) resulted in temporary improvement. Surgery was refused by the patient. Her condition soon deteriorated with increasing obtundation of consciousness. She expired on December 12, 1967.

COMMENT:
This patient certainly presented a syndrome characterized by disturbance in concept of body image with a marked neglect of the left side, a denial of illness, and a marked constructional apraxia. The various laboratory studies indicated a large lesion in the right posterior temporal parietal area. In many cases, the location of the lesion may appear to be predominantly posterior temporal. Such large posterior temporal lesions would certainly compromise the cortex and subcortical white matter of the adjacent inferior parietal area.

In this case, marked deficits in perception of the cortical modalities of sensation were present. In other cases, such involvement is much less marked. In some cases, involvement of the motor cortex is evident with an actual left hemiparesis accompanied by an increase in deep tendon reflexes and an extensor plantar response. At times there may be several indications on the clinical examination and in the laboratory studies that the involvement of the frontal lobe areas is more prominent than the parietal involvement.

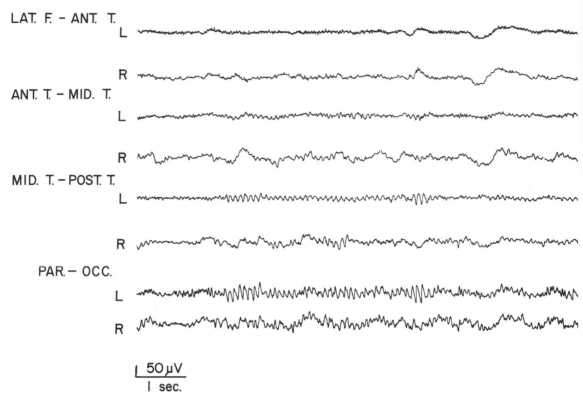

LAT. F. – ANT. T.

L

R

ANT. T. – MID. T.

L

R

MID. T. – POST. T.

L

R

PAR. – OCC.

L

R

50 μV

1 sec.

Figure 21–14 Case History 4. Electroencephalogram demonstrating focal slow wave active in right temporal and parietal areas. In the temporal lobe, the slow wave activity is more prominent in middle temporal (Mid. T.) and posterior temporal (Post. T.) than the anterior temporal (Ant. T.) areas. The left hemisphere demonstrates normal alpha activity of 10 cps.

We have already indicated that the neglect components of this syndrome may be noted in lesions of the anterior premotor area (area 8). The premotor area has been described as receiving long association fibers from many sensory association areas. It is possible that in some cases the posterior temporal–inferior parietal location of the lesion may be critical in interrupting these association fibers. For these several reasons, it is perhaps more appropriate to use the term, syndrome of the nondominant hemisphere, rather than the more localized designation, nondominant inferior parietal syndrome.

With lesions of the nondominant hemisphere, there is a significant alteration of the patient's awareness of his environment. The behavior of an individual is in part determined by his own particular perception of the environment. If that perception is altered or disorganized, his behavioral responses may appear inappropriate to others. Obviously not all individuals will respond in the same manner to a given environmental situation; part of the response will be determined by the past experience and personality of the individual.

In the following case of an infarct in the nondominant hemisphere, the apparent inappropriateness of behavior was quite evident.

Case History 5. Walson Army Hospital. Date of admission: 3/65.

A 62-year-old, right-handed, retired army colonel was brought to the emergency room of Walson Army Hospital by his wife in March 1965. Hospital personnel recalled that prior to his retirement the patient had been an efficient and forceful officer in the inspector general's office.

Shortly after arising, the patient had been noted by his wife to have a weakness of the left arm; he was clumsy and dropping objects. The patient denied any problems. Shortly thereafter he fell to the floor in the bathroom. It was evident to the patient's

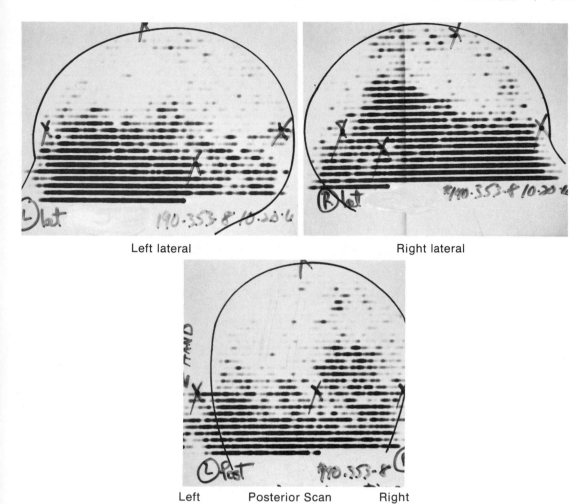

Left lateral   Right lateral

Left   Posterior Scan   Right

Figure 21–15 Brain Scan, Case History 4. A large uptake of radioisotope is demonstrated in the right parietal and adjacent posterior temporal area. This is seen in both the posterior scan and the right lateral scan. (Courtesy of Dr. Bertram Selverstone.)

wife, but not to the patient, that he had sustained a paralysis of his left arm and leg.

NEUROLOGICAL EXAMINATION:

Mental status:

Examination several hours later indicated an alert but impersistent patient. The patient was unaware as to why he had been brought to the hospital.

Cranial nerves:

The patient tended to look to the right although head and eyes were not markedly deviated to the right. He ignored the left visual field and failed to look to the left on command. Unilateral finger movements by the examiner were not perceived in the periphery of the patient's left visual field, and in the more central portions extinction of simultaneously presented stimuli occurred on the left. A marked left supranuclear facial weakness was present.

Motor system:

A marked hemiparesis of left arm and leg was present.

Reflexes:

Deep tendon reflexes were increased on the left. A left Babinski sign was present.

Sensory System:

The patient was aware of single, tactile, and painful stimuli in an inconsistent manner. Some position sense was preserved at the left fingers and toes for gross and medium amplitude movements. However, with simultaneous left and right tactile stimuli, the patient neglected (extinguished) stimuli on the left side of the face, arm, and leg. Graphesthesia was defective over the left face, hand, and leg. When the patient's left arm was passively brought across the midline into his right visual field, the patient denied that this was his own hand and arm. When recumbent in bed, the patient failed to cover the left side of the body with the sheet. The hospital gown covered only the right half of the body.

SUBSEQUENT COURSE:

Little improvement occurred over the next week. The patient soon began to complain to visitors and to various officials that there must be a conspiracy between the doctors and his wife to forcibly keep him in the hospital since so far as he was concerned he was perfectly healthy and did not require hospitalization.

OCCIPITAL LOBE (Visual Cortex)

The occipital lobe in the numerical scheme of Brodmann consists of areas 17, 18, and 19. Area 17, the striate cortex, the principal visual projection area in man, is found primarily on the medial surface of the hemisphere occupying those portions of the cuneus (above) and lingual gyrus (below) which border the calcarine sulcus. For this reason it is often termed calcarine cortex. Much of this cortex is located on the walls and in the depths of this fissure. In man very little of area 17 extends around the occipital pole onto the lateral surface, as opposed to the monkey where a considerable portion of area 17 is found on the lateral surface.

Area 18 (also termed the parastriate area) and area 19 (the preoccipital or prestriate area) form concentric bands about area 17 and are found on both the medial and lateral surfaces. From a cytoarchitectural standpoint area 17 represents a classic example of specialized granular cortex or koniocortex. Areas 18 and 19 represent progressive modifications from koniocortex towards homotypical cortex (Figs. 17–7, 17–8, 20–9, 20–10).

Area 17 is the primary visual projection area—the termination of the geniculocalcarine (or optic) radiation. This projection is arranged in a topographic manner with the superior quadrant of the contralateral visual field represented on the inferior bank, and the inferior quadrant of the contralateral visual field on the superior bank of the calcarine fissure. The macula has a large area of representation which occupies the posterior one-third of the calcarine cortex.

Except for the geniculocalcarine tract all communication with area 17 occurs through area 18. Area 17 receives and sends fibers to area 18 but does not receive or send any direct callosal or long association fibers to other cortical areas. Area 18, on the other hand, has been demonstrated, in both the earlier strychnine neuronography studies and the more recent silver degeneration studies, to send callosal fibers to the opposite hemisphere and to communicate with the premotor and inferior temporal areas by the superior longitudinal and inferior longitudinal fasciculi.

In addition both areas 18 and 19 send fibers to the tectal area of the superior colliculus. Such connections are necessary if visual fixation and accurate following of a moving visual stimulus are to occur. These conjugate eye movements in relation to a moving visual stimulus should be distinguished from the independent phenomenon of voluntary conjugate eye movements. The latter phenomenon does not require a visual stimulus and does not depend on any connections to area 18. Rather this is dependent on area 8 which sends fibers to the lateral gaze center of the pons.

Areas 17, 18, and 19: Stimulation. Stimulation of areas 17, 18, or 19 in conscious man (as in the studies of Penfield) produces visual sensations (Fig. 21–16). These images do not represent elaborate hallucinations but rather are described as flickering lights,

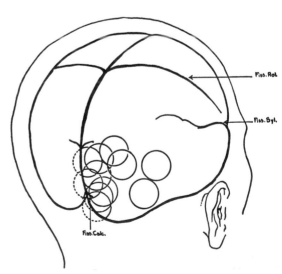

Figure 21–16 Focal discharge in occipital lobe. Location of the lesions at surgery in 11 patients with focal seizures consisting of visual sensations. (From Penfield, W., and Kristiansen, K.: *Epileptic Seizure Patterns.* Springfield, Charles C Thomas, 1951, p. 47.)

stars, lines, spots, and so forth. Often the images are described in terms of color. Movement of the image is often noted. The images are usually localized to the contralateral field, at times to the contralateral eye. At times the patient cannot determine laterality. In addition stimulation of areas 18 and 19 will produce conjugate deviation of the eyes to the contralateral field and at times vertical conjugate movements.

Area 17: Ablation. Complete unilateral ablation of area 17 will produce a complete homonymous hemianopsia (the same one-half field in each eye will have no vision) in the contralateral field. With partial lesions, a partial defect will result. For example, if only the superior bank of the calcarine fissure is involved, the visual field defect will be limited to the inferior quadrant of the contralateral field. With such calcarine cortex lesions, the field defects are similar in the two eyes (termed congruous) as compared to optic tract lesions which may produce somewhat unequal (noncongruous) homonymous field defects in the two eyes. Vascular lesions, in particular occlusion of the posterior cerebral artery, often result in a homonymous hemianopsia in which macular sparing is said to occur. That is, vision in the macular area of the involved field remains intact. Such preservation of macular vision probably occurs because the macular area has a large representation in the most posterior one-third of the calcarine cortex and is the area nearest the occipital pole. This area, then, is best situated to receive some leptomeningeal anastomotic blood supply from the middle cerebral artery.

In vascular insufficiency or occlusion of the basilar artery infarction may occur in the distribution of both posterior cerebral arteries, producing a bilateral homonymous hemianopsia and a syndrome of "cortical blindness." Such patients show a loss of all visual sensation but have a preservation of pupillary constriction in response to light.

Areas 18 and 19: Ablation. These areas have often been referred to as visual association areas, and it has been stated that lesions of these areas have produced deficits in visual associations. This would include, for example, defects in visual recognition and reading. The problem of analysis in man relates to the fact that in a unilateral lesion, one is almost never dealing with disease limited to areas 18 and 19. Rather one finds that either adjacent portions of the inferior par-

ietal lobule (angular and supramarginal gyri) are involved or that the lesion extends into the deeper white matter of the lateral occipital area involving association and callosal fibers. Such more extensive lesions will of course produce the deficits previously noted in the discussion of parietal function. A limited unilateral ablation might produce defects in visual following, as tested by means of opticokinetic nystagmus. (The nystagmus generated in following moving vertical black lines on a white background or the moving train-telephone pole situation.)

Bilateral lesions limited to areas 18 and 19 have not occurred through the process of disease in man. Although Lashley (as discussed in the more recent paper of Mishkin) failed to find evidence for deficits in visual discrimination in monkeys, the effects in man might be quite different. Such a lesion would deprive the speech areas of the dominant hemispheres of all visual information. The patient would presumably see objects but be unable to recognize them or to place these visual sensations into the context of previous experience. He would be, moreover, unable to relate these visual stimuli to tactile and auditory stimuli.

The following case history will return our discussion to the former ground of clinical reality since it illustrates some of the more common symptoms of focal disease involving the occipital lobe.

Case History 6. NECH #191–262. Dates of admission: 12/3/67–12/23/67; 1/3/66–2/17/68.

This 47-year-old white, right-handed, real estate salesman (Mr. A.T.) was referred for evaluation of headache and visual disturbance. One month prior to admission the patient had a cough with some blood present in the sputum (hemoptysis). Five days prior to admission the patient developed a generalized headache which would awaken him from sleep and which would be precipitated by coughing or straining. Two days prior to admission, the patient noted blurring in the left inferior quadrant of his field of vision. The day prior to admission, he noted complete loss of vision in this quadrant. On the day of admission, headache increased and the patient was unable to see anything in the left visual field. The patient had experienced no weakness, no disturbance of memory, and no language disturbance.

Past History was significant. The patient

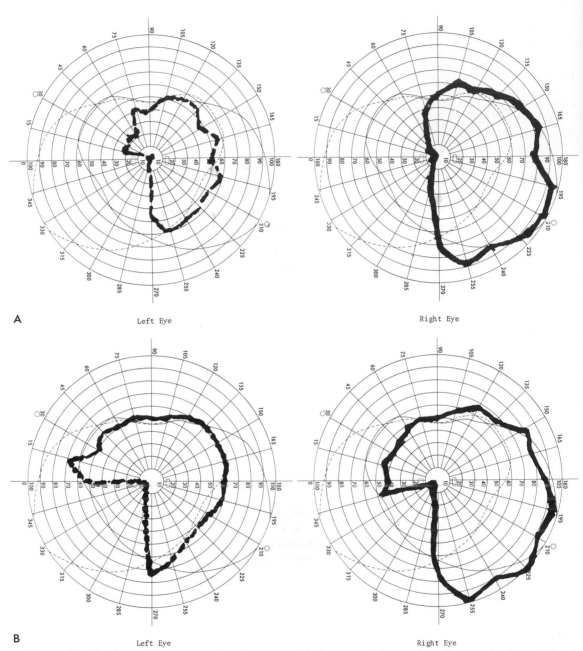

A

Left Eye

Right Eye

B

Left Eye

Right Eye

Figure 21–17 Case History 6. Brain abscess, occipital area. (Right) Perimetric examination of visual fields.

A, Fields on 12/6/67, demonstrating a left homonymous hemianopsia which is somewhat asymmetrical (termed incongruous). The defect being less in the left eye than the right. The fields are shown from the patient's point of view.

B, Fields on 12/22/67: with antibiotic therapy, an improvement had occurred. An incongruous, quadrantanopsia was now suggested as opposed to the previous defect which was more of a complete homonymous hemianopsia.

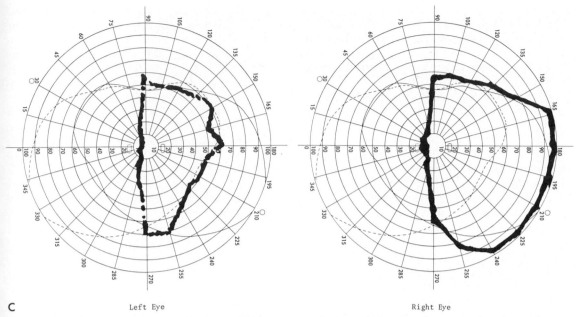

C

Left Eye   Right Eye

Figure 21–17 Continued. C, Fields on 2/15/68: a relatively complete homonymous hemianopsia was present at the time of hospital readmission when abscess had progressed. This same deficit persisted following surgery as shown above. Note that to a certain extent macular sparing is present.

had multiple pulmonary infections, treated with antibiotics in the past.

NEUROLOGICAL EXAMINATION:

1. Blood pressure 110/60. Pulse 68. Temperature 99° (F.) orally.

2. Mental status and language function, including reading and writing, were intact.

3. *Cranial nerves* were intact except for:
   a. Funduscopic examination: blurring of disc margins was present bilaterally with venous engorgement indicating early papilledema.
   b. A left homonymous hemianopsia was present (Fig. 21–17*A*).

4. *Motor system:*
   a. Strength and gait were intact.
   b. Cerebellar tests were normal.

5. *Reflexes:*
   a. Deep tendon: a minimal asymmetry was present with a slight increase on the left compared to the right.
   b. Plantar responses. On the right side, the response was flexor; on the left, possibly extensor.

6. *Sensation:* No deficits were present as regards pain, touch, position, vibration, left and right simultaneous stimulation, and point localization.

LABORATORY DATA:

1. Skull x-rays were normal.

2. Chest x-rays revealed resolving pneumonitis in the right costophrenic angle.

3. Sinus x-rays indicated a possible inflammation (sinusitis) of right frontal sinus (opacification without definite fluid level).

4. Electroencephalogram: The record was abnormal because of frequent focal 3 to 4 cps, slow waves in the right occipital area and to a lesser degree, in the right posterior parietal area. Consistent with focal damage in the right occipital area (Fig. 21–18*A*).

5. Right brachial arteriogram was normal.

6. Cerebrospinal fluid:
   a. Pressure was elevated to 210 mm.
   b. Number of white blood cells was increased 97 lymphocytes.
   c. Protein was increased to 75 mg./100 ml. (upper limit of normal is 45 mg./100 ml.)
   d. Glucose was 75 mg./100 ml. (normal when compared to blood sugar of 95 mg./100 ml.)

7. Brain scan: on December 4, 1967 this study was normal. On December 6, 1967 there was a diffuse uptake in the posterior and medial aspect of the right hemisphere (occipital and adjacent parietal).

SUBSEQUENT COURSE:

The patient was treated with antibiotics (Keflin, penicillin, and streptomycin) with an improvement in visual fields, EEG, and spinal fluid findings. By the time of discharge on December 23, 1967 the field defect had resolved to an incongruous (not entirely homonymous) left inferior quadrantanopsia (Fig. 21–17B).

The patient was readmitted to the hospital on January 3, 1968 with a three day history of right eye pain, sweats, and chills. Neurological examination now revealed a recurrence of blurred optic disc margins, a left homonymous hemianopsia, and a slight increase in deep tendon reflexes on the left. The electroencephalogram showed an increase in focal slow wave activity in the right occipital area indicating increasing damage (Fig. 21–18C). The brain scan now indicated a well-defined focal uptake of isotope in the right occipital region extending to the occipital pole and measuring 6 × 4 × 5 cm., consistent with an abscess (Fig. 21–19). Pneumoencephalogram now revealed a large space-occupying lesion in the right parietal occipital region, displacing the right lateral ventricle forward and downward. Following treatment with antibiotics (penicillin and streptomycin) a craniotomy was performed on January 12, 1968 by Dr. Bertram Selverstone. A mass could be palpated medially in the right occipital and adjacent posterior parietal area. A collection of approximately 15 cc. of purulent material was found at 1.5 cm. below the surface in a multiloculated thin-walled abscess which extended along the medial aspect of the hemisphere to the occipital pole. The abscess and a large surrounding area of hard granulomatous cortex and white matter were removed. (The etiologic organism was subsequently found to be streptococcus: microaerophilic.)

Postoperatively, the patient continued on treatment with penicillin. Neurological examination was intact except for the left homonymous hemianopsia (Fig. 21–17C). This deficit was still present at the time of follow-up evaluation 6 months following surgery.

COMMENT:

The rapid evolution of neurological signs and symptoms in this case accompanied by the early development of papilledema and by progressive changes in electroencephalogram and brain scan is consistent with the diagnosis of brain abscess. The primary infection in this case was probably in the lung. The initial visual symptoms of inferior field involvement (quadrantanopsia) suggested that the abscess in its early stages involved predominantly the superior portion of the optic radiation in the posterior parietal-occipital area or the superior bank of the calcarine fissure. With progression of the lesion, the entire optic radiation or the entire calcarine cortex was involved by the lesion. The lesion found at surgery does not allow a differentiation of the terminal portion of optic radiation or calcarine cortex since the lesion destroyed or damaged both these areas.

The treatment of a brain abscess requires not only surgical drainage and removal of the abscess but also the adequate pre- and postoperative use of antibiotics.

Although this patient has not yet developed focal seizures, many of these patients do develop this problem at some time after successful surgical treatment of the abscess. Prophylactic anticonvulsant medication is therefore routinely administered. This patient received diphenylhydantoin (Dilantin).

It is important to note in this case, as a negative finding, that at no time did the patient experience any language disturbance. Reading and writing remained intact as did capacity for construction of drawings. This case involving the right occipital lobe should be compared to case 10 on page 531 in which a focal lesion of the left occipital lobe was present.

TEMPORAL LOBE

In considering the functions of the temporal lobe and the effects of disease involving the temporal lobe, one must first consider that the temporal lobe has several structural, phylogenetic, and functional subdivisions. Thus one may distinguish the archicortex of the hippocampal formation and the dentate gyrus, the paleocortex of the anterior parahippocampal gyrus, the transitional mesocortex bordering this area, and finally the neocortex which occupies all of the lateral surface and the more lateral portions of the inferior temporal areas. The non-neocortical subdivisions are also parts of the rhinencephalon or limbic system. The structure and connections of these areas will be considered in greater detail in a separate section on the rhinencephalon.

It must, however, be indicated that these areas have significant anatomical connections with the amygdaloid complex, the

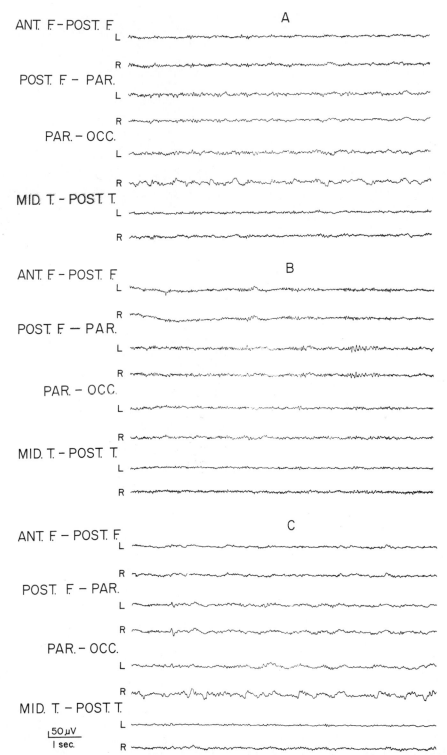

Figure 21-18 Case History 6. Brain abscess, right occipital, electroencephalograms. (Bipolar) ANT. F. = anterior parasagittal frontal; POST. F. = posterior parasagittal frontal; PAR. = parietal parasagittal; OCC. = occipital; MID. T. = midtemporal; POST. T. = posterior temporal.

A, Record of 12/4/67, shortly after admission, demonstrating focal 3–4 cps slow waves in right occipital area and to lesser degree right parietal area.

B, Record of 12/15/67: following treatment with antibiotics, significant improvement occurred. Only a minor degree of abnormality is now present in the right occipital area.

C, Record of 1/3/68, with progression of the abscess, a recurrence of focal 2–3 cps slow wave activity in right occipital area is noted.

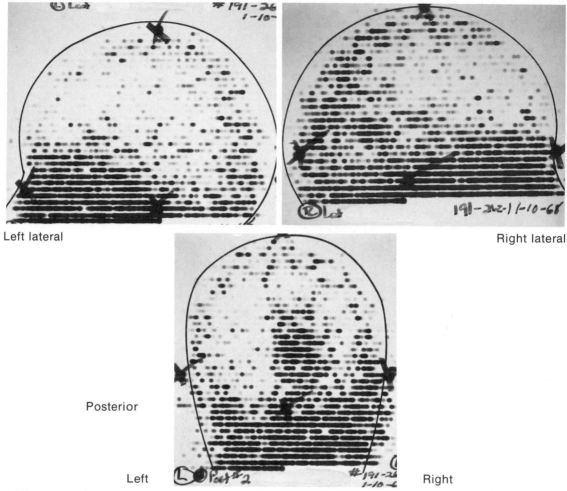

Left lateral

Right lateral

Posterior

Left   Right

Figure 21–19 Brain Scan, Case History 6. Brain abscess, right occipital. A large, well-defined uptake of radioisotope is present in the right occipital area and right posterior-inferior temporal area. This is demonstrated in both the posterior and lateral scans. (Courtesy of Dr. Bertram Selverstone.)

septal nuclei, the preoptic area, the hypothalamus, the anterior thalamic nuclei, and the midbrain tegmental nuclei. These rhinencephalic or limbic areas then have a significant role in emotion, autonomic and visceral function, motivation, and instinctive behavior. On the other hand, these rhinencephalic structures have significant connection with the neocortex of the lateral and inferior temporal areas and of the orbital-prefrontal areas. The rhinencephalon, then, is in a position to provide transmission for these neocortical higher association areas and for complex sensory perceptions which have been processed at the neocortical level, to the diencephalic and midbrain areas involved in more primitive

visceral, autonomic, emotional, and instinctive motor activities (Fig. 18–7).

As regards the neocortical areas, area 41, the primary auditory projection area, is located on the more anterior of the transverse gyri of Heschl (Fig. 21–20). This area is granular (konio) cortex similar to but considerably thicker than areas 17 and 3. Area 41 receives the main projection from the medial geniculate nucleus of the thalamus. Within this projection area there is a tonotopic representation, with the lowest frequencies, projecting to the more rostral area (in monkey and chimpanzee).

The remaining neocortical areas of the temporal lobe, from a cytoarchitectural standpoint, are homotypical. Area 42 surrounds area 41 and receives association fibers from this area. Area 22, in turn, surrounds area 42 and communicates with areas 41 and 42. Both areas 42 and 22 are often designated as auditory association areas. In the dominant hemisphere these auditory association areas are of importance in the understanding of the spoken word. The role of the other lateral temporal neocortical areas may best be considered in terms of disease processes. The inferior temporal areas have significant connections with area 18 providing a pathway by which visual perceptions, processed at the cortical level, may be then related to the limbic areas.

When one comes to consider disease processes affecting the temporal lobe it is evident that the symptoms and signs do not follow the precise subdivisions that have been outlined above. There are several reasons for this: (1) The basic lesion (e.g., a glioma) often involves both neocortical and non-neocortical areas of the temporal lobe. (2) The threshold of the hippocampus for seizure discharge is relatively low, that of the neocortical areas on the lateral surface is relatively high. Since connections from the lateral temporal and inferior temporal area to the hippocampus exist, seizure discharges beginning in the lateral temporal neocortex will often activate discharge in the hippocampus. (3) Lesions in the more posterior temporal areas often involve the adjacent posterior parietal areas, that is, the inferior parietal lobule. In contrast anteriorly placed lesions of the temporal lobe often involve the adjacent inferior frontal gyrus. Lesions spreading into the deeper white matter of the temporal lobe (particularly in its middle and posterior thirds) will involve part or all of the optic radiation.

Temporal Lobe: Stimulation. Seizures involving the temporal lobe produce a variety of symptoms: (a) auditory sensation, (b)

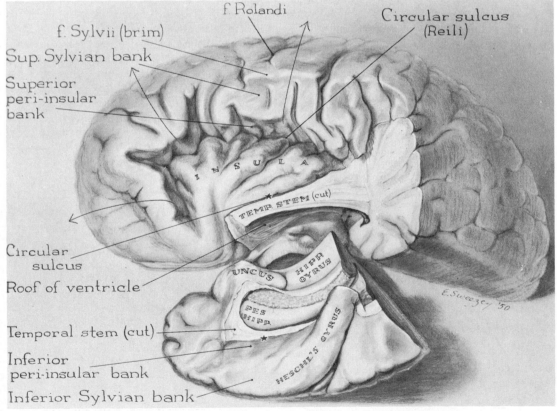

Figure 21–20 The superior and medial surfaces of the temporal lobe. The transverse gyrus of Heschl and the relationships of the temporal lobe to the gyri of the other structures surrounding the Sylvian fissure are demonstrated. The temporal stem refers to the core of white matter relating the temporal lobe to the remainder of the cerebral hemisphere. (From Penfield, W., and Jasper, H.: *Epilepsy and the Functional Anatomy of the Human Brain.* Boston, Little, Brown and Company, 1954, p. 52.)

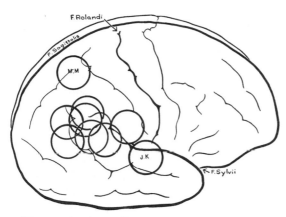

Figure 21-21 Effects of focal discharge in superior temporal gyrus. The location of the discharging lesion at surgery in nine patients with focal seizures beginning with a sensation of vertigo is demonstrated to be primarily superior temporal gyrus. (From Penfield, W., and Kristiansen, K.: *Epileptic Seizure Patterns.* Springfield, Ill., Charles C Thomas, 1951, p. 49.)

vestibular sensation, (c) alterations in perception, (d) fear, (e) hallucinations in the auditory, visual, or olfactory spheres, (f) arrest of speech, (g) repetitive movements of a complex type—automatisms, (h) complex emotional behavior, and (i) confusion with defects in memory recording. Keeping in mind the reservations listed above concerning strict localization, it is possible to make certain anatomical correlations based on the studies of Penfield (Penfield and Perot, 1963).

Crude auditory sensation. Tinnitus (a tone, buzzing, or knocking) is best produced by stimulation of the primary auditory projection area, the anterior transverse gyrus (Fig. 21-20). At times an auditory sensation will be produced from the adjacent superior temporal gyrus, but this is considered to represent an alteration in the interpretation of sound rather than an actual auditory sensation.

Vestibular sensations (vertigo, dizziness) are at times produced by stimulation in the superior temporal gyrus adjacent to the auditory cortex (Fig. 21-21).

Arrest of speech is produced by stimulation in the dominant hemisphere of area 22 of the superior and adjacent middle temporal gyri (Wernicke's receptive aphasia area). In addition, arrest of speech also occurs on stimulation of the posterior temporal region which extends into the angular and supramarginal inferior parietal areas of the dominant hemisphere. As we have previously indicated, arrest of speech is not specific for these areas, since such arrest of speech also occurs on stimulation of "Broca's area" (the inferior frontal gyrus) and of the supplementary motor areas of the dominant hemisphere (Fig. 21-22).

Alterations in perception (illusions) are produced by stimulation of the lateral temporal surface in patients already subject to temporal lobe seizures. Penfield has referred to the nonspeech areas of the lateral temporal

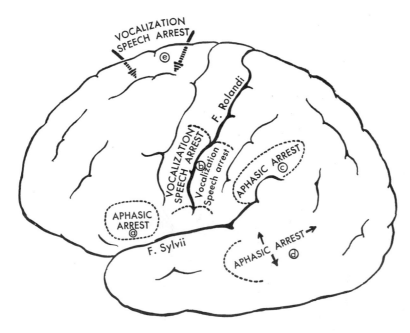

Figure 21-22 Arrest of speech on stimulation of dominant hemisphere at surgery. The following cortical areas are indicated: (a) Broca's areas 44 and 45 of inferior frontal gyrus; (b) Rolandic motor and sensory areas related to face, lips, and tongue; (c) inferior parietal cortex—angular and supramarginal gyri; (d) posterior temporal lobe; (e) supplementary motor cortex. See Figure 21-26. (From Penfield, W., and Rasmussen, T.: *The Cerebral Cortex of Man.* New York, The Macmillan Company, 1955, p. 107.)

surface as the interpretive cortex and to the illusions as interpretive illusions. Several types may occur during seizure discharges originating from the temporal lobe or during stimulation at the time of surgery (Fig. 21–23). *Auditory illusions* (sounds seem louder, fainter, more distant, or nearer) occur on stimulation of the superior temporal gyrus in either hemisphere. *Visual illusions* (objects are nearer, farther, larger, smaller) occur predominantly on stimulation in the nondominant temporal lobe. *Illusions of recognition* [present experience seems familiar (referred to as deja vu), or strange, unreal, and dreamlike] occur predominantly in relation to stimulation of the nondominant temporal lobe. Emotional illusions (feeling of fear, loneliness, or sorrow) may occur on stimulation of either temporal lobe.

Hallucinations of previous experiences (experiential responses of Penfield) occur on stimulation of the lateral temporal surface in some patients who are already subject to temporal lobe seizures. These hallucinations, which may also occur spontaneously during temporal lobe seizures, are of several types. *Auditory hallucinations* (a familiar voice or voices, familiar music) occur predominantly in relation to stimulation of the superior temporal gyrus of either hemisphere. *Visual hallucinations* (a familiar street scene, familiar people such as mother, father, doctor, nurse) occur predominantly but not exclusively in relation to stimulation of the lateral surface of the nondominant temporal lobe.

The visual responses may be produced from the posterior temporal areas (and adjacent inferior parietal areas) as well as from the superior and middle temporal gyri (Fig. 21–24). Usually both the auditory and visual hallucinations are identified by the patient as recollections of familiar past experiences.

In interpreting this data, a certain degree of caution is essential. One should not jump to the conclusion that specific memory traces are localized to the specific areas stimulated during surgery. Certain points should be kept in mind: (1) The memory remains after ablation of the area which has been stimulated. (2) Moreover, these experiential responses are not obtained on stimulation of the "normal" temporal lobe during surgery directed at disease in other cortical areas; they are obtained only in patients who already have disease of the temporal lobe. (3) Although some of the patients with temporal lobe seizures have disease involving the neocortex on the lateral surface, others have pathology involving the mesial temporal areas, that is, the hippocampus and parahippocampal gyri.

The following components of seizures originating in the temporal lobe have been related to the mesial non-neocortical areas of the temporal lobe rather than to the lateral neocortical surface:

a. *Olfactory hallucinations* are relatively common during temporal lobe seizures particularly where such seizures are secondary to a tumor (glioma usually) of the temporal

INTERPRETIVE ILLUSIONS

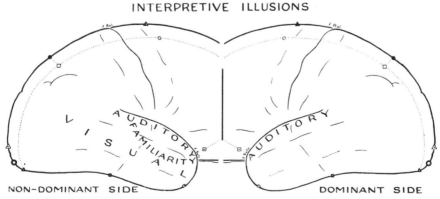

NON-DOMINANT SIDE　　　DOMINANT SIDE

Figure 21–23 Interpretive illusions (disturbances of perception) produced by stimulation at surgery of temporal lobe cortex in patients with temporal lobe seizures. Visual illusions were produced predominantly in the minor (that is, nondominant) hemisphere. Auditory illusions were produced on both sides chiefly in the superior temporal gyrus. Illusions of familiarity (deja vu) were produced predominantly from the nondominant hemisphere. Sensations of fear, unreality, loneliness, or of detachment were produced from stimulation in either temporal region. (From Penfield, W., and Perot, P.: Brain, *86*: 599, 1963. After Mullan and Penfield: Archives of Neurology Psychiatry, *81*:269, 1959, p. 269.)

EXPERIENTIAL RESPONSES

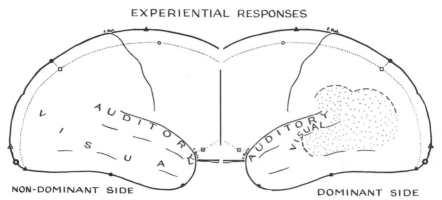

Figure 21-24 Experiential responses (hallucinations) to stimulation at surgery of temporal lobe and adjacent inferior parietal area in patients with temporal lobe seizures. Auditory responses occur from stimulation in either dominant or nondominant hemisphere, (primarily superior temporal gyri). Visual responses occur primarily from stimulation of the nondominant hemisphere. The posterior speech area of the dominant hemisphere is indicated by the stippled area within the interrupted lines. No experiential responses occur on stimulation of this speech area in the dominant hemisphere. (From Penfield, W., and Perot, P., Brain, *86*:676, 1963.)

lobe. The olfactory hallucination is usually termed an unpleasant odor: rarely does the patient identify the odor as familiar. Rarely, during surgery, are these olfactory hallucinations produced by direct stimulation in or near the cortex of the uncus.

b. *Automatisms* (repetitive complex movements, e.g., repetitive rubbing of an ear, repetitive chewing, repetitive smoothing of the bed sheet or of clothing) are considered to represent spread of discharge into the amygdaloid-hippocampal zone. The automatisms are invariably accompanied by some degree of confusion; the patient is amnesic for the events. These automatisms are often modified by or appropriate to a specific stimulus which has been introduced into the environment. Thus the patient may continue certain actions that he was performing at the onset of the seizure but in an imperfect repetitive manner. If an object touches the back of the neck or ear, the patient may brush this away repetitively. If attempts are made to restrain the patient, he may resist, assault those restraining him, ·or attempt to flee. There is at times a strong emotional flavor to many of the automatisms. At times, these represent emotional gestures accompanied by laughter, crying, anger, and the like.

c. *Confusion with amnesia* reflects the interference effect of hippocampal stimulation on the capacity for recording new memories. During this time, relatively complex but familiar behavior, such as the driving of an automobile, may be continued. The problem

of memory recording will be discussed at greater length in a separate section. For perhaps the best illustration of the phenomenon the reader is referred to the original case reports of Hughlings Jackson concerning "dreamy states" in which a physician, subject to temporal lobe seizures, was able to perform a relatively complete physical examination and to begin appropriate treatment during such an episode (Taylor, 1958).

In general as we have indicated there is a mixture of symptomatology during a temporal lobe seizure. The following case history illustrates many of the points just discussed.

Case History 7. NECH #186–890.
Dates of admission: 5/11/67–6/6/67; 8/3/67–8/16/67.

This 56-year-old, white right-handed, male baker (Mr. A.S.) was referred for evaluation of a seizure disorder. In February 1967, the patient had the onset of episodes of vertigo and tinnitus, each episode lasting 4 minutes and unrelated to position. The patient then noted increasing forgetfulness and later in February developed a generalized convulsive seizure that occurred without any warning. The patient then developed episodes of confusion and unresponsiveness, followed by the development of a left frontal headache. Various studies—EEG, pneumoencephalogram, and carotid arteriogram—were all negative at this time. In April 1967, minor episodes began, characterized by lip smacking and a vertiginous sensation.

During these episodes the patient was able to report that he had seen various well-formed colorful scenes. At times he had visions of "loaves of bread being laid out on the wall." In addition to these visual hallucinations the patient, at times in relation to these minor episodes, would have a disturbance of perception—objects would appear larger than normal. The patient also reported at this time that he had associated "terrifying dreams."

General physical examination: not remarkable.

NEUROLOGICAL EXAMINATION:

The patient was observed to have frequent transient episodes of distress characterized by saying, "oh, oh, oh my." On occasion these were accompanied by automatisms: fluttering of the eyelids, smacking of the lips, and repetitive picking at the bed clothes with his right hand. Consciousness was not completely impaired during these episodes which lasted from 30 seconds to 3 minutes and the patient was able to report afterwards having seen "loaves of bread on the wall" and at times of having had an "unpleasant odor" which was poorly described. At times the olfactory hallucination was described as pleasant resembling the odor of baked bread.

1. *Mental status:*
   a. The patient was oriented to person but not to dates.
   b. He could not recall his street address.
   c. He was unable to pronounce the name of the hospital correctly.
   d. Calculations were correctly performed.
2. *Cranial nerves:*
   a. There was a suggestion of a deficit in the periphery of the right visual field.
   b. There was a minor right central facial weakness.
3. *Motor system:*
   a. No weakness was present.
   b. Gait was normal.
4. *Reflexes:*
   a. Deep tendon reflexes were symmetrical and physiologic.
   b. Plantar responses: A right Babinski response was present.
5. *Sensation:* All modalities were intact.

LABORATORY DATA:

1. *Skull and chest x-rays:* Negative
2. *Electroencephalogram:* The recording of May 12, 1967, indicated a frequent focal spike discharge throughout the left temporal and parietal areas, consistent with a focal seizure disorder originating in the left temporal parietal areas (Fig. 21–25).

The recording of May 18, 1967 indicated a decrease of focal spikes (i.e., a decrease in seizure activity) but the presence now of frequent focal slow wave activity in the left temporal area (almost continuous 3 to 5 cps slow wave activity) suggesting that focal damage was also present in the left temporal area.

3. *Brain scan* (Hg^{197}): Normal
4. *Left carotid arteriogram:* This study suggested an avascular space-occupying lesion in the left posterior frontal area. (The only abnormality was a 4 mm. shift of the anterior cerebral artery to the right.)

SUBSEQUENT COURSE:

The patient continued to have multiple short episodes characterized by the sensation of odor and a sensation that he was looking at objects upon the wall. These episodes were eventually controlled with anticonvulsant medication: diphenylhydantoin (Dilantin) and primidone (Mysoline). However, in July 1967 the patient had a day in which he had many episodes during which he noted "crazy things," i.e., colorful visions and terrifying nightmares.

The patient was readmitted to the hospital in August 1967. On the day of admission he had a seizure characterized by an aura of unpleasant odor followed by a generalized convulsive seizure. He then had 4 or 5 subsequent seizures of a somewhat different character. These were characterized by deviation of the head and eyes to the right, then tonic and clonic movements of the right hand spreading to the arm, foot, and leg and lasting approximately 1 to 2 minutes, followed by a postictal right hemiparesis.

Neurological examination now indicated a marked expressive aphasia with little spontaneous speech. The patient had marked difficulty in naming objects. There was a dense right homonymous hemianopsia, a flattening of the right nasolabial fold and a right hemiparesis with a right Babinski response. During a 2-week hospital period the patient continued to have minor seizures characterized by sensory phenomena on the right side of the body. A moderate degree of expressive aphasia persisted throughout the 2-week hospital course, although the right homonymous hemianopsia in large part disappeared. The symptoms and findings suggested that the basic disease process may well have spread to involve the adjacent

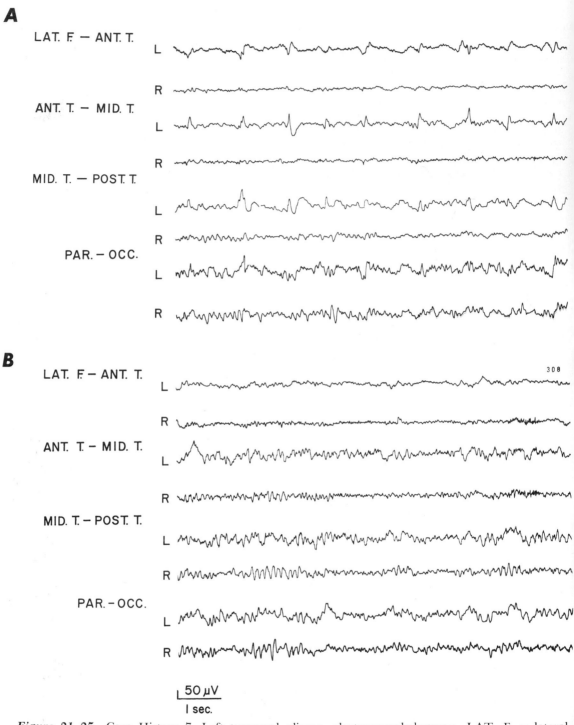

A

LAT. F. — ANT. T.

ANT. T. — MID. T.

MID. T. — POST. T.

PAR. — OCC.

B

LAT. F. — ANT. T.

ANT. T. — MID. T.

MID. T. — POST. T.

PAR. — OCC.

50 µV
I sec.

Figure 21–25 Case History 7. Left temporal glioma, electroencephalograms. LAT. F. = lateral frontal; ANT. T. = anterior temporal; MID. T. = midtemporal; POST. T. = posterior temporal; PAR. = parietal; OCC. = occipital.

A, Bipolar recording of May 12, 1967, demonstrating frequent focal discharge of blunt spikes in the left temporal area.

B, Bipolar recording of May 18, 1967, demonstrating focal 2–5 cps slow wave activity in left temporal and parietal areas.

areas across the Sylvian fissure, the speech areas of the inferior frontal convolution; the premotor areas; and the sensory motor cortex.

The patient developed increasing expressive aphasia and right hemiparesis, with increasingly severe headache. Arteriogram now indicated a large space-occupying tumor of the left temporal lobe (Fig. 21–26) and surgery was undertaken on June 5, 1968 by Dr. Robert Yuan. The anterior and middle portions of the superior temporal gyrus were widened, and the anterior temporal area (the temporal tip) had an abnormal and discolored appearance. At a depth of 1 to 2 cm. within the superior temporal gyrus, obvious necrotic glial tissue was found involving all of the deeper temporal areas. The process had extended superficially under the Sylvian fissure to involve the adjacent posterior portion of the inferior frontal gyrus. A temporal lobectomy was performed (from the anterior temporal pole posteriorly for a distance of 6 cm.). The operative impression of a ma-

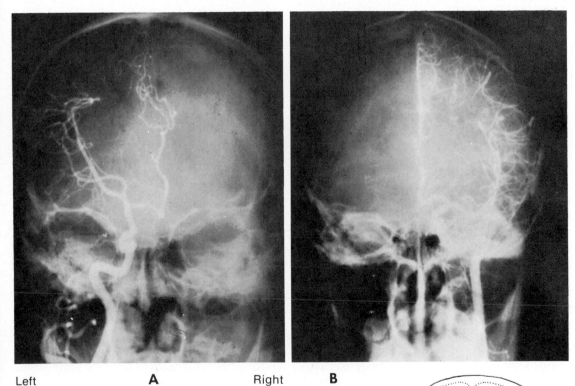

Left   **A**   Right   **B**

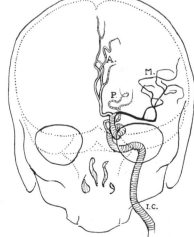

Figure 21–26 Temporal lobe tumor: angiographic appearance. *A*, A relatively avascular mass in the temporal lobe has elevated and displaced medially the middle cerebral artery. The anterior cerebral artery has also been displaced across the midline. *B*, Normal carotid arteriogram for comparison. (Courtesy of Dr. John Hills and Dr. Samuel Wolpert.) *C*, Diagram of normal carotid arteriogram. (From Ranson, S. W., and Clark, S. C.: *The Anatomy of the Nervous System.* Philadelphia, W. B. Saunders, 1959, p. 87.)

C

lignant glial tumor (glioblastoma) was confirmed by histological examination.

COMMENT:

This patient presented, at one time or another during his seizures, most of the phenomena associated with temporal lobe seizures: vertigo, tinnitus, visual perceptual distortions, visual hallucinations, olfactory hallucination, fear, automatisms involving the lips and hands, and episodes of confusion. The visual and olfactory hallucinations are of interest in that both reflected the patient's occupation (experience) as a baker. The later progression clearly indicated spread of the process across the Sylvian fissure to involve the motor association areas. This patient had a highly malignant tumor which clearly involved both the cortex of the lateral surface, the deeper white matter, and presumably the medial temporal areas including the amygdaloid-hippocampal regions. His clinical picture is highly reminiscent of the original case described in 1887 by Hughlings Jackson of Emily M., a cook who experienced visual and olfactory hallucinations and who had a tumor arising in the "temporal-sphenoidal lobe," (the uncus). Such seizures have subsequently been referred to as *uncinate epilepsy.* As we have indicated, the disease invariably involves more than just the uncus.

Temporal Lobe: Ablation. From a clinical standpoint, unilateral lesions limited to the auditory projection area in the temporal lobe do not cause any significant alteration in hearing. This is consistent with the fact that multiple decussations occur in the auditory pathway at a brain stem level so that each auditory projection area receives impulses from both left and right cochlea. The studies of Penfield and Evans have suggested that unilateral temporal lobe ablation may produce a disturbance in the ability to locate a source of sound to the left or right of the midline. Bilateral lesions of the auditory projection, from a theoretical standpoint, would result in "cortical deafness." Such limited bilateral lesions are unlikely, but bilateral destruction of these areas would of course occur with more extensive bilateral cortical lesions.

Lesions which deprive the receptive aphasia area of Wernicke in the dominant temporal lobe (area 22) of information from the auditory projection areas of the right and left hemispheres would result in a syndrome of pure word deafness. Such a patient would hear sounds and words but would be unable to relate these sounds to previous sound associations. As indicated by Geschwind such a lesion would have to destroy the primary auditory projection area of the dominant hemisphere or the thalamic projection to that area in addition to the callosal radiation from the temporal lobe of the nondominant hemisphere. In some cases the same effect would be achieved by bilateral lesions. A more common symptom picture is that which results from destruction of area 22 in the dominant hemisphere (Wernicke's receptive aphasia). Such a patient not only has difficulty in interpreting words which he hears but also, in a sense, has lost his ability to make use of previous auditory associations. The patient, then, also has difficulty in using his own speech. His verbalizations often resemble nonsense words and make little sense to listeners.

Unilateral lesions of the temporal lobe which involve the subcortical white matter often produce damage to the geniculocalcarine radiations. Since the most inferior fibers of the radiation often are the first to be involved, the initial field defect may be a contralateral superior field quadrantanopsia. As the lesion moves towards the inferior parietal area, the entire radiation may be involved, producing a homonymous hemianopsia in the contralateral field.

Bilateral ablation of the temporal lobes of the monkey in the studies of Kluver and Bucy (1939) produced a preparation characterized by a release of oral automatisms—a tendency to mouth and touch all visible objects. The animal showed marked deficits in visual discriminations, particularly in regard to visual stimuli related to various motivations. Thus, objects which would normally evoke fear in the monkey no longer did so. Sexual behavior was no longer released only in heterosexual situations. Rather, a marked increase in all types of sexual activity occurred. Various food objects, usually rejected, were now eaten. The original ablations of Kluver and Bucy had involved all of the temporal lobe, including the neocortex, hippocampus, and amygdala. More recent studies summarized by Mishkin have suggested that much of the impairment of visual discrimination in these situations may be attributed to damage to the inferior temporal areas (inferior and middle temporal gyri). Such damage would serve to disconnect the visual association areas from the hippocampal areas, producing what has been described by Geschwind (1965) as the visual-limbic disconnection syndrome.

In man, bilateral temporal lobectomy has been performed on rare occasions for relief of temporal lobe seizures. The most striking effects of bilateral temporal lobectomy relate to the marked impairment in the ability to learn new associations, that is, an inability to establish new memories at a time when remote memory is well preserved. A similar syndrome may be seen when unilateral temporal lobectomy is performed in a patient with already existing disease in the contralateral temporal lobe. This syndrome relates primarily to hippocampal damage and may be found in situations where the damage has been relatively restricted to hippocampal areas with relative preservation of neocortical areas of the temporal lobe, e.g., hypoglycemia and anoxia. This syndrome of impairment of recent memory (the Wernicke-Korsakov syndrome) will be discussed in greater detail in the section on learning and memory.

Another aspect of temporal lobe dysfunction is apparent in patients with seizures originating in the temporal lobes, as opposed to patients with focal seizures originating in other cortical areas or patients with nonfocal seizure disorders. These patients have a high incidence of psychiatric disturbance often expressed as a severe personality disorder or, somewhat less often, as an actual psychosis. The psychiatric disturbance is apparent in periods between seizures (the interictal period) and is often most severe during periods when the seizure disorder is well under control. At times in low-grade tumors of the temporal lobe, certain long-standing disturbances of personality may be reported by relatives of the patient. The occurrence of such psychiatric disturbances should not be surprising when one considers the role of the limbic system in emotion and motivation and the role of the temporal lobe in relating various environmental stimuli to motivational systems.

SPEECH, LANGUAGE, AND CEREBRAL DOMINANCE

In the preceding sections, we have alluded to various areas in the dominant hemisphere concerned with speech and language. The reader may well have been confused by the introduction of such terms as aphasia, apraxia, agnosia, and dyslexia. It is well to warn the student beginning the study of language function that this is indeed an area of much confusion, with much disagreement and multiple hypotheses. Some of these hypotheses have a solid anatomical base, others do not. This discussion will be limited to the more practical problems of anatomical localization.

We should indicate at the onset that we are not concerned here with the problem of dysarthria. *Dysarthria* refers to a difficulty in articulation of speech from weakness or paralysis or from mechanical difficulties. Dysarthria may have many causes at many levels of the peripheral or central nervous system:

a. Local disease of the larynx, tongue, or lips, e. g., laryngeal carcinoma.

b. Disease of the muscles affecting the tongue and the lips of pharynx, e. g., oculopharyngeal dystrophy.

c. Disease affecting the neuromuscular junction in the muscles of the tongue, lips, and pharynx, e.g., myasthenia gravis.

d. Disease affecting the peripheral nerve supply of the tongue, lips, or pharynx, e.g., compression of hypoglossal nerve during carotid artery surgery, compression of the recurrent laryngeal nerve during thyroid surgery.

e. Disease of the brain stem motor nuclei, e.g., a lateral medullary infarction producing destruction of the nucleus ambiguus, or amyotrophic lateral sclerosis involving the motor neurons (so called progressive bulbar palsy), or bulbar poliomyelitis which also involves these same motor neurons.

f. Bilateral damage to the corticobulbar fibers descending to the brain stem motor nuclei, producing a pseudobulbar palsy. This damage may occur at the cortical level, at the capsular level, or at the midbrain level.

There are, however, more complex disturbances of language function, as regards verbal expression, that occur at a time when the basic motor and sensory systems for articulation are intact. Similarly there are complex disturbances in language function, as regards comprehension of written and spoken symbolic forms, that occur at a time when the basic auditory and visual receptor apparatus is intact. We refer collectively to these more complex disturbances of language function as *aphasias or dysphasias*. In general, it is possible to relate these language disturbances to disease of the dominant cerebral hemisphere, involving the cerebral cortex or cortical association fiber systems.

CEREBRAL DOMINANCE

It is perhaps appropriate at this point to consider the question of cerebral dominance. Most individuals are right handed (93 per cent of the adult population), and such individuals almost always are left-hemisphere dominant. A minority of individuals (some on a hereditary basis) are left-hand dominant: some of these are right-hemisphere dominant but a certain proportion are left-hemisphere dominant. It has been estimated that 96 per cent of the adult population are left-hemisphere dominant for speech.

One might inquire as to why the majority of humans are right handed. Although hand preference does not become apparent until one year of age, the studies of Yakolev and Rakic would suggest that there is even before this age an underlying anatomical basis for the dominance of the right hand. In the study of the medullae and spinal cords of a large number of human fetuses and neonates, the fibers of the left pyramid were found to cross to the right side of the spinal cord at a higher level in the decussation than fibers of the right pyramid. Moreover, more fibers of the left pyramid crossed to the right side of the spinal cord than vice versa. Although the majority of pyramidal fibers decussated, a minority of fibers remained uncrossed. It was more common for fibers from the left pyramid to decussate completely to the right side of the spinal cord. The minority of fibers which remained uncrossed were more often those descending from the right pyramid into the right side of the spinal cord. The end result, in the cervical region at least, was for the right side of the spinal cord and presumably the anterior horn cells of the right side of the cervical cord to receive the greater corticospinal innervation. There is then an anatomical basis for the preference or dominance of the right hand. Since the majority of fibers supplying the right cervical area have originated in the left hemisphere, on this basis alone one could refer to the dominance of the left hemisphere.

The recent studies of Geschwind and Levitsky suggest that an actual anatomical asymmetry may be found in the adult brain between the two hemispheres in an area significant for language function. That area of the auditory association cortex, posterior to Heschl's gyrus on the superior-lateral surface of the temporal lobe (areas 22 and 42) and including the speech reception area of Wernicke, was found to be larger in the left hemisphere. Whether similar differences would be found in the brain of the child is not certain. It is clear that from a functional standpoint a considerable degree of equipotentiality exists in the child as regards dominance for language function. Thus in a child under the age of 5 years, destruction of the speech areas of the dominant left hemisphere does not result in a significant language disturbance. If the damage to the speech areas in the dominant hemisphere occurs before the age of 12 years a temporary aphasia occurs; but recovery of language usually occurs within a year. In these cases the right hemisphere must assume a dominant role in mediating those learned associations important in language and in the use of symbols. If total destruction of the speech area of the dominant hemisphere occurs in adult life only a limited recovery of language functions will occur.

APHASIA

In approaching the patient with aphasia it is well to keep in mind that text book discussions of this problem are often artificial, in the sense that such discussions tend to deal with relatively isolated pure types of language disturbance which have relatively specific localization. The actual patient with aphasia more often presents a mixed disturbance with damage to several areas. This is not unexpected when one realizes that all of the major speech areas of the dominant hemisphere fall within the central cortical supply area or border zone area of the middle cerebral artery.

Three cortical areas of the dominant hemisphere are of importance in language disturbances (Fig. 21-27):

1. *Broca's motor aphasia or expressive speech center:* The opercular and triangular portions of the inferior frontal convolution (areas 44 and 45).

2. *Wernicke's receptive aphasia area:* The auditory association area on the superior and lateral surface of the posterior portion of the superior temporal gyrus (area 22 and adjacent portions of area 42).

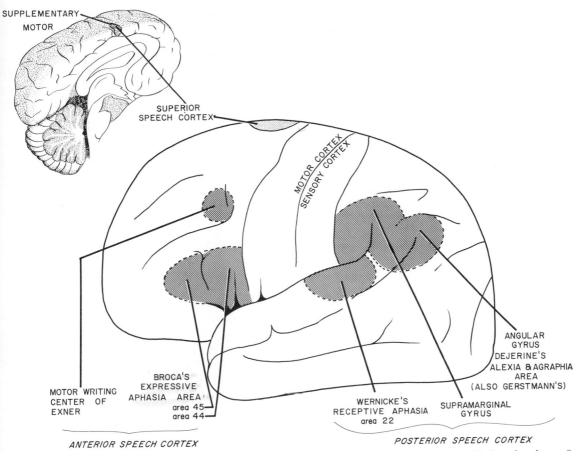

Figure 21-27 Speech areas of the dominant hemisphere. Summary diagram combining the data of pathological lesions and stimulation studies. The borders of the speech areas are indicated in an approximate manner. Precise sharp borders are not implied. Thus, the motor writing center simply implies an area of premotor cortex anterior to the area of hand representation in the precentral gyrus. The area for the alexia and agraphia of Dejerine and the Gerstmann syndrome refers to both the angular and supramarginal gyri. The designations of Penfield and Roberts (*Speech and Brain Mechanisms*, Princeton University Press, 1959, p. 201) have been followed as regards the use of the terms "anterior speech area," "posterior speech area," and "superior speech cortex."

3. *Inferior parietal lobule:* The angular and supramarginal gyri (area 39 and 40), at times associated with Gerstmann's syndrome of dysgraphia, dyscalculia, left-right confusion, and finger agnosia.

Other cortical areas such as the supplementary motor cortex may also play a minor role in language function. In addition to these cortical areas, the association fiber systems relating these areas to each other and to other cortical areas are of considerable importance for certain types of language disturbance, as we will indicate later.

From a practical localization standpoint we can, in a general sense, speak of patients as presenting an anterior or posterior type of aphasia (anterior or posterior to the central sulcus) (Fig. 21-27). *The anterior type of aphasia* relates to Broca's motor aphasia area. The patient's speech may be described in a general sense as nonfluent with little spontaneous verbalization. On the other hand, patients with *posterior types of aphasia* are fluent and do have spontaneous speech. Their lesions involve Wernicke's area in the posterior portion of the superior temporal gyrus or the inferior parietal lobule. Since these posterior areas are relatively close to one another it is not unusual for a single disease process to involve both areas.

Now let us consider in greater detail these various centers and their related language functions:

AREA FOR MOTOR APHASIA

This area is essentially a continuation of premotor cortex and may be considered a specialized motor association area with regard to the tongue, lips, pharynx, and larynx. This area is adjacent to the motor cortex representation of the face, lips, tongue, and pharyngeal muscles. It is not, therefore, unusual for these patients to have also a supranuclear type weakness of the right side of the face. This by itself is not sufficient to explain the problems in speech which these patients manifest, since lesions involving the face area of the nondominant motor cortex do not produce the speech disturbance. Moreover, tongue and pharynx receive a bilateral corticobulbar supply, so that a unilateral cortical lesion involving the motor cortex in this area is not a sufficient explanation. These patients appear to have lost the motor memories of the sequence of skilled coordinated movements of tongue, lips, and pharynx which are required for the vocalization of understandable single words, phrases, and sentences. They are usually able to vocalize sounds. At times they may be able to vocalize single words but are unable to arrange these words into a proper grammatical sequence for sentences.

In the patient with a relatively pure form of Broca's motor asphasia, the capacity to formulate language and to select words in a mental sense is intact. The student might logically inquire as to whether the patient has also lost his motor memories or motor associations for making a nonverbal sequence of movements of the tongue and lips. Frequently this is the case, as will be demonstrated in the illustrative case history. We may refer to this defect in skilled sequential motor function (at a time when no paralysis is present, when sensory and cerebellar function are intact, and when the patient is alert and understands what movements are to be performed) as a *motor apraxia*. We have mentioned apraxia previously. There are several types of apraxia with different localization. In general, we may relate the more purely motor forms of apraxia to the motor association areas of the premotor cortex. One could then refer to patients with

Broca's motor aphasia as patients with a motor apraxia of speech.

Case History 8. NEMC #75–80–63. Date of admission: 4/15/69.

This 55-year-old, right-handed, white housewife (Mrs. E. C.) while working in her garden at 10:00 a. m. on the day of admission suddenly developed a weakness of her right side and was unable to speak. Apparently the right-sided weakness affected predominantly the face and arm since the patient was able to walk.

The past history was significant. In 1960, the patient had been admitted to the hospital with a three-year history of progressive congestive heart failure secondary to rheumatic heart disease (mitral stenosis with atrial fibrillation). An open cardiotomy was performed with a mitral valvuloplasty (the valve opening was enlarged). A thrombus found in the left atrial appendage was also removed. Postoperatively the patient was given an anticoagulant, bishydroxycoumarin (Dicumarol). She did well until the day of admission, although atrial fibrillation continued. Prothrombin time at the time of admission was close to normal; that is, the patient was not in a therapeutic range for anticoagulation.

GENERAL PHYSICAL EXAMINATION:
1. Blood pressure was moderately elevated to 170/80. Pulse was 110 and irregular (atrial fibrillation).
2. Examination of the heart revealed the findings of mitral stenosis: a loud first sound, a diastolic rumble, and an opening snap at the apex.

NEUROLOGICAL EXAMINATION:
1. *Mental status and language function:*
   a. The patient was alert.
   b. She had no spontaneous speech and could not use speech to answer questions and could not even use yes or no answers. She could not repeat words.
   c. The patient was, however, able to indicate answers to questions by nodding or shaking her head if questions were posed in a multiple choice situation. In this manner it was possible to determine that she was grossly oriented for time, place, and person.
   d. The patient was able to carry out spoken commands and simple

written commands, such as, "hold up your hand, close your eyes." She had significant difficulty in performing voluntary tongue movements (such as "wiggle your tongue;" "stick out your tongue") on command.

2. *Cranial nerves:*
   a. The patient tended to neglect stimuli in the right visual field.
   b. She was unable to look to the right on command although the head and eyes were not grossly deviated to the left at rest.
   c. A marked right supranuclear (central) type facial weakness was present.
   d. The patient had difficulty in tongue protrusion. When the tongue was protruded it deviated to the right. The patient was unable to wiggle the tongue.

3. *Motor system:*
   a. Strength of voluntary movement: there was a marked deficit in the right upper extremity, most marked distally. Some shoulder movements were possible; no hand or finger movements could be made. There was a minor degree of weakness involving the right lower extremity (75 per cent of normal).
   b. No definite spasticity was present.

4. *Reflexes:*
   a. Deep tendon reflexes were increased on the right in the arm and leg.
   b. Plantar responses were both extensor; the right more marked than the left.
   c. The abdominal reflex was absent on the right; present on the left.

5. *Sensory system:*
   a. Pain, touch, and vibration were intact.
   b. It was difficult to test other modalities but tactile localization appeared to be intact.

LABORATORY DATA:
1. Skull x-rays were normal
2. EEG was normal (48 hours after admission)
3. Cerebrospinal fluid was normal
4. Electrocardiogram revealed atrial fibrillation

HOSPITAL COURSE:
Within 24 hours a significant return of strength in the right hand had occurred; independent finger movements could be made. Within 48 hours after admission the patient was able to repeat single words but still had almost no spontaneous speech. She appeared aware of her speech disability and would manifest some frustration. She was able to carry out two- or three-stage commands although tongue movements and perseveration remained a problem. Within 6 days of admission the patient used words, phrases, and occasional short sentences spontaneously. She was better able to repeat short sentences. At this time strength in the right arm had returned to normal, but a right central facial weakness was still present.

More detailed language evaluation two weeks after admission indicated the persistence of expressive disabilities consisting of word-finding and apraxic components. The apraxic components were evident on tongue placement and alternating tongue movements. Although complete sentences were used, sentence formulation in spontaneous speech was slow and labored with word-finding difficulties. Repetition was better performed. In reading sentences aloud, substitutions or word omissions were made. The patient did well in naming common pictures and in matching printed words to spoken words or printed words to pictures. She could write from dictation and would often respond preferentially in writing when difficulty in speaking was encountered. No left-right confusion was present. Minor difficulties with simple arithmetic were reported. A right central facial weakness was still present.

COMMENT:
There would appear little doubt that this patient had the sudden passage of an embolus (presumably from the left atrial appendage) into the left middle cerebral artery. In view of the selective face and arm weakness with a predominant expressive aphasia the involved vessels must have been cortical branches such as the prerolandic and rolandic. From the onset, it was clear that although some receptive components might be present, these were minor. The major problem was rather that of a severe nonfluent aphasia. As the hand weakness disappeared, the only other residual neurological findings were those of a right central facial weakness and an apraxia of tongue movements. Such findings would of course be consistent with a relatively selective in-

volvement of Broca's area in the inferior frontal gyrus.

WERNICKE'S RECEPTIVE APHASIA AREA

Geschwind has indicated that this area may be viewed as a center or storehouse of auditory associations. With destruction of this area, the patient not only has difficulty in understanding symbolic sounds, i. e., words which have been heard (he is unable to carry out verbal commands), but also is unable to use those same auditory associations in the formulation of his own speech. Moreover he is essentially unable to monitor his own spoken words as he talks, since he lacks the ability to interpret and to compare the sounds which he himself is producing to previous auditory association. The end result is a patient who is fluent but who uses words combined into sentences which lack any meaning to the listeners. Word substitution (paraphasia) is frequent. The patient however is usually unaware of his errors. The patient usually fails to show the frustration which is characteristic of patients who have Broca's motor aphasia and are aware of their errors. At times the patient shows some awareness that his verbal responses are failing to deal with the environment. In severe cases, not only are phrases and words combined into meaningless sentences but the patient combines syllables into words which have no meaning (jargon aphasia).

We have indicated previously in discussing the auditory cortex, that there is a related problem which may on rare occasions occur in pure form—word deafness. In cases of pure word deafness, the center of auditory word association appears to be intact but auditory information is unable to reach this center from the auditory projection cortex; in a sense disconnection has occurred. The auditory word association center is intact. Previous auditory associations may be used in the formulation of the patient's own speech.

It should be evident to the student that the distinctions which have been made here between Wernicke's receptive aphasia and word deafness are to some extent artificial. In general, lesions in this area do not respect such artificial distinctions and often destroy not only the center for auditory word associations but also the inputs into this area from the auditory projection areas.

Both Wernicke's receptive aphasia and word deafness are often grouped under the general term of auditory *agnosias*. An agnosia may be defined as a failure to recognize stimuli presented within a particular sensory modality at a time when the specific pathways from the periphery and the specific primary cortical projection areas are intact. Agnosias may occur with regard to audition, vision, or tactile sensation. We will discuss later a specific type of visual agnosia—word blindness (dyslexia).

DOMINANT INFERIOR PARIETAL AREAS: ANGULAR AND SUPRAMARGINAL GYRI

Geschwind has indicated the important critical location of the inferior parietal lobule in man situated between the visual, auditory, and tactile association areas. As such it may act as a higher association area between these adjacent sensory association areas. Geschwind has suggested that correlated with the development of this area in the human (the angular and supramarginal gyri cannot be recognized as such in the monkey and are present only in rudimentary form in the higher apes) there has developed the capacity for cross modality sensory-sensory associations without reference to the limbic system. He contrasts this situation with that in subhuman forms where the only readily established sensory-sensory associations are those between a nonlimbic (visual, tactile, or auditory) stimulus and a limbic stimulus: those stimuli related to primary motivations such as hunger, thirst, sex. (Such considerations of course do not rule out the establishment of limbic-nonlimbic stimuli associations in man, particularly during infancy and childhood.) These theoretical concepts would suggest the underlying basis for man's language functions.

It is not surprising then that those aspects of language function which are most dependent on association between auditory and visual stimuli and auditory-visual-tactile stimuli (reading and writing) are most disturbed by lesions of angular and supramarginal gyri. In the words of Geschwind, "It is a region which turns written language into spoken language and vice versa."

The component parts of the resultant syndrome are not constant. The patient will have a varying degree of difficulty in writing *(dysgraphia)*, particularly as regards spontaneous writing. Often the ability to copy letters, words, and sentences will be relatively well preserved. In contrast the patient will usually have difficulty writing from dictation, although at times this function may be less affected than spontaneous writing. There is often an associated deficit in reading (dyslexia) although this is not invariable.

Significant defects in spelling and in calculations (*dyscalculia*) may be present. There may be an associated left-right confusion. Errors may be made in finger identification, with confusion as to index, ring, and middle fingers (*finger agnosia*).

From the standpoint of localization, several points of caution should be indicated. Dysgraphia may also result from disease involving the premotor cortex anterior to the motor cortex representation of the hand. It is likely that information is conveyed from the inferior parietal area to the premotor motor association cortex and then to the precentral motor cortex. This area of premotor cortex (sometimes termed the writing center of Exner) must function in a manner analogous to Broca's area. It would be reasonable to consider dysgraphia from a lesion in this premotor location as essentially a motor apraxia due to destruction of an area concerned in the motor association memories for writing.

Pure dyslexias may occur without actual involvement of the angular supramarginal areas. The basic lesion as we will indicate, is a lesion which deprives the inferior parietal cortex of information from the visual association areas.

Finally, many lesions in the inferior parietal area extend into the subcortical white matter involving the long association fiber system. An association fiber system of importance in this area is the arcuate fasciculus (Fig. 20-19). Information is conveyed from Wernicke's area in the superior temporal gyrus to Broca's area in the inferior frontal gyrus by this fiber system which arches around the posterior end of the sylvian fissure to join the superior longitudinal fasciculus. Damage to this fiber system produces what has been termed a *conduction aphasia* or *repetition aphasia*. Essentially the patient understands spoken commands and is able to carry out complex instructions that do not require a language response. He is unable, however, to repeat verbally the information received although he is able to speak spontaneously and has no evidence of a Broca's motor type aphasia. The patient, however, is unable to repeat test phrases and sentences and is unable to write from dictation.

Patients with dominant inferior parietal lobule lesions often demonstrate problems in drawing (constructional drawing). Whether this reflects damage to the cortex of the angular and supramarginal gyri or a disconnection of these areas from the more anterior motor areas because of involvement of subcortical association fibers is usually uncertain.

The following case demonstrates many of the language disturbances which have been discussed in relation to the angular and supramarginal gyri. The apparent involvement of the subcortical association fiber system (the arcuate fasciculus) will be evident. The later development of a classic Wernicke's type receptive aphasia following dominant temporal lobe ablation at surgery is clearly demonstrated.

Case History 9. NECH #188–493. Date of admission: 7/20/67.

This 42-year-old, right-handed truck driver (Mr. D. M.) 6 to 8 weeks prior to admission noted fatigue and a mild personality change (he was more easily irritated by his children). Three to four weeks prior to admission the patient noted that he was speaking words which he did not mean to use. He noted that certain words would not come to him. During the week prior to admission, the patient had experienced two generalized convulsive seizures, each preceded by a ringing sensation in the ear.

NEUROLOGICAL EXAMINATION:
1. *Mental status:*
   a. The patient was alert and oriented for time, place, and person.
   b. He was cooperative and able to carry out a series of a three-step command: "Stick out your tongue, close your eyes, hold up your hand, and touch the thumb to your ear." There was, however, evidence of a significant left-right confusion when laterality was introduced, e.g., "left hand to right ear."
   c. Ability to do even simple calculations was markedly impaired. The patient was unable to do even simple subtraction, with or without paper (e.g., $100 - 9 = 99$).
   d. Memory was impaired with imme-

diate object recall of 2-out-of 5 objects and delayed recall of 0-out-of 5 objects in 5 minutes. Digit span was limited to 2 forward and 0 in reverse.

e. There was little evidence of an expressive aphasia. Flow of speech was slow with only minor mispronunciation. Reading was slow but with few errors. The patient did have minor difficulty in naming objects (a mild nominal aphasia). The patient's greatest difficulty was in the repetition of simple test phrases. There were moderate defects in drawings — a house and a clock (constructional apraxia) — but few errors in copying simple figures. There was a significant dysgraphia with marked difficulties in writing a simple sentence spontaneously or in writing from dictation. The patient was better able to copy a simple sentence.

Significant errors were made in spelling.

2. *Cranial nerves:*

Intact except for a mild right facial weakness of supranuclear type.

3. *Motor system:*
   a. Strength was intact with normal tone.
   b. Gait was intact.

4. *Reflexes:*
   a. Deep tendon reflexes were symmetrical and physiologic.
   b. Plantar responses were flexor but slightly asymmetrical, the left slightly more flexor than the right.

5. *Sensory system:*
   a. Pain, touch, and vibration were intact.
   b. Point localization was impaired on the right side but stereognosis, simultaneous stimulation, graphesthesia, and position sense were all intact.

LABORATORY DATA:

1. *Skull and chest x-rays* were normal.

2. *Electroencephalogram:* Abnormal because of focal 4 to 5 cps slow wave activity in the left parietal and posterior temporal area, suggesting focal damage in these areas.

3. *Brain scan:* There was a relatively discrete uptake of radioisotope (Hg^{197}) in the left posterior temporal parietal area measuring 4×5 cm. Findings were consistent with an infiltrating intrinsic tumor.

4. *Left carotid arteriogram:* A moderately vascular space-occupying tumor was demonstrated in the area of the angular gyrus with tumor stain in this area.

SUBSEQUENT HOSPITAL COURSE:

Early papilledema soon developed and since severe language difficulties were already present, partial resection of the tumor was performed by Dr. Robert Yuan on August 1, 1967. At surgery, although the cortex appeared externally normal, a firm mass could be palpated in the area, slightly above and posterior to the angular gyrus. At 2 cm. below the cortical pial surface, firm yellow tissue was encountered. Removal of all visible tumor and adjacent cortex of the angular and supramarginal gyri was performed, in addition to a partial left temporal lobectomy.

Histological examination disclosed a malignant tumor arising from the glia with evidence of active mitosis and necrosis (a malignant astrocytoma, essentially a glioblastoma).

Postoperatively a marked expressive and receptive aphasia was apparent. By the time of hospital discharge on September 1, 1967 some improvement had occurred as regards fluency of speech, but the patient was frequently unable to carry out simple commands. His responses, however, were usually appropriate. Speech was mumbling and incoherent, with nonsense words and neologisms (new words composed by the patient). He appeared unaware of his speech deficits and did not appear frustrated by his failure to follow directions. The patient was unable to repeat words of two syllables. Calculations could not be performed. Although the patient had no significant motor or sensory deficits, he made marked errors in copying a drawing such as a daisy flower and a cube. He was unable to write his name or to write any numbers on the face of a clock.

The patient received radiation therapy but his status worsened with the development of a marked expressive and receptive aphasia and of a progressive right hemiparesis. Consciousness became obtunded with respiratory difficulties and pupillary changes. Death occurred on February 8, 1968.

COMMENT:

The early language and mental status disturbances in this patient were clearly most severe in those tasks requiring repetition: thus the patient could repeat no more than two digits, was unable to repeat any of the test phrases, and was unable to write from dictation at a time when he could copy a sentence. Any expressive aphasia was minor and there was little evidence of any receptive aphasia. Reading was relatively well preserved compared to writing and calculations.

This repetition problem certainly suggests that the speech reception area was disconnected from the motor association areas for speech and writing—areas 44, 45, and related premotor areas. The lesion, as described by the neurosurgeon, certainly involved the white matter deep to the angular and supramarginal area, the known location of the arcuate fasciculus. The left-right confusion, dyscalculia, and constructional apraxia must have reflected damage to the dominant angular-supramarginal area or to the underlying white matter.

The state seen following surgery clearly indicated presence of a severe receptive aphasia undoubtedly due to the extensive ablation of the temporal lobe. The patient's preoperative findings were accentuated as well (constructional apraxia, writing, and repetition deficits) undoubtedly due to the operative ablation of the supramarginal angular areas and their subjacent white matter.

The later development of severe expressive aphasia and right hemiparesis indicated the infiltration of the posterior frontal areas by this malignant glial tumor.

The patient's initial seizure should be recognized as probably originating in the transverse gyrus of Heschl, which is situated relatively far posteriorly in the temporal lobe and thus not far from the lesion in the angular gyrus.

VISUAL AGNOSIA AND SELECTIVE DYSLEXIA (ALEXIA WITHOUT AGRAPHIA)

Visual agnosia may be defined as a failure to recognize visually presented material. *Dyslexia or alexia* represents a more selective deficit: a failure to recognize visually presented words (this is sometimes also called word blindness). The student may conceptualize the basic disturbance as a disconnection of the visual areas from the speech areas of the posterior temporal and inferior parietal areas. This disturbance could result from bilateral lesions or from a unilateral lesion. As we have previously indicated, bilateral destruction of the visual association cortex (areas 18 and 19) would theoretically produce this effect. An alternate combination of lesions would involve destruction of the primary visual cortex (area 17) of the

dominant left hemisphere and the visual association cortex of the right hemisphere.

A large unilateral lesion producing essentially this same effect has been implicated in dyslexia. This lesion has usually destroyed the visual cortex of the dominant left hemisphere and at the same time damaged the posterior portion or, at least, the splenium of the corpus callosum (or the fibers radiating from the splenium). The fibers conveying visual data from the right hemisphere must presumably reach the speech areas of the dominant hemisphere by passing through the posterior segment of the corpus callosum. The following case would suggest this type of unilateral lesion producing a transient and partial but selective type of dyslexia.

Case History 10. NECH #177–905. Date of admission: 3/12/66. (Patient of Dr. John Sullivan.)

On March 5, 1966, this 15-year-old, right-handed, white, male, high school student (Mr. W.E.) had the onset of a 48-hour period of sharp pain in the left jaw and the supraorbital area, following a period of athletic activity. On March 6, 1966, the patient began to complain of blurring of vision and the following day had the onset of vomiting. On March 8, 1966, the patient noted that he was unable to read and to translate his Latin lessons. No definite aphasia was apparent. On March 10, 1966, patient had the sudden onset of severe left facial pain accompanied by tingling paresthesias of the right leg. The patient became stuporous and then unresponsive for approximately 90 minutes. An examination of spinal fluid at that time revealed pressure elevated to 290 mm. of water with 250 fresh blood cells.

NEUROLOGICAL EXAMINATION:

1. *Mental status:* All aspects, including language function, were intact.

2. *Cranial nerves:*
   a. Examination of the fundus showed several small flame-shaped hemorrhages. Visual fields were intact.
   b. A slight, right, supranuclear-type (central), facial weakness was present.

3. *Motor system* was intact.

4. *Reflexes:* Deep tendon reflexes and superficial reflexes were symmetrical and physiologic.

5. *Sensory system:* Primary and cortical modalities were intact.

6. A slight degree of resistance was present on flexion of the neck (nuchal rigidity)

consistent with the presence of blood in the subarachnoid space.

LABORATORY DATA:

1. *Arteriograms:* An arteriovenous malformation was present in the left occipital region. The main arterial supply was the posterior temporal branch of the left posterior cerebral artery. The malformation drained into the lateral sinus. The posterior portion of the anterior cerebral artery was shifted across the midline, indicating a hematoma as well as the malformation.

SUBSEQUENT COURSE:

During the evening of March 12, 1966 the patient had the sudden onset of a bifrontal headache. For a 2- to 3-minute period, the patient was unconscious with deviation (repetitive driving) of both eyes to the right, sweating, and slowing of the pulse rate. Over the next two days an increase in blurring of the optic disc margins was noted (early papilledema). On March 16, 1966 the patient suddenly complained of being unable to see from his right eye. He became restless and agitated. Additional headache and neck pain with numbness of right arm and leg were reported. Examination now disclosed a dense right visual field defect (homonymous hemianopsia). The deep tendon reflexes were now slightly more active on the right. Funduscopic examination suggested that recent additional subarachnoid bleeding had occurred: new retinal hemorrhages were present. On March 17, 1966 the patient was noted to have a significant reading disability (dyslexia), although other language functions were intact.

Because of the progressive evolution of neurological findings with the possibility of an expanding intracerebral hematoma, craniotomy was performed by Dr. Robert Yuan on March 18, 1966. Blood was present in the subarachnoid space. The lateral occipital cortical surface had numerous areas of bluish discoloration indicating an intracerebral clot. The main arterial vessel was a lateral and inferior branch of the posterior cerebral artery, bearing no relationship to the calcarine region. The draining vein was located in the occipital-temporal area, close to the tentorium. At a depth of 1 cm., a hematoma of 50 cc. of clot was found. The clot extended down to the occipital horn of the lateral ventricle but did not enter the ventricle. The malformation, hematoma, and related cerebral tissue of the lateral occipital area were removed. The calcarine area remained intact at the end of the procedure.

Over a period of several days, the visual field deficits disappeared.

Detailed language and psychological testing approximately two weeks after surgery indicated that language function was intact except for reading. Oral reading was very slow (4 times slower than normal for a test paragraph), halting, and stumbling. Comprehension of the material read was good. Minor errors were made in the visual recognition of letters. This was reflected in occasional errors in spelling.

Visual recognition and naming of objects was intact. Auditory and tactile recognition of sounds, words, letters, sentences, questions, commands, and so forth was intact. Calculations were intact. No right-left confusion or finger agnosia was present. Writing and drawing were intact but slow. Repetition speech and spontaneous speech were intact.

Follow-up evaluation at 20 and 30 months indicated that, although the patient was doing well in school, receiving A's and B's with excellent grades in mathematics, he still was described as slow in reading compared to his level prior to illness. No actual errors were made in reading when this was tested.

COMMENT:

The arteriovenous malformation in this case had involved and eventually required surgical removal of the lateral occipital area of the dominant hemisphere. The hematoma in the occipital lobe extending in from the lateral surface to the occipital horn would be so located as to compress the optic radiation passing to the calcarine cortex or perhaps even to indirectly compress the calcarine cortex. Such a hematoma would also interfere with association fibers passing from left occipital areas to temporal parietal areas and with callosal radiation fibers passing from the occipital region (area 18) of the right hemisphere to the occipital and parietal areas of the dominant hemisphere. Following surgery the patient had a relatively good recovery with the minor difficulties in reading; a selective dyslexia was perhaps the only indication of any damage to these fiber systems.

The complaint of the patient at the time that the right homonymous hemianopsia appeared was of blindness in the right eye. It is not uncommon for patients to localize field defects in this manner to the eye of the same side. The same may sometimes be true of patients with discharging lesions in the occipital area; the flashing lights and lines may be localized to the contralateral eye rather than to the contralateral visual field.

The episode on the night of March 12, 1966 is of interest because it suggests a focal adversive seizure, in this case presumably originating in areas 18 and 19 of the left hemisphere.

Geschwind has reviewed many of the previously reported cases of selective dyslexia. It is uncertain whether the information from area 18 of the nondominant hemisphere passes to the nondominant angular gyrus and then crosses to the dominant temporal parietal areas or whether these fibers pass instead directly to area 18 of the dominant hemisphere with information then conveyed to the dominant temporal parietal areas. He finally concludes that both pathways are probably operative. The relatively minor nature of the final residual deficit in the present case would be consistent with such multiple pathways.

It should be noted that a relatively selective dyslexia in the absence of a severe general visual agnosia may occur. Geschwind has suggested that whether a general visual agnosia or a dyslexia occurs may depend on the degree of disconnection of the dominant speech areas from the parietal and occipital areas of the nondominant hemisphere. In the patient who already has left occipital cortex damage, dyslexia may require only damage to the splenium, whereas visual agnosia may require more extensive damage to the posterior body of the corpus callosum as well. As noted bilateral visual association lesions (areas 18 and 19) would also produce a visual agnosia.

NOMINAL APHASIA

There remains a variety of aphasia—nominal aphasia—which is commonly encountered but which is not as readily localized to a particular cortical area. Nominal aphasia is often noted as part of other aphasic syndromes. The patient recognizes objects when these are present in the visual or tactile sphere but is unable to name the object. He will tell the examiner that he certainly does know the name but is unable to verbalize this name. He certainly will select the name in a multiple-choice situation. At times, he will substitute other names; more often he will describe the use of the object as a means of naming it, e.g., for a light switch—"That's the thing that makes the light go on and off."

At times, associated findings suggest localization to the dominant posterior temporal parietal area; at times there is some association with a Broca's area motor aphasia.

APRAXIA

As we have previously indicated this term may be defined as an impairment in motor performance in the absence of a paralysis or sensory receptive deficit and at a time when cerebellar function is intact. In the carrying out of a skilled movement on command there are several stages which are similar to those considered under language function. The command, if auditory, must be received at the cortical auditory projection area of the dominant hemisphere. The information must then be relayed to the auditory association areas for the words of the command to be comprehended, that is, to evoke the appropriate auditory associations. From these areas information must be relayed, presumably via association fiber systems such as the arcuate fasciculus, to the motor association areas in the premotor cortex of the dominant hemisphere. Information must then be conveyed from the dominant premotor cortex to the dominant motor cortex. At the same time information must also be conveyed to the premotor and motor areas of the nondominant hemisphere so that the nondominant hand can also perform learned skilled movements on command.

Apraxia then could result from damage at any point in this series of association centers and their interconnections. Depending on the point of disruption in the circuit, the type of impairment will vary. Thus a lesion of the anterior one half of the corpus callosum will result in an apraxia limited to the nondominant hand. In contrast, a lesion of the dominant premotor association areas would be more likely to produce a bilateral impairment in certain tongue and hand movements.

The concept that many varieties of apraxia represent a disconnection between various cortical areas, as recently reintroduced by Geschwind, provides a more anatomically based approach than the use of terms such as motor kinetic (motor association areas) or ideomotor apraxia (parietal lobe apraxia).

The student will also encounter the term ideational apraxia. This term has generally been used to refer to the patient with diffuse disease, such as presenile dementia, who carries out a completely different act than the one requested or begins the act and then goes to some other activity. In a sense the patient may be unable because of recent memory deficits to retain the command in memory long enough for the series of acts to be carried out. Some would suggest that this type of dysfunction really represents not an apraxia but a deficit in recent memory and would require among the defining conditions of apraxia that dementia not be present.

NONDOMINANT HEMISPHERE FUNCTIONS

As we have previously indicated certain symptoms appear to follow damage to the nondominant parietal areas such as lack of awareness of hemiplegia, neglect syndrome, defects in spatial construction, and in perception of three-dimensional space. Some have questioned whether a true dominance of these functions actually exists in the hemisphere which is nondominant for speech. Certainly neglect syndromes may also follow lesions of the dominant parietal area or of either premotor area. Deficits in construction may also follow lesions of the dominant parietal area. As regards concepts of visual space, there is some evidence from the studies of Gazzaniga et al. on section of the corpus callosum that the dominant left hemisphere is dependent on information which must be conveyed from the right hemisphere. Moreover, the studies of Penfield suggest that in patients with temporal lobe seizures visual hallucinations are more likely to arise from stimulation of the right hemisphere than of the left. (Refer to preceding discussion of temporal lobe.)

ROLE OF CORPUS CALLOSUM IN TRANSFER OF INFORMATION

As we have indicated in the discussion of selective dyslexia, the corpus callosum allows the nondominant hemisphere access to the special language centers of the dominant hemisphere. Thus the intact right-handed individual can name an object, such as a key, independent of whether the object is placed in the left or right hand. Following section of the corpus callosum, the object can be named when placed in the right hand but not when placed in the left hand. In a similar manner, the corpus callosum allows the dominant hemisphere access to those specialized areas of the nondominant hemisphere concerned with concepts of visual space.

There is also evidence that the corpus callosum is involved in the transfer of information concerned with learned sensory discriminations. Thus the intact monkey or man, who has been trained to press a key with the right hand only when a particular visual pattern appears in the right visual field, has no difficulty in performing the same discrimination without additional learning when the left visual field and left hand are employed. Section of the corpus callosum interferes with such transfer of learned information. There is evidence, however, that some sensory information and learned sensory discrimination is transferred between hemispheres via noncallosal pathways. (Refer to Ettlinger, 1965.)

References

Bignall, K. E., and Imbert, M.: Polysensory and cortico-cortical projections to frontal lobe of squirrel and rhesus monkeys. Electroenceph. clin. Neurophysiol., 26:206–215, 1969.

Corkin, S., Milner, B., and Rasmussen, T.: Effects of different cortical excisions on sensory thresholds in man. Trans. Amer. neurol. Ass., 89:112–116, 1964.

Dusser De Barenne, J. G., and McCulloch, W. S.: Suppression of motor response obtained from area 4 by stimulation of area 4S. J. Neurophysiol., 4:311–323, 1941.

Ettlinger, F. G. (ed.): Function of the Corpus Callosum. Boston, Little, Brown, and Company, 1965.

Evarts, E. V.: Representation of Movements and Muscles by Pyramidal Tract Neurons of the Precentral Motor Cortex In Yahr, M. D., and Purpura, D. P. (eds.): Neurophysiological Basis of Normal and Abnormal Motor Activities. Hewlett, N.Y. Raven Press, 1967, p. 215–253.

Fangel, C., and Kaada, B. R.: Behavior "attention" and fear induced by cortical stimulation in the cat. Electroenceph. clin. Neurophysiol., 12:575–588, 1960.

Foerster, O.: The motor cortex in the light of Hughlings Jackson's doctrines. Brain, 59:135–159, 1936.

Fulton, J. F.: Physiology of the Nervous System, 3rd. Edition. New York, Oxford University Press, 1949.

Gazzaniga, M. S., Bogen, J. E., and Sperry, R. W.: Observations on visual perception after disconnections of the cerebral hemispheres in man. Brain, 88:221–236, 1965.

Geschwind, N.: Disconnection syndromes in animals and man. Brain, 88:237–294, 585–644, 1965.

Geschwind, N., and Levitsky, W.: Human brain: Left-right asymmetries in temporal speech region. Science, 161:186–187, 1968.

Harlow, J. M.: Recovery from the passage of an iron bar through the head. Mass. Med. Soc. Publ., 2:327–346, 1868.

Hecaen, H.: Clinical Symptomatology in Right and Left Hemispheric Lesions In Mountcastle, V. B. (ed.): Interhemispheric Relations and Cerebral Dominance. The Johns Hopkins Press. Baltimore, 1962.

Hubel, D. H., and Wiesel, T. N.: Receptive fields and functional architecture of monkey striate cortex. J. Physiol. (Lond.), *195*:215–243, 1968.

Kennard, M. A., and Ectors, L.: Forced circling in monkeys following lesions of the frontal lobes. J. Neurophysiol., *1*:45.-54, 1938.

Kluver, H., and Bucy, P.: Preliminary analysis of functions of the temporal lobes in monkeys. Arch. Neurol. Psychiat., *42*:979–1000, 1939.

Lewis, R., and Brindley, G. S.: The extrapyramidal motor map. Brain, *88*:397–406, 1965.

Marcus, E. M., Watson, C. W., and Simon, S. A.: Behavioral correlates of acute bilateral symmetrical epileptogenic foci in monkey cerebral cortex. *Brain Res.*, *9*:370–373, 1968.

Maynard, C. D., and Janeway, R.: Radioisotope Studies in Neurodiagnosis. *In* Toole, J. F. (ed.): *Special Techniques for Neurologic Diagnosis.* Philadelphia, F. A. Davis, 1969, pp. 71–91.

Mishkin, M.: Visual Mechanisms Beyond the Striate Cortex *In* Russell, R. W. (ed.): *Frontiers in Physiological Psychology.* New York, Academic Press, 1966, p. 93–119.

Nauta, W. J. H.: Some Efferent Connections of the Prefrontal Cortex in the Monkey, *In* Warren, J. M., and Akert, K. (eds.): *The Frontal Granular Cortex and Behavior.* New York, McGraw Hill, 1964, p. 397–409.

Nielsen, J. M.: Agnosias, Apraxias, Speech and Aphasia *In* Baker, A. B. (ed.): *Clinical Neurology,* New York, Hoeber-Harper, 1955, Vol 1, p 352–378.

Nielsen, J. M.: *Agnosia, Apraxia, Aphasia: Their Value in Cerebral Localization.* 2nd Edition. New York, Hafner Publishing, 1962.

Penfield, W.: Speech, Perception and The Uncommitted Cortex *In* Eccles, J. C. (ed.): *Brain and Conscious Experience.* New York, Springer-Verlag, 1966, p. 217–237.

Penfield, W., and Evans, J. P.: Functional Defects Produced by Cerebral Lobotomies. Res. Publ. Ass. nerv. ment. Dis., *13*:352–377, 1934.

Penfield, W., and Jasper, H.: *Epilepsy and the Functional Anatomy of the Human Brain.* Boston, Little Brown, 1954, p 41–154, 350–539.

Penfield, W., and Perot, P.: The brain's record of auditory and visual experience. *Brain,* *86*:595–696, 1963.

Phillips, C. G.: Changing Concepts of the precentral Motor Area *In* Eccles, J. C. (ed.): *Brain and Conscious Experience.* New York, Springer-Verlag, 1966, p. 389–421.

Taylor, J. (ed.): *Selected Writings of John Hughlings Jackson.* New York, Basic Books, Inc. 1958, p. 1–36, 385–405, 406–411, 458–463.

Twitchell, T. E.: The restoration of motor function following hemiplegia in man. *Brain,* *74*:443–480, 1951.

Weiskrantz, L., Liharlovic, L. J., and Gross, G. G.: Effects of stimulation of frontal cortex and hippocampus on behavior in the monkey. *Brain,* *85*:487–504, 1962.

Welch, K., and Stuteville, P.: Experimental production of unilateral neglect in monkeys. *Brain,* *81*:341–347, 1958.

Wilkins, R. H., and Brody, I. A.: The thalamic syndrome. Arch Neurol., *20*:559–562, 1969.

Wilkins, R. H., and Brody, I. A.: Jacksonian epilepsy. Arch. Neurol., *22*:183–188, 1970.

Wilkins, R. H., and Brody, I. A.: Wernicke's sensory aphasia. Arch. Neurol., *22*:279–282, 1970.

Williams, D.: Man's Temporal Lobe. *Brain,* *91*:639–654, 1968.

Yakolev, P. I., and Rakic, P.: Patterns of decussation of bulbar pyramids and distribution of pyramidal tracts on two sides of the spinal cord. *Trans. Amer. neurol. Ass.,* *91*:366–367, 1966.

22

Clinical Considerations of the Cerebral Hemispheres and a General Survey of Neuropathology

ELLIOTT M. MARCUS

The course and nature of some of the more common diseases affecting the cerebral hemispheres are already familiar to the student on the basis of those case histories presented in the previous chapter on cortical localization. We will refer back to some of those case histories. However, we will not limit our discussion simply to the neocortex but will discuss the cerebral hemispheres in a more general sense. It will also be convenient at this point to consider several broad categories of diseases, not previously discussed, which do not necessarily restrict themselves to the cerebral hemispheres.

Diseases affecting the cerebral hemispheres account for the largest proportion of central nervous system diseases encountered in medical practice. These diseases may be focal or diffuse in nature. There is also a third or intermediate category of multifocal (that is, comprised of many focal events). At times the end result of an apparent multifocal process may be difficult to

distinguish from a diffuse process. Our major concern will be with focal processes but we will consider diffuse and multifocal diseases as well.

VASCULAR DISEASES OF THE CEREBRAL HEMISPHERE

Vascular problems account for the largest category of diseases affecting the cerebral hemispheres. Several types must be considered: (1) atherosclerosis with ischemia—occlusion (by far the most frequent), (2) embolism, (3) intracerebral hemorrhage, (4) subarachnoid hemorrhage, and (5) traumatic hemorrhage. These various categories are not mutually exclusive. Thus occlusive vascular disease usually occurs in relation to the process of atherosclerosis—the deposition of fatty material (cholesterol) in the walls of arteries. However, emboli produce their effect essentially by occlusion of cere-

536

bral arteries. Such emboli generally originate in relation to clots within the chambers of the heart. At times, however, such embolic material has originated at an area of occlusive disease when atheromatous material or an overlying thrombus (clot) has broken loose to be carried into the more distal circulation. There is, on the other hand, an overlap between ischemic occlusive disease and intracerebral hemorrhage. Thus certain areas of tissue damage resulting from ischemia may become hemorrhagic secondarily. The symptoms and signs which then evolve may resemble those of intracerebral hemorrhage.

ISCHEMIC-OCCLUSIVE DISEASE

The basic process is that of atherosclerosis involving the large- and medium-sized extracranial and intracranial portions of the cerebral arteries. With increasing deposition of fatty material at points of bifurcation or angulation, a progressive narrowing (stenosis) of the lumen occurs (Fig. 22–1). Eventually, a decrease in cerebral blood flow through this point of narrowing in the vessel will occur (the actual relationship may be calculated according to Bernoulli's principle). The area supplied by this vessel may then at some point receive less than the required amount of blood (oxygen, glucose, and so forth). When this occurs, we may speak of cerebral ischemia.

A dysfunction of the involved area then occurs with focal symptoms of weakness, numbness, and the like. This dysfunction may be only temporary in nature or it may be prolonged with actual tissue death (infarction) and residual neurological deficit. As progressive narrowing of the lumen occurs, eventually a point of total occlusion is reached. The narrowing of the lumen is moreover accentuated by several additional processes: (a) thrombus formation—the formation of a clot of platelets, fibrin, and blood cells due to stasis, change in intimal surface, and so forth, (b) ulceration of the intimal surface at the locus of the atherosclerotic plaque, and (c) subintimal hemorrhage in relation to this area of deposition. The process of ulceration of the intimal wall may produce an originating site for emboli composed of the atheromatous material. Such an ulcerated intimal wall is a likely site of thrombus formation producing additional

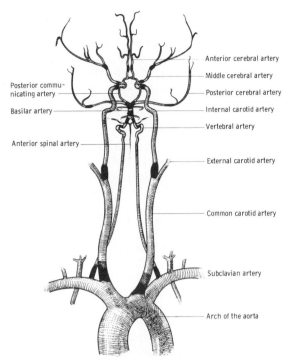

Figure 22–1   Major sites of atherosclerosis involving the cerebral blood vessels. The darkened areas represent the common sites. (From McDowell, F.: In Beeson, P. B., and McDermott, W.: *Textbook of Medicine*, 13th Edition, Philadelphia, W. B. Saunders, 1971, p. 191.)

stenosis. Fragments of the clot may also travel as emboli into the distal circulation.

We have used the joint term, atherosclerotic ischemic-occlusive vascular disease, since there is no one-to-one relationship between actual occlusion of a vessel and tissue death (infarction or encephalomalacia) in the region supplied by that artery. Thus, total occlusion of a vessel may occur without the development of significant neurological symptoms and signs. On the other hand, one may have very significant focal symptoms and signs. There may be at times persistent symptoms and signs correlated with significant tissue destruction. At other times, with stenosis, there may be only episodes of transient symptomatology without actual tissue destruction. These transient episodes, related to vascular insufficiency, are referred to as *transient ischemia attacks*.

Several factors account for this lack of close correspondence between the state of a particular artery and the vascular status of the region supplied by that vessel.

1. There are significant variations in the capacity of the circle of Willis to provide

collateral circulation. Thus, in a particular individual, total occlusion of the left carotid artery may have no significant effect because the left anterior cerebral and left middle cerebral artery receive adequate supply via the anterior communicating artery, essentially from the right carotid artery. Occlusion of the right carotid artery of course in such an individual might well produce significant damage in the left cerebral hemisphere. In some individuals, the posterior cerebral artery is actually a continuation of the posterior communicating artery originating from the internal carotid artery. In such cases occlusion of the carotid artery might produce not only the classic carotid symptoms to be discussed later but also posterior cerebral symptoms. Obviously then in any particular case it is important to know the status of all the major cerebral vessels.

2. There are significant leptomeningeal anastomoses over the surface of the cerebral cortex between the anterior, middle, and posterior cerebral arteries of a given hemisphere. In addition, anastomotic loops occur across the corpus callosum between the anterior cerebral arteries of the two cerebral hemispheres.

With regard to each cerebral artery one may then speak of its area of central supply and its area of peripheral supply. This latter peripheral area usually receives also the peripheral supply of adjacent vessels and is in a sense a border zone. Thus one may speak of a central area of supply of the middle cerebral artery.

In the dominant hemisphere this corresponds to the cortical area of representation of the face, mouth, and tongue and includes Broca's motor speech area. While part of the area of representation of the hand falls within this central area, the hand representation is predominantly within the peripheral area of the middle cerebral supply. This peripheral area also receives collateral circulation from the anterior cerebral artery via leptomeningeal anastomoses. The hand would therefore show less symptomatology than the face and Broca's area, with a pure middle cerebral artery occlusion. On the other hand, a process which decreased blood flow but did not eliminate blood flow in both the middle and anterior cerebral arteries would produce its greatest effects in relation to this border zone between the middle and anterior cerebral middle arteries, i.e., the

area which is the peripheral field of supply of both these vessels—the area of hand representation.

The student will at once realize that such a process must involve the carotid artery, for a decrease in the blood flow of this artery would be the basic cause of a decreased blood flow in both the middle and anterior cerebral arteries. We may then assume that vascular disease producing focal symptoms in the hand is presumptive evidence of disease of the carotid artery.

Similarly, there is a border zone which represents the joint peripheral supply regions of the anterior, middle, and posterior cerebral arteries. This area corresponding to the posterior parietal (inferior parietal lobule) lateral occipital area would suffer most if the blood flow in all three vessels was reduced simultaneously. Such a condition does occur under conditions of hypotension when blood pressure falls. The resultant lesions are found in this triple border zone area. Similar border zone areas are present in the spinal cord and cerebellum between overlapping arterial supplies.

3. To a variable degree, anastomoses are present between the external and internal carotid arteries. One such area is around the orbit with blood from the external carotid vessels passing into the ophthalmic artery. Such anastomoses may serve to avert damage when the internal carotid artery is occluded.

4. Finally, a considerable variability occurs because of certain general systemic and metabolic factors. Thus a narrowed vessel may still deliver sufficient blood when the systemic blood pressure is 190/100 but fails to do so when the blood pressure falls to 120/70. Such a fall in blood pressure may occur during sleep, on sudden standing after a long period of recumbency, and in relation to treatment with various agents which are designed to lower blood pressure. Similarly, stenotic blood vessels may deliver a sufficient blood flow when metabolic conditions such as serum sodium and temperature are at normal levels but this blood flow may fail to meet essential requirements when metabolic conditions have changed. Thus under conditions of hyponatremia or fever, significant focal symptoms may develop. Changes in oxygenation, as in patients with pulmonary disease, and in blood glucose, as in diabetics using insulin, may also be factors in the production of focal vascular symptomatology.

INFARCTION (ENCEPHALOMALACIA)

It is appropriate at this point to briefly summarize the gross and microscopic changes which occur when ischemia has been of a sufficient degree to produce tissue death. The neuropathologist generally distinguishes between pale and hemorrhagic infarction. Most infarcts following ischemia are "pale" and are not complicated by hemorrhage. During the first 4 to 6 hours no gross or microscopic changes are apparent. Between 8 and 48 hours swelling of gray and white matter is noted; the white matter may appear somewhat granular. After 48 hours the infarcted area feels soft and mushy; the descriptive term necrosis may be used. This state may be generally recognized by visual inspection. Over the next 10 days a decrease in swelling occurs. Through enzymatic processes, liquefaction occurs. By 3 weeks, in larger lesions a gross cavity begins to appear. Within a period of several months, all of the necrotic tissue is replaced by a fluid-filled cavity.

From the microscopic standpoint indistinct staining of the neurons (which are more sensitive to anoxia than other elements, e.g., capillaries, and glia) may be noted as early as 12 hours. Within 1 to 3 days, swelling or shrinkage or alteration in the distribution of Nissl substance (chromatolysis) may be noted. Within 2 to 4 days disintegration of cells occurs. As these neuronal changes are developing, alterations are also occurring in the appearance of axons (swelling of myelin sheaths, poor staining, and disintegration) and of glial cells (swelling of astrocytes with fragmentation of processes).

While this process of necrosis is underway, various histological responses to the infarction are also taking place. Within 24 to 36 hours, the area of infarction is infiltrated by neutrophilic polymorphic leukocytes (the acute response cells). Within 24 hours of infarction, phagocytic cells (macrophages) begin to appear. These macrophages arise from various sources: microglia, blood vessel walls, circulating blood cells. By 48 hours of infarction, macrophages, filled with fatty debris (from myelin and cell breakdown), are noted. These cells remain the predominant repair cell from the period 5 days to 30 days (Fig. 22–2). Some of these cells may be found years later at the edge of the infarct. If some hemorrhagic component has also been present, products from the breakdown of the blood may also be present in these cells. This removal of debris by the macrophages will eventually result in the

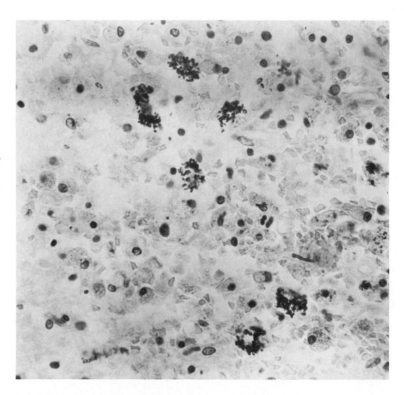

Figure 22–2 Macrophage stage of reaction in an area of necrosis. Approximately 28 days after a hemorrhagic infarct of the brain stem. Many macrophages are filled with heme pigment. (H & E × 400). (Courtesy of Dr. John Hills, New England Center Hospitals.)

appearance of the cavity which may be seen grossly.

At the same time that macrophages are removing the debris, the capillaries and astrocytes are beginning to engage in repair processes. Within several days to weeks after the infarct, new capillaries are noted at the edge of the lesion. There is also a thickening of the capillary walls with increased cellularity and the appearance of mesodermal fibrils in the adjacent tissue. There also occurs in this adjacent tissue a proliferation of astrocytes (first noted at 3 days) with the formation of reaction astrocytes containing large amounts of pink cytoplasm (in H & E stains). There is a correlated proliferation of astroglial fibers. By 4 to 5 weeks a meshwork wall has been formed about the cavity by these mesodermal and glial fibers.

The syndromes associated with ischemic-occlusive disease of each of the vessels supplying the cerebral hemispheres will now be considered in greater detail. The student, however, should interpret this material keeping in mind those limitations of correlation which have been indicated above.

INTERNAL CAROTID ARTERY

The carotid artery may be involved by atherosclerosis in its extracranial or intracranial portions (Fig. 22–1). A favorite location for stenosis in this system is at the origin of the vessel at the bifurcation of the common carotid artery into the internal and external carotid branches. Another favorite location is at the carotid siphon. The branches of the internal carotid artery are in order as follows: the ophthalmic, posterior communicating, anterior choroidal, anterior cerebral, and middle cerebral. With stenosis of the internal carotid artery, a variable symptomatology and pattern of infarction may develop (Fig. 22–3). The pattern is dependent on the availability of collateral circulation.

One syndrome involves the occurrence of repeated *episodes of monocular blindness* on the side of the involved carotid artery with the later development of motor and sensory symptoms involving the contralateral extremities.

The episodes of monocular blindness are referred to as *amaurosis fugax*. In such cases, when symptoms are limited to monocular blindness we may presume that there is ischemia predominantly in the ophthalmic artery distribution with the more distal branches temporarily receiving adequate collateral supply from the posterior communicating and anterior communicating arteries and via leptomeningeal anastomosis over the cortical surface. With progression of the occlusive process even this collateral supply becomes inadequate and additional symptoms develop.

One of the most common patterns of ca-

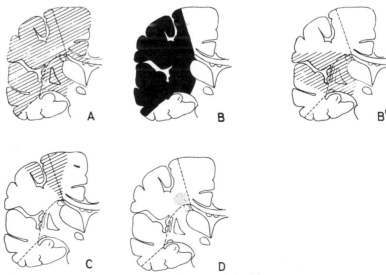

Figure 22–3 Various types of infarcts in total occlusion of carotid artery. (Autopsy sample of 52 cases of occlusions with 40 cases of infarction.) *A*, Total middle and anterior cerebral artery territory infarct—37.5%. *B*, Total middle cerebral artery territory infarct—13%. *B,'* Proximal middle cerebral territory infarct—21%. *C*, Water shed infarct—19%. *D*, Terminal infarct—5%. (Modified from Torvik, A., and Jörgensen, L.: J. Neurol. Sci., *3*:415, 1966.)

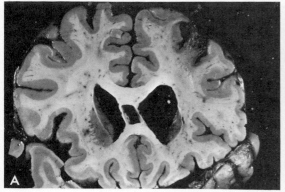

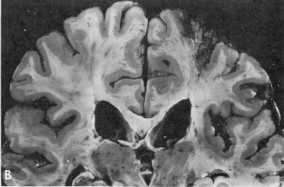

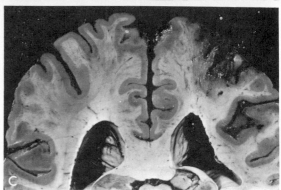

Figure 22–4 Left carotid stenosis with old infarction predominantly within the border zone between anterior and middle cerebral arteries. The major neurological deficit in this 72-year-old male related to a persistent paralysis of the right upper extremity with defective position sense at fingers. (Courtesy Dr. John Hills, New England Center Hospitals; and Dr. Jose Segarra, Boston Veterans Administration Hospital.)

See Filmstrip, Frame 44.

rotid artery insufficiency is the *carotid border-zone syndrome* (Fig. 22–4). As we have indicated, with ischemia of the carotid artery, symptoms will initially develop in the upper extremity. The patient will experience numbness and weakness involving the hand. The upper extremity corresponds to the cortical border zone between the middle and anterior cerebral arteries. With increasing stenosis and increasing ischemia there will be involvement of the face with numbness and a supranuclear type weakness. If the ischemia involves the dominant hemisphere an expressive aphasia will develop due to involvement of Broca's motor speech area. These symptoms indicate the progression to *involvement of the more central cortical supply area of the middle cerebral artery.* As a general rule, one may assume that carotid ischemia will occur predominantly over the areas of cerebral cortex within the peripheral and central supply area of the middle cerebral artery (Fig. 22–5). Involvement of the area supplied by the anterior cerebral artery is usually less marked since the anterior cerebral artery is more likely to receive a collateral supply via the anterior communicating artery and via

leptomeningeal anastomosis over the corpus callosum from the opposite anterior cerebral artery. At times, however, both the middle and anterior cerebral areas will be equally involved and infarcted.

The following case histories indicate these patterns of disease in patients with stenosis of the carotid artery. In both cases the disease was in the extracranial portion of the vessel; thus an opportunity for surgical correction of the stenotic lesion was presented. Of course, similar symptoms could have occurred with disease of the intracranial portion of the carotid artery, e.g., with stenosis at the siphon. However, in evaluating patients presenting these symptoms, the student should remain alert to the possibility that surgically remedial disease is present. The aim should be recognition of such disease when insufficiency symptoms alone are present, that is, prior to the development of actual infarction. It also should be noted that in some cases no premonitory symptoms will be present but the patient will present with the sudden onset of cortical motor and sensory disturbances involving the contralateral arm and face and to a

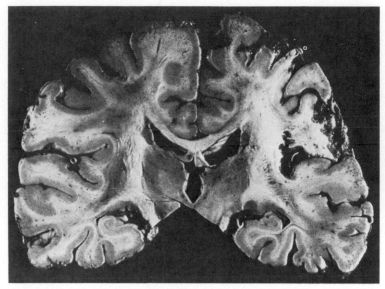

Figure 22-5 Left carotid occlusion with old infarction, predominantly of left middle cerebral territory with lesser involvement of anterior cerebral territory. This 69-year-old, right-handed male expired in 1965. The patient, in 1961 and 1963, had experienced transient episodes of right hemiparesis and aphasia, both followed by complete recovery. In 1964, a more persistent right hemiparesis and aphasia had developed. Evaluation in 1965 had revealed, in addition, an absent left carotid pulsation. Speech was nonfluent with only a small verbal output, although comprehension of spoken language was good. A marked apraxia was present in addition to a significant nominal aphasia with paraphasias. Reading was limited. Note that minor cortical infarcts are also present involving cortex of right hemisphere. (Courtesy of Dr. John Hills, New England Center Hospitals; and Dr. Jose Segarra, Boston Veterans Administration Hospital.) (See also Figure 22–10.)

lesser and variable extent the lower extremity. In some individuals, there will be marked anterior as well as middle cerebral symptoms.

Case History 1. NECH #75–66–64. Date of admission: 3/31/69.

This 54-year-old, right-handed, white male (Mr. C.B.) had experienced intermittent episodes of blurring and blacking out of vision in the left eye for at least 7 years. Each episode would last 30 to 60 seconds and would occur twice per month. Ten days prior to admission, the patient had the onset of numbness of the right side of the face accompanied by minor weakness of the right face, arm, and leg. There was also a transient difficulty in speech (possibly dysarthria, possibly difficulty in word finding). Symptoms cleared completely in 45 to 60 minutes with the exception of residual numbness of the right side of the face.

PAST HISTORY:

The patient's mother died of a "stroke" at age 66 years, and his father, of heart disease at age 57.

GENERAL PHYSICAL EXAMINATION:

1. Blood pressure was slightly increased to 160/100 in both arms.

2. Bruits (murmurs) were present over each carotid artery.

3. The retinal artery pulsation was easily obliterated by pressure on the globe of the left eye. No significant changes occurred on compression of the right globe.

4. Peripheral pulses were poor in the lower extremities.

5. Heart was normal with a normal sinus rhythm.

NEUROLOGICAL EXAMINATION:

1. *Mental status* was intact with no aphasia.

2. *Cranial nerves* were intact except for a minor right central facial weakness.

3. *Motor system* was intact as regards strength and gait.

4. *Deep tendon reflexes* were symmetrical. Plantar responses were flexor.

5. *Sensory system* was intact.

LABORATORY DATA:

1. *Hemoglobin* was normal at 15.3 grams. Serological tests (Hinton and VDRL) were

negative. Cholesterol was normal at 284 mg./100 ml.

2. *Skull and chest x-rays* were normal.

3. *Electroencephalogram* was normal.

4. *Brain scan* was normal.

5. *Arteriography* (aortic arch study) demonstrated a complete occlusion at the origin of the left internal carotid artery. A right brachial arteriogram demonstrated filling of the left anterior and middle cerebral arteries by cross flow through the anterior communicating artery from the right side. Additional studies also demonstrated filling of the intracranial portion of the left internal carotid artery from the left posterior communicating artery.

SUBSEQUENT COURSE:

A left carotid endarterectomy was performed by Dr. Allan Callow on April 10, 1969 with a restoration of blood flow following removal of the occlusive lesion (atherosclerosis with recent thrombosis) at the carotid bifurcation.

COMMENT:

The location of disease in the left carotid artery was clearly indicated by the episodes of left eye visual disturbances followed by symptoms on the contralateral side of the body. The development of symptoms in the face, with disturbance of speech is consistent with total occlusion of the carotid artery, with greater involvement of the middle cerebral territory than of the anterior cerebral territory. The fact that this patient, with progressive stenosis of the carotid artery for many years, had symptoms only in the ophthalmic-retinal artery distribution, is explained by the excellent collateral flow into the anterior and middle cerebral arteries from the anterior communicating bypass. In addition collateral flow would enter the common carotid artery from the posterior communicating artery above the take off of the ophthalmic artery.

It should be apparent that the final complex of neurological symptoms and signs, occurring with occlusion of the carotid artery, will depend on the total pattern of cerebral blood flow in the individual patient. In many patients total occlusion of the carotid artery will produce an infarction of that portion of the cerebral hemisphere supplied by the carotid artery (primarily the middle cerebral territory).

In this particular case, earlier evaluation of the patient might well have resulted in a demonstration of occlusive disease of the extracranial portion of the carotid artery prior to total occlusion. For such patients surgical therapy is feasible. To restore blood flow 20 days after occlusion as in this case is unusual.

Case History 2.   NECH #75–86–46.
Date of admission: 4/22/69.

This 52-year-old, white, right-handed priest (Mr. J.L.) had noted occasional episodes of numbness of the fingers of the right hand during the one year prior to admission. One month prior to admission the patient had a 10-minute episode of numbness (tingling, pins-and-needles sensation) from the right elbow down into the right hand, accompanied by loss of movement of the right wrist, hand, and fingers. Two days prior to admission, he had a similar episode lasting 30 minutes and had difficulty closing the right eye for 5 minutes.

PAST HISTORY:

1. The patient had sustained a myocardial infarction in 1964, (presumed coronary artery occlusion) and had been receiving anticoagulants since that time.

2. He had also been receiving medication for a high blood cholesterol level.

3. Both parents had died of heart disease.

GENERAL PHYSICAL EXAMINATION:

1. Blood pressure right arm 70/60; left arm 140/70.

2. Bruits (murmurs) were present over both carotid arteries in the neck.

3. The left retinal artery pulse was easily extinguished by pressure on the globe.

4. Peripheral pulses (posterior tibial and dorsalis pedis) in the lower extremities were reduced.

NEUROLOGICAL EXAMINATION:

1. *Mental status:* Intact.

2. *Cranial nerves:* Intact.

3. *Motor system:* Intact.

4. *Reflexes:* Intact.

5. *Sensory system:* Intact.

LABORATORY DATA:

1. Hemoglobin was normal at 14.3 grams. Serology (Hinton) was nonreactive. Cholesterol was normal at 263 mg./100 ml. Two hour postprandial blood sugar was 120 mg./100 ml.

2. Skull and chest x-rays were normal.

3. Electroencephalogram was normal.

4. Arteriograms (aortic arch study) demonstrated a narrowing (stenosis) of the left

common carotid artery at its bifurcation into the internal and external carotid arteries. In addition, a complete obstruction of the innominate artery was present. Blood from the intracranial circulation was being shunted in a retrograde manner down the right vertebral artery to supply the right subclavian artery as it passed into the right arm (termed a subclavian steal syndrome).

SUBSEQUENT COURSE:

During hospitalization the patient had several short episodes, particularly after smoking a cigarette, of numbness in the right arm. On one occasion this was accompanied by aphasia.

COMMENT:

This patient certainly had stenosis of the left carotid artery. The episodes of ischemia experienced by the patient certainly indicated primary involvement of the carotid border zone, that area between the primary supplies of the middle and anterior cerebral arteries—the area of hand representation. It is evident, however, that in this case, as in many cases of cerebral vascular disease, one cannot understand the development of symptoms simply in relation to the state of one vessel. Rather the development of symptoms is dependent on the total pattern of cerebral blood supply.

The occlusion of the innominate artery in this case or of the proximal subclavian artery in other cases may result in a situation in which blood is shunted down the vertebral artery in a retrograde manner to supply the portion of the subclavian artery distal to the point of obstruction. The central nervous system symptoms which develop under these circumstances may be variable, at times reflecting shunting of blood from the brain stem, at times reflecting shunting of blood from the carotid circulation via the posterior communicating artery.

This patient also demonstrates another point of importance; patients with atherosclerotic disease involving the large and medium sized cerebral vessels do not have disease simply limited to their extracranial and intracranial cerebral vessels, but also have disease involving vessels in other parts of the body, e.g., coronary arteries, femoral arteries, and so forth.

MIDDLE CEREBRAL ARTERY

As we have indicated the middle cerebral artery is the final branch and, in a sense, the direct continuation of the internal carotid artery. One of the classic internal carotid artery syndromes is essentially a syndrome of the cortical branches of the middle cerebral artery.

Depending on the point of occlusion of the middle cerebral artery and its branches several syndromes are possible. Essentially these syndromes reflect disease of the lenticulostriate penetrating branches or the cortical branches. In some cases, the clinical picture reflects involvement of the territory of both penetrating and cortical branches.

Syndrome of the Lenticulostriate Penetrating Branches. These branches (Fig. 22–6) supply the putamen, most of the caudate nucleus, the outer portion of the globus pallidus, and most of the adjacent internal capsule (particularly the anterior half of the posterior limb). These vessels ascend with no anastomotic loops between adjacent branches.

The classic clinical picture associated with occlusion of these branches is that of the pure motor syndrome, relatively rapid in onset, involving equally the face, arm, and leg in a spastic hemiplegia (so-called capsular hemiplegia). As discussed by Fisher and Curry (1965), there are often no sensory symptoms and no aphasia. These hemiplegic symptoms, reflecting capsular damage, tend to predominate initially over any extrapyramidal symptoms, although portions of the basal ganglia may also be infarcted. The patient may demonstrate a rapid improvement, so that within months, there is little if any residual motor disability.*

Additional penetrating branches, however, tend to be occluded in the same or the contralateral hemisphere. The patient then begins to manifest a typical clinical syndrome which has been assigned the name "lacunar state," based on the findings at the time of pathological examination of multiple small cavities (Fig. 22–7). The patient begins to manifest an apraxia of gait, and a release of grasp reflex occurs as a result of damage to the descending fibers from the premotor areas. An extrapyramidal type of rigidity and a slowness of movement develop with, at times, a minor degree of tremor. These symptoms may reflect the damage to the

---

*As indicated in Figure 22–6, however, larger infarcts, involving the lenticulostriate territory, may result in a persistent spastic hemiplegia with considerable motor deficits.

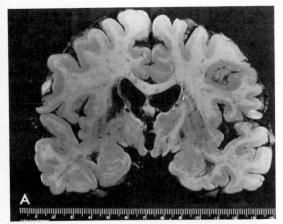

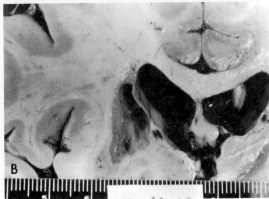

Figure 22–6 Lenticulostriate penetrating branches of the middle cerebral artery. *A,* The pattern of an old infarction within the distribution of these branches is indicated. *B* is a close-up of the areas of infarction demonstrating the details of the cavity formed in the late stage of infarction. This 73-year-old white male, in relation to hypertension at age 53, had sustained a right hemiplegia with persistent and dense motor deficits involving the right central face, arm, and leg. (Courtesy of Dr. John Hills, New England Center Hospitals; and Dr. Jose Segarra, Boston Veterans Administration Hospital.)

See Filmstrip, Frame 45.

putamen and globus pallidus or, perhaps, damage to the descending fibers from the premotor areas.

This aspect of the syndrome has sometimes been designated as arteriosclerotic Parkinson's disease. There may be a variable degree of dementia. This dementia probably reflects the fact that the basic pathological process involves as well small infarcts in subcortical white matter. However, as Fisher (1965) has indicated, the patients are often elderly, and a coincidental senile dementia with loss of cortical neurons may be present in some cases. (Refer to Chapter 27.)

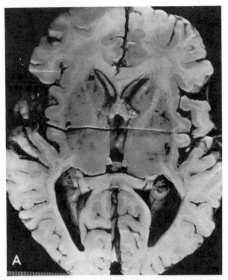

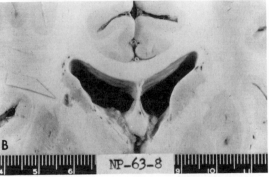

Figure 22–7 Lacunar state. *A,* Multiple small infarctions in territories of the middle cerebral penetrating branches are demonstrated. This 71-year-old hypertensive (210/116) had episodes of right hemiparesis and dysarthria 11 years and 8 years prior to death in 1965. The patient had frequent dizzy spells with loss of consciousness and 2 years prior to death became wheelchair bound. Evaluation in 1965 demonstrated significant dysarthria without actual naming defects. An inappropriate jocularity and incontinence of urine was present. Apraxia of lips, limbs, and gait was present. Bilateral limb weakness was present with bilateral hyperreflexia, hyperactive jaw jerk, and bilateral extensor plantar responses. A bilateral grasp reflex was present. (Courtesy of Dr. John Hills, and Dr. Jose Segarra, *B,* Detail of a small lacune from another patient, a 48-year-old white male, with severe hypertension (250/140). (Courtesy of Dr. John Hills, New England Center Hospitals; and Dr. Jose Segarra, Boston Veterans Administration Hospital.)

The basic pathological process is termed segmental fibrinoid arterial degeneration. The walls of these small vessels become thickened and converted into a hyalinized material. Invariably this occurs on a background of long-standing hypertension and atherosclerosis. The lenticulostriate branches rising as the initial branches of the middle cerebral artery are under relatively high pressure; not only may these vessels become occluded, they may be the site of large intracerebral hemorrhages also complicating the process of hypertension. We shall have cause to discuss these vessels again later in this chapter.

Syndromes of the Cortical Branches.
(Figs. 22–8 and 22–9). The main stem of the middle cerebral artery divides into two main cortical divisions: a superior division and an inferior division. At the point of division, the smaller lateral orbital frontal and temporal polar arteries originate. The superior division has pre-Rolandic branches (to inferior frontal gyrus and premotor area including Broca's area in dominant hemisphere), Rolandic branches (to pre- and postcentral gyri), and anterior parietal branches (to postcentral gyrus). The inferior division includes anterior temporal, posterior parietal, angular and posterior temporal branches, named after the areas supplied. The syndrome which results from occlusion will depend on whether the main stem, the superior or inferior division, or the branches thereof have been involved.

In general, the most commonly encountered syndrome relates to occlusion of the main stem, producing a mixed motor cortical sensory syndrome involving the contralateral face (supranuclear) and arm; this is termed a faciobrachial paralysis. If this occurred in the dominant hemisphere a mixed type of aphasia would also be present with expressive and receptive components. Face and language involvement would be greater to a variable degree than hand involvement.

The degree to which the hand is involved would depend on the degree of collateral circulation. Thus only the central cortical territory or the entire cortical territory of the middle cerebral artery could be involved.

Occlusion of the superior division in the dominant hemispheres would produce a mixed motor-cortical sensory syndrome involving again predominantly the face and hand plus an expressive Broca's type aphasia. This syndrome is well illustrated in Chapter 21 by case history #8 (Mrs. E.C.) in which superior division branches (predominantly preRolandic and Rolandic) were occluded by embolic material. It should be noted that the cortical branches of the left middle cerebral artery are a frequent site for the lodgment of embolic material. This probably follows from the relatively direct vertical take-off of the left common carotid artery from the arch of the aorta and the fact that the middle cerebral artery is the direct continuation of the internal carotid artery; the cortical branches are the direct continuation of the main middle cerebral trunk.

For the clinical manifestations of occlusion of the inferior division branches, which occur less frequently, the reader should refer back to the chapter on cortical localization.

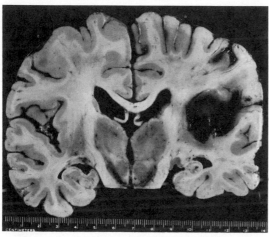

Figure 22–8 Cortical branches of the middle cerebral artery. Acute hemorrhagic infarction of the central cortical territory. This 74-year-old, right-handed, white male, 5 days prior to death, had the sudden onset of pain in the left supraorbital region and lost consciousness. Upon regaining consciousness, the patient had a right central facial weakness and a right hemiparesis. He was described as responsive, e.g., able to follow commands, but mute. Speech was never regained and the patient subsequently lost the ability to follow verbal commands. At autopsy, the left carotid artery was found to be occluded at the bifurcation, but in addition, calcific material was present occluding the lumen of the left middle cerebral artery (possibly embolic). (Courtesy of Dr. John Hills, New England Center Hospitals; and Dr. Jose Segarra, Boston Veterans Administration Hospital.)

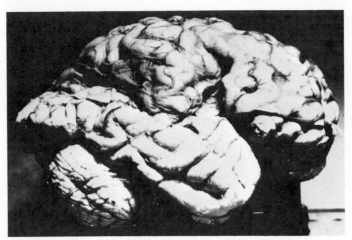

Figure 22–9 Cortical branches of the middle cerebral artery. Old infarcts involving much of the total cortical territory of the right middle cerebral artery. This 72-year-old, right-handed male with severe hypertension and auricular fibrillation expired in 1963. In 1960 he had a sudden episode of left central facial weakness and left hemiplegia. In 1962, the patient experienced another episode of left hemiparesis with more severe involvement of arm and face than of leg. In 1963, the patient developed focal seizures of the left arm with worsening of the paralysis of the left arm. (Courtesy of Dr. John Hills, New England Center Hospitals; and Dr. Jose Segarra, Boston Veterans Administration Hospital.)

See Filmstrip, Frame 46.

Combined Syndrome: Total Occlusion of Initial Segment of Middle Cerebral Artery. (Fig. 22–10). The resultant syndrome in this case will be the summation of the lenticulostriate and cortical branches syndrome. The following case history illustrates such an occlusion with massive infarction of the entire territory of the middle cerebral artery.

Case History 3.   NECH #197–686.
Date of admission: 10/13/68.

This 61-year-old, right-handed Negro housewife (Mrs. B.W.), one week prior to admission, suddenly fell to the floor while taking a bath and lost consciousness. She was picked up off the floor by her son who found that she was unable to move her left arm and leg. She was unable to walk and had regained no function in these extremities. Her speech had been thick, but no aphasia had been present. No headache had been noted.

PAST HISTORY: Hypertension had been present for three years. Five days prior to admission, she had been switched to a new antihypertensive medication. There was no history of heart disease. Both parents had died of heart disease and hypertension.

GENERAL PHYSICAL EXAMINATION:
Blood pressure was 150/100, the pulse was 84 and regular.

NEUROLOGICAL EXAMINATION:

1. *Mental status:* The patient was obtunded and slow to respond. However, she was grossly oriented to time, place, and person.
2. *Cranial nerves:*
   a. The head and eyes were deviated to the right. On vestibular stimulation, the eyes could be moved to the left; however, the patient could not move the eyes to the left on command.
   b. The patient neglected stimuli in the left visual field. The pupils did respond to light.
   c. Papilledema was present bilaterally particularly in the right fundus where a recent hemorrhage was present.
   d. There was a decrease in pain sensation or a neglect of painful stimuli on the left side of the face.
   e. A marked left central facial weakness was present.
3. *Motor system:*
   a. A complete flaccid paralysis of the left arm and leg was present.
   b. The patient was unable to sit up without support.
4. *Reflexes:*
   a. Deep tendon reflexes were increased on the left compared to the right.

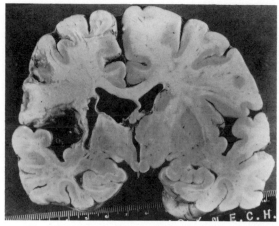

Figure 22–10 Left carotid occlusion: combined syndrome of middle cerebral artery; cortical and lenticulostriate branches. An old infarct has involved almost all of the territory of the cortical and deep branches of the left middle cerebral artery. This 62-year-old, left-handed, white male expired in April 1964. In August 1963, during a left radical neck dissection for treatment of epidermoid carcinoma of the tongue, the left common carotid artery was clamped and excised. The patient regained consciousness without an apparent hemiparesis but 8 hours later a weakness of right hand grip was noted. Over the next 24 hours, a complete right hemiparesis with right central facial weakness gradually evolved. Two weeks later, right facial weakness was more marked. There was no effective function of the right hand, although the right lower extremity showed only minimal deficits. Speech was limited to grunts, related in part to the surgical involvement of the tongue and recurrent laryngeal nerve. The patient was unable to comprehend spoken speech, wrote jargon with his left hand, but was able to copy. (Courtesy of Dr. John Hills, New England Center Hospitals; and Dr. Jose Segarra, Boston Veterans Administration Hospital.)

See Filmstrip, Frame 47.

b. The left plantar response was extensor.

5. *Sensory system:*

All modalities of sensation were decreased on the left side of the body.

LABORATORY DATA:

1. *Chest and skull x-rays* were negative.

2. *Electrocardiograms* showed left ventricular hypertrophy.

3. *Electroencephalogram* on October 15, 1968 indicated focal damage throughout the right hemisphere—most prominent in the right frontal area, (focal 3 to 5 cps slow waves). In addition there was a relative absence of electrical activity in the right temporal area (Fig. 22–11).

4. *Brain scan* on October 16, 1968 showed a significant but diffuse uptake of isotope (Hg^{197}) in the right hemisphere. A repeat brain scan on October 22, 1968 showed a more marked uptake measuring $11 \times 6 \times 6$ cm., extending from the right frontal area to the posterior parietal area. Uptake extended from the surface to the deep midline (Fig. 22–12).

5. Cerebrospinal fluid contained no significant cells. Protein was moderately increased to 57 mg./100 ml. Pressure at the lumbar area was 150 mm. of water.

6. Right brachial arteriogram revealed a complete occlusion of the right middle cerebral artery at its origin (Fig. 22–13).

HOSPITAL COURSE:

The patient showed no significant improvement during a 4-week hospital course.

COMMENT:

The patient had a sudden occlusion of the right middle cerebral artery with massive infarction of the entire area of the right hemisphere supplied by the middle cerebral artery. Such massive infarctions are often, as in this case, associated with a significant degree of cerebral edema with the development of papilledema. At times the degree of swelling of the cerebral hemisphere may be sufficient to displace the pineal or the anterior cerebral artery. It is also possible in this case that the infarct was secondarily hemorrhagic. In many cases of hemorrhagic infarction the spinal fluid does not contain red blood cells.

The equal involvement of face, arm, and leg was consistent with the involvement of the penetrating branches of the middle cerebral artery with resultant infarction in the posterior limb of the internal capsule. The deviation of head and eyes to the right indicates destruction of area 8 of the right hemisphere or of the fibers descending from this area, through the corona radiata. Involvement of the cortex in addition to the internal capsule is also indicated by the findings on the brain scan and electroencephalogram and by the neglect of visual and tactile stimuli on the left side.

ANTERIOR CEREBRAL ARTERY

In our clinical experience occlusive disease of the anterior cerebral artery is much less

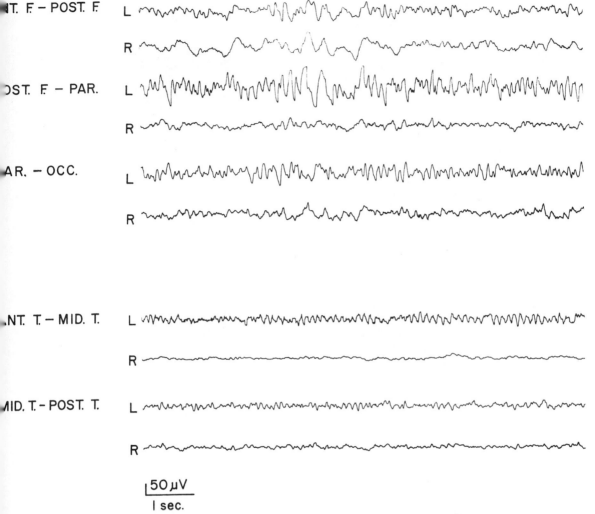

ANT. F. – POST. F.

POST. F. – PAR.

PAR. – OCC.

ANT. T. – MID. T.

MID. T. – POST. T.

50 μV

I sec.

Figure 22–11 Case History 3. Right middle cerebral artery occlusion: electroencephalogram. Bipolar recordings of 10/15/68 demonstrating focal 3–5 slow wave activity throughout right hemisphere, most prominent in right frontal area. In addition, a relative absence of electrical activity is demonstrated in the right temporal area. Note that there is some spread of slow wave activity into left frontal parasagittal areas. ANT. F. = anterior frontal (parasagittal); POST. F. = posterior frontal (parasagittal); PAR. = parietal; OCC. = occipital; ANT. T. = anterior temporal; MID. T. = midtemporal; POST. T. = posterior temporal.

common than that involving the internal carotid or middle cerebral arteries. The antomical explanation for this is evident. Each anterior cerebral receives collateral circulation from several possible sources: (a) leptomeningeal anastomotic end-to-end loops from the middle cerebral artery of the same side, (b) leptomeningeal anastomotic loops from the contralateral anterior cerebral artery over the corpus callosum, and (c) anterior communicating artery from the contralateral anterior cerebral artery. Finally, at postmortem examination atherosclerotic plaques are found less frequently in the anterior cerebral than in the larger, internal carotid, middle cerebral, basilar, and vertebral arteries. The branches of the anterior cerebral artery (the penetrating, the orbital, frontal, frontal polar, callosal marginal, and pericallosal arteries) supply the anterior limb of the internal capsule, the anterior head of the caudate nucleus, much of the corpus callosum (genu and body), and the orbital frontal cortex, the medial aspects of the frontal and parietal lobes including the sensory motor areas of the para-

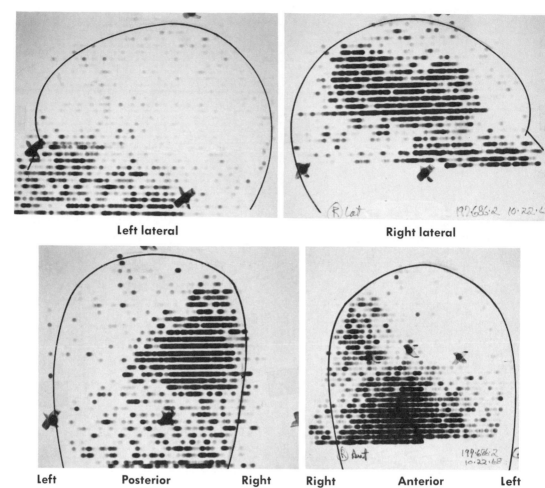

Left lateral　　　　　　　　　　　**Right lateral**

Left　　　Posterior　　　Right　　　Right　　　Anterior　　　Left

Figure 22–12 Brain scan. Case History 3. Right middle cerebral artery occlusion: 10/22/68. A marked uptake of isotope (Hg^{197}) is found throughout the territory of the right middle cerebral artery. This is demonstrated in the posterior, anterior, and right lateral scans. (Courtesy of Dr. Bertram Selverstone.)

central lobule. Symptoms then when they occur will be most severe in the contralateral lower extremity with minor involvement of the contralateral upper extremity and no involvement of the face.

At times both anterior cerebral arteries may be essentially branches of the same proximal segment. Occlusion of this proximal anterior cerebral artery segment will then result in infarction of the medial frontal-parietal areas of both hemispheres. The resultant syndrome will include a change in personality and affect (due to involvement of the prefrontal and anterior cingulate areas), an akinetic and mute state (due to involvement of the prefrontal and premotor areas), urinary incontinence (due to involve-

ment of the paracentral lobule, medial premotor, and supplementary motor areas), and a sensory motor syndrome involving both lower extremities (due to involvement of paracentral lobule) (Figs. 22–14 and 22–15). There may also be a significant apraxia of the nondominant hand from damage to the corpus callosum depriving the premotor and motor areas in the nondominant motor hemisphere of information from the dominant hemisphere. A bilateral release of the grasp reflex is present because of the bilateral involvement of the premotor and supplementary motor areas. An example of infarction in the distribution of the anterior cerebral arteries complicating aneurysm surgery is provided in case history #6 (p. 563).

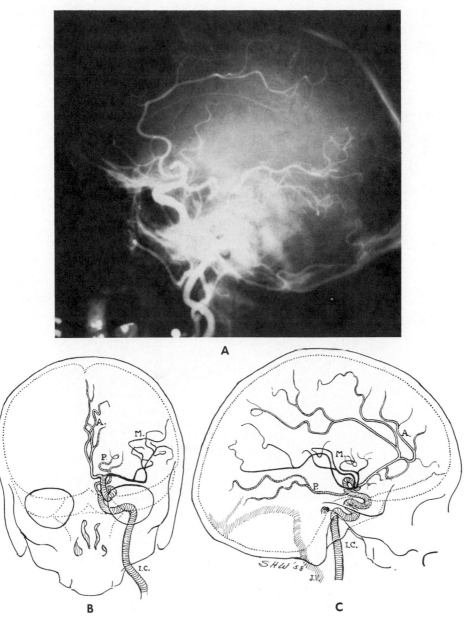

Figure 22–13 Case History 3. Total occlusion, right middle cerebral artery. *A*, Right brachial arteriogram (lateral view). Selective common carotid injection reveals total right middle cerebral artery occlusion. (Courtesy of Dr. Samuel Wolpert.) *B*, Reference diagram of the major branches of the internal carotid artery. Anterior and lateral views of the head showing the main divisions of the internal carotid artery traced from x-ray plates of a patient following intra-arterial injection of a radiopaque suspension. *IC*, internal carotid artery (cross-banded); *A*, anterior cerebral artery (outlined); *P*, posterior cerebral artery (cross-banded); *M*, middle cerebral artery (solid black). In the lateral view posteriorly (shown in cross banding with no outline) are seen the transverse sinus and sigmoid sinus extending downward into the internal jugular vein, *JV*. (From Ranson, S. W., and Clark, S. L.: *The Anatomy of the Nervous System*. Philadelphia, W. B. Saunders, 1959, p. 63.)

Note that in all illustrations the posterior cerebral artery is supplied directly from the carotid artery.

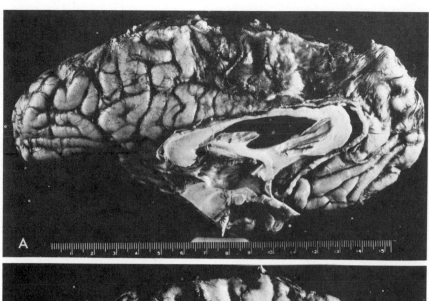

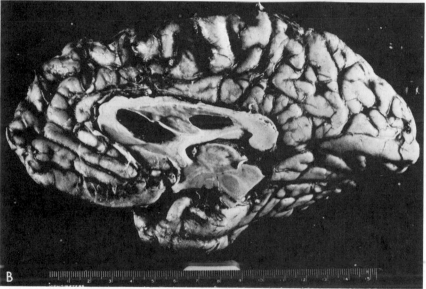

Figure 22–14 Anterior cerebral arteries: old bilateral infarcts. Left hemisphere involvement was marked (*A*), with a lesser involvement of the right hemisphere (*B*). This 61-year-old, right-handed female expired in October 1964. In June 1963, the patient had the onset of difficulty in speech, right-sided weakness, and an apraxia of hand movements. Several days later she developed a difficulty in walking and became mute. Shortly thereafter, urinary incontinence and stupor developed. The akinetic mute state became more prominent after an episode of fever. The patient was described as remaining in bed with eyes open and unable to move extremities or to comprehend. At autopsy, there was severe atherosclerosis of all vessels at the base of the brain (Fig. 22–15). The right anterior cerebral artery was completely occluded. (Courtesy of Dr. John Hills, New England Center Hospitals; and Dr. Jose Segarra, Boston Veterans Administration Hospital.) See Filmstrip, Frame 48.

ANTERIOR CHOROIDAL ARTERY

This is the only branch of the internal carotid artery which has not yet been discussed. This vessel supplies the inner portion of the globus pallidus and a small adjacent section of the internal capsule (the area occupied by the ansa and fasciculus lentic-ularis). At the present time in the clinical situation, no definite syndrome has been associated with occlusion of this vessel. However, the initial surgical procedures of Cooper indicated that occlusion of this vessel in the patient with Parkinson's disease resulted in a relief of tremor and rigidity in the contralateral limbs. No significant focal deficits,

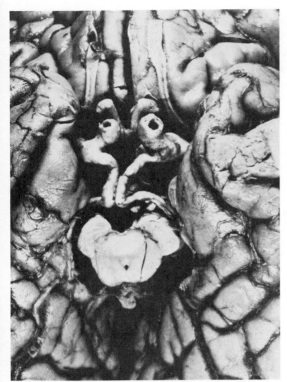

Figure 22–15 Severe atherosclerosis of all arteries of circle of Willis at base of brain. (Refer to Figure 22–14.) As indicated in this case the anterior cerebral arteries were severely involved with occlusion of right anterior cerebral and bilateral infarcts in the anterior cerebral territories. (Courtesy of Dr. John Hills, New England Center Hospitals; and Dr. Jose Segarra, Boston Veterans Administration Hospital.) **See Filmstrip, Frame 43.**

such as hemiparesis, developed. This procedure was soon superseded by the less complicated and more effective operation of stereotaxic chemopallidectomy and chemo- or cryothalamectomy. The rationale for these various surgical procedures will be discussed in the chapter on the motor system (p. 682).

POSTERIOR CEREBRAL ARTERY

The posterior cerebral arteries originate as the direct continuation of the basilar artery following its bifurcation. At times, then, occlusive disease of the vertebral or basilar artery will be manifested by the development of symptoms within the posterior cerebral territory. At times, a mixture of brain stem and cerebral hemisphere symptoms will be present. At times, bilateral posterior cerebral artery symptoms will be present. More-

over, since the cortical and penetrating vessels of the posterior cerebral artery are the distal branches of the basilar vertebral circulation, they will at times be subject to embolization from extracerebral sources or from occlusive disease in the more proximal sections of the basilar artery. Essentially two categories of posterior cerebral symptomatology may be recognized: (a) syndromes of the penetrating branches, and (b) syndromes of the cortical branches. With main trunk occlusions, a mixture of these two syndromes may be present.

Syndromes of the Penetrating Branches The penetrating or perforating branches of the posterior cerebral artery supply the rostral portion of the midbrain and the thalamus. Those syndromes following occlusion of the more medially placed penetrating vessels to the midbrain have been discussed previously in the consideration of brain stem disease. These syndromes reflect damage to the cerebral peduncle, the third cranial nerve, and the red nucleus. Several syndromes of occlusion of the perforating branch supplying the subthalamus and ventrolateral nucleus of the thalamus may result in contralateral movement disorders: hemichorea or hemiballismus. (These syndromes will be discussed in greater detail in Chapter 24: Basal Ganglia.) Occlusion of the penetrating branch to the ventral posterior nucleus (the thalamogeniculate artery) results in a loss of contralateral sensation. With repetitive tactile stimulation, painful sensations (dysesthesias) often result; spontaneous pains may also occur in the contralateral extremities. This "thalamic syndrome" is also termed the Dejerine-Roussy syndrome.

Syndromes of the Cortical Branches (Fig. 22–16). Various branches (anterior temporal and posterior temporal) supply the inferior and medial surfaces of the temporal lobe. The posterior cerebral artery then divides into a parieto-occipital branch (which usually follows the parietal occipital sulcus) and the calcarine artery which follows the calcarine sulcus to supply the visual (calcarine) cortex. Those medial areas of the temporal lobe within the posterior cerebral territory are concerned with the learning of new information (recent memory). With bilateral posterior cerebral disease marked impairment of recent memory may occur, with a significant degree of confusion and

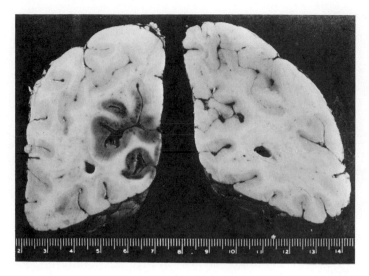

Figure 22–16 Posterior cerebral artery: acute hemorrhagic infarction has occurred predominantly within the distribution of the right calcarine branch. This 53-year-old male had a right frontal-anterior temporal glioma. Tentorial herniation occurred with compression of the right posterior cerebral artery (in addition to brain stem structures). (Courtesy of Dr. John Hills, New England Center Hospitals; and Dr. Jose Segarra, Boston Veterans Administration Hospital.)

See Filmstrip, Frame 49.

disorientation. (At times, a confusional state may follow unilateral posterior cerebral disease if the dominant temporal lobe is involved.) This resultant amnestic confabulatory syndrome will be considered in greater detail in the chapter on memory. It should be noted that at times the occurrence of this syndrome in disease of the posterior cerebral arteries may reflect damage to the medial thalamic areas. The role of this area in recent memory will also be discussed later (Chapter 27).

The effect of ischemia or infarction within the calcarine artery territory is a contralateral homonymous hemianopsia. There is often a sparing of the macular area due to collateral circulation to that portion of the area of macular representation at the occipital pole.

The following case history illustrates many aspects of ischemia within the cortical distribution of the posterior cerebral arteries. Bilateral posterior cerebral ischemia was present transiently at the onset with more severe residual symptoms reflecting unilateral posterior cerebral disease.

Case History 4. NECH #15–86–24. Date of admission: 5/25/67.

This 75-year-old, white, right-handed widow (Mrs. M.U.) developed sudden headache on the day prior to admission, with nausea, vomiting, and a poorly described bilateral disturbance of vision. She was found by a relative the morning of admission complaining of total blindness and of severe headache. She was noted to be confused and incoherent (believed she was in New Jersey rather than Massachusetts). She was able to walk only with assistance.

PAST HISTORY: A minor degree of hypertension had been noted several days prior to admission.

PHYSICAL EXAMINATION:

1. Blood pressure was slightly elevated at 170/100.

2. Examination of the heart revealed no significant findings.

3. The patient was obese.

4. She was holding her head complaining of headache.

NEUROLOGICAL EXAMINATION:

1. *Mental status:*

a. The patient was restless and disoriented for time and place.

b. There were difficulties in cooperation so that detailed testing of mental status could not be performed.

c. Simple calculations were poorly performed.

d. Digit span was markedly limited.

e. There was no left-right confusion and no evidence of aphasia.

2. *Cranial nerves:*

a. Initially the patient was unable to detect objects (e.g., a face or lights) in either visual field. Within six hours, a change had occurred. Although conjugate extraocular movements were full, the patient tended to keep her eyes deviated to the right and failed to follow objects introduced from the periphery of the left visual field. The eyes could be deviated to the left on command.

   c. The pupils responded to light.

3. *Motor system:*

   a. Strength was grossly intact.

   b. A slight unsteadiness (ataxia) of gait was present.

4. *Reflexes:*

   a. Deep tendon reflexes were grossly symmetrical.

   b. A Babinski response was present on the left; a probable Babinski sign was also present on the right.

5. *Sensory system:*

All modalities were intact.

LABORATORY DATA:

1. Hematocrit was normal.

2. Total cholesterol was slightly elevated to 312 mg./100 ml.

3. The glucose tolerance test was consistent with diabetes mellitus.

4. Chest and skull x-rays were normal.

5. The electrocardiogram was normal.

6. The electroencephalogram demonstrated focal 3 to 4 cps slow waves in the right posterior parietal occipital area with rare slow waves in the right posterior temporal area consistent with focal damage in this area (Fig. 22–17).

7. Lumbar puncture indicated clear spinal fluid with no cells and a normal protein of 18 mg./ml.

HOSPITAL COURSE:

The patient had a significant improvement in headache and a clearing of confusion with a return of mental status to her normal level. Her hospital stay was prolonged by the development of thrombophlebitis of the left femoral vein. At the time of hospital discharge, one month after admission, there was still a residual left field defect (homonymous hemianopsia) with preservation of vision in the macular area (macular sparing). Follow-up evaluation approximately 14 months after discharge indicated no significant neurological findings except for the residual left field defect (homonymous hemianopsia with macular sparing) (Fig. 22–18).

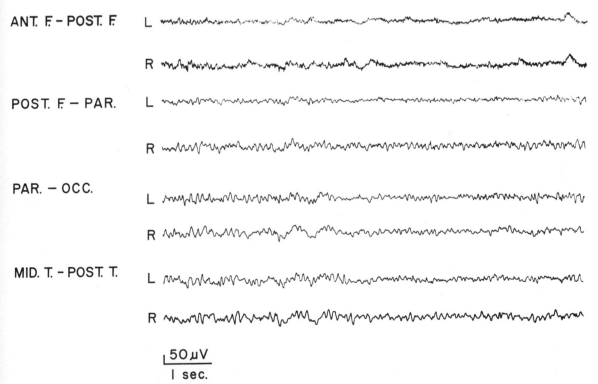

ANT. F. – POST. F. L   R

POST. F. – PAR. L   R

PAR. – OCC. L   R

MID. T. – POST. T. L   R

50 μV

1 sec.

Figure 22–17 Case History 4. Occlusion of right posterior cerebral artery. Electroencephalogram: May 5, 1967 (Bipolar). Occasional focal slow waves were noted in right parietal occipital and right posterior temporal areas. ANT. F. = anterior parasagittal frontal; POST. F. = posterior parasagittal frontal; PAR. = parietal; OCC. = occipital; MID. T. = midtemporal; POST. T. = posterior temporal.

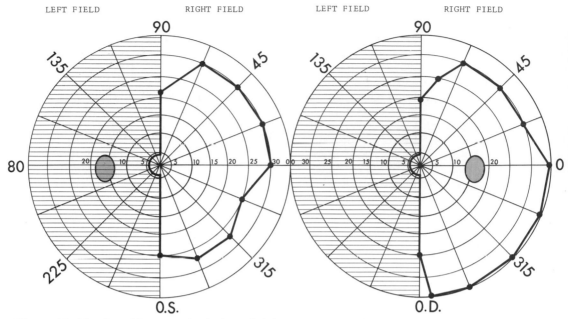

Figure 22–18 Case history 4. Occlusion of right posterior cerebral artery. Tangent screen examination of visual fields. Fields on August 26, 1968, demonstrating a residual left homonymous hemianopsia with macular sparing. O.S. = left eye; O.D. = right eye.

COMMENT:

The initial symptom of total blindness suggested bilateral posterior cerebral ischemia. The development of confusion and disorientation is also consistent with bilateral posterior cerebral ischemia. The nausea, vomiting, and minor ataxia of gait may well have indicated ischemia of the brain stem, suggesting that the basic occlusive process may have originated at a lower point in the basilar artery. The residual and most severe degree of involvement was certainly within the territory of the right calcarine artery.

The occurrence of severe headache is not usually considered in connection with ischemic-occlusive disease. A review of our cases of posterior cerebral occlusion indicates that the occurrence of severe headache is often a prominent symptom. Often in these cases prior to lumbar puncture, the diagnosis of subarachnoid hemorrhage was considered.

As regards management of patients with atherosclerotic ischemic-occlusive disease the student should consult texts such as Harrison or Merritt or the following references: Bauer et al., 1969; Browne and Poskanzer, 1969; Fields, 1970; Toole and Patel, 1967. For most patients who have suffered infarcts, there are no specific curative ther-

apies. Some patients with transient ischemic episodes will have treatable extracranial vascular disease (particularly in the carotid distribution) which will benefit from surgical correction of the stenosis or occlusion. Some with vertebral basilar transient ischemic episodes will benefit from anticoagulation therapy. (For a discussion of ischemic-occlusive disease involving the basilar-vertebral circulation, the student should refer to Chapter 15.)

CEREBRAL EMBOLISM

In general, cerebral embolism is a complication of cardiovascular disease. However, as we have indicated, at times embolization of atheromatous material may occur from areas of stenosis in the aorta or extracranial vessels. Rarely emboli may be composed of tumor cells or, following trauma, of fat or air. The embolus in most cases is a fragment of thrombus (clot, platelets, fibrin, and blood cells) which has become detached from a larger thrombus within the heart. The causes of such a thrombus within the heart are several: (a) a clot will often form in the left auricular appendage when atrial fibrillation is present. This is often the case when a relative stasis of blood in this area occurs as in mitral stenosis. (b) A "mural thrombus" may form on the endocardium in relation to an area of myocardial infarction. (c) Thrombus may collect on heart valves (so called valvular vegetations), usually the mitral valve, when these valves are the subject of infection and inflammation as in bacterial endocarditis. Sudden changes in cardiac rhythm as may occur when the fibrillating heart returns to a normal sinus rhythm may result in embolic material breaking off and entering into the circulation.

Multiple small emboli may occur to many cerebral vessels to produce a syndrome of multiple small vessel occlusion with a resultant clinical picture of dementia, alteration in personality, and so forth. Patients with multiple cerebral emboli also have embolization to extracerebral areas as well, such as the femoral artery, the kidney, the spleen, and the skin. Emboli to the kidney will often be detected following the sudden appearance of red blood cells in the urine (hematuria).

From the standpoint of anatomical localization we are more concerned with a single larger embolus. Such emboli occlude vessels and produce syndromes which follow the patterns indicated in the section above on ischemic-occlusive disease. As we have already indicated certain vessels are particularly the target of cerebral emboli. The cortical and, to a lesser extent, the penetrating branches of the middle cerebral artery (particularly the left middle cerebral artery) are perhaps the most frequent site of lodgement for the reasons we have cited. In this regard the student may wish to review Case History 8 (Mrs. E.C.) in Chapter 21. In the posterior circulation the posterior cerebral artery and its penetrating branches are the favored sites of embolization.

Several points should be considered in differentiating embolic from true ischemic-occlusive disease:

a. Perhaps most important is the fact that embolic occlusion of a vessel is sudden. In general there are no preceding transient ischemic events. At times the event may be so sudden that the patient stops speaking in midsentence with a complete loss of speech. One should of course note that the same vessel may be subject to several episodes of embolization; each of these episodes, however, would represent a sudden event. On the other hand, infarction due to ischemic-occlusive disease is often preceded by one or more transient episodes of ischemia.

b. Since embolic occlusions are sudden, the event is often accompanied by a loss of consciousness or a seizure which may be focal or generalized.

c. Embolic occlusions may occur during any time of the day and often during periods of activity. Ischemic-occlusive infarctions tend to occur during sleep when blood pressure is relatively lower or shortly after arising in relation perhaps to transient falls in blood pressure.

d. Infarction due to embolic occlusion of a vessel is more likely to be hemorrhagic than a nonembolic infarction. (Most embolic infarctions, however, do not result in a hemorrhagic infarction.) The development of secondary hemorrhage into an area of infarction may relate to the disintegration of the embolic material with its subsequent passage into more distal branches. However, there will then be perfusion of an area of recent necrosis. In such an area, the walls of blood vessels have also been ischemic and recently damaged. Such vessels when again perfused under a normal head of pressure will then leak blood into the surrounding tissues. Evidence of this hemorrhage may appear in the spinal fluid as red blood cells or discoloration caused by products resulting from the breakdown of blood (xanthochromia).

e. Infarctions due to embolic occlusions are also often subject to rapid improvement because with the disintegration of embolic material blood flow is restored.

The treatment of cerebral emboli involves the prevention of additional embolic episodes. Assuming that hemorrhagic infarction has not occurred, this may involve the use of anticoagulants. At times, cardiac surgery may be considered to remove a large thrombus in the atrial appendage. At times, following anticoagulation, attempts will be made to restore the cardiac rhythm to normal sinus.

INTRACEREBRAL HEMORRHAGE

Hemorrhage into the brain may occur as a complication of various hematological problems which are characterized by bleeding disorders, e.g., leukemia. Bleeding into the brain may also occur in relation to intracranial tumors (such as glioblastomas or metastatic malignancy) or as the complication of the rupture of a saccular aneurysm with extension of blood from the subarachnoid space into the substance of the cerebral hemisphere. In general, however, the term intracerebral hemorrhage is applied to those massive and medium-sized hemorrhages which occur in patients with hypertension (elevated blood pressure). Occasionally, blood pressure is normal. Patients with intracerebral hemorrhages are seen less commonly on general neurological and neurosurgical services than patients with occlusive vascular disease and those with subarachnoid hemorrhage. Patients with intracerebral hemorrhage are, however, not uncommon when acute general medical admissions and autopsies are considered.

The basic pathogenesis involved in intracranial hemorrhage is not certain. There is certainly a predilection for certain areas of the brain. Approximately 60 per cent involve the lenticular nucleus, particularly the putamen (Fig. 22–19). (These are termed lateral ganglionic mass hemorrhages.) There is often spread to involve the internal and external capsules. The bleeding is pre-sumed to occur from penetrating branches of the middle cerebral artery (the lenticulo-striate branches). We have noted previously that these same vessels are involved in a process of occlusion in hypertension—segmental fibrinoid necrosis with the development of a pure motor syndrome involving the face, arm, and leg. The second most common site within the cerebral hemisphere is the thalamus, particularly the posterior portion where hemorrhage occurs, from penetrating branches of the posterior cerebral artery. A third area is the subcortical white matter particularly at the origin of the temporal lobe or in the occipital lobe. Other sites are the tegmentum of the pons and the cerebellum.

The fact that the lenticulostriate arteries, which are the most common sites of hemorrhage, are also involved in occlusion with infarction in hypertension has led to several hypotheses concerning the etiology of the hemorrhages:

a. The vessel wall may be weakened by this process and may dilate and rupture (the miliary aneurysm of Bouchard and Charcot).

b. The vessel may occlude with infarction;

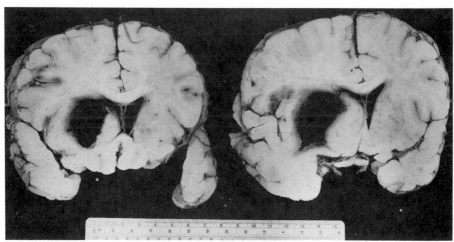

Figure 22-19 Intracerebral hemorrhage—putamen. A large mass of hemorrhage has disrupted the substance of the putamen, displaced adjacent structures, and ruptured into the lateral ventricle. The hemorrhage presumably originated from the penetrating (lenticulostriate) branches of the right middle cerebral artery. This 46-year-old, Negro housewife with severe hypertension (230/130) had a sudden episode of left central facial weakness, left hemiplegia, and left field defect. Over a 72-hour period she experienced a remarkable degree of recovery. She then had a rapid deterioration of neurological status with lethargy, ptosis of the eyelids, and fixed dilated pupils. Eye movements could not be elicited by dolls' head maneuvers or by caloric stimulation, signifying significant brain stem compression with compromise of brain stem functions (See Fig. 15–4, Chapter 15). This sequence of events with apparent initial recovery suggested possible hemorrhage into previous area of penetrating branch ischemia. (Courtesy of Pathology Department, New England Medical Center Hospital.)

See Filmstrip, Frame 50.

when collateral flow is then introduced into the acutely necrotic area, hemorrhage occurs.

c. Related to this hypothesis is the concept of fluctuations in blood pressure. Certainly such wide fluctuations may occur in some hypertensive patients. With a fall in blood pressure, infarctions would occur. With restoration of elevated blood pressure, these necrotic vessel walls would be unable to take the stress of the increased pressure and would bleed.

In both explanations (b) and (c) there is implied a concept of hemorrhagic infarction. In some cases of premonitory ischemia, symptoms will be noted. Our own experience with carotid artery surgery would suggest that hemorrhagic infarction certainly is a complication of the restoration of blood flow by a carotid endarterectomy when this procedure is performed shortly after an occlusion, which has resulted in acute infarction.

d. Another explanation suggests that in some cases venous occlusion may have occurred. Venous occlusions are usually hemorrhagic.

e. It is also possible that in some cases bleeding has occurred from an arterio-venous malformation, the evidence of which has been destroyed by the massive hemorrhage.

The pathological features to be found with an intracerebral hemorrhage may be briefly summarized. Within a few hours of cessation of the hemorrhage, clotting occurs. In general with hypertensive hemorrhages, bleeding does not again occur into the same area. The blood is not quickly removed from the brain parenchyma. If this hemorrhage is actually a complication of infarction, then in the early stages, the changes of ischemic infarction will be noted with infiltration of adjacent ischemic tissue by polymorpho-nuclear leukocytes.

The actual clot of a hemorrhage will remain as a red or reddish black mass for a matter of several weeks. Macrophages which may have been already abundant in adjacent necrotic tissue begin to digest red blood cells at the periphery of the hemorrhage producing the yellow-brown iron pigment hemosiderin. At three weeks, this produces at the periphery, a rim of orange. The more central area of hemorrhage never undergoes phagocytosis but is converted to a semiliquid mass after several additional weeks or months.

When the brain is examined many months after a hemorrhage, there will be found a residual cleft or cavity with orange-stained walls. The staining is due to the persistence of hemosiderin-containing macrophages. The wall, in general, is similar to that surrounding the cavity which results from an ischemic infarct. A proliferation of capillaries has occurred with the formation of connective tissue fibers. In adjacent tissue, proliferation of astrocytes has occurred with the formation of glial fibers.

The clinical manifestations will depend on the location and size of the hemorrhage. In general with the most common variety—those into the putamen—there is the sudden onset of headache, followed by hemiparesis, and then within a period of minutes to hours of hemianesthesia, confusion, and coma develop. The progression of symptoms is due to the progressive enlargement of the hematoma and to dissection of the hemorrhage along fiber pathways. Displacement of midline brain stem structures and tentorial herniation often occur. With these brain stem complications and with extension of the hemorrhage into the ventricular system, a decerebrate state and a compromise of respiratory functions develop. Death occurs in a high percentage of such patients (75 per cent) within hours to days.

With hemorrhages into the thalamus, hemianesthesia and an impairment of upward gaze may be early symptoms. The posterior thalamic location often results in compromise of the adjacent pretectal area and of the superior colliculus.

Hemorrhages into the white-matter stem of the temporal lobe may be characterized by the signs of a progressive mass lesion in the temporal lobe with involvement of adjacent areas of subcortical white matter and eventual tentorial herniation.

Pontine hemorrhages are characterized by the rapid onset of coma, quadriplegia, and early arrest of respiratory functions. Death occurs within minutes to hours.

Cerebellar hemorrhages are characterized by the sudden onset of headache, vomiting, ataxia, and vertigo; as progression and compression of the brain stem occur, extraocular findings emerge.

The diagnosis of intracerebral hemorrhage may be made on the basis of the sudden onset of symptoms. The onset occurs during a period of activity as opposed to the pattern for arteriosclerotic ischemic-occlusive disease where onset during sleep or shortly after awakening is more characteristic. Occasionally warning prodromal symptoms are present; such warning symptoms, however, are more characteristic of ischemic-occlusive disease.

In general, the cerebrospinal fluid is under increased pressure and contains red blood cells. The total number of such cells, however, is usually less than that found in subarachnoid hemorrhage.

As regards treatment, the deep location of hemorrhages into the putamen, thalamus, and pons means that surgical evacuation of these massive hemorrhages is not feasible. Moreover, with pontine hemorrhages, death rapidly ensues. With extension of hemorrhages of the putamen or thalamus into the ventricle, death usually occurs within a short time. However, expanding masses of hematoma within subcortical white matter, e.g., temporal lobe, offer the possibility of surgical therapy. Cerebellar hematomas when diagnosed prior to brain-stem compromise also may be evacuated.

Case History 5. NECH #193–731. Date of admission: 5/15/68.

This 33-year-old white, right-handed, male linotype operator (Mr. E. H.), at approximately 8:30 p.m. on May 14, 1968 had the sudden onset of numbness of the left side of his mouth. At 10:30 p.m. he developed a severe right frontal headache and noted sudden onset of numbness of the left upper extremity. This rapidly spread to involve the left half of the body, including the left lower extremity. Marked weakness of the left face, arm, and leg rapidly developed. Evaluation that evening at his local community hospital revealed a dense left homonymous hemianopsia, a marked left central facial weakness, an absence of any voluntary movement of the left arm and leg, and no awareness of painful stimulation of the entire left side. A left Babinski sign was present. Lumbar puncture revealed opening pressure elevated to 235 mm. of water; 50 fresh red blood cells per cubic mm. were present in the spinal fluid. The patient was subsequently transferred to the neurosurgical service at New England Center Hospital.

PAST HISTORY: There were no remarkable features as regards hypertension, renal disease, or diabetes mellitus.

PHYSICAL EXAMINATION:
1. The patient was moderately obese.
2. Blood pressure was normal at 110/85.
3. Examination of the heart revealed no abnormalities.
4. No rigidity of the neck was present.
5. There were no murmurs over the cranium.

NEUROLOGICAL EXAMINATION:
1. *Mental status:*
   a. The patient was oriented for time, place, and person.
   b. Speech was intact.
   c. The patient could provide a coherent history of the events of the present illness.
2. *Cranial nerves:*
   a. Examination of the fundi showed no hemorrhage or papilledema.
   b. A dense left homonymous hemianopsia was present.
   c. Sensation was defective on the left side of the face, as on the left side of the body.
   d. A left central facial weakness was present.
   e. The tongue deviated to the left.
3. *Motor system:*
   a. A dense paralysis of the left arm and leg was present.
   b. There was no resistance to passive motion in the left arm and little in the left lower extremity (that is, a flaccid paralysis was present).
   c. Cerebellar tests were negative.
4. *Reflexes:*
   a. Deep tendon reflexes were absent in the left upper extremity. In the lower extremities, the quadriceps and Achilles deep tendon reflexes were increased on the left compared to the right.
   b. A Babinski sign was present on the left. The plantar response on the right was flexor.
   c. No grasp reflexes were present.
5. *Sensation:*
   a. There was no perception of pinprick or of tactile stimuli on the entire left side of the body.
   b. Position and vibratory sensation were absent on the left.

LABORATORY DATA:
1. Hematocrit, white blood count, and

differential were all within normal limits. Sedimentation rate was normal.

2. Tests of bleeding time, clotting time, and prothrombin time were all within normal limits.

3. Urinalysis and blood urea nitrogen were within normal limits.

4. Skull x-rays revealed a shift of the pineal, 7 mm. from right to left.

5. Electroencephalogram revealed frequent focal 4 to 5 cps slow waves in the right hemisphere most prominent in the frontal and parietal areas consistent with focal damage in these areas.

6. Arteriograms (right common carotid) revealed a 12 mm. shift of the pericallosal branch of the anterior cerebral artery from right to left. The internal cerebral vein was also shifted 8 mm. from right to left. The middle cerebral branches emerging through the sylvian fissure were depressed. There was no evidence of an abnormal arteriovenous shunt or of an aneurysm. Cortical vessels and veins in the suprasylvian area were stretched over a relatively avascular area. The conclusion was a space-occupying mass in the right posterior frontal area consistent with an intracerebral hematoma.

SUBSEQUENT COURSE:

On the day of admision, the patient was taken to the operating room. A right parietal burr hole was made. The underlying cortex was noted by the neurosurgeon, Dr. Robert Yuan, to bulge prominently. A needle was inserted to a depth of 1 cm. into the cortex where 25 cc. of old, dark red blood under pressure was expelled. Free drainage of blood continued through a catheter which remained in place for 2 days.

Return of voluntary movement in the left lower extremity at the hip and knee was noted on the day following surgery. Re-evaluation of neurological status 2 weeks after surgery revealed continued improvement. The left homonymous hemianopsia was no longer present but the patient did have some difficulty in reading (losing the left half of the line of print). A left central facial weakness was present; voluntary hand-foot movements on the left were still not possible. Proximal muscle groups (shoulder, hip, knee) had returned to 60 per cent of normal strength. Deep tendon reflexes were now hyperactive in the upper and lower left extremities with a left Babinski sign. A dense sensory deficit remained on the left side with no perception of pain, touch, vibration, and position in the upper and lower extremities. Re-evaluation 4 weeks after surgery revealed a return of pain and temperature sensation but continued deficits in proprioception. Re-evaluation by Dr. Yuan 4 months after surgery indicated a return of strength in the left hand with a strong grip. The gait was typical of a spastic hemiplegia. Reflexes were unchanged. Sensory examination revealed a return of primary modalities such as vibration and pain, but marked errors in cortical modalities, such as position sense, were made. Follow-up 7 months after surgery indicated an excellent return of strength on the left side but continued incoordination in the left hand due to deficits in proprioception.

COMMENT:

This patient from several standpoints presents a number of unusual features not seen in the typical case of intracerebral hemorrhage. The patient was relatively young (33 years old) and had no history of hypertension. He had none of those conditions such as leukemia, bleeding disorders, and the like which predispose to intracerebral hemorrhage. The arteriogram provided no evidence of an intrinsic or a secondary metastatic brain tumor. Moreover, histological examination of the tissue and drainage material obtained at the time of surgery failed to reveal tumor cells. The site of the intracerebral hemorrhage makes the rupture of an aneurysm unlikely (see later discussion regarding common sites of aneurysm). Although no arteriovenous malformation was demonstrated at the time of arteriography, such a malformation may have been present previously but destroyed in the process of hemorrhage. The significance of the minor prodromal sensation of numbness of the face remains uncertain. This may have reflected an initial small area of ischemia with secondary hemorrhage.

Where was the initial site of hemorrhage? This question remains unanswered. Although the putamen is the most common site of intracerebral hemorrhage, in this case, the hemorrhage may have originated in the subcortical white matter of the parietal lobe. The pattern of initial evolution of symptoms and the final pattern of sensory deficit is perhaps more consistent with such a parietal lobe location. The patient is certainly atypical from the prognostic standpoint. He did not lapse into coma and did not have compromise of brain stem functions as so often occurs when there is tentorial hernia-tion or an extension of the hemorrhage into the ventricular system. Moreover this patient survived. The usual mortality in large intracerebral hemorrhages is 75 to 80 per cent. That these various events did not occur, may in part relate to the drainage of the hematoma by the neurosurgeon with removal of this supratentorial mass lesion.

SUBARACHNOID HEMORRHAGE

The diagnosis of subarachnoid hemor-rhage is made on the basis of gross blood present in the cerebrospinal fluid in the absence of primary intracerebral hemor-rhage. As we have indicated, the majority of primary intracerebral hemorrhages result in the leakage of some blood into the sub-arachnoid space. In the majority of cases of subarachnoid hemorrhage in the adult, the source of bleeding is a ruptured saccular aneurysm. A less common cause of bleeding is an angioma (arteriovenous malformation) involving the cerebral cortex.

The basic pathology in the saccular or berry aneurysm relates to a defect in the media and internal elastic membrane of the vessel wall. Since the media of cerebral arteries develops in a multicentric manner, adjacent sections meet at arterial bifurcations where clefts or gaps in the media are com-mon. These developmental defects in the media probably occur to some extent in all individuals. When later in life thinning or loss of the internal elastic membrane is superimposed at this point of defect, the thin layer of intima bulges out and is covered only by the loose connective tissue of the adventitia. The ballooned protrusion is re-ferred to as a saccular aneurysm.

The unruptured saccular aneurysm is usually asymptomatic. Unruptured saccular aneurysms occur as an incidental finding in 2 per cent of routine autopsies. Occasionally, however, symptoms may be noted prior to rupture. Thus, an enlarging aneurysm of the posterior communicating artery may com-press the third nerve. At times an aneurysm of the cavernous portion of the carotid artery may invade the pituitary fossa or compress the optic chiasm. At times, an aneurysm of the anterior communicating artery may attain large size and act as a tumor, compressing the optic chiasm, nerves, and orbital prefrontal areas.

In general, however, the initial symptoms are those related to rupture. The usual symptoms are those of sudden severe head-ache, vomiting, neck pain, and stiffness. The latter symptoms are due to meningeal irritation. The headache is often precipi-tated by sudden straining, exercise, or sexual activity. Consciousness is often well pre-served. Often no specific focal symptoms are present, and it may then be difficult to deter-mine, on the basis of the clinical findings alone, the actual site of rupture. At times, the presence of minor focal signs will allow a clinical diagnosis as to where the aneurysm is located. Those cases where consciousness has been preserved and where few focal signs are present can of course be readily distinguished from cases of primary intra-cerebral hemorrhage. In intracerebral hemorrhage, secondary leakage of blood into the subarachnoid space may occur, but consciousness is usually poorly preserved, and well-developed focal signs are present, e.g., hemiparesis, hemianesthesia, hemi-anopsia, and quadriparesis.

At times in ruptured aneurysm, significant focal or bilateral signs of cerebral involve-ment will be present. In some cases coma will be an early sign. In some of these cases there has occurred extension of the hemorrhage into the substance of the cerebral hemisphere. At times, rupture from the base of the brain into the third ventricle has occurred. At times, the vessel beyond the point of rupture has been deprived of blood, and infarction has occurred within its territory. At times, spasm of the artery distal to the point of aneurysm will occur, related perhaps to the presence of blood in the subarachnoid space. Such arterial spasm may produce sufficient vasoconstriction, apparently via adrenergic mechanisms, to result in ischemia and in-farction.

Those red blood cells which have entered the subarachnoid space undergo a series of changes. Within a few hours, disruption of red blood cells has begun with a yellow discoloration (so called xanthochromia) of the spinal fluid. At this time oxyhemo-globin and methemoglobin may also be detected in the spinal fluid. After 48 hours, increasing amounts of bilirubin pigment may be noted with an increase in the degree of xanthochromia. The red blood cells have usually been completely disrupted by 10 days. The bilirubin product of this disruption disappears more slowly. The spinal fluid does not become colorless for 15 to 30 days after the hemorrhage. In tissues adjacent to the subarachnoid blood, hemosiderin-filled macrophages may be seen for several weeks after the acute episode of bleeding. Initially in the spinal fluid obtained by lumbar puncture, the number of white blood cells are in the same proportion to red blood cells as in the peripheral blood. With the passage of time, after the acute hemorrhage, as red blood cells decrease due to disruption and as meningeal reaction occurs, a relative increase in white blood cells will be noted.

In considering the location of the aneurysm, certain statistics should be considered (Fig. 22–20). Approximately 90 to 95 per cent of aneurysms occur in relation to the anterior portion of the circle of Willis at the base of the brain and its main branches. Only 10 per cent occur in relation to the basilar-vertebral system. In 15 per cent of cases, multiple aneurysms are present.

We may specify three major general locations for single aneurysms within the anterior circulation:

a. The junction of the posterior communicating and internal carotid arteries (30 per cent).

b. The initial bifurcation or trifurcation of the middle cerebral artery (20 per cent) within the sylvian fissure.

c. The anterior communicating-anterior cerebral junctional area (30 per cent).

In general the neurologist faced with the problem of subarachnoid hemorrhage will select the location from essentially these three main anatomical areas. His clinical diagnosis will be more specific if certain focal findings are also present. The following series of cases will illustrate these diagnostic points:

POSTERIOR COMMUNICATING INTERNAL CAROTID (Figs. 22–21 and 22–22)

Case History 6.   NECH #182–302.
Date of admission: 10/2/66.

This 66-year-old white housewife (Mrs. E. S.), five days prior to admission, had the sudden onset of a severe bioccipital-bifrontal headache associated with vomiting. The headache was constantly present for 3 days but was increased by coughing. At the same time, she noted an alteration of vision in the right eye. She noted also a drooping of the right eyelid. The headache subsided, only to recur one night prior to admission as a severe occipital headache associated with vomiting. There was no past history of hypertension. The patient was admitted to her community hospital. A lumbar puncture revealed the presence of subarachnoid blood.

GENERAL PHYSICAL EXAMINATION: The patient was an obese female with blood pressure of 140/80 and complaints of severe headache. Her temperature was normal.

NEUROLOGICAL EXAMINATION:

1. *Mental status:* The patient was alert with mental status intact.

2. *Cranial nerves:*

a. Fundus: Blurred discs were present bilaterally, being greater on the right. No venous pulsations were present on the right.

b. Nerve III: The right pupil measured 4 mm. and was not reactive to light on direct or consensual stimulation. The left pupil measured 2 mm. and responded to light. Ptosis of the right eyelid was present. At rest on forward gaze there was outward deviation of the right eye. The patient was unable to adduct the right eye on left lateral gaze and failed to move this eye on upward or

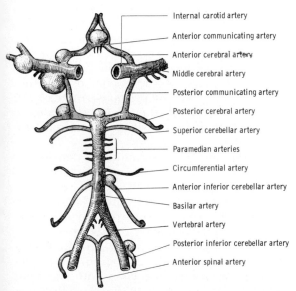

Internal carotid artery

Anterior communicating artery

Anterior cerebral artery

Middle cerebral artery

Posterior communicating artery

Posterior cerebral artery

Superior cerebellar artery

Paramedian arteries

Circumferential artery

Anterior inferior cerebellar artery

Basilar artery

Vertebral artery

Posterior inferior cerebellar artery

Anterior spinal artery

Figure 22–20 The common sites of saccular (berry) aneurysms. The size of the aneurysm at these various sites has been drawn in direct proportion to the frequency at that site. (From McDowell, F.: *In* Beeson, P. B., and McDermott, W.: *Textbook of Medicine*, 13th Edition. Philadelphia, W. B. Saunders, 1971, p. 209.)

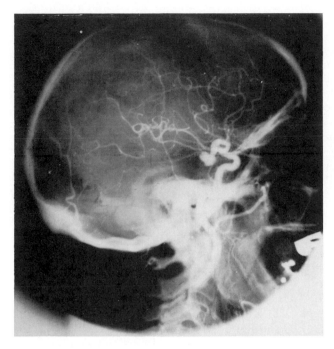

Figure 22–21 Saccular aneurysm, arising from junction right internal carotid artery and posterior communicating artery demonstrated by right carotid arteriogram. This 70-year-old widow, 18 months previously, had the sudden onset of severe pain in the right eye and complete third nerve paralysis which had partially improved in the interim. (Courtesy of Dr. Samuel Wolpert, New England Center Hospitals.) (Compare to Fig. 22–13 for nonaneurysm reference.)

downward gaze. Other extraocular movements were intact.

c. Nerve VII: Minimal flattening of the right nasal labial fold was present.

3. *Motor system*: Strength, coordination, and gait were intact.

4. *Reflexes*: Deep tendon: A minimal relative increase was present on the right. Plantar responses: The left was flexor, the right was equivocal.

5. *Sensation:* All modalities were intact.

6. *Neck*: Mild nuchal rigidity was present (resistance to passive flexion of head onto chest).

LABORATORY DATA:

1. Skull and chest x-rays were normal.

2. Studies of bleeding time, clotting time, and prothrombin time were all within normal limits.

3. Arteriograms revealed an aneurysm of the right internal carotid artery just below its junction with the posterior communicating artery. There was no left-to-right flow through the anterior communicating artery. There was narrowing of the anterior cerebral arteries near their origin bilaterally. This suggested to the radiologist the possibility of spasm, secondary to the presence of subarachnoid blood.

HOSPITAL COURSE:

Because the history suggested several episodes of bleeding, surgical therapy was selected. A right temporal craniotomy was performed on October 5, 1966 by Dr. Robert Yuan with clipping of the neck of the aneurysm. The temporal lobe was retracted revealing a 13 mm.-long saccular aneurysm, arising from the internal carotid artery close to the junction with the posterior communicating artery. Distally the aneurysm enlarged into a large sac which was hidden behind the oculomotor nerve. This nerve was bulging at the point where the aneurysm was impinging. The neck of the aneurysm, which was clipped, was well formed. The more distal sac of the aneurysm was thin and showed signs of previous rupture with yellow staining of the adjacent meninges. The sac of the aneurysm was covered with gelfoam.

Postoperatively, significant deficits as compared to the preoperative neurological status were evident. The level of consciousness waxed and waned with periods of alertness alternating with periods of apathy and drowsiness. Twenty days after surgery, she was described as sitting with both eyes closed, continuously grasping and palpating the arm of the chair with the right hand, less frequently with the left. There was a marked bilateral release of an instinctive grasp reflex. There was increased resistance in both upper extremities, at times described as plastic rigidity, at times as the "Gegenhalten," associated with bilateral frontal lobe disease. No spontaneous voluntary

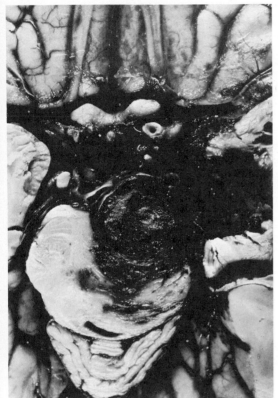

Figure 22-22 Large saccular aneurysm arising from junction left internal carotid posterior communicating artery with compression of and rupture into the brain stem. This 51-year-old white male in September 1962 had a subarachnoid hemorrhage and underwent common carotid artery ligation for an aneurysm arising from junction of left internal carotid and posterior communicating arteries. The patient did well, except for a residual left third nerve palsy, until March 1965 when he began to have transient episodes of right-sided weakness. On November 15, 1965 the patient complained of a sudden severe bifrontal headache, slumped to his right side with a dense right hemiplegia and became unresponsive. Examination of cerebrospinal fluid revealed elevated pressure and grossly bloody fluid. Condition rapidly deteriorated with the development of periodic respiration, fluctuating blood pressure, and irregular pulse. (Courtesy of Dr. John Hills, New England Center Hospitals; and Dr. Jose Segarra, Boston Veterans Administration Hospital.)

See Filmstrip, Frame 51.

with infarction in the territory of the anterior cerebral arteries and additional involvement of the basal ganglia. The complete paralysis of the right third nerve remained at preoperative level. At the time of hospital discharge, one month after surgery, the frontal lobe findings and the weakness in the left leg remained prominent.

COMMENT:

The presence of a severe headache in association with a mild degree of nuchal rigidity suggests meningeal irritation. Such irritation could indicate a subarachnoid hemorrhage or a meningitis (inflammation of the meninges due to bacterial or viral infection). The sudden onset of the headache is more consistent with a subarachnoid hemorrhage. The lack of fever and of accompanying or prodromal systemic findings is also against the diagnosis of meningitis. Finally, the clearly focal third nerve findings are more in favor of the diagnosis of subarachnoid hemorrhage (although focal or multifocal neurological findings may develop as complications of a bacterial meningitis).

In this case, the significant findings on neurological examination related to the right third cranial nerve. The third cranial nerve is particularly subject to compression by aneurysms of the posterior communicating artery because having emerged from the midbrain it pursues an anterior course towards the cavernous sinus in a close parallel relationship to the posterior communicating artery. In general, compressive lesions of the third nerve produce initially an alteration in pupillary constrictor functions, then involvement of the levator palpebrae, and finally involvement of the superior, medial and inferior rectus, and inferior oblique muscles. The initial alteration in vision in the right eye and and ptosis of the right eyelid at the onset of headache are then consistent with a compressive lesion. The patient at the onset of symptoms did not report a diplopia.

The third nerve as it emerges from the midbrain also passes in close relationship to the posterior cerebral and superior cerebellar arteries, but aneurysms of these vessels are much less common than those which occur in relation to the posterior communicating artery and internal carotid artery.

These findings with extrinsic compressive disease of the third nerve are to be contrasted with the pattern of intrinsic brain stem involvement of the third nerve nucleus

movements of the left leg occurred. Bilateral Babinski signs were present. A bilateral resting tremor of the hands and of the head was also present. At times inappropriate jocularity was present. All of these findings suggested a bilateral frontal lobe syndrome where medial rectus or superior rectus function is more likely to be initially compromised.

The patient had minimal findings suggesting involvement of the left corticospinal and cortiobulbar tracts: minimal right central facial weakness, minimal increase in deep tendon reflexes on the right side, and an equivocal right plantar response. The findings may have been produced by a slight shift of the brain stem to the left due to the small mass of aneurysm on the right side of brain stem. With such a shift, compression of the left cerebral peduncle against the tentorium might occur. In any case, these findings were minimal. The significant findings in this case clearly related to the third cranial nerve and it is these findings which allowed localization of the lesion prior to arteriography.

As regards the postoperative course, it is evident that this patient had severe involvement of the frontal lobes presumably as a result of bilateral infarction within the territory of the anterior cerebral arteries. In retrospect, the narrowing of the anterior cerebral arteries at their origin, presumed secondary to "spasm" noted at the time of arteriography, may have provided a clue as to the development of this complication. The neurosurgeon, faced with the decision as to the best time to intervene, would prefer as the ideal situation, the moment when arterial spasm is no longer present but bleeding has not yet recurred. The student may perhaps raise the question "Why operate at all?" The answer relates to the overall mortality in cases of ruptured aneurysm. We will survey prognosis and results of treatment after reviewing the additional examples below.

MIDDLE CEREBRAL BIFURCATION

Case History 7. NECH #179–881.
Date of admission: 6/10/66.
This 46-year-old, right-handed, white, married male (Mr. H. P.), 10 days prior to admission, had the sudden onset of a severe, throbbing, supraorbital and vertex headache. The headache began while the patient was in bed in the early stages of sexual intercourse. The patient noted no weakness except that his tongue "felt funny" in articulation for approximately one minute. There was a transient difficulty in speech during this period.

PAST HISTORY: Mild hypertension had been present.
GENERAL PHYSICAL EXAMINATION: Blood pressure was 160/100.
NEUROLOGICAL EXAMINATION:
1. *Mental status* was intact.
2. *Cranial nerves* were intact.
3. *Motor system* was intact.
4. *Sensory system* was intact.
5. *Headache* could be precipitated by head movement.
6. With flexion of the head, pain in the neck and lumbar area occurred.
LABORATORY DATA:
1. Skull and chest x-rays were normal.
2. Electroencephalogram revealed focal damage in the lateral aspect of the left hemisphere (focal 3 to 5 cps slow waves) (Fig. 22–23).
3. Lumbar puncture on May 11, 1966 revealed opening pressure elevated to 270 mm. of water and closing pressure to 210 mm. of water. The fluid was xanthochromic (yellow discoloration). In addition 38 fresh red blood cells per cubic mm. were present. Protein was elevated to 80 mg./100 ml. Hinton was negative.
4. Arteriography revealed a bilobed aneurysm at the trifurcation of the left middle cerebral artery measuring 8×4 mm. Spasm and narrowing of the proximal anterior and middle cerebral arteries were noted.
HOSPITAL COURSE:
On June 11, 1966, the patient complained of a few-minute episodes of numbness in the right face, tongue, and right upper extremity with thickness of speech. Examination now revealed right central facial weakness and slight slurring of speech. The patient also now complained of additional neck pain on extreme forward flexion. On June 12, 1966, the patient had another short episode beginning with numbness over the right thumb, spreading to the right hand and then to the angle of the mouth.
Because of the several episodes which occurred, following hospital admission, involving the right face, tongue, and hand in association with the finding of fresh red blood cells in the spinal fluid, it was considered likely that bleeding from the aneurysm was continuing to occur. Surgical therapy was therefore considered necessary to prevent additional (and possibly fatal) subarachnoid hemorrhage. On May 20, 1966 a left frontotemporal craniotomy was

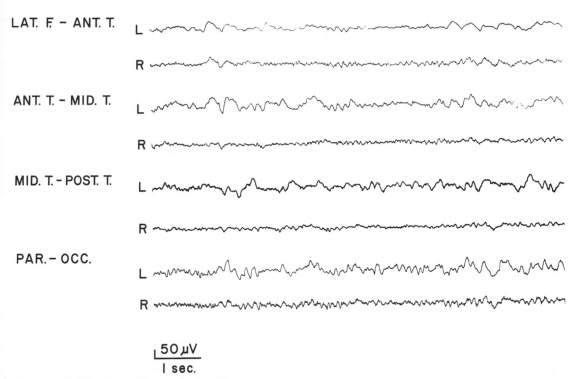

LAT. F. – ANT. T.

ANT. T. – MID. T.

MID. T. – POST. T.

PAR. – OCC.

50 μV
I sec.

Figure 23–23 Case History 7. Middle cerebral artery aneurysm with subarachnoid hemorrhage. Preoperative electroencephalogram. (Bipolar recordings on 6/13/66.) Focal 3–5 cps slow waves were present throughout left temporal, left lateral frontal, and left parietal areas indicating focal damage in these areas. LAT. F. = lateral frontal; ANT. T. = anterior temporal; MID. T. = midtemporal; POST. T. = posterior temporal; PAR. = parietal; OCC. = occipital.

performed by Dr. Robert Yuan with subsequent plastic coating of the entire aneurysm to reinforce its wall. There was evidence of recent hemorrhage in the subarachnoid space with yellow discoloration of the meninges. In order to expose the aneurysm, it was necessary to remove the anterior tip of the temporal lobe back to a distance of 2.5 cm. There was a small amount (5 to 10 cc.) of intracerebral blood clot in the superior temporal region close to the aneurysm. The aneurysm itself had no actual neck that could be clipped. Several middle cerebral branches appeared to arise from the dome or lateral wall of the aneurysm.

In the postoperative period, the patient initially did well. A minor expressive aphasia was present, but the patient was alert and well oriented. However, fever and jaundice developed. With the development of significant alterations of liver functions approximately 7 days after surgery, the patient became confused and agitated. The prothrombin time fell to 3 per cent of normal

and there was evidence of bleeding into the gastrointestinal tract at this time. The prothrombin deficit was corrected by administration of vitamin K. It was unclear, however, as to whether any minor intracranial bleeding occurred during this time. Some improvement in liver functions occurred, and the patient became more alert but continued to manifest inappropriate behavior, emotional lability, and disturbance of memory. He left the hospital against medical advice one month after surgery, on July 20, 1966.

The patient was readmitted to the hospital approximately one month later on August 13, 1966. For two days, the patient had been less active, appeared confused, glassy eyed, and failed to communicate. The degree of obtundation cleared when adequate dosage of the anticonvulsant medication, Dilantin, was administered. This fact taken in conjunction with the electroencephalogram, which demonstrated frequent focal spikes (excessive neuronal discharge) in the left temporal area (Fig. 22–24) led to the conclusion that the episode which precipitated

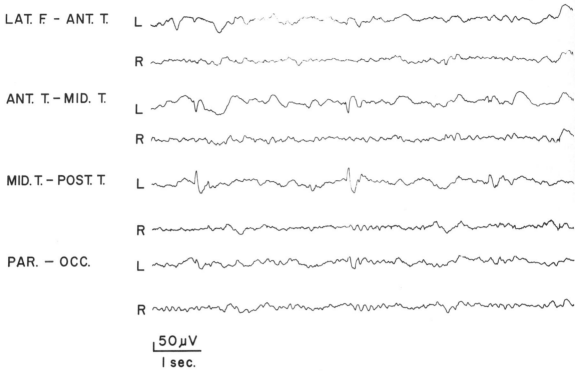

LAT. F. - ANT. T.   L

R

ANT. T. - MID. T.   L

R

MID. T. - POST. T.   L

R

PAR. - OCC.   L

R

50 μV

1 sec.

Figure 22-24 Case History 7. Middle cerebral artery aneurysm with subarachnoid hemorrhage. (Bipolar recording on 8/17/66, two months following surgery.) Focal blunt spikes are demonstrated with phase reversal at the left midtemporal electrode, consistent with focal discharge originating in left temporal lobe. (For designation of channels, see Figure 22–23.)

his readmission might well have represented a prolonged seizure discharge. The electroencephalogram also demonstrated an increase in slow wave activity in the left hemisphere, particularly the left temporal area indicating a possible increase in damage in the left temporal area. This appeared to be correlated with apparent progression of the patient's aphasia which was now receptive as well as expressive in nature. At the time of discharge, a severe expressive aphasia was still present.

COMMENT:

The sudden onset of severe headache during exercise or exertion (sexual intercourse in this case) is characteristic of subarachnoid hemorrhage. The location of the aneurysm was suggested by the symptoms relevant to the tongue and speech during the initial episode. The episode on June 11, 1966, involving numbness of the right face, tongue, and right upper extremity, could only indicate disease within the territory of the left middle cerebral artery. The lumbar puncture at this time indicated not only evidence of the initial leakage of blood

10 days prior to admission (an elevation of cerebrospinal fluid protein and a xanthochromia), but also fresh red blood cells suggesting that additional leakage of blood had occurred.

The nature of the episodes which occurred on June 11 and 12 is not certain. Most likely these were ischemic in nature related to decrease in blood flow as a result of clot formation within the aneurysm or from spasm of the adjacent portion of the middle cerebral artery. At times, however, symptoms such as rapidly spreading numbness occurring in episodes may suggest focal epileptic discharge. The development of an area of excessive discharge would not be unusual since this aneurysm involves those middle cerebral artery branches which are supplying the cerebral cortex.

The patient's course following surgery was complicated by the development of severe liver dysfunction. The etiology of this problem was never clear, the various studies suggesting either a toxic hepatitis related to various drugs and anesthetic agents or a variety of obstructive jaundice. What the patient's eventual recovery would have been had this problem not developed is uncertain. It is clear, however, that during this postoperative period the patient did develop significant impairment of language functions, possibly related to infarction or oozing of blood in areas supplied by the middle cerebral artery. It is also evident that a seizure focus had developed in this area. Such seizure foci may have developed in relation to the preoperative hematoma noted in the temporal lobe, in relation to the surgical manipulation of the area, or in relation to the postoperative complications.

ANTERIOR COMMUNICATING ANTERIOR CEREBRAL (Figs. 22–25 and 22–26)

Case History 8. NECH #174–025. Date of admission: 9/7/65. (Patient of Dr. John Sullivan.)

This 49-year-old, right-handed truck driver (Mr. C. F.) was transferred from his local community hospital for evaluation of subarachnoid hemorrhage.

The patient had experienced occasional frontal headaches for the previous 5 years. In June, 1965, while changing a tire, he had a severe throbbing frontal headache which cleared after thirty minutes. Since that time he had experienced daily throbbing frontal headaches, usually present on arising in the morning. On September 4, 1965, the patient had the onset of a particularly severe headache which began while he was engaged in heavy work on a boat. There was associated stiffness of the neck, nausea, vomiting, and a general sensation of weakness.

Evaluation at his local community hospital revealed papilledema (blurred optic disk margins on funduscopic examination). Nuchal rigidity was present. The lumbar puncture demonstrated grossly bloody cerebrospinal fluid.

PAST HISTORY:

1. Hypertension had been noted in June, 1965.

2. The patient's father had died at age 59 of a cerebrovascular accident.

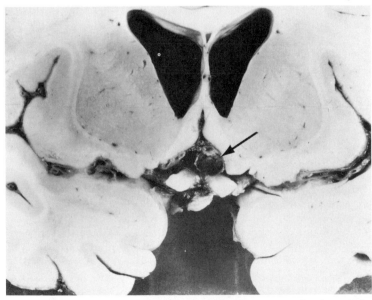

Figure 22–25 Saccular aneurysm at junction of anterior communicating–left anterior cerebral artery. The relationship of an aneurysm in this location to the optic chiasm is clearly demonstrated. This 52-year-old, white male had the sudden onset one evening of headache, nausea, and vomiting. The following morning he could not be roused. On admission to the hospital, the patient was stuporous, inattentive, and disoriented but could move all of his extremities and would occasionally turn his head when his name was called. A bilateral Babinski sign was present, in addition to the release of a strong grasp reflex. Urinary and fecal incontinence were present. Cerebrospinal fluid contained greater than 100,000 red blood cells per cu. mm., the supernatant fluid was xanthochromic. (Courtesy of Dr. John Hills, New England Center Hospitals; and Dr. Jose Segarra, Boston Veterans Administration Hospital.)
See Filmstrip, Frame 52.

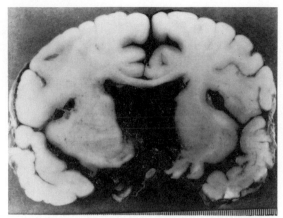

Figure 22–26 Saccular anterior communicating aneurysm with rupture into ventricular system. This 65-year-old white male, 14 days after a confirmed subarachnoid hemorrhage without definite localizing findings, had a generalized seizure followed by quadriplegia and coma. Death from pneumonia occurred 6 days later. (Courtesy of Dr. John Hills, New England Center Hospitals; and Dr. Jose Segarra, Boston Veterans Administration Hospital.)

GENERAL PHYSICAL EXAMINATION:

1. Blood pressure was moderately elevated to 180/100. Pulse was 60.

2. No bruits (murmurs) were present over the skull.

3. A significant degree of nuchal rigidity was present. The neck could not be actively or passively flexed.

NEUROLOGICAL EXAMINATION:

1. *Mental status*:
   a. The patient was somnolent but could be aroused, although attention span was noted to be shortened.
   b. He was oriented for place and situation but confused as to time.
   c. Digit span was shortened to 5 forward and 4 in reverse.
   d. The patient was unable to do calculations.

2. *Cranial nerves*:
   a. Sense of smell was decreased on the right side.
   b. Disk margins were indistinct on examination of the fundus. Arterioles were tortuous and irregular.

3. *Motor system*:
   a. Strength and tone were intact.
   b. Cerebellar tests were normal.

4. *Reflexes*:
   a. Deep tendon reflexes were symmetrical.
   b. Plantar responses were flexor.

5. *Sensory system*: All modalities were intact.

LABORATORY DATA:

1. Bleeding, clotting, and prothrombin times were all normal. Platelets were normal on smear.

2. Chest and skull x-rays were normal.

3. Arteriograms demonstrated an aneurysm of the anterior communicating artery which extended posteriorly and to the right. The aneurysm filled from the left carotid circulation.

HOSPITAL COURSE:

During the evening of September 11, 1965, the patient became lethargic and would not speak or obey commands. Blood pressure rose to 240 mm. systolic. The patient became totally unresponsive with pupils fixed and dilated and with incontinence of urine. Deep tendon reflexes were exaggerated with plantar responses extensor. Within minutes, the patient became responsive again; pupils were reactive, although the right remained sluggish. The patient made purposive movements and obeyed commands. Lumbar puncture subsequently indicated grossly bloody spinal fluid. The patient remained confused and less alert with a tendency to fall asleep.

On September 17, 1965, the patient again suddenly complained of violent headache and lost consciousness for approximately 30 minutes. The right pupil became dilated, and the right eye deviated to the right suggesting a right medial rectus weakness. The blood pressure again rose to 240/140. As previously, the patient regained consciousness. Although confused, he had no clearly lateralizing signs. Subsequent lumbar puncture again revealed the presence of fresh red blood cells.

Because repeated episodes of bleeding had occurred, surgical therapy was undertaken. On September 21, 1965 a left frontal craniotomy was performed by Dr. Robert Yuan. The left frontal pole was resected exposing the left anterior cerebral artery and the aneurysm which arose from the anterior communicating artery. The medial surface of the right frontal lobe was cystic and contained 20 cc. of hematoma. The hematoma was evacuated. The aneurysm was reinforced by spraying with a plastic coating.

Neurological examination approximately 1 week after surgery indicated that the patient was confused and disoriented, with a "rather negative response" refusing to follow directions and to speak to examiners. Blood pressure was noted to be extremely labile with a drop of 50 mm. of mercury systolic when the patient moved from prone to sitting position. Equivocal Babinski signs were present, and the patient was incontinent of urine and feces.

Re-evaluation on November 17, 1965, approximately two months after surgery, indicated that although the patient was ambulatory and able to take care of his daily needs, he remained confused for time and place. When the patient was examined 6 months after surgery, confusion was no longer present; intellectual functions were consistent with his education.

Approximately 2 years after surgery, the patient, who had recently been married, reported that he was impotent, unable to obtain an erection.

COMMENT:

In this case, the history of sudden onset of severe headache and stiffness of the neck, precipitated by exertion, clearly suggested a subarachnoid hemorrhage originating from the rupture of an intracranial aneurysm. While the clinical findings of somnolence and confusion with a decrease in olfaction on the right may have suggested the possibility of an anterior communicating-anterior cerebral artery location, these were certainly not firm diagnostic clues. The episodes characterized by sudden alteration in blood pressure, while nonspecific, might have raised the question of orbital-frontal, anterior cingulate, or hypothalamic effects (areas within the distribution of the anterior-cerebral arteries).

The negativity of the patient following surgery undoubtedly indicated preoperative and operative damage to the orbital and prefrontal areas. The bilateral Babinski signs and the incontinence of urine and feces in the postoperative period probably reflected damage to the parasagittal motor and premotor areas within the distribution of the anterior cerebral arteries.

TREATMENT OF INTRACRANIAL ANEURYSMS

Each of the three patients presented in the preceding illustrative case histories was subjected to surgical therapy. Surgical therapy has as its primary objective the prevention of additional subarachnoid hemorrhage. The prevention of additional sub-

arachnoid hemorrhage is a desirable goal from the standpoint of preventing the following types of complications of subarachnoid hemorrhage:

a. Massive rupture into the subarachnoid space with sudden shifts of the temporal lobe or cerebellar tonsils resulting in brain stem compression and death.

b. Rupture into the ventricular system with brain stem compression and death (Fig. 22–26).

c. Rupture into the substance of the brain with the development of focal neurological deficits and the possibility of residual neurological disability (morbidity) (Fig. 22–22).

d. The development of vasospasm (of uncertain etiology) with resultant infarction in the territory of the involved vessels. Alternatively, other mechanisms of occlusion with resultant infarction may be considered. The end result is focal, often massive infarction, with significant residual disability.

e. Obliteration of the subarachnoid cisterns and channels due to the presence of blood with the subsequent development of hydrocephalus.

f. Development of radicular pain due to the collection of blood in the lumbar subarachnoid space (through gravity).

A secondary aim of surgical therapy is the prevention of the compressive effects of an enlarging aneurysm with regard to the optic chiasm, the third nerve, and so forth (Figs. 22–21 and 22–25).

These complications in the untreated patient must be balanced against the risks of surgery. These risks include both the operative and postoperative mortality and morbidity. The use of the term "morbidity" refers to the disability relevant to the destruction of cerebral tissue incurred during the process of exposing the area of the aneurysm and during the process of obliterating the aneurysm by clipping its neck, or in the process of reinforcing the wall of the aneurysm by spraying it with plastic or wrapping it with gauze or muscle. During these procedures, operative occlusion of the parent vessel may be necessary with the risks of subsequent infarction. In addition to these intracranial operative procedures, occlusion of the carotid artery in the neck may be employed.

Controversy regarding the management of patients with subarachnoid bleeding from intracranial aneurysm relates to the relative value of conservative therapy (strict bed rest for 3 to 6 weeks) compared to surgical therapy.

For a realistic comparison, the natural history of the disease should be known, and the two groups to be compared should be in an equivalent clinical state prior to the beginning of the treatment trial. The two groups also should be equivalent as regards location of the aneurysm. Such statistics were not available until the recent reports of Mc-Kissock and of the Cooperative Intracranial Aneurysms Study (Nishioka, 1966; Skultety, 1966).

Several general conclusions may be drawn from these studies. Approximately 15 to 22 per cent of patients die in relation to the first episode of bleeding. In general, these deaths represent patients who dic prior to reaching the treatment center, or who arrive at the treatment center in a clinical state that does not allow for the performance of x-ray studies or surgery.

Of those patients who survive the initial episode of bleeding, the risk of rebleeding has been variously estimated at 30 to 50 per cent during the first year following the initial hemorrhage (usually within the first several weeks after the initial hemorrhage). The mortality associated with the repeated episodes of bleeding is relatively high. In the cooperative study, 42 per cent of the patients who had a second episode of bleeding expired. In the studies of Mc-Kissock, an even higher mortality was noted for recurrent bleeding—77 to 80 per cent.

At all stages, patients who are unconscious or poorly responsive have a poor prognosis whether conservative or surgical management is employed. In this category (category A of McKissock) are also included patients who are too ill for arteriography and surgery. The overall mortality in such patients approaches 67 to 95 per cent. If these poor-risk patients are eliminated, the overall mortality and morbidity in the remainder of patients (category B of Mc-Kissock) do not greatly differ when surgical and nonsurgical therapy are considered. When particular sites of aneurysm are considered, however, there is some indication that particular surgical procedures represent the treatment of choice. Thus, in aneurysms at the posterior communicating-internal carotid junction, common carotid artery ligation in the neck provides results superior to those achieved by conservative management. Intracranial surgery in middle cerebral

artery aneurysms reduces the mortality compared to conservative management. Whether a significant disability follows surgery may in part relate to where the middle cerebral artery aneurysm is located in relation to the dominant hemisphere. With regard to the anterior cerebral-anterior communicating location, at this point no significant benefit of surgery has been demonstrated.

In general, most would agree that where rupture of an intracranial aneurysm has resulted in an expanding and accessible intracerebral hematoma, surgical evacuation of the hematoma is indicated. Hydrocephalus also requires neurosurgical therapy to decompress the ventricular system.

OTHER CAUSES OF SUBARACHNOID HEMORRHAGE

Among the cases of subarachnoid hemorrhage reported to the central registry of the cooperative study, 51 per cent could be attributed to an identifiable aneurysm. In 33 per cent of the cases, a subarachnoid hemorrhage had clearly occurred, but neither an aneurysm nor an arteriovenous malformation could be identified. In some cases of this latter group, the aneurysm or malformation could have been the source of bleeding but was destroyed by the bleeding. In the case of aneurysms, spasm or clot within the sac of the aneurysm may have prevented the clear angiographic demonstration of this pathology. In general, this group of cases has a relatively favorable prognosis.

Arteriovenous malformations accounted for 8 per cent of the cases submitted to the central registry of the cooperative study. Included within this diagnostic category of vascular malformations are a variety of pathological entities, such as telangiectasis, varices, cavernous hemangiomas, arteriovenous anomalies, and angiomas. In general these represent developmental tangles of abnormal vessels within the substance of the brain (less often involving meningeal vessels). These abnormal vessels provide arteriovenous shunting of blood. Since the vessels are abnormal with defects in their walls, bleeding into the substance of the brain (producing an intracerebral hematoma) or into the subarachnoid space may occur. Moreover, these abnormal vessels are also prone to occlusion with the development of local infarction of cerebral tissue. These malformations are found predominantly within the posterior one-half of the cerebral hemisphere (Fig. 22–27). Case history 10 in Chapter 21, page 531 (Mr. W. E.) provides an illustration of the problem. In general, these malformations produce symptoms earlier in life than do saccular aneurysms. They are moreover less often fatal. Thus several episodes of subarachnoid hemorrhage may occur without loss of life. In the majority (50 per cent) of cases, the first manifestation is a seizure, often focal. In 20 per cent of the cases, the intracerebral hematoma with focal deficits is the initial manifestation. Only 20 per cent present a subarachnoid hemorrhage as their initial manifestation.

TRAUMATIC DISEASES OF THE CEREBRAL HEMISPHERE

In the era of the automobile, trauma to the head constitutes one of the most frequent neurological problems presented to emergency room physicians. Not all head injuries

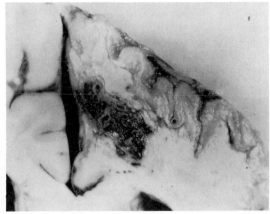

Figure 22–27 Arteriovenous malformation in the right parietal area demonstrating the abnormal tangle of vessels and infarction of the surrounding cerebral cortex and white matter. In this case, the malformation was fed mainly by the right anterior cerebral artery and drained into the superior sagittal sinus. This 46-year-old widow had, as a primary problem, multiple saccular aneurysms: anterior-communicating, left posterior communicating, and right superior cerebellar. Subarachnoid hemorrhage had occurred from the anterior communicating aneurysm and surgical treatment had been attempted. (Courtesy of Dr. John Hills, New England Center Hospitals.)

involve the brain. Thus significant scalp lacerations and simple skull fractures may be present without the development of significant neurological deficits. On the other hand, closed head injuries may be present with significant neurological signs but without major external signs of head trauma (i.e., scalp and skull appear intact).

Concussion. Perhaps the most common neurological syndrome occurring in relation to head trauma is the cerebral concussion, a syndrome characterized by a transient alteration of consciousness and of higher cerebral functions lasting a matter of minutes to hours following a blow to the head. Consciousness may or may not be lost transiently at the onset. The patient complains of "being in a dazed state" with blurring of vision and a sense of unsteadiness. Memory is often impaired for events during this period following the injury: posttraumatic amnesia. In addition, memory for events which occurred minutes, hours, or even several days prior to the injury may be impaired: retrograde amnesia.

No definite pathology has been associated with cerebral concussion; the pathophysiology remains unclear. There is some indication that differential acceleration or deceleration of the brain and skull may force the cerebral cortex against the hard surface of the skull producing a transient neuronal dysfunction.

Contusions and Lacerations. More serious injuries of the cerebral hemisphere involve contusions and lacerations. Contusions (local areas of swelling and capillary hemorrhage resembling bruises) are found particularly at the anterior poles and under surfaces of the frontal and temporal lobes. These contusions of the cerebral cortex occur as a result of the sudden impact of the cortex against the bony wall of the skull. The anterior portions of the anterior and middle fossa provide relatively constricting compartments favoring the development of such contusions. Contusions may directly underlie the site of the blow to the skull (*so-called coup injuries*) or may be across from the site of skull injury (*so-called contre coup injuries*). When examined at autopsy years later, the brain may show small orange-yellow colored areas of depression on the orbital-frontal and anterior-temporal areas (plaques jaunes).

Lacerations of the brain involve actual tears in the cortical surface (Fig. 22–28). Both lacerations and contusions may result

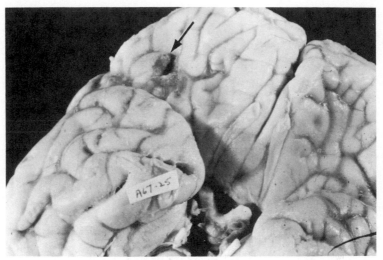

Figure 22–28 Old contusion and laceration of the right orbital frontal area (*arrow*). This 59-year-old white male expired with carcinoma of the tongue. He had a long history of heavy alcohol intake and had been admitted to the Boston V. A. Hospital in 1961 with a well-developed Wernicke-Korsakoff syndrome including recent memory deficits, disorientation, and confabulation. In addition to the traumatic lesion shown above, the patient had evidence of an old Wernicke's encephalopathy involving the mammillary bodies and of alcoholic cerebellar cortical degeneration. (Courtesy of Dr. Jose Segarra, Boston Veterans Administration Hospital.)

in the appearance of some red blood cells in the subarachnoid space. In general, patients with contusion and laceration have a loss of consciousness in relation to the injury. This is then followed by a state of drowsiness and confusion which is more prolonged than that noted in a concussion. Residual alterations in mental function, memory, and personality are often noted. Such alterations are uncommon with a simple concussion. Focal neurological findings may be present during the acute stage, at times remaining as residual deficits. Severe focal deficits such as hemiparesis or aphasia are, however, usually absent.

Complications of Skull Fractures. Certain types of skull injuries provide serious problems as regards the brain and require surgical attention. Thus, depressed skull fracture may compress the cerebral cortex, with bony splinters lacerating the dura and cortex. *Penetrating head injuries* (the object causing trauma has penetrated the skin, bone, and meninges) may introduce contaminated material into the brain, producing abscess formation and meningitis. Fractures involving the cribriform plate with laceration of the overlying dura and arachnoid may result in *cerebrospinal rhinorrhea:* the drainage of spinal fluid through the nose. The presence of such a pathway, of course, allows for the ready entry of bacteria from the nasopharynx into the cerebrospinal fluid spaces, providing recurrent episodes of meningitis. Air may also enter the intracranial cavity through this passageway. Both air and infection may also enter when skull fractures extend into any of the paranasal sinuses or the middle ear. In the latter instance a cerebrospinal fluid *otorrhea* may occur: drainage of spinal fluid from the external ear canal.

EXTRADURAL HEMATOMAS AND SUBDURAL HEMATOMAS

Of great importance from the neurological standpoint are these two traumatic conditions in which progressive compression of the cerebral hemispheres occurs.

These are conditions where early recognition and treatment will produce excellent results. The failure of recognition will result in progressive deterioration of neurological status with death as the eventual outcome.

Extradural Hematoma. Extradural hematoma is a complication of skull fractures which extend across a meningeal artery, usually the middle meningeal artery. Less often the skull fracture has torn a large venous sinus. Since the bleeding is usually arterial and brisk into the narrow extradural space (normally the dura is closely applied to the skull), compression of the cerebral hemisphere soon results with the rapid development and progression of neurological symptoms. The classic description is usually that of a short period of unconsciousness related to the acute trauma, then a short lucid interval, which is followed by progressive confusion and coma. A rapidly progressive hemiparesis is often noted with the development of a fixed dilated pupil on the side of the hematoma indicating uncal herniation by the mass which may be placed laterally over the temporal lobe. At other times as in the following case history, these lateralized findings may be overshadowed by the rapid progression to a stage of functional midbrain transection.

Case History 9. W.A.H.
Date of admission: 12/64.

This twenty-two-year-old, white airman, during a winter storm, was involved in an auto accident at 11:30 P.M. in which he struck his head against the windshield. He also sustained minor abrasions of the shoulder, hands, and chest.

The patient apparently was dazed, perhaps unconscious for a matter of seconds to minutes. He was taken by ambulance to the emergency room of the nearby army hospital where a brief evaluation indicated that the patient was alert, without definite neurological findings, and apparently without significant injuries. Skull x-rays did indicate a linear fracture over the right temporal area not, however, definitely crossing the major groove of the middle meningeal artery. The patient was therefore admitted to the intensive care ward for head injury observation.

The patient was apparently alert upon his arrival on the ward. It should be noted that the major attention of the physicians in the emergency room and of the nurses on the intensive care ward was given to four other patients from the same accident who had sustained very severe and obvious injuries. However, by 5 A.M., the patient was reported by the nurses to be agitated and confused.

NEUROLOGICAL EXAMINATION: 8:00 A.M.

1. *Mental status:* The patient was agitated and unable to cooperate. He was sitting up in bed, holding his head, and moaning and hyperventilating to a marked degree. He answered only occasional questions and then with a yes or no answer.

2. *Cranial nerves:*
   a. Fundi: The examination was negative but incomplete.
   b. Pupils: There was a bilateral but sluggish response to light. A minimal asymmetry was present. The right pupil was perhaps slightly larger and slightly more sluggish than the left.
   c. The remainder of cranial nerves: Intact.

3. *Motor system:*
   a. All limbs were moved spontaneously.
   b. There was a variable increased resistance to passive motion, but this was apparently due to the patient's inability to cooperate.

4. *Reflexes:*
   a. Deep tendon reflexes were increased bilaterally.
   b. Plantar responses were equivocal but apparently flexor.

5. *Sensation:* Pain sensation appeared to be intact.

6. *Neck:* There was variable resistance to attempted flexion.

7. *Head:* The patient moaned when palpated over left or right temporal areas.

SUBSEQUENT COURSE:

The patient was to be evaluated by the civilian neurosurgical consultant, whose arrival was delayed by several other emergencies and a snowstorm. In the meantime, progression occurred.

NEUROLOGICAL EXAMINATION at 4 P.M. now indicated fixed bilaterally dilated pupils. The four limbs were now extended in a decerebrate posture with significant spasticity on passive motion. The degree of spasticity in the upper limbs could be modified by tonic neck maneuvers. The plantar responses were bilaterally extensor. Spontaneous respirations were now irregular and infrequent, and the patient required the assistance of a mechanical respirator.

Immediate and definitive therapy was undertaken by the general surgeon with a significant improvement in the patient's status. Bilateral burr holes were placed. An epidural hematoma over the right temporal-parietal area was evacuated and the bleeding middle meningeal artery branch was coagulated.

Follow-up examination approximately two months later indicated that the patient had returned to active duty but was experiencing some problems related to changes in recent memory and to changes in motivation and personality. No significant motor or sensory findings were present. Minor and inconsistent asymmetry of deep tendon reflexes was present.

COMMENT:

This patient followed the usual pattern of a short lucid period followed by the rapid progression of confusion, agitation, and coma. As indicated by Plum and Posner, the development of hyperventilation is often indicative of a midbrain-upper pontine stage of damage from an expanding supratentorial lesion. The early appearance of hyperventilation followed by bilaterally fixed dilated pupils and a decerebrate state may well indicate that the supratentorial lesion was producing a more central downward compression of the midbrain and less of a lateral uncal-type compression. In any case, it is evident that brain stem compromise was progressing rapidly. So rapidly in fact that therapy had to be undertaken immediately. In such a case, there was no longer time for the transfer of the patient to a specialized treatment center and no longer any time for specialized laboratory studies such as arteriography.

Subdural Hematomas. Subdural hematomas (Fig. 22–29) represent the accumula-

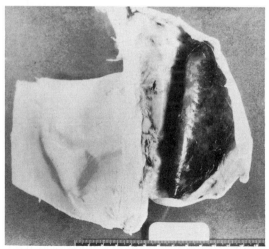

Figure 22–29 Subdural hematoma. This 69-year-old patient with Parkinson's disease had many dizzy spells and had fallen frequently. The specific manifestations of this relatively acute lesion were unclear at the time he was admitted with pulmonary edema and pneumonitis. (Courtesy of Dr. John Hills, New England Center Hospitals; and Dr. Jose Segarra, Boston Veterans Administration Hospital.)

tion of blood within the subdural space overlying the cerebral convexities. Such hematomas may be acute, subacute, or chronic. The acute and subacute types are clearly associated with trauma. The chronic variety may appear after closed-head trauma, often trivial; at times there may be no definite history of trauma.

The acute type is usually associated with other significant injuries of the brain such as cerebral contusion and laceration. With tears in the arachnoid, blood from the lacerations passes into the subdural space. Moreover, small bridging veins from the pia arachnoid to the superior sagittal sinus are also likely to be torn. The clinical picture of the acute subdural hematoma is often then modified by the clinical manifestations of these associated injuries. At times, however, the typical picture of a rapidly progressive supratentorial space-occupying lesion with progressive obtundation of consciousness and the signs of tentorial herniation will develop in acute (24 to 48 hours) relationship to the head injury.

The subacute and chronic subdural hematomas develop after a variable latent period of days, weeks, or months following the injury. The bleeding is venous from small bridging veins passing from the pia arachnoid to the superior sagittal sinus. The resultant accumulation of blood then is relatively slow. Associated injuries to the brain are usually not present. The blood in the subdural space is not readily removed and remains adherent to the dura. Instead, a growth of fibroblasts and blood vessels occurs from the dura at the edges of the clot, producing a thin membrane which separates the clot from the arachnoid. At the same time a thicker layer of connective tissue and blood vessels is forming a membrane where the clot is adherent to the inner layer of the dura. The hematoma often continues to increase in size apparently for several reasons: continued venous oozing may occur; moreover, bleeding may occur from the blood vessels which are growing into the hematoma from the dural surface. Finally it has been suggested that as some breakdown occurs within the clot, a fluid with high protein content is produced. The resultant fluid of high osmotic pressure then attracts more fluid into the hematoma.

The clinical manifestations are those of a progressive supratentorial mass lesion. At times progressive focal symptoms and signs are present; for example, hemiparesis, aphasia, and focal seizures. Eventually alterations in consciousness occur, often of a fluctuating nature. With eventual tentorial herniation, a fixed dilated pupil and the signs of a progressive functional midbrain transection are noted. Often, however, a syndrome is present in which focal symptoms and signs are not prominent, perhaps reflecting the fact that bilateral subdural hematomas are present in a high percentage of cases. The resultant picture then is that of a progressive state of confusion with fluctuating alterations in consciousness. A bilateral grasp reflex is often present. Eventually, if untreated, coma and the signs of tentorial herniation develop. In both types of syndrome progressive headache may be present although this complaint as well as the past history of head trauma may be difficult to elicit when the patient is admitted to a hospital in a confused state.

The following case illustrates a subacute subdural hematoma occurring in clear relationship to head trauma.

Case History 10. NECH #74–76–01–8. Date of admission: 10/28/69. (Patient of Dr. George Robertson and Dr. Huntington Porter.)

This 73-year-old white businessman (Mr. P.M.) was involved in an auto accident approximately ten days prior to admission, in which his auto was struck by a logging truck. The patient walked out of his car but was dazed and amnesic for approximately the next fifteen minutes. This condition, however, then cleared. Subsequent skull x-rays were normal and the patient was found to have no significant injuries except for ecchymosis (bruises) about the right eye and knee. The patient, however, did note a steady bilateral frontal-temporal headache which would on occasion awaken him from sleep and which gradually became worse.

Five days prior to admission, some fogginess in thinking was noted and the patient's family reported some personality change. The patient reported weakness of both legs getting out of a bath tub and felt that this was predominantly right-sided.

Two days prior to admission, the patient was noted to be sleeping longer.

On the day of admission, the patient and his physician noted a more persistent left-sided weakness, and the patient was admitted to the neurology service.

PAST HISTORY:

Was not remarkable except for hyperthyroidism under treatment since 1966. The patient had been evaluated in 1966 for a minor episode of dizziness which had occurred in relation to bradycardia and a transient fall in blood pressure. Note was made at that time of a normal neurological status including mental status. The right carotid pulse was noted to be decreased compared to the left.

NEUROLOGICAL EXAMINATION: October 28, 1969

1. *Mental status:*
   a. The patient was alert.
   b. He was oriented for time, place, and person.
   c. His knowledge of current events was intact.
   d. Memory was intact. The patient could remember 4-of-5 objects in 5 minutes. Digit span was 8 forward and 5 in reverse.

2. *Cranial nerves:* All were intact except for a questionable left-central facial weakness.

3. *Motor system:*
   a. A decrease in strength, predominantly distal, was noted in the left leg. To a lesser degree, a mild weakness of the left upper extremity was present.
   b. The patient dragged the left leg in walking.

4. *Reflexes:*
   a. Deep tendon reflexes were symmetrical but increased bilaterally.
   b. Plantar responses were flexor.

5. *Sensory system:* Intact.

6. The right carotid pulse was decreased as noted previously in 1966.

LABORATORY DATA:

1. *Electroencephalogram:* Frequent focal 3 to 5 cps slow wave activity was present throughout the right hemisphere, being most prominent in the frontal area, suggesting focal damage.

2. *Brain scan (Hg^{197}):* Normal.

3. *Arteriogram:* A right carotid study indicated a shift of the anterior cerebral vessels to the left and a depression downward of the middle cerebral vessels. The terminal cortical branches of the right middle and anterior cerebral arteries failed to reach the inner table of the skull, suggesting an avasc-

ular area overlying the cortex: for example, a subdural hematoma.

HOSPITAL COURSE:

A progressive change in neurological status was soon evident.

Twenty-four hours after admission, the patient was intermittently lethargic. If roused, he was able to answer questions. Mental status testing was not possible except to ascertain that the patient was disoriented for time. Deep tendon reflexes were now asymmetrical and increased on the left, and a left Babinski sign was now present. Later that day increasing weakness of the left arm and leg were now present. The patient was unable to raise his arm at the shoulder, or the leg, at the hip. The patient became more lethargic and approximately 30 hours after admission, the right pupil was noted to be sluggish in response to light. A significant pupillary asymmetry was now present. The right measured 3.5 mm., the left 2.5 mm.; previously the pupils had been symmetrical. The right carotid arteriogram was immediately performed. Shortly thereafter, under local anesthesia, Trephine (burr) holes were placed in the right frontal and parietal areas by Dr. Bertram Selverstone and Dr. Peter Carney of the neurosurgical service. A 1.5 cm. thickness of dark chocolate fluid blood with a thin covering membrane was evacuated from the right frontal-parietal subdural space. The cortex which had been depressed from the inner table re-expanded to fill the space previously occupied by the subdural hematoma. The cortical surface appeared normal.

The patient made a rapid recovery. Examination ten hours after surgery disclosed an alert and well-oriented patient who was able to lift his leg off the bed and had only a minimal weakness in the left upper extremity. The pupils were equal. The deep tendon reflexes were symmetrical and the plantar responses were flexor.

At the time of discharge on November 11, 1969, 13 days after surgery, the neurological examination was completely normal.

COMMENT:

The relatively sudden development of a hemiparesis in a man of 73, taken in isolation, probably would have resulted in a diagnosis of cerebral vascular disease with cerebral infarction. The history of trauma 10 days previously and the history of some change in personality and fogginess in thinking proc-

esses 5 days prior to admission, raised the question of a possible subdural hematoma. The subsequent progression in the hemiparesis following his hospital admission and the fluctuating state of alertness made further investigation mandatory.

It should be noted that the preliminary laboratory studies in this case (skull x-ray, electroencephalogram, and brain scan) were not helpful as regards the diagnosis of subdural hematoma. At times, however, such studies may be more helpful. Thus the skull x-rays may reveal displacement of a calcified pineal gland. The electroencephalogram may reveal a focal reduction in amplitude (voltage suppression) suggesting that a nonviable mass of tissue is separating the recording electrodes from the electrically active tissue of the cerebral cortex. The electrically inactive tissue does not always have to be a subdural hematoma. Swelling of the scalp, an epidural hematoma, a subdural effusion, a large intracerebral hematoma, or a porencephalic cyst close to the cortical surface could also produce this effect. At times the brain scan may be helpful in demonstrating a crescent-shaped area close to the inner table; at times, an avascular area, at times, a border of increased uptake of dye.

In the present case, the arteriogram certainly indicated a space-occupying mass in the right hemisphere. More important, from a diagnostic standpoint, was the suggestion of an avascular area overlying the right frontal-parietal area.

Even without the results of the arteriogram, the next step, the placement of Trephine holes, would have been indicated on the basis of the progressive but fluctuating impairment of alertness. The development of the sluggish pupil on the right suggesting tentorial herniation of the right temporal lobe required that this procedure be performed as an emergency. In some instances there may be insufficient time for arteriography to be performed. In other instances, it is clear that the risks of arteriography are greater than the minor risks of burr hole placement. In any case, the risks of the operative procedure are minor compared to the clinical state which will result following tentorial herniation. The prompt recovery in the present case confirmed these guide lines.

The following case history illustrates a chronic subdural hematoma. The relationship to trauma was not clear cut. There were only minor findings of a focal nature. Rather the predominant findings were those related to progressive confusion and lethargy.

Case History 11. NECH #129–538.
Date of admission: 9/16/59.

This 67-year-old, right-handed, retired, divorced, male insurance broker (Mr. L.J.) was referred for evaluation of headaches and confusion. The patient lived by himself, and the history was obtained from the patient's landlady.

Three months prior to admission, the patient began complaining of frontal headache relieved by recumbency. Three weeks before admission, the onset of minor confusion in conversation was noted. One week prior to admission, the patient became very lethargic and more confused. The lethargy improved somewhat over the two days prior to admission. During the week prior to admission, the patient remained in bed complaining of an inability to walk.

PAST HISTORY: There was a questionable history of minor head trauma perhaps 3 to 5 months prior to admission. This information, however, only emerged later during his hospitalization. There was no significant intake of drug or of ethanol. There was a 7-year history of apathy and depression.

GENERAL PHYSICAL EXAMINATION:

There were no remarkable findings except for diffuse rhonchi and wheezes throughout both lungs.

NEUROLOGICAL EXAMINATION:

1. *Mental status:*
   a. The patient was drowsy but could be aroused, at which time a marked vulgarity of speech was present, indicating a significant preoccupation with feces and the anal genital area.
   b. The patient was grossly disoriented for time and place (March 1, 1938, Springfield, Massachusetts).
   c. Store of information was fair and calculations were relatively well performed.
2. *Cranial nerves:*
   a. On funduscopic examination, the disk margins were slightly indistinct.
   b. The pupils were equal and responded to light.
   c. A slight left facial asymmetry was present—? actual weakness.
3. *Motor system:*
   a. The patient moved all four limbs with no definite weakness.
   b. The patient claimed he was unable to sit or stand by himself. When assisted to his feet, he was able to walk in a staggering manner, using small steps. His gait improved once he had started off.
   c. Cerebellar tests were negative.
4. *Reflexes:*
   a. Deep tendon reflexes were all hyperactive and slightly increased on the left.
   b. The plantar response was flexor on the right, extensor on the left.
   c. Strong grasp reflexes were present bilaterally.
5. *Sensation:* Pain was intact. Other modalities could not be tested.
6. *Skull:* There was no definite local tenderness.

LABORATORY DATA:

1. Complete blood count and sedimentation rate were normal.
2. Skull x-rays were normal. The pineal was not calcified. Chest x-rays revealed apical blebs suggesting emphysema. There was no evidence of tumor.
3. Electroencephalogram was abnormal because of generalized slow wave activity suggesting a generalized damage.

HOSPITAL COURSE:

Examination on the day following admission demonstrated progression of neurological findings. The patient was incontinent of urine and somewhat less alert. By 5 days after admission, the patient's verbal responses were limited to yes and no answers. Unintelligible mumbling was prominent. Simple directions were followed in an inconsistent manner. On September 22, 1959, 6 days after admission, several observers now noted a slightly larger pupil on the right. Because of increasing lethargy and a "catatonic state," bilateral burr holes were produced in the temporal-parietal areas under local anesthesia by Dr. Samuel Brendler. The underlying dura was dark and when incised 100 to 125 cc. of old dark blood was ejected in a pulsatile manner under pressure. Significant amounts of hematoma were washed out of the anterior areas overlying the frontal lobes. The underlying brain was covered by a smooth glistening yellow-tinged membrane.

The surface of the cortex which had been depressed 2 cm. pulsated well. During the procedure, after the hematomas had been removed, the patient began to move about actively. He spoke fluently and clearly when the operation was completed. In marked contrast to his preoperative status of semi-coma, he now appeared somewhat agitated.

It was noted, incidentally, in shaving the skull for the operative procedure, that a depression was present in the right parietal area. This may have reflected the remote trauma which precipitated the subdural hematomas.

By the third postoperative day, the patient was described as alert and totally oriented with significant improvement in memory and concentration. The patient was discharged from the hospital on the seventh postoperative day with neurological status intact.

COMMENT:

When admitted to the hospital, the location of the lesion appeared relatively clear. The predominant findings were those of bilateral frontal lobe involvement with confusion, bilateral grasp reflexes, and a frontal lobe apraxia of gait. The latter undoubtedly explained the patient's complaint of an inability to sit or stand at a time when no actual weakness was present.

The nature of the pathological process involving the frontal lobes, however, was uncertain. The history of trauma emerged only later during his hospitalization. Although the possibility of subdural hematoma was considered, this diagnosis did not rate high on the differential diagnostic list. More likely possibilities were metastatic disease from the lung, either a carcinoma or abscess, in view of the pulmonary findings and a past history of heavy cigarette smoking. Also in view of the 7-year history of a late onset depression and personality change, the possibilities of a frontal parasagittal meningioma or of a frontal glioma were raised. The subsequent historical information, the fluctuations in the level of consciousness with progressive obtundation of consciousness, and the minor pupillary change then suggested the possibility of subdural hematomas. The burr holes were diagnostic as well as therapeutic.

General Comment Concerning Subdural Hematomas. Certain general comments should be made regarding subdural hematomas. The history of trauma may be lacking. In some cases, the actual trauma may have been trivial. This is particularly the case in patients who may be regarded as being at special risk: patients receiving anticoagulant medications following coronary artery occlusion or cerebral vessel insufficiency, or in patients with bleeding disorders, e.g., as in leukemias. The problem is more common in the elderly and in chronic alcoholics, perhaps because such population groups are more prone to ataxia and falls.

The problem also exists during the first year of infancy; the picture presented, however, differs significantly from that seen in the adult because in the infant, separation of the sutures may occur, allowing the intracranial cavity to expand. The onset is then often nonspecific and nonfocal: an enlargement of the head, a failure to thrive, a failure to gain weight, a failure to reach developmental landmarks. At times generalized seizures, vomiting, and papilledema may be noted. The etiology often relates to presumed birth trauma.

A related problem may also be seen in infants following meningitis. This is the problem of *subdural effusions* usually occurring in relation to hemophilus influenza meningitis. The diagnosis of both subdural hematoma and subdural effusions may be made in the infant by needle punctures into the subdural space at the lateral margin of the still-open anterior fontanelle. The cerebrospinal fluid in these cases is often found to be abnormal with the presence of blood or xanthochromia and an elevated protein content.

It is clear then that the manifestations and the latent period of a subdural hematoma may well depend on the potential subdural space available before compression of the cerebral cortex occurs. In the infant, separation of sutures may occur, and tentorial herniation is unlikely. In the elderly adult when senility is present with marked cortical atrophy, a considerable volume of hematoma may collect after trauma before symptoms are noticeable. One may comment in retrospect that perhaps case #10 developed symptoms so soon after trauma because, although age 73, he did not have atrophy of the cerebral cortex.

Several less common traumatic problems involving the vasculature of the brain should be mentioned. Thus, occasional rupture of the cavernous portion of the carotid artery into the cavernous sinus may occur—more particularly if an aneurysm is present in this location. The resultant syndrome involves a unilateral pulsating exophthalmos (outward protrusion of the eye) with an audible bruit (pulsatile sound) over the eye.

There is, in addition, involvement of those cranial nerves passing through the wall of the cavernous sinus—most often the ophthalmic division of the trigeminal nerve and the oculomotor. Often cranial nerves VI and IV are involved as well.

The student should also bear in mind that occasionally trauma involving the neck will result in compression and occlusion of the carotid artery with the production of acute infarctions within the territory of this vessel.

LATE EFFECTS OF HEAD TRAUMA

Posttraumatic Epilepsy. Seizures are common, but minor head trauma is even more common. Frequently when a history is being taken from a patient with seizures, the patient or his relatives will mention a minor head injury weeks, months, or years prior to the onset of the seizures. Often the history of head trauma in itself is irrelevant, but there are other factors in the history suggesting another etiology for the seizures, e.g., strong family history of a seizure disorder, birth trauma, long-standing mental retardation, previous meningitis, or encephalitis. Under certain circumstances, however, there is a relationship of the head trauma to the seizures. These seizures may be termed posttraumatic epilepsy. They may be focal or generalized.

Penetrating injuries of the head, as in wartime wounds from bullets or shrapnel, are likely to be associated with posttraumatic seizures. In the World War II series of Watson, 41.6 per cent of such patients developed seizures within 3 years of the injury, the majority within 6 to 12 months. There is some evidence that factors such as the location of the wound within the cerebral hemisphere and the complication of abscess may influence the incidence of such posttraumatic seizures.

Most head injuries in civilian life, however, are not penetrating missile wounds but rather blunt and nonpenetrating injuries (closed head trauma), and under these circumstances, seizures are much less common. Thus, in the series of Jennett, the overall incidence of seizures in 1000 consecutive blunt head injuries was approximately 5 per cent over a 4-year period. The risk of late seizures was definitely increased by several factors:

a. Depressed skull fractures with penetration of the dura had a 50 per cent risk, but simple fractures only a 3 per cent risk.

b. Intracranial hematomas had a 25 to 33 per cent risk.

c. Patients who had seizures associated with the acute injury had a 25 to 33 per cent risk of posttraumatic epilepsy.

d. Patients who had prolonged periods of unconsciousness associated with the injury were more likely to have posttraumatic seizures.

When the factors of acute seizures, depressed fractures, and intracranial hematomas were disregarded, the overall risk for posttraumatic seizures in this group fell to 1 per cent. This does not differ greatly from the overall risk of seizures in the general population. In summary, the posttraumatic seizures are more likely to occur in those head injuries where actual structural damage of the cerebral cortex has occurred.

Postconcussion Syndrome. Another relatively common late complication of head trauma is the posttraumatic or postconcussion syndrome consisting of recurrent episodes of headache and dizziness (vertigo or light-headedness). The episodes often appear to be precipitated by exercise or change in posture from the recumbent to the upright. The severity and duration of the syndrome bears no relationship to the severity of the trauma; the episodes may continue for years after a trivial injury. In a few cases, the vertigo may be related to a traumatic disturbance of the labyrinthe. In many cases, the dizziness is actually a light-headedness related to anxiety and hyperventilation. In general, no actual pathology is found. As a general rule, stable, well-motivated individuals who are anxious to return to their previous occupation or studies, do not experience this syndrome in severe degree. On the other hand, individuals with disorders of personality or psychoneurosis or with problems in adjusting to studies or employment appear to be severely affected.

INFECTIONS AFFECTING THE CEREBRAL HEMISPHERES

The central nervous system may be involved by all of the general types of organisms which infect other systems of the body: bacteria, viruses, rickettsiae, fungi, protozoa, and helminths. Certain organisms do have a predilection for the central nervous system and often for particular segments or certain systems of the neuroaxis. Thus we have already seen that the virus of poliomyelitis involves predominantly the motor neurons of the anterior horn and brain stem. Bacteria such as meningococcus and Hemophilus influenzae involve predominantly the meninges. In most instances when infectious agents involve the central nervous system, they also involve to a variable degree other systems of the body in a general or focal manner. The student should bear in mind that the clinical and pathological manifestations of an infectious disease reflect not only the direct effects of the invading organism but also those effects which reflect the body's defensive responses to invasion.

Infections involving the nervous system may be considered under two broad categories:

1. Those infections which involve the central nervous system or subdivisions of the central nervous system in a general or diffuse manner.

2. Those infections which involve the central nervous system in a focal (or multifocal) manner.

GENERAL OR DIFFUSE INFECTIONS

The first category of diseases is usually considered in more detail in microbiology courses and in the infectious disease sections of internal medicine. We will, however, outline several common syndromes. In a broad sense such infections may be subdivided into

a. those involving primarily the leptomeninges (pia and arachnoid) producing leptomeningitis. Generalized infection of the dura (pachymeningitis) is uncommon.

b. those involving primarily the parenchyma of the brain, producing encephalitis.

There are some infections, often viral, where a combined involvement is produced, a meningoencephalitis.

MENINGITIS

The manifestations of meningitis depend on the organism involved, the age of the patient, and the underlying physical status of the patient. Acute, subacute, and chronic forms may be considered.

Acute Purulent (Bacterial or Septic) Meningitis. This is the most common form of infection of the central nervous system (if one omits from consideration certain in-

frequent epidemics of encephalitis). In each case, a specific bacterial organism may be isolated from the cerebrospinal fluid in the subarachnoid space. In addition the spinal fluid shows evidence of an acute inflammatory reaction. The fluid is cloudy and under increased pressure with large numbers of white blood cells, predominantly polymorphonuclear leukocytes, e.g., 90 to 98 per cent of 500 to 40,000 white blood cells per cubic mm. The sugar content is markedly reduced.

The specific responsible organism will depend on the age of the patient. During the first month of life the gram negative rod Escherichia coli — normally found in the gastrointestinal tract — accounts for most of these cases. During the period 6 months to 4 years of age, Hemophilus influenzae (a small gram negative bacillus occurring in rod or coccoid form) is the major offender.

In older children and young adults, Neisseria meningitidis (intracellularis) — meningococcus (a gram negative diplococcus) — predominates. Sporadic cases occur but the majority of cases probably occur during epidemics when overcrowded conditions exist. Such conditions are likely to exist in school dormitories or in military barracks. The agent is present in the nasopharyngeal secretions, and spread probably occurs through droplet contamination. In this age group, those cases not due to the meningococcus are invariably due to the pneumococcus (a lancet-shaped, gram positive diplococcus), an agent more commonly responsible for infections in the respiratory tract (lung, middle ear, and paranasal sinuses).

It should be noted that both the meningococcus and the pneumococcus may produce meningitis in the 6 months to 4 years age group, although the more common etiological agent in that age group is Hemophilus influenzae. At all ages, acute meningitis due to trauma (associated with compound skull fractures or with dural tears allowing communication of the subarachnoid space with the paranasal sinuses) is usually due to the pneumococcus, or less often to the staphylococcus.

The method of invasion of the central nervous system in other cases may involve the direct extension of a purulent infection involving the middle ear or paranasal sinuses or bone of the skull. Rarely, retrograde infection from these areas may involve the dural venous sinuses in a thrombophlebitis and, then, in a retrograde manner, may spread to involve the leptomeninges. On rare occasions a congenital dermal sinus tract is present, permitting skin bacteria to invade the meninges. In the large majority of cases of bacterial meningitis, however, the organism has infected the meninges after entering the blood stream from a primary focus in the respiratory tract or gastrointestinal tract. The circumstances that allow such blood borne infection to involve the meninges only in particular cases are not certain. Thus most patients with a bacteremia do not develop a meningitis.

The pathological features on postmortem examination of the brain reflect the cere-

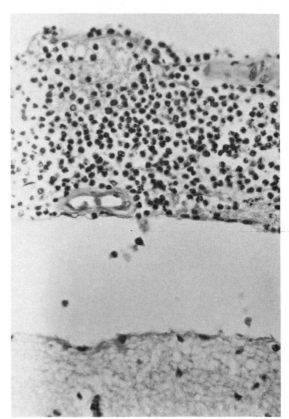

Figure 22–31 Acute meningitis (pneumococcal). The subarachnoid space is filled with inflammatory cells, predominantly polymorphonuclear leukocytes. There has been artifactual detachment of the pia from the cortical surface. (H & E × 400.) (Courtesy of Pathology Department, Tufts University School of Medicine.)

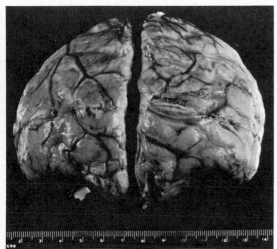

Figure 22–30 Acute meningitis (pneumococcal). This 57-year-old white male had been living in a nursing home with a diagnosis of chronic undifferentiated schizophrenia. He had always been withdrawn and uncommunicative, but 2 weeks previously had become less responsive than usual. Three days prior to admission, he developed a temperature of 104° and was given penicillin for the "grippe." On the day of admission, the patient fell out of bed and became comatose. A left and then bilateral fixed dilated pupils developed followed by Cheyne-Stokes periodic respirations, decerebrate posture, and death. Cerebrospinal fluid was cloudy with 11,861 white blood cells (80% polymorphonuclears) and a sugar of 36 mg./100 ml. Culture of the cerebrospinal fluid subsequently revealed D. pneumococcus. At autopsy, the brain was swollen with a yellow-green purulent exudate present in the subarachnoid space. (Courtesy of Dr. John Hills, New England Center Hospitals; and Dr. Jose Segarra, Boston Veterans Administration Hospital.)

See Filmstrip, Frame 53.

brospinal fluid findings. Grossly, the pia-arachnoid is congested and cloudy (Fig. 22–30). Creamy colored purulent material may be visualized in the subarachnoid space particularly within the sulci and subarachnoid cisterns. Microscopic examination reveals that the subarachnoid space is filled with an exudate of polymorphonuclear leukocytes with infiltration of the pia and arachnoid (Fig. 22–31). Within the exudate, bacteria may be present in an intracellular or extracellular manner. The exudate is also noted within the Virchow-Robin spaces—that extension of the subarachnoid space about the blood vessels as they pass into the substance of the brain. The subpial areas of the cortex usually appear otherwise quite normal. Infiltration of the outer adventitial sheath of the blood vessels within the subarachnoid space may be noted. If the inflammatory process continues as when treatment has been delayed, these vessels may be occluded with infarction of the cerebral cortex. Also, with time, the character of the exudate changes; mononuclear cells appear, fibrin is deposited, and eventually (after 3 to 4 weeks) fibroblastic proliferation occurs. This latter process may result in compression of the cranial nerves at the base of the brain and obliteration of the subarachnoid cisterns.

The clinical picture of acute purulent meningitis depends on the age of the patient. An infant under 6 months of age may be febrile, listless and drowsy and may vomit and fail to take feedings. The anterior fontanelle of an infant will be under increased pressure and bulging. An older infant or a child is likely to have nuchal rigidity (resistance to passive flexion of the neck) in addition to fever, convulsions, and coma. A posture of opisthotonos may be present (extreme extension of head, neck, trunk, and limbs).

The older child and adult with meningococcal meningitis will usually have a prodromal period characterized by symptoms of an upper respiratory infection, low grade fever, and various body aches. With septicemia and, then, the subsequent involvement of the meninges, the symptoms of chills, vomiting, severe headache, and neck stiffness occur, often followed by an alteration in consciousness. The signs of central nervous system involvement often appear relatively abruptly. A skin rash is common in the stage of bacteremia. Small or large areas of skin hemorrhage (petechiae and purpura) due to involvement and occlusion of the skin capillaries occur during the process of septicemia and are caused either directly by the organism or indirectly as a result of disseminated aggregation of platelets into small thrombi.

The early recognition of acute purulent meningitis is of importance. If it is untreated, serious intracranial complications develop and death is the usual outcome. Prior to the era of specific antimicrobial therapy, the mortality was close to 90 per cent. With specific therapy this figure has been markedly reduced so that the actual mortality in meningococcal and H. influenzae meningitis is now under 10 per cent. In the case of meningococcal meningitis, with adequate treatment and early recognition, complications and morbidity are now uncommon.

The drugs of choice at the present time are chloramphenicol and sulfadiazine for Hemophilus influenzae; penicillin for meningococcus; penicillin for pneumococcus; and chloramphenicol for E. coli. At times when identity of the microbial agent is uncertain or bacterial culture reports are not yet available, triple therapy with penicillin, chloramphenicol, and sulfadiazine will be employed. Alternatively a single broad spectrum semisynthetic penicillin, such as ampicillin, may be used. At times hydrocortisone may also be administered to counter adrenal cortical exhaustion and to reduce meningeal inflammatory response. The student should consult appropriate references as regards dosage and duration of treatment.

There are several possible complications of meningitis. While these are more likely to occur in delayed or untreated cases, some may occur in those patients receiving adequate treatment. With a marked increase in intracranial pressure (at times lumbar subarachnoid cerebrospinal fluid pressure at lumbar puncture may be 600 mm. of water compared to a normal pressure of 150 mm.) herniation of medial temporal areas through the tentorium may occur with compression of the third cranial nerve and midbrain. With involvement of blood vessel walls, occlusion of cortical arteries and veins may occur with resultant infarction. Venous involvement may lead to dural sinus occlusion. The occlusion of cortical veins and superior sagittal sinus may lead to hemorrhagic infarction of the parasagittal frontal parietal areas with a resultant weakness of the lower extremities and focal seizures. In addition, a further increase in intracranial pressure may occur.

As we have already indicated, a thick exudate at the base of the brain (somewhat more likely to occur in pneumococcal meningitis) may damage cranial nerves and also obliterate the subarachnoid cisterns. The end result may be a significant degree of hydrocephalus since cerebrospinal fluid will be unable to pass up over the hemispheres to the areas of absorption. In the child, a progressive enlargement of the head occurs.

Another complication in the infant (usually in relation to H. influenzae meningitis) may also result in progressive drowsiness and a progressive enlargement of the head: subdural effusions. This complication can be ascertained through the use of the electroencephalogram, translumination of the skull, and, more specifically, subdural taps through the lateral corners of the anterior fontanelle.

Acute Aseptic Meningitis. In these cases, the clinical signs and symptoms of meningitis are present in the sense that the patient complains of headache and stiffness of the neck. Vomiting and nuchal rigidity are present. These findings are usually less fulminating than those in acute purulent meningitis, e.g., sudden coma and purpura in the adult is unlikely; consciousness is usually well preserved. The spinal fluid, moreover, is often clear or only minimally cloudy (often described as opalescent). A relatively small number of white blood cells is present (5 to 2000 per cubic mm. and usually less than 500 per cubic mm.) in comparison to acute purulent meningitis. Moreover, the white blood cells are predominantly mononuclear (lymphocytes and monocytes). The sugar content of the spinal fluid is normal. Moreover, smears and bacteriological cultures of the spinal fluid fail to reveal a responsible organism. In general the causative organism is a virus: ECHO, Coxsackie, nonparalytic poliomyelitis, mumps, and lymphocytic choriomeningitis.

In general these viral meningitides are self-limited, nonfatal, and without significant complication. The student should note, however, that a similar cerebrospinal fluid reaction may also characterize certain diseases where a secondary meningeal reaction occurs: subdural empyema, brain abscess, and venous sinus thrombosis. At times a similar spinal fluid formula may be noted in a viral encephalitis. The aforementioned viral agents may of course at times present a combined syndrome of meningoencephalitis.

Moreover, at times several more significant subacute infections in their early stages may present a predominantly mononuclear reaction in the spinal fluid: tuberculous and cryptococcal (fungal) meningitis. Bacterial organisms will be absent on routine smears and cultures of the cerebrospinal fluid. However, both of these infections are characterized by a low spinal fluid sugar, and appropriate stains and cultures will eventually disclose the organisms. These infections, although not common at the present time, are of importance because specific therapy is required.

Differentiation of the various types of viral meningitis may be made by specialized immunological techniques for the measurement of neutralizing antibodies.

Viral meningitis is a self-limited disease. No specific treatment is available. Recovery is in general complete.

Subacute and Chronic Forms of Meningitis. Within this group the following may be included: tuberculous meningitis (Mycobacterium tuberculosis), fungal meningitis, (usually Cryptococcus neoformans), and the meningovascular form of neurosyphilis (Treponema pallidum). Chronic meningitis may also occur on a noninfectious basis when a metastatic carcinoma, a sarcoma, or a glioblastoma involves the meninges. Each of these infections is associated with a mononuclear reaction in the cerebrospinal fluid. The protein content is increased. The sugar content is low in the tuberculous and fungal forms, but usually normal in the meningitis-complicating neurosyphilis. The chloride content is often low in the tuberculous and fungal varieties. Each of these diseases is characterized from the pathological standpoint by a more chronic type of inflammatory reaction designated as granulomatous and characterized by aggregates of mononuclear cells, altered elongated mononuclear cells (epithelioid cells), multinucleated giant cells, and fibroblasts. In both the tuberculous and syphilitic varieties, inflammatory involvement of blood vessel walls is prominent.

Tuberculous Meningitis. In general, tuberculous meningitis occurs in young children or young adults and is usually indicative of miliary dissemination from a primary focus in the lung (less often the primary focus is gastrointestinal). It is still uncertain whether direct hematogenous spread to the meninges occurs or whether there is a prodromal stage of hematogenous spread resulting in tubercles (chronic granulomatous infection) involving the meninges or the surface of the cortex, with secondary meningeal dissemination then occurring from these areas.

The picture on pathological examination is that of a thick, gray, fibrous, gelatinous, and necrotic exudate at the base of the brain. Areas of caseation (cheese-like necrosis) may be found in addition to small firm yellow-white nodules (tubercles). Microscopic examination reveals a dense exudate composed of lymphocytes, histocytes, fibrin, local areas of necrosis, and surrounding epithelioid cells. Infrequent giant cells are noted. The acid fast tubercle bacillus may be demonstrated with special stains. Involvement of the walls of an artery by this inflammatory reaction is common, with a resultant occlusion of the vessel and infarction of the areas supplied by the vessel.

The pathophysiology involves, however, not only this vascular process but also the local compression and invasion of cranial nerves at the base of the brain. Thus, extraocular palsies may be frequent and persistent. This thick exudate at the base of the brain also serves to obliterate the subarachnoid cisterns; hydrocephalus then is not an infrequent complication in cases which survive.

The diagnosis is made on the basis of the clinical picture of subacute ill health, weight loss, vomiting, headache, confusion, and extraocular palsies, plus chest x-ray findings, plus spinal fluid findings, plus or minus a positive tuberculin skin test in a young child or young adult. The organism may be demonstrated in acid fast (Ziehl-Neelsen) stains of smears of the spinal fluid sediment or of smears of the fibrin clot which often forms in a test tube of cerebrospinal fluid. The results of the smear may be confirmed by special cultures and guinea pig inoculation.

Untreated, the disease, in the past, was usually fatal in 3 to 8 weeks. With modern treatment—isoniazid, plus streptomycin, plus paraminosalicylic acid, plus or minus hydrocortisone (to reduce the inflammatory response)—the mortality rate in young children has been reduced to 25 per cent. If early treatment is undertaken, significant permanent morbidity may often be avoided. If treatment is delayed, the patient will survive but with significant residual deficits of the types previously indicated.

Fungal Meningitis. The most common form of fungal meningitis is that caused by *Cryptococcus neoformans.* This is a relatively uncommon disease. It occurs occasionally in an otherwise intact individual. Most of the cases have occurred in patients with alterations in immunological defenses, e.g., patients with leukemia or lymphomas—particularly those treated with immunosuppressive drugs or with high dosages of corticosteroids. Cases have also been reported in patients under treatment for pulmonary tuberculosis or for sarcoid, the latter a chronic granulomatous disease often treated with corticosteroids.

The clinical picture is that of a chronic headache, with signs of meningeal irritation and increased intracranial pressure. The process is often present for weeks to months prior to the establishment of a diagnosis. From a gross pathological standpoint, a chronic granulomatous exudate is found at the base of the brain. This often contains nodules and foamy gelatinous cysts which may involve the superficial layers of the cortex and ventricular system as well. The exudate contains mononuclear cells, giant cells, and the thick encapsulated organism.

The diagnosis is made on the basis of the clinical picture of chronic meningitis occurring in special-risk patients (patients with diseases of the reticuloendothelial systems), plus the characteristic cerebrospinal fluid findings, plus or minus the demonstration of the thickly encapsulated organisms on India Ink stains of the spinal fluid, plus isolation of the organism by culture of the cerebrospinal fluid on Sabouraud's medium or after animal inoculation of the spinal fluid.

The untreated disease is often fatal within months; however, it is not unusual to find cases where the disease has been present for several years. A significant improvement will occur following treatment with the antifungal agent, amphotericin B. This agent must be administered intravenously; various side effects commonly occur.

Meningovascular Syphilis. The nervous system may be involved by syphilis (Treponema pallidum) in a variety of syndromes, grouped under the term *neurosyphilis.* Invasion of the central nervous system by Treponema pallidum may occur within a few weeks or months of the original infection. Rarely, abnormalities may be noted in the cerebrospinal fluid during the primary (focal) stage of the infection (the stage of the primary cutaneous or mucus membrane chancre). Abnormalities do occur in the spinal fluid in one-third of the patients during the secondary stage (a stage of a generalized rash when generalized dissemination of the disease has occurred). Some patients will present clinical evidence of an acute meningitis at this time, but more often the onset of neurological symptoms is delayed for a number of years until the tertiary stage.

It should be pointed out that the majority of patients who have had syphilis do not have actual invasion of the central nervous system. Thus, in the era before the use of specific antibiotic therapy (penicillin), Merritt, Adams, and Solomon found clinical or serological evidence of involvement of the nervous system in only 29 per cent of 2263 cases examined after the secondary stage infection. At the present time, adequate treatment with penicillin during the primary or secondary stage will prevent the development of significant central nervous system involvement.

In the past, when invasion of the central nervous system had occurred, several clinical syndromes resulted: (a) *asymptomatic* cases (abnormalities in the spinal fluid without clinical symptoms or signs of nervous system damage), (b) *meningovascular* cases (chronic meningitis with inflammatory involvement and occlusion of cerebral and spinal blood vessels), (c) *parenchymatous-tabetic* cases (involvement of posterior roots with secondary degeneration of the posterior columns producing the syndrome of tabes dorsalis), (d) *parenchymatous-paretic* cases (invasion of cerebral cortex in an encephalitis producing the personality changes, dementia, and psychosis of general paresis). In the neurosyphilis series of Merritt, Adams, and Solomon, 31 per cent of the cases were asymptomatic, 16 per cent were meningovascular, 30 per cent were tabetic, and 12 per cent were paretic.

Tabes dorsalis has been considered in Chapter 8, p. 191; general paresis will be considered later in this chapter.

The asymptomatic cases represent inadvertent early discovery of instances where tertiary parenchymatous involvement of the cardiovascular or central nervous system may occur at a later point in time. The spinal fluid changes—a positive serological test and a minor cellular response—probably indicate subclinical meningeal inflammation. The blood serological tests also are usually positive. These cases are of importance because prompt treatment with penicillin will prevent the development of such late complications.

The meningovascular form of neurosyphilis usually appears within the first 2 years of the infection. As noted, however, meningitis may occur during the time of the secondary stage rash. Moreover, the vascular occlusive component of meningovascular syphilis may continue to occur many years after the symptoms of the meningitis have subsided.

As with the other forms of chronic meningitis, chronic inflammation of the meninges (mononuclear infiltration, fibrosis, and some granuloma—so-called gumma formation) at the base of the brain results in several complications: (a) obliteration of subarachnoid cerebrospinal fluid pathways with the production of hydrocephalus and increased intracranial pressure (reflected in an increased pressure at the time of lumbar puncture), (b) cranial nerve palsies, or (c) inflammatory involvement of the vessels at the base of the brain and of those smaller vessels present in the pia arachnoid supplying the cortical surface of the cerebral convexity.

The development of focal symptoms such as hemiplegia or aphasia is not unusual. In some patients the meningeal and vascular pathology appear to involve the spinal cord predominantly with lesser involvement of the cerebral hemispheres.

The diagnosis of meningovascular syphilis is made on the basis of a subacute meningitis, plus characteristic cerebrospinal fluid findings (increased pressure, cell count of 100 to 1000 lymphocytes per cubic mm., increased protein, normal sugar, and positive serology), plus positive blood serology, plus or minus a past history and findings of focal or multifocal infarcts involving the cerebral cortex, brain stem, and spinal cord.

The primary meningeal symptoms of headache, stiff neck, and vomiting usually subside even without treatment within several weeks. These are, however, likely to be residuals reflecting the involvement of cranial nerves and occlusion of multiple vessels. These complications and the later development of the parenchymatous forms of neurosyphilis can be avoided through the prompt administration of penicillin.

ENCEPHALITIS

At the present time significant diffuse inflammatory involvement of the parenchyma of the brain produced by infectious agents is probably less common as a clinical problem than those diseases considered under the category of meningitis. This statement should, however, be modified to indicate that during particular epidemics certain infectious agents involving the central nervous system have produced a large number of cases with encephalitis. Moreover, subclinical or minor diffuse involvement of the central nervous system probably occurs in the course of a number of common viral diseases.

In general, most cases falling into this category reflect viral infection. With the exception of the spirochete, bacteria do not produce a diffuse encephalitis, although bacteria may produce multiple areas of abscess formation. Other infectious agents may produce encephalitic involvement of the nervous system. The rickettsiae (intermediate in size between bacteria and viruses) usually produce signs of a meningoencephalitis in addition to a characteristic skin rash (e.g., Typhus, Rocky Mountain spotted fever). Moreover, certain protozoal parasites may invade the central nervous system producing a subacute encephalitis (e.g. toxoplasmosis or trypanosomiasis—the latter referred to as African sleeping sickness).

Encephalitis may be acute or chronic. Most cases fall into the acute category; most viral and rickettsial diseases are acute. On the other hand, the spirochetal infection and protozoal infections of the central nervous system are, in general, chronic or subacute processes. Recently, however, several viruses have been implicated in chronic diffuse progressive processes (previously considered to be of an unknown etiology) involving the nervous system.

ACUTE ENCEPHALITIS: ACUTE VIRAL INFECTIONS

The pathology of viral invasion of neural parenchyma may be described in general terms as involving a viral invasion of neurons with the production of intranuclear or intracytoplasmic inclusions and the acute degeneration and destruction of nerve cells. There is a cellular infiltration of neural tissue and an accumulation of inflammatory cells about the degenerating nerve cells, in a perivascular location (Fig. 22–32). The cells are usually mononuclear although in some processes, e.g., acute poliomyelitis or in a severe case of encephalitis, there is often noted a significant number of polymorphonuclear leukocytes at times involved in neuronophagia. A microglia proliferation is often noted in the involved neural parenchyma. To a variable degree infiltration of adjacent meninges by inflammatory cells is usually present. Depending on the degree of meningeal infiltration and on the severity to which the underlying parenchyma is involved, a variable increase in cells (predominantly lymphocytes) will be noted in the spinal fluid. Occasionally a normal cell count may be present, more often 100 to 500 cells per cubic mm. are present. The protein content is usually increased; the sugar and chloride content are normal. The differentiation of the particular virus involved depends on:

a. The specific clinical pattern of the disease: some viruses involve particular areas

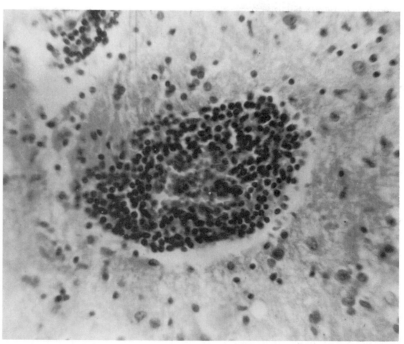

Figure 22–32 Encephalitis (herpes simplex). A significant collection of mononuclear cells is present in the perivascular space with infiltration of adjacent cerebral cortex. This 32-year-old patient had the acute onset of fever, headache, and generalized convulsions. Over a 30-day period, he developed increasing stupor, bilateral extensor plantar responses, and dilated pupils. (H & E × 320.) (Courtesy of Dr. John Hills, New England Center Hospitals.)

of the central nervous system; some have associated involvement of other organ systems.

b. Virus isolation studies: inoculation of blood, nasal washings, excretions, cerebrospinal fluid, or fresh postmortem brain tissue into susceptible animals. In some specialized centers, tissue culture techniques may be employed.

c. Application of acute and chronic serological tests to measure antibody levels (complement fixation or antibody neutralization tests).

It is customary to divide those viral infections involving the nervous system into a *neurotropic group* (primary involvement of the central nervous system) and a *non-neurotropic group* (involvement of the central nervous system in man is secondary to or less prominent than involvement of other organ systems).

Neurotropic Group. The neurotropic group is usually subdivided into those viral infections which are epidemic and those which are nonepidemic.

EPIDEMIC GROUP. Within the *epidemic* group several infections may be grouped together because they share common characteristics:

a. Equine encephalomyelitis (eastern U.S.A., western U.S.A., and Venezuelan subtypes are distinguished.)

b. Japanese B. encephalitis.

c. Russian tick encephalitis.

d. St. Louis encephalitis.

In each of these infections a relatively diffuse involvement of the cerebral cortex, diencephalon, brain stem, and cerebellum occurs. In each, an *arthropod*, e.g., mosquito, has been implicated as a vector of transmission. A species of bird or mammal has often served as a reservoir of infection. For these reasons cases have occurred predominantly in a seasonal manner. (In northeastern United States, for example, most cases of Eastern Equine encephalitis have occurred in the late summer or early fall months, a time when mosquitoes are frequent.)

The clinical syndrome in most cases is characterized by the sudden onset of headache, vomiting, drowsiness, convulsions, coma, fever, and stiffness of the neck. Evidence is often present on examination of the patient of both diffuse and multifocal involvement at multiple levels of the neural axis, e.g., hemiplegia, aphasia, decorticate rigidity, coma, cranial nerve palsies, and cerebellar findings. The duration of the disease is a matter of days to several weeks.

A variable mortality occurs related in part to the age of the affected patients. The mortality in Eastern Equine encephalitis, which has affected children predominantly, has approached 75 per cent, with significant residuals in those recovering. A similar pattern has been noted for Japanese B. encephalitis. On the other hand, Western Equine encephalitis and St. Louis encephalitis have been characterized by a lower mortality (10 to 20 per cent) and a lower incidence of residual neurological deficits.

In addition to the arthropod-borne infections, two other acute epidemic neurotropic viral infections of the central nervous system must be discussed as presenting contrasting clinical syndromes: encephalitis lethargica and poliomyelitis.

Encephalitis lethargica (Von Economo's encephalitis) occurred as an epidemic in the years 1916–1926. A viral etiology was suspected but never confirmed; the means of transmission remained uncertain. This infection differed from the previously described varieties of encephalitis in the sense that although diffuse, the pathology tended to be concentrated in a periventricular location with severe involvement of structures bordering the aqueduct and third and fourth ventricles. The periaqueductal region and other structures of the midbrain were particularly affected. Reflecting the significant involvement of the midbrain and of the associated structures of the extrapyramidal system, disorders of eye movement and movement disorders of various types were prominent symptoms—in addition to the more general symptoms of lethargy, headache, and fever. Since the involvement of the cortex was less severe, seizures and focal cortical deficits were infrequent. The mortality approached 25 per cent. Among those who survived, postencephalitic residuals were common. In contrast to other forms of encephalitis, Parkinson's disease and other disorders of extrapyramidal function were frequently noted; the Parkinson's disease usually appeared to emerge or evolve as a symptom after the clearing of the acute symptoms (p. 685).

Acute anterior poliomyelitis, the other member of this epidemic group of neurotropic viruses, has already been discussed in relation to the spinal cord. The portal of entry is the gastrointestinal tract. The central nervous system is involved either by spread along the axis cylinders or via a generalized viremia. The virus involves predominantly the large motor neurons of the anterior horn and of the brain stem with lesser involvement of other neurons in the spinal cord. With the development of effective vaccines (the Sabin live attenuated and the Salk killed virus types), poliomyelitis has become a preventable disease.

NONEPIDEMIC NEUROTROPIC VIRUS INFECTIONS. The two most familiar members of this group—herpes zoster and rabies—do not have their major effects at the level of cerebral cortex.

In *herpes zoster,* discussed earlier in relation to the spinal cord, the inflammatory changes involve the posterior root ganglion cells with somewhat lesser involvement of the posterior and anterior horns and the anterior and posterior roots, at one or several adjacent segments. On occasion, the corresponding components of cranial nerves such as nerves V and VII may be involved. Rarely, an encephalomyelitis may occur, under condition of an altered immune system, e.g., in patients with lymphomas or in patients receiving glucocorticoids. The responsible virus is in many respects similar to the varicella virus responsible for chickenpox. The clinical symptoms of severe radicular pain, which is usually present, is clearly related to the segmental involvement of the posterior root ganglion. At times significant segmental weakness is present as well, indicating involvement of the anterior horn and anterior root. In addition, a vesicular eruption similar to that of chickenpox occurs in the skin overlying the involved segments.

The virus of *rabies* is present in the saliva of rabid animals and invades the central nervous system several weeks to months after a bite from an infected animal (dog, cat, wolf, fox, squirrel, or bat). The virus travels to the central nervous system along peripheral nerves. The symptoms relate to the characteristic involvement of nuclei of the brain stem, Purkinje cells of the cerebellum, and pyramidal cells of the hippocampus (Ammon's horn). In addition there is a significant inflammation and necrosis of the spinal cord or brain stem at the segmental site corresponding to the radicular dermatome involved by the bite.

The initial symptoms consist of numbness and tingling in the distribution of the involved peripheral nerve, followed by head-

ache, vomiting, and a stage of agitation. This latter stage is characterized by restlessness, generalized convulsions, and at times visual and auditory hallucinations. Marked alteration in emotions occurs: unreasonable fear, rage, and depression. In this stage laryngeal and pharyngeal spasm (with fear of water, "hydrophobia") is prominent. In a later stage of flaccid paralysis, impairment of vocal cords and of respiratory centers develops.

Death occurs within 2 to 5 days of onset of central nervous system symptoms. At autopsy, the diagnosis may be established in man or other infected animals by the findings of characteristic acidophilic (eosinophilic) inclusions within the cytoplasm of hippocampal pyramidal cells (Negri bodies).

Because of the long incubation between exposure to the virus and the development of neurological symptoms, prophylactic treatment is possible. Thus, the administration of a vaccine containing the attenuated virus induces the production of antibodies and will prevent the development of neurological symptoms. This active immunization, first introduced by Pasteur, may be supplemented by passive immunization with antiserum containing antibodies to rabies. Once symptoms have developed, no effective treatment is available.

Another agent of this group, *lymphocytic choriomeningitis,* has been previously discussed under viral meningitis (aseptic meningitis).

Non-Neurotropic Viral Infections. These viruses usually do not produce significant symptoms of central nervous system involvement although indirect evidence suggests that some of these viruses (mumps and measles) do invade the central nervous system in a much greater percentage of otherwise asymptomatic cases. In some of these diseases, e.g., herpes simplex, there is evidence of direct invasion of the central nervous system when the syndrome of acute encephalitis occurs. In other viral infections, e.g., mumps and measles, it is often unclear when central nervous system symptoms develop, whether one is dealing with an actual viral invasion of the central nervous system producing an acute encephalitis, or whether one is observing an immunological reaction to infection elsewhere producing an acute allergic postinfectious encephalomyelitis.

The clinical symptoms of these various diseases are variable; some (mumps and infectious mononucleosis) produce minor central nervous system symptoms, with an excellent recovery to be expected. In other infections of this group (herpes simplex and measles) evidence of severe involvement of the central nervous system is present (convulsions, myoclonic jerks, coma, decorticate or decerebrate state) with a poor prognosis for life. Among those who live, significant neurological residuals, related to the severely destructive pathological process, are frequently present.

In a general sense, these diseases differ from the neurotropic viral infections as regards pathological involvement. Thus, these diseases often demonstrate significant damage to white matter with perivenous demyelination in addition to the direct invasion and destruction of neurons.

In addition to those viruses already mentioned—herpes simplex, measles, mumps, and infectious mononucleosis—there are several other viruses which are often classified within this group. These viruses, however, produce predominantly an aseptic meningitis and have been discussed previously: ECHO and Coxsackie.

CHRONIC ENCEPHALITIS

Spirochetal: Dementia Paralytica, General Paresis. As indicated in our earlier discussion of syphilis, evidence of involvement of the parenchyma of the central nervous system may emerge as a tertiary manifestation of the infection, many years (10 to 25) after the primary infection. Of the parenchymal varieties of infection, tabes dorsalis has been discussed previously. The problem of general paresis is pertinent for the present discussion.

From a pathological standpoint, several features are noted:

1. A chronic mononuclear meningoencephalitis with greatest involvement of the frontal and anterior temporal cortex.

2. A granular ependymitis.

3. Diffuse loss of neurons most prominent in the frontal and anterior temporal areas, resulting in a gross cortical atrophy.

4. Microglial proliferation in the form of rod cells.

5. With special stains, the presence of spirochetes within the cortex.

6. Characteristic deposition of iron pigment in the involved areas.

The clinical manifestations are those of a progressive alteration in personality and a progressive dementia (reflecting the major involvement of the frontal or temporal areas) with progression to a fully psychotic and a terminal bedridden state. Tremors, dysarthria, generalized convulsions, increased deep tendon reflexes, and bilateral Babinski signs are often noted during the course of the disease.

These causes may be differentiated from other causes of a progressive dementia by the positive serological test for syphilis in the blood and by the characteristic cerebrospinal fluid findings (a positive serological test for syphilis, an increased cell count of mononuclear cells, an increased protein content with an abnormal colloidal gold test—first zone or paretic curve—reflecting the alterations in spinal fluid globulins) plus or minus a past history of infection by syphilis.

Untreated, the disease will progress over a period of several years. In the preantibiotic era, such cases constituted a significant proportion of the patients in the state mental hospitals. With the use of penicillin, the disease can be arrested in most patients and significant improvement produced in those patients with mild symptoms. Where significant cortical atrophy has occurred, significant frontal and temporal lobe findings will persist.

Subacute or Chronic Viral Infections
Herpes Simplex and Syndrome of Subacute Dementia. We have already indicated that the herpes simplex infection of the central nervous system may produce an overwhelming rapidly fatal acute encephalitis with generalized convulsions, myoclonic jerks of the extremities, coma, and decorticate rigidity (Fig. 22–32). Another syndrome may, however, be encountered in herpes simplex infection of the nervous system—that of a progressive subacute involvement of the limbic system: orbital frontal and medial temporal (hippocampus). Even in acute cases, the more severe involvement of these limbic structures is evident (Fig. 22–33). The resultant clinical picture is characterized by a progressive confusional state with defects in recent memory and temporal lobe seizures. The diagnosis is made on the basis of a cellular response in the spinal fluid, an increase in antibody levels to herpes simplex virus and isolation of the specific virus from the brain in fatal cases.

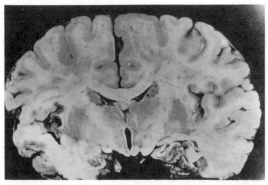

Figure 22–33 Herpes simplex encephalitis. Predominant involvement of medial and inferior temporal structures (and of insula) by an acute necrotic process is evident, although a generalized encephalitis was also present. Same case as Figure 22 32. (Courtesy of Dr. John Hills, New England Center Hospitals.)

See Filmstrip, Frame, 54.

Measles Virus and Syndrome of Subacute Inclusion Body Encephalitis (Subacute Sclerosing Panencephalitis). This is a progressive (months to years) disease of children and adolescents characterized by a progressive impairment of memory (dementia), generalized seizures, myoclonic jerks, and ataxia with the eventual development of a bedridden, decorticate state. Recent evidence suggests that the disease represents a reactivation of measles virus within the central nervous system in patients who have had uncomplicated measles infections several months or years previously. The pathological findings are those of a chronic encephalitis with mononuclear infiltration of the cortex and white matter, inclusion bodies within the neurons, and degeneration of neurons. White matter is also involved; spotty demyelination occurs.

Polyoma-Papova Virus and Progressive Multifocal Leukoencephalopathy. This is a rare syndrome occurring in patients with chronic disease of the reticuloendothelial system, e.g., Hodgkin's disease or leukemia. Multiple areas of demyelination occur in the central nervous system over the course of several months. The clinical picture consists of multifocal signs such as hemiplegia, cranial nerve palsies, and dementia.

The possibility of a viral etiology has been suggested by the presence of a perivascular inflammatory cell infiltration and by the presence of virus-like particles in astrocytes on electron microscopy.

Slow Virus Infection and Other Degenerative Diseases. The recent research of Gajdusek has raised the possibility of chronic viral infection as an explanation for several chronic and progressive diseases of the nervous system previously classified as degenerative in nature. Examples are Kuru, a progressive cerebellar degeneration found in a particular tribal group in New Guinea, and Jakob-Creutzfeldt disease. The latter is a subacute progressive syndrome characterized by dementia, generalized convulsions, myoclonic jerks, ataxia, extrapyramidal findings, and fasciculations suggesting a diffuse central nervous system involvement. Both of these diseases have been transmitted from human patients to chimpanzees with an incubation period of 1 to 2 years after inoculation of brain suspensions from the affected patients.

Chronic Diffuse Protozoal Infections of the Central Nervous System. Although central nervous system symptoms may occur during the course of malaria, the diseases usually considered under this category are trypanosomiasis and toxoplasmosis. *Trypanosomiasis* has an African form transmitted by the tsetse fly (African sleeping sickness) and a South American form (Chagas' disease) transmitted by a blood sucking insect. The African form presents the picture of a chronic meningoencephalitis with fever, lethargy, convulsions, and coma. The South American form presents the picture of a disseminated multifocal granulomatous process with multifocal neurological symptoms. The organisms are sensitive to pentavalent arsenical drugs.

Infections with *toxoplasmosis* occur predominantly *in utero*, producing disseminated but multifocal areas of chronic inflammation and granuloma formation within the cerebral hemispheres. Ependymal involvement is frequent; granulomas in this location may result in blockage of the ventricular system with hydrocephalus. The areas of granuloma formation are often calcified and may be visualized on x-rays of the skull. In addition, involvement of the retina is frequent producing a characteristic chorioretinitis. Involvement of liver and spleen is frequent.

Microscopic sections demonstrate the characteristic organisms within the epithelioid cells of the granulomas and often, as well, within neurons and blood vessels.

The congenital form presents the clinical picture of an infant who fails to thrive and manifests generalized convulsions and decorticate and decerebrate states, with abnormalities of eye, retina, liver, and spleen.

Less frequently an "acquired" form of toxoplasmosis is seen in children or adults. The adult form may present a picture of focal or multifocal granulomas (see below). The diagnosis may be established by demonstrating a rising antibody titer. The organism has some sensitivity to sulfa drugs.

Intrauterine Infections Producing Malformations. Intrauterine infections have been implicated in a small percentage of congenital diseases of the nervous system. Toxoplasmosis has been discussed. Several viral agents should also be considered.

Rubella (German measles) virus infection during the first trimester of pregnancy may result in defects in the eye, deafness, and severe malformations of the heart. In some cases malformations of the cerebral hemisphere, such as microcephaly, have occurred.

Cytomegalic inclusion body disease (salivary gland virus), occurring during intrauterine development, has resulted in hydrocephalus and microcephaly with severe retardation and seizures. The encephalitis and ependymitis produce a periventricular calcification which may be demonstrated on x-rays of the skull. Still births, premature births, or death shortly after birth is frequent. There is often significant involvement of liver, spleen, and the hemopoietic system with the presence of jaundice and thrombocytopenia.

Mumps virus infection in the fetus or neonate has recently been implicated by the studies of Johnson and Johnson as a possible cause of aqueduct stenosis producing hydrocephalus.

FOCAL INFECTIONS OF THE NERVOUS SYSTEM

The problem of focal infections of the nervous system has an importance far out of proportion to the actual frequency of occurrence of such cases. These focal infections represent, in general, rapidly progressive and compressive space-occupying lesions, and they often require emergency neurosurgical intervention.

We have already seen that at the level of spinal cord, focal infections are essentially extradural in location. The favorite site of acute focal infection is the fatty tissue of the epidural space. The resultant clinical picture is that of a rapidly progressive extradural compressive lesion of the spinal cord. The symptoms and signs are due both to the direct damage from compression and the indirect destruction of tissue produced by vascular compression and occlusion. At the level of the spinal cord also, spinal cord compression may result from the involvement of and collapse of vertebral bodies by chronic tuberculosis.

Above the foramen magnum, focal infections involve not the epidural space (the outer layer of dura is actually the periosteum of the skull bone), but the subdural space and the parenchyma of the brain. Infections involving the subdural space are referred to as *subdural empyema*. The subdural space in relation to the cerebral convexity is usually involved. Focal infections involving the parenchyma of the brain may be subdivided into *acute purulent brain abscesses* and *chronic granulomas*. Both may be solitary or multiple; both may involve cerebral hemisphere or cerebellum.

SUBDURAL EMPYEMA

In general, subdural empyema occurs as a result of direct extension of purulent infection from an adjacent focus of infection in the nasal sinuses or middle ear or following compound skull fractures. The nasal sinuses are now implicated as the major source of infection. Osteomyelitis of the intervening bone is a frequent finding; thrombophlebitis of the venous sinuses and of the feeding cortical veins is not unusual as a complication. The pus is present in a space which offers very little resistance to the expansion of this purulent mass. The mass is apparently never well-encapsulated although in older cases after the removal of the pus, a fibrinous exudate will be found on the inner surface of the dura and the inner surface of the arachnoid. The responsible organism is most commonly the Staphylococcus aureus. A sterile secondary inflammation is usually present in the subarachnoid space. This results in spinal fluid findings on lumbar puncture of moderate increase in cells and protein but a normal sugar and negative culture.

The effects produced by the collection of pus are similar to those resulting from a subdural hematoma or other rapidly expanding intracranial mass: headaches, hemiparesis, focal or generalized seizures, confusion, and eventual uncal herniation with brain stem compression. Papilledema is often present, reflecting the rise in intracranial pressure. Some of the focal cortical findings such as hemiparesis, aphasia, and focal seizures may reflect phlebitis of the cortical veins with hemorrhagic infarction of tissue — in addition to the direct compressive effects of the mass lesion. If untreated by surgical evacuation of the pus, death is the usual outcome 3 to 14 days after the onset of focal symptoms. Prompt surgical evacuation of the pus and appropriate antibiotic therapy will prevent these complications. The extent of neurological recovery will depend on whether focal infarction has occurred due to venous occlusion.

The subdural effusion in infants complicating H. influenzae meningitis does not represent a subdural empyema. The effusion is sterile and nonpurulent in contrast to the positive bacterial culture obtained from the purulent material in an empyema.

The following case history presents an example of subdural empyema.

Case History 12. NECH #175–169.
Date of admission: 11/9/65.

This forty-eight-year-old, right-handed, white male (Mr. J.M.) was referred for evaluation of headaches and papilledema. For 3 weeks prior to admission the patient had severe bifrontal headaches which were constantly present and interfered with sleep. One week prior to admission the patient developed a fever of 105° with a white blood count (WBC) of 25,000. X-rays indicated "sinusitis." The patient was hospitalized at his local community hospital. Confusion soon developed. Three days prior to admission to NECH, the patient had a series of seizures characterized by turning of the head and eyes to the left. Lumbar puncture then indicated clear cerebrospinal fluid with pressure of 300 mm. and protein increased to 65 mg./100 ml. The patient was transferred to NECH for neurological evaluation.

PAST HISTORY:

1. Chronic right nasal discharge for ten years.

2. Eight weeks prior to admission, the patient, while stooping down, struck his right frontal area but was not unconscious. A right periorbital ecchymoses developed, and the patient also had the onset of bilateral frontal headaches.

GENERAL PHYSICAL EXAMINATION:

1. Temperature was elevated to 101°.

2. There was right periorbital edema.

3. Excoriation of right nasal mucosa was present.

NEUROLOGICAL EXAMINATION:

1. *Mental status:*
   a. The patient was alert but irritable and slightly confused.
   b. He was poorly attentive and failed to persist in carrying out motor activities.
   c. He was oriented grossly for time, place, and person.
   d. Calculations were poorly performed.
   e. Delayed recall was defective.

2. *Cranial nerves:* All were intact with the exception of the fundi. Papilledema (low-grade) was present with absence of venous pulsations.

3. *Motor system:*
   a. Strength was intact, but there was a slight drift of outstretched left arm.
   b. Gait was intact.
   c. Cerebellar tests were negative.

4. *Reflexes:*
   a. Deep tendon reflexes were somewhat brisker at the left arm and leg (3+) as compared to the right (2+).
   b. Plantar responses were flexor.
   c. A bilateral grasp reflex was present.

5. *Sensation:* All modalities were intact.

6. *Skull:* There was slight tenderness at the right periorbital area. Minimal nuchal rigidity (resistance to passive flexion of neck) was present.

LABORATORY DATA:

1. The WBC was increased to 14,350 cells per cubic mm., and the sedimentation rate was increased to 110 mm. in one hour.

2. Chest x-rays were negative.

3. Sinus x-rays: Bilateral maxillary and frontal sinusitis was present with resorption of bone.

4. *Electroencephalogram* (11/9/67):
   a. Focal 4 to 7 cps slow wave activity was present in the right parietal area suggesting focal damage.
   b. However, focal voltage suppression (reduction of voltage) was present in the right anterior frontal area suggesting a possible subdural collection.

5. *Right Carotid Arteriogram* showed an apparent slight shift of the anterior cerebral vessels to the left suggesting a right hemisphere space-occupying lesion.

HOSPITAL COURSE:

On November 10, 1965, a right frontal Trephine (burr) hole was placed by Dr. Robert Yuan. When the dura was incised, 5 cc. of yellow purulent material escaped from the subdural space and additional purulent drainage was aspirated. Additional burr holes were placed in the right occipital area where a few drops of subdural pus were encountered. No pus was obtained from the left subdural area. Subsequent cultures demonstrated Staphylococcus aureus as the responsible organism. The dura and cortex otherwise appeared unremarkable although cerebral edema was present. The patient was subsequently treated with an appropriate antibiotic (Keflin). His temperature gradually subsided to normal and his mental status cleared.

On November 30, 1965, a bilateral frontal sinusotomy was performed by Dr. Thomas Klein with drainage of the sinus. Histological examination of a section of sinus mucosa removed demonstrated intense chronic inflammation.

The patient continued to improve. Papilledema had subsided by the time of follow-up examination in March 1966. No neurological findings were present except for a slight reflex asymmetry (slightly increased on the left).

COMMENT:

This patient presented a definite history of chronic nasal sinus infection with a recent exacerbation. The role of trauma in the exacerbation is uncertain. It is clear, however, that the sinusitis had produced involvement of the adjacent bone with subsequent spread to the adjacent frontal subdural space. The severe headache experienced by the patient reflected not only the process of infection involving sinus and meninges but presumably also the increase in intracranial pressure. The initial involvement of the right frontal area was suggested by the initial symptoms of confusion and by the occurrence of focal seizures characterized by turning of the head and eyes to the left. The findings of the electroencephalogram suggested a subdural collection of fluid or pus in the right frontal area. These clinical and laboratory impressions were confirmed by the subsequent surgical observations.

As we have already indicated, the purulent material in the subdural space does not remain limited but tends to spread over the convexity of the cerebral hemisphere. It is therefore not surprising that the electroencephalogram demonstrated some damage in the right parietal area as well and that some pus was obtained from the right occipital burr hole. In the present case the arteriogram suggested only a nonspecific space-occupying lesion in the right frontal area. The more specific finding in these cases would involve the displacement of distal branches of the anterior and middle cerebral artery from the inner table of the skull as in a subdural hematoma.

PURULENT BRAIN ABSCESS

A brain abscess (Fig. 22–34) reflects the spread of purulent infection to the brain by several pathways. Direct extension may occur from a nearby focus of infection in the nasal sinuses or mastoid or middle ear. For this reason many solitary brain abscesses tend to be located in the frontal or temporal lobe of the cerebral hemisphere or in the cerebellar hemisphere. Direct introduction of infected material may occur in relation to trauma, e.g., compound skull fractures, or in relation to neurosurgical procedures. Finally hematogenous spread may occur in patients with a primary source in the lung, in patients with bacterial endocarditis, and in patients with cyanotic congenital heart disease where the blood may bypass the screening system of the lungs. Such hematogenous spread is more likely to result in multiple abscesses rather than a solitary abscess.

Since the introduction of antibiotics, there has been a significant decrease in the overall number of patients presenting with brain abscess particularly those secondary to sinusitis and mastoiditis. Moreover, among the remaining patients there has been a decrease in the percentage of cases with an identifiable primary focus of infection and an increase in cases without an identifiable primary focus from which direct or hematogenous spread could have occurred. These latter cases may reflect instances where partial antibiotic therapy has eradicated the primary focus but not the brain abscess.

As might be expected, the most common organism is Staphylococcus aureus. Streptococci and pneumococci are also commonly encountered as responsible organisms. Rarely, under special circumstances, a fungus may be implicated, e.g., *mucormycosis* (Mucorales) in severely debilitated diabetics and

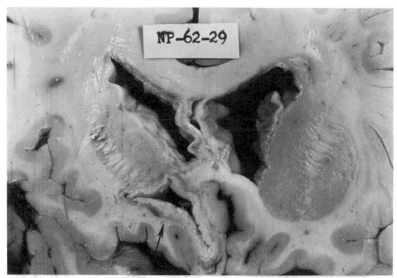

Figure 22–34 Subacute brain abscess (arrow) with associated ventriculitis. This 41-year-old white male, as a child, had a fibroma of the right maxillary sinus which had been treated with surgery and radon implants. In December 1961, the patient developed headache, nuchal rigidity, fever, and chills; cerebrospinal fluid contained 495 white blood cells (75% polymorphonuclear) and a CSF-sugar of 40 mg./100 ml. Despite antibiotic therapy and temporary improvement, three recurrences of this syndrome occurred. On his final admission in March 1962, pus and crusts were present in the right nostril and chronic sinusitis of right maxillary and ethmoid sinuses was apparent on x-rays. The patient expired following a craniotomy for repair of a defect in the bone dura in relation to the right ethmoid sinus. (Courtesy of Dr. John Hills, New England Center Hospitals; and Dr. Jose Segarra, Boston Veterans Administration Hospital.)

See Filmstrip, Frame 55.

aspergillosis (Aspergillus) in patients receiving immunosuppressive therapy after renal transplantation.

From a pathological standpoint the initial stage of infection is a local purulent encephalitis (local cerebritis with polymorphonuclear infiltration and necrosis). As necrosis proceeds, a mesodermal connective tissue and vascular proliferation begins at the margin. Beyond this area in the adjacent tissue, microglial and astroglial proliferation begins to occur. Eventually the picture is that of a liquefied mass of purulent material surrounded by a fibrous capsule which in turn is surrounded by a zone of astroglial cells and fibers. There is often significant edema in the surrounding tissue.

As the abscess expands, it acts as a space-occupying lesion producing compression of adjacent structures and eventually uncal herniation, with brain stem compression. This is a particular danger in an abscess involving the temporal lobe where early herniation may occur. An abscess in the cerebellum of course provides the risk of tonsillar herniation with compression of the lower brain stem.

The reactive effort to wall off the abscess is often not successful; additional necrosis of adjacent tissue may occur and rupture into the ventricular system or subarachnoid space may occur with the development of a purulent ventriculitis and meningitis. In such cases organisms will be present in the cerebrospinal fluid on lumbar puncture. In general, however, when rupture has not occurred the cerebrospinal fluid is sterile with a normal sugar content although pressure, protein, and cell count are elevated.

The clinical symptoms will correspond to that area of the cerebral hemisphere involved with focal seizures and focal neurological deficits as the prominent features.

The clinical and laboratory picture is usually that of a rapidly progressive space-occupying lesion. The electroencephalogram is likely to show continuous focal 0.5 to 2 cps slow wave activity indicating severe focal damage.

In general the outcome in the untreated brain abscess is fatal. Treatment consists of surgical drainage and total excision of the abscess cavity. In addition appropriate antibiotic therapy must be administered. In the series of Loeser and Scheinberg, surgical therapy in the 1940–1944 period was associated with a 47 per cent mortality. By 1949–1956, an era of specific antibiotic, this mortality had dropped to 19 per cent.

A brain abscess involving the right parietal-occipital area has already been presented in Chapter 21 (Case history 6, p. 509). The student should review this case at this time.

In reviewing this case, the student should keep in mind that events in a more anteriorly placed abscess may proceed at a much more rapid pace as regards tentorial herniation with third nerve and brain stem compression.

The following case history demonstrates the problem of temporal lobe abscess.

Case History 13. BFH #41573.

Date of admission: 5/15/61. (Patient of Dr. Samuel Brendler.)

This 14-year-old, white female (Miss. S.K.) was admitted with chief complaint of "draining left ear" and left frontal headache.

Approximately 4 weeks prior to admission the patient had the onset of pain in the left ear region which increased in severity and was accompanied by fever up to 104°. Four days later, a discharge from the left ear developed. Three days later (3 weeks prior to admission) a "total" left-sided facial paralysis developed. The patient was evaluated at the Massachusetts Eye and Ear Infirmary where a drainage of the left middle ear was performed (yielding additional purulent material). Culture of this drainage revealed Staphylococcus aureus. The patient was treated with antibiotics: erythromycin and Chloromycetin with a complete resolution of symptoms. One week prior to admission the patient developed a severe and constant left frontal headache with swelling about the left eye. Discharge of a thick green purulent material occurred from the left ear. Two days prior to admission confusion and delirium developed. The patient was noted to have marked difficulties in language function and in calculations.

GENERAL PHYSICAL EXAMINATION: Temperature was 98.6°. The patient appeared chronically ill. Gauze soaked with purulent drainage was present in the left external auditory canal.

NEUROLOGICAL EXAMINATION:

1. *Mental status:*
   a. The patient was unable to give the month but was able to provide the day and the year.
   b. Calculations were poorly performed.
   c. There was significant confusion as to past and recent events.
   d. There was a marked deficit in naming objects. Even when the name of an object was supplied, the patient was unable to recognize the name as correct. Paraphrasing was evident. The patient was able to carry out spoken commands. Reading of isolated words was defective. Simple writing and spelling were intact.
   e. There was no left-right confusion.
   f. The patient was able to identify and to point out the various parts of her body with the exception of the thumb.
   g. At times, the patient acted in a silly manner and would giggle without any clear pertinence to the questions asked.

2. *Cranial nerves:*
   a. Papilledema was present with elevation of the disk on the right. A recent hemorrhage was present just below the disk of the right fundus.
   b. The pupils were regular and equal and responded to light.
   c. There was a minor peripheral facial weakness on the left side, most prominent in the left frontalis muscle.
   d. Hearing was decreased on the left.

3. *Motor system:* Strength and gait were intact.

4. *Reflexes:*
   a. Deep tendon reflexes were symmetrical.
   b. The left plantar response was flexor; the right was equivocal.

5. *Sensation:* Was intact.

LABORATORY DATA:

1. *White blood count and differential* were normal.

2. *Skull and mastoid x-rays* indicated an acute mastoiditis on the left with an increased density throughout the left mastoid, extending into the medial aspect of the petrous ridge.

3. *Electroencephalogram* (5/15/61): Was abnormal because of 2 to 3 cps slow wave activity throughout the left hemisphere but most prominent in the left frontal-temporal area suggesting focal damage (Fig. 22–35).

LAT. F. – ANT. T.

ANT. T. – MID. T.

MID. T. – POST. T.

PAR. – OCC.

L

R

L

R

L

R

L

R

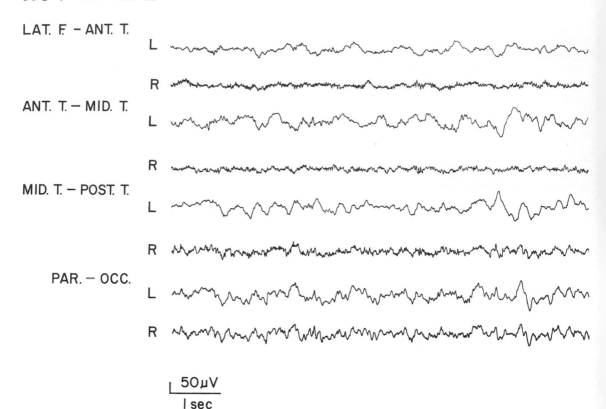

50 μV

1 sec

Figure 22–35 Case History 13. Brain abscess, left temporal lobe. Electroencephalogram. (Bipolar recording of May 15, 1961.) Focal 2–3 cps slow wave activity was present in the left lateral frontal and temporal areas indicating focal damage in these areas. LAT. F. = lateral frontal; ANT. T. = anterior temporal; MID. T. = midtemporal; POST. T. = posterior temporal; PAR. = parietal; OCC. = occipital.

4. *Arteriograms* (5/25/61): Demonstrated anterior displacement and elevation of the left middle cerebral artery. The findings were consistent with large avascular mass in the left temporal lobe.

HOSPITAL COURSE:

On May 15, 1961, a left mastoidectomy and exploration of the epidural space was performed by Dr. Daniel Miller of the ENT service. Pus was present in the softened mastoid cells. Purulent granulation tissue extended into the adjacent epidural area. Cultures of this material subsequently revealed Staphylococcus aureus. The lateral sinus was uncovered and was found to be uninvolved. Therapy with erythromycin was reinstituted.

Over the next 4 days, improvement occurred as regards clinical and electroencephalographic findings. Electroencephalogram 7 days after admission demonstrated progression of the abnormalities in the left temporal area and the aforementioned arteriogram was performed.

On May 26, 1961, with a presumptive diagnosis of brain abscess, a burr hole was placed over the left temporal lobe by Dr. Samuel Brendler. A needle was inserted into the posterior-inferior aspect of the temporal lobe, and at a depth of 3 cm., 10 cc. of thick yellow pus was obtained. A catheter was then placed within the cavity of the abscess to facilitate drainage and irrigation with bacitracin solution (bactericidal antibiotic).

The patient remained stable until May 28, 1961, when she began to complain of bifrontal headache. The next morning she was somewhat lethargic. At 1:30 p.m. on May 29, 1961, when rounds were being made, she was noted to be less alert with an increase in her degree of nominal aphasia. The patient would speak to examiners and did respond to painful stimuli. A white blood count was elevated to 22,000 with an increase in polymorphonuclears. Within 2 hours, there was a decrease in arousal even to painful stimulus. Within 5 hours of these initial events, additional progression had occurred. The left pupil was now 1.5 mm. larger than the right. The left eye remained in a divergent position. The patient failed to move the right arm and leg. A Babinski response was now present on the right side. The patient failed to respond to pinprick on the right side of the body, but she did respond on the left. The patient received intravenous urea to reduce brain swelling and was immediately taken to the operating room where a left temporal craniotomy was performed by Dr. Samuel Brendler.

Since the dura was markedly tense with the danger of brain herniation, a separate left frontal burr hole was placed. A needle was inserted into the frontal horn of the lateral ventricle to decompress the ventricular system. At a depth of 0.5 cm. in the middle-posterior portion of the inferior temporal gyrus, a thin abscess cavity was encountered. Within this was a layer of a thick gummy yellow tissue. The entire abscess content was excised down to what appeared to be normal brain. The remainder of the inferior temporal gyrus was retracted to allow exposure of the tentorium which was then sectioned to its free edge. As the incision in the tentorium was made, an "enormous gush" of cerebrospinal fluid was encountered. Examination of the tissue removed revealed hemorrhagic, necrotic, and inflamed cortex and white matter.

Following surgery, there was a slow but progressive improvement. By the fifth post-operative day, the patient was described as alert and oriented, although a residual right homonymous hemianopsia and a mild right hemiparesis were present in addition to the persistence of a severe but relatively selective nominal aphasia.

At the time of discharge on June 25, 1961, the nominal aphasia and right homonymous hemianopsia were still present to a significant degree (Fig. 22–36).

Examination 1 year after discharge revealed that language function had improved although a deficit in naming objects was still evident. The visual field defect was less marked involving predominantly the right upper fields with sparing of the macular and the lower fields.

Examination 3 years after discharge revealed no actual language impairment. A right visual field defect was still present.

Anticonvulsant medication had been used

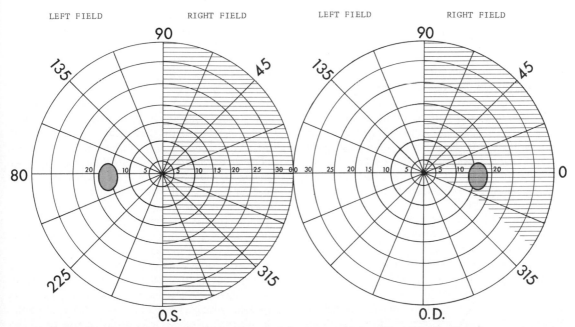

Figure 22–36 Case History 13. Brain abscess, left temporal lobe. Visual fields 6 weeks postoperative. (Tested by Dr. Howard Blazer.) A residual right homonymous hemianopsia was present on tangent screen examination. This was noncongruous with some preservation of vision in the macular area and the lower quadrant. The greater involvement of the upper quadrants is consistent with the greater involvement of the more inferior fibers of the geniculocalcarine radiation to be expected in a lesion of temporal lobe. O.S. = left eye; O.D. = right eye.

following surgery (Dilantin and Mebaral), but these were gradually discontinued over the intervening years. The patient did experience a single generalized convulsive seizure in December, 1967, and the medications were re-instituted.

A final follow-up evaluation 7 years following surgery indicated that the patient had completed two and a half years of college and had married. Her only deficit in speech was a slight hesitation and stumbling over a word when excited. The right visual field defect was unchanged.

COMMENT:

In this case, it was clear at the time of hospital admission that the purulent infection in the left middle ear and mastoid had spread to produce a significant acute intracranial process. The severe deficits in naming, calculations, and reading suggested a possible posterior temporal-posterior parietal location of the lesion. The papilledema and electroencephalographic findings suggested a space-occupying lesion such as an abscess. This was confirmed by the arteriogram which pinpointed a left temporal lobe location.

The initial needle aspiration of the abscess failed to eliminate the process. Progression of the necrotic purulent and edematous process in the left temporal lobe subsequently occurred with tentorial herniation of the medial aspect of temporal lobe; compression of the left oculomotor nerve resulted with the development of an enlarged pupil and an apparent impairment of medial rectus function (the left eye was divergent).

Such a recurrence of infection and expansion of the abscess is not unusual after simple aspiration of a brain abscess. Definitive treatment generally requires total excision of the abscess and of the involved cortex. Moreover, the incidence of seizures is much higher in those cases treated by aspiration and drainage alone as opposed to total excision.

In the present case, seizures were a minor problem. A single generalized convulsive seizure occurred at a time when the patient was not receiving anticonvulsants.

The severe but relatively selective nominal aphasia shown by the patient after surgery is consistent with the posterior temporal location of the resected lesion. The excellent eventual recovery probably reflects in part the relatively young age of the patient. The field defect, which was most severe in the right upper quadrant with less marked involvement of the lower quadrant, was consistent with the involvement of optic radiation fibers within the white matter of the temporal lobe.

The initial left peripheral facial weakness experienced by the patient undoubtedly reflected the involvement (possibly only edema) of the facial nerve in the facial canal which is in close anatomical relationship to the mastoid air cells and to the middle ear.

CHRONIC FOCAL INFECTIONS: GRANULOMAS

Those agents which have been considered under the heading of chronic meningitis, tuberculosis, cryptococcus, and syphilis may all produce chronic focal infections of the brain (in a sense a chronic focal nonpurulent abscess). These may be single or multiple. In addition other agents may be implicated in focal or multifocal granulomas. For example, in the adult, toxoplasmosis may on rare occasions produce a focal space-occupying lesion.

In some parts of the world, e.g., Latin America, infection of the brain by the larva of the pork tapeworm, *Taenia solium*, is relatively common producing a chronic state referred to as *cerebral cysticercosis*. The ova occur as cyst-like structures within the substance of the cerebral hemisphere and the ventricular system. Most die and become calcified. Focal seizures are a common manifestation. Occasionally the cysts within the ventricular system produce obstruction and hydrocephalus.

Less frequently and in other geographic areas, e.g., Japan, China, and the Philippines, infection of the brain by the ova of the *Trematoda schistosomia japonicum* may occur producing *cerebral schistosomiasis*. Other species of schistosomes are found commonly in other areas of the world, producing intestinal and bladder involvement and on rare occasions involving the brain. The ova elicit a large granulomatous lesion which is characterized by a large number of eosinophils, necrosis, and calcification. Involvement of the cerebral cortex is characterized by focal seizures and cortical deficits such as aphasia. Rarely a focal or multifocal granulomatous process may involve the brain in addition to other organ systems without a definite infectious agent established as an etiology, e.g., *Boeck's sarcoid*.

In general, when solitary, these various chronic focal infections have presented as space-occupying lesions. (The student should note that the suffix "oma" is always used to refer to a tumor or a tumor-like mass.) Often it has been impossible to distinguish such chronic granulomas from more common space-occupying lesions such as brain tumors. The diagnosis has then only been established at the time of surgery when histological examination of the tissue has been performed. Even then, more precise diagnosis has often required the information produced by special cultures of the tissue obtained at the time of surgery.

Tuberculomas. The tuberculoma should be discussed in somewhat greater detail. In contrast to the granuloma of syphilis (the gumma) and that of cryptococcus infection (the toruloma), both of which were rare as intracranial space-occupying tumors, the tuberculoma once was relatively common as an intracranial tumor. In parts of the world where tuberculosis remains as an endemic problem, tuberculoma is still a common intracranial mass lesion. In the series of Asenjo, from Chile, tuberculomas accounted for 3.2 per cent of all neurosurgical admissions in the period 1940 to 1949. This lesion constituted almost 20 per cent of all intracranial tumors treated by his service during that period. In the recent series of Dastur and Desai from Bombay, India, tuberculomas formed 30.5 per cent of all verified brain tumors in the period 1957 to 1963. In contrast, gliomas accounted for 28.6 per cent of all tumors in this series. At the present time in most neurosurgical centers in the United States and Western Europe, tuberculomas and other granulomas account for less than 1 per cent of all tumors.

The pathological picture of the tuberculoma is similar to that encountered when tuberculosis affects other organs. There is a central area of caseous material (cheese-like necrosis). This is surrounded by aggregates of mononuclear cells, modified elongated mononuclear cells (epithelial cells), and some multinucleated giant cells. Surrounding this mass is a fibrous capsule. Calcification of the lesion is common. In contrast to the purulent abscess, arrest of the process may occur spontaneously.

The majority of tuberculomas are solitary and occur in the cerebral hemisphere, usually in a relatively superficial location involving the cerebral cortex. In the series of Asenjo, approximately 47 per cent involved the cerebral hemisphere, 33 per cent the cerebellum, 10 per cent the brain stem, and 10 per cent multiple sites. A greater proportion of cerebellar lesions occurred in the series of Dastur and Desai. In a more limited series of 18 cases from the New York Neurological Institute reported in 1956, Sibley and O'Brien found 16 of the 18 lesions to have a supratentorial location. Only one of the 18 cases had a clinical diagnosis of tuberculoma established prior to surgery for a space-occupying lesion. The usual presenting symptoms related to seizures and increased intracranial pressure. (Seizures were present in 13 of 16 supratentorial cases.) Fever was usually not present, and 50 per cent of the patients had normal chest x-rays. The spinal fluid usually contained no cells but the protein content was increased.

As regards treatment before the era of antibiotics, attempted resections usually resulted in tuberculous meningitis and death. With the combined use of surgery and antituberculous agents, the mortality has been significantly reduced. In the recent series of Dastur and Desai, 60 per cent of the patients had a complete neurological recovery; 23 per cent were alive but had residual neurological signs.

NEOPLASMS

GENERAL CONSIDERATIONS

The student has already encountered in the previous case histories some of the more common problems of neoplasia of the central nervous system and has already formed some concepts of the biological behavior of such tumors. While any of the tissues or cell types found within or surrounding the central nervous system may undergo neoplasia, certain cell types in particular locations and at particular ages in life may be identified as common tumor types. Thus it is evident that in childhood most intracranial tumors are infratentorial; in adult life, the larger proportion are supratentorial. It is also evident that at particular ages in life, particular cell types are subject to neoplasia. Thus meningiomas, pituitary adenomas, acoustic nerve schwannomas (or neurinomas), and metastatic carcinomas are tumors of the adult. On the other hand, medulloblastomas and ependymomas are primarily tumors of childhood.

It is also evident that identity of the cell

type of a tumor does not necessarily enable the observer to predict the future biological and clinical behavior of the tumor. Identity of the cell type and knowledge of the location of the tumor allow for a higher order of prediction. Thus glial tumors may arise in the cerebral hemisphere, the brain stem, and the cerebellum.

The biological behavior of the tumor in each location is quite different. Thus most glial tumors of the cerebral hemispheres— cortex and subcortical white matter—in the adult are highly malignant in the sense of being rapidly growing invasive necrotic tumors with variable cell morphology and frequent nuclear mitotic figures. The brain stem glioma, on the other hand, is slower growing and has a more constant cellular and nuclear pattern. The cerebellar astrocytoma is a limited cystic and encapsulated tumor of low histological grade which can be removed in its entirety with essential cure of the patient.

The clinical manifestations of a particular tumor are not only determined by the cell type of the tumor (astrocytoma, meningioma) and the biological activity of the particular tumor (benign meningioma, low-grade astrocytoma, or highly malignant astrocytoma). Much more important in the determination of clinical signs and symptoms is the location of the tumor. This applies to both the local symptoms and signs (focal cortical symptoms and signs) and the general symptoms (headache, vomiting, drowsiness—those effects relevant to increased intracranial pressure resulting from a space-occupying lesion, from cerebral edema, or from a ventricular system blockage).

It should be evident that there is no one-to-one correlation between how benign a lesion is and the eventual clinical outcome. Thus a benign lesion such as a meningioma may by virtue of its location produce significant shifts of intracranial contents or brain stem compression with significant neurological disability and death. Consider, for example, the ease with which serious compressive effects may be produced by a meningioma of the foramen magnum or tentorium.

Essentially three general types of tumor affect the cerebral hemispheres:
  I. Primary intrinsic tumors
      a. Astrocytomas, including glioblastomas
      b. Oligodendrogliomas
      c. Ependymomas
 II. Primary extrinsic tumors
      a. Meningiomas
      b. Pituitary adenomas
      c. Craniopharyngiomas
      d. Epidermoids
      e. Dermoids
III. Secondary tumors
      a. Metastatic
        1. Intracerebral predominantly
        2. Dural and leptomeningeal
      b. Local Invasive

The overall relative frequency of the various types of tumors affecting the central nervous system varies from series to series depending on whether a surgical or autopsy series is being reported (Table 22–1). In addition, the particular interests of the neurosurgeon have often resulted in a specialized tumor type being referred to a particular neurosurgeon.

Table 22–1   Relative Frequency of Verified Intracranial Tumors

Type of Tumor	Combined Neurosurgical Series: (Grant and Cushing)* Total Cases: 4349. Per cent of Total	Autopsy Series: (Courville) Total Cases: 3010 Per cent of Total
Gliomas	43.0	41.5
Meningiomas	15.0	11.6
Metastatic Tumors	6.5	23.7
Pituitary Adenomas	13.0	3.4
Acoustic Neuromas	6.5	2.5
Congenital Tumors	4.0	3.5
Blood Vessel Tumors	3.0	7.8
Miscellaneous (Granulomas, Sarcomas, Papillomas)	9.0	5.7

*After Merritt, 1967.

*Table 22–2   The Overall Incidence of Various Types of Verified Gliomas**

Type of Glioma	NEUROSURGICAL SERIES (CUSHING) TOTAL NUMBER: 862 Per cent	AUTOPSY SERIES (COURVILLE) TOTAL NUMBER: 1259 Per cent	Average Survival in Months Following Onset of Symptoms (after Merritt, 1967)
Astrocytoma (Astrocytoma I)	30.0	23.0	76
Astroblastoma (Astrocytoma II)	4.0	1.0	28
Glioblastoma (Astrocytoma III & IV)	24.0	52.0	12
Polar spongioblastoma	4.0	2.0	46
Ganglioglioma	0.3	2.0	—
Oligodendroglioma	3.0	1.0	66
Ependymoma	3.0	6.5	32
Medulloblastoma	10.0	6.0	17
Pinealoma	2.0	1.0	—
Unclassified	20.0	4.0	—

*The series are not restricted to the cerebral hemispheres but include all intracranial lesions.

Thus metastatic tumors which are usually not considered amenable to surgery are under-represented in the operative series. Pituitary adenomas were of particular interest to Cushing and thus are over-represented in the operative series. The true clinical frequencies are somewhere between the operative and autopsy incidences.

PRIMARY INTRINSIC TUMORS

The most frequent tumors affecting the cerebral hemispheres are those arising from glia. Those of the astrocytic series are by far the most frequent (see Table 22–2). Oligodendrogliomas are relatively infrequent and ependymomas involving the cerebral hemispheres are rare.

ASTROCYTOMAS

The astrocytomas have been subdivided into various types. According to the classification of Kernohan and his associates these tumors are subdivided into four grades based on their degree of malignancy. This classification has, to a variable degree, replaced the older nomenclature of Bailey and Cushing which classified the glial tumors on an embryological basis, the tumor being called after the actual or hypothetical embryological cell of closest resemblance.

Grade I Astrocytomas. This grade of astrocytoma (Fig. 22–37) corresponds to the older term *astrocytoma* and consists of an in-

creased number of mature astrocytes of relatively normal appearance with no evidence of mitosis. At times, on viewing a biopsy of such a lesion, particularly from the cerebral hemisphere, it may be difficult to decide whether this area really differs from an area of reactive gliosis. Those arising in the cortex are composed predominantly of protoplasmic astrocytes; those arising in the white matter are composed predominantly of fibrillary astrocytes. The protoplasmic variety is sometimes referred to as "gemistocytic;" the cells resemble reactive astrocytes. The fibrillary variety is sometimes referred to as "piloid." Grossly, the lesion is nonencapsulated, firm, and granulous and gray. Cysts may be present. At times, the only hint of the lesion may be a lack of distinction between gray and white matter.

Grade 2 Astrocytoma. These astrocytomas correspond to the older term *astroblastoma.* The cells are nearly all adult astrocytes but appear larger than normal. Rare mitotic figures are present and the cells are at times arranged in the form of pseudorosettes around the vessels.

Grades 3 and 4 Astrocytomas. These two grades of astrocytomas (Figs. 22–38 and 22–39) correspond to the older terms *glioblastoma multiforme* and *spongioblastoma multiforme.* The term glioblastoma multiforme remains in common usage. Essentially, both of these grades have all of the characteristics which are usually cited as indicating a significant degree of malignancy. A high degree

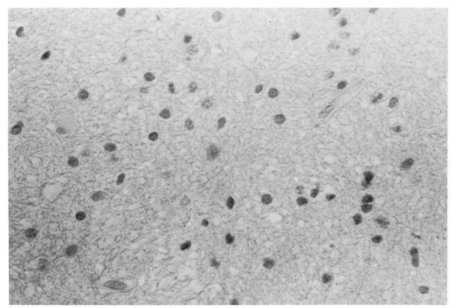

Figure 22–37 Low-grade astrocytoma. (H & E × 400). (Courtesy of Dr. David Cowen, Columbia-Presbyterian, Neuropathology.)

of cellularity is present. There is a marked variability of cellular and nuclear appearance.

In the Grade 4 variety almost no normal astrocytes are noted. Multinucleated giant cells are often noted. Mitotic figures are prominent; in the Grade 3 tumor, one figure per every two high-power fields; in the Grade 4 lesion, 4 or 5 figures per every high-power field.

Zones of necrosis often surrounded by a pseudopallisade of tumor cells are frequently present, and at times hemorrhage into the tumor may occur. The necrosis and hemorrhage are usually evident on gross examination of the brain (Fig. 22–40).

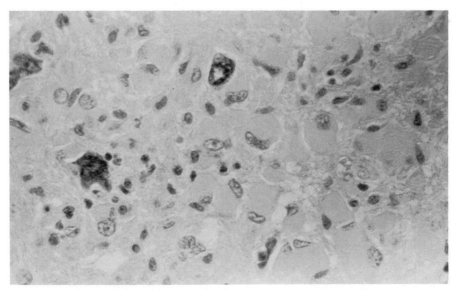

Figure 22–38 Gemistocytic astrocytoma, demonstrating a relatively high grade of malignancy. Swollen astrocytes are present. The nuclei which are displaced to the periphery are often bizarre and, in this case, multinucleated. (H & E × 400.) (Courtesy of Dr. David Cowen, Columbia-Presbyterian, Neuropathology.)

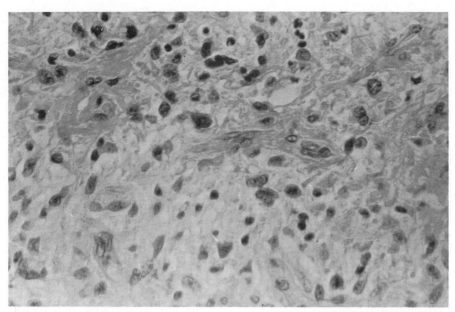

Figure 22–39 Glioblastoma multiforme. A marked variability of cellular and nuclear appearance is apparent. Multinucleated cells and mitotic figures are apparent. Hyperplasia of small vessels is apparent. (H & E × 400.) (Courtesy of Dr. David Cowen, Columbia-Presbyterian, Neuropathology.)

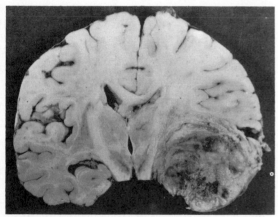

Figure 22–40 Glioblastoma multiforme of left temporal lobe. Compression of brain stem and ventricular system is evident. This 43-year-old white male began to experience, in August 1961, short "dreamy" states preceded by a distinctive taste and a sensation of familiarity. Despite a craniotomy and radiation therapy, in December 1961 the patient developed a progressive right hemiparesis, a nominal aphasia, and a severe receptive aphasia. Examination in February 1962 demonstrated, in addition, a right upper quadrant homonymous field defect. In June 1962 the patient developed increasing disorientation, lethargy, headache, vomiting, and papilledema. Despite temporary improvement with steroid therapy, the patient expired with pneumonitis in October 1962. (Courtesy of Dr. John Hills, New England Center Hospitals; and Dr. Jose Segarra, Boston Veterans Administration Hospital.)

See Filmstrip, Frame 56.

A prominent feature is the presence of hyperplasia of the adventitia and endothelium of the capillaries and small vessels. At times in the Grade 4 tumor this process may be so striking as to suggest that the malignancy may be arising in part from the mesodermal components of the vessel wall (e.g., as a sarcoma). Both the hyperplasia of the blood vessel wall and the rapid growth of the tumor often result in a tumor which outgrows its blood supply with resultant necrosis within the tumor.

A word of caution should be introduced at this point. Histological grading according to degree of malignancy is often based on a small biopsy specimen. It is not unusual for an astrocytoma in one section or at a periphery to show a relatively low-grade of malignancy while another sector of the tumor (which may not have been included in the biopsy) shows quite clearly the findings of a highly malignant tumor (a glioblastoma). Moreover, it is not unusual for astrocytomas which were of relatively low-grade at the time of initial evaluation to show, at a later point in time, a marked increase in degree of malignancy.

The glioblastoma is by far the most common type of intrinsic tumor affecting the cerebral hemisphere in adults (Table 22–2). Although at times they arise superficially in the cerebral cortex, more often they seem to originate in the subcortical white matter. They then appear to infiltrate widely throughout the cerebral hemisphere, often along white matter systems to involve other areas of the brain (e.g., via the corpus callosum to involve the opposite hemisphere). At times a multicentric origin may be suspected. Necrosis and hemorrhage are frequent; and progression of neurological deficit is often rapid. At times the episodes of necrosis and hemorrhage may suggest vascular accidents. The majority of cases are fatal within one year of onset (Fig. 22–41). Surgery may be employed for purposes of decompression, but cure is not to be expected. Although the significant degree of anaplasia might lead to the expectation of radiosensitivity, this is not the case.

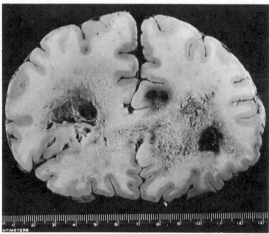

Figure 22–41 Glioblastoma multiforme with acute onset and rapid progression. A necrotic and hemorrhagic tumor has involved the subcortical white matter of both frontal lobes (in a butterfly manner) infiltrating across the corpus callosum, producing a thickening of this structure. This 53-year-old white male, 5 months prior to death, had the sudden onset of weakness of the right leg. Within 3 days, he had become lethargic and apathetic. Speech was initially normal but within an additional 2 days, a receptive aphasia, right visual field defect, and right central facial weakness had developed. Brain scan suggested a deep lesion near the midline. Despite a left hemisphere biopsy (which revealed only hemorrhage and neutrophilic reaction), left temporal bone flap decompression, and radiation therapy, rapid progression continued to occur with the development of a quadriparesis, coma, and bilateral third nerve paralysis. (Courtesy of Dr. John Hills, New England Center Hospitals; and Dr. Jose Segarra, Boston Veterans Administration Hospital.)

See Filmstrip, Frame 57.

The clinical course of the glioblastoma should be familiar to the student from his study of the following cases in Chapter 21: Case #1 (Mr. H.G.), p. 488; Case #7 (Mr. A.S.), p. 518; and Case #9 (Mr. D.M.), p. 529. These cases should be reviewed at this time.

Less often a low-grade astrocytoma is encountered in the cerebral hemisphere of the adult with a history that has often stretched back over a number of years. Many times the patient has received treatment for several years for a focal or generalized seizure disorder before the presence of a space-occupying lesion has become evident. At times these lesions have been discovered fortuitously in patients subjected to temporal lobectomy for treatment of intractable temporal lobe seizures.

The clinical course of a low-grade astrocytoma is illustrated in the following case history.

Case History 14. NECH #186–873.
Date of admission: 5/10/67.

This 41-year-old, right-handed widow (Mrs. A.V.D.) was admitted to the hospital for evaluation of increasing frequency of seizures. In 1956, at the age of 30, (11 years prior to admission) the patient experienced her first generalized convulsive seizures. The electroencephalogram at the time was normal. The seizures were relatively well-controlled on anticonvulsant medication (Dilantin and phenobarbital). There was an apparent increase in seizure frequency following the death of the patient's husband in 1958.

In 1963, the patient had a change in the character of her seizures; she began to experience focal seizures involving the right arm and leg. These focal seizures would begin with a sensation of a chill or a stiffening of the right leg which would spread to the lower back. At the same time, a sensation of "numbness" (tingling) and weakness was present in the right leg. There was then a repetitive clonic movement of the right arm. During this time, the patient would be unable to talk distinctly but would be aware of her surroundings. The episodes would last several minutes and would not be accompanied by loss of consciousness.

Examination by Dr. John Hills in 1963 indicated some slowness of response but no definite neurological defects. The electroencephalogram was again normal. Follow-up in 1966 indicated that focal seizures were continuing to occur once every 2 to 4 weeks. Neurological examination was again unremarkable. Evaluation in March, 1967, however, did reveal a minor and inconsistent increase in deep tendon reflexes in the right lower extremity and an equivocal plantar response on the right side. In May, 1967, the patient reported that the seizures were becoming more severe as regards the weakness experienced in the right leg; hospital admission was therefore advised.

GENERAL PHYSICAL EXAMINATION: The patient was thin with an appearance of chronic debilitation.

NEUROLOGICAL EXAMINATION:

1. *Mental status:*
   a. The patient was anxious and tremulous with moderate psychomotor retardation.
   b. She was oriented for time, place, and person.
   c. Memory and delayed recall (object retention) were intact.
   d. Digit span, however, was limited to 5 digits forward and 4 in reverse, perhaps reflecting a decrease in attention span.
   e. Calculations were intact.
2. *Cranial nerves* were all intact.
3. *Motor system:* Strength and gait were intact.
4. *Reflexes:*
   a. Deep tendon reflexes were slightly increased on the right side.
   b. The plantar response on the right was equivocally extensor.
5. *Sensory system* was intact except for a minimal bilateral decrease in position sense at the toes.

LABORATORY DATA:

1. *Chest and skull x-rays* were normal.
2. *Electroencephalogram* was now borderline due to minor focal abnormalities (occasional focal sharp waves in the left parietal area).
3. *Brain scan* (Hg[197]) was normal.
4. *Left carotid arteriogram* revealed no definite abnormality.
5. The *pneumoencephalogram* revealed a slight downward displacement of the left lateral ventricle and suggested a possible lesion in the left parasagittal area.
6. *Cerebrospinal fluid protein* was 25 mg./100 ml.; no cells were present.

SUBSEQUENT COURSE:

The patient's anticonvulsant medication was altered. Since the brain scan and arteriogram were negative, a meningioma was considered unlikely. A low-grade glioma was felt to be the most likely diagnosis. However, since the dominant hemisphere was involved and the patient was relatively free of neurological deficit, neurosurgical exploration was not considered to be indicated at this time. Instead, the patient was discharged from the hospital.

Frequent office evaluations by Dr. John Hills indicated that significant progression was occurring. In September, 1967, the patient noted weakness of the right leg. At the same time, she noticed difficulty with handwriting, mainly an inability to form the letters and words clearly. She also experienced occasional slurring of speech. The patient was readmitted to the hospital where neurological examination (September 27, 1967) now indicated a right central facial weakness and a mild right hemiparesis with greater weakness in the arm than the leg. Deep tendon reflexes were now clearly increased on the right with a definite Babinski response on the right. Speech was dysarthric, hesitant, and slurred with a minor degree of misnaming or inability to name objects. A left carotid arteriogram now indicated a deep left posterior frontal mass lesion, depressing the upper branches of the middle cerebral vessels as they emerged from the sylvian triangle. There was also a suggestion of abnormal vascularity in the region of the pericallosal and callosal marginal arteries. The venous phase of the arteriogram suggested flattening of the left lateral ventricle from above downward.

Surgical exploration of the left frontal area was undertaken on November 7, 1967 by Dr. Samuel Brendler. The cortex of the left frontal lobe appeared to be slightly discolored and the gyri were widened. Probe counting located an area of increased uptake of radioisotope (P[32]) estimated at 16 × normal in the mid- and posterior frontal area. A partial frontal lobectomy was performed from the level of the sphenoid wing laterally and forward. However, tumor was noted remaining in the posterior aspect of the lobectomy. (The lobectomy was of necessity limited posteriorly by the presence of the speech areas of the dominant hemispheres.) Histological examination of the tissue revealed an astrocytoma, grade I or II. Postoperatively in the recovery room, speech showed no change from the previous level. The patient's right-sided weakness progressively improved.

Following hospital discharge, the patient received a course of super voltage irradiation (7500 roentgens to the left frontal-parietal area over a 3-month period).

Re-evaluation 1 year after surgery revealed a moderate degree of disorientation (particularly for time) and a nominal aphasia. Serial subtractions were poor. There was also a moderate right central facial weakness and a clumsiness of the right hand. Focal seizures continued as prior to surgery. Examination 18 months after surgery revealed a slowness in following commands with perseveration of speech and performance. Otherwise findings were unchanged.

COMMENT:

The occurrence of seizures for the first time at the age of 30 or 40 or 50 usually raises the question as to whether a tumor is present. As a general rule, if the seizures are generalized without focal onset and if the neurological examination is normal and the electroencephalogram does not demonstrate focal abnormality, there is little danger that the patient has a brain tumor. If the patient with adult onset of seizures does have focal components to the seizure or has focal findings on neurological examination or has focal abnormality in the electroencephalogram, then the chances of a brain tumor being present are significantly increased. In such a patient additional diagnostic tests and close follow up are clearly indicated.

In the present case, when the patient began to experience generalized convulsive seizures, the probabilities for the eventual emergence of a brain tumor were extremely low. When the focal components appeared as a seizure phenomenon 7 years later, the odds were markedly altered. Even so, an additional 4 years passed before the low-grade astrocytoma, which had presumably been present for 11 years, became evident from a clinical and laboratory standpoint. Perhaps for reasons unknown, there was some alteration in the basic biological behavior of the lesion.

The relative absence of abnormality in the electroencephalogram and the lack of uptake of radioisotope in the preoperative period is not unusual for a low-grade astrocytoma.

Polar Spongioblastoma. This term is no longer in common usage. In general the cases described under this heading in Table 22–2 were grade I astrocytomas arising in the pons, optic chiasm, or diencephalon (perithird ventricular). The predominant cell was a relatively uniform elongated astrocyte often infiltrating along white matter tracts. These tumors are now usually included under the category of astrocytoma and are described as piloid or fibrillary. As we have already indicated, the biological behavior of these astrocytomas often differs from that of the glioblastoma—the most frequent astrocytoma of the cerebral hemisphere. The average survival of such patients is considerably longer; moreover, these lesions often appear to have some response to radiation therapy.

Ganglioglioma or Neuroastrocytoma. The use of this term implies that a neoplasia of both neurons and astrocytes is present. There is some doubt whether neoplasia of neurons within the central nervous system ever occurs. Many of these tumors (which are rare in any case) are now considered to represent the diffuse infiltration by a low-grade astrocytoma among neurons of the cerebral cortex—basal ganglia or diencephalic nuclei. At times this type of histological picture has been noted in the lesion of tuberous sclerosis.

OTHER TYPES OF GLIAL TUMORS

Oligodendrogliomas. This variety of glioma is found in the cerebral hemisphere of young adults. Although various grades have on occasion been applied to this tumor type, invariably the tumor consists of an almost uniform field of relatively normal appearing oligodendrocytes. There is a mosaic pattern of cells with a small dark nucleus surrounded by a clear halo of cytoplasm which has failed to stain. The mosaic effect is achieved because the cell membrane does stain (Fig. 22–42). The clinical course of this slow growing tumor is similar to that of the grade I astrocyte. In almost 50 per cent of the cases, the lesion is calcified. Plain x-ray of the skull will then provide a clue as to the presence of this lesion as opposed to the grade I astrocytoma which usually is not calcified. Rarely a mixed astrocytoma and oligodendroglioma will be found.

Ependymomas. These tumors arise from the ependymal cells lining the ventricular

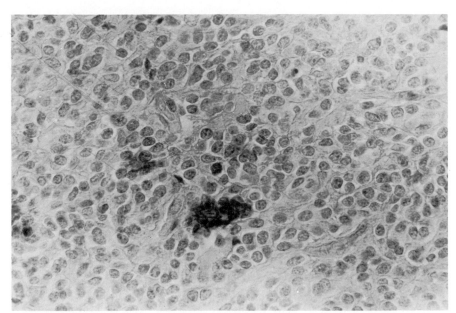

Figure 22–42 Oligodendroglioma. A relatively uniform mosaic pattern of cells with a small nucleus surrounded by a clear halo of cytoplasm is evident. A small area of calcification is present in this field; much larger areas of calcification were evident in other fields. (H & E × 400.) (Courtesy of Dr. David Cowen, Columbia-Presbyterian, Neuropathology.)

system or from nests of ependymal cells which have lost their original continuity with the ventricular system. These tumors are found predominantly in relation to the floor of the fourth ventricle occurring primarily in children and young adults. Less often they may occur in the sacral spinal cord. (Ependymomas are, however, the most common variety of "glial" tumor of the lower one-third of the spinal cord; lumbar, sacral, conus medullaris.) Rarely they may occur in relation to the lateral ventricle presenting a differential problem of a space-occupying supratentorial lesion.

The more common variety in relation to the fourth ventricle has been already introduced in Chapter 15, p. 340. Grossly this variety presents as a fleshy mass protruding into the fourth ventricle, blocking the flow of spinal fluid, and pressing upward against the midline cerebellum. The microscopic appearance is variable. The ependymal cells may be arranged in a rosette forming primitive neural canals. In other areas pseudo-rosettes about blood vessels may be formed (Fig. 22–43). At other times sheets of ependymal cells may be formed or the tumor may consist of masses of ependymal cells. The actual appearance of the cells may be variable. At times a mixture of ependymoma and astrocytoma may be apparent, particularly

in the subependymal areas. At times a transition to a more malignant ependymoblastoma is apparent. (The ependymal tumors are sometimes graded in the same manner as astrocytomas.)

At times extracranial metastases have been noted, usually following surgery. The clinical manifestations of the fourth ventricular variety reflect: (a) the blockage of the ventricular system with the development of increased intracranial pressure and (b) the midline cerebellar compression—truncal and gait ataxia. The manifestations then are similar to those of the more common tumor in this location in childhood, the medulloblastoma. Treatment involves shunting of the ventricular system and radiation. There is a moderate degree of response to radiation therapy. In general those rare ependymomas which originate in the cerebral hemisphere appear to have a relatively good prognosis in comparison to the more typical variety involving the fourth ventricle.

Medulloblastomas. This tumor arises from the cerebellum in the roof of the fourth ventricle. Usually it is midline, originating in the vermis and projecting downward as a gray mass to block the ventricle and to compress the brain stem. The symptoms—truncal ataxia and severe papilledema accompanied by vomiting—relate to the midline cerebellar

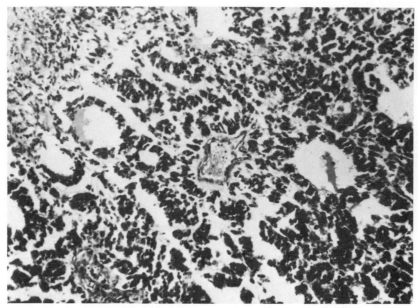

Figure 22–43 Ependymoma of the fourth ventricle. Clusters of ependymal cells are arranged as rosettes or as perivascular pseudorosettes. (H & E × 125.) (Courtesy of Dr. John Hills, New England Center Hospitals.)

involvement and the increased intracranial pressure. The tumor is relatively limited to the pediatric age group.

The microscopic appearance is characteristic. The tumor is packed with small cells with densely staining nuclei containing mitotic figures. At times the cells resemble lymphocytes; at times they are somewhat elongated into a carrot shape (Fig. 22–44). Background stroma and blood vessels are sparse. When blood vessels are noted, there will also be observed a clustering of tumor cells about the vessel to form a pseudorosette. The origin of the cells is uncertain since they lack the appearance of the usual glioma. The cells, however, do bear some resemblance to those cells found in the external granular layer of the developing cerebellar cortex of the infant.

Although this is the classic example of a posterior fossa tumor of childhood, symptoms and signs may occur in relation to the cerebral hemispheres, spinal cord, and nerve roots as a result of the marked propensity of

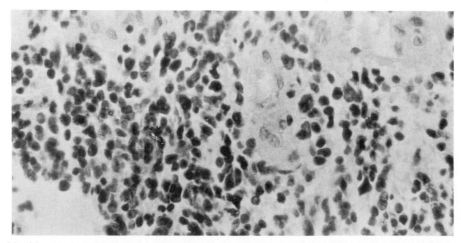

Figure 22–44 Medulloblastoma. Clusters of small cells with densely staining nuclei are present. (H & E × 400.) Refer to p. 340, Chapter 15 for illustration of a gross specimen. (Courtesy of Dr. David Cowen. Columbia-Presbyterian, Neuropathology.)

the tumor to spread along the cerebrospinal fluid pathways. Such spread at times follows attempted surgery or biopsy and might in a sense be predicted on the basis of the lack of stroma. Such seeding may result in focal cortical seizures or radicular pain. Rarely extracerebral spread may occur following surgery. Complete surgical removal cannot be achieved. Radiation has a significant effect on the tumor. It does not produce a cure but does increase the period of survival of the patient. In general the entire central nervous system must be radiated. (Refer to Case #1, Chapter 25, p. 702.)

Pinealomas. These tumors of the pineal have been considered already in relation to the brain stem. These lesions are relatively rare. Although not clearly justified from a histological standpoint these tumors have usually been classified with the gliomas. In the tumor of the pineal, two cellular types are present: clusters of small cells resembling lymphocytes and large cells with vesicular nuclei. At times these latter cells may have some resemblance to neuronal or glial elements. The pineal may also be the site of congenital lesions: the *teratoma*. Moreover, the true pinealoma may occur in an ectopic location: pituitary or hypothalamic region. It is uncertain whether such ectopic lesions represent congenital nests or more recent seeding from a primary pineal location via the cerebrospinal fluid. The usual pinealoma occurs in an adolescent male; occasionally, they will appear in the adult. The location of the lesion results in early compression of the pretectal area, the superior colliculus and the aqueduct of Sylvius. (Refer to Fig. 15–3).

The resultant syndrome involves a paralysis of upward gaze (Parinaud's syndrome) and the early development of severe papilledema. With additional compression of the midbrain, additional impairment of eye movement and of hearing will result. Eventually a decorticate or decerebrate state reflects severe functional midbrain transection. The tumor also exerts pressure on the superior aspect of the cerebellum; ataxia is common. The extension of the tumor into the third ventricle and the invasion of the hypothalamus often result in various hypothalamic syndromes such as diabetes insipidus and precocious puberty.

Although apparently encapsulated, the tumor has some tendency to invade adjacent structures: midbrain, cerebellum, and hypothalamus. This tendency plus the relatively inaccessible position of the tumor in the human brain (from the neurosurgical standpoint) has resulted in a treatment based on shunting procedures (to bypass the aqueductal block of the ventricular system) and on radiation therapy. (Refer to Case #3, Chapter 15, p. 344.)

OTHER PRIMARY INTRINSIC TUMORS

Primary intrinsic tumors of nonglial origin are not common. In this group are included those tumors arising from blood vessels. While large saccular aneurysms or arteriovenous malformations may at times present as "tumor masses," they are not true neoplasms. Probably the only true vascular neoplasm intrinsic to the central nervous system is the *hemangioblastoma*. Thus the angiomas or arteriovenous malformation of the brain and meninges are composed of adult vascular elements.

The *hemangioblastomas* on the other hand are composed of embryonic vascular elements. This tumor has been rarely reported affecting the cerebral hemisphere. The usual site is the cerebellum in a paramedian location. (Less often the tumor arises in the lateral cerebellar hemisphere.) The tumor is often present as a cyst containing a mural nodule of tissue. There may be in the solid tumors some infiltration of adjacent cerebellar tissue. The neurological symptoms are those of a progressive cerebellar ataxia and headache. While relatively uncommon in the overall sense, these tumors within the limited group of cerebellar neoplasms developing in the adult are relatively common. Typical examples have been presented in Chapter 25, Case #4, p. 707 and Chapter 15, Case #2, p. 340. Although these tumors may present as isolated problems, certain associations have been described: (a) with vascular malformations of the retina —*Hippel-Lindau disease*, (b) with a secondary type of polycythemia, and (c) in association with neoplasms of the kidney. Treatment involves complete surgical resection of the tumor, with relatively total resolution of symptoms.

EXTRINSIC TUMORS

MENINGIOMAS

The most common example of this group above the tentorium is the *meningioma*. Meningiomas constitute over 20 per cent of all types of brain tumors above the tentorium. Below the tentorium, the most common type of tumor extrinsic to the neural axis is the *schwannoma* of the acoustic nerve.

Meningiomas are tumors of the adult population 30 to 70 years of age. They arise from arachnoidal cells embedded in the dura. Normally arachnoidal villi invaginate into the venous sinuses as arachnoidal or pacchionian granulations. In addition, arachnoidal cells may be embedded in the dura. In addition, fibrous and vascular elements are, to a variable degree, also included in these tumors.

The variable composition has resulted in a histological classification according to the following main types:

1. A *syncytial* or *meningiothelial* variety composed of clusters of cells similar to the outer layer of arachnoid arranged in nests or whorls and surrounded by layers of elongated or flattened cells.

2. A *fibrous* variety in which interlacing bundles of fibroblastic elements predominate.

3. A *psammomatous* variety (probably the most common type) consisting of the same type of arachnoidal cells, arranged in a whorl. In the center of the whorl is an area of hyalinization arranged in concentric lamellae and calcified (psammomatous granules). The calcification is often visible on plain x-rays of the skull.

4. A less common *angioblastic* variety, presenting from both a gross and a microscopic standpoint, a spongy structure due to multiple small vascular channels.

5. A mixed or transitional variety. Considerable overlap is apparent as demonstrated in Figure 22–45.

These tumors are in general slow growing. Almost all occur external to the brain with a dural attachment—compressing, displacing, and occasionally invaginating into the brain. Rarely the tumors may be found without a dural attachment within the ventricle or within the sylvian fissure. Although not invading the brain, the otherwise benign meningioma may invade the overlying bone of the skull. Others excite an osteoblastic reaction in the overlying bone with a marked local thickening of the bone (*hyperostosis*).

These tumors are important because they are in general readily amenable to neurosurgical removal. Since the symptoms are due to the local and general effects of an extrinsic compression, a marked relief of

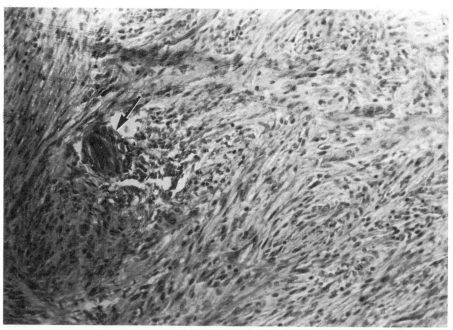

Figure 22–45 Meningioma. Histological appearance of a mixed or transitional type meningioma. Interlacing fibrous bundles and whorls of meningothelial cells are present in addition to a calcified psammoma body (arrow). (Courtesy of Dr. David Cowen, Columbia-Presbyterian, Neuropathology. H & E × 100.)

neurological symptoms and signs may be achieved in contrast to the gliomas. It must, of course, be noted that some meningiomas are small and apparently asymptomatic and may be discovered incidentally on skull x-ray in an elderly patient or on autopsy. In cases of this type, the risks of surgery may have to be balanced against the medical condition of the patient.

What is important about meningiomas is not their histological cell type (sarcomatous degeneration is rare) but their location. Meningiomas tend to occur in certain specific locations. The most common location is the parasagittal region where the tumor arises in relation to the superior sagittal sinus (and less often in relation to the falx) (Fig. 22–46). Taveras and Wood (1964) estimate that one-third to one-half of all meningiomas occur in this location. Most other series estimate that 21 to 23 per cent occur in this location. The symptoms and signs are those of involvement of the parasagittal sectors—of the

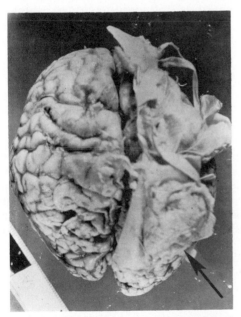

Figure 22–46 Parasagittal meningioma arising from the superior sagittal sinus in relation to the dura overlying the *right parietal-occipital cortex.* The dura and tumor (arrow) have been reflected back onto the contralateral hemisphere revealing the local cortical atrophy which has occurred in the underlying cortex, secondary to the compressive effects of the tumor. This 72-year-old male had developed a left hemiparesis two months prior to death. (Courtesy of Dr. Jose Segarra, Boston Veterans Administration Hospital.)

prefrontal, premotor, motor, or parietal cortex. Unilateral or bilateral involvement may predominate. Those parasagittal lesions overlying the motor cortex have a very high incidence of focal seizures.

The second most common location is in relation to the lateral convexity of the cerebral hemisphere accounting for 17 per cent of cases (series of Cushing and Eisenhardt and of Courville). These cases merge into the parasagittal lesions as regards location and symptomatology. Their manifestations are related to focal-cortical neurological deficits and focal seizures.

The third most common location is the sphenoid ridge accounting for 9 to 17 per cent of cases. The manifestations depend on the portion of the sphenoid ridge involved. Three syndromes have been distinguished:

Inner Third Syndrome. Because of involvement of the anterior clinoid area there is unilateral loss of vision with optic atrophy and unilateral exophthalmos (protrusion of eye). There is often papilledema of the contralateral eye. The combination of ipsilateral optic atrophy and contralateral papilledema is referred to as the *Foster Kennedy syndrome.* Some involvement of the lateral aspect of the optic chiasm or the optic tract may also occur, producing a contralateral homonymous hemianopsia. Involvement of the nerves passing through the adjacent superior orbital fissure may result in extraocular palsies and numbness in the distribution of the ophthalmic nerve.

Middle Third Syndrome. Bilateral papilledema is more common at the onset (as opposed to unilateral optic atrophy). As the tumor extends into the inner third sector, the findings previously indicated will be noted.

Outer Third or Greater Wing of Sphenoid Syndrome. (Fig. 22–47). The symptoms and signs in this location reflect the involvement of the temporal lobe, particularly its medial and inferior portion. Focal temporal lobe seizures with olfactory or visual hallucinations and/or generalized seizures are frequent.

Almost equal in frequency to the sphenoid ridge as a location is the floor of the anterior fossa, accounting for 8 to 18 per cent of these cases. Essentially two sublocations are included: the olfactory groove and the tuberculum sellae. Those arising from the olfactory groove often present as large subfrontal mass lesions, producing damage to

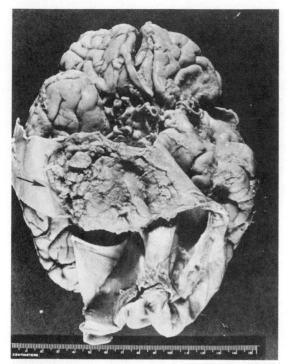

Figure 22–47 Sphenoid wing meningioma (outer third). The dura overlying the sphenoid wing has been reflected, revealing a large meningioma (arrow) compressing but not invading the inferior surface of temporal lobe and the adjacent orbital frontal area. This 73-year-old Negro male had experienced "grand mal" (generalized convulsions) and "psychomotor" seizures since 1951. In 1962–1963, the patient became increasingly incapacitated by these seizures complaining of increasing weakness. In March 1964, sudden difficulty in walking and lethargy developed. In August 1964, focal motor seizures involving the right leg, hand, and face occurred. On examination, the patient was stuporous and severely dehydrated. Cerebrospinal fluid protein was elevated to 124. Although brain scan and arteriogram suggested the nature of the lesion, therapy could not be undertaken because of severe medical complications: gram negative septicemia, dehydration, and gastrointestinal bleeding. (Courtesy of Dr. John Hills, New England Center Hospitals; and Dr. Jose Segarra, Boston Veterans Administration Hospital.)

the prefrontal areas. In addition, unilateral anosmia (loss of olfactory sensation) is an early finding. The aforementioned Foster Kennedy syndrome is also not infrequent when the tumor remains predominantly unilateral.

Those arising from the tuberculum sellae may produce a syndrome that mimics a pituitary tumor, with compression of the optic chiasm resulting in a bitemporal hemianopsia.

A posterior fossa location is noted in approximately 7 per cent of cases. Three favorite sites may be indicated: tentorial, the cerebellar-pontine angle, and the foramen magnum (basilar groove).

Other less common sites are peritorcular (compressing occipital lobe), deep sylvian fissure, and intraventricular.

The course of several meningiomas is indicated in the following illustrative case histories.

Parasagittal Meningioma

Case History 15.   NECH #100–123. Date of admission: 5/27/68.

This 69-year-old white housewife (Mrs. E.N.), in July 1966, visited a relative in Israel whom she had not seen in a number of years. This relative then wrote to the patient's physician (an old family friend) indicating her concern over the change in the patient's personality. The patient was described as apathetic, and her reactions as silly. The patient's husband indicated in retrospect that this alteration in personality had begun insidiously a number of years previously.

In May 1967, the relative in Israel again wrote to the patient's physician indicating that letters received from the patient were incoherent. These letters became less frequent and eventually the patient stopped writing letters.

In July 1967, the patient was noted to have a left central facial weakness. In September 1967, a decreased swing of the left arm was noted. In December 1967, the patient's husband noted that she was purchasing things for which she had no need — 24 pairs of shoes, 15 brassieres. Subsequently, she had become careless in housework. On several occasions, the patient had lost her purse. The patient's ability to play bridge had decreased over the last year, although her golf game was unchanged.

NEUROLOGICAL EXAMINATION (May 23, 1968):   The patient was right-handed.
  1. *Mental status:*
    a. The patient was oriented × 3.
    b. There was a marked impersistence in motor activities and coordination. Answers were often irrelevant. (Her husband stated this had been present for many years — "all of her life.")
    c. There was inappropriate joking.
    d. Delayed recall was 2-out-of-5 objects

in 5 minutes without help and 5-out-of-5 objects with help. Digit span was decreased to 5 forward, 3 in reverse.

e. There were marked deficits in serial 7 subtractions. At times the patient began to subtract other numbers; at times she added rather than subtracted.

f. There was a significant spatial disorientation. There was marked impairment of ability to copy a cube and deficits in drawing a house. There was disorientation in locating cities on a map.

2. *Cranial nerves:*

a. There was a significant neglect of single stimulus objects in the left visual field. This was possibly greater when bilateral simultaneous stimuli were used.

b. A left central facial weakness was present.

c. At times limitation of voluntary gaze to the left was noted.

3. *Motor system:*

a. There was a minimal weakness of the left arm and leg.

b. Resistance to passive motion at the left wrist and elbow was present (?) inconsistent spasticity, (?) rigidity, (?) "Gegenhalten" of frontal lobe disease.

c. Gait: There was poor swing of the left arm. The gait was initially broad-based, but improved as the patient picked up speed.

4. *Reflexes:*

a. Deep tendon: increased on left.

b. Left. Babinski sign.

c. Bilateral release of grasp reflex.

5. *Sensory system:* Intact.

LABORATORY DATA:

1. *Skull x-ray:* There was a shift of the calcified pineal gland 5 mm. to the left. Demineralization of the sella turcica from pressure effects was present. Chest x-ray was normal.

2. *Electroencephalogram:* Focal 3–4 cps slow waves were present in the right frontal-

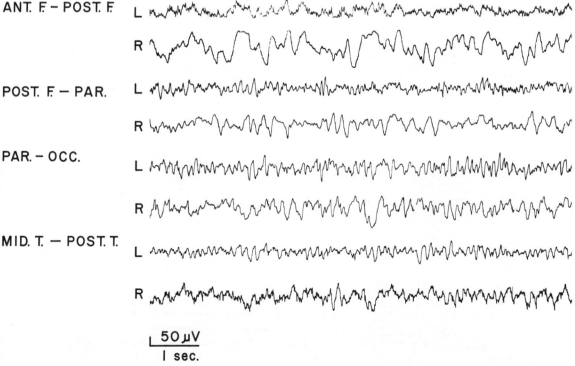

Figure 22–48 Case History 15. Parasagittal meningioma: right frontal. Bipolar electroencephalogram. Focal 2–5 cps slow waves were present in the right frontal-parietal area: most prominent right parasagittal frontal. ANT. F. = anterior frontal (parasagittal); POST. F. = posterior frontal (parasagittal); PAR. = parietal (parasagittal); OCC. = occipital; MID. T. = midtemporal; POST. T. = posterior temporal.

parietal area suggesting focal damage. Abnormality was most prominent in right frontal area close to the midline where continuous 2–5 cps slow waves occurred (Fig. 22–48).

3. *Brain scan (Hg*[197]*):* There was a very heavy uptake in the right frontal area, somewhat deep and towards the midline and measuring $5 \times 5 \times 4$ cm. (Fig. 22–49).

4. *Arteriograms:* There was evidence of a parasagittal tumor in the right posterior frontal region (Fig. 22–50). The left anterior cerebral artery was displaced downward and was shifted from the right to the left side. A diffuse tumor stain was present. On both the arterial and venous phases the cortical vessels were draped around the tumor mass. The vascular supply to this tumor, a probable meningioma, was derived from the left and right middle meningeal arteries and from the left anterior meningeal artery.

HOSPITAL COURSE:

Following the arteriogram on May 29, 1968, the patient began vomiting, and showed signs of lethargy and papilledema. (The borders of the optic disks became indistinct.) These symptoms improved with the use of Decadron (a glucocorticoid used to reduce cerebral edema). Prior to definitive surgery, ligation of the right external carotid artery was performed since the tumor appeared to have a significant blood supply from this source. A bilateral frontal craniotomy was performed on June 11, 1968 by Dr. Samuel Brendler. Bulging of the dura

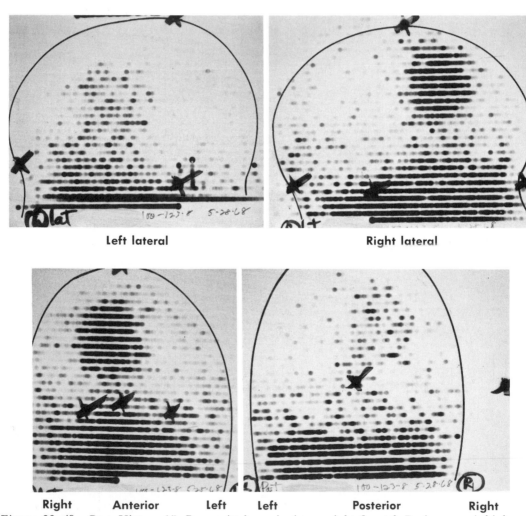

Left lateral   **Right lateral**

Right   Anterior   Left   Left   Posterior   Right

Figure 22–49   Case History 15. Parasagittal meningioma, right frontal. Brain scan. A high uptake of isotope (Hg[197]) is demonstrated in the right frontal parasagittal area, close to the midline. This is most prominent in the anterior and right lateral scans, but is also noted to a lesser degree in the posterior and left lateral scans.

In general, meningiomas and metastatic lesions are characterized by a dense focal uptake. (Courtesy of Dr. Bertram Selverstone.)

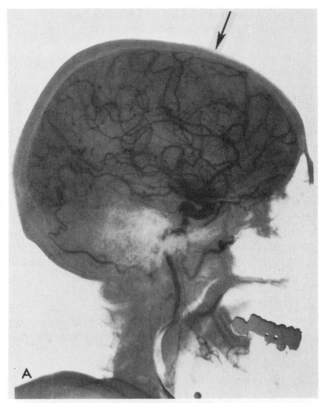

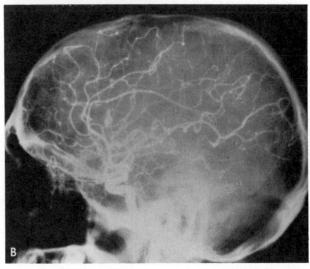

Figure 22–50 Case History 15: Para-sagittal meningioma. *A,* Right carotid arteriogram. In this lateral view, a square-shaped area may be outlined, formed by anterior cerebral arterial branches displaced by and draped around the tumor mass. *B,* Normal carotid arteriogram in the same approximate phase for comparison. (Courtesy of Dr. Samuel Wolpert, New England Center Hospitals, Neuroradiology.)

was present bilaterally, requiring the administration of a hyperosmotic agent (20% Mannitol solution). Following reduction of brain swelling, the dura was opened, revealing a large right posterior frontal parasagittal meningioma measuring 8 cm. in anteroposterior diameter and 8 cm. in transverse diameter. The tumor was attached to the right side of the superior sagittal sinus. During the course of removing the tumor, it was necessary to ligate several bridging veins entering the superior sagittal sinus in addition to arteries feeding the tumor. Histological sections revealed a fibrous and meningothelial meningioma.

At the conclusion of the procedure, it was noted that the right pupil was larger than the left; neither pupil reacted to light. The patient failed to regain consciousness following surgery. She remained in a state of coma with bilateral extensor plantar responses and with decerebrate postures on stimulation.

On June 12, 1968, section of the tentorium

was performed because it was suspected that midbrain compression had occurred as a result of tentorial herniation of the temporal lobe during the period of cerebral edema. No significant improvement occurred. The pupils remained nonreactive and dilated. Respiratory assistance was required. After several episodes of cardiac arrest, the patient expired on June 24, 1968.

COMMENT:

It is difficult even in retrospect to decide when the patient's symptoms began. We may presume that the changes in personality were relatively insidious extending possibly over several years prior to 1966. As this large lesion in the posterior frontal area progressed, there was involvement not only of the premotor area (resulting in the release of grasp reflex) and of the prefrontal areas (resulting in the personality alterations) but also of the motor cortex (resulting in the appearance of a left central facial weakness and the increased deep tendon reflexes on the left side).

The neglect of stimuli in the left visual field may have reflected compromise of the premotor cortex or may have indicated involvement of the nondominant parietal cortex. The lesion was large enough to have produced compromise of both these areas in the right hemisphere.

The brain scan and arteriographic findings in this case were in general consistent with the diagnosis of a meningioma. The extremely dense uptake of radioisotope is seen predominantly in meningiomas and metastatic lesions. The electroencephalogram in a meningioma usually does not show the severe degree of slow wave activity seen in the present case.

There is little question that surgical removal of the tumor was required at this time. The patient was beginning to develop increasing symptoms of increased intracranial pressure. In such cases, a minor event may add to a sufficient degree of brain swelling and result in tentorial herniation and brain stem compression. Such events may include a minor degree of anoxia or hypoventilation during induction of anesthesia or a minor degree of over-hydration in the administration of intravenous solutions. These are events which may be tolerated in the normal patient but are not well tolerated in the patient with a large supratentorial mass. We should also note that the operative procedure of removing a parasagittal meningioma arising from the superior sagittal sinus often requires the ligation of bridging veins passing into this sinus. It is not unusual for some degree of hemorrhagic infarction and cerebral edema to develop in relation to the ligation of these vessels.

Sphenoid Wing Meningioma
Case History 16. NECH #76–29–63–2. Date of admission: 6/15/69. (Patient of Dr. Huntington Porter.)

This 53-year-old, white, right-handed housewife (Mrs. A.C.) was referred for evaluation of progressive right-sided headache and decreasing vision in the right eye. For 20 years the patient had experienced right supraorbital pain and headache. This had progressively increased in the 2 years prior to admission. Over the 2 year period prior to admission, the patient had experienced decreasing visual acuity in the right eye. This had progressed to the point of almost total unilateral blindness. During the 3 years prior to admission intermittent tingling parasthesias had been noted in the left face, arm, or leg. One and one-half years prior to admission the patient had a sudden loss of consciousness. The patient was then amnesic for the events of the next 48 hours. She was hospitalized at that time; an explanation for the episode was not clearly established. Cerebrospinal fluid protein at the time was reported as elevated to 200 mg./100 ml.

The patient and her family reported some personality changes over a period of several years, with a loss of spontaneity and increasing apathy.

GENERAL PHYSICAL EXAMINATION: This was not remarkable except for a minor degree of proptosis (downward protrusion) of the right eye.

NEUROLOGICAL EXAMINATION:

1. *Mental status:*
   a. The patient was, in general, alert. At times she would become lethargic.
   b. Her affect was flat.
   c. At times, she would laugh or joke in an inappropriate manner.
   d. The patient was oriented for time, place, and person.
   e. Delayed recall was intact.
   f. Calculations were intact.
   g. The ability to do abstractions was intact.

2. *Cranial nerves:*
   a. There was anosmia for odors, such as cloves, on the right and a reduced detection on the left.
   b. Pallor of the right optic disk was present indicating optic atrophy. Visual acuity in the right eye was markedly reduced. The patient had only a small crescent of vision in the temporal field of the right eye. Even in this sector only vague outlines of objects could be seen.
   c. Marked papilledema was present in the left eye with marked elevation of the disk.
   d. A slight left central facial weakness was present.
3. *Motor system:*
   a. Strength was intact although movements on the left side were slow.
   b. In walking, there was a decreased swing of the left arm.
4. *Reflexes:*
   a. Deep tendon reflexes were symmetrical.
   b. Plantar responses were flexor.
   c. A release of grasp reflex was present on the left side.
5. *Sensory system:* All modalities were intact.

LABORATORY DATA:

1. *Skull x-rays* demonstrated erosion of the dorsum sellae. In addition, special *lamniograms* demonstrated hyperostosis of the sphenoid bone (planum sphenoidale) suggesting a meningioma originating in this area.

2. *Electroencephalogram* demonstrated focal 2–4 cps slow waves in the right anterior frontal area and to a minor degree, left anterior frontal. Damage in the right frontal area was suggested (Fig. 22–51).

3. *Brain scan* (Hg^{197}) revealed a heavy uptake of isotope in the right posterior subfrontal area (Fig. 22–52).

4. *Carotid arteriograms:* The anterior cerebral arteries were shifted upward, posteriorly, and across the midline to the left (Fig. 22–53). The lateral ventricles were shifted back and upwards. A 6 × 8 cm. tumor blush was present in the right subfrontal area (Fig. 22–54). The posterior portion of this tumor blush extended back to the right optic nerve groove. The major feeding vessel was the right ophthalmic artery. These findings were felt to be most consistent with an olfactory groove meningioma.

HOSPITAL COURSE:

On June 24, 1969 a bifrontal craniotomy was undertaken by Dr. Samuel Brendler. A small, right, prefrontal lobectomy was performed, exposing a well-encapsulated smooth tumor attached to the sphenoid wing on its medial third. After intracapsular removal of 90 to 95 per cent of the tumor, the right optic nerve could be visualized. The small portion of tumor attached to the bone could not be removed because of considerable bleeding from the bone. At the end of the procedure, the patient was moving all extremities and responding to verbal stimulus. Histological examination of the tissue removed indicated a meningioma.

The postoperative course was complicated by low-grade fever, mental obtundation, and a fluctuating left hemiparesis. Some of the obtundation may have reflected acute renal failure in the postoperative period (acute renal tubular necrosis). This latter problem was successfully treated with peritoneal dialysis. At the time of hospital discharge on September 15, 1969 residual right anosmia and right optic atrophy were present. Follow-up one month later indicated essentially the same findings.

COMMENT:

If one considered only the patient's primary complaint—that of decreasing vision in the right eye—and the findings of right optic atrophy and left-sided papilledema (the Foster Kennedy syndrome), then the most probable diagnosis was that of inner third sphenoid wing meningioma. The small temporal crescent of preservation of some vision is consistent with compression of the optic nerve on its lateral surface. By the time of hospitalization, the lesion was quite large and had extended into the subfrontal area, producing anosmia on the right and some changes in personality. At this point the various diagnostic studies suggested only a subfrontal mass and did not clearly differentiate between an olfactory groove meningioma and a sphenoid wing meningioma. One might suggest in retrospect that the degree of involvement of the right optic nerve was far out of proportion to any change in prefrontal function and therefore the inner third sphenoid wing location was more likely.

The surgical approach in any case was the same. The actual origin of the tumor was evident at surgery. The eventual prospects for recovery of vision in this case remain

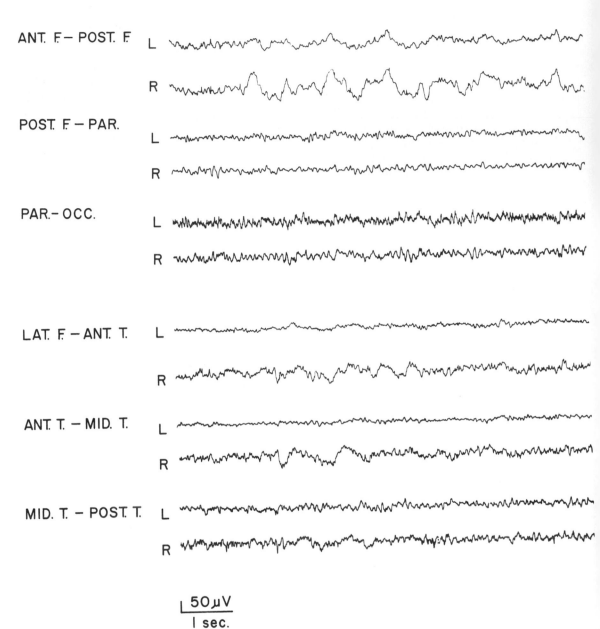

ANT. F. – POST. F. L

R

POST. F. – PAR. L

R

PAR. – OCC. L

R

LAT. F. – ANT. T. L

R

ANT. T. – MID. T. L

R

MID. T. – POST. T. L

R

50 μV

1 sec.

Figure 22–51 Case History 16. Sphenoid wing meningioma. Bipolar electroencephalogram. Focal 2–4 cps slow wave activity was present in right anterior frontal area (prefrontal parasagittal) and to a lesser degree left anterior frontal and right anterior temporal. These findings were consistent then, with a large subfrontal tumor which was mainly producing damage to the right prefrontal area but was also, because of its mass, producing some involvement of the right anterior temporal and left prefrontal area. ANT. F. = anterior frontal (parasagittal prefrontal); POST. F. = posterior frontal (parasagittal); PAR. = parietal (parasagittal); OCC. = occipital; LAT. F. = lateral frontal; ANT. T. = anterior temporal; MID. T. = midtemporal; POST. T. = posterior temporal.

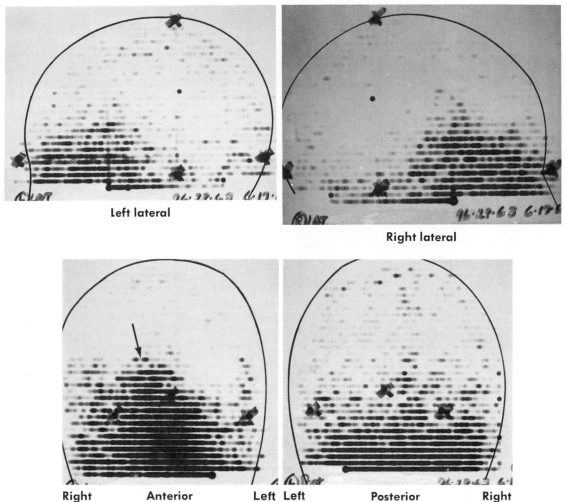

Left lateral

Right lateral

Right   Anterior   Left Left   Posterior   Right

Figure 22–52　Case History 16. Sphenoid wing meningioma. Brain scan. A dense uptake of isotope is present in the right subfrontal area, close to the midline. This is best seen on the anterior scan (arrow) but is also noted to a lesser degree on the right lateral scan.

In the anterior scan, in addition to a dense uptake close to the midline (arrow), a less marked uptake is present more laterally. The midline X in this scan indicates the nose, the lateral X's, the orbits. (Courtesy of Dr. Bertram Selverstone.)

uncertain. The optic nerve is actually an extension of the central nervous system. The effects of compression often are not reversible.

Olfactory Groove Meningioma. The student should review Case 2 in Chapter 21, p. 496 and compare the clinical course to the sphenoid wing meningioma illustrated above.

PITUITARY ADENOMAS

This group of extrinsic brain tumors, arising in the anterior lobe of the pituitary gland within the sella turcica, is second to meningiomas in frequency. These tumors are of interest both to the endocrinologist and to the neurologist. In many instances the endocrine manifestations are primary and the neurological manifestations are absent. When neurological manifestations occur, it is because the tumor has extended out of the pituitary fossa to compress the structures at the base of the diencephalon—classically the optic chiasm.

It is customary to divide these histologically benign tumors into three varieties based on the dominant cell type: (1) chromophobe adenoma (the most common), (2) acidophilic adenoma, and (3) basophilic adenomas.

Basophilic Adenomas. The basophilic variety, from the clinical standpoint, is the least common. These lesions do not grow to

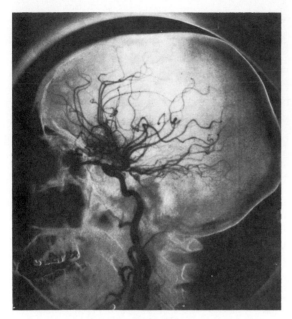

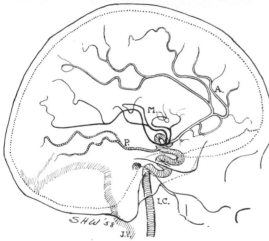

Figure 22–53 Case History 16: Sphenoid wing meningioma. Carotid Arteriogram. *Top;* Lateral view—subtraction technique—demonstrating upward and posterior displacement of both anterior cerebral arteries by a subfrontal mass. (Courtesy of Dr. Samuel Wolpert, New England Center Hospitals, Neuroradiology.)

Bottom, Diagram of a lateral view in a normal carotid arteriogram for comparison. *A,* Anterior cerebral artery (outlined); *P,* posterior cerebral artery (cross-banded); *M,* middle cerebral artery (solid black); *JV,* jugular vein. (From Ranson, S. W., and Clark, S. C.: *The Anatomy of the Nervous System.* Philadelphia, W. B. Saunders, 1959, p. 87.)

sufficient size to produce enlargement of the sella turcica and do not have any extrasellar extension.

In 1932 Cushing described a syndrome of adrenal hyperfunction which he related to the presence of a basophilic adenoma of the pituitary (*pituitary basophilism*). The syndrome has since carried his name. It is evident, however, that most cases of Cushing's syndrome are due to primary overactivity of the adrenal cortex owing to hyperplasia or a tumor (adenoma or adenocarcinoma). In some instances there has been an association with malignant tumors involving the lung and rarely other organs. The clinical and laboratory findings of Cushing's syndrome may be reproduced by administering ACTH (corticotropin) or cortisone.

The typical patient is a female, 25 to 50 years of age, with hypertension, obesity, elevated blood sugar, amenorrhea, and infertility. There is a characteristic plethoric facies and a "buffalo hump" dorsal kyphosis. The obesity is in contrast to the extremity weakness and actual muscle atrophy experienced by the patient. Dermatological manifestations include increased growth of hair on the face and extremities (hypertrichosis), and purple abdominal striae. Psychiatric disturbances are common with alterations in personality. Laboratory studies of urine and blood indicate increased output of steroids derived from the adrenal cortex. Therapy relates to surgical resection of the tumor or hyperplastic tissue of the adrenal.

Acidophilic Adenoma. The acidophilic (or eosinophilic) adenoma presents predominantly the endocrine manifestations of increased secretion of growth hormone. The specific manifestations of this hyperactivity depend on the age of the patient. When the hyperfunction begins in childhood before closure of the epiphyseal lines, the result is gigantism owing to a generalized increase in size of the bones, particularly the long bones of the extremities. When the hyperactivity begins in the adult, after closure of the epiphyses of the long bones, the characteristic skeletal overgrowth produces a progressive enlargement of hands, feet, skull, and mandible (*acromegaly*). Nonskeletal tissues are affected as well with enlargement of the tongue, lips, and nose.

As the tumor enlarges, the remainder of the pituitary gland is compressed and destroyed. The additional endocrine manifestations then are those of anterior pituitary

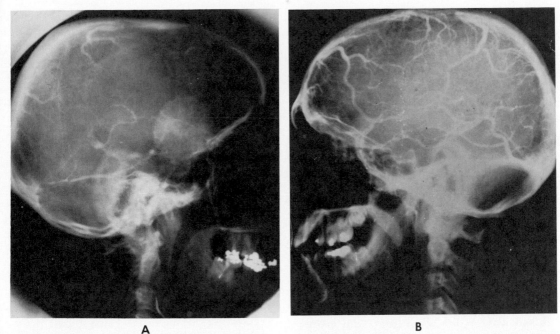

Figure 22–54 Case History 16: Sphenoid wing meningioma. *A*, Right carotid arteriogram venous phase. A large tumor blush is apparent in the subfrontal area of the anterior fossa—extending back into middle fossa. *B*, Normal venous phase for comparison. (Courtesy of Dr. Samuel Wolpert, New England Medical Center Hospitals, Neuroradiology.)

hypofunction. Only late in the course does this tumor extend outside of the sella to produce compression of the optic chiasm.

The general rules for treatment are those considered for the chromophobe adenoma. It should be noted that it is not unusual to find on histological examination of the adenoma in a patient with acromegaly that the dominant cell type is chromophobic rather than acidophilic.

Chromophobe Adenomas. These adenomas (Fig. 22–55) are by far the most frequent tumor within the pituitary. Their course is characterized by progressive enlargement. The resultant ballooning of the sella turcica may be visualized on plain x-ray of the skull (Fig. 22–56). As the tumor enlarges, it exerts pressure on the anterior pituitary, destroying the normal secreting tissue with resultant secondary hypofunction of the target organs—thyroid, adrenals, ovaries, or testes. Supra - or extrasellar extension is common with resultant compression damage to:

a. the *optic chiasm* (or the adjacent optic nerves and tracts depending on the variable anatomical relationship of the chiasm to the sella and the direction of spread). The classic defect is a bitemporal impairment of the

visual field from pressure on the chiasm—the syndrome of the optic chiasm.

b. the *hypothalamus* and the supraoptic-hypophyseal tract. Many of the endocrine and metabolic alterations usually attributed to pituitary damage may reflect combined destruction of the pituitary and hypothalamus. Destruction of the supraoptic-hypophyseal pathways will result in diabetes insipidus.

c. the *third ventricle* with resultant block of the ventricular system.

d. the *third and sixth nerves* passing in the wall of the cavernous sinus with resultant diplopia.

e. the *temporal lobe* as a result of lateral extension with resultant temporal lobe seizures.

The actual extension of the tumor outside of sella is often preceded by severe headache, attributed to the pressure of the tumor upward against the diaphragm of the sella.

It must be noted that the actual critical compromise of the optic chiasm with impairment of vision may, in some cases, occur in a sudden manner, because of hemorrhage into and necrosis of the adenoma (a form of so-called pituitary apoplexy). The hemorrhage and necrosis result in a sudden in-

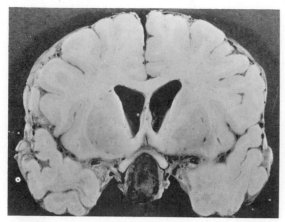

Figure 22–55 Chromophobe adenoma. A large chromophobe adenoma has extended upward out of the sella to compress the optic chiasm. Hemorrhage has occurred within the tumor. Meningitis has occurred as a late complication of therapy. This 53-year-old white male who expired in February 1962, had the onset in March 1961 of difficulty in reading small print, with greater involvement of the right eye than the left. At the same time, pain in the right eye was noted. In September 1961, vision became definitely worse and pain more severe. By November 1961, no vision was present in the right eye and only limited vision in the left eye. Shortly thereafter, vision suddenly was lost in the left eye. Neurological examination revealed total bilateral blindness, an absence of pupillary responses, and a bilateral anosmia. Some improvement in vision then occurred. A greater degree of recovery followed partial surgical removal and x-irradiation. Death followed the development of meningitis. (Courtesy of Dr. John Hills, New England Center Hospitals; and Dr. Jose Segarra, Boston Veterans Administration Hospital.)

See Filmstrip, Frame 58.

crease in the mass of the tumor causing a sudden increase in the degree of compression of the optic chiasm.

The treatment of chromophobe and acidophilic adenomas of the pituitary involves radiotherapy or surgical resection. If visual defect is not present, radiation therapy is used because the tumor is radiosensitive. If visual impairment is present, surgical resection is the treatment of choice. This is particularly indicated when the visual defect appears to be evolving rapidly.

The chiasmatic syndrome (bitemporal hemianopsia) is not always due to a pituitary adenoma. Other tumors in this area may invade and compress both the pituitary and the optic chiasm. The more common ex-amples are aneurysms of the internal carotid artery, craniopharyngiomas, tuberculum sellae meningiomas, and optic chiasm gliomas. Thorough diagnostic evaluation, then, must be undertaken prior to surgery. The dangers of biopsy of an aneurysm in the belief that one is dealing with a solid chromophobe adenoma are obvious.

The following case history illustrates the problem of pituitary adenomas.

Case History 17. NECH #154–327. Date of admission: 2/8/63.

This 51-year-old, white, married, lumber company salesman (Mr. A.G.) was admitted for evaluation of a progressive disturbance of vision. Approximately 8 years previously, the patient noted blurring of print on the labels of paint cans. Glasses were obtained and produced improvement, but within a short time, symptoms recurred. During the succeeding years, the glasses had to be changed eight times.

For 6 to 7 months, the patient had noted diplopia, especially on right lateral gaze when driving at night. For 3 to 4 months, a left frontal-parietal and left orbital headache had been present.

One month prior to admission, progression of visual symptoms occurred. The patient had a marked decrease in visual acuity — he was unable to find objects on shelves. He reported also that he was unable to drive his automobile because he was unable to see the sides of the road. The patient consulted an ophthalmologist who noted visual field defects and referred the patient for neurological evaluation.

PAST HISTORY:

The patient denied any significant change in physical appearance, appetite, or fluid intake. The patient's sexual interests had declined. He had had no sexual intercourse since 1945.

GENERAL PHYSICAL EXAMINATION:

1. The patient was obese with large puffy hands and feet, a prominent jaw, and prominent frontal skull areas.

2. Pallor of skin and mucous membranes was noted.

3. Blood pressure was 140/60; pulse was 88.

4. Axillary hair was absent; pubic hair was normal.

5. Testes were of normal size but were described as soft.

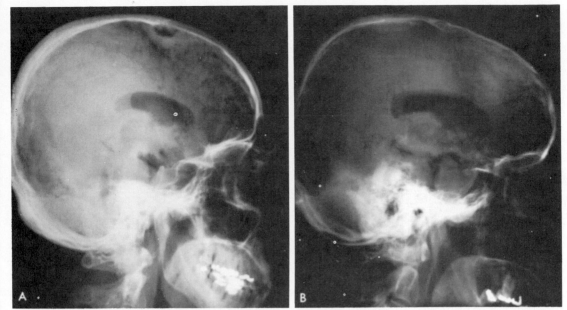

Figure 22–56 Chromophobe adenoma. *A,* Normal lateral skull x-ray. *B,* Ballooned-out sella turcica from a case of chromophobe adenoma. In both cases air has been injected at time of lumbar puncture to outline the ventricular system and the subarachnoid cisterns (pneumoencephalogram). Note the significant suprasellar extent of the chromophobe adenoma which has been outlined by the air. (Courtesy of Dr. Samuel Wolpert, New England Center Hospitals, Neuroradiology.)

NEUROLOGICAL EXAMINATION:

1. *Mental status:* No defects were present as regards orientation, general information, calculations, memory, and delayed recall. No language disturbances were present.

2. *Cranial nerves:*
   a. Visual acuity was reduced bilaterally; however, the patient could read 1 cm. of print at 14 inches.
   b. On visual field examination a complete bitemporal defect was present, cutting the central vision (Fig. 22–57).
   c. Examination of the fundi revealed pallor of the left optic disk, suggesting optic atrophy.
   d. On testing extraocular movements, a diplopia was present in a pattern which suggested bilateral medial rectus involvement (that is, bilateral third nerve damage).

3. *Motor system:* Strength, gait and cerebellar tests were intact.

4. *Reflexes:* Deep tendon and plantar reflexes were intact.

5. *Sensory system:*
   a. Pain and touch were intact.
   b. Rare errors were made in fine movement perception at the toes.
   c. Vibratory sensation was moderately decreased at the toes.

6. *Head:*
   a. Tenderness was present over the left orbit.
   b. No bruits (murmurs) were heard over the head or orbits.

LABORATORY DATA:

1. The patient had a slight degree of anemia with a hemoglobin of 11.2 grams and a hematocrit of 35%. Total white blood cell count was normal at 6500 but the relative proportion of lymphocytes was increased to 51%.

2. Thyroid studies indicated borderline low function with a protein bound iodine of 4.0 microgram/100 ml. (normal = 4–8 microgram/100 ml.) and radioactive iodine of 23.3% in 24 hours (normal = 20–50%).

3. Adrenal function studies indicate subnormal values. *Urinary 17 hydroxysteroids* were 2.1–2.3 mg./24 hr. (normal = 3–10 mg./24 hr.).

4. *Urinary 17 ketosteroids* were 4.0 mg./24 hr. (normal = 10–25 mg./24 hr.), reflecting decreased output of adrenal and gonadal steroids.

5. Despite these low urinary steroid levels, no FSH was detectable in the urine.

Temporal Field   Nasal Field   Nasal Field   Temporal Field

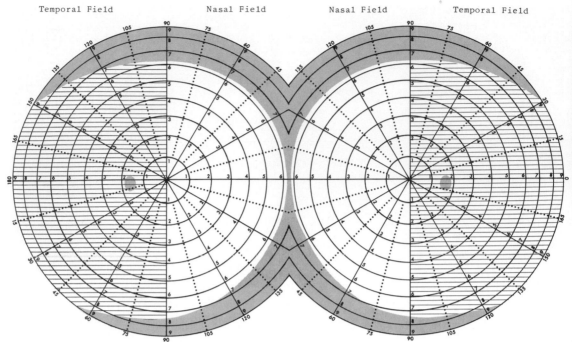

Figure 22–57   Case History 17. Chromophobe adenoma. Visual fields. Perimetric examination of February 5, 1963. A bitemporal hemianopsia is demonstrated. O. S. = left eye; O. D. = right eye.

6. *Skull x-ray* revealed a marked enlargement of the sella turcica (length was 3 cm., depth, 2 cm.). No calcification was present.

7. *Electroencephalogram* was abnormal because of bilateral frontal, 5 cps slow waves suggesting a bilateral frontal dysfunction.

8. *Bilateral carotid arteriograms* demonstrated a marked elevation of the distal segment of the internal carotid arteries with elevation of the origins of both anterior and middle cerebral arteries. These findings were consistent with a large tumor within the pituitary fossa growing superiorly.

9. *Pneumoencephalogram* demonstrated upward and backward midline displacement of the third ventricle. A large lesion of the pituitary fossa was again demonstrated.

10. *Cerebrospinal fluid* protein was elevated to 85 mg./100 ml.

HOSPITAL COURSE:

Replacement therapy with cortisone acetate and thyroid was begun.

On February 25, 1963, a right frontal craniotomy was performed by Dr. Bertram Selverstone. The right frontal lobe was elevated, exposing a cystic gray-purple tumor arising from the sella turcica and elevating

and stretching the optic nerves and chiasm. On aspiration, 15 cc. of dark yellow fluid was obtained. The capsule of the pituitary was then opened and soft tumor tissue was completely removed. Histological sections of the tissue revealed necrotic chromophobe adenoma.

Postoperatively, the patient made an uneventful recovery, except for a partial left-sided third nerve palsy (pupil dilated, responding sluggishly to light with ptosis of the left lid and weakness on upward, downward, and medial movements). This had improved by the time of discharge on March 9, 1963. Moreover, improvement in the visual fields had occurred, and central sectors of the temporal fields were now present, particularly in the right temporal field.

Following hospital discharge, supravoltage radiation therapy was administered (4000 roentgens to the pituitary over 30 days). In addition, the patient continued to receive thyroid cortisone and testosterone replacement therapy. Visual fields, 6 months, 1 year, and 3 years after surgery showed the continued presence of a left temporal field defect and a lesser right temporal field defect (lower quadrant partially spared). Visual acuity remained poor in all quadrants of the left eye.

COMMENT:

It is not unusual for patients in the middle years of life to develop a decrease in visual acuity, so that correction by glasses is required. What was unusual in this case was the continued progression of the deficit in visual acuity, presumably reflecting compression of the optic nerves. Although the patient did not emphasize an acute history of a bitemporal hemianopsia, he did mention that his ability to drive had been limited not only by the decrease in visual acuity, but also by his inability to see the road at the sides of the car, that is, the peripheral temporal fields. Although the patient presented many of the physical stigmata of acromegaly, he claimed that many of these were long-standing; i.e., he had had large hands, feet, jaw, and so forth for all of his adult life. Changes in libido had apparently been present for at least 18 years. Axillary hair had never been present. One may only speculate that perhaps a mixed tumor of the pituitary had been present almost all of the patient's life, only becoming symptomatic once extrasellar (that is suprasellar) extension with compression of optic nerves and chiasm had occurred. The diplopia prior to surgery undoubtedly reflected compression of the third nerves in the wall of the cavernous sinus resulting from lateral enlargement of the pituitary. The more severe but transient third nerve palsy following surgery may have reflected damage to the third nerve in the process of resection of the tumor. The removal of the adenoma of course did not restore the normal pituitary which had been destroyed previously by the growth of the adenoma and the removal of its remnants at the time of surgery. Continuous replacement therapy was therefore required. The deficits in vision which follow compression of the optic nerve and chiasm are often, as in this case, largely nonreversible. Additional progression of the visual defect was of course prevented.

OTHER EXTRINSIC TUMORS INVOLVING THE CEREBRAL HEMISPHERES

Craniopharyngioma. In general, these are relatively uncommon tumors arising usually from various congenital rests. Within this group, by far the most frequent example in both surgical and autopsy series is the craniopharyngioma, which is also referred to as Rathke's pouch tumors, hypophyseal duct tumors, and adamantinomas. They arise from remnants of the hypophyseal duct (the pathway along which the nonneural tissue, which was to give rise to the anterior lobe of pituitary, originated from the primitive oral gut, i.e., the oral pharynx).

A variable histological appearance has been described reflecting the origin of the lesion: squamous epithelium with cystic degeneration; mucoid-filled cysts lined with ciliated columnar epithelium; and epithelial masses forming a sheet of cells resembling the enamel pulp of developing teeth (thus the term adamantinoma). Essentially the importance of these tumors lies in the fact that they present enlarging solid or cystic masses in a suprasellar location. From this anatomical standpoint, they are so situated as to produce compressive destruction of the pituitary and compression of the optic chiasm and hypothalamus with extension upward to block the third ventricle. At times they may also extend as expanding lesions into the subfrontal area.

Usually symptoms begin in childhood or adolescence. However, we have seen occasional patients where symptoms began in adulthood. In approximately 80 per cent of cases, the tumor is calcified. Diagnosis can then be made on the basis of plain skull x-rays demonstrating suprasellar calcification. Treatment involves evacuation of cysts and partial resection of the tumor, followed by radiation. As with pituitary adenomas, appropriate endocrine replacement therapy is necessary.

Epidermoids or Cholesteatoma. Epidermoids or cholesteatomas represent epidermal (stratified squamous epithelium and keratin) inclusions within the bone of the skull or in relation to the dura. Favorite locations are the cerebellar pontine angle, the suprasellar area (where these lesions are essentially indistinguishable from craniopharyngiomas), and the fourth ventricle. They are calcified, well-encapsulated, and noninvasive. Surgical removal is usually possible.

Dermoids and Teratomas. Dermoids and teratomas tend to occur along the midline of the neural axis at points where nonneural tissue grows in close relationship to the nervous system (or closing neural tube), pineal, pituitary, fourth ventricle, and distal end of spinal cord.

Chordomas. Chordomas arise from the remnants of the primitive notochord, the cartilaginous origin of the nucleus pulposus of the intervertebral disks. Originally, this structure extended from the dorsum sellae to the last coccygeal segment. Tumors arising from remnants are usually found at the upper end in relation to the clivus. The clivus is that downward continuation of the dorsum sellae and sphenoid bone in fusion with the occipital bone which is found anterior to the brain stem. Chordomas arising in this location will then produce displacement of the brain stem and cranial nerves, in addition to involvement of structures about the dorsum sellae including the carotid artery and temporal lobe. They are highly locally invasive, often extending into the nasopharynx. A less common location is at the lower end of the neural axis where compression of the cauda equina occurs. The tumors on section resemble soft cartilage. Histological examination reveals large vacuolated cells containing mucin. Treatment consists of limited surgical resection and radiotherapy.

Colloid Cysts. Colloid (paraphysical) cysts of the third ventricle are rare, but may have an importance far out of proportion to their rarity. Because of their location, these benign masses may act as a ball valve in relation to postural changes, producing a sudden obstruction of the ventricular system. The symptoms consist of sudden intermittent attacks of headache, vomiting, dizziness, and weakness. Sudden death is not unusual. It is often uncertain whether the cyst originates from ependyma or represents an old developmental pouch, (the paraphysis) which has failed to disappear.

OTHER EXTRINSIC TUMORS LIMITED TO THE POSTERIOR FOSSA

Schwannoma. The Schwannoma or neurinomas, the most frequent extrinsic tumor of the posterior fossa, has been discussed in relation to the brain stem in Chapter 15, case history #1, p. 337.

Almost all of these tumors, which arise from the Schwann cells of the cranial nerve root, occur at the cerebellar pontine angle, in relation to cranial nerve VIII. Less often, the tumor occurs in relation to the trigeminal or glossopharyngeal roots. Multiple tumors may occur as in Von Recklinghausen's disease (neurofibromatosis). It should of course be pointed out that solitary Schwannoma occur commonly as extramedullary, intradural tumors arising from spinal sensory nerve roots. (Refer to Chapter 8, case #7, p. 174). Similar tumors may also arise in relation to peripheral nerves.

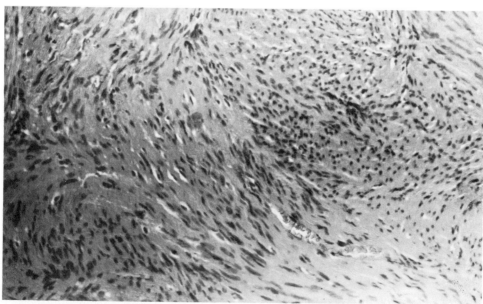

Figure 22–58 Acoustic neuroma or neurofibroma or schwannoma. Microscopic examination of these tumors usually indicates two tissue types: interwoven bundles of spindle-shaped cells with alignment of nuclei in the form of palisades; and looser, somewhat cystic areas. (H & E ×100.) (Courtesy of Dr. David Cowen, Columbia-Presbyterian, Neuropathology.)

Microscopic examination of the acoustic neuroma reveals two types of tissue (Fig. 22–58): type A tissue of Antoni composed of compact interwoven bundles of large spindle-shaped cells, at times showing an alignment of nuclei in the form of palisades, and type B tissue of Antoni composed of a loose structure with cystic areas.

The course and treatment of these benign lesions has been previously discussed. Although the tumor can be easily approached from a neurosurgical standpoint, there is considerable morbidity due to the fact that cranial nerve VII must often be sacrificed in the process of removing the tumor.

SECONDARY TUMORS

Metastatic Tumors. The greatest number of secondary tumors of the central nervous system are spread from a distant site via the blood stream. The majority spread to the cerebral hemisphere or to the cerebellar hemisphere. Metastatic lesions may be solitary or multiple. These secondary metastatic tumors represent a significant percentage of patients seen with intracranial tumors in a general hospital population (24 per cent in the series of Courville).

The most frequent site of primary tumor is the lung (bronchogenic carcinoma) accounting for almost a third of the cases. It has been estimated that 26 per cent of patients with bronchogenic carcinoma will have cerebral metastasis. The second most frequent site of primary lesion is the breast. Several examples have been presented in Chapter 21, Cases 3 and 4, pp. 499 to 501 and 503 to 506. Certain tumors although occurring with a lower overall frequency than carcinoma of the lung and breast have a particularly high frequency of metastatic spread to the brain: (a) malignant melanoma (usually multiple) (Fig. 22–59), (b) hypernephromas (often solitary), and (c) choriocarcinoma.

Solitary metastatic lesions may be subjected to surgical removal. At other times, e.g., in multiple metastasis, radiation therapy or hormonal therapy may be employed, often with a significant reduction in symptoms.

Metastatic spread to the leptomeninges or dura is less common. Carcinomatous meningitis involves multiple metastatic implants on nerve roots and meninges with multiple root symptoms.

Local Invasive Tumors. Direct extension of tumors to involve the brain is less common

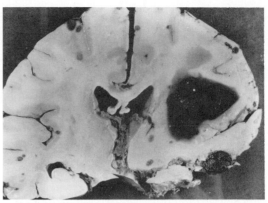

Figure 22–59 Multiple metastatic tumors to cerebral hemisphere from malignant melanoma, with secondary hemorrhage into several of the pigmented lesions. This 40-year-old white female, in 1957, 5 years prior to death, had excision of a melanoma of the left knee with dissection of the left groin. Two years later, in 1959, tumor recurred at the left knee and was excised. In May 1962, excision of a metastatic melanoma to the right breast was performed. Multiple cutaneous nodules then appeared. Despite chemotherapy, the patient developed, in November 1962, right temporal headache, nausea, and vomiting. Two weeks later, the patient suddenly became unresponsive and incontinent. Examination revealed a comatose patient with sluggish pupillary responses, bilateral papilledema, and bilateral extensor plantar responses. Despite removal of a hemorrhagic cystic tumor of the right temporal lobe, coma deepened and a decerebrate state appeared. (Courtesy of Dr. John Hills, New England Center Hospitals, Neuropathology.)

than metastatic disease. Common primary sites are carcinomas originating in the nasopharynx and nasal sinuses. These tumors may erode the base of the skull or spread through the foramina at the base of the skull to involve cranial nerves such as nerves V and VI. Treatment involves local radiation; results are dependent on the capacity for response of the primary lesion.

DEGENERATIVE DISEASES

A variety of degenerative processes may involve the central or peripheral nervous system. In this section we will consider these problems in a general manner. Since many of these diseases have as their major manifestations a progressive impairment of memory (dementia) or a progressive impairment of motor function, they will be considered only briefly in the present section.

A more detailed discussion with illustrative case histories will be found in the chapters dealing with memory and the motor system.

In considering this category of disease, several general rules should be listed:

1. Systems are involved. At times, the primary involvement is of neurons—for example, the large motor neurons in amyotrophic lateral sclerosis. At times, the primary involvement is of axons and myelin sheaths, as in Friedreich's ataxia where posterior columns, spinocerebellar pathways, and pyramidal tracts are primarily involved. At times, the degenerative process is limited to the central nervous system; at times, to the peripheral nervous system. At times, as in certain spinocerebellar degenerations, both peripheral and central nervous systems are involved.

Degenerative diseases have been classified on the basis of the system(s), of neurons, or of fibers primarily involved. In clinical practice, one often encounters cases that correspond to the classic entities. However, one also encounters a significant proportion of cases that combine aspects of several degenerative diseases and do not fit conveniently into a single diagnostic pigeon hole. To a certain extent, then, there is a continuum or spectrum of degenerative diseases.

2. The system involvement is bilateral and, in general, symmetrical.

3. Onset is usually insidious; the course is slowly progressive. In general these are chronic diseases; a few are characterized by a subacute course.

4. A clear understanding of the basic etiology in most degenerative diseases remains uncertain. Some are clearly genetic with well-defined patterns of transmission, e.g., autosomal dominant inheritance of high penetrance in Huntington's chorea. The term genetic presumes that an underlying biochemical defect might well be present. The actual nature of this defect usually remains unknown.

It should be evident to the student that this diagnostic category is actually a catch-all basket in which progressive diseases of unknown etiology have been included. A number of diseases previously included in this degenerative category have been found to have a specific metabolic etiology. Thus cases of combined system disease or posterior lateral sclerosis were once included in this category, until the actual cause was discovered: a nutritional deficiency of vitamin B 12, owing to a lack of the intrinsic factor required for absorption of this compound. Similarly, Wilson's disease, hepatolenticular degeneration, has now a clearly established etiology—the toxic effects resulting from unbound copper in the blood, passing into the brain, liver, and kidneys and binding to tissue proteins because of a deficiency of the normal copper-binding plasma protein, ceruloplasmin. Formerly, this disease was classified within the degenerative category as pseudosclerosis.

Several diseases resulting from exogenous toxins may also mimic degenerative disease of the nervous system. Thus, chronic exposure to manganese may produce a Parkinsonian syndrome because of damage to the basal ganglia. Chronic exposure to mercury (as once was the case in the hatting industry) may produce a progressive cerebellar syndrome with a prominent component of upper extremity tremor. Chronic heavy alcohol intake (with a possible additional nutritional deficiency) may be associated with a severe cerebellar degeneration (anterior superior portions) with a prominent truncal and gait ataxia that may be indistinguishable from a late onset of familial cerebellar degeneration.

A chronic peripheral neuropathy may occur on a familial basis, but might also reflect a chronic vitamin deficiency, (thiamine or B 12 deficiency), chronic exposure to arsenic or lead, or diabetes mellitus.

Thus the student, faced with a patient manifesting a progressive disease syndrome, should, before diagnosing the condition as degenerative disease, rule out the possible treatable causes of that syndrome—nutritional, toxic, and metabolic. (The term degenerative otherwise implies that no specific treatment of the disease is available.)

In addition to the remediable metabolic problems previously cited, it has recently become evident that other possible etiologic factors must be searched for in these degenerative diseases. Thus as we have indicated, a slow virus infection has been recently implicated in several rare chronic progressive diseases formerly classified as degenerative: subacute sclerosing parencephalitis; kuru, and Jakob-Creutzfeldt syndromes.

The development of the postencephalitic

variety of Parkinson's disease in relation to Von Economo's encephalitis has already been noted as a form of a degenerative disease evolving following an infectious process.

5. In general, the pathological picture, at a histological level, is characterized by a loss of neurons or axons in the particular system involved or in related systems. Surviving neurons in the involved system may show various degenerative changes, including lipid inclusions. To a variable degree, some proliferation of glia and glial fibers may be present. Cellular response, however, is never prominent. Grossly, the loss of neurons and axons is often indicated by the loss of bulk of the involved areas—atrophy.

CLINICAL SYNDROMES

Since several levels of the neural axis (and one or more systems) may be involved in these diseases, the best approach is to group these disorders according to the predominant clinical features. In each of these syndromes, a predominant involvement of one or several systems will of course be evident to a large extent. The following classification of clinical syndromes follows, in general, that of Richardson, Torvik, and Adams (Harrison et al., 1966.)

Syndromes in which Dementia Predominates. In these conditions involvement of the cerebral cortex is predominant. Other neurological signs are absent. (These conditions will be discussed in greater detail in Chapter 27.)

DIFFUSE CEREBRAL ATROPHY. The major subdivisions within this category are: Senile Dementia and Presenile Dementia (*Alzheimer's disease*). These are essentially the same disease. The use of differing terminology is arbitrary. The presenile variety begins before age 60 to 65; the senile variety, after this age. Although diffuse cortical involvement is present, the process is most prominent in the frontal, temporal, and hippocampal areas.

CIRCUMSCRIBED CEREBRAL ATROPHY: (PICK'S DISEASE). In this rare condition, the atrophy is relatively restricted to the frontal and temporal poles.

Dementia Combined With Other Neurological Signs. In these conditions, involvement of neurons in the cerebral cortex is combined with involvement of neurons in the basal ganglia or brain stem or retina. This catetory may be subdivided.

VARIETIES OCCURRING PRIMARILY IN THE ADULT. *Huntington's chorea,* in which dementia and psychosis are combined with a disorder of gait and movement (due to involvement of the cerebral cortex and caudate nucleus).

CHILDHOOD AND YOUNG ADULT VARIETIES

The Lipidoses. In lipidosis abnormal accumulations of lipid occur in neurons. The best known example is probably *Tay-Sachs disease* or *infantile amaurotic familial idiocy,* in which dementia is combined with blindness, seizures, and a spastic quadriparesis.

The Leukodystrophies. In these conditions a diffuse breakdown of myelin into abnormal lipid products occurs, that is, products not normally found in the usual breakdown of myelin in trauma or infarcts. Dementia (owing to involvement of cerebral white matter—association, projection, and commissural fibers) is combined with a spastic quadriparesis and variable cerebellar findings. Obviously, both the lipidosis and the leukodystrophies represent, in a sense, biochemical disorders involving primarily the nervous system, rather than degenerative diseases of unknown cause. Similarly a progressive impairment of psychomotor function occurs in the aminoacidurias (e.g., phenylketonuria), but these represent metabolic disorders of known and treatable etiology.

Progressive Development of Disturbances of Posture and of Movement (Extrapyramidal Disorders). The major subdivisions within this category are:

PARKINSON'S DISEASE (PARALYSIS AGITANS). This is a relatively common disorder characterized by rigidity, tremor, and akinesia (a slowness or lack of movement).

DYSTONIA MUSCULORUM DEFORMANS. This is a relatively uncommon disorder characterized by bizarre posture of the trunk and limbs.

The pathology in both cases involves the basal ganglia or those structures connected to the basal ganglia, e.g., substantia nigra.

The biochemical nature of the pathology in Parkinson's disease has now been elaborated in sufficient degree, that this disease may soon be shifted into the category of known metabolic disturbance. (These syndromes will be discussed in greater detail in Chapter 24.)

Progressive Ataxia (Unsteadiness of Trunk, Gait, or Movement). Within this category, characterized by unsteadiness of trunk, gait, and movements, three major subdivisions may be distinguished (with considerable overlap).

PARENCHYMATOUS CEREBELLAR DEGENERATION. The atrophic process involves mainly the cerebellar cortex: primarily the Purkinje cells of the anterior superior portions. The predominant symptom, an ataxia of gait with involvement of the lower extremities but little involvement of the upper extremities, occurs primarily in middle-aged or older adults. (Refer to Chapter 25 for a more detailed discussion.)

OLIVOPONTOCEREBELLAR DEGENERATION. In this condition in which there is combined degeneration of the cerebellum, pontine nuclei, and olivary nuclei the cerebellar involvement and the cerebellar symptomatology are more diffuse. The trunk, extremities, speech and eye movements are affected. Adolescents and adults are primarily affected.

PREDOMINANT SPINAL CORD INVOLVEMENT (FRIEDREICH'S ATAXIA). In this disease there is degeneration of the posterior columns and the spinocerebellar and corticospinal pathways and at times the peripheral nerves. Those primarily affected are children and adolescents. The prominent symptoms are ataxia of gait, absent deep tendon reflexes, and loss of position and vibration sensation. Posterior column involvement is always more prominent than lateral column involvement. (This problem has been illustrated in Chapter 8).

Slowly Developing Weakness and Spasticity (Hereditary Spastic Paraplegia). This disease, which affects children and adolescents, may be related to Friedreich's ataxia. The lateral column involvement, however, is most prominent.

Syndromes With Slowly Developing Muscular Weakness and Muscle Atrophy Due to Motor Neuron Involvement, But Without Sensory Changes. Within this category, two diseases may be cited:

a. The various forms of motor system disease affecting the adult in middle age or later years: (*amyotrophic lateral sclerosis*) progressive muscular atrophy, progressive bulbar palsy, and primary lateral sclerosis.

b. Infantile muscular atrophy (*Werdnig-Hoffmann disease*). These problems have been illustrated and discussed in Chapter 8, Diseases Affecting the Spinal Cord.

Progressive Muscular Weakness And Muscle Atrophy Due to Disease of Peripheral Nerve, but with Less Marked Sensory Involvement. The major example is *peroneal muscular atrophy (Charcot-Marie-Tooth disease).* This is a not uncommon syndrome occurring in adolescent or young adult males. The muscles of the legs and the lower one-third of the thighs are primarily affected. The sensory involvement may suggest posterior column involvement. There may be considerable overlap with the spinocerebellar degenerations.

A less common variety with more pronounced sensory findings is *hypertrophic interstitial neuritis (Dejerine-Sottas disease),* which occurs in childhood. The name is derived from the characteristic thickening of the nerves.

Progressive Sensory Peripheral Neuropathy. These are relatively uncommon. The major example is the hereditary sensory neuropathy described by Denny-Brown with pathology in the posterior root ganglion. The syndrome is characterized by a dissociated sensory loss. Pain and temperature sensation are markedly impaired compared to position, vibration, and touch.

Progressive Muscle Weakness and Atrophy Due to Muscle Disease. The muscular dystrophies (see Chapter 6).

Progressive Loss of Vision. The major examples are: *hereditary optic atrophy of Leber* resulting from degeneration of the retinal ganglion cells and *pigmentary degeneration of the retina (retinitis pigmentosa)* owing to degeneration of rods and cones with displacement of cells from the pigment epithelium to the more superficial layers of the retina.

NUTRITIONAL, TOXIC, AND METABOLIC DISEASES

These are all, in a sense, diseases involving the metabolic activities of the brain. Nutritional deficiencies may remove certain vitamins required as coenzymes in vital metabolic energy transformations. Particular toxins may have their effects by interfering with specific enzymatic processes. We can consider most of these problems only briefly. The student should refer to the standard textbooks of clinical medicine and clinical biochemistry for a more thorough presentation.

In beginning the study of these diseases we should first consider several general principles:

1. The central and peripheral nervous systems have only a limited number of pathological responses. Different disease states may produce a similar clinical and patho-

logical picture. Thus a distal symmetrical peripheral neuropathy may reflect several nutritional deficiencies (thiamine, B12, pyridoxine), or diabetes mellitus, or chronic degenerative disease, or the toxic effects of arsenic. Other examples already have been cited in relation to degenerative disease.

2. These diseases may then mimic degenerative or familial diseases of the nervous system. As we have already indicated, several diseases previously considered to be of unknown degenerative cause have now been shown to have a specific metabolic or nutritional deficiency, e.g., combined systems disease of vitamin B12 deficiency and hepatolenticular degeneration.

3. The metabolic disturbance is usually not limited to the nervous system but involves many systems of the body. In some instances the nervous system appears to be predominantly involved. In several rare problems (the lipidoses and the leukodystrophies), the metabolic disturbance is relatively limited to the nervous system.

4. Not all levels of the neural axis are equally affected. In specific metabolic disturbances a selective vulnerability of particular segments is often evident. This selective vulnerability is often based on selective enzymatic or specific metabolic requirements of the affected areas. Thus the neocortex and hippocampus are the first areas affected by anoxia or hypoglycemia.

5. These diseases may produce physiological function and pathological changes at one or several levels of the neural axis: peripheral nerve, spinal cord, diencephalon, or cerebrum. In a given patient one level of involvement may predominate although in another patient with the same deficiency a different level of involvement may be most prominent. Although we have spoken in terms of anatomical levels, it is perhaps more correct to speak in terms of systems. Since these diseases often are system diseases, the involvement is usually symmetrical.

6. These diseases have an importance far out of proportion to their actual frequency in a modern industrialized society. Specific treatment will arrest the progress of the disease and disordered function will often be corrected. However, we should keep in mind that any disordered metabolic function, if it persists and progresses, will usually result in structural changes which will be visible at a gross or microscopic level (degeneration and loss of neurons, degeneration of myelin and axons). Structural changes and their associated clinical changes will, moreover, usually be irreversible (particularly in the central nervous system).

7. At times, in nutritional problems, a specific deficiency has not been established but a general relationship to nutritional deficiency has emerged (e.g., cerebellar degeneration and central pontine myelinolysis).

NUTRITIONAL DEFICIENCY DISEASE SYNDROMES

The following classification has been derived from a similar classification by Victor (1965). The classification is based on predominant anatomical levels or the systems involved.

SYNDROMES WITH CEREBRAL MANIFESTATIONS

Pellagra. Pellagra results from a deficiency of nicotinic acid. Daily requirements are 10 to 30 mgm. per day but tryptophan in the diet may serve as a precursor of nicotinic acid. Cerebral nicotinic acid derivatives are found in the form of nicotinamide adenine dinucleotides (NAD, NADP), which are of crucial importance in the energy yielding oxidative phosphorylations of the tricarboxylic acid cycle. The clinical syndrome may be considered as a triad consisting of mental changes, dermatitis, and diarrhea.

The earliest symptoms are usually related to the disturbance in cerebral function: depression, irrational fears, agitation, hallucinations, disorientation, and delirium. The characteristic histological change is that of central chromatolysis in large pyramidal cells of the cerebral cortex, particularly the motor cortex. Motor neurons in the brain stem and spinal cord horn will also demonstrate these same changes. The central chromatolysis may well reflect metabolic injury to axons in the peripheral nerve or spinal cord.

The dermatological manifestations occur on those skin surfaces exposed to sunlight (hands, face, neck). Characteristically, the mouth, lips, and tongue are also involved.

The neurological, dermatological, and gastrointestinal effects of the deficiency are rapidly reversed by the administration of nicotinic acid or nicotinamide.

Pyridoxine (Vitamin B6) Deficiency in Infants. Pyridoxine deficiency may involve the nervous system at several levels. In the adult the deficiency occurs predominantly in patients receiving the antituberculous agent, isoniazide (INH, isonicotinic hydrazide), an antagonist of pyridoxine. The result is a peripheral neuropathy. In infants, however, the effects relate predominantly to alterations in the excitability of the hippocampus and neocortex, with the production of convulsions. That alterations in threshold for convulsions might occur would not be unexpected in view of the known metabolic activities of pyridoxal phosphate as a coenzyme. Thus the decarboxylation of glutamic acid to gamma aminobutyric acid (Gaba, an inhibitor of excitatory synapses) requires the presence of the coenzyme, pyridoxal phosphate. Pyridoxal phosphate also is the coenzyme required for the decarboxylation which yields serotonin from 5-hydroxytryptophane. Pyridoxal phosphate also functions in the vital transamination reaction which yields aspartate and alpha ketoglutarate from glutamic acid and oxaloacetate.

Pyridoxine deficiency is not common as a cause of convulsions in infants. However, a group of otherwise normal infants who were fed a manufactured baby food deficient in pyridoxine did develop severe convulsions and myoclonic seizures with rapid improvement on administration of this vitamin. In general, a normal infant or child has sufficient reserves of pyridoxine to continue on a pyridoxine-deficient diet for eight weeks before the development of convulsions. However, a small group of newborn infants have been found to have need for pyridoxine far beyond the normal daily requirements (15 mgm., compared to normal requirements of 1.5 mgm.). These infants (referred to as pyridoxine-dependent) develop intractable seizures: generalized convulsions and myoclonic jerks which are rapidly controlled by administration of the agent.

Progressive Dementia of Vitamin B12 Deficiency. Vitamin B12 (Cobalamin) deficiency in almost all cases reflects a failure to absorb this vitamin because of a deficiency of the intrinsic factor secreted by the gastric mucosa. A similar failure may occur as a result of gastrectomy. In some cases, the deficiency is a result of a malabsorption syndrome.

Vitamin B12 is utilized as a coenzyme in the formation of methionine and of the nucleotide, thymidine. The resultant disordered synthesis of deoxyribonucleic acid (DNA) leads to a failure of normal maturation of cells. From a clinical standpoint, this is manifested as the megaloblastic anemia of pernicious anemia. However, since the neurological manifestations of Vitamin B12 deficiency are not always present in pernicious anemia and since these neurological manifestations may exist when the anemia is only of minor or minimal degree, the specific enzymatic role of Vitamin B12 in the nervous system remains unclear. For example, folic acid will correct the megaloblastic anemia by restoring the normal synthesis of DNA in the erythropoietic system, yet folic acid is unable to prevent the development of neurological symptoms.

The neurological symptoms of Vitamin B12 deficiency relate primarily to the involvement of the posterior and lateral columns of the spinal cord. These symptoms occur in 30 to 70 per cent of patients with pernicious anemia. In addition, however, a significant percentage of patients also demonstrate changes in cerebral function (which are unrelated to the degree of anemia). In some cases, these cerebral symptoms are minor, consisting of instability, lassitude, and mild depression. In other cases (formerly, perhaps as many as 16 per cent of cases of pernicious anemia), the symptoms are severe, consisting of a severe psychosis or a significant degree of dementia. At times, the cerebral symptoms may be far out of proportion to the degree of spinal cord involvement. The neuropathological correlate of these changes in mental function is found in the cerebral white matter where destruction of myelin and axons has occurred. This is the same pathological change which will be noted in the posterior and lateral columns of spinal cord. The progression of symptoms can be prevented by parenteral administration of Vitamin B12.

Primary Degeneration of the Corpus Callosum: Marchiafava-Bignami Disease. This is a rare disease involving demyelination and necrosis of axons in the central portions of the corpus callosum and the anterior commissure. Most of these cases have occurred in older Italian males who have consumed large amounts of crude Italian red wine. A toxic or nutritional etiology was suspected but never proven. The symptoms and signs consist of convulsions, dementia, psychosis, and multifocal cortical findings.

The diagnosis is usually only established at the time of postmortem.

NUTRITIONAL DEFICIENCY DISEASES AFFECTING THE DIENCEPHALON AND BRAIN STEM

Wernicke-Korsakoff Encephalopathy. Wernicke, in 1881, described a syndrome which is of relatively acute onset, occurs in alcoholics or nutritionally deficient patients, and consists of a triad: mental disturbance (confusion and drowsiness), paralysis of eye movements, and ataxia of gait. The basic cause of the syndrome is a deficiency of thiamine. Since a deficiency of thiamine and of the other B complex vitamins also results in a peripheral neuropathy, symptoms relevant to degeneration of peripheral nerves will often be present as an associated finding.

Thiamine pyrophosphate functions as a coenzyme (cocarboxylase) in the decarboxylation of pyruvic acid. The step is the initial reaction in the energy producing tricarboxylic acid cycle. Thiamine also participates in the oxidative decarboxylation of alpha ketoglutaric acid at a later point in this cycle. In addition, thiamine pyrophosphate functions in the transketolase reaction which is involved in the pentose phosphate pathway (hexosemonophosphate shunt) for the breakdown of glucose, particularly for the conversion of ribose-5 phosphate to sedoheptulose-7 phosphate.

The pathological findings involve the grey matter surrounding the third ventricle (anterior and medial thalamus and hypothalamus), the aqueduct (the periaqueductal gray matter and third nerve nuclei), and the fourth ventricle (nucleus of cranial nerve VI, dorsal motor nuclei, and vestibular nuclei). To a degree, pathological changes also occur in the anterior superior portion of the midline cerebellum. The basic pathology consists of a necrosis of neural parenchyma and a prominence of blood vessels due to a proliferation of adventitial and endothelial cells. Petechial hemorrhages often occur about these vessels. The lesions in general are usually most prominent in the mammillary bodies and the medial thalamic areas.

As regards the correlation of clinical symptoms with pathological lesions, the ophthalmoplegia which is predominantly a bilateral involvement of cranial nerve VI (i.e., lateral rectus) clears rapidly on parenteral administration of thiamine.

Since pathological changes in the extraocular nuclei are often minimal, it has been postulated that the extraocular palsies are a reflection of a biochemical disturbance that has not yet progressed to permanent structural damage. The drowsiness, which also clears on treatment, may reflect damage to the periaqueductal gray matter. The ataxia which involves gait and trunk usually resolves to a significant degree. This symptom undoubtedly reflects the involvement of the anterior superior portion of the cerebellum. The symptom and the pathology in this location are noted to a more severe degree in the "alcoholic" cerebellar degeneration.

As the drowsiness clears with treatment, it will often be evident that a severe deficit in recent memory is present. This will be the case particularly if the patient has delayed seeking medical diagnosis and treatment. The patient will be unable to learn new material although he will have little difficulty recalling events of the distant past. The patient often provides imaginary answers for questions concerning the recent past and for questions involving material he has been requested to learn by the examiner (*confabulation*).

The deficits in memory for recent events may be transient, clearing with continued treatment, or may be more persistent. The persistence of these disorders of recent memory and the state of confusion as a chronic phenomenon is referred to as *Korsakoff's psychosis.* In these cases, pathological examination of the brain reveals persistent lesions in the dorsomedial and anterior nuclei of the thalamus. In contrast, cases coming eventually to autopsy after a history of Wernicke's encephalopathy but without the persistent memory deficits have not shown pathological changes in these thalamic nuclei (although lesions have been present in hypothalamic structures).

This problem will be discussed in greater detail and illustrated in the section on memory and memory disturbances (Chapter 27).

Central Pontine Myelinolysis. This is a rare disease in which a diagnosis is usually established only at the time of autopsy. The basic pathology involves an area of demyelination with a relative preservation of axis cylinders and neurons in the central area of basilar and adjacent tegmental portions of pons. Most cases have occurred in chronic alcoholics; in a few cases, severe nutritional deprivation or malabsorption was present without the alcoholism.

NUTRITIONAL DEFICIENCY DISEASES AFFECTING THE CEREBELLUM

"Alcoholic" Cerebellar Degeneration. This problem has already been mentioned in relation to Wernicke's encephalopathy in thiamine deficiency. The basic pathological change consists of an atrophy of cerebellar cortex with a relative selective loss of Purkinje's cells in the anterior superior portions of the cerebellar vermis. The symptoms relate primarily to an ataxia of gait. There is little involvement of the upper extremities and nystagmus is usually not present. Although most cases have occurred in chronic alcoholics, rare cases have been reported in nonalcoholics with severe nutritional problems due to absorption deficits. The specific nutritional deficiency is not clear. In general, progression of symptoms in the chronic alcoholic has ceased when alcohol was discontinued.

NUTRITIONAL DEFICIENCY DISEASES AFFECTING THE SPINAL CORD

Subacute Combined System Disease: Vitamin B12 Deficiency. This is the most common of the nutritional myelopathies. The metabolic aspects of Vitamin B12 deficiency have been previously discussed under the cerebral manifestations. As we have already indicated, the symptoms and signs of spinal cord involvement occur in a high percentage of patients with pernicious anemia.

It cannot be emphasized enough that the spinal cord pathology may be present and progressive at a time when the degree of anemia is minimal. The basic pathological change is a loss of myelin and a degeneration of axons. The loss may be so profound that a spongy appearance results. In such cases a significant gliosis is generally present.

Although the myelopathy is referred to as combined system disease or posterior lateral sclerosis, it is not entirely in the strict sense a system disease. Thus the demyelination is often somewhat patchy. Moreover, within the lateral columns the process is often not limited to the lateral cortical spinal tract but involves adjacent tracts as well. The pathological changes usually begin in the posterior columns.

The initial clinical manifestations then usually consist of bilateral paresthesias involving the toes and fingers. A sensory type ataxia develops after a variable interval. Examination at this point will usually reveal an absence of vibration and position sensation in the lower extremities and, to a lesser degree, in the fingers. A positive Romberg test will be present. Deep tendon reflexes are usually absent, but plantar responses are often extensor. The absence of deep tendon reflexes probably indicates the early involvement of large diameter IA fibers involved in the monosynaptic stretch reflex as these fibers pass from the posterior root through the posterior horn to their synapse with the anterior horn cell. (The fibers of the posterior column are of course of a similar diameter and both are presumably affected by the same metabolic disturbance early in the disease.)

The bilateral extensor plantar responses reflect early involvement of lateral funiculi; later, weakness of the legs will develop. Spasticity may develop but a severe degree is unusual in untreated cases. To a minor extent, in addition to the marked changes in sensation as regards position and vibration, a distal decrease in pain and temperature sensation may also be noted, probably reflecting a degree of peripheral neuropathy.

The diagnosis can be made on the basis of the characteristic neurological picture, plus or minus the peripheral blood findings of a macrocytic anemia, plus or minus the bone marrow findings of a megaloblastic type of anemia. Free acid is generally absent on gastric analysis. Moreover, the Schilling test to measure absorption of orally administered radioactive B12 demonstrates a low absorption (as reflected subsequently in a low urinary excretion). Normal values for urinary excretion are 7 to 22 per cent of the orally administered dose. The serum level of Vitamin B12 may also be measured and will be found to be low.

Other diseases which may present a clinical syndrome of posterior and lateral column involvement must be differentiated: (a) Friedreich's ataxia, (b) cervical spondylosis with midline compression by osteophytes on the ruptured disk, and (c) multiple sclerosis.

Adequate treatment to prevent progression of the disease requires the life-long parenteral administration of Vitamin B12. In mild cases, an almost complete remission of symptoms will occur; in more severe cases, the improvement will be less marked.

An illustrative case history has been presented in Chapter 8 on the spinal cord and should be reviewed at this time (p. 195).

Other Nutritional Myelopathies are not common but may occur in pellagra. In addition, a syndrome of spastic paraplegia, of uncertain etiology, has been reported from Jamaica.

NUTRITIONAL DEFICIENCY DISEASES AFFECTING THE PERIPHERAL NERVES

Thiamine or Multiple B Vitamin Deficiencies. A peripheral neuropathy of variable degree is commonly encountered in patients on nutritionally inadequate diets, e.g., chronic alcoholics. The neuropathy is in general a distal symmetrical polyneuropathy of mixed sensory motor type. Often the neuropathy is mild, predominantly sensory, involving a loss of vibration sense at the toes, a minor decrease in pain sensation and an absence of Achilles and quadriceps deep tendon reflexes. At times the full-blown peripheral neuropathy of "neuritic beri-beri" may be present. Although thiamine deficiency will produce a distal peripheral neuropathy, many patients, such as chronic alcoholics, have been on diets which are deficient in many of the B complex vitamins, e.g., niacin, pyridoxine, pantothenic acid, and cobalamin (B12) each of which by itself may under experimental conditions produce a peripheral neuropathy. Diets high in carbohydrates may increase the requirements for thiamine and may precipitate symptoms.

From a clinical standpoint, severe cases present with distal and symmetrical sensory symptoms of tingling, paresthesias, numbness, sensory loss, and dysesthesias. (The feet are often described as burning and painful to the touch.) A distal weakness is usually present in the lower extremities with the development of drop foot. The gait reflects not only the foot drop but also the severe loss of proprioception due to an absence of sensory input with a resultant sensory ataxia. Deep tendon reflexes and plantar response are usually absent. As the disease progresses, the level of sensory and motor involvement gradually ascends. The upper border of involvement is usually not sharp but rather fading.

Pathologically, both axons and myelin are destroyed. The involvement is most severe distally. The level of myelin involvement is usually greater and at a higher proximal extent than the involvement of the axons. In addition to the Wallerian degeneration described in Chapter 3, a segmental loss of myelin (Gombault's type) may be noted in areas where axons are still intact. Secondary changes of central chromatolysis may be noted in the motor neurons of the anterior horn.

The treatment consists of the oral or parenteral administration of the multiple B vitamins to include a thiamine dosage of at least 10 mg. per day. In very severe cases where Wernicke's encephalopathy, or the cardiac involvement of beri-beri is also present, the parenteral administration of 20 to 30 mg. of thiamine three times a day has been recommended. The usual human requirement of thiamine is 0.4 mg. per 1000 calories.

When one considers the pathological change in the peripheral nerve, it is not surprising that there is often (particularly in severe cases) only a slow response to treatment. Peripheral nerve regenerates at a rate of 1 to 2 mm. per day. Severe Wallerian degeneration involving the sciatic nerve would then require a regeneration period of many months. In such cases some degree of weakness of the lower extremities and sensory symptoms may be expected a year after onset of treatment. Deep tendon reflexes may still be absent several years after the episode.

Pyridoxine Deficiency. As previously indicated the patients receiving INH (isoniazid), a pyridoxine antagonist for treatment of tuberculosis, may develop a distal, symmetrical, predominantly sensory, peripheral neuropathy. This may be prevented by the concurrent administration of pyridoxine.

An outline of the Differential Diagnosis of Peripheral Neuropathies is presented in Table 22–3.

NUTRITIONAL DEFICIENCY DISEASES AFFECTING THE OPTIC NERVE

Nutritional or Tobacco Amblyopia Syndrome of Bilateral Retrobulbar Neuropathy. In these patients there is a bilateral degeneration of the myelinated fibers of the optic nerve involving primarily the fibers coursing from the macula to the optic disk (the papillomacular bundle). Since the

Table 22–3   Classification of Peripheral Neuropathies**

I. *Acute symmetrical ascending polyneuropathy (predominantly motor)* but with variable sensory involvement.
   A. Acute polyneuritis
     *1. Idiopathic of Guillain-Barré syndrome
     2. Complicating infectious mononucleosis
     3. Complicating hepatitis
     4. Rarely complicating LE or periarteritis
   B. Diphtheritic polyneuropathy (Diphtheria exotoxin)
   C. Porphyric polyneuropathy (as manifestation of acute intermittent porphyria—abdominal pain, confusion, and convulsion)
   D. Toxic: Triorthocresyl phosphate
II. Subacute distal symmetrical polyneuropathy
   A. Sensory motor
     *1. Beri Beri, of thiamine deficiency or multiple B vitamin deficiency of alcoholism
     2. Arsenical poisoning
     3. Furadantin therapy
     4. Isoniazid therapy (pyridoxin deficiency)
   B. Predominantly motor
     1. Lead poisoning
     2. Idiopathic
   C. Predominantly sensory:
     *1. Diabetic distal polyneuropathy
     2. B12 deficiency
III. Chronic sensory motor polyneuropathies
   A. Nonfamilial sensory (motor)
     *1. Carcinoma and myeloma (remote complication of malignancy)
     2. Uremia
     3. Amyloidosis
     4. Idiopathic chronic progressive or recurrent
   B. Nonfamilial predominantly sensory
     *1. Diabetes mellitus
     2. Rheumatoid arthritis
     3. Sensory type carcinomatous neuropathy (Denny-Brown's syndrome)
   C. Familial
     1. Peroneal muscular atrophy (Charcot-Marie-Tooth-Hoffmann syndrome)—distal motor
     2. Progressive hypertrophic interstitial (Déjérine-Sottas syndrome) predominantly sensory at onset
     3. Refsum's Disease (sensorimotor and deafness and retinitis pigmentosa)
     4. Peripheral neuropathy and spinocerebellar degeneration
     5. Hereditary sensory neuropathy (Denny-Brown syndrome—degeneration of posterior root ganglion with loss of pain and temperature sensation)

macula is concerned with acute central vision, there is a decrease in visual acuity and the presence of central or cecocentral scotoma on examination. In far advanced cases, progression to the pale optic disk of optic atrophy may occur.

The syndrome may occur in isolation but is more often noted in association with a peripheral neuropathy or in association with Wernicke's syndrome. The specific nutritional deficiency is unknown. Thiamine, riboflavin, or Vitamin B12 may be involved. In this country the syndrome has been described primarily in alcoholics, but a similar syndrome occurred in prisoner of war camps in the Far East during World War II.

The treatment consists of administration of therapeutic dosage of multiple vitamins.

Strachan's Syndrome. This syndrome is seen less commonly among nutritionally deficient populations than many of the preceding entities. This syndrome is composed of a sensory peripheral neuropathy (apparently due to the involvement of the dorsal root ganglion), retrobulbar neuritis (due to involvement of the papillomacular bundle), and deafness and vertigo (due to the involvement of cranial nerve VIII). The specific deficiency involved is uncertain.

TOXIC DISEASES

METALLIC POISONS

Lead. Lead poisoning may result in the adult from industrial exposure, from accidental exposure to the fumes of burning batteries containing lead, or from the ingestion of whiskey which has been illicitly distilled in stills containing lead condensers and connecting pipes. In the child, lead poison-

Table 22–3   Classification of Peripheral Neuropathies** (Continued)

IV. Mononeuropathy
- A. Etiological Classification
  - 1. Traumatic section
  - 2. Chemical injury (e.g., penicillin injection into peripheral nerve)
  - *3. Compression or traction (see below for details)
  - *4. Infection (Herpes Zoster)
  - 5. Vascular occlusion: sciatic most common (as in painful proximal mononeuropathy of diabetes mellitus)
  - 6. Neoplastic local neuroma or compression by adjacent tumor tissue
- B. Anatomical classification of common compression or traction type injuries
  - 1. Radial (Saturday night) humerus ⎫ (idiopathic)
  - * 2. Median (carpal tunnel) often bilateral ⎬ (myxedema)
  - * 3. Ulnar (olecranon groove) ⎭ (acromegaly)
  - * 4. Brachial plexus (thoracic outlet)
  - 5. Upper brachial plexus (C5, C6) Erb-Duchenne syndrome—birth injury
  - 6. Lower brachial plexus (C7-T1) Déjérine Klumpe syndrome—birth injury
  - 7. Long thoracic (serratus anterior weakness)
  - * 8. Lateral femoral cutaneous (meralgia paresthetica)
  - 9. Obturator (obstetric trauma, dislocation of hip, hernia)
  - *10. Common peroneal (leg crossing pressure of nerve over head of fibula)
  - 11. Tibial nerve
  - 12. Sciatic (pelvis fractures)
  - *13. Facial (CN VII—Bell's palsy—fallopian canal)
V. Mononeuropathy multiplex
- A. Vasculitis (periarteritis nodosa)
- †B. Infection (leprosy)
- C. Tumor
  - 1. Multiple neurofibromatosis
  - 2. Carcinomatosis or lymphomatosis
- D. Sarcoidosis
- E. Familial mononeuropathy multiplex (often precipitated by pregnancy, trauma, fever)

---

*Frequent—most common.
†Frequent—when considered on a worldwide basis.
**Modified from Adams, R. D., and Perlo, V. P.: *In* Harrison, T. R.: Principles of Internal Medicine. New York, McGraw-Hill, 5th Edition, 1966, p. 1122.)

ing usually results from the ingestion of paints containing lead. Layers of old paint containing lead are often found on the walls of older houses and tenements in the lower socioeconomic sections of the inner city. Moreover, the children of economically disadvantaged groups are more likely to be unattended and thus more subject to pica (the ingestion of inorganic materials).

The specific action of lead on the brain is not clear. Apparently interference with various intracellular enzymes occurs, with damage to capillary endothelium and neurons. In the child, the result is an acute encephalopathy with massive cerebral edema, coma, and convulsions. Associated symptoms of constipation, abdominal pains, and anemia reflect the effects of lead on the gastrointestinal and hematopoietic systems. The morbidity and mortality from lead encephalopathy are high despite acute treatment designed to reduce brain edema (steroids, intravenous urea, and surgical decompression) and despite later treatment designed to mobilize lead from soft tissues for excretion (the chelating agent, Calcium Disodium Versenate). Most of those surviving the acute encephalopathy will manifest a significant degree of mental retardation.

The encephalopathy of lead poisoning must be differentiated from the other causes of acute toxic encephalopathy of infancy and childhood (acute cerebral edema of childhood). This latter syndrome occurs as a complication of acute febrile illness, such as viral infections of the upper respiratory or gastrointestinal tract. The specific etiology is uncertain. Meningitis and encephalitis must also be differentiated. Diagnosis of lead poisoning is based on the level of lead in the blood and urine, the presence of an increased amount of coproporphyrin in the urine, the presence of basophilic stippling of red blood cells, and the presence of lead lines at the epiphyses in x-rays of the extremities in children.

In the adult, chronic lead poisoning is much more likely to result in a peripheral neuropathy than in central nervous system involvement. The peripheral neuropathy is predominantly motor, often involving the extensors of the hand, producing a characteristic wristdrop. Calcium Disodium Versenate is employed in treatment.

Arsenic. Arsenicals are employed (as arsenates) in insecticides and were formerly used in the organic form in the treatment of syphilis. Arsenic binds to sulfhydryl group in proteins and thus interferes with a number of enzyme systems. Either the central or peripheral nervous system may be involved. An acute hemorrhagic encephalopathy manifested by headache, confusion, convulsions, drowsiness, and coma may occur in cases of severe acute poisoning. More chronic cases or less severe acute exposures are more likely to result in a distal symmetrical polyneuropathy. This is a mixed sensory-motor neuropathy with distal paresthesias and dysesthesias as prominent symptoms. Associated symptoms reflect involvement of skin, mucosa, and the gastrointestinal tract.

Diagnosis is based on determination of arsenic levels in the hair and urine.

Treatment employs the agent BAL (British anti-lewisite; 2, 3 dimercapto-1-propanol) which combines with metallic ions such as arsenic and mercury. The BAL has such a strong affinity for these metallic ions, that these metals are removed from their binding to tissue sulfhydryl groups.

Mercury. *Acute* poisoning with mercury usually occurs in relation to the ingestion of soluble salt such as mercuric chloride. The symptoms reflect the predominant involvement of the gastrointestinal tract, the mucus membranes, and the renal tubules.

Chronic mercury poisoning from metallic mercury vapor does result in neurological symptoms. Exposure to mercury in industrial processes was common in the jewelry and hatting industries prior to the introduction of alternate manufacturing processes during the 1930's. The expression "mad as a hatter" suggests the changes in personality and mood which were often noted among hatters, presumably due to the cerebral effects of the agent. Much more prominent and equally frequent as a symptom was the occurrence

of the "hatter shakes"—a mixed type of tremor, present in the outstretched hands and present on movement and intention. The appearance of the tremor may be correlated with the occurrence of neuronal loss in the cerebellar cortex particularly involving the granule cells. In some cases alterations in basal ganglia and anterior horn cells have also been reported.

Recent attention has focused on the high levels of mercury (as methylmercury) in marine fish such as tuna and swordfish ingested by man. It has been suggested that such high levels may reflect the concentration by these fish of mercury dumped into the environment through industrial and agricultural pollution (refer to discussion of Hammond, 1971).

Treatment of mercury poisoning involves removing the patient from the offending environment and using BAL, as previously discussed.

Copper. Exogenous copper poisoning is uncommon. Endogenous copper poisoning does occur in Wilson's disease (hepatolenticular degeneration) and is discussed in relation to diseases of the basal ganglia (Chapter 24).

Manganese. A Parkinsonian syndrome has been noted in manganese miners. These patients demonstrate a loss of neurons in the substantia nigra. (Additional discussion of Parkinson's disease will be found in Chapter 24.)

PHARMACOLOGICAL AGENTS

A variety of pharmacological agents have effects on the central nervous system. The use and abuse of some of these agents has been known for centuries (e.g., alcohol and opiates). Modern technology has made possible the development of many additional agents with neuropharmacological action: anesthetics, sedatives, anticonvulsants, analgesics, tranquilizers, and antidepressants. This same modern technology has produced alterations in our culture and society. There has been a shift from the relatively nonstressful extended family unit of rural society to the small nuclear family living in the more stressful urban and suburban environment. With stress and the greater availability of the neuropharmacological agents has come increasing use and abuse of these agents to alter central nervous system function.

A detailed account of these agents is beyond the scope of this textbook; the reader is referred to the standard textbooks of pharmacology.

We will, however, delineate certain of the neurological syndromes which may complicate the use of these agents. In some cases these syndromes represent the effects of excessive amounts of the particular agent. In some instances, a selective sensitivity of the individual to otherwise therapeutic dose level has occurred due to abnormalities in enzymatic detoxification processes (e.g., defects in parahydroxylation of diphenylhydantoin and phenobarbital).

Alcohol. Several neurological syndromes complicate the use of alcohol.

Acute intoxication in mild cases produces frontal-lobe and cerebellar dysfunction. The latter is manifested by the characteristic ataxia of gait, trunk, and limbs: movements lack coordination and speech is slurred. In severe intoxication, coma will occur (refer to Chapter 26 for discussion of coma).

Various syndromes relevant to *nutritional deficiency* have already been discussed. These include peripheral neuropathy, Wernicke-Korsakoff syndrome, optic neuropathy, central pontine myelinolysis, degeneration of the cerebellum, and degeneration of the corpus callosum.

Chronic alcoholism represents a complex physiological, psychological, and socioeconomic problem. A detailed discussion of alcohol addiction is beyond the scope of this survey.

Alcohol withdrawal after chronic ingestion produces a syndrome characterized by generalized convulsive seizures and delirium tremens (refer to Chapter 26 for discussion).

Barbiturates (Sedatives) and the Minor Tranquilizers: Chlordiazepoxide (Librium), Diazepam (Valium) and Meprobamate. All of these agents may produce *chronic toxicity* manifested by symptoms of cerebellar system involvement: ataxia of gait, nystagmus, slurring of speech, and tremor. At times a drowsy confusional state may be present. Severe *acute overdosage,* as in a suicide attempt, will result in coma (see discussion, Chapter 26). *Sudden withdrawal* after chronic use may produce a typical withdrawal state, characterized by convulsions and delirium tremens.

Diphenylhydantoin (Dilantin). The toxicity produced by this anticonvulsant reflects involvement of the cerebellar system with ataxia of gait, nystagmus, slurring of

speech, and tremors. The symptoms usually disappear on reduction of dosage. In severe and chronic overdosage, significant cell loss in the cerebellum may actually occur.

In some patients chronic therapy with this agent may result in a mild peripheral neuropathy manifested by loss of deep tendon reflexes and a decrease in vibratory sensation in the lower extremities.

Bromides. Chronic use of bromides (which were formerly widely employed as sedatives) may frequently result in a confusional state characterized by disorientation, hallucination, agitation, ataxia, and tremor. This state has in the past often been mistaken for a functional psychosis, resulting in admission to a chronic psychiatric hospital.

Phenothiazides and Reserpine. The tonic effects of these tranquilizers relate to the extrapyramidal system. Depending on the age of the patient, a Parkinsonian syndrome or a dystonic syndrome may develop. These problems are discussed in Chapter 24.

Morphine and Heroin. *Acute severe intake* of these narcotic agents may produce drowsiness, coma, and respiratory arrest. Characteristically the pupils are pinpoint prior to any onset of coma. During deep coma, the pupils may be dilated.

There have been recent reports of neurological complications resulting from the intravenous administration of impure mixtures of heroin by narcotic addicts. These complications, which may consist of a hemiplegia or a myelitis, may represent an allergic vascular response to some of the impurities contained in these mixtures.

Chronic narcotic addiction represents a complex physiological and psychological problem. A complete discussion is beyond the scope of this book.

Withdrawal from morphine or heroin after chronic administration in the addicted state produces a characteristic syndrome which is characterized by tremors, agitation, cramps, diarrhea, vomiting, and anorexia. Convulsions usually do not occur, unlike the syndrome which results from alcohol and barbiturate withdrawal. Whether the withdrawal syndrome will occur and how intense the withdrawal symptoms will be often appear to be related to the level of expectation of the patient; that is, there appear to be psychological determinants in addition to the physiological aspects of withdrawal.

Hallucinogens. The effects of LSD, mescaline, and related hallucinogens on sensory and other central systems are reviewed by Smythies (1962).

OTHER AGENTS

Carbon Monoxide. Accidents or suicide attempts with acute carbon monoxide poisoning result in significant neurological defects. The patient is usually found to be in deep coma. If survival occurs, significant deficits in mentation and motor function will often be present. These deficits reflect the significant interference of the carbon monoxide with proper oxygenation of the cerebral cortex and basal ganglia among other central nervous system structures. The effects of carbon monoxide are due to its ability to form a stable compound with hemoglobin, thus reducing the oxygen-carrying capacity of the blood. At pathological examination loss of neurons in the cerebral cortex may be noted, often in a laminar pattern. Significant destruction of basal ganglia may also be present, with particular involvement of the globus pallidus.

Chronic exposure to relatively smaller doses of carbon monoxide may produce headache and confusion. Such symptoms may be noted in garage workers and traffic policemen so exposed.

COMPLICATIONS OF SYSTEMIC METABOLIC DISEASE

A variety of metabolic diseases may affect the central and peripheral nervous system. We may summarize these briefly into several syndromes.

Acute or Subacute Impairment of Consciousness (Confusion, Stupor, and Coma). The more frequent metabolic diseases in this category are: hypoxia, hypercapnia, hypoglycemia, acidosis (as in diabetes), uremia, hepatic failure, and Addison's disease. The differential diagnosis of coma and stupor is discussed in Chapter 26.

Chronic Dementia or Mental Retardation Plus or Minus Extrapyramidal or Cerebellar Motor Deficits or Seizures or Myoclonus. These disorders are discussed in relationship to the differential diagnosis of dementia in Chapter 27 and in relationship to the basal ganglia in Chapter 24. The following disorders fall into this category: hepatolenticular degeneration, chronic encephalopathy of hepatic failure, acute intermittent porphyria, chronic hypercapnia (confusion, tremor, and myoclonus), hypoparathyroidism (tetany, convulsions, and cerebral calcifications), hypothyroidism, chronic uremia (confusion plus or minus myoclonus). In addition, several disorders seen primarily in childhood present as progressive retardation of intelligence: the aminoacidurias and the lipid storage diseases. An additional syndrome should be added into this category: the Kornzweig-Bassen syndrome consisting of cerebellar and sensory ataxia, acanthocytosis (of red blood cells) and a deficiency of serum beta lipoproteins.

Neurological Complications of Diabetes Mellitus. Diabetes mellitus is widespread. The neurological complications are frequent. The most frequent complication is a distal symmetrical peripheral neuropathy. In addition a painful mononeuropathy or radiculopathy, usually proximal motor, may occur, involving most frequently the sciatic nerve. This mononeuropathy is due to vascular occlusion of the blood supply of the nerve. Cranial neuropathies involving the sixth and seventh nerves are also more frequent in diabetics. Autonomic neuropathy also occurs in severe diabetics producing a severe syndrome of diarrhea. Degeneration of cervical and lumbar intervertebral disks appears to occur more frequently in diabetics than in the general population, producing significant root and spinal cord compressions due to cervical spondylosis. In addition we, of course, should note that atherosclerosis occurs at a younger age and more frequently among diabetics, producing coronary and cerebral vascular occlusive disease which results in central nervous system complications.

Neurological Complications of Thyroid Disease. Primary manifestations of *hyperthyroidism* include psychomotor hyperactivity and accentuation of physiological tremor. In addition, ophthalmoplegias may be noted in relation to the exophthalmos which characterizes the disease. Thyrotoxic myopathies have been reported. Myasthenia gravis may also be exacerbated. Periodic paralysis may also occur in relation to hyperthyroidism.

Hypothyroidism (myxedema) also is associated with a number of neurological symptoms. Myxedema may present as a chronic dementia or depression. Hoarseness is frequently noted. The patient also complains of a general sense of muscle weakness, of muscle pains and of paresthesias. The deep tendon reflexes are often delayed in their relaxation phase (referred to as pseudomyotonic). There is often an accentuation of myasthenia gravis. Ataxia has on occasion been noted. In severe cases, coma may result.

Remote (Nonmetastatic) Neurological Complications of Carcinoma. In these instances either the central or peripheral systems may be involved. Presumably the lesions represent a toxic or immunological complication of the malignancy. The most frequent neurological manifestation is a combination of peripheral neuropathy and myopathy. The most frequent site of the primary lesion is the lung. A pseudomyasthenic syndrome has also been noted primarily with bronchiogenic carcinoma of the lung. Encephalopathies, myelopathies, and cerebellar degenerations have also been reported. The primary malignancy again has been usually in the lung, although on occasion ovary and breast have been the primary sites. Another variety of encephalopathy, multifocal leukoencephalopathy, complicates malignant diseases which involve the lymphatic and reticuloendothelial system (lymphomas, lymphocytic leukemia, reticuloendotheliosis and sarcoid). In this disease multifocal lesions rather than a diffuse process are noted.

DEMYELINATING DISEASE

We have already discussed demyelinating disease in relationship to the spinal cord and brain stem. As we have indicated, there are essentially two types of diseases that affect myelin.

Destruction of Normal Myelin. In Type I a primary destruction of normally formed myelin occurs with the usual breakdown products of myelin resulting. In this category are included: (1) the most frequent variety, multiple sclerosis; (2) acute disseminated encephalomyelitis (often a postinfectious type illness); (3) diffuse cerebral sclerosis, Schilder's disease (a diffuse demyelinating disease involving primarily the cerebral hemispheres and affecting children as a degenerative disease).

Leukodystrophies. In the Type II group of diseases, there is a diffuse loss of myelin. The loss, however, involves the destruction of defectively formed myelin. The leuko-

dystrophies are a rare group of diseases which occur primarily in infancy and childhood. Several varieties have been described:

Metachromatic leukoencephalopathy in which breakdown of myelin and engorgement of nerve cells with a metachromatic lipid occurs. The metachromatic lipid is chiefly composed of cerebroside sulfatides. The basic biochemical abnormality is an absence of the enzyme, cerebroside sulfatase.

Krabbe's disease, a form of leukodystrophy in which there are large multinucleated giant cells containing lipid-breakdown products (so-called globoid cells containing cerebroside). The enzyme which is deficient is cerebroside sulfotransferase (which normally acts to bind sulfate to cerebroside).

Pelizaeus-Merzbacher syndrome, a familial disease, in which there is a long chronic course with the white matter lesions distributed in a patchy manner but significantly affecting the cerebellum and brain stem out of proportion to other structures.

Multiple Sclerosis. As we have indicated previously there are in the early stages of multiple sclerosis several predominant clinical syndromes: the spinal cord form, the brain stem-cerebellar form, the cerebral form, and the optic nerve form. We have indicated that in most patients seen late in their disease course, a mixture of these various clinical syndromes is present. In general, a predominant cerebral form is less common than the other varieties. It should be noted, however, that the cerebral form tends to have a poor prognosis: significant progression tends to occur and remissions are less likely. The development of a significant and progressive dementia is not unusual. A typical example of a cerebral form of multiple sclerosis is demonstrated in Figure 22–60. The case history of this patient is included in the legend.

As we have indicated in our earlier considerations of multiple sclerosis, this is a disease of unknown etiology. At times a slow virus infection has been suspected but never confirmed. A possible auto-immune etiology has often been suggested, with the development of demyelinating antibodies postulated.

As discussed previously (Chapters 8, 15) not all cases are progressive. A significant proportion of cases with noncerebral involvement follow a relatively benign course. There is no specific treatment. In particular cases involving the optic nerve and chiasm,

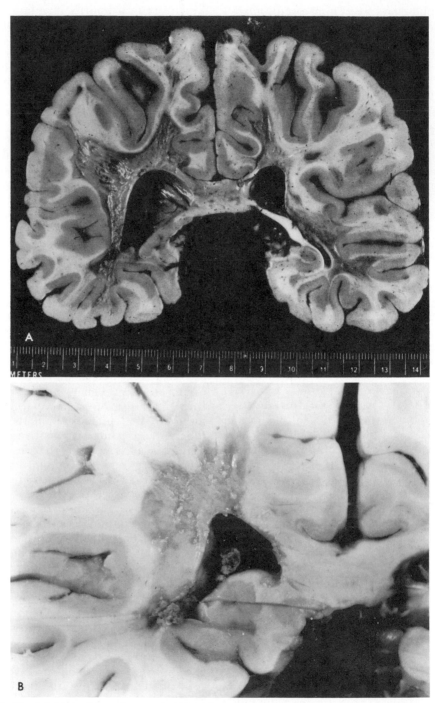

Figure 22–60   Multiple sclerosis: cerebral involvement.

A, Severe involvement of the cerebral white matter has occurred in this patient. Although multifocal gray sclerotic lesions are present, it is also apparent that large confluent lesions have occurred in a periventricular location. The large confluent lesions and the relative sparing of the arcuate fibers is reminiscent of Schilder's diffuse sclerosis. It is also evident that destruction of axons, as well as of myelin, has occurred in the larger lesions. The case history is as follows:

Legend continues on opposite page.

the use of adrenal steroids may be of value for the treatment of acute exacerbations.

References

GENERAL

Adams, R. D., and Sidman, R. L.: *Introduction to Neuropathology.* New York, McGraw-Hill, 1968.

Blackwood, W., Dodds, T. C., and Sommerville, J. C.: *Atlas of Neuropathology,* 2nd edition. Baltimore, Williams and Wilkins, 1964.

Farmer, T. W. (ed.): *Pediatric Neurology.* New York, Hoeber Medical Division, Harper and Row, 1964.

Harrison, T. R., Adams, R. D., Bennett, I. L., Resnik, W. H., Thorn, A. W., and Wintrobe, M. N.: *Principles of Internal Medicine,* 5th edition. New York, McGraw-Hill, 1966, pp. 180–281, 1107–1330.

Merritt, H. H.: *A Textbook of Neurology.* Philadelphia, Lea & Febiger, 1967.

VASCULAR DISEASES

Bauer, R. B. et al.: Joint study of extracranial arterial occlusion: III. Progress report of controlled long-term survival in patients with and without operation. JAMA, 208:509–518, 1969.

Browne, T. R. III, and Poskanzer, D. C.: Treatment of strokes. New Engl. J. Med., 281:594–602, 650–657, 1969.

Fields, W. S. et al.: Joint study of extracranial arterial occlusion: V. Progress report of prognosis following surgery or nonsurgical treatment for transient cerebral ischemia attacks and cervical carotid artery lesions. JAMA, 211:1993–2003, 1970.

Fisher, C. M.: Occlusion of the carotid arteries. Arch. Neurol. Psychiat., 72:187–204, 1954.

Fisher, C. M., Gore, I., Okabe, N., and White, P. D.: Atherosclerosis of the carotid and vertebral arteries — extracranial and intracranial. J. Neuropath. Exp. Neurol., 24:455–76, 1965.

Fisher, C. M.: Pure sensory stroke involving face, arm and leg. Neurology, 15:76–80, 1965.

Fisher, C. M.: Lacunes: small deep infarcts. Neurology, 15:774–784, 1965.

Fisher, C. M., and Adams, R. D.: Observations on brain embolism with special reference to the mechanism of hemorrhagic infarction. J. Neuropath. Exp. Neurol., 10:92–94, 1951.

Fisher, C. M., and Curry, H. B.: Pure motor hemiplegia of vascular origin. Arch. Neurol., 13:30–44, 1965.

Fogelholm, R.: Occlusive lesions of the cervical arteries in patients with ischemic cerebrovascular disease. Acta Neurol. Scand. Suppl., 42:1–64, 1970.

Hass, W. K. et al.: Joint study of extracranial arterial occlusion. II Arteriography, techniques, sites and complications. J.A.M.A., 203:159–166, 1968.

McKissock, W., Paine, K. W. E., and Walsh, L. S.: An analysis of the results of treatment of ruptured intracranial aneurysms: report of 772 consecutive cases. J. Neurosurg., 17:762–776, 1960.

McKissock, W., Richardson, A., and Walsh, L.: Middle cerebral aneurysms: further results in the controlled trial of conservative and surgical treatment of ruptured intracranial aneurysms. Lancet, II:417–421, 1962.

McKissock, W., Richardson, A., and Walsh, L.: Posterior communication aneurysms: a controlled trial of the conservative and surgical treatment of ruptured aneurysms of the internal artery at or near the point of origin of the posterior communicating artery. Lancet, 1:1203–1206, 1960.

McKissock, W., Richardson, A., and Walsh, L.: Anterior communicating aneurysms. Lancet, 1:873, 1965.

Mutlu, N., Berry, R. G., and Alpers, B. J.: Massive cerebral hemorrhage: clinical and pathological correlations. Arch. Neurol., 8:74–91, 1963.

Nishioka, H.: Report of the cooperative study of intracranial aneurysms and subarachnoid hemorrhage, Section VII: 1. Evaluation of the conservative management of ruptured intracranial aneurysms. J. Neurosurg., 25:574–592, 1966.

Ojemann, R. G.: The surgical treatment of cerebrovascular disease. New Engl. J. Med., 274:440–448, 1966.

Romanul, F. C. A., and Abramowicz, A.: Changes in brain and pial vessels in arterial border zones. Arch. Neurol., 11:40–65, 1964.

Stein, B. M., McCormick, W. F., Rodriquez, J. N., and Taveras, J.: Postmortem angiography of the cerebral vascular system. Arch. Neurol., 7:83–97, 1963.

Skultety, F. M., and Nishioka, H.: Report on the cooperative study of intracranial aneurysms and subarachnoid hemorrhage, Section VIII: 2. The results of intracranial surgery in the treatment of aneurysm. J. Neurosurg., 25:683–704, 1966.

Toole, J. F., and Patel, A. N.: *Cerebrovascular Disorders.* New York, McGraw-Hill, 1967.

Wells, C. E.: Cerebral embolism. Arch. Neurol. Psychiat., 81:667–677, 1959.

Wylie, E. J., Hern, M. F., and Adams, J. E.: Intracranial hemorrhage following surgical revascularization for treatment of acute strokes. J. Neurosurg., 21:212–215, 1964.

Figure 22–60 Continued.
This white housewife at age 26 first developed an episode of numbness of the left leg. At age 28, she developed incontinence of urine and loss of bladder sensation along with ataxia and diplopia. In addition to neurological findings relevant to brain stem, spinal cord, and optic nerve, the patient, at this time, had some difficulty in mental status as regards delayed recall and calculations. Progression occurred in all areas affected, so that by age 30, the patient was essentially bedridden with paralysis of all four extremities, marked impairment of vision, and a marked internuclear ophthalmoplegia. Re-evaluation at age 33 indicated severe impairment of mental status with marked deficits in delayed recall (0-out-of-5 in 3 minutes), information, and calculations. Death occurred at age 39.

B, A more typical area of demyelination in the periventricular subcortical white matter is demonstrated in this coronal section from another case of multiple sclerosis. (Courtesy of Dr. John Hills, New England Center Hospitals.) **See Filmstrip, Frame 59.**

TRAUMA

Brock, S. (ed.): *Injuries of the Brain and Spinal Cord and Their Coverings,* 4th Edition. Baltimore, Williams and Wilkins, 1960.

Caveness, W. F., and Walker, A. E.: *Head Injury.* Philadelphia, J. B. Lippincott, 1966.

Jennett, W. B.: *Epilepsy After Blunt Head Injuries.* London, William Heinemann Medical Books, 1962.

Plum, F., and Posner, J. B.: *The Diagnosis of Stupor and Coma.* Philadelphia, F. A. Davis, 1966.

Watson, C. W.: Incidence of epilepsy following craniocerebral injury, II. Three year follow-up study. Arch. Neurol. Psychiat., *68:*831–834, 1952.

INFECTIONS

Asenjo, A., Valladares, H., and Fierro, J.: Tuberculoma of the brain. Arch. Neurol. Psychiat., *65:*146–160, 1951.

Dastur, H. M., and Desai, A. D.: Comparative study of brain tuberculomas and gliomas based on 108 case records of each. Brain, *88:*375–396, 1965.

Farmer, J. W.: Neurologic complications during meningococcal meningitis treated with sulfonamide drugs. Arch. Intern. Med., *76:*201–209, 1945.

Gajdusek, D. C.: Slow virus infections of the nervous system. New Engl. J. Med., *276:*392–400, 1967.

Gibbs, C. J., Jr., and Gajdusek, D. C.: Infection as the etiology of spongiform encephalopathy (Creutzfeldt-Jakob disease). Science, *165:*1023–1025, 1969.

Harter, D. H., and Petersdorf, R. G.: A consideration of the pathogenesis of bacterial meningitis: review of experimental and clinical studies. Yale J. Biol. Med., *32:*280–309, 1960.

Hitchcock, E., and Andreadis, A.: Subdural empyema: a review of 29 cases. J. Neurol. Neurosurg. Psychiat., *27:*442, 1964.

Johnson, R. T., and Johnson, K. J.: Hydrocephalus following viral infection: the pathology of aqueductal stenosis developing after experimental mumps virus infection. J. Neuropathol. Exp. Neurol., *27:*591–606, 1968.

Johnson, R. T., and Johnson, K. J.: Slow and Chronic Virus Infections of the Nervous System *In* Plum, F. (ed.): *Recent Advances in Neurology.* Philadelphia, F. A. Davis, Vol. 6, pp. 33–78, 1969.

Johnson, R. T., and Mims, C. A.: Pathogenesis of viral infections of the nervous system. New Engl. J. Med., *278:*23–30, 84–92, 1968.

Kubik, C. S., and Adams, R. D.: Subdural empyema. Brain, *66:*18–42, 1943.

Liske, E., and Weikers, N. J.: Changing aspects of brain abscesses: review of cases in Wisconsin, 1940 through 1962. Neurology, *14:*294–300, 1964.

Loeser, E. Jr., and Scheinberg, L.: Brain abscesses – A review of ninety-nine cases. Neurology, 7:601–609, 1957.

Merritt, H. H., Adams, R. D., and Solomon, H. C.: *Neurosyphilis.* New York, Oxford University Press, 1946.

Payne, F. E., Baublis, J. V., and Itabashi, H. H.: Isolation of measles virus from cell cultures of brain from a patient with subacute sclerosing panencephalitis. New Engl. J. Med., *281:*585–589, 1969.

Sibley, W. A., and O'Brien, J. L.: Intracranial tuberculoma: a review of clinical features and treatment. Neurology, 6:157–165, 1956.

Swartz, M. N., and Dodge, P. R.: Bacterial meningitis – A review of selected aspects. New Engl. J. Med., *272:*725–731, 779–787, 842–848, 898–902, 954–960, 1003–1010, 1965.

Watson, C. W., Murphey, R., and Little, S. C.: Schistosomiasis of the brain due to schistosoma japonicum. Arch. Neurol. Psychiat., *57:*199–210, 1947.

Wilkins, R. H., and Brody, I. A.: Neurological classics IV: Encephalitis lethargica. Arch. Neurol., *18:*324–328, 1968.

NEOPLASMS

Cook, A. W., and Browder, E. J.: Total removal of acoustic neuroma: immediate and long term results. Arch. Neurol., *21:*7–14, 1969.

Courville, C. B.: Intracranial Tumors. Bull. Los Angeles, Neurological Societies, #2: Supplement #2:1–80, 1967.

Cushing, H., and Eisenhardt, L.: *Meningiomas.* Springfield, Ill., Charles C Thomas, 1938.

Grant, F. C.: A study of the results of surgical treatment in 2326 consecutive patients with brain tumors. J. Neurosurg., *13:*479–488, 1956.

Hoessly, G. F., and Olivecrona, H.: Report on 280 cases of verified parasagittal meningiomas. J. Neurosurg., *12:*614–626, 1955.

Jelsma, R., and Bucy, P. C.: Glioblastoma multiforme: its treatment and some factors affecting survival. Arch. Neurol., *20:*161–171, 1969.

Kernohan, J. W., and Sayre, G. P.: *Tumors of the Central Nervous System.* Washington, D.C., Armed Forces Institute of Pathology, 1952.

Russell, D. S., and Rubinstein, L. J.: *Pathology of Tumors of the Nervous System.* Baltimore, Williams and Wilkins, 1963.

Taveras, J. M., and Wood, E. H.: *Diagnostic Neuroradiology.* Baltimore, Williams and Wilkins, 1964.

Zulch, K. J.: *Brain Tumors: Their Biology and Pathology.* New York, Springer Publishing Company, 1965.

NUTRITIONAL, TOXIC, AND METABOLIC DISEASES

Aita, J. A.: *Neurological Manifestations of General Diseases.* Springfield, Ill., Charles C Thomas, 1964.

Barr, D.: Problems in the appraisal and use of tranquillizers, analgesics, and hypnotics *In* Williams, D. (ed.): *Modern Trends in Neurology,* London, Butterworth & Company, 1962, Vol. 3, pp. 336–352.

Brody, I. A., and Wilkins, R. H.: Neurological Classics IX: Wernicke's encephalopathy. Arch. Neurol., *19:*228–232, 1968.

Drachman, D. B.: Myasthenia gravis and the thyroid gland. New Engl. J. Med., *266:*330–333, 1961.

Freedman, D. X.: The psychopharmacology of hallucinogenic agents. Ann. Rev. Med., *20:*409–418, 1969.

Hammond, A. L.: Mercury in the environment: natural and human factors. Science, *171:*778–789, 1971.

Neal, D. A., and Jones, R. R.: Chronic mercurialism in the hatters' fur-cutting industry. JAMA., *110:*337, 1938.

Smythies, J. R.: Hallucinogenic Drugs *In* Williams, D. (ed.): *Modern Trends in Neurology.* London, Butterworth & Company, 1962, Vol. 3, pp. 353–366.

Sullivan, J. F.: The neuropathies of diabetes. Neurology, *8:*243–249, 1958.

Victor, M.: Alcoholism *In* Baker, A. B. (ed.): *Clinical Neurology.* New York, Harpers, 1962, Vol II, 1084–1129.

Victor, M.: The effects of nutritional deficiency on the nervous system *In* Brain, Lord, and Norris, F. H. (eds.): *The Remote Effects of Cancer on the Nervous System.* New York, Grune and Stratton, 1965.

Wilker, A.: Drug addiction *In* Baker, A. B. (ed.): *Clinical Neurology.* New York, Harpers, 1962, Vol. II, pp. 1054–1083.

DEMYELINATING DISEASES

(Refer also to the references in Chapters 8 and 15.)

Bauer, H. J.: History, facts, problems and clinical aspects of multiple sclerosis. *In* Burdzy, K., and Kallos, P.: *Pathogenesis and Etiology of Demyelinating Disease.* Basel, S. Karger, 1969.

Cumings, J. N.: Genetically determined neurological diseases in children *In* Cumings, J. N., and Kremer, M.: *Biochemical Aspects of Neurological Disorders.* Series 3, Philadelphia, F. A. Davis, 1968.

Kurtze, J. F.: Neurological impairment in multiple sclerosis and the disability status scale. Acta Neurol. (Scand.), *46*:493–512, 1970.

Norman, R. M.: Lipid diseases of the brain *In* Williams, D. (ed.): *Modern Trends in Neurology.* London, Butterworth & Company, 1962, Vol. 3, pp. 173–199.

Patterson, P. Y.: Immune processes and infectious factors in central nervous system disease. Ann. Rev. Med., *20*:75–100, 1970.

Walsen, J.: Genetically determined neurological diseases in children *In* Cumings, J. N., and Kremer, M. (eds.): *Biochemical Aspects of Neurological Disorders.* Series 3. Philadelphia, F. A. Davis, 1968, pp. 250–267.

DEGENERATIVE DISEASES

(Refer to the references in Chapters 24, 25, and 27.)

APPENDIX TO CHAPTER 22

ELLIOTT M. MARCUS

DIAGRAM LESIONS

For each diagram list the structures involved. If cortex is involved specify the cortical area. If the lesion appears to be vascular in etiology indicate the relevant blood vessel. For each structure or area involved, list the specific clinical effects which would be found on neurological examination. Be certain to lateralize the findings as to left or right.

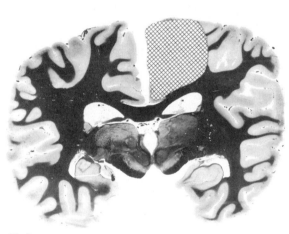

Right   *Figure 22A–1.*   **Left**   **Left**   *Figure 22A–3.*   **Right**

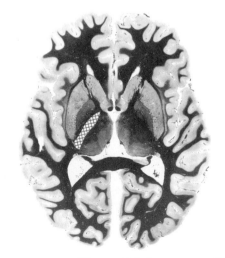

Left   *Figure 22A–2.*   **Right**   **Left**   *Figure 22A–4.*   **Right**

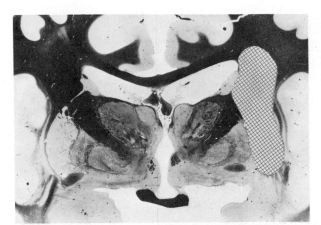

Figure 22A-5.

Right　　　　　　　　　　　　　　　　　　　　Left

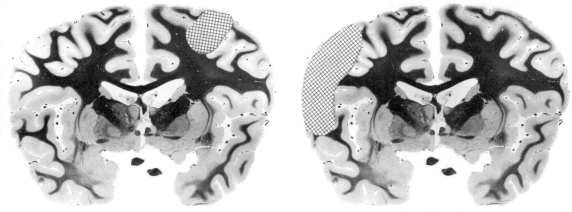

Right　　　　　　*Figure 22A-6.*　　　　　　Left　　Right　　　　　*Figure 22A-7.*　　　　　　Left

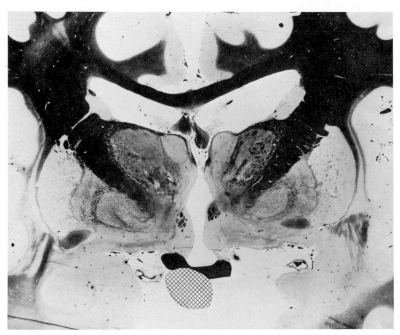

Right　　　　　　　　*Figure 22A-8.*　　　　　　　　Left

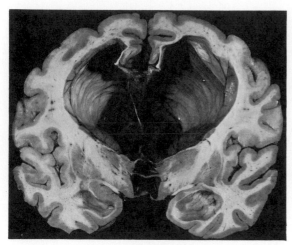

Figure 22–A9 (From Robbins, S. L.: *Pathology*. 3rd Edition. Philadelphia, W. B. Saunders, 1967, p. 1379.)

PROBLEM SOLVING EXERCISES: CEREBRAL HEMISPHERES

These cases represent the gamut of disease affecting the cerebral hemispheres. The pathology represented may be tumor, infarction, or hemorrhage. Some of the lesions are intrinsic; others are extrinsic. The nature of the pathology may be uncertain; the location of the pathology, however, should be evident to you.

Diagram each lesion. If the etiology appears to be vascular, attempt to identify the vessel involved.

Case History 1A. NECH #129–292. Date of admission: 9/3/59.

This 39-year-old, right-handed, white, male mechanic (Mr. R.M.) was admitted for evaluation of headache and visual disturbances. On June 11, 1959 the patient had the first of repetitive episodes characterized by "vertical wavy lines" in his left visual field. The initial episode lasted 30 minutes; subsequent episodes, 1 to 2 minutes. The patient had been seen by an ophthalmologist during the first of these episodes and a left visual field defect, which would disappear at the end of the episode, was detected. An electroencephalogram revealed no definite abnormality. Approximately 1 month later, the left visual field defect remained as a permanent deficit. At this time the patient also noted the onset of a numbness in his left hand. In July 1959 the patient noted the

onset of bitemporal and bifrontal headaches precipitated by any motion of the head. One week prior to admission there was an onset of vomiting.

PAST HISTORY: Not remarkable.

GENERAL PHYSICAL EXAMINATION: Not remarkable.

NEUROLOGICAL EXAMINATION:
1. *Mental status:*
   a. The patient was oriented as to time, place, and person.
   b. Delayed recall was intact.
   c. The chronology for events in the present illness was somewhat vague.
   d. No aphasia was present; reading and writing were intact.
2. *Cranial nerves:*
   a. A complete left homonymous hemianopsia was present.
   b. Funduscopic examination indicated bilateral papilledema with venous engorgement, arteriovenous nicking, and a recent hemorrhage in relation to the right disc. Visual acuity, however, was well-preserved.
   c. Both pupils demonstrated a sluggish response to light.
   d. A left central (supranuclear) type of facial weakness was present with a droop of the left corner of the mouth.
3. *Motor system:*
   a. Strength was intact.
   b. The patient tended to lean slightly to the left when walking.
   c. Cerebellar tests were negative.
4. *Reflexes:*
   a. Deep tendon reflexes were asymmetrical, being slightly more active on the left than on the right.
   b. Plantar responses were flexor. Abdominal reflexes were present bilaterally.
   c. No release of grasp and suck reflexes had occurred.
5. *Sensory system:*
   a. Pain, touch, and vibration were intact.
   b. Position sense for fine amplitude movements at the fingers and toes was decreased on the left.
   c. On simultaneous tactile stimulation of left and right side; extinction of stimuli on the left occurred.
   d. Errors were made in object identification in the left hand.
   e. Occasional errors were made in the

identification of numbers drawn on the fingers of the left hand.

LABORATORY DATA:
The electroencephalogram and arteriogram suggested a single lesion.

QUESTIONS:
1. Where was the lesion initially located at its onset?
2. Which areas are now involved by the lesion?
3. What is the pathological nature of the lesion?

In your consideration as to the location of the lesion, you will wish to indicate the localizing significance of the following:
a. the initial episodes of "vertical wavy lines"
b. the homonymous hemianopsia
c. the pattern of findings on sensory examination.

Case History 2A. NECH #176–582.
Date of admission: 1/14/66.
This 35-year-old, right-handed, white male (Mr. I.C.) in June 1964 had the onset of a sudden pins-and-needles sensation which began in the left foot and then spread within a few seconds to involve the entire left side of the body including the arm and the face. The total episode lasted for 8 minutes. Similar episodes then recurred once or twice weekly beginning most frequently on the left side of the face or tongue and less often on the left foot or hand. In October 1964 the patient had a similar episode but fell to the floor with a loss of consciousness of several minutes duration during which observers reported some clonic movements of the left arm and leg. Neurological examination, lumbar puncture, and electroencephalogram at that time were reported as normal. The episodes were temporarily controlled with anticonvulsant medication, diphenylhydantoin (Dilantin), but then recurred with increasing frequency. At the time of hospital admission, these episodes of numbness were occurring 3 to 4 times per day.

PAST HISTORY:
There was no history of significant head trauma. There was no family history of seizures.

NEUROLOGICAL EXAMINATION:
1. *Mental status:* Orientation and memory were normal.

2. *Cranial nerves:* No abnormalities were present.
3. *Motor system:* No relevant findings were present. The patient had fallen during the seizure in 1964, sustaining a fracture of the left humerus and dislocation at the left shoulder. Since that time he had a poor swing of the left arm due to limitation of left shoulder movement. A slight atrophy of the hypothenar eminence with some weakness in the ulnar distribution had also been present since that injury.
4. *Reflexes:* Deep tendon reflexes were symmetrical; plantar responses were flexor.
5. *Sensory system:* All modalities were intact except for errors in graphesthesia in the left hand outside the distribution of the ulnar nerve.

LABORATORY DATA:
1. Skull x-rays: Calcified pineal was shifted 4 to 5 mm. compared to shift of 2 mm. in films obtained 1 year previously.
2. Electroencephalogram: Focal slow wave activity of 4 to 6 cycles per second was present.
3. Cerebrospinal fluid: Normal pressure and protein (21 mg./100 ml.) were present.
4. Arteriogram was consistent with a single focal lesion.

QUESTIONS:
1. Where is the lesion?
2. What is the most likely pathological diagnosis? In answering this question you should keep in mind that the patient is of middle age (35) and that the episodes are clearly focal. These facts alone, even without the confirmatory laboratory data, should lead to certain suspicions.

Case History 3A. NECH #184–346.
Date of admission: 1/6/67.
A 66-year-old, right-handed, white widow (Mrs. A.B.) developed changes in affect and lack of interest in her surroundings over a 1-month period. Although previously she had been alert, caring for herself, doing her own shopping, and interested in her relatives, she now took to her bed and became disheveled in appearance. She would talk little if at all. She complained of a vague weakness in her legs, was unwilling to walk, but was able to walk to the bathroom without assistance.

PAST HISTORY:

Myocardial infarct had occurred in April 1966. There was a 10-year history of Paget's disease involving the bones of the lower extremities.

NEUROLOGICAL EXAMINATION:

1. *Mental status:*
   a. The patient was apathetic with a dull appearance.
   b. The patient was disoriented for person and time. She knew that she was in a hospital in the state of Massachusetts but did not know the city.
   c. She was unable to recall her birth date or to name any presidents. She could give no account of her illness.
   d. She was unable to add 5 and 5 and could not do multiplication or substractions.
   e. She repeated 4 digits forward and none in reverse.
   f. Spontaneous speech was scanty but without a definite dysarthria or dysphasia. She could name 3-out-of-6 objects, could repeat 6-out-of-6, and could read aloud 4-out-of-6. She was able to perform slowly a two-step command. She was apparently unable to write.

2. *Cranial nerves:* II-XII were intact except that the left disc margin was blurred on funduscopic examination.

3. *Motor system:*
   a. No focal weakness was present.
   b. There was a variable resistance in both lower extremities described as a "Gegenhalten."
   c. The patient was very hesitant and very fearful of sitting, standing, or walking. There was some retropulsion (a tendency to fall backwards when attempting to sit or walk). When she walked her right foot appeared to be glued to the floor.

4. *Reflexes:*
   a. Deep tendon reflexes were symmetrical and active.
   b. An equivocal plantar response was present on the right; that on the left was flexor.
   c. Strong grasp reflexes were released at hands and feet. Visual and tactile suck reflexes were also released.

5. *Sensory system:*
   a. Pain, touch, and position sense were intact.
   b. There was a minor decrease in vibratory sensation at the toes which may well have related to the patient's general nutritional status.

LABORATORY DATA:

1. Sedimentation rate elevated to 98 mm. in one hour.

2. Skull x-rays: An osteolytic lesion (area of bone destruction) was present.

3. Lumbar spine x-ray: A suspicious, probably osteolytic lesion was seen in the body of the L1 vertebra.

4. Stool Guaiac: A small amount of occult blood was present. Hematocrit and hemoglobin were normal. Rectal and proctoscopic examination revealed a firm mass at approximately 9 cm. above the anus.

5. Electroencephalogram indicated a focal lesion having the quality of damage (continuous focal 2 to 4 cps slow waves).

6. Arteriogram and brain scan were consistent with a single focal lesion.

7. A lumbar puncture 3 weeks prior to admission had revealed pressure increased to 220 mm. of H_2O and protein elevated to 59 mg./100 ml.

QUESTIONS:

1. Where is the lesion? (Assume a single central nervous system lesion.)

2. What is the most likely pathology?

3. How would you manage this problem as regards more specific diagnosis and therapy?

In considering these question you will wish to keep in mind the following points:

1. As regards the location of the lesion: (a) the personality change, accompanied by impairment of all areas of mental function, (b) the release of strong grasp reflexes in both upper and lower extremities, in addition to suck reflexes, (c) the apparent inconsistent findings as regards resistance to passive motion, (d) the disturbance of sitting posture and of gait.

2. As regards the type of pathology: (a) the elevation of sedimentation rate, (b) the apparently rapid onset of symptoms, (c) the presence of occult blood in the stool, (d) the presence of osteolytic lesions, (e), the mass noted on examination of the rectum.

Case History 4A. NECH #192–665. Date of admission: 3/26/68.

This 62-year-old right-handed, white, male civil engineer (Mr. O.L.) was noted by his wife on the evening prior to admission to have the gradual onset of slurred speech associated with a drooping of the left side of the face. The patient denied that these symptoms were present. The following morning he was examined by his brother who confirmed the presence of slurred speech and weakness of the lower one-half of the left side of the face. His brother, a physician, also noted a weakness of the left arm and leg.

PAST HISTORY:

Gout present since age 20. Apparent coronary artery occlusion in 1964.

NEUROLOGICAL EXAMINATION:

1. *General:* blood pressure 130/80; pulse 85 and regular.

2. *Mental status:*

   a. The patient was oriented for time, place, and person.

   b. Memory for recent and remote events was intact. Immediate and delayed recall was intact.

   c. The patient could do simple calculations but had difficulty with more complex problems.

   d. These results may have been influenced by the fact that the patient demonstrated a marked impersistence in following commands. The patient was somewhat apathetic and yawned frequently during the examination. There was a flattening of mood.

   e. The patient denied that he had any particular problems requiring hospitalization. He denied illness and stated he was as healthy now as he had been one week prior to hospitalization.

   f. Abstract reasoning was intact, as tested in proverb interpretation (used abstract concepts).

   g. No aphasia was present.

   h. A distinct deficit in the construction of three-dimensional drawings was present.

3. *Cranial nerves:* All were intact except for

   a. a significant left facial weakness of supranuclear type.

   b. an inconstant neglect of left field on simultaneous stimuli to left and right visual fields.

4. *Motor system:*

   a. Strength and gait were intact.

   b. Cerebellar tests were negative.

5. *Reflexes:*

   a. Deep tendon reflexes were symmetrical.

   b. Plantar responses were flexor.

   c. No pathological grasp reflex was present.

6. *Sensation:*

   a. Pain and touch were intact.

   b. Stereognosis, two-point discrimination, and tactile localization were normal. However, position sense was decreased at toes and fingers on the left. There was a tendency to ignore tactile stimuli on the left face, arm, and leg when simultaneous left and right stimulation was carried out. Graphesthesia was intact in the right hand, but defective on the left.

LABORATORY DATA:

1. Blood serological test for syphilis was negative.

2. Skull x-rays were normal.

3. Electroencephalogram: abnormal because of focal 2–5 cps slow waves.

4. Brain scan: A diffuse focal uptake was present.

SUBSEQUENT COURSE:

Over the next 3 months, significant improvement occurred. The patient was able to do complex calculations. He had no difficulty in drawing or in locating points on a map. Sensory examination was normal. The patient still had difficulty in maintaining his concentration. Psychological testing in June 1968 now indicated verbal IQ of 123, performance IQ of 104, with full scale IQ of 116, compared to much lower scores of 111, 87, and 101 respectively at the time of his acute illness.

QUESTIONS:

1. Where is the lesion (be specific)?

2. What is the nature of the lesion?

Case History 5A. NECH #156–287. Date of admission: 5/22/63.

This 52-year-old housewife (Mrs. H.L.) was referred for evaluation of episodic "twitching of the left thumb and forefinger" beginning 2 weeks prior to admission. The patient had noted the sudden onset of a numbness of the left thumb, followed in seconds by twitching of the left eyelid and then almost immediately by a twitching of the distal segment of the left thumb. This soon spread to the left forefinger, then to the middle finger, and then involved the hand in repetitive clonic movements. According to observers, the clonic movements then spread into the left arm. The twitching about the eyelid spread to the entire face. This initial episode lasted a total of 15 minutes; there was, however, a residual numbness of the left thumb and index finger: "as though they had fallen asleep." There was also a transient weakness of those areas first involved. Since the first episode, the patient had experienced minor recurrences of "tingling" of the left thumb and index finger.

PAST HISTORY:

Six years prior to admission the patient underwent a right radical mastectomy for scirrhous carcinoma of the breast. Regional lymph nodes were reported as negative. The patient's mother and sister also had carcinoma of the breast.

NEUROLOGICAL EXAMINATION:

1. *Mental status:* intact with no evidence of aphasia. No deficits were noted in drawing.

2. *Cranial nerves:* A minimal left supranuclear central facial weakness was present.

3. *Motor system:*
   a. A mild weakness was present in the left upper extremity.
   b. Rapid alternating movements of the left hand were slowly performed perhaps related to the mild weakness.

4. *Reflexes:*
   a. Deep tendon reflexes were increased on the left.
   b. An equivocal plantar response was present on the left; that on the right was flexor.
   c. No grasp reflex was present.

5. *Sensory system:*
   a. Pain, light touch, position, and vibration were normal.
   b. There was a slight disturbance in graphesthesia over the left hand and face. There was minor impairment of two-point discrimination over the left thumb and forefinger.

QUESTIONS:

1. Indicate the location of the lesion in this case.

2. Indicate the most likely pathology.

3. Attach a label to the twitching which began in the left thumb, then spread to the other fingers, then to left hand, arm, and face.

CASE HISTORY 6A. NECH #76–29–77. Date of admission: 6/16/69.

This 19-year-old, right-handed, white, male pharmacy student (Mr. M.D.A.) was referred for evaluation of frequent minor seizures. At age 18 months, the patient had fallen striking his head against a concrete floor and within hours had lapsed into coma.

Later that day he required emergency neurosurgical treatment at the Children's Medical Center for a "skull fracture and a bleeding vessel which the neurosurgeon had to tie." The patient apparently made an excellent recovery. However, from 3 years of age until 5 years of age he experienced "large convulsions" (apparently generalized convulsive seizures). During this time he also experienced minor episodes characterized by the sensation that objects were becoming smaller or larger. The patient recalled that at times, he had the sensation that bright geometric patterns were shrinking in size. Almost invariably the patient experienced the sensation of fear with these episodes. The patient had no seizures from age 5 years until age 16 years. Since age 16 the patient had had frequent minor episodes of several types occurring as frequently as 15 to 30 times a day.

One type of episode was accompanied by dreamy sensations lasting a few seconds; at times things looked unreal. At the same time the patient would feel that the whole episode was somehow very familiar, that objects looked very familiar in a manner that could not be described. There was an accompanying sensation of fright. During such an episode the patient would be able to continue driving or walking.

A second type of episode, lasting 30 to 120 seconds, was characterized by an inability to talk properly, a babbling of speech, and an inability to understand speech. During this time a sensation of vague familiarity and fatigue and at times a sense of re-incarnation would exist.

A third variety was characterized by the visual sensation of looking down a long dark corridor with a light at the other end. There was no concept of time: at times the corridor seemed to move from right to left. At the end of such an episode things would not look as they should; objects appeared distorted, and color altered. Objects were seen as black and white. The whole scene would seem unworldly. Sounds would be perceived but would fail to be registered and would not make sense.

NEUROLOGICAL EXAMINATION:

Mental status, cranial nerves, motor-system reflexes, and sensory system were all intact except for a minimal lag of the left side of the face in smiling. During the examination, the patient had a minor episode; his head dropped and he appeared out of contact for 20 to 30 seconds. He did not answer questions directly but replied by saying "What was that then, what was that then?"

QUESTIONS:

1. The electroencephalogram indicated a stable focus of discharge. Indicate the location of that focus.

2. Speculate concerning the events which occurred at age 1½ years.

Case History 7A. NECH #185–056. Date of admission: 2/10/67.

A 44-year-old, right-handed, white housewife (Mrs. F.M.) awoke 2 weeks prior to admission with numbness of the left hand and arm, extending to the level of the elbow. At the same time a left wristdrop was noted. Symptoms gradually cleared except for residual numbness in the left middle, ring, and little fingers and some clumsiness and weakness of the left fingers.

On the morning of admission the patient awoke with numbness of the left side of the face and some exacerbation of symptoms in the left hand. The numbness was intermittent and could be precipitated by turning the head to the right.

PAST HISTORY:

In 1963 several hours after awakening, the patient had had the onset of weakness of the right hand and paresthesias of the fingers of the right hand, lasting a total of 2 days. At the same time numbness and weakness of the face (right central) was noted and lasted a matter of minutes. No definite aphasia was present at that time although some difficulty in handwriting was experienced.

FAMILY HISTORY:

The patient's mother was diabetic.

NEUROLOGICAL EXAMINATION:

Blood pressure 150/80. Pulse 90. Cardiac status was normal.

1. *Mental status:* normal
2. *Cranial nerves:* normal
3. *Motor system:* Strength was decreased in left upper extremity as follows: shoulder abduction 100 per cent normal; triceps 50 per cent normal; elbow flexors 90 per cent normal; wrist extensors 50 per cent normal; finger flexors 50 per cent normal; long thumb abductors 40–50 per cent normal; short thumb abductors 40 per cent normal; opponens of thumb 50 per cent normal; digiti quintiabductors 40 per cent normal. Gait intact.

4. *Reflexes:*
   a. Deep tendon reflexes were asymmetrical as follows:
   Biceps: right, 2+; left, 3++
   Triceps: right, 2+; left, 3++
   Radial: right, 2+; left, 3++
   Quadriceps: right, 3+; left, 3+
   Achilles: right, 1–2+; left, 1–2+
   b. Plantar responses were asymmetrical —right down; left equivocal.

5. *Sensation:* Pain, touch, and vibration were intact. Position sense: errors were made in fine movement perception in left fingers. Graphesthesia: errors were made in number recognition: fingertips of the left hand. In addition occasional errors were made in number recognition on the left side of face.

6. *Carotid arteries:* A minimal bruit (murmur) was heard over the right carotid. Pulse on right high in neck was less than on left.

7. Compression of left carotid artery produced light-headedness and blurring of vision in the left eye. Similar effects occurred to a lesser degree following compression of the right carotid artery.

HOSPITAL COURSE:

Patient continued to experience episodes of numbness on the left side of the face and the left hand with minimal increase in weakness of the left hand.

QUESTIONS:

1. Where is the lesion with regard to the present episode?

2. Where was the lesion which was responsible for the previous episode? (You should be aware that lesions disseminated in time and space may represent multiple vascular problems rather than the more classic problem of multiple sclerosis.)

3. Assume a vascular etiology and indicate the vessel involved in the present episode. Indicate the vessel involved in the previous episode.

4. In the present case a contrast study was performed. Which contrast study would you perform?

5. Contrast this case to the patient who has sudden onset of pure motor paralysis of the right face, arm, and leg with *no* aphasia and no visual or sensory deficits. Examination showed findings limited to right central facial weakness and right hemiparesis (with increased deep tendon reflexes on right and right Babinski response). EEG was normal. The patient had significant improvement over several weeks. In this latter case where is the lesion likely to be located (assume a

vascular etiology)? Indicate, in addition to location of the lesion, the vessel involved.

Case History 8A.

Date of office visit: 1/8/68.

This 20-year-old white male (Mr. K.B.) had been admitted to Boston City Hospital at age 9 months with acute right hemiplegia and acute right-sided hemiconvulsions associated with a fever. A right hemiplegia was present for several days. Several additional seizure episodes occurred between age 1–3 years. No additional episodes occurred until age 17 when the patient had a focal seizure characterized by tonic posture of the right arm—abducted at the shoulder and flexed at the elbow—followed by turning of the head and eyes to the right. Consciousness was impaired but not completely lost. For several minutes the patient was unable to speak. Upon regaining speech, he was able to follow commands.

Treatment with anticonvulsants (Eskabarb —long-release form of phenobarbital) was relatively effective in preventing seizure recurrence. Once a month the patient did experience a few seconds of "weakness or limpness" of the right hand with a possible small jerk of the right hand. Approximately two weeks before his office visit in January 1968, the patient discontinued his medications. Four days prior to this visit, at a time of sleep deprivation, the patient had a focal seizure with tonic movement of the right arm and deviation of the head and eyes to the right followed by a generalized convulsive seizure.

Since age 9 months, residual weakness of the right arm had been present.

NEUROLOGICAL EXAMINATION:

1. The patient was left-handed with long-standing smallness of the right side of the face, the right arm, and the right leg.

2. *Mental status* was intact with no aphasia.

3. *Cranial nerves* were intact except for slight lag on the right in smiling.

4. *Motor system:*
   a. There was a mild weakness of the right upper extremity, most marked distally and particularly marked in the thumb abductor.
   b. Gait: A minimal circumduction of the right leg was noted.

5. *Reflexes:*
   a. Deep tendon reflexes were increased on the right.
   b. Plantar response was equivocal on the right.

6. *Sensation:* Minor deficits were present in the right upper extremity characterized by errors in fine-movement perception of the right fingers and errors in graphesthesia of the right hand. Pain and touch were intact.

QUESTIONS:

1. Locate the lesion.

2. Where are the focal seizures originating (tonic posture of the right arm with deviation of the head and eyes to the right and with arrest of speech)?

3. The patient has a right hemiplegia and yet he does not have an aphasia. Explain.

4. In view of the acute onset of the hemiplegia at age 9 months and the subsequent lack of progression, speculate concerning the etiology.

5. Why was the weakness most prominent in the distal muscles of the upper extremity (particularly the thumb)?

6. Why did seizures recur?

7. Why has the smallness of the right side occurred?

8. What is the nature of the sensory deficit?

9. How would you manage the seizure problem?

10. Does the recurrence of seizures at age 17, after no seizures since age 3, indicate that a progressive pathology is present?

Case History 9A.   NECH #179–501.

Dates of admissions: 5/27/66 and 10/6/67.

This 65-year-old, right-handed housewife (Mrs. A.R.) was referred for evaluation of two loss-of-speech episodes on the day of evaluation. Approximately 1 hour after arising, the patient had difficulty in speaking for 1 or 2 minutes. She was unable to produce any words. A second episode occurred 10 minutes later, again of 1 to 2 minutes duration. Thirty minutes after this the patient's daughter-in-law arrived and found that although speech had returned there was a definite hesitancy in using words. Within 90 minutes of the second episode, symptoms cleared completely. The patient noted no lateralized weakness of the face, arm, or leg; no lateralized numbness of the face, arm, and leg; and no visual symptoms. The patient, however, had complained of a general feeling of tiredness or weakness for 10 to 15 days. She apparently had had an upper respiratory infection during the preceding 4 to 5 days with a temperature of 102, but on the day of evaluation she was afebrile.

PAST HISTORY:

1. The patient had had a large retrosternal and suprasternal goiter for a number of years.

2. Three to four months previously the patient had experienced an episode of sudden tachycardia; this was treated with quinidine (drug used in cardiac arrhythmias) for several days. The patient had also been treated with thyroid, 120 mg. a day, beginning three to four months prior to evaluation; she had received none, however, in the last month. The thyroid was discontinued when irregular pulse (atrial fibrillation) was noted. (An electrocardiogram one year previously apparently was normal with no evidence of an arrhythmia.)

3. Several years previously, the patient had passed renal stones.

FAMILY HISTORY:

The patient's mother had expired at age 84 of hypertension and a cerebral vascular accident. The patient's sister died of cancer.

NEUROLOGICAL EXAMINATION:

1. Blood pressure was 120/80; temperature, 98.6; pulse, 130 with irregular irregularity (probable atrial fibrillation). Chest examination revealed a loud, opening snap with a grade III/IV diastolic rumble at the apex, consistent with mitral stenosis. A large goiter was present.

2. The patient presented a relevant history.

3. There was no evidence of a nominal aphasia. Reading was not impaired and writing was intact. The patient could write her address and could write from dictation.

4. *Cranial nerves:* Nerves II through XII were intact except for a minimal weakness of the right central area of the face.

5. *Motor system:*
   a. Strength was intact.
   b. Gait was intact except for a minimal decrease in swing of the right arm.
   c. Cerebellar findings were within normal limits.

6. *Reflexes:*
   a. There was a minimal increase in deep tendon reflexes at the right biceps, triceps, knee jerk, and ankle jerk.
   b. Plantar responses were flexor.

7. *Sensation:* Pain, position, and touch were within normal limits. There was no extinction on simultaneous stimulation. There

was a minimal decrease in vibratory sensation at the toes as compared to the ankles.

8. *Carotid pulses* were present bilaterally. The left carotid pulse high in the neck was slightly less than that on the right side; otherwise the pulses were strong. There were bruits on auscultation of the carotids. There were no bruits on auscultation of the cranium. Brief carotid compression for 10 seconds produced no symptoms on the right and no symptoms on the left side.

LABORATORY DATA:

1. Hct 45; WBC 6800; sedimentation rate 8 mm.

2. PBI 8.2 mg./100 ml. (normal 4–8 mg./100 ml.).

3. *Chest x-rays:* The heart was enlarged. Chest fluoroscopy showed evidence of mitral valvular disease.

4. *Skull x-rays* were normal.

SUBSEQUENT COURSE:

The patient was treated with digitalis and with anticoagulants. She was discharged from the hospital on June 7, 1966. She did well until October 6, 1967 when she had the sudden onset of pain, numbness, and paralysis of the left lower extremity. Examination indicated that the right popliteal pulse was present but the left was absent. The left leg was cold and pale with demarcation above the knee and no pain sensation below this level. Atrial fibrillation was still present. An endarterectomy was immediately performed with a return of pulses, sensation, and movement.

On October 16, 1967, the 9th postoperative day, at 10 A.M. the patient suddenly stopped speaking in midsentence and was noted to have a complete right hemiplegia.

NEUROLOGICAL EXAMINATION:

1. *Mental status:* The patient was somnolent but could be aroused. She was unable to produce any intelligible words and was unable to follow any verbal commands.

2. *Cranial nerves:*
   a. No response to visual threat on the right occurred.
   b. Head and eyes deviated to the left. Eye movements were full in response to head turning.
   c. A right central facial weakness was present.
   d. There was a decreased response to pin prick on the right side of the face.

3. *Motor system:*
   a. The right arm and leg were im-

mobile. Only minimal movement occurred even on painful stimulation.

b. A minor degree of spasticity was present on the right side.

4. *Reflexes:*
  a. Deep tendon:
Biceps:	right, 2; left, 2+
Triceps:	right, 1; left, 2
Radial:	right, 1; left, 2
Quadriceps:	right, 3; left, 2+
Achilles:	right, 3; left, 2+

  b. Plantar responses: extensor on the right, flexor on the left. Grasp was absent on the right.

5. *Sensation:*
  a. The patient responded to pain over the left side of the body. There was a questionable response on the right.
  b. The patient was described as "ignoring" the right side.
  c. Carotid pulses were strong in the neck.

Lumbar puncture revealed probable traumatic tap: Tube #1, 2000 RBC; #3, 135 RBC.

Heparin and 5% CO_2 were given with no definite improvement.

Neurological follow-up examination in February 1968 revealed little return of language function. Almost no spontaneous speech was present. Patient was able to answer yes and no to some questions. She had return of certain automatic gestures and speech; e.g., in responding to greeting she would smile and say hello. At conclusion of examination she would grasp hand of doctor and say thank you. Patient was able to understand simple one-stage commands but was unable to carry out more complex commands. Perseveration was evident. Other findings were unchanged.

QUESTIONS:

1. Where is the lesion?

2. Indicate the specific vessel involved.

3. What is the nature of the pathology?

4. What significance do you attach to the spinal fluid findings?

5. What is the anatomical significance of the language disturbance?

6. What was the nature of the symptoms involving the left leg?

7. The deep tendon reflexes at the biceps, triceps, and radial on the right never became particularly hyperactive. What prognosis do you attach to this?

8. In a patient who has suffered a dense hemiparesis is the absence of spasticity several days after the stroke a good or bad prognostic sign?

9. What is the neurological interpretation of the episode on May 27, 1966? Be specific.

Case History 10A. NECH #101–504. Date of admission: 6/12/66.

This 65-year-old, right-handed, white male (Mr. T.M.) was in good health until the night prior to admission when he was noted to have slurred speech. In retrospect, he was also noted to be clumsy in the use of his hands as in lighting cigarettes and in driving an automobile. The following morning (the day of admission) on walking to the bathroom, he fell down and was noted to have a left-sided weakness and a slurring of speech. The patient denied any headache, diplopia, or numbness of any part of his body.

PAST HISTORY:

There was no relevant history of diabetes, hypertension, or heart disease.

PHYSICAL EXAMINATION:

1. The patient was an obese man who was confused but easily aroused. Blood pressure was 120/80, pulse 76 and regular.

2. A grade II/VI basilar systolic ejection murmur was present.

3. There was no nuchal rigidity.

NEUROLOGICAL EXAMINATION:

1. *Mental status:*
  a. The patient was oriented for time, place, and person. However, the patient often muttered disconnected sentences.
  b. General information was intact.
  c. There was no evidence of aphasia or apraxia.
  d. The patient was able to carry out one-step or two-step commands.

2. *Cranial nerves:*
  a. Nerve II—a left homonymous hemianopsia was present.
  b. Nerves III, IV, and VI—pupils were equal and responded to light and accommodation. There was a question of a gaze palsy with inability to look voluntarily to the left.
  c. Nerve VII—a left central facial weakness was present.
  d. Nerves IX and X—uvula deviated to the right. Gag was depressed on the left.

3. *Motor system:* A left hemiparesis was

present with greater distal than proximal weakness. Both arm and leg were equally involved.

4. *Reflexes:*
   a. Deep tendon reflexes were slightly more active on the left.
   b. Plantar stimulation revealed a left Babinski sign.
5. *Sensation:*
   a. All modalities were intact except for a questionable and variable decrease in pain sensation on the left side.
6. *Carotid arteries:* Strong pulses were present without bruits.

LABORATORY DATA:
1. Skull x-rays: Normal
2. Lumbar puncture (day of admission)
   a. Opening pressure was elevated to 240 mm. of water and closing pressure to 235 mm. of water.
   b. Cells: Tube #1 revealed 6100 RBC (62% crenated)/cu. mm. and tube #4 revealed 6650 RBC (54% crenated)/cu. mm.
   c. Protein was increased to 63 mg./100 ml.

SUBSEQUENT COURSE:
Shortly after admission (at approximately 10 P.M.) the patient's condition suddenly deteriorated. He became obtunded and poorly responsive to stimuli. Eyes deviated to the right. Pupils became sluggish in response to light. Blood pressure was elevated to 240/105 and Cheyne-Stokes periodic respirations were noted. The pupils became pinpoint. Bilateral Babinski signs were now noted and spasticity was now present on the right side. Approximately 2½ hours later, the patient's condition further deteriorated. He required respiratory assistance. Pupils became dilated and fixed in response to light. A decerebrate posture developed. There was no meaningful response to painful stimuli. His condition remained unchanged until his death on June 20, 1966.

QUESTIONS:
1. The initial weakness, with equal involvement of face, arm, and leg without significant numbness, represents, in a sense, a relatively pure motor hemiplegia and might suggest the initial location of the lesion. Indicate the location.
2. Present a differential diagnosis as to the pathology.
3. Outline the pathophysiology of the sequence of events following hospital admission. Would one usually expect such prodromal symptoms with this type of lesion, e.g., the hypertensive patient who developed this problem?
4. Indicate the findings to be expected at autopsy.
5. What is the usual prognosis in this problem?
6. Discuss the findings on spinal fluid examination. Does this pattern suggest a "traumatic tap"?

Case History 11A. NECH #72–48–24.
Date of admission: September 1970.
This 59-year-old, white male (Mr. S.C.) had an 8-year history of diabetes mellitus and mild hypertension. Approximately 2 days prior to admission, the patient complained of a general sensation of ill health. The day prior to admission, the patient was unable to get out of bed but apparently was responsive. On the morning of admission, the patient was brought by his family to the emergency room because of a transient period of unresponsiveness.

GENERAL PHYSICAL EXAMINATION:
1. The blood pressure was 190/105; the pulse was 64 and regular.
2. The neck was stiff.
3. There was a marked fluctuation in the level of consciousness. During periods when the patient was able to answer questions appropriately, he complained of a severe right-sided headache and of a severe pain in the back of the neck.

NEUROLOGICAL EXAMINATION:
1. *Mental status:*
   a. As previously mentioned there was a marked fluctuation in the level of consciousness. At times the patient would respond only to deep pain; at other times, however, the patient was able to answer questions appropriately and to follow a verbal command.
2. *Cranial nerves:*
   a. The fundi were not remarkable.
   b. The pupils were 3 mm. in diameter and reacted well to light.
   c. A left central facial weakness was present.
3. *Motor system:*
   a. A flaccid left arm was present; however, strength in the lower extremities appeared normal.

4. *Reflexes:*
   a. Deep tendon reflexes were slightly asymmetrical; being more active on the right than on the left.
   b. Plantar response on the left was definitely extensor; that on the right was equivocal.

5. *Sensory system:* The patient neglected stimuli on the left side in an inconsistent manner. Otherwise, all modalities were intact.

LABORATORY DATA:

Lumbar puncture demonstrated an elevated cerebral spinal fluid pressure of 420 mm. of water. The spinal fluid was grossly bloody with no evidence of clearing between the first and third tubes.

SUBSEQUENT COURSE:

Several hours following admission, the patient's condition deteriorated. He became sweaty and his pulse rate increased to 160 per minute. Pupillary responses now became sluggish. Doll's eyes movements, however, were preserved. Twelve hours later, the patient had a respiratory arrest and expired.

QUESTIONS:

1. Present a differential diagnosis and indicate the most likely diagnosis in this case.

2. Indicate the location of the lesion and if vascular, indicate the vessel involved. (Be specific.)

3. Outline your diagnostic and therapeutic management of this problem.

4. Review the expected prognosis.

23

The Motor System and the Integration of Reflex Activity

ELLIOTT M. MARCUS

INTRODUCTION

In studying the motor system we will consider two interrelated aspects: posture and movement. Under posture we will be studying static or tonic reactions. Under movement we will be studying short duration phasic reactions. We should keep in mind, as Sherrington has indicated, that the reflexes involved in posture and movement are the same. There are no reflexes exclusively for the maintenance of a correct posture as opposed to those reflexes involved in a movement. We should note that with more detailed microelectrode studies we may find that some neurons in the cerebral cortex or spinal cord are predominantly involved in phasic activities and others predominantly in tonic activities. Additional aspects of movement will be considered in subsequent chapters on the basal ganglia (Chapter 24) and the cerebellum (Chapter 25).

The use of the term *reflex* has several implications. There is implied a definition of the adequate stimulus. For example, is the stimulus a nociceptive (painful) stimulus? Is the stimulus a proprioceptive (a stretch type) stimulus? Is the stimulus tactile? Is the stimulus visual?

A definition of a reflex also implies a definition of the synapses involved. Are the synapses monosynaptic? Are the synapses polysynaptic? We should note that the stretch reflex, as already indicated, is a monosynaptic pathway. The flexion reflex is polysynaptic.

A definition of a reflex also involves a definition of the segments involved in the reflex pathway. Is the reflex segmental; that is, are the afferent input, the interneurons, and the efferent anterior horn cell all located at the same segment? Or perhaps the reflex is intersegmental, involving the coordination of several segments of the spinal axis. Perhaps the reflex is suprasegmental; that is, there is the exercise of supraspinal control over motor activities at a spinal cord level.

The definition of a reflex also implies the definition of the movement or response. For example, one may speak of flexion reflexes, extension reflexes, or righting reflexes. We also speak in terms of the grasp response, the avoidance response, placing, and hopping. We also speak in terms of projection of the limb in visual space.

In addition to these aspects of the definition of the term reflex, some scientists would add that the definition should also include

661

the aim of the reflex. This statement implies that reflexes are purposive. This implies a relationship of the behavior of the organism to the environment.

It is important to realize that motor functions are represented and rerepresented at successively higher physiological and anatomical levels of the neural axis. As we go higher in the neural axis, we are utilizing and modifying mechanisms that have been integrated at a lower level of the neural axis.*

TYPES OF ANIMAL PREPARATIONS

The capacity for motor activity will depend on the animal preparation employed (Fig. 23–1).

1. The *low spinal preparation* involves a transection at the midthoracic level.

2. The *high spinal preparation* involves a transection at a high cervical level, usually the cervical medullary junction.

3. The *decerebrate preparation* has undergone a transection at some level between the vestibular nuclei and the red nucleus. The transection is usually performed between the superior and inferior colliculi. This is referred to as an *intercollicular section*. The preparation is sometimes referred to as a "low midbrain" animal. Less often, the transection is performed at the junction between the pons and the inferior colliculus. This preparation is sometimes labeled a *pontine preparation*.

4. The *midbrain preparation* involves a transection above the superior colliculus. This is sometimes referred to as a *precollicular section*. The red nucleus is usually intact. Portions of the subthalamus and posterior hypothalamus may be intact. At times this animal preparation is referred to as the *high midbrain preparation*.

5. The *thalamic preparation* has had a transection at a higher level. The thalamus is intact. The cerebral cortex and basal ganglia, however, have been removed.

6. The *decorticate preparation* is one in which the cerebral cortex alone has been removed. This is essentially the same preparation as the thalamic preparation, but it varies as regards the presence of basal ganglia. From a functional standpoint, this preparation is the same as the thalamic preparation.

In considering each of these preparations, one must also evaluate the phylogenetic factor; that is, there is a progressive encephalization of function. Thus, we should consider the colloquial reference to the chicken who ran around the barnyard for a short period after his head was cut off. The chicken, obviously, has considerably more integration of motor function at a brain stem and spinal cord level than does the human or the infrahuman primate. Thus, a midbrain chicken is able to walk around with no particular difficulty. On the other hand, it would be very unlikely that a monkey or man with transection at the level of the midbrain would ever be able to walk.

The student should be alert to the fact that the comparison of acute animals earlier in the study of motor function did result in overemphasis on some of these phylogenetic differences, since such a comparison tended to underestimate the return of certain functions in man or monkey after spinal cord transection or decortication. We should note that the results in a chronic animal who has had good postoperative care may provide a better index of the actual capacity of the various preparations. Thus, one must consider the factors of spinal shock and cortical shock.

THE SPINAL PREPARATION

The immediate effects of transection of the spinal cord reflect the factors of spinal shock and of release of function. The course of recovery following transection of the spinal cord is characterized by changes in flexion and stretch reflexes. The changes in stretch reflexes are reflected in the deep tendon reflexes and in the resistance to passive motion. There are, in addition, during the course of recovery, changes in bladder and bowel control which must be considered.

SPINAL SHOCK

The nature of spinal shock is still not certain. This phenomenon is progressively more profound in higher forms. In the frog, it is fleeting. In the cat it is a matter of minutes to hours in duration. In the dog, it is a matter of several hours duration. In the monkey and man, spinal shock may endure for a matter

---

*The present chapter approaches the motor system from the standpoint of integration of reflex activity. The student, however, should note that certain complex patterns of movement may occur without apparent sensory input. As discussed in the recent papers of DeLang (1971) and Burke (1971) increasing attention has been given to these types of central patterning and to their interaction with reflex activity.

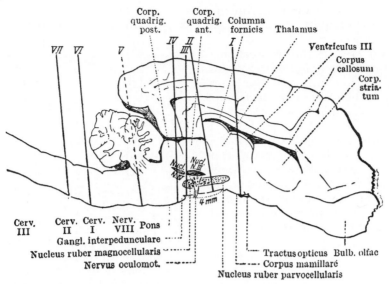

Figure 23–1 Levels of transection in experimental preparations.
Diagram of cat's brain, showing various levels of transection of brain stem used by Magnus, and also by Rademaker, in their analysis of decerebrate rigidity.

Section I. Thalamus animal possessing heat regulation and normal posture.
Section II. Midbrain animal. Posture normal, thermal regulation abolished.
Section III. Excluding red nucleus level brings on decerebrate rigidity.
Section IV. If unilateral gives homolateral rigidity.
Section V. Just above level of vestibular nuclei. Rigidity still present.
Section VI. Rigidity absent.
Section VII. Neck reflexes absent. True spinal animal.

(From Fulton, J. F.: *Physiology of the Nervous System*, 2nd Edition, New York, Oxford University Press, 1943, p. 146.)

of days or weeks. Spinal shock involves a depression of those reflex activities which are integrated at a spinal cord level. Thus, there is a marked loss of stretch reflexes and of flexion reflexes. There is a loss of those reflexes, triggered by the stretch of the bladder and the bowel, which result in evacuation of bladder and bowel.

The nature of spinal shock, as we have indicated, is still not certain. At the alpha motor neuron level in the anterior horn, a hyperpolarization of the membrane has been found. It is uncertain whether this type of hyperpolarization derives from a withdrawal of facilitation with a correlated decrease in excitatory postsynaptic potentials or from an increase in tonic inhibition, that is, an increase in inhibitory postsynaptic potentials. It is also uncertain whether the source of the hyperpolarization is supraspinal or segmental.

In the cat and the dog, spinal shock appears to relate to section or damage to the vestibulospinal tract and to the ventral reticulospinal tract. In the primates, spinal shock does not occur when there is damage to the vestibulospinal tract but depends much more upon damage to the corticospinal tract, that is, pyramidal tract damage.

The depth and duration of spinal shock depend on the rapidity and completeness of section of the spinal cord. Thus, slowly expanding chronic compressive lesions of the spinal cord *do not* result in the appearance of spinal shock. Acute traumatic transections of the spinal cord *do* result in the appearance of spinal shock. The depth and duration also depend on the occurrence of fever and infection and upon the nutritional status of the individual. Thus, bladder infection will often prolong the duration of spinal shock. Moreover, once some recovery from spinal shock has taken place the occurrence of fever or infection results in a regression to an earlier stage of more severe spinal shock.

TRANSECTION OF THE SPINAL CORD IN THE CAT OR DOG

Effects of spinal cord transection obviously will depend upon the species studied. We will contrast the effects of transection and the course of recovery from transection in the cat and dog as opposed to man. Let us first consider the cat and dog (animals which have been employed in many experimental studies). We can distinguish the immediate effects and the recovery stage.

Immediate Effects. If the transection is above the outflow to the diaphragm—that is, C3, C4, and C5, as in a high spinal preparation where the section has been performed between the medulla and these levels of the spinal cord—it is found that the animal is unable to breathe; assisted respiration is necessary. If the section has been made below this level of the midcervical cord, then spontaneous respiration will continue since the connections between the medullary respiratory centers and those spinal cord anterior horn cells giving rise to the phrenic nerve outflow remain intact.

There are significant *changes in reflex activity.* There is a depression of stretch reflexes with a resultant flaccidity. The deep tendon reflexes (the phasic component of the stretch reflex) are difficult to obtain although they are usually not completely lost. The flexion reflex is present; this is the flexion withdrawal to a painful stimulus. The flexion reflexes become, as we will note, progressively more enhanced. The crossed extension reflex is usually markedly depressed. This reflex usually results in the extension of the contralateral hind limb when the ipsilateral hind limb has been withdrawn from a painful stimulus. The purpose is, obviously, to maintain the organism in a standing posture. The scratch reflex is present in fragments, but poorly coordinated. The scratch reflex occurs when a moving contact to the skin or trunk leads to a repetitive scratching movement much as a dog might make in attempting to rid itself of fleas on the skin of the trunk.

Sensation is abolished as regards all modalities below the level of the lesion. *Bladder and bowel control* are lost. Urinary and fecal incontinence is the rule in the cat and the dog.

As regards *movement,* there is no brain stem or cerebral control. There is no movement in relation to visual, auditory, or olfactory stimuli. Control of *temperature regulation* below the level of the transection is lost.

Recovery Phase. The *recovery phase* may be outlined as follows: The nociceptive (pain induced) flexion reflex recovers first and remains prepotent (Fig. 23–2). The afferent input for this polysynaptic reflex consists of type III and IV fibers from free nerve endings. In the initial stages of recovery, a painful stimulus to the plantar surface of the foot

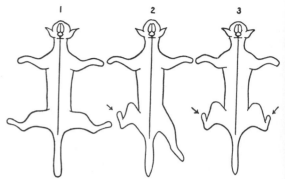

Figure 23–2 High spinal cat: flexion and crossed extension reflexes. *1,* The initial posture of the animal. *2,* Nociceptive stimulation of the left hind foot produces flexion of the left hind limb and crossed extension of the right hind limb. *3,* Nociceptive stimulation of both right and left hind limbs leads to flexion of both hind limbs. *Flexion reflex then remains prepotent.* (From Sherrington, C.: *The Integrative Action of the Nervous System.* New Haven, Yale University Press, 1947, p. 226.)

leads to abduction of the thigh and then to withdrawal of the entire limb. The initial withdrawal is relatively stereotyped.

As recovery continues *local sign* becomes evident. Local sign may be defined as a differential movement to a differential location of stimulus. Thus, if a painful stimulus is delivered to the inner border of the foot one notes an eversion of the foot, a flexion of the foot and thigh, and an abduction of the leg. On the other hand, if a painful stimulus is delivered to the outer border of the foot there is a combination of inversion and flexion of the foot in addition to a flexion and adduction of the thigh. In the cat and dog, local sign becomes evident as the after discharge of the flexion reflex and the diffuseness of the flexion reflex decreases. In the earlier stages of recovery of the flexion reflex one may find that a bilateral flexion of hind limbs occurs prior to the development of local sign.

As local sign develops, however, one finds that a *crossed extension reflex* (Fig. 23–2) becomes evident as well. Thus, in addition to the limited flexion of the ipsilateral hind limb to a painful stimulus delivered to the plantar surface, one finds a crossed extension of the contralateral hind limb. The recovery of the crossed extension reflex provides early evidence of the recovery of extensor capacities.

At this time there is also evidence of recovery of some of the *extensor proprioceptive mechanisms* as seen in the hyperactivity of the deep tendon reflexes and the development of spasticity. The spastic resistance to passive motion, of course, is an indication of the hyperactivity of the stretch reflexes. Another indication of the return of stretch reflexes is the occurrence of the positive *support reaction*, also called the extensor thrust response. The adequate stimulus for this response is a pressure stimulus delivered to the plantar surface of the limb. This results in some spread of the toes and stretch of the relevant muscles. The stretch then triggers a strong stretch reflex in the quadriceps; the result is a limb which provides a firm support for the body.

In additional recovery, alternate stepping — that is, alternate flexion and extension with crossed extension and flexion in the contralateral limb — may occur. As additional recovery continues, one finds that there is a modification of these *proprioceptive reflexes* by a tactile stimulus. The extensor thrust, for example, becomes triggered by a light stroke to the plantar surface of the foot. One also finds that tactile stimuli to the buttock or the side of the thigh, as in contact of these areas with a surface of a sheet, produces changes in resistance in passive motion.

Thus, *the pattern of recovery has been a progression from purely nociceptive flexion reflexes to proprioceptive triggered reflexes to modification of the proprioceptive reflexes by tactile stimuli.* As additional recovery occurs, one may see the development of *coordination of reflexes at intersegmental levels.* Thus, components of reflex figures may be seen.

The classic form of the reflex figure will best be seen in the decerebrate preparation and we will discuss this later. In addition, the coordination at intersegmental levels allows for the complete recovery of the scratch reflex. As we have indicated, the adequate stimulus is a moving contact to the skin of the trunk. This leads to a repetitive scratching movement by the ipsilateral hind limb. Scratching is delivered to the correct spot. There is, then, a local sign.

The scratch reflex depends on unilateral long propriospinal fibers running along the border of the grey matter. These fibers end on small internuncial neurons at the base of the posterior horn (the internuncials of the zona intermedia). The pathway for the scratch reflex is diagrammed in Figure 23–3.

In some animals, following spinal tran-

Figure 23–3 The scratch reflex.
A, The "receptive field," as revealed after low cervical transection, a saddle-shaped area of dorsal skin, whence the scratch reflex of the left hind-limb can be evoked. *lr* marks the position of the last rib.
B, Diagram of the spinal arcs involved. *L,* receptive or afferent nervepath from the left foot; *R,* receptive nervepath from the opposite foot; *Rα, Rβ,* receptive nervepaths from hairs in the dorsal skin of the left side; *PC,* the final common path, in this case the motor neurone to a flexor muscle of the hip; *Pα, Pβ,* propriospinal neurones. (From Sherrington, C.: *The Integrative Action of the Nervous System.* New Haven, Yale University Press, 1947, p. 123.)

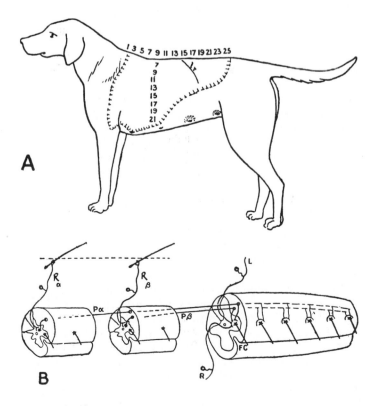

section, cutaneous stimulation of the genital area and of the medial thighs will produce certain of the postural adjustments involved in the coitus reflex. Distention of the bladder may also lead to certain of the postural adjustments characteristic of the animal during urination or defecation.

TRANSECTION OF THE SPINAL CORD IN MAN

We may again consider the effects of spinal cord transection in terms of immediate effect and those effects noted during the recovery of spinal cord reflex activity.

Immediate Effects. The immediate effects involve a complete loss of deep tendon reflexes below the level of the lesion with an accompanying flaccid paralysis. There is no resistance to passive motion at the joints below the level of the lesion. These effects are, of course, indicative of the state of spinal shock. There is a complete loss of sensation of all modalities of sensation below the level of the lesion. There is a dry skin below the level of the lesion reflecting the loss of autonomic control. There is a depression of bladder and bowel reflexes with a retention of urine and feces.

Recovery Phase. The course of recovery may be outlined as follows: At some time within 1 to 5 weeks after a complete transection, the *flexion reflex* appears. The receptive field for the flexion reflex becomes more extensive. Eventually, an activity described as the *mass reflex* predominates. This is a stage when a massive flexion reflex occurs without any evidence of local sign. This massive flexion is triggered by any stimulus to the lower extremities or to the abdomen or trunk below the level of section. The response involves a massive spasm of flexor muscles of the trunk and lower extremities with sweating, emptying of the bladder, penile erection, and ejaculation. As recovery continues, the mass reflex becomes less prominent and local sign with regard to the flexion reflex develops. We should, however, note that the mass reflex is likely to return if fever and infection develop.

As recovery continues the *stretch (proprioceptive) reflexes* return. We therefore find that deep tendon reflexes return and become hyperactive. Extensor postures and reflexes return. This may take a year if a complete transection has occurred. These extensor reflexes may appear earlier if the transection is incomplete.

The extensor capacities in man may include, in addition to hyperactive deep tendon reflexes, the crossed extension reflex and the alternate flexion extension of the mark time reflex, that is, alternate stepping. The extensor capacities may result in fragments of standing. We should note that standing with support is not unusual in the "spinal" cat or dog. The extensor thrust may allow sufficient extensor tone for the animal to stand on the limbs. Of course, the cat or dog will tumble over if such support is withdrawn. In man, this state usually is never reached. There usually is not sufficient extensor tone for actual standing when the transection has been complete. The bladder emptying and rectal evacuation reflexes return 3 to 4 weeks after injury. The initial "atonic" bladder then becomes a spastic bladder. Sweating below the level of transection may not return for 2 to 3 months.

Additional aspects of recovery from spinal cord transection, spinal cord compression, and other diseases involving the spinal cord will be found in Chapter 8.

THE DECEREBRATE PREPARATION

The decerebrate preparation, as we have earlier indicated, involves a transection of the brain stem at some point between the vestibular nuclei and the red nucleus. In general this is performed between the superior and inferior colliculi and such a preparation is often referred to as an intercollicular section. In discussing the decerebrate preparation it is important to distinguish between the acute preparation and the chronic preparation. Most studies have dealt with the acute preparation and much of the information available in the standard textbooks relates to the acute preparation.

In man the decerebrate state may reflect several pathological processes such as basilar artery thrombosis with brain stem infarction, temporal lobe herniation with midbrain compression, or massive destruction of both cerebral hemispheres.

ACUTE DECEREBRATE PREPARATION

Decerebrate Rigidity. A state described as decerebrate rigidity develops almost immediately. Decerebrate rigidity may be defined as the exaggerated posture of extension of the antigravity muscles due to the enhancement of proprioceptive stretch reflexes. In four-legged animals, such as the cat and dog, the enhancement of these stretch reflexes results in extensor posture in all four limbs with extension of the tail and arching of the back and neck. This posture is also referred to as *opisthotonos* (Fig. 23–4.)

Sherrington has described the posture of decerebrate rigidity as "an exaggerated caricature of standing." This is most intense in those muscles which normally counteract the effect of gravity. In an animal such as the sloth which normally hangs upside down, it is the flexor posture that is exaggerated. It is important to realize that with transection of the brain stem, the decerebrate rigidity develops almost immediately. Spinal shock does not result.

It is important to note that though the extensor tone is sufficient to allow the animal to stand, the animal is pillar-like. The pillar-like limb seen in this extensor posture is indicative of the positive supporting reaction already seen in the "spinal" cat and dog. This is the tonic form of the extensor thrust reaction previously noted. The extension is sufficient to allow the animal to stand. The animal, however, is pillar-like with no reaction to sudden displacement. The animal lacks righting reflexes.

Modification of Decerebrate Rigidity. The posture of decerebrate rigidity may be modified by several influences: tonic neck reflexes, tonic labyrinthine reflexes, and noxious stimuli.

By Tonic Neck Reflexes (Fig. 23–5). Tonic neck reflexes are studied best after destruction of the labyrinth or after bilateral section

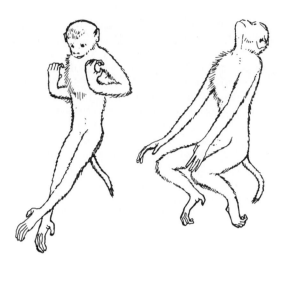

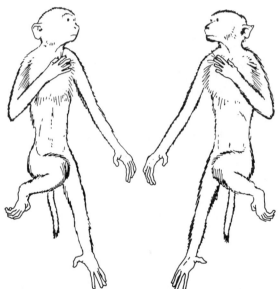

Figure 23–5 Tonic neck reflexes modifying rigidity in the decerebrate monkey preparation. *Upper Figures,* Flexion of head results in flexion of upper extremities. Extension of head results in extension of upper extremities. *Lower Figures,* Rotation of head produces extension of upper limb on side to which face is turned and flexion of contralateral upper limb. Correlated adjustments occur in the lower extremities. (From Twitchell, T. E.: J. Amer. Phys. Ther. Ass., *45:* 413, 1965.)

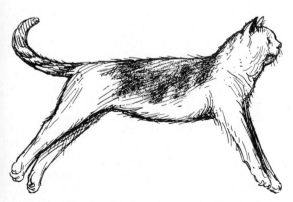

Figure 23–4 The posture of the decerebrate cat when suspended. The hyperextended, rigid posture of neck, back, limbs, and tail is to be noted (opisthotonus). (From Pollack, L. J., and Davis, L.: J. Comp. Neurol., *50:*384, 1930.)

of nerve VIII. These procedures eliminate various labyrinthine influences. The afferents for the tonic neck reflexes are conveyed via the upper cervical dorsal root from joint receptors—for example, those located in the atlanto-occipital joint.

The tonic neck reflexes produce several types of modification of the decerebrate posture. Rotation of the head produces a fencer's posture with extension of the forelimb on the side to which the face (chin, nose, eyes) has rotated with flexion of the forelimb on the contralateral side. Correlated interlimb adjustments may occur in the lower extremities. Extension of the head at the neck produces extension of the forelimbs and flexion of the hindlimbs. One may imagine the posture of a cat who is attempting to look at objects upon a table. Flexion of the head onto the chest produces flexion of the fore-

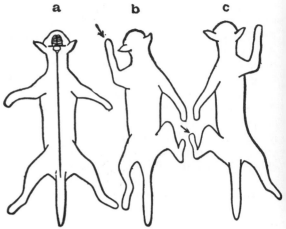

Figure 23–7 Reflex figures in the decerebrate cat preparation. Effects of nociceptive stimulation.
  a. Position under decerebrate rigidity.
  b. Change of attitude from *a* evoked by stimulation of left fore foot.
  c. Change of attitude from *a* evoked by stimulation of left hind foot. (From Sherrington, C. S.: *The Integrative Action of the Nervous System.* New Haven, Yale University Press, 1947, p. 167.)

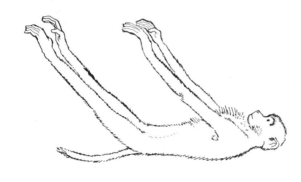

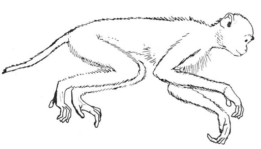

Figure 23–6 Tonic labyrinthine reflexes modifying rigidity in the decerebrate monkey preparation. *Upper Figure,* With the animal held in the supine position and the head facing upwards, the limbs extend. *Lower Figure,* With the animal held in the prone position (face downwards) the limbs flex. It is presumed through this series of maneuvers, that tonic neck influences have been eliminated by immobilization of the neck or by section of the upper cervical dorsal roots.

Note that in man with neurological disease, the opposite pattern may occur so that a flexion posture predominates when the patient is supine and an extensor posture when prone. (From Twitchell, T. E.: J. Amer. Phys. Ther. Ass., *45:* 414, 1965.)

limbs and extension of the hindlimbs. One may imagine the posture of a cat who is attempting to look under a shelf or door.

By Tonic Labyrinthine Reflexes (Fig. 23–6). These tonic labyrinthine reflexes are studied best after the head has been immobilized in a plaster cast or after section of the upper cervical dorsal roots. The afferents are conveyed from the otoliths via the vestibular nerves to the vestibular nuclei. The pattern of postural adjustment which is induced varies in different species. If the cat, dog, or monkey is on his back in a horizontal supine position the extremities are maximally extended. When the animal is turned prone with his snout extended 45 degrees to the horizontal plane, extension is minimal.

By Noxious Stimulus to a Limb (Classic Reflex Figures) (Fig. 23–7). The classic reflex figures are best seen in the decerebrate preparation although they may occur in a high spinal preparation. A noxious stimulus to a hindlimb produces flexion of this limb. In addition, crossed extension of the contralateral hindlimb occurs. At the same time, extension of the ipsilateral forelimb occurs and flexion of the contralateral forelimb. As shown in Figure 23–7, stimulus to a forelimb produces an altered pattern which is consistent with the pattern previously outlined.

One may imagine that the purpose of the reflex figure is to allow the animal to remove the limb stimulated by the nociceptive stimulus from that stimulus. At the same time the animal, by extending the contralateral hindlimb, is able to maintain his upright posture. The adjustments in the forelimb allow the animal to escape from the painful stimulus.

Comparison of Acute Decerebrate Preparation and Spinal Preparation. The decerebrate preparation is capable of a number of responses not noted in the high spinal preparation. In the decerebrate preparation, for example, the animal is capable of swallowing; and there is control of respiration as regards rate and depth, and control of blood pressure. There are a number of significant differences as regards *static reactions*, that is, *postural reflexes*. In this regard, we are concerned primarily with comparisons employing the cat as the spinal or decerebrate preparation.

As regards *local static reactions*, the high spinal animal has stretch reflexes which may be prominent. He has an extensor thrust but has no well-developed support of body parts. In contrast, in the decerebrate preparation there are well-developed, positive supporting reactions sufficient to support the body.

As regards *segmental static reflexes*, the high spinal preparation has crossed extensor reflexes. These are also noted in the decerebrate preparation. As regards *intersegmental reflexes*, fragments of reflex figures are noted in the high spinal preparation. In contrast, reflex figures are well-developed in the decerebrate preparation.

As regards *general static reflexes*, minor fragments of tonic neck reflexes may be noted in the high spinal or bulbospinal preparation. However, in the decerebrate preparation, tonic neck reflexes are well-developed. In addition, tonic labyrinthine reflexes are well-developed. Neither the spinal nor the decerebrate preparation has righting reflexes.

Anatomical Basis of Decerebrate Rigidity (Fig. 23–8). The studies of Sherrington demonstrated that the corticospinal tracts — that is, pyramidal tracts — were not involved in decerebrate rigidity since with hemisection of the brain stem at the intercollicular level the unilateral rigidity which occurred was ipsilateral to the hemisection. Sherrington also was able to indicate that deafferentation decreased rigidity in a limb. Decerebrate

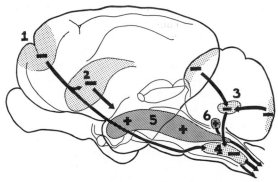

Figure 23–8 Reconstruction of the cat's brain showing the suppressor and facilitatory systems concerned in spasticity. Suppressor pathways are 1, corticobulboreticular; 2, caudatospinal; 3, cerebelloreticular; and 4, reticulospinal. Facilitatory pathways are 5, reticulospinal and 6, vestibulospinal. (From Lindsley, D. B., Schreiner, L. H., and Magoun, H. A.: J. Neurophys., *12*:198, 1949.)

rigidity was conceived to be a release phenomenon.

The studies of Magoun and Rhines (1946) demonstrated that stimulation of the reticular formation in a ventromedial area of the medullary tegmentum produced a decrease in decerebrate rigidity, a decrease in the quadriceps deep tendon reflex, and a decrease in the movement which could be elicited by simultaneously stimulating the motor cortex. This area was labeled the *bulbar reticular inhibitory area.* From an anatomical standpoint the inhibitory area of the medulla corresponds to the nucleus reticularis gigantocellularis. The neurons of this nucleus give rise to the reticulospinal tract which is found in the lateral column of the spinal cord.

In contrast, stimulation of a region of the reticular formation in the pons and midbrain resulted in an increase in the degree of decerebrate rigidity. In addition, the quadriceps deep tendon reflex (the knee jerk) was increased and responses to stimulation of the motor cortex were facilitated. This facilitatory area extends into the subthalamus, the adjacent hypothalamus, and the intralaminar areas of the thalamus (e.g., centrum medianum). This area in the more lateral tegmental reticular formation in the pons and midbrain may be termed a *brain stem* (or *bulbar reticular*) *facilitatory area.* From an anatomical standpoint the facilitatory area of the pons corresponds to the nucleus reticularis pontis oralis and caudalis.* The neurons of this nucleus give rise to that reticulospinal tract found in the anterior column.

It is important to note that the inhibitory area of the medulla is driven from other inhibitory areas. Among these are the anterior portions of the cerebral cortex (the suppressor areas already indicated as areas 4S and 8) and the caudate nucleus. The anterior lobe of the cerebellum also exerts an inhibitory driving influence although it is uncertain whether this cerebellar influence is as significant in primates and man as in the cat. It is now recognized that flexors and extensors are not equally affected by these facilitatory and inhibitory systems. Rather, it is more proper to speak of these areas as bulbar reticular extensor inhibitory area (since actually flexor tone is increased by stimulation of these areas) and bulbar reticular extensor facilitatory area (since flexor tone is decreased by stimulation of this area). In the decerebrate animal the effects of the extensor facilitatory system predominate because the extensor inhibitory system must be driven from higher centers. These higher centers, of course, are disconnected from the inhibitory area in the brain stem by the section through the brain stem. On the other hand, the facilitatory center is driven by afferent inputs from below, that is, the collaterals of ascending sensory fibers (refer to Fig. 23–8) derived from the spinothalamic tracts and the trigeminal system.

These brain stem reticular areas give rise to reticulospinal pathways which descend to the spinal cord level to influence stretch reflexes. In addition, vestibular centers give rise to facilitatory vestibulospinal pathways which may also influence to some degree stretch reflexes.

As regards the effects of these brain stem reticular centers on stretch reflexes, one may postulate two possible mechanisms of action. There might well be a facilitation or inhibition of large alpha motor neurons. On the other hand, these centers might exert their effects through a facilitation or inhibi-

tion of the small gamma neurons. This latter situation would alter tension on the spindle and change the rate of discharge of the muscle spindle.

Granit and Kaada have demonstrated that stimulation of the facilitatory area did augment the spindle discharge. Stimulation of the inhibitory area reduced the spindle discharge. Both effects, then, were exerted via the gamma system. Classic decerebrate rigidity may be considered essentially "*gamma rigidity.*"

Alpha rigidity is less common and results when the cerebellum, particularly the anterior cerebellum, is destroyed in the decerebrate preparation (anemic decerebrate preparation) produced by vascular occlusion. The facilitatory effect may be exerted on the alpha motor neuron by the vestibulospinal tract. There is some evidence that although alpha rigidity may occur in the cat, this is probably not a significant form of rigidity in the primate or in man.

THE CHRONIC DECEREBRATE PREPARATION

Much of the information concerning decerebrate preparation and many of our concepts of the decerebrate preparation are based on observation of the acute animal. It is evident, however, that when the decerebration is performed under aseptic conditions and the animal is allowed to survive for several days, significant changes occur. The degree of rigidity decreases and the animal begins to show righting reflexes. Thus, in a *pontine decerebrate preparation* at 7 to 10 days one notes that the animal begins to right its head in response to a nociceptive stimulus. At 17 days after section the animal rights the shoulder and responds to a nociceptive stimulus and shows some hopping and proprioceptive placing although these are poorly executed. If one studies the *intercollicular preparation* one finds that at 7 to 14 days with a nociceptive stimulus the animal will right, that is, change from a position on the side to a crouching position. At a later time the animal will right spontaneously. This then indicates a modulation of the proprioceptive stretch reflexes by the effects of asymmetrical cutaneous and subcutaneous tactile and pressure stimuli. An intercollicular preparation, at a later point, when provided with a sufficiently strong stimulus, will not only right but will show some walking activity.

---

*As discussed previously (p. 290), the nucleus gigantocellularis and the nucleus reticularis pontis oralis and caudalis may be considered as a relatively continuous cell column within the reticular formation, with a major role in reticulospinal motor activities. The other major cell groupings are the paramedian cell groups (paramedian reticular nuclei and reticulotegmental nucleus) concerned with cerebellar relationships and the lateral reticular nucleus. This lateral area of reticular formation is the major relay area for afferent collateral input to the reticular formation.

THE MIDBRAIN PREPARATION

As previously indicated, this preparation is produced by a section above the level of the red nucleus. Usually included within the brain stem are small amounts of the sub-thalamus and posterior hypothalamus. In this preparation there is noted a definite *modification of proprioceptive reactions triggered by contactual stimuli.* In the cat or dog midbrain preparation, although there is some increase in extensor tone, the animal lacks the marked extensor rigidity seen in the decerebrate preparation. The various local static and segmental static reactions already discussed with regard to decerebrate preparation are also noted in the midbrain preparation. There are, however, several general static reactions in the midbrain preparation not noted in the acute decerebrate preparation although fragments of righting reflexes are noted in the chronic decerebrate preparation.

Righting Reflexes. It is perhaps appropriate at this time to discuss in a general sense the righting reflexes which are found in the intact animal (Figs. 23-9 and 23-10). First let us consider a situation in an intact, blindfolded animal dropped from a position upside down in midair several feet above the ground. The righting reflexes to be noted in this animal will also be found in the midbrain preparation. Initially, the head rotates because of labyrinthine influences (termed the *labyrinthine righting reflex*). Then, because of *neck righting reflexes* there is a rotation of the upper body to align with the altered position of the head. There is then a rotation of the lower body to align with the altered rotated position of the upper portion of the body. We may term this a *body righting reflex* acting on the body. Finally, the animal will manifest certain reflex responses to labyrinthine acceleration, *the vestibular placing response,* that is, the four limbs are extended as the animal descends, ready to place the paws of these limbs on the expected surfaces.

The situation noted in a nonblindfolded, intact animal would be relatively similar. However, there would also be the possibility of the visual placing reaction as the animal comes close to the surface and is able to make use of visual cues. Moreover, at the onset, the optical righting reflex would also be intact. These visual reactions would not be present in the midbrain preparation.

Now let us consider the situation of righting reflexes in an intact but blindfolded animal,

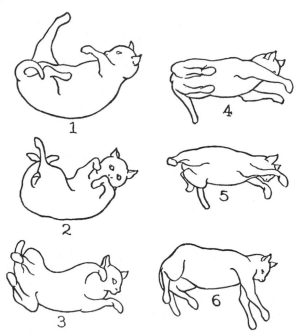

Figure 23–9 Righting reflexes in intact cat. Diagram showing series of maneuvers which a cat executes in order to turn itself in the air: 1, free fall; 2, head turns, forelimbs drawn in, hindlimbs extended; 3, 4, 5, continued turning with gradual extension of forelimbs while hindlimbs are drawn closer to axis of rotation; 6, turning completed. (Redrawn from Marey, C. R. *Acad. Sci. Paris,* 1894, *119*:714–717: From Fulton, J. F.: *A Textbook of Physiology,* 17th Edition. Philadelphia, W. B. Saunders, 1955, p. 221.)

recumbent on its side. These same responses would also be noted in a midbrain cat preparation. Initially, the head rotates to a horizontal position as a result of labyrinthine righting reflexes. This righting of the head will occur even if the body contact is symmetrical; that is, if one placed a board on the upright side of the cat to counteract the tactile stimuli delivered to the undersurface in contact with the table counter. In addition, there is in this situation, a *body-on-head righting reflex.* Thus, if the labyrinths are destroyed and the body contact is asymmetrical, i.e., the animal is in contact only on one side (the undersurface), the head tends to right and to be held upright. In the intact, blindfolded preparation, of course, the righting of the head is produced both by labyrinthine influences and by the asymmetrical body contact. In any case, turning of the head, as previously discussed, stimulates the neck muscle proprioceptors and joint receptors. The body, then, tends to be brought into a hori-

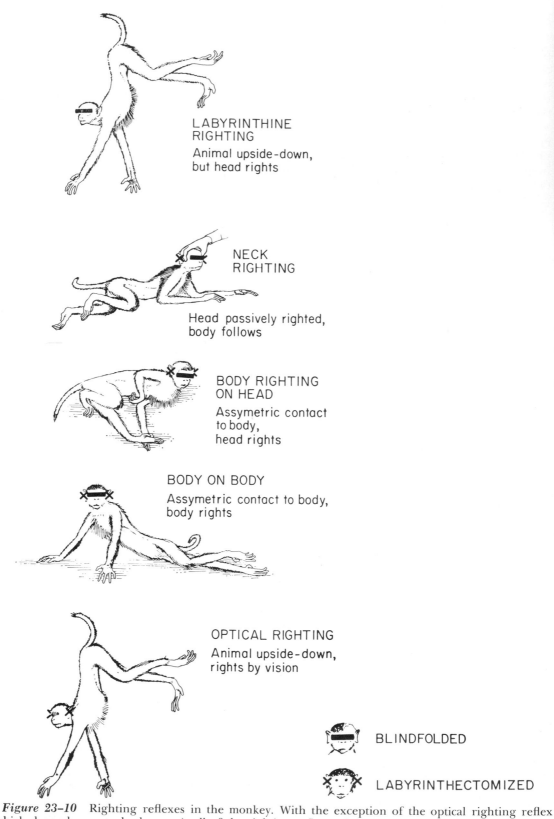

LABYRINTHINE RIGHTING
Animal upside-down, but head rights

NECK RIGHTING
Head passively righted, body follows

BODY RIGHTING ON HEAD
Assymetric contact to body, head rights

BODY ON BODY
Assymetric contact to body, body rights

OPTICAL RIGHTING
Animal upside-down, rights by vision

BLINDFOLDED

LABYRINTHECTOMIZED

Figure 23–10 Righting reflexes in the monkey. With the exception of the optical righting reflex (which depends on cerebral cortex), all of the righting reflexes demonstrated above are within the capacity of the midbrain preparation. (From Twitchell, T. E.: J. Amer. Phys. Ther. Ass., *45*:415, 1965.)

zontal position. This may be termed the *neck righting reflex*. Other righting reflexes also act on the body. Thus, asymmetrical contact or pressure to the upper half of the body—for example, the shoulders—leads to righting of the lower half. We may term these *body righting reflexes acting on the body.*

Kinetic Reactions. The midbrain cat preparation not only manifests righting reflexes but also shows kinetic reactions. The preparation can stand "spontaneously" and walk "spontaneously." This may require several days of recovery and is much better developed if the subthalamus is also intact. The overall activity of the midbrain preparation is often subject to marked swings. Thus, one may find that after a prolonged period of relative immobility in a specific posture, the animal spontaneously stands and begins to walk. He often continues to walk even though he encounters a wall. He then shows in a sense an obstinate progression.

Primate Midbrain Preparation. The capacities for the midbrain preparation previously discussed refer primarily to the cat and the dog. In the primate midbrain preparation (this applies also to the decorticate or "thalamic primate"), although some body contact righting occurs, one finds that the animal is unable to stand. In the primate, asymmetrical body contact produces flexion in the uppermost fore and hind limb. There are, then, fragments of righting (Fig. 23-11). In addition there is seen in the midbrain primate a response which occurs when the

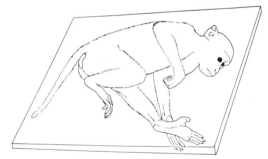

Figure 23–11 The "thalamic" reflex pattern. This posture may also be noted in the midbrain primate or decorticate primate preparation. The actual preparation illustrated has undergone bilateral removal of motor and premotor cerebral cortex. Note that the lowermost extremities are extended and the uppermost flexed. When the animal is turned over, the condition reverses itself. (From Breber, I., and Fulton, J. F., Arch. Neurol. Psychiat., *39*:448, 1938.)

adductors of the shoulders have been stretched by pulling up on the hand. This results in an adduction at the shoulder; in most cases, with flexion at the elbow, wrist, and fingers. The synergistic flexion is called the *traction response.* Fragments of this traction response may also occur in the chronic decerebrate primate preparation. Refinements of the traction response will be noted at higher levels and termed the *tonic grasp reflex* and the *instinctual grasp response.* In man, the midbrain preparation usually reflects severe bilateral damage to the cerebral cortex and cerebral hemispheres as in anoxia, cardiac arrest, and carbon monoxide poisoning.

The Hypothalamus. The hypothalamus, when included within the brain stem, in continuity with the descending neural axis provides little additional motor capacity. Bard has shown that the integrity of the hypothalamus is essential for the sham-rage reaction of the decorticate animal. It should be noted, however, that the actual motor responses for rage are represented at the brain stem levels. Thus, Graham-Brown and Sherrington had previously demonstrated that stimulation of a point on the cut surface of the decerebrate cat midbrain (that portion of the midbrain distal to the section) produced a reflex imitation of anger: lashing of the tail, protrusion of the claws, piloerection, and an increase in the arterial pressure.

THE DECORTICATE OR THALAMIC PREPARATION

The cat or dog, following decortication, acts similar to the midbrain preparation except that the intact subthalamus provides for more regular righting. In the primate, reflex capacities of the decorticate preparation extend beyond those noted at the midbrain level. Thus, a tonic grasp reflex may be noted (sometimes referred to simply as the grasp reflex). This reflex is elicited by a tactile stimulus to the palmar surface, most prominently to the first interosseous space. A rapid flexion of the fingers results. As the stimulus continues to move across the palm and encounters the flexed fingers, stretch of these flexed fingers results which then triggers proprioceptive traction response previously described under the traction response ("traction grasp"). The tonic grasp reflex is often long-lasting.

The decorticate preparation may also show

the *tonic avoiding response*. In this case, a contactual stimulus to the palm or outer border of the hands results in an abduction of the hand and arm with spreading of the fingers. In the decorticate preparation this is a tonic response—that is, long-lasting. The decorticate preparation lacks the reaction listed below under the animal with intact cerebral cortex. It should be noted that the decorticate primate or human manifests often a considerable degree of spasticity, often referred to as decorticate rigidity (refer to Fig. 23–12). The decorticate posture involves extension of the lower extremities and flexion of the upper extremities. In a sense this is a double hemiplegic posture. The decorticate primate or human is not capable of walking. We should note that the decorticate cat and dog are capable of such activities.*

REACTIONS DEPENDENT ON CEREBRAL CORTEX

The cerebral cortex analyzes afferent information from many sources and utilizes

---

*This is not to imply that the walking of the decorticate cat and dog is identical to that of the intact animal. Particular defects are noted in the placing of the paws of the forelimbs upon the floor as the animal progresses.

reactions which have been integrated at lower levels of the neural axis.

The cerebral cortex may be considered as providing for a more complex reaction to the external environment. Thus, the presence of the cerebral cortex allows for the projection of the limb in space and for the interaction of various reflex activities with visual and tactile stimuli. The *optical righting reflex* results in the righting of the head in relation to a visual stimulus. This response occurs after elimination of the labyrinths and dorsal roots from the upper cervical neck proprioceptors. The response can still be demonstrated after bilateral ablation of the motor and premotor areas in the primate. We should, of course, note that righting of the head when the head has been turned on to the side is dependent not only on visual cues but on labyrinthine cues and asymmetrical body contact stimuli.

A number of *placing reactions* are also noted in the intact animal. When the animal approaches a visible edge, the forelimb is advanced to be placed on the surface. This is termed the *visual placing reaction*. On the other hand, if the animal is blindfolded and the dorsum of the foot or hand touches the edge of a surface, appropriate adjustments are then made to place the plantar or palmar surface of the extremity on the surface. This is termed the *tactile placing reaction*. Also

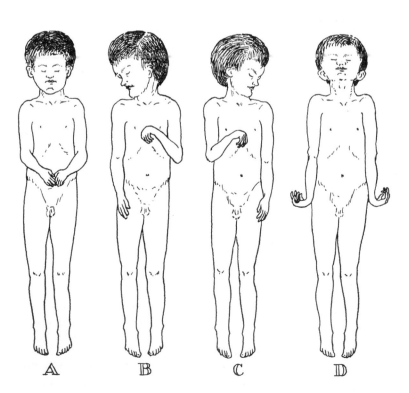

Figure 23–12 Decorticate rigidity in the human. Diagram illustrating differences in man between decorticate rigidity (*A*) and true decerebrate rigidity (*D*). *A*, lying prone with head unturned; note that both forelimbs are flexed. *B* and *C*, note changes of position with head turning. *D*, true decerebrate rigidity in man with arms rigidly extended and pronated. Effects of tonic neck reflexes on decorticate rigidity *B* and *C*. (From Fulton, J. F., *A Textbook of Physiology*. Philadelphia, W. B. Saunders, 1955, p. 217.)

A   B   C   D

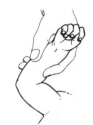

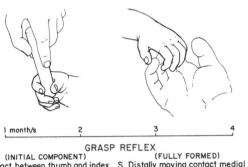

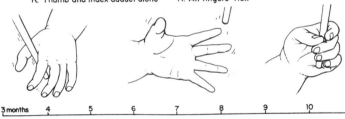

AT BIRTH
TRACTION RESPONSE
Stimulus: Stretch shoulder adductors and flexors
Response: All joints flex

Figure 23–13 Evolution of the automatic grasping responses of infants. (From Twitchell, T. E., Neuropsychologia, *3*:251, 1965.)

1 month/s   2   3   4

GRASP REFLEX
(INITIAL COMPONENT)   (FULLY FORMED)
S. Contact between thumb and index   S. Distally moving contact medial palm
R. Thumb and index adduct alone   R. All fingers flex

3 months   4   5   6   7   8   9   10   11

INSTINCTIVE GRASP REACTION
S. Contact radial or ulnar side   S. Contact hand (any part)   S. Contact hand (any part)
R. Hand orients   R. Hand gropes   R. Hand grasps

noted in the intact preparation is a *hopping response*. If the animal's body is displaced to one side, the animal abducts the leg to that side to regain stability.

The instinctive tactile grasping reaction (Fig. 23-13) is triggered by a tactile (or contactual) stimulus to the hand. The hand orients so as to grasp the object. Often the hand follows a moving object making moment-to-moment adjustments so as to grasp onto the object. This instinctive tactile grasping reaction provides for the exploration by the hand directed in space. The instinctive tactile grasping reaction is, of course, seen normally when the intact individual attempts to grasp onto an object. It is not surprising that intact motor and parietal cortex is required. The movements involve distal finger and thumb movement and require precise feed-back information.

At times, however, the reaction is seen to be released in abnormal form and degree and to occur in a context where voluntary grasping is not desired. It is found that these patients usually have damage to the premotor cortex (areas 6 and 8) and the adjacent supplementary motor cortex and cingulate area on the medial surface of the hemisphere. The instinctive tactile grasp reaction, then, although requiring an intact motor and parietal cortex is released in an abnormal form by lesions of the premotor, supplementary motor, and cingulate areas. This is a form of transcortical release. The same lesion, of course, also acts to release various subcortical areas.

The instinctive tactile grasp reaction is to be compared to the *instinctive tactile avoiding reaction* (Fig. 23-14). The stimulus for this reaction is a distally moving tactile stimulus to the outer (ulnar) border of the hand or to the palmar surface of the hand or to the dorsum of the hand. This stimulus leads to a nontonic orientation of the hand away from the stimulus. This is a more precise form of the tonic avoiding response noted in a decorticate preparation. The instinctive tactile avoiding response does not require the pyramidal system. The integrity of the cingulate area, area 8, and the supplementary motor cortex are required. The reaction is released in abnormal degree by damage to the parietal lobe (and adjacent motor cortex). (Various avoiding reactions are noted in Fig. 23-14.) The instinctive grasp and avoidance responses normally are in equilibrium from an anatomical and physiological standpoint.

In addition to these tactile instinctive grasp and instinctive avoiding responses, various

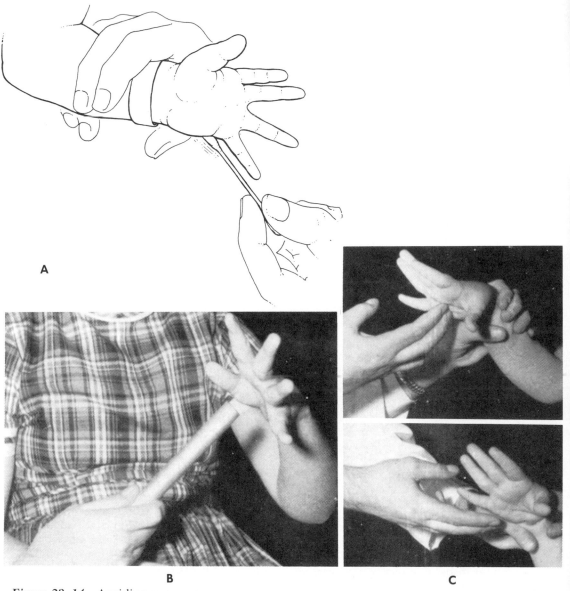

A

B

C

Figure 23–14 Avoiding responses.

A, Elicitation of the avoiding response by contact stimulus of ulnar border of hand as normal response in infant of 4 to 6 weeks. (From Twitchell, T. E.: Neuropsychologia, *3*:250, 1965.)

B, Avoiding response as a pathological phenomenon. Overextension and abduction of fingers as hand approaches object. (Child with infantile spastic hemiparesis.)

C, Avoiding response as a pathological phenomenon in another patient with infantile spastic hemiparesis. Reaction of hand to contact stimulation of the palm. (*B* and *C* from Twitchell, T. E.: Neurology, *8*:17, 1958.)

visual triggered responses of a similar nature may be seen. One may speak of a visual instinctive grasp reaction. This requires the integrity of the posterior parietal areas, the visual mechanisms, and the motor cortex. Damage to the temporal lobe releases this reaction in an abnormal form. The response does occur, of course, in a normal form as one normally reaches for an object, using visual stimuli. The reaction as we have indicated is released by a lesion of the temporal lobe. This type of phenomenon occurred in the Klüver-Bucy syndrome which followed the production of bilateral lesions of the temporal lobe in the monkey. The release of various visual automatisms occurred. The animals tended to pick up all objects which appeared in their field of vision and to bring these objects to their mouth.*

Another variety of visually cued reaction is the *visual instinctive avoiding reaction.* This requires the integrity of the temporal lobe and visual mechanisms. The response apparently is independent of the pyramidal system. Again, in the intact individual, an equilibrium of grasp and avoidance is to be noted.

ABLATION OF PRECENTRAL CORTEX: PATTERN OF RECOVERY

Many aspects of the integration of reflex activity at successive levels of the neural axis are illustrated if the recovery from ablation of the motor cortex is studied.

Monkey. Complete ablation of the precentral gyrus in the monkey, to include all of the area 4 motor cortex, results in an immediate flaccid hemiplegia involving the contralateral lower half of the face and the arm and the leg. The weakness of the hip muscles is only partial. Within hours the animal begins to use the proximal muscles of the lower limb. Within 2 to 3 days the affected arm is used in climbing if the animal is frightened. The hand and foot are hooked onto the cage wire. At this time also, recovery from cortical shock is indicated by the fact that deep tendon reflexes are becoming more active.

*As discussed previously in Chapter 21, page 522, such a lesion (particularly when inferior and middle temporal gyri are involved) serves to disconnect the visual association areas from the hippocampal (limbic) areas. A marked disruption of visual discrimination results, particularly as regards the relation of visual stimuli to various motivations relevant to the limbic system.

Within 1 to 2 additional weeks, a traction grasp reaction is noted. At approximately 1 week, spasticity in the flexors of the upper limb and the extensors of the lower limb appears. In the lower limb the appearance of the traction response is associated with a positive support reaction. In the upper limb the return of extensor posture is delayed so that the end result at this time is a typical hemiplegic posture with flexion of the upper extremities and extension of the lower extremities. In addition, there is external rotation at the hip in the lower extremity.

Within 2 to 3 additional days, with a strong stimulus, and the other limbs restrained, the animal will make gross movements of the limb to bring the object to the mouth. This movement is facilitated by turning the neck. The animal soon learns to utilize these tonic neck responses. At the same time, one might also note that the traction grasp can be facilitated by placing the animal on his side. This triggers body contact reflexes with an increasing flexion of the uppermost limbs as noted in Figure 23-11.

The true grasp reflex does not appear for several weeks. This reflex is triggered by a moving tactile stimulus. Its appearance is soon associated with some measure of ability to flex the wrist or fingers independently of the proximal joints. (It should be noted that of course the traction response involves a synergistic movement of all of these joints.) After some moves the hand may close in response to a simple coarse contact but it does not make any orienting response to the stimulus, that is, the instinctive tactile grasp reaction does not return. Though the hand closes on a stimulus object it does not make the moment-to-moment adjustments to follow the stimulus object.

Eventually, the thumb may be approximated to the other fingers, but never to the extent possible prior to the ablation. With the appearance of the true grasp reflex, spasticity, especially in the flexors of the fingers and toes, lessens considerably. It should be noted that with complete ablation of the precentral motor cortex the instinctive tactile grasp reaction never recovers.

Man. A similar sequence of recovery of voluntary movement in hemiplegia in man has been found by Twitchell following partial precentral or capsular lesions. The sequence varies slightly from that noted in the monkey. Initially flaccidity is present in the contralateral arm and leg. This soon gives way to a return of deep tendon reflexes and to the appearance of spasticity.

It should be noted that in man, following massive lesions of the motor cortex, a long delay may occur before spasticity develops and deep tendon reflexes return. Such a long delay in the reappearance of stretch reflexes usually signifies a poor prognosis for complete recovery. Following the return of stretch reflexes, variation in the relative degree of spasticity in the flexor and extensor muscles in relation to tonic neck reflexes may be noted. With the return of tonic neck reflexes one will begin to note proximal limb movements. The next stage of recovery involves the return of the traction response. Abduction of the arm and shoulder will result in stretch of the adductors. There will then be an adduction of the arm at the shoulder. In addition, synergistic flexion of the arm at the elbow, wrist, and fingers will occur, and objects may be grasped in this manner. This flexion synergy, however, results in a whole hand grasp; all of the fingers flex together.

The next stage of recovery involves a more selective grasp of the entire hand albeit a tonic grasp. There is some dissociated synergy so that the hand alone tends to grasp. Finger and thumb opposition begin to return. The next stage of recovery relates to the return of the instinctive tactile grasp reaction with the capacity of projective movement. It should be noted that for a return of instinctive grasp reaction to occur the destruction of motor cortex must not be complete; rather, the lesion must have been a partial lesion.

From a physiological and anatomical standpoint, the logic of this pattern of recovery should be evident. One sees in this sequence a recovery of spinal reflex activities and of brain stem reflex activities as noted in the decerebrate preparation, then of activities noted in the midbrain preparation, then those noted in the decorticate preparation, and finally those reflexes integrated at a cortical level.

Postnatal Development of Motor Reflexes. A similar sequence of reflex activities is noted in the developing human infant as regards the use of hands and fingers (Fig. 23-13). Thus, a traction response with brief holding of objects may be noted at birth. At 4 to 8 weeks, one sees a grasp reflex involving a contactual stimulus with a palmar grasp and brief holding. All the fingers, however, tend to flex as a unit. The next stage of development is that of the instinctive grasp reaction. This results in a projected grasp of objects. The instinctive grasp reaction initially involves all the fingers and the thumbs and is noted at 4 to 5 months. With increasing development, one finds at 6 to 8 months of age a projected grasp of objects in the form of a pincer grasp. There is a fractionation of finger movement with thumb and finger opposition, and soon a voluntary control of the grasp reflex is attained.

It should be noted that the newborn infant also shows tonic neck reflexes and these may be prominent for several weeks after birth. By 3 to 4 months of age, however, it is unusual to find that tonic neck reflexes are still persistent.

As regards other relatively gross developmental motor landmarks, we may note that normally an infant sits unsupported at 6 to 7 months, stands with support at 8 to 9 months, and walks with support at 10 to 11 months. By 12 months the infant walks by himself.

THE PYRAMIDAL TRACT

We have previously indicated that the student should consider as the primary manifestations of an upper motor neuron lesion a spastic paralysis with increased deep tendon reflexes and the sign of Babinski. A more detailed analysis indicates that the effects of selective pyramidal tract damage are not quite the same or equivalent to those which follow, in a general sense, upper motor neuron lesions. We should note that section of the pyramidal tract in the medullary pyramid or in the cerebral peduncle does not have the same anatomical and physiological effects as ablation of the motor cortex, which has been previously summarized. We should note that the ablation of the motor cortex destroys not only the origin of the pyramidal tract (the corticospinal tract) but also the origin of the corticoreticular, the corticorubral, the corticothalamic, and the corticostriatal fibers. The effects of such a cortical ablation are to release these various brain stem centers from cortical control and to produce the effects of damage to the corticospinal tract.

We should also note that selective section of the pyramidal tract or cerebral peduncle may yield different effects than section of the lateral column in the spinal cord. The descending rubrospinal and the lateral reticulospinal tract (from the bulbar inhibitory center of the medulla) are closely related to the corticospinal tract in the lateral column. We should note that the medial reticulospinal tract from the pontine extensor facilitatory center descends in the anterior column and thus would be left undamaged by a lesion of the lateral column.

The studies of Bucy suggest that both man and the monkey are capable of useful movements after section of the pyramidal tract in the cerebral peduncle. Thus, locomotor abilities returned. The monkey could use his hand in feeding and in manipulating small objects. With bilateral section, however, the hand was used as a claw with some deficiency in independent finger movements. It should be stressed that spasticity and increased deep tendon reflexes were not noted. The sign of Babinski was found in the human patient. In the human patient the retention of discrete finger movements was remarkable.

Somewhat different results were obtained by Denny-Brown following section of the pyramidal tract in the medullary pyramid. There was a moderate increase of deep tendon reflexes and a mild spasticity. What was clearly defective after section was the discrete fractionated distal finger movements required for the instinctive tactile grasp reaction that allowed the precise orientation of fingers to a moving three-dimensional stimulus. We should note that the pyramidal tract fibers mediating cortical control of these distal muscles make direct connection to the anterior horn cell. These direct fibers of the corticospinal system elicit predominantly flexor facilitation and extensor inhibition. In contrast, the indirect corticospinal fibers (those which do not synapse directly on anterior horn cells) synapse predominantly in relation to interneurons which make synaptic contact with anterior horn cells innervating more proximal muscles.*

CORTICORUBRAL SPINAL SYSTEM

In the monkey and cat, if the pyramidal tracts are intact, destruction of the rubral spinal system produces no definite motor deficit. However, in monkeys and cats who have already had bilateral section of the pyramidal tract (a section which has produced very little qualitative change in limb movement) a complete loss of distal limb movement may occur after additional bilateral destruction of the rubrospinal tract.

In the intact monkey, complex coordinated movements may be evoked by stimulation of the red nucleus. Flexor excitation predominates with extensor inhibition.

References

Motor System

Bizzi, E., and Evarts, E. V.: Translational mechanisms between input and output. Neurosciences Research Program Bulletin, 9:31–59, 1971.

Bucy, D. C., Ladpli, R., and Ehrlich, A.: Destruction of the pyramidal tract in the monkey. J. Neurophysiol., 25:1–20, 1966.

Burke, R. E.: Control systems operating on spinal reflex mechanisms. Neurosciences Research Program Bulletin, 9:60–85, 1971.

DeLong, M.: Central patterning of movement. Neurosciences Research Program Bulletin, 9:10–30, 1971.

Denny-Brown, D.: Motor mechanism introduction, the general principles of motor integration. *Handbook of Physiology*, Section 1, Neurophysiol., 2:781–796, Washington, D.C., American Physiological Society, 1960. (Should be read by all students.)

Denny-Brown, D.: The midbrain and motor integration (Sherrington Memorial Lecture). Proc. Roy. Soc. Med., 55:527–538, July 1962.

Denny-Brown, D.: *The Cerebral Control of Movement*, Springfield, Ill., Charles C Thomas, 1966.

Eldred, E., and Buchwald, J.: Central nervous system motor mechanisms. Ann. Rev. Physiol., 29:573–606, 1967.

Fulton, J. F.: *Physiology of the Nervous System*, 3rd Edition. New York, Oxford University Press, 1951.

Granit, R., and Kaada, B. R.: Influence of stimulation of central nervous structures on muscle spindle in cat. Acta physiol. Scand., 27:130–160, 1952.

Landau, W. M.: Spasticity and rigidity. *In* Plum, F. (ed.): *Recent Advances in Neurology.* Philadelphia, F. A. Davis, 1969, pp. 1–32.

Magoun, H. W., and Rhines, R.: An inhibitory mechanism in the bulbar reticular formation. J. Neurophysiol., 9:161–171, 1946.

McCulloch, W. S., Graf, C., and Magoun, H. W.: A cortical bulbar reticular pathway from area 4S. J. Neurophysiol., 9:127–132, 1946.

Rhines, R., and Magoun, H. W.: Brain stem facilitation of cortical motor response. J. Neurophysiol., 9:219–229, 1946.

Ruch, T. C.: Transection of Spinal Cord (Chapter 8), and Pontobulbar Control of Posture and Orientation in Space (Chapter 9), pp. 207–214, 215–225. *In* Ruch, T. C., and Patton, H. D. (Eds.): *Physiology and Biophysics*, Philadelphia, W. B. Saunders, 1965. (Should be read by all students. Some may wish to read Chapters 6 and 7 on Spinal Reflexes and Synaptic Transmission, pp. 153–180, 181–206.)

---

*We have not considered in our discussion the possible role of the pyramidal tract in modifying transmission of sensory information at the spinal cord (posterior horn) and brain stem levels (nucleus gracilis and nucleus cuneatus). The various recent studies which have suggested such a role are considered in the review of Bizzi and Evarts (1971).

Rushworth, G.: Muscle tone and the muscle spindle in clinical neurology. Mod. Trends in Neurol., *3*:36–56, 1962.

Sherrington, C.: *The Integrative Action of the Nervous System.* New Haven, Yale University Press, 1947.

Twitchell, T. E.:* The restoration of motor function following hemiplegia in man. Brain, *74*:443–480, 1951.

Twitchell, T. E.: The grasping deficit in infantile spastic hemiparesis, Neurol., *8*:13–21, 1958.

Twitchell, T. E.: Attitudinal Reflexes, J. Amer. Phys. Ther. Ass., *45*:411–418, 1965. (Should be read by all students.)

Twitchell, T. E.: The automatic grasping responses of infants. Neuropsychologia, *3*:247–259, 1965.

Twitchell, T. E.: Mechanisms for Motor Recovery Following Cerebral Lesions. *Conference on Mechanisms in Restitution of Function After Brain Damage Proceedings.,* 1966, NINDB, Bethesda.

*The author wishes to gratefully acknowledge the advice of Dr. Thomas Twitchell in the preparation of this chapter.

24

The Relationship of the Basal Ganglia to Movement

ELLIOTT M. MARCUS

ANATOMICAL BACKGROUND

The term "basal ganglia" originally included the caudate and lenticular nuclei and the claustrum. As additional studies of these nuclei and of their connections have been undertaken, additional structures have been included within this anatomical group: the substantia nigra, the subthalamic nucleus, the red nucleus, and the ventrolateral and ventral anterior nuclei of the thalamus. The *lenticular nucleus* is composed of the putamen and the globus pallidus. The putamen actually, as we have noted previously, has the same structure as the caudate nucleus and the two are often grouped together as the *striatum*. The caudate, putamen, and globus pallidus are often grouped together as the *corpus striatum*.*

The known anatomical circuits involving these various nuclei of the basal ganglia must be reviewed since these provide a clear suggestion as to the role of the basal ganglia as a complex feedback circuit which modifies movement. (Refer to Figures 17–12, 13 and 14, pages 406 and 407.) In a sense, these circuits provide a somewhat circuitous loop, off the main high-speed highway.†

It is important to note that we study the functions of the basal ganglia primarily in terms of the dysfunction of the basal ganglia. It is easier to talk of the relationship between a particular abnormality of movement and a particular portion of the basal ganglia than it is to speak in terms of the known function of that area as regards movement. We should note that the effects of dysfunction of the basal ganglia are expressed via the motor cortex. It is not surprising then, that surgical section of the major pathway from the motor cortex (the pyramidal tract) in the cerebral peduncle will often eliminate certain disorders of movement.

It should be noted that the nuclei of the basal ganglia, the circuits involving the basal ganglia, the cortical areas projecting to the basal ganglia, the cerebellar nuclei relating to the basal ganglia, and the reticular formation (which has connections with both the cortex and the basal ganglia) are often grouped together as an extrapyramidal system. It is important to note, however, that

---

*The caudate nucleus and putamen are sometimes referred to as the neostriatum. The globus pallidus is sometimes termed the paleostriatum, and the amygdala, the archistriatum.

†For a detailed discussion of the basic neuroanatomy refer to Nauta and Mehler (1966) and Haymaker, Mehler, and Schiller (1969).

the cortical areas giving rise to this extra-pyramidal system are also, in large part, the same areas giving rise to the pyramidal system.

The major input into the basal ganglia enters the *caudate nucleus* and *putamen.* This input arises from the cerebral cortex, primarily from the premotor and motor cortices (areas 8, 6, and 4). However, the projection from the neocortex occurs from many other areas. In general, precentral, frontal, and occipital areas project to the caudate nucleus. Temporal and parietal areas project to the putamen.

The major outflow from the caudate-putamen passes to the *globus pallidus.* There is a lesser outflow of fibers from the striatum to the substantia nigra, but the major outflow, however, is to the inner segment of the globus pallidus. From the inner segment of the globus pallidus the major outflow is to the ventrolateral nucleus of the thalamus and to a lesser extent the ventral anterior nucleus of the thalamus.

This outflow passes via two fiber systems: the fasciculus lenticularis and the ansa lenticularis. The fasciculus lenticularis penetrates through the posterior limb of the internal capsule; the ansa lenticularis loops around the undersurface of the most inferior part of the internal capsule and then passes upward to join the fasciculus lenticularis (Fig. 24–1).

These two fiber systems join at a point known as the Field H_2 of Forel, then curve back towards the thalamus in the Field H_1 of Forel where they are known as the thalamic fasciculus. This fasciculus then enters the ventrolateral and ventral anterior nuclei of the thalamus. The major projection of the ventrolateral and ventral anterior nuclei of the thalamus, as we have noted previously, is to the motor and premotor cerebral cortex. This, then, completes the loop: cerebral cortex to striatum to globus pallidus to ventrolateral and ventral anterior thalamus back to premotor and motor cortex.

Several additional loops and connections must now be considered. In addition to its major input from the cerebral cortex, the caudate-putamen also receives a lesser afferent input from the nucleus centrum medianum (C.M.). It should be noted that the C.M. represents a major interlaminar nucleus of the thalamus and is the main thalamic extension of the ascending reticular formation.

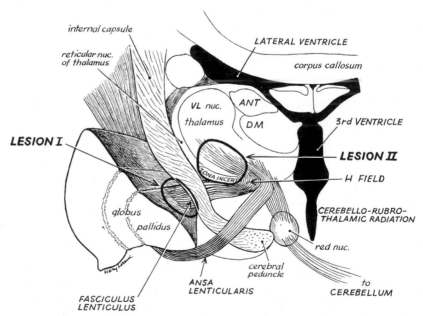

Figure 24–1 Major connections of the basal ganglia with sites of surgical lesions for the relief of resting tremor. The fasciculus lenticularis and the ansa lenticularis join at the field of Forel (H field), then curve back toward the ventral lateral nucleus of the thalamus at the field H_2 of Forel as the thalamic fasciculus. (From Lin, F. H., Okumura, S., and Cooper, I. S.: Electroenceph. clin. Neurophysiol., *13*:633, 1961.)

The centrum medianum, however, also receives fibers from the globus pallidus and from the precentral motor cortex.

It should also be noted that some fibers leave the ansa lenticularis and, rather than passing into the thalamus, descend to nuclei within the tegmentum of the mesencephalon and pons, constituting the rostral reticular formation (an area giving rise to a reticulo-spinal pathway). Some fibers also apparently descend via the central tegmental tract to the inferior olivary nucleus. There is, then, another loop involving the motor cortex, the basal ganglia, the reticular formation, and the centrum medianum of the thalamus.

An additional small loop may be identified in the sense that some fibers leave the lateral globus pallidus and pass to the subthalamic nucleus. The major outflow from the subthalamic nucleus is back to the medial sector of the globus pallidus.

We have already indicated that, although the major outflow of the striatum is to the globus pallidus, some fibers leave this fiber system and end in the substantia nigra. The major efferent pathway from the substantia nigra is to the ventrolateral nucleus and to the ventral anterior nucleus of the thalamus. There is, however, also considerable evidence that some of the cells in the substantia nigra project to the striatum.

These pathways involve the neurotransmitter, dopamine (dihydroxyphenylethylamine). There is a high content of dopamine in the substantia nigra and a high content of this transmitter also in the caudate nucleus and putamen. The caudate nucleus, however, also contains particularly high levels of acetylcholine, cholineacetylase and acetylcholine esterase.

Spontaneous release of acetylcholine from the caudate can be enhanced by stimulating the thalamic nuclei as well as the anterior (motor) portion of cerebral cortex — for example, the anterior sigmoid cortex in the cat. Some of these acetylcholine esterase-containing fibers, however, apparently also originate in the tegmentum of the mesencephalic reticular formation.

There is considerable evidence that the dopamine-containing terminals and their related synapses and the cholinergic synapses in the caudate are essentially antagonistic. Normally, however, they remain in a particular balance. We will discuss the problem of an imbalance when we come to discuss Parkinson's disease (Duvoisin, 1967; Hornykiewicz, 1970).

In considering the basal ganglia-thalamic-cortical interrelationships it is also important to remember that the major outflow from the cerebellum (via the superior cerebellar peduncle) terminates in relation to the same ventrolateral and ventral anterior nuclei of the thalamus. These thalamic nuclei, then, receive an overlapping projection from both the cerebellum (predominantly the dentate nucleus) and the globus pallidus. The information from the cerebellum, then, is projected through these same thalamic nuclei to the same areas of cerebral cortex, predominantly the premotor and motor cortices.

It should be noted that the dentate nucleus of the cerebellum also has some outflow (via the superior cerebellar peduncle) to the red nucleus. After synapsing at the red nucleus, fibers are also conveyed to the ventrolateral and ventral anterior nuclei of the thalamus. The major outflow, however, apparently is directly to these thalamic nuclei from the dentate and, to a lesser degree, from the emboliform nucleus of the cerebellum.

An understanding of these basic anatomical interrelationships will aid in an understanding of the effects of the various medical and surgical modalities of treatment in Parkinson's disease. Thus, when dysfunction develops in the circuit, disconnection of the entire modifying or modulating side circuit by a lesion in the globus pallidus or, better still, at the crucial ventrolateral thalamic entry area allows restoration of function in the main highway.

We must then consider the circuits through the basal ganglia as a side loop which normally modifies movement. The modification, however, represents a focused equilibrium of opposing influences. When one of these influences acts to a disproportionate degree, dysfunction in the main circuit from the motor cortex to the anterior horn cells and to the reticular formation will result. Disconnecting the entire side loop will restore a significant degree of function in the main pathway.

The usual location of surgical lesions for the relief of the tremor and rigidity of Parkinson's disease are shown in Figure 24–1. Thus, once dysfunction in this circuit has developed, a destructive lesion within the globus pallidus will eliminate the outflow from the globus pallidus to the thalamus and thus interrupt the circuit. A much more effective lesion is placed in the thalamic fasciculus since this interrupts not only the fasciculus lenticularis but also the ansa lenticularis.

It should be evident that this lesion in the ventrolateral nucleus of the thalamus would also be extremely effective in eliminating disturbances originating in the cerebellum since such a lesion would prevent a disordered cerebellum from acting on the circuits passing through the ventrolateral thalamus and would prevent this disordered cerebellum from influencing motor activities originating at a cortical level (Sarma et al., 1970).

As we have previously indicated the function of the basal ganglia is best studied in terms of its dysfunction. Dysfunction of the basal ganglia often results in a release of various automatisms or a disequilibrium of opposing mechanisms. The progressive dysfunctions involving the system often are characterized early in the disease by swings of posture. Late in the disease course, extremes of maintained posture often are noted. The early disturbances and swings of posture are often referred to as *movement disorders*. The latter fixity of posture is referred to as *dystonia*. A number of different types of movement disorders will be discussed in the sections that follow.

THE PARKINSONIAN SYNDROME

The most common disease involving the basal ganglia is Parkinson's disease. Parkinson's disease represents a syndrome of variable etiology. A certain mixture of symptoms is present in varying degrees. The essential signs and symptoms consist of: tremor, rigidity, akinesia, and defects in righting reflexes.

The *tremor* occurs at rest and is a rhythmical, alternating type, initially fine and then, as the disease progresses, often coarse. The tremor disappears on movement, but may re-emerge when a posture is maintained. The alternate movements of thumb against opposing index finger are often referred to as "pill rolling." The tremor affects not only the extremities, but also the eyelids and the tongue.

Clinical rigidity should be differentiated from decerebrate rigidity (p. 666). Decerebrate rigidity is primarily spasticity with the jack-knife quality of spasticity; that is, a sudden resistance is encountered, which, as additional force is applied, suddenly gives way. Clinical rigidity, however, is a plastic lead-pipe variety in which the resistance is relatively constant throughout the range of motion. As with spasticity, rigidity may reflect increased activity of the gamma system.

The term *akinesia* applies to the lack of spontaneous movement and the difficulty in initiating movement. A corollary term is *bradykinesia* which refers to a slowness of spontaneous movement. This lack of spontaneous movement is seen in the fixed facies of the Parkinsonian patient and in the lack of spontaneous blinking. There is also a loss of associated movements (the swing of the arms in walking).

The *defects in righting reflexes* are best noted as the patient walks and attempts to turn. Normally, as an individual turns, his eyes move initially in the direction of the turn, his head moves, then shoulders and arms, and the body then follows. The patient with Parkinson's disease, however, turns "en bloc." He has lost the righting reflexes (p. 671). The Parkinsonian patient in walking also at times develops a forward propulsion and seems to tilt forward and develop increasing speed. At times, this results in loss of balance with falls and injuries. The patient also shows unsteadiness in turning.

Several types of Parkinson's disease may be specified. The most common variety is the *idiopathic*, a degenerative disease arising insidiously in the patient of age 40, 50, or 60. At times, there is a family history of the same disease. The basic pathology involves a loss of the pigmented nerve cells of the substantia nigra (Fig. 24–2). (The student will recall that both melanine and dopamine are steps in the metabolic pathway involving phenylalanine.)

Other pathological processes also will produce many of the symptoms of Parkinson's disease. Thus, akinesia may follow bilateral necrosis of the globus pallidus. Such a necrosis could occur in carbon monoxide poisoning, or anoxia, or in relation to infarction. Rigidity in flexion may also follow bilateral necrosis of the putamen or the globus pallidus. A tremor at rest may occur with destructive lesions involving the ventromedial tegmentum of the midbrain. Such

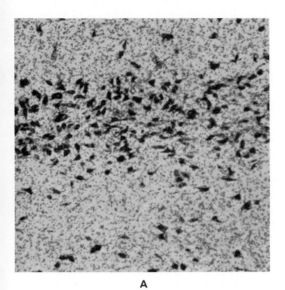
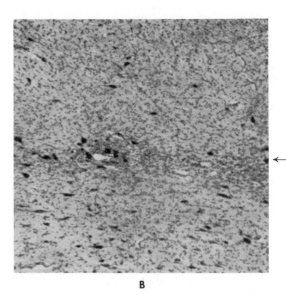

A   B

Figure 24-2 The substantia nigra in Parkinson's disease. *A,* Normal substantia nigra. The nerve cells are darkly stained because of their melanin content. (Thionine ×60). *B,* Similar region in case of idiopathic Parkinson's disease (paralysis agitans). A marked loss of pigmental neurons with a replacement by astrocytic gliosis is evident. (Thionine ×60). (From Blackwood, W., Dodds, T. D., and Sommerville, J. D.: *Atlas of Neuropathology.* Baltimore, Williams and Wilkins, 1960, p. 128.)

lesions apparently interrupt the pathway from the substantia nigra to the striatum. A degeneration of neurons in the substantia nigra and a decrease in dopamine in the corpus striatum occurs.

Another type of Parkinson's disease, then, is the *arteriosclerotic* variety in which bilateral infarcts occur in the putamen. Usually, this is an accompaniment of a lacunar state in which multiple small infarcts have occurred in the basal ganglia and internal capsule.

A certain proportion of cases may be termed *postencephalitic.* These cases had a clear onset in relation to the epidemic of Von Economo's encephalitis in the years 1916–1926. In addition to the aforementioned symptoms and signs these patients present other evidence of involvement of the central nervous system. In addition to the involvement of the substantia nigra, they present other evidence of multifocal pathology of the central nervous system.

Aside from the previously mentioned causes, a relatively rare cause of a Parkinsonian syndrome is manganese poisoning. Manganese apparently accumulates in the melanin containing neurons of the substantia nigra and interferes with the enzyme systems involved in the production of dopamine (Mena et al., 1970).

A significant percentage of patients also will develop symptoms of Parkinson's disease in relation to the use of the tranquilizers, phenothiazides (chlorpromazine) and reserpine. Reserpine interferes with the storage of dopamine within the nerve cells and thus depletes the brain of this neurotransmitter. Phenothiazides, on the other hand, block the postsynaptic receptors for dopanergic synapses. In general, with the symptoms produced by these agents, the rigidity and tremor will disappear when the agent has been cleared from the body. However, in some cases the extrapyramidal symptoms appear to remain as a permanent deficit. In such patients, one may find evidence in the family history of other cases of Parkinson's disease (Schmidt and Jarcho, 1966).

When one considers that the basic pathology in Parkinson's disease represents a loss of dopamine-containing neurons in the substantia nigra and a decrease in the amount of dopamine in the corpus striatum leaving unopposed the actions of the cholinergic system in the corpus striatum, then the types of treatment that may be considered are evident. For many years, the standard treatment involved the use of anticholinergic compounds such as belladonna and atropine or of synthetic analogues (Artane). The anticholinergic compounds affect primarily the rigidity of Parkinson's disease and in many cases may produce some improvement. Various surgical procedures were attempted in the 1940's and 1950's, involving limited ablations of area 4 or area 6 or section of the cerebral peduncle.

In 1952, while attempting to section the cerebral peduncle, Cooper occluded, by accident, the anterior choroidal artery, and the Parkinsonian patient showed a significant improvement in his contralateral symptoms, presumably as a result of infarction of the inner section of the globus pallidus. Cooper soon came to employ stereotaxic techniques for the direct production of lesions in the globus pallidus (Fig. 24–1, lesion 1). The procedure produced a significant reduction in contralateral tremor and to a lesser extent, a decrease in the contralateral rigidity. Cooper was able to demonstrate later that lesions in the ventrolateral thalamus were much more effective for the reasons previously cited (Fig. 24–1, lesion 2). Initially, the stereotaxic lesions were produced by the injection of alcohol or coagulation. In later procedures, a freezing cannula was employed.

With the increasing knowledge of the neurotransmitters involved in the substantia nigra and corpus striatum and with reports of deficits of dopamine in these structures in patients with Parkinson's disease, the use of replacement therapy with L-Dopa (dihydroxyphenylalanine) has developed (Cotzias et al. 1967, 1969). As we have indicated, the anticholinergic drugs appear to benefit primarily the rigidity; surgery benefits primarily the tremor; the use of L-Dopa, which is more a physiological technique, has improved the severe akinesia in addition to decreasing the tremor and rigidity.

The following case history illustrates the course in an idiopathic case of Parkinson's disease.

Case History 1. NECH #173–828. Date of admission: 8/27/65.

This 50-year-old, white housewife (Mrs. R.C.) had noted the onset of a tremor of the right hand 13 years prior to admission. This was relatively stable and not incapacitating until 1958, 7 years prior to admission, when in relation to intake of tranquilizer drugs, a definite progression occurred. At the same time, the patient had the onset of a stiffness of movement. Approximately 4 years prior

to admission, a tremor and stiffness of the right leg had been noted. Three years prior to admission, the left leg had also been involved. Four to 5 months prior to admission, an exacerbation occurred. The patient, however, had been able to do her housework until 1 week prior to admission, when a definite additional progression of symptoms occurred with an increase in degree of rigidity. The patient now required aid in rising from a chair, showed a definite unsteadiness when she was able to walk, had been depressed and anorexic, was unable to go to sleep, and had lost some weight.

PAST HISTORY:

There was no past history of encephalitis. There was no family history of neurological disease. The patient had received treatment with Artane (trihexyphenidyl), a total of 6 mgs. per day for approximately 7 years.

GENERAL PHYSICAL EXAMINATION:

The patient was a thin, well-developed white female. There were, however, no significant findings.

NEUROLOGICAL EXAMINATION:

1. *Mental status:* There was a significant degree of anxiety and a moderate depression of mood. However, detailed testing of mental status revealed no remarkable findings.

2. *Cranial nerves:* There were no remarkable findings.

3. *Motor system:*

   a. Strength was everywhere intact.

   b. The patient was unable to get out of a chair from a sitting position. She was unable to walk unaided. She had marked difficulty initiating even the slightest movement. When she was assisted to a standing position, propulsion and retropulsion were noted on walking. The patient turned with great difficulty. When she did so, the turns were *en bloc*.

   c. The cogwheel rigidity was present in all limbs but most marked in the right upper extremity.

   d. A masked facies was present with a relatively unbreaking expression. On tap of the forehead, a tremor and spasm of the eyelids occurred.

   e. A tremor of approximately 6 per second was present in both upper extremities, more marked on the right side. This was coarse in nature. It was a flexion-extension, supination-pronation, pill-rolling, distal type tremor. The tremor was absent

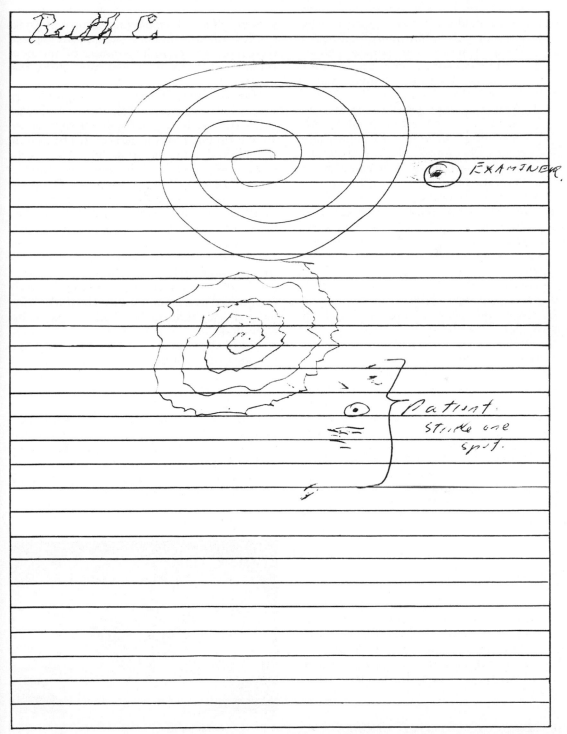

Figure 24–3 Case History 1: Parkinson's disease. Handwriting and concentric circle drawing demonstrate significant degree of tremor. The marked deficit in attempted repetitive tapping at same spot is also shown.

on complete relaxation and was exaggerated with anxiety. The tremor was also present when the hands were held in a fixed posture. The tremor was significantly dampened by movement. The patient's handwriting showed a significant degree of tremor without definite micrographia (Fig. 24–3).

    f. Repetitive tapping movements were markedly impaired (Fig. 24–3). Alternating movements were also markedly impaired; for example, finger tapping or alternate hand movements.

    g. Cerebellar testing was intact.

4. *Reflexes:* Deep tendon reflexes and plantar responses were within normal limits. A minor bilateral grasp reflex was present.

5. *Sensory system:* No remarkable features were present.

LABORATORY DATA:

1. *Hemogram* was normal.

2. *Thyroid function tests* were within normal limits.

3. *Skull x-rays* were normal.

HOSPITAL COURSE:

The patient's anticholinergic medication was gradually increased to a maximum therapeutic dose. With this, the patient's akinesia lessened and with the assistance of some physiotherapy she began to walk unaided and to get out of bed and out of a chair by herself. She was able to feed herself. The tremor remained unchanged, but her rigidity and akinesia showed some considerable improvement at the time of discharge on September 8, 1965.

CHOREA

Chorea may be defined as a sudden, random coordinated but involuntary movement occurring at a proximal or distal part of the extremities. Two distinct types of process must be distinguished: the bilateral generalized type of chorea and lateralized hemichorea.

BILATERAL GENERALIZED CHOREA

Bilateral generalized chorea may occur as a progressive, chronic entity, indicating degenerative disease (Huntington's chorea or senile chorea) or may occur in an acute episode as one aspect of rheumatic fever (Syden-

ham's chorea). Considerable interest has been generated by the observation that choreiform movements frequently occur as a toxic effect of levodopa therapy in Parkinson's disease. Such observations should contribute to an understanding of the neurochemical basis of these movement disorders.

Huntington's Chorea. Huntington's chorea is a progressive, degenerative disease of clearly established genetic etiology (autosomal dominant inheritance) beginning in the middle years of adult life. The major symptoms are chorea, dementia, and alterations of personality with psychosis. The pathology (Fig. 24–4) reflects these major symptoms. There is a marked atrophy with loss of nerve cells in the caudate nuclei and to a lesser extent in the putamen and pallidum. In addition, there is a significant atrophy of the cerebral cortex with the frontal regions involved most severely. Although clearly established as a genetic entity, the underlying biochemical abnormality has not been ascertained.

The following case history illustrates the problem of Huntington's chorea.

Case History 2. NECH #185–092. Date of admission: 2/24/67.

This 49-year-old, white, male physician had been hospitalized on the psychiatric service for treatment of a depression which had been present for approximately 3 years. Neurological consultation was requested for evaluation of an unsteadiness of gait and

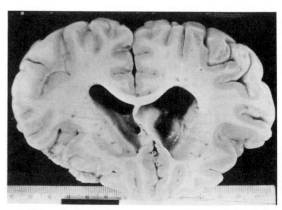

Figure 24–4 Huntington's chorea. Marked atrophy of the caudate and putamen with secondary dilatation of the lateral ventricles is evident. Cortical atrophy was less prominent in this case. (Courtesy of Dr. Emanuel Ross, Chicago).
See Filmstrip, Frame 60.

dysarthria present for approximately 2 to 3 years. During the last 3 years, the patient had been taking relatively excessive amounts of various medications such as diazepam (Valium).

FAMILY HISTORY: A maternal uncle had been depressed and disoriented several years prior to his death by suicide at age 65. This relative also had choreiform movements. Two of the uncle's sons had developed similar symptoms in their 40's. Of the patient's four siblings, ages 51 to 70, one sister, age 61, according to some accounts, had a similar disease. Of four sons, ages 14 to 24, one was mentally retarded.

GENERAL EXAMINATION:
Blood pressure was 110/70. No hepatomegaly was present.

NEUROLOGICAL EXAMINATION:
1. *Mental status:*
   a. The patient was oriented for time, place, and person.
   b. There was an adequate fund of general information.
   c. Digit span was limited to 5 forward and 3 in reverse.
   d. Delayed recall was limited to 2 objects out of 4 after 5 minutes.
   e. Calculations were poorly performed.
2. *Cranial nerves:* All were intact except for
   a. Occasional facial grimacing
   b. Mild bilateral decrease in hearing
   c. Restless movements of the tongue
3. *Motor system:*
   a. Strength was intact.
   b. Resistance to passive motion was normal.
   c. All movements were abrupt. Occasional random sudden movements of the hands occurred while the patient was talking and more particularly when he was walking. When hands were extended at wrists, rare interruptions of sustained posture were noted. Rapid alternating movements of the hands were disorganized. Heel to shin test was negative.
   d. Gait was stiff—described by some observers as "jerky." Occasional adventitious hand movements occurred.
4. *Reflexes:*
   a. Deep tendon reflexes were 3–4+ bilaterally.
   b. Plantar responses were flexor.
   c. No grasp was present.

5. *Sensation:* Intact. Romberg's test was negative.
6. No Kayser-Fleischer ring was present.
LABORATORY DATA:
1. Skull x-rays were normal.
2. EEG demonstrated diffuse 6–8 cps slow wave activity.
3. On slit lamp examination, no Kayser-Fleischer ring was present. Thus hepatolenticular degeneration (Wilson's disease) was unlikely.
4. No bromides or barbiturates were detected in the blood.
5. Blood Hinton was nonreactive.
6. Cerebrospinal fluid (CSF): no cells were present; protein was normal at 27 mg./100 ml.
7. Total plasma proteins was 7.2 grams /100 ml. with albumin of 4.5 grams/100 ml. and alkaline phosphatase was 2.3 units, indicating normal liver function.
8. Pneumoencephalogram revealed dilation of the lateral ventricles and prominence of the air pattern in the sulci over the convexities. The latter suggested cortical atrophy.

SUBSEQUENT COURSE:
Follow-up evaluation by Dr. Charles Kunkle approximately 7 months later indicated that an additional slow progression had occurred. The gait was slightly more "jerky" and there was now a faint chorea of the hands at rest or in extension.

COMMENT:
This patient presents a typical example of Huntington's chorea. The initial symptoms developed in the late 30's and consisted primarily of alteration in mental capacities. This was followed by an alteration of mood (depression) and the subsequent emergence of sudden random choreiform movements. Rigidity was not present. A significant degree of rigidity may be seen late in the disease course in these adult onset patients. In some families, the disease begins in childhood or adolescence. In such cases, rigidity is a prominent early symptom. A similar pattern is noted in Wilson's disease as regards age-related variations in the degree of rigidity.

There could be little doubt as regards genetic pattern in this case. Eugenic advice must, of course, be conveyed to other family members (the children in this case) regarding the advisability of having offspring. This is a complex problem, since the individual receiving the advice will not know whether he is to develop the disease until age 35 or 40.

HEMICHOREA

This disorder of lateralized movement develops contralateral to a lesion in the ventrolateral nucleus of the thalamus or the subthalamic nucleus. This area is supplied by penetrating branches of the posterior cerebral artery, more specifically, the thalamo-perforating artery. The basic pathological process is that of occlusion with resultant infarction. At times, the occlusion is secondary to an embolic process. At times, a small hemorrhage in this area of the diencephalon has occurred. Symptoms may begin suddenly at the time of the vascular accident or may be delayed for several weeks or months, emerging and evolving as the hemiparesis or hemianesthesia is disappearing as in the following illustrative case history. There is often no clear distinction between hemichorea and hemiballismus. As in the case history which follows, the movement disorder may consist of both hemichorea and hemiballismus. The essential lesion location for the latter disorder is the subthalamic nucleus.

Case History 3. NECH #171–044. Date of admission: 4/22/65. (Patient of Dr. John Sullivan and Dr. Huntington Porter.)

This 67-year-old, white, right-handed, retired school teacher (Miss M.G.S.) awoke one morning in December 1964, with numbness over the entire right side of her body. The right corner of her mouth drooped. She was able to go to a family physician but was unsteady on her feet. She had no diplopia or dysphasia. Numbness disappeared gradually over a 2-week period, but as the numbness subsided the left hand became restless and would move in a jerky up and down movement. The hand and arm would take on abnormal postures and tend to trail behind her. One week later this involuntary movement came to affect the left foot. The foot became restless with constant motion, seriously interfering with the ability to walk. There may have been numbness of the left foot at this time. Over the next several weeks, the movement disorder in the left hand disappeared.

PAST HISTORY: Not remarkable except for menopause at age 30.

FAMILY HISTORY: Mother died at age 63 of

heart attack. Father died at age 72 of a "shock."

GENERAL PHYSICAL EXAMINATION: Blood pressure 160/100, heart negative with normal sinus rhythm.

NEUROLOGICAL EXAMINATION:

1. *Mental status:* All areas were intact with no evidence of aphasia.
2. *Cranial nerves:*
   a. A slight droop of the left corner of the mouth was present.
   b. There was an unsustained nystagmus on far lateral gaze.
3. *Motor system:*
   a. Strength was intact with good retention of skilled movements of the hands.
   b. In the left leg, there was an almost constant play of movement, smooth and rhythmical, consisting of eversion-inversion of foot and ankle with flexion-extension movements of toes. In the left arm, the same type of movement was present. This movement was not synchronized with that in the foot and was often absent for periods of time. As the patient used the right arm, the movement disorder became apparent in the left hand. When the patient performed repetitive movements of the left fingers, mirrored movements of the right fingers occurred.
   c. Gait: The body was twisted to the left. The left hand trailed behind with the index finger pointing down and the other fingers clenched. The gait was unsteady. Walking did not dampen the movement in the left leg, in fact, at times the left leg would suddenly buckle.
4. *Reflexes:*
   a. Deep tendon reflexes were symmetrical and physiological.
   b. Plantar responses were flexor bilaterally.
   c. There was no grasp and no repellent apraxia.
5. *Sensation:* Pain, touch, position, and other discriminative modalities were intact. There was a slight decrease in vibration at the toes.

SUBSEQUENT COURSE:

The patient did well for approximately one month. Then she began to have sudden "jerky movements" of the left arm, causing the arm to strike her in the face. The left arm also began to posture in a position of relative flexion at the elbow, wrist, and fingers. The patient also reported occasional violent flinging movements of the arm. To some extent numbness had returned to the right upper extremity.

NEUROLOGICAL EXAMINATION: (April 22, 1965)

Certain changes had occurred in the movement disorder. A distal fluid, flowing 2–4 cps, movement was still noted at the fingers, toes, hand, and foot, alternating between flexion-supination and extension-pronation. There was now also the appearance of this movement at more proximal joints and some spread of movement into the face was reported. In addition, there were sudden pronation and posterior rotatory movements at the shoulder. At times, this was described as a wild swinging movement of the left upper extremity.

A minor deep tendon reflex asymmetry was noted with a slight increase on the right as compared to the left. A minor side-to-side terminal tremor was noted on the right in finger-to-nose testing.

LABORATORY DATA:

1. Fasting blood sugar 250 mg./100 ml.

2. CSF: Opening pressure 60; no cells; protein 45 mg./100 ml.

3. Chest and skull x-rays were negative except for calcification of the carotid siphon

4. Brain scan was negative

5. Sedimentation rate, 17 mm. in 1 hour

SUBSEQUENT COURSE:

Neurology follow-up visit June 4, 1965 showed that no improvement had occurred. Movements of any of the four limbs would induce wild excursion movements at the proximal joints of the upper and lower left extremities.

At the time of a subsequent visit in October 1965, significant improvement had begun to occur. By the time of follow up in December 1965, there was little evidence of any movement disorder, occasional distal movements occurring only when the patient was emotionally excited.

COMMENT:

The specific location of the lesion is uncertain in this case. There are, however, clear indications that the posterior circulation was involved. Thus, the initial numbness involving the right face, arm, and leg, with no actual weakness of the arm or leg, suggested ischemia of the left thalamus. The initial episode of hemichorea was accompanied by numbness of the left foot. The bilaterality of involvement then would suggest disease of the basilar vertebral circulation. The presence of nystagmus on lateral gaze would be consistent with brain stem involvement as well.

At the time of the exacerbation of symptoms, an increase in deep tendon reflexes was present on the right side. At the same time, a cerebellar intention tremor was present in the right hand. This would suggest a disease process involving the superior cerebellar peduncle (the brachium conjunctivum, above the level of its decussation) — for example, possibly at a midbrain or thalamic entry level. The movement disorder in the left upper extremity had now evolved into a rotatory flinging movement at the shoulder (hemiballismus).

As is often the case, the movement disorder in this case gradually subsided spontaneously.

HEMIBALLISM

As we have previously indicated, the movements of hemichorea may evolve or merge into more violent, uncoordinated, rotatory, flinging movements at the shoulder joint and other proximal joints; termed hemiballistic. The responsible lesion is located in the subthalamic nucleus (Fig. 24–5). In most cases, a hemorrhage has occurred. Less often, an infarction or metastatic lesion is present. The following case history illustrates this movement disorder. It is important to note that both hemichorea and hemiballism are relatively rare disorders.

Case History 4. NECH #117–009. Date of admission: 10/18/59. (Patient of Dr. John Sullivan.)

This 79-year-old, right-handed, white housewife (Mrs. C. M. A.) had the abrupt onset in the early morning hours, 2 days prior to admission, of almost constant flinging movements of the right arm over which she had no control. At the same time, she noted that her right arm felt numb and heavy. Over the next 2 days the movements decreased markedly and she regained more control over the arm.

PAST HISTORY:

The patient had been a known diabetic

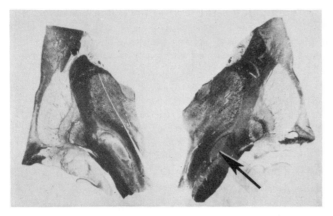

Figure 24-5 Hemiballismus. Myelin stain of basal ganglia of a 75-year-old man with sudden onset of flinging movements of the left extremities due to a discrete hemorrhage into the right subthalamic nucleus. The arrow points to the subthalamic nucleus of the normal left hemisphere. Note that the corresponding area of the right hemisphere has been destroyed by the hemorrhage. (From Luhan, J. A.: *Neurology.* Baltimore, Williams and Wilkins, 1968, p. 334.)

for 21 years, receiving insulin—most recently lente insulin, 25 units each morning.

GENERAL PHYSICAL EXAMINATION:
Pulse was 85: blood pressure was 125/60.

NEUROLOGICAL EXAMINATION:
1. *Mental status:*
    a. The patient was alert and well-oriented.
    b. There was no aphasia present.
2. *Cranial nerves:* All were intact.
3. *Motor system:*
    a. Weakness was present in the right upper extremity at the elbow, wrist, and fingers but was of minor degree.
    b. Alternating movements of the right hand were markedly impaired. Finger-to-nose testing was impaired on the right.
    c. Gait was intact.
    d. Occasional involuntary flinging movements occurred at the right shoulder.
4. *Sensory system:* Pain, touch, vibration, and position sense were all absent in the right upper extremity to the elbow and decreased in this extremity above the elbow.

LABORATORY DATA:
1. Chest and skull x-rays were normal.
2. EEG was normal.
3. Cerebrospinal fluid was normal.

SUBSEQUENT COURSE:
The flinging movements of the right arm subsided spontaneously, shortly after admission. Position sense returned and pain sensation showed a mild improvement. The ataxia on finger-to-nose testing disappeared.

COMMENT:
The loss of pain, touch, vibration, and position sense in the right upper extremity at the onset of symptoms in this case would suggest a lesion involving the ventral posterior lateral nucleus of the thalamus, presumably as a result of occlusion of the penetrating branches of the posterior cerebral artery. Presumably the subthalamic nucleus was affected as well.

DOUBLE ATHETOSIS

Athetosis may be described as an instability of posture, a relatively continuous alternation or swing between two positions. For example, in the hand, this would involve a swing from hyperextension of the fingers and thumb with pronation at the wrist to full flexion of the fingers with flexion and supination of the wrist. In a sense, there is an alternation between grasp and avoidance. Occasionally, athetosis may occur as a unilateral phenomenon admixed with hemichorea. In general, athetosis occurs as a bilateral phenomenon with involvement not only of the upper extremities but also of the lips, tongue, and lower extremities.

The pathology of double athetosis is found in the putamen where a marbled or mottled appearance may be present as a result of the presence of excessive numbers of abnormally situated myelin sheaths. To a lesser degree, the thalamus may also be involved. The etiology is not certain; anoxia at birth or other perinatal insults are considered the likely cause. Some of the cases can be related to kernicterus—the rise in bilirubin which occurs in the perinatal period owing to hemolysis of red blood cells when an Rh factor or other incompatibilities of blood type have been present. The basic pathology in these latter cases is more often a loss of myelin in the corpus striatum, globus pallidus, or thalamus. In general, the symptoms of athetosis with associated rigidity usually begin during the first year of life.

There is often an additional admixture of symptoms and signs with the other varieties of cerebral palsy. *Cerebral palsy* may be defined as a congenital abnormality of motor function. There are also included in this disease category, however, cases of motor dysfunction, acquired in infancy. The basic types of cerebral palsy are the following: (a) spastic diplegia (bilateral hemiplegia with greatest involvement of the lower extremities), (b) double athetosis, (c) ataxic variety, and (d) hemiplegic variety (usually acquired). There is often some overlap of symptoms and signs. In addition, many cases also present mental retardation, disorders of perception, or deficits in higher sensory function, or seizure disorders.

DYSTONIA MUSCULORUM DEFORMANS

This is a relatively rare, progressive disorder (at times familial) beginning in childhood or adolescence. The early symptoms are essentially those of athetosis; rigidity and fixity of postures (dystonia) soon become prominent. The pathology and its location are in general similar to those noted in double athetosis. Significant improvement may be produced by stereotaxic lesions in the ventrolateral nucleus of the thalamus. (See previous discussion of Parkinson's disease.)

HEPATOLENTICULAR DEGENERATION (WILSON'S DISEASE)

This is a familial disorder (recessive inheritance) which affects, to a variable degree, the liver and the central nervous system. In the latter, the most severe involvement occurs in the basal ganglia: the putamen and globus pallidus (loss of neurons, cavitation, and an increased number of swollen astrocytes). To a lesser extent, the cerebellum and cerebral cortex are involved.

The basic etiology has now been clearly established as a metabolic defect. There is a deficient plasma level of the circulating copper-binding globulin, ceruloplasmin. As a result, there is an excessive serum level of unbound copper. Normally, the binding of copper to ceruloplasmin prevents the passage of copper out of the serum. In Wilson's disease, however, the increased amount of unbound copper results in passage of this metal into the brain, liver, and kidney. In some cases, the symptoms of liver involvement predominate. Wilson's disease should always be suspected when hepatocellular disease develops in a child or adolescent. In other cases, the central nervous symptoms predominate and hepatic disease may be only minor. Deposition of copper also occurs in the cornea at the scleral junction. The resultant greenish brown pigmentation is referred to as the *Kayser-Fleischer ring*. This ring is almost always present when central nervous system involvement is present.

The actual symptoms referable to the neurological involvement relate to the age of the patient. In early onset cases (late childhood and early adolescence) rigidity predominates. When cases begin in early adult life, movement disorders predominate (tremor and choreoathetosis). The tremor is coarse and best described as sustained postural. The term "wing beating" is often used. The copper also produces damage to the renal tubules, resulting in glycosuria and aminoaciduria.

The treatment of Wilson's disease is dependent on a reduction of copper in the diet or the administration of an agent which will bind copper. Penicillamine (β,β-dimethylcysteine) is an effective chelator of copper. It is well absorbed on oral administration and promotes the urinary excretion of copper, resulting in a decreased level of copper in the serum, central nervous system, and liver. Previously, another chelating agent, dimercaprol (BAL, British Anti-Lewisite) was employed as the major therapeutic agent.

The following case history illustrates the clinical problem of hepatolenticular degeneration.

Case History 5. NECH #93–644. Dates of admission: 1/15/55, 1956, 1960, 1962. (Patient of Dr. Huntington Porter.)

This 22-year-old, single, white, female shoeworker (Miss T. V.) in January 1954 had the onset of a "shaking," or trembling of the fingers and hands which progressed to involve both arms and legs. The degree of involvement increased sufficiently to force her to give up her work. In September 1954, she began to note increasing difficulty with balance and coordination and a slurring of speech. She had also noted increasing weakness and difficulty in doing repetitive tasks. In December 1954, the patient noted blurring of vision, occasional diplopia, and periods of "staring." She also had experienced increasing urgency and occasional urinary incontinence.

FAMILY HISTORY:

A brother of the patient had died in 1952 at age 16 of a disease with manifestations similar to this patient's. Evaluation of this sibling in 1950 by Dr. John Sullivan, Dr. Raymond Adams, and Dr. D. Denny-Brown had indicated the presence of choreoathetosis with lapses in posture of the hands. In addition a brownish green ring at the corneal-scleral junction was noted. Liver disease was present in this sibling and possibly other members of the family.

NEUROLOGICAL EXAMINATION:

1. *Mental status:*
   a. The patient was anxious, at times crying, at other times, euphoric.
   b. Digit span was limited to 6 forward, 3 in reverse.
   c. Serial 7 subtractions were poorly performed.
2. *Cranial nerves:*
   a. A brown ring was present at the limbus of the cornea, more evident inferiorly and superiorly.
   b. Extraocular movements were impaired by involuntary jerk movements and an inability to track the moving finger smoothly.
   c. Facial expression was masklike.
   d. Speech was dysarthric and of a nasal quality with slurring and slowness of articulation.
3. *Motor system:*
   a. No actual weakness was present. However, this patient had difficulty maintaining the limbs in a fixed posture.
   b. There was a rigidity to passive movement of the limbs.
   c. A coarse arrhythmic tremor was present which was most marked proximally and more marked on sustained posture and on movement than at rest.
   d. Alternating movements were poorly performed.
   e. Gait was ataxic. Romberg test was negative.
4. *Reflexes:*
   a. Deep tendon reflexes were hyperactive.

b. Plantar responses were flexor.
5. *Sensation:* Intact.

LABORATORY DATA:
1. Liver function tests were normal.
2. Glucose tolerance test indicated that blood levels were normal, but glycosuria occurred.
3. Total plasma copper 52 mg./100 ml. (normal 115 mg./100 ml.). Direct reacting copper (unbound to cerulosplasmin) 31 mg./100 ml. (normal 10 mg./100 ml.). Indirect copper (ceruloplasmin bound) 21 mg./100 ml. (normal 105 mg./ml.).

SUBSEQUENT COURSE:

The patient did relatively well following the use of the chelating agents, BAL and calcium versenate and the institution of a copper free diet. A liver biopsy performed at the time of a cesarean section in August 1956 was compatible with perihepatitis with a question of postnecrotic cirrhosis.

Re-evaluation in 1960 revealed, in addition to the earlier findings, the presence of "continual spontaneous involuntary movements of the limbs; at the feet, characterized by alternating flexion and extension at the ankle and a waving of the toes." A broad amplitude coarse tremor was noted when the patient was asked to abduct arms, flex elbows, and hold hand just before her nose. A side-to-side tremor of the head was also present. The gait was slightly wide-based and associated with continual dystonic movements of the hands and arms. Treatment with d-penicillamine was begun in 1960. Urine copper excretion increased from 700 mg. per 24 hours to 3240 mg. per 24 hours. Neurological symptoms had shown improvement from the previously noted status. The patient had been able to do her housework and take care of her children.

Follow-up in 1962 indicated significant improvement as regards the findings noted in 1960: dystonic facies and dysarthria were less marked. No tremor was present in the left hand; that in the right hand was evident only when under tension. Dystonic posturing of the hands was present only to a minimal degree. At last report in 1966, the patient continued to do well. She had remarried and was expecting another child.

COMMENT:

This patient presents a typical case of Wilson's disease with onset in the young adult years and with a definite familial background. The copper levels were consistent with the diagnosis with an increased unbound fraction and a decreased bound fraction. Early establishment of a specific diagnosis in this case allowed for specific therapy with improvement of neurological symptoms and the prevention of progression of hepatic disease. With a specific diagnosis established in the patient, periodic blood tests were performed on her offspring to determine whether they also had inherited this genetic disease. (The child born in 1956 had not.)

References

Brody, I. A., and Wilkins, R. H.: Neurological classics I: Huntington's chorea. Arch. Neurol., *17*:331–333, 1967.

Carman, J. B.: Anatomic basis of surgical treatment of Parkinson's disease., New Eng. J. Med., *279*:919–930, 1968.

Cooper, I. S.: *Involuntary Movement Disorders.* New York, Hoeber Medical Division, 1969.

Cotzias, G. C., Papavasiliou, P. S., and Gellene, R.: Modification of parkinsonism—Chronic treatment with L-Dopa. New Eng. J. Med., *280*:337–345, 1969.

Cotzias, G. C., Van Woert, M. H., and Schiffer, L. M.: Aromatic amino acids and modification of parkinsonism. New Eng. J. Med., *276*:374–379, 1967.

Denny-Brown, D.: Diseases of the Basal Ganglia and Subthalamic Nuclei, *In* Christian, H. A. (ed.): *Oxford Loose-leaf Medicine,* 6:261–302, 1945.

Denny-Brown, D.: *The Basal Ganglia and their Relation to Disorders of Movement.* London, Oxford University Press, 1962.

Duvoisin, R. C.: Cholinergic-anticholinergic antagonism in parkinsonism. Arch. Neurol., *17*:124–136, 1967.

Haymaker, W., Mehler, W. F., and Schiller, F.: Extrapyramidal motor disorders *In* Haymaker, W. (ed.): *Bing's Local Diagnosis in Neurological Disease.* St. Louis, C. V. Mosby, 1969, pp. 404–440.

Hoehn, M. M., and Yahr, M. D.: Parkinsonism: Onset, progression and mortality. Neurology, *17*:427–442, 1967.

Hornykiewicz, O. D.: Physiological, biochemical, and pathological backgrounds of levodopa and possibilities for the future. Neurology, *20* (Part 2):1–13, 1970.

Keenen, R. E.: The Eaton collaborative study of levodopa therapy in parkinsonism. Neurology, *20* (Part 2):46–59, 1970.

Mena, I., Court, J., Fuenzalida, S., Papavasiliou, P. S., and Cotzias, G. C.: Chronic manganese poisoning: treatment with L Dopa or 5-OH tryptophane. New Eng. J. Med., *282*:5–10, 1970.

Nauta, W. J. H., and Mehler, W. R.: Projections of the lentiform nucleus in the monkey. Brain Res., *1*:3–42, 1966.

Sarma, K., Waltz, J. M., Riklan, M., Koslow, M., and Cooper, I. S.: Relief of intention tremor by thalamic surgery. J. Neurol., Neurosurg. Psychiat., *33*:7–15, 1970.

Schmidt, W. R., and Jarcho, L. W.: Persistent dyskinesias following phenothiazide therapy. Arch. Neurol., *14* 369–377, 1966.

Walshe, J. M., and Cummings, J. N.: *Wilson's Disease: Some Current Concepts.* Springfield, Ill., Charles C Thomas, 1961.

Wilkins, R. H., and Brody, I. A.: Neurological classics XVI: Sydenham's chorea. Arch. Neurol., *20*:330–331, 1969.

Wilkins, R. H., and Brody, I. A.: Neurological classics XVII: Parkinson's syndrome. Arch. Neurol., *20*:440–445, 1969.

25

The Cerebellum and Movement

ELLIOTT M. MARCUS

ANATOMICAL CONSIDERATIONS

SUBDIVISION OF THE CEREBELLUM

A number of schemes for dividing the cerebellum into various lobes and lobules have been devised. From a functional stand-point, it is perhaps best for the student to visualize the cerebellum as composed of various longitudinal and transverse divisions. In order to visualize these subdivisions, it is necessary to unfold and to lay out flat the surface of the cerebellum as in Figure 25-1.

Longitudinal Divisions. The major lon-

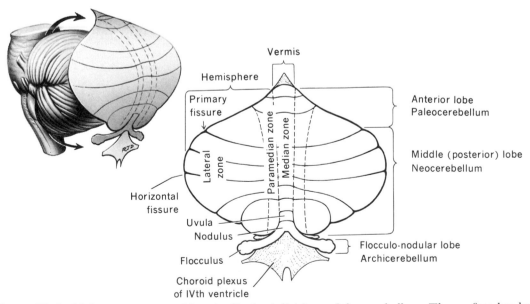

Figure 25–1 Major transverse and longitudinal subdivisions of the cerebellum. The surface has been unfolded and laid out flat. (From Noback, C. R.: *The Human Nervous System.* New York, McGraw-Hill Book Company, 1967, p. 146.)

Table 25–1 *Longitudinal Subdivisions of the Cerebellum*

Median (Vermal cortex)	*Paramedian* (Paravermal)	*Lateral* (Remainder of cerebellar hemisphere)
Projects to Fastigial nucleus	*Projects to* Interpositus nuclei (globus and emboliform)	*Projects to* Dentate nucleus (lateral)
Role in Posture and movements of whole body (axial)	*Role in* Discrete ipsilateral extremity movements (appendicular)	*Role in* Discrete ipsilateral extremity movements. Coordinated with cerebral cortex, thalamus, and red nucleus

gitudinal divisions are the *median* (vermal cortex), the *paramedian* (paravermal), and *lateral* (remainder of the cerebellar hemisphere). The major projections and functional correlations may be outlined as in Table 25–1.

Transverse Divisions. The transverse subdivisions are essentially phylogenetic divisions. The *archicerebellum* is composed of a flocculus and nodulus and is related primarily to the vestibular nerve and vestibular nuclei. The *paleocerebellum* or anterior lobe relates primarily to the spinocerebellar system and to its analogue for the upper extremities, the cuneocerebellar pathway (the lateral cuneate nucleus is the analogue of the dorsal nucleus of Clarke). Its major function, however, appears more related to the lower extremities than to the upper extremities. The primary fissure separates the anterior lobe from the middle or posterior lobe. The middle or posterior lobe, *neocerebellum*, relates primarily to the neocortex. The function of the neocerebellum relates primarily to the coordination of discrete movements of the upper and lower extremities. (See Table 25–2).

CYTOARCHITECTURE OF THE CEREBELLUM

In contrast to the cerebral cortex, all areas of the cerebellar cortex have the same basic cytoarchitectural pattern. The basic pattern in molecular, granule cell, and medullary layers is indicated in Figure 25-2. The arrangement of cells and the basic synaptic connections are indicated in Figure 25-3.

Afferent fibers enter the cerebellar cortex as *mossy fibers*. These fibers are so named because each terminates in a series of moss-like glomeruli where axodendritic synaptic contacts are made with granule cells. The mossy fibers have already been encountered as spinocerebellar, cuneocerebellar, corticopontocerebellar, vestibulocerebellar, or reticulocerebellar pathways.

The *granule cell axon* is sent into the molecular layer where a division into two long branches occurs. These branches travel (as *parallel fibers*) parallel to the long axis of the cerebellar folium, making synaptic contact with the dendrites of *Purkinje* and *basket cells*. The basket cells are inhibitory to the Purkinje cells via axosomatic synapses (Fig. 25-3C). The axons of the Purkinje cells are projected

Table 25–2 *Transverse Divisions of the Cerebellum*

Archicerebellum (Floccular nodular)	*Paleocerebellum* (Anterior lobe)	*Neocerebellum* (Middle or posterior lobe)
Connections Vestibular	*Connections* Spinocerebellar (+ cuneocerebellar) Exteroceptive	*Connections* Neocortex (Inferior olive)
Role Equilibrium – Axial (Trunk primarily) Posture Muscle tone	*Role* Equilibrium Posture Muscle tone (Lower extremities primarily)	*Role* Limb coordination in phasic movements Upper and lower extremities

to the *deep intracerebellar nuclei* (dentate, emboliform, globose, fastigial); the resultant axosomatic synapses are inhibitory in nature (Fig. 25–3*C, D*). The axons of the neurons in these deep cerebellar nuclei are the major outflow from the cerebellum to the brain stem and thalamus.

Several additional systems must be considered. The climbing fibers are excitatory to the Purkinje cell dendrites (Fig. 25–3*A, D*). Their origin remains uncertain. Some researchers (Eccles and Szentagothai) have suggested that these fibers originate in the olivary nuclei representing a long latency pathway from the spinal cord or cerebral cortex to the cerebellum (spino-olivocerebellar). Others have suggested an origin for these fibers as collaterals of the axons of neurons in the deep cerebellar nuclei.

The parallel fibers also have excitatory synapses in the molecular layer in relation to the dendrites of the *Golgi cells.* The Golgi cell in turn is inhibitory to the granule cell (Fig. 25–3*B*).

The parallel fibers also excite in the molecular layer other interneurons (small stellate cells) which in turn are apparently inhibitory to the Purkinje cells.

With the outflow from the cerebellar cortex occurring via the axons of Purkinje cells and with this outflow being inhibitory to the deep cerebellar nuclei, it is logical to inquire as to what excitatory influences drive the neurons of these deep nuclei. The answer is not cer-

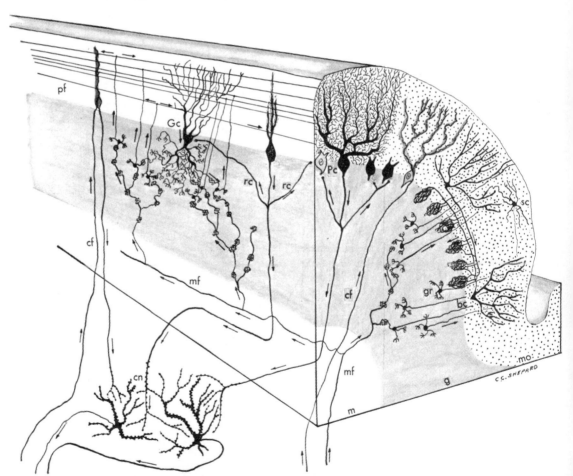

Figure 25–2 Schematic view of a cerebellar folium demonstrating the relationships of mossy fibers mf) to granule cells (gr) and the various synaptic relationships of the axons of granule cells as parallel fibers (pf), with Purkinje cells (Pc), Golgi cells (Gc), and basket cells (bc). The Purkinje cells also receive excitation from climbing fibers (cf). The major outflow from cerebellar cortex occurs via the axons of Purkinje cells to the deep cerebellar nuclei (cn). Other abbreviations: m = medullary layer, g = granule cell layer, mo = molecular layer. (From Fox, C. A.: The Structure of the Cerebellar Cortex, *In* Crosby, F. C., Humphrey, T., and Lauer, E. W.: *Correlative Anatomy of the Nervous System.* New York, Macmillan, 1962, p. 196.)

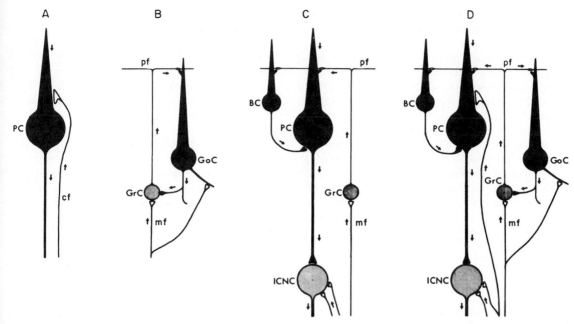

Figure 25–3 Synaptic interrelationships within the cerebellum. Diagrams of the most significant cells and their synaptic connections in the cerebellar cortex. The component circuits of *A, B,* and *C* are assembled together in *D.* Arrows show lines of operation. Inhibitory cells are shown in black. PC, Purkinje cell; cf, climbing fiber; GrC, granule cell; pf, parallel fiber; GoC, Golgi cell; mf, mossy fiber; BC, basket cell; ICNC, intracerebellar nuclear cell. (From Eccles: Postsynaptic Inhibition in the Central Nervous System. *In* Quarton, G. C., Melnechuk, T., and Schmitt, F. O. (eds.): *The Neurosciences: A Study Program.* New York, The Rockefeller University Press, 1967, p. 425.)

tain but apparently collaterals of the mossy fibers and climbing fibers serve this function.

AFFERENTS

The inputs into the cerebellum in relation to the various cerebellar peduncles may be summarized as follows:
A. Via the inferior cerebellar peduncle (restiform body)
   1. Uncrossed dorsal spinocerebellar and cuneocerebellar
   2. Crossed olivocerebellar
   3. Uncrossed reticulocerebellar (from lateral reticular and paramedian nuclei)
B. Via the middle cerebellar peduncle (brachium pontis)
   1. Crossed corticopontocerebellar
C. Via the juxta restiform body
   1. Uncrossed from vestibular nuclei
   2. Uncrossed from vestibular nerve (note that some fibers from the vestibular nerve bypass the vestibular nuclei and enter the cerebellum directly.

D. Via the superior cerebellar peduncle (brachium conjunctivum)
   1. Crossed ventral spinocerebellar
   2. Tectal cerebellar
The superior cerebellar peduncle, then, serves only a minor role as regards input to the cerebellum. Its major role is as the efferent pathway.

RELATION OF AFFERENT INPUT TO CEREBELLAR TOPOGRAPHY

These have already been summarized. The vestibular cerebellar inputs are predominantly to the floccular nodular lobe, the archicerebellum. The spinocerebellar input is primarily to the anterior lobe (paleocerebellum) and the intermediate area of the paraflocculus. The corticopontocerebellar input (via the pontine nuclei) is primarily to the neocerebellum of the lateral hemisphere.

EFFERENTS

From the dentate nuclei and interpositus (globose and emboliform) nuclei there is a major projection via the crossed brachium conjunctivum (superior cerebellar peduncle) to the ventral lateral (and ventral anterior) nuclei of the thalamus and to the red nucleus (dentato-rubral-thalamic). In addition, the descendens division of the brachium conjunctivum conveys impulses to the paramedian reticular nuclei.

The archicerebellum projects directly from the floccular nodular lobe and via the fastigial nuclei to the vestibular and reticular areas of the brain stem. The fastigioreticular and fastigiovestibular pathways hook around the superior cerebellar peduncle as the uncinate fasciculus. In addition, impulses are also conveyed via the juxta restiform body.

TOPOGRAPHIC PATTERNS OF REPRESENTATION IN CEREBELLAR CORTEX

Stimulation of tactile receptors or of proprioceptors results in an evoked response in the cerebellar cortex. There is a topographic pattern of representation. Visual and auditory stimuli also evoke responses. Stimulation of the specific areas of the cerebral cortex also evokes responses from the cerebellar cortex in an appropriate topographic manner. Moreover, direct stimulation of the cerebellar cortex in the decerebrate animal will produce, in a topographic manner, movement or changes in tone of flexors or extensors. The general pattern of representation is consistent with the pattern of sensory and cortical representation previously noted.

A possible pattern of somatotropic representation in the primate cerebellum is shown in Fig. 25–4.

It is important to recall that there is *no* conscious perception of stimuli at the cerebellar level.

FUNCTIONS OF THE CEREBELLUM

The cerebellum acts as a servomechanism: essentially a feedback loop which acts to dampen movement and motor power. As such, it tends to prevent overshoot and oscillations (that is, tremor) during movements. It acts to maintain stability of movement and posture.

The *effects on posture and equilibrium of the trunk* are mediated via interconnections with the lateral vestibular nuclei (vestibulospinal tracts) and reticular nuclei (reticulospinal tracts) from the archicerebellum and paleo-cerebellum. The pathways involved are the fastigiovestibular, fastigioreticular, and the descendens of the brachium conjunctivum.

The *effects on discrete movement of the appendages* are mediated via the dentate (and interpositus) nuclei from the neocerebellum to the contralateral ventrolateral nucleus of the thalamus (or via the dentatorubral thalamic circuit). The major projection of the ventrolateral thalamus is to the motor and premotor cerebral cortex. These cortical areas not only give rise to the corticospinal and corticoreticular fiber systems but also project to the corpus striatum and to the pontine nuclei. From the pontine nuclei, the circuit back to the topographically appropriate areas of the neocerebellum is completed by the brachium pontis.

The cerebellum then may be viewed as a machine processing information from many sources (sensory receptors, vestibular nuclei, reticular formation, cerebral cortex) and then acting to smooth out the resultant movements or postures of response. Sudden displacements, sudden lurches are prevented. The large number of inhibitory feedback circuits in the cerebellum (with the major influence of Purkinje cells on deep cerebellar nuclei being inhibitory) in a sense well qualifies the cerebellum for this role.

LESIONS OF THE CEREBELLUM

The cerebellum functions as a feedback loop which acts to dampen sudden oscillations and displacements with a variety of inhibitory circuits. It is not designed for the direct, fast conduction, control, or initiation of movements. Thus, it is not surprising that in the monkey, total ablation may produce little effect, although some deficit in contact placing may be evident. In man, extensive destruction of cerebellum may be present with little deficit evident. Moreover, cerebellar symptoms if present in a "static" disease process may often disappear with time.

While we will discuss from an anatomical standpoint three distinct syndromes of cerebellar disease (the floccular nodular lobe, the anterior lobe, and the lateral hemisphere) it should be pointed out that many diseases which affect the cerebellum are not limited by these strict anatomical borders. Moreover, the cerebellum is positioned in a relatively tight compartment with bony walls and a relatively rigid tentorium cerebelli above. An

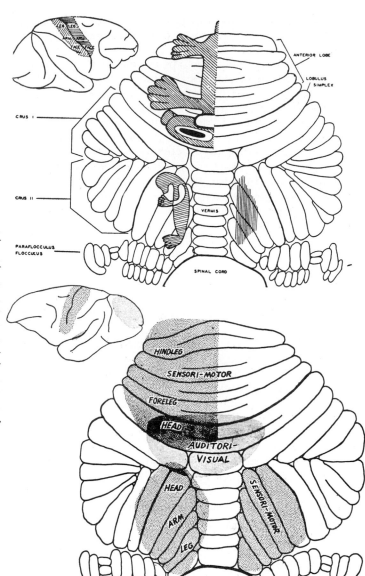

Figure 25–4 Topographic localization in cerebellum. *A*, Summary of projections from sensory area and motor area in monkey; *B*, Summary of corticocerebellar projections in the monkey. Note that there is a unilateral representation on the dorsal surface and a representation within each paramedian lobule on the ventral surface. At the lateral margin the division between crus I and crus II is essentially the border between dorsal and ventral surface. See Figure 25-5 for terminology in human cerebellum. (From Snider, R. S.: *Arch. Neurol. Psych., 64*:204, 1950.)

expanding lesion in the posterior fossa then may produce a generalized compression of the cerebellum. In such clinical situations, it may be possible to differentiate only between midline (vermal) involvement and lateral (cerebellar hemisphere) involvement. Midline lesions produce disorders of equilibrium and axial ataxia; lateral lesions produce appendicular ataxia and tremor.

SYNDROME OF THE FLOCCULAR NODULAR LOBE

The major findings in man, monkey, cat, and dog relate to a loss of equilibrium and to an ataxia of trunk, gait, and station. Thus, the patient, when standing on a narrow base with eyes open, has a tendency to fall forward, backwards, or to one side. He may be unable to sit or stand. The patient walks on a broad base often reeling from side to side and often falling. Despite the loss of equilibrium, the patient usually does not complain of a rotational vertigo. When recumbent in bed, the patient often fails to show any ataxia or tremor of limbs. Thus, the finger-to-nose and heel-to-shin tests are performed without difficulty.

With unilateral disease of the floccular nodular lobe, a head tilt may be present. In addition, spontaneous horizontal nystagmus may be present as a transitory phenomenon.

In man, the most frequent cause of this syndrome is neoplastic. The type of neoplasm is dependent on the age of the patient. The most likely cause in an infant or child is a medulloblastoma, a tumor arising in cell nests of external granular cells in the nodulus. In older children and young adults, the ependymoma, arising from ependymal cells in the floor of the fourth ventricle may cause this syndrome, pressing upward against the nodulus. In middle-aged adults, the most common cause is probably the midline hemangioblastoma.

The course of the medulloblastoma is indicated in the following case history.

Case History 1. BFH #74–67–82. Date of admission: 1/3/69. (Patient of Dr. Peter Carney.)

This 27-month-old, white female was referred for evaluation of ataxia. The mother had noted that the child had been unsteady in gait with poor balance, falling frequently since the age of 13 months when she began to walk. In October 1968, in relation to a viral infection manifested by fever and diarrhea, the patient developed increasing anorexia and lethargy. In December 1968 vomiting increased and the patient also became more irritable.

PAST HISTORY: Negative. Perinatal history had been normal.

GENERAL PHYSICAL EXAMINATION: Head circumference was normal.

NEUROLOGICAL EXAMINATION:

1. *Mental status:* The child was irritable but cooperative.
2. *Cranial nerves:* All were intact.
3. *Motor system:*
   a. Strength was intact.
   b. A significant ataxia of the trunk was present when sitting or standing. Bobbing of the head was present when sitting.
   c. Gait was broad-based and unsteady. Assistance was required.
   d. No ataxia of the extremities was present. No tremor was present.
   e. Muscle tone was normal.
4. *Reflexes:*
   a. Deep tendon reflexes were symmetrical.
   b. Plantar responses were flexor.
5. *Sensory system:* All modalities were intact.

LABORATORY DATA:

1. Left brachial arteriogram indicated an avascular area in the posterior fossa. The superior cerebellar artery was elevated, the inferior cerebellar arteries were depressed.
2. Air contrast ventriculogram demonstrated enlargement of the lateral and third ventricles. The cerebral aqueduct was displaced forward to a marked degree. The fourth ventricle was deformed with a mass overlying the posterior wall.

HOSPITAL COURSE:

On January 14, 1969 a suboccipital craniotomy was performed by Dr. Peter Carney. The dura was bulging. The cerebellar tonsils were herniated to a minor degree. Upon gentle retraction of the inferior posterior vermis, a pinkish gray tumor was visualized at the obex, originating from a higher point in the fourth ventricle. Limited biopsies of this tumor were taken, revealing a medulloblastoma. Samples of cerebrospinal fluid obtained at surgery revealed the presence of many malignant cells. The placement of a permanent shunt from the lateral ventricle to the jugular vein therefore could not be performed because of the possibility of spread of tumor cells into systemic circulation. Instead, a catheter was connected from the lateral ventricle to a small reservoir inserted under the skin of the scalp to allow daily drainage. Radiation therapy to the entire central nervous axis was begun on January 16, 1969.

By the time of hospital discharge on February 23, 1969 the patient was able to walk unassisted with only a moderate degree of ataxia.

On April 15, 1969 the patient was readmitted because of recurrent irritability and vomiting. A mild degree of papilledema was present. Horizontal nystagmus was present on lateral gaze bilaterally. A wide-base ataxic gait was still present. Various antineoplastic agents were employed (methotrexate into the cerebrospinal fluid, and vincristine intravenously) without significant improvement. On May 15, 1969 respirations became slow, deep, and irregular. Death occurred shortly thereafter. The findings at autopsy are demonstrated in Figure 25-5.

COMMENT:

This patient had a severe degree of ataxia which involved the trunk when she attempted to walk and poor equilibrium; but she had no specific ataxia or tremor of the upper or lower extremities. The tumor arising from

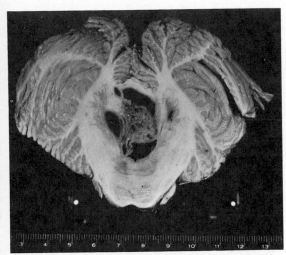

Figure 25–5 Medulloblastoma. Case History 1. Syndrome of the floccular nodular lobe. Vomiting and truncal ataxia were present without tremor or ataxia of the extremities. (Courtesy of Dr. John Hill, New England Center Hospitals.) **See Filmstrip, Frame 24.**

the floccular nodular lobe and projecting into the fourth ventricle produced a block of the ventricular system and early evidence of increased intracranial pressure: vomiting, lethargy, and irritability in this case. Surgery in these cases is strictly limited to decompression and biopsy to establish a histological diagnosis. Radiation may produce a significant remission of symptoms. Dissemination of tumor cells throughout the cerebrospinal fluid is frequent because of the friable, cellular, nonstromal nature of the lesion. Radiation must therefore be delivered to the entire neural axis to deal with any implants.*

SYNDROME OF THE ANTERIOR LOBE

Significant changes in tone may be produced by stimulation or ablation of the anterior lobe in the cat or dog. This stimulation of the midline anterior lobe will result in a decrease in spindle discharge and will inhibit gamma rigidity of the decerebrate preparation. Stimulation of the intermediate area of the anterior lobe produces an increased

---

*An additional case history illustrating truncal ataxia as a result of a midline cerebellar tumor (hemangioblastoma) can be found in Chapter 15, p. 340.

spindle discharge (facilitating gamma rigidity in the decerebrate preparation). Actual ablation of the anterior lobe in these animals or functional ablation (cooling) produces an increase in decerebrate rigidity without a change in the gamma system (alpha rigidity).

However, *in man*, ablation of the anterior lobe does not change tone. The major symptoms are an ataxia of gait with a marked side-to-side ataxia of the lower extremities as tested in the heel-to-shin test. The upper extremities in contrast are unaffected or affected to only a minor degree.

A typical example of this syndrome may be seen in cases of alcoholic cerebellar degeneration (Fig. 25–6*A* and 25–6*B*). Although occurring primarily in alcoholics, the basic etiology may be a nutritional deficiency (the specific factor is unknown). The following case history illustrates this problem.

Case History 2: NECH #144–514.
Date of admission: 10/18/61.

This 64-year-old, white male (Mr. M. F.) was admitted with a chief complaint of a slowly progressive incoordination of gait present for 8 years. The patient and others had noted that his gait was staggering. The patient denied weakness, numbness, diplopia, vertigo, or memory difficulty.

The patient admitted the consumption of one half pint (8 oz.) of brandy every 4 nights. He indicated that he used to drink more in his younger days, at least 6 to 8 beers per night.

FAMILY HISTORY: There was no history of pes cavus or neurological disease.

NEUROLOGICAL EXAMINATION:

1. Blood pressure was 140/80. Liver was down 2 fingerbreadths beyond the costal margin. Face was red with dilation of vessels.
2. *Mental status:*
   a. The patient was slightly disoriented for time. He gave the date as September 31, 1961. The date was actually October 19, 1961.
   b. Delayed recall was 0-out-of-5 objects in 5 minutes.
   c. He was unable to give the date of his birth, but he knew his phone number.
   d. Digit span was 7 forward, 4 in reverse.
   e. Calculations: The patient was unable to subtract 7 from 100 or 3 from 30; he could not add 14 and 13, although he had had a fourth grade education.

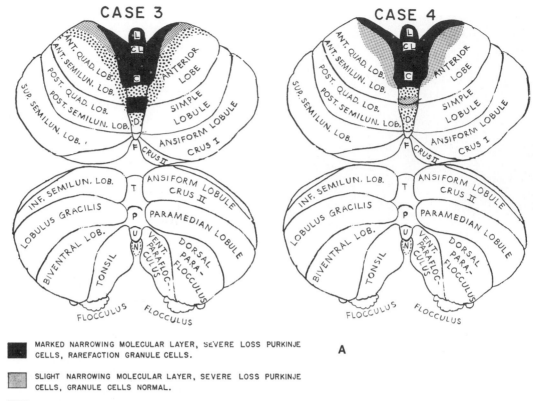

CASE 3

CASE 4

MARKED NARROWING MOLECULAR LAYER, SEVERE LOSS PURKINJE CELLS, RAREFACTION GRANULE CELLS.

SLIGHT NARROWING MOLECULAR LAYER, SEVERE LOSS PURKINJE CELLS, GRANULE CELLS NORMAL.

◆ MODERATE LOSS PURKINJE CELLS ONLY.

A

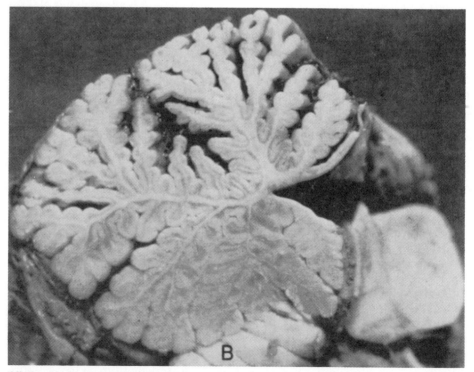

B

Figure 25–6 Alcoholic cerebellar degeneration: the anterior lobe syndrome. There is a loss of Purkinje cells with atrophy of the cerebellar folia. Relatively selective involvement of the anterior lobe occurs. *A*, Schematic representation of the neuronal loss. *B*, Atrophy of the anterior superior vermis is shown in this sagittal section. (From Victor, M., Adams, R. D., and Mancall, E. L.: *Arch. Neurol., 1:*579, 599, 600, 1959.)

3. *Cranial nerves:* All were intact. No nystagmus was present.

4. *Motor system:*

a. Strength was intact.

b. Gait was broad-based with an ataxia of trunk. The patient was unable to walk a tandem gait. His ataxia was accentuated by rapid walking. Small lateral nodding movements of the head were noted.

c. There was a minimal tremor at rest. In addition, there was, to a minor degree, a resistance to passive motion at the wrists and elbows with a suggestion of a cogwheel component.

d. There was a minor tremor on finger-to-nose testing and a minor impairment of alternating hand movements.

e. There was, however, a very significant heel-to-shin ataxia which was out of proportion to any tremor or ataxia involving the upper extremities.

5. *Reflexes:*

a. Deep tendon reflexes were physiological and symmetrical (2–3+).

b. Plantar responses were flexor bilaterally.

6. *Sensory system:*

a. Position, pain, and touch were intact.

b. There was a moderate decrease in vibratory sensation at the toes and ankles.

LABORATORY DATA:

1. Cerebrospinal fluid was normal with pressure of 140; no cells; protein 43 mg./100 ml.

2. Skull and chest x-rays were normal.

3. Sedimentation rate: 12, Hct 43, albumin 4 gm./100 ml., total protein 6.4 gm./100 ml.

SUBSEQUENT COURSE:

The patient was advised to discontinue any intake of alcohol. Neurological re-evaluation over the next 6 years indicated that no essential progression had occurred.

COMMENT:

The major findings of the broad-based, staggering gait with truncal ataxia and heel-to-shin ataxia may be related to the anterior lobe of the cerebellum. In view of the absence of progression after the discontinuation of alcohol, a toxic or nutritional factor may be postulated. The minor extrapyramidal findings of cogwheel rigidity may have represented unrelated disease. The minor degree of dementia may have related to previous nutritional problems with minor Wernicke-Korsakoff's syndrome or may have reflected a minor unrelated dementia.

In other cases, this syndrome is the result of a chronic degenerative disease, of unknown etiology, but often occurring on a familial background. As discussed in Chapter 22, there are a variety of degenerative diseases involving the cerebellum. These diseases vary as regards the areas of cerebellum involved, the involvement of brain stem structures, the age of onset, and the degree of hereditary background.

In the following case history, the major involvement was primarily of the anterior lobe. There was a definite family history with evidence of consanguinity as well. The case in general corresponds to cases of familial cortical cerebellar atrophy reported by Holmes and to the cases presented by Andre Thomas, Marie, Foix, and Alajounine. As in alcoholic cerebellar degeneration, the predominant histological change is the loss of Purkinje cells in the anterior lobe. Reference to the diagram of topographic representation will indicate that this area corresponds to the representation of the lower extremities and to the area of projection of the spinocerebellar pathways.

Case History 3. September, 1968. (Office patient of Dr. E. M. Marcus.)

A 45-year-old, single, white, male carpenter (Mr. A. C.) presented with a 4-year history of progressive unsteadiness in walking present during daytime as well as nocturnal hours. He had during this period noted some loss of coordinated movements in his hands, but felt that his greatest deficit related to unsteadiness. The patient had noted no actual weakness but reported some numbness at the toes. He had also noted some minor difficulty in swallowing.

FAMILY HISTORY:

The patient lived in a small town in Virginia. His mother and father were second cousins. Several aunts and uncles had "trouble with their legs" in later life resulting in a difficulty in walking.

PAST HISTORY:

The patient admitted to some minor intake of alcohol in the past. He had recently been under the care of a naturopath and had experienced a 7-lb. weight loss.

NEUROLOGICAL EXAMINATION:

1. *Mental status:* Findings were consistent with his grade-school education.

2. *Cranial nerves:* Intact except for minimal dysarthria.

3. *Motor system:*
   a. Strength was intact.
   b. The patient walked on a broad base with an ataxia of trunk as though intoxicated, reeling from side to side with marked unsteadiness on turns. He was unable to walk a tandem gait with eyes open. The patient was able to sit without significant ataxia of the trunk.
   c. A mild intention tremor was present with minimal disorganization of alternating movements. A marked ataxia and tremor were evident on heel-to-shin test. Horizontal nystagmus was present on lateral gaze, vertical nystagmus on upward gaze.

4. *Reflexes:*
   a. Deep tendon reflexes were intact except for a relative decrease in ankle jerks compared to knee jerks.
   b. Plantar responses were flexor.

5. *Sensation:* All modalities were intact except for a minimal decrease in vibration at toes.

LABORATORY DATA:

Pneumoencephalogram had been performed at the University of Virginia Hospital in June, 1965 (Dr. Stewart) and had revealed superficial cerebellar atrophy. Cerebrospinal fluid and other laboratory data at that time had been normal.

SYNDROME OF THE LATERAL CEREBELLAR HEMISPHERES (NEOCEREBELLAR OR MIDDLE POSTERIOR LOBE SYNDROME) (FIG. 25-7)

A number of disease entities may produce symptoms relevant to the lateral hemisphere. Some of these same disease entities; e.g., intrinsic or metastatic tumors, may also involve midline structures. The diagnostic problem, moreover, is complicated by the fact that involvement of the cerebellar peduncles may possibly produce many of the same symptoms which result from direct involvement of the cerebellar hemisphere. The student will recall that the lateral medullary infarct produces an ipsilateral intention tremor and an impairment of alternating movements of the ipsilateral upper extrem-

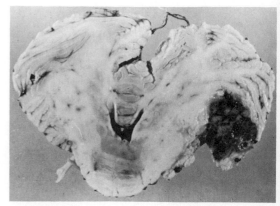

Figure 25-7 Hemangioblastoma of cerebellum: syndrome of the lateral hemisphere. This 72-year-old male had a 2-year history of vertex headache (worse on coughing), blurring of vision, and diplopia. He presented, among other findings, papilledema and a lateralized intention tremor on finger-to-nose testing. (Courtesy of Dr. Jose Segarra, Boston Veterans Administration Hospital.) **See Filmstrip, Frame 25.**

ity.* Of course, it may be noted that the lesions of vascular disease or of demyelinating disease may involve, in a specific case, both brain stem and cerebellum in a multifocal manner.

Cases presenting relatively pure focal involvement of the lateral hemisphere are those patients surviving after gunshot or shrapnel wounds. Such cases have been studied by Holmes (1922, 1939); they are not encountered frequently in civilian practice.

The major findings in lateral hemisphere lesions are as follows: intention tremor involving the extremities, disorganization of alternating movements of the extremities (dysdiadochokinesis), dysmetria, and ataxia of the extremities, hypotonia of the extremities, and overshoot on rebound. The *intention tremor* may be described as a tremor perpendicular to the line of motion, often becoming more prominent on slower movements and as the target is approached. This intention tremor may be noted in the finger-to-nose test. One may also demonstrate a similar tremor in the lower extremities as the patient attempts to raise the foot off the bed

---

*The interpretation of such lesions, however, is often cloudy on this point. The posterior inferior cerebellar artery does supply a portion of the cerebellum (posterior inferior), as well as the lateral medulla. (Refer to Mettler and Orioli, 1958.)

to touch the examiner's finger. As with the other signs of cerebellar disease, intention tremor is usually ipsilateral to the hemisphere involved.

At times, in addition to an intention tremor, a sustained postural tremor may be evident, more particularly if the superior cerebellar peduncle is involved. This will be discussed later. The intention tremor represents a defect in the ability to dampen oscillations and to dampen overshoot. In the lower extremities, a similar side-to-side ataxia may be noted when the patient attempts the heel-to-shin test.

Repetitive movements may be tested by having the patient slap his own knee with his hand at a particular rhythm. One can also test for repetitive movement in the lower extremities by having the patient tap the toes or the heel on the floor.

Alternating movements are tested by having the patient slap his own hand on his knee or on his opposite hand, alternating between the palmar and dorsal surface of the hand. In disease of the cerebellar hemisphere a *marked disorganization of repetitive and alternating movements occurs*. This is almost always ipsilateral to the hemisphere involved.

These patients are also said to demonstrate *dysmetria*. This may be defined as a defect in the force and rate of movement necessary for an extremity to reach a target. The result, then, in the finger-to-nose test is that the patient fails to accurately touch the finger to the nose. The finger may overshoot its goal or fail to reach the goal.

The affected limbs often show a *hypotonia* which is ipsilateral to the hemisphere involved. In addition, there is often a failure to properly adjust force when pulling against an opposing force so that as this force suddenly gives way, the patient fails to break the action of an arm and he tends to have a rebound overshoot.

Finally, patients with cerebellar hemisphere disease are said to have a *dyssynergia,* a disturbance in the synergy of movements, e.g., the coordination required at the joints of the arm in reaching out for an object.

The patient with disease of the cerebellar hemisphere also has a disturbance of gait. This tends to be an ipsilateral disturbance of gait with a tendency to fall to the affected side of the lesion. In these patients, however, balance is often well maintained in distinction to the lesions of the floccular nodular lobe previously described where a disturbance of

gait also occurs. The following case history illustrates a focal lesion of the lateral hemisphere.

Case History 4   NECH #181–341. Date of admission: 8/22/66. (Patient of Dr. John Sullivan.)

This 36-year-old, white, male attorney (Mr. M. I.) was referred with a chief complaint of headaches and vomiting. The patient had had frontal and biparietal headaches for approximately 1 month. These headaches were precipitated by coughing, sneezing, or bending. On at least one occasion the patient had been awakened by the headache. The patient had had nausea and vomiting independent of the headaches. At times, the vomiting would occur suddenly without preceding nausea.

For several weeks prior to admission the patient had been unsteady on his feet with a tendency to fall to the right. On several occasions he admitted to clumsiness of his right hand. For several days prior to admission, the patient had had double vision and he had had to keep one eye closed. During the week prior to admission he had been excessively drowsy and constantly tired. The headaches had increased in frequency so that they were now occurring 3 to 4 times per day. Past history was not remarkable except for an unrelated episode of rheumatic fever in 1940.

GENERAL PHYSICAL EXAMINATION: There were no abnormalities.

NEUROLOGICAL EXAMINATION:

1. *Mental status:* All areas were intact.
2. *Cranial nerves:*
   a. On funduscopic examination there was evidence of bilateral papilledema.
   b. A bilateral paralysis of the sixth nerve was present.
   c. Horizontal nystagmus was present on right lateral gaze.
3. *Motor system:*
   a. Strength was everywhere intact.
   b. The patient's gait was wide-based. In walking the patient tended to veer to the right. The patient was unable to stand on his right leg. The Romberg test, however, was negative.
   c. There was a significant intention tremor of the right upper extremity on finger-to-nose test and of the right lower extremity on heel-to-shin test. Alternating movements of the right hand were disorganized.

4. *Reflexes:*
   a. Deep tendon reflexes were symmetrical and physiologic.
   b. Plantar responses were flexor.
5. *Sensory system:* All modalities were intact.

LABORATORY DATA:
1. Complete blood count was normal.
2. Skull x-rays were normal.
3. Right brachial arteriogram revealed in the late arterial phase a density in the right cerebellar hemisphere relatively inferior and posterior. This blush during the arteriogram was consistent with hemangioblastoma of the right cerebellar hemisphere.
4. Pantopaque ventriculogram revealed a dilated third ventricle and a dilated aqueduct leading from the fourth ventricle. There was obstruction to outflow from the fourth ventricle. The fourth ventricle and aqueduct were shifted to the left. The aqueduct was shifted to a lesser degree than the fourth ventricle. These findings were consistent with a right cerebellar mass displacing and obstructing the fourth ventricle.
5. Brain scan was negative.

HOSPITAL COURSE:
Following admission, because of the finding of increased intracranial pressure, the patient was placed on high dosage of Decadron (a steroid given to relieve increased intracranial pressure). On August 22, 1966 a suboccipital craniectomy was performed by Dr. Samuel Brendler. When the dura was opened, bulging of the lower portion of the right cerebellar hemisphere was noted with widening of the cerebellar folia. The widest area of the folia was tapped with a needle and yellow cystic fluid was removed. A transcortical incision was then made revealing a large cyst with a small strawberry-shaped angioma located within. The angiomatous stalk was ligated and the angioma separated from the cystic capsule. Histological examination of the tumor revealed a hemangioblastoma.

Postoperatively the patient did well. His headache and diplopia disappeared. There was then improvement in the patient's tremor and ataxia although there was a slight slowness on finger-to-nose testing on the right. A minor side-to-side tremor was present on right heel-to-shin testing. There was a tendency to veer to the right in walking but tandem gait indicated only a minor dysmetria on right heel-to-shin testing.

Evaluation 6 months after surgery in February 1967 indicated only a minimal unsteadiness on tandem walking . Evaluation in May 1967 indicated no significant neurological findings. Re-evaluation in December 1969 again indicated a completely intact neurological status.

COMMENT:
The headaches experienced by the patient suggested a space-occupying lesion in relation to the ventricular system or meninges with pain occurring on coughing, sneezing, or mechanical changes. This tumor had produced a block of the ventricular system. and relatively early in its course it had produced an increase in intracranial pressure with headache, vomiting, and papilledema. The bilateral sixth cranial nerve weakness was of moderate degree and its occurrence would not be unusual in a situation where intracranial pressure had rapidly increased.

The cerebellar symptoms experienced by the patient were lateralized in the sense that the patient was falling to the right side and had noted clumsiness of his right hand. On examination, these findings of lateralized cerebellar disease were confirmed in the sense that an intention tremor of the arm and leg was present on the right with disorganization of alternating movements on the right side.

In this case the hemangioblastoma was in the lateral cerebellar hemisphere. In other cases of hemangioblastoma (p. 340), the lesion is much more midline in location and the symptoms may be those of a midline cerebellar tumor. Thus, the patient may complain of essentially an ataxia of gait and truncal ataxia without clearly lateralized symptoms involving the appendages. Thus, one may find in other cases of hemangioblastoma that the patient has an ataxia of gait and trunk without actual intention tremor and without any ataxia on heel-to-shin testing.

The hemangioblastoma is a surgically curable lesion. The nodule of tumor often exists within a non-neoplastic cystic cavity. It is therefore possible to remove the tumor without sacrificing a large amount of the cerebellum. In some cases both the mural nodule and the cyst are removed. In almost all cases a complete cure may be obtained; recurrences are unlikely and the patients usually have a relatively complete resolution of symptoms with absence of any residual disability.

In some cases, hemangioblastomas of the cerebellum are associated with angiomatous malformations of the retina (Lindau-von

Hippel's disease). In some cases, there is an association with a secondary increase in red blood cell production (polycythemia). In rare cases, there is an association with tumors of the kidney.

Other neoplasms may also involve the cerebellar hemispheres: cystic astrocytomas and metastatic tumors (Fig. 15–2B, p. 343).

LESIONS OF THE CEREBELLAR PEDUNCLES

As we have indicated, some patients demonstrating cerebellar symptoms and findings actually have damage to the cerebellar peduncle rather than direct involvement of the cerebellum. Lesions of the *inferior cerebellar peduncle* result in an ataxia of the extremities on the side of the lesion with falling to the side of the lesion and nystagmus.

Lesions of the *superior cerebellar peduncle*, the brachium conjunctivum, produce a unilateral ataxia of limbs, with intention tremor and hypotonia. Symptoms are essentially those outlined for the cerebellar hemisphere. The clinical symptomatology is ipsilateral if the lesion occurs between the dentate nucleus and the decussation of the brachium conjunctivum. If above this decussation, the clinical findings are contralateral. Moreover, if the lesion is above the decussation, the tremor often is more than a pure intention tremor. Thus the tremor will often be of a sustained postural type. At times with involvement of this area within the midbrain, a resting tremor results as well as discussed in relation to the basal ganglia. It is not unusual to have an evolution of the tremor with a relatively pure intention tremor initially present and the resting tremor emerging as a later finding. At times, a minor degree of hemichorea may also be present. This is not unusual when one considers that these closely adjacent areas of the midbrain, the subthalamus, and the ventrolateral nucleus of thalamus are all supplied by penetrating branches of the posterior cerebral artery.

The effects of isolated lesions of the *middle cerebellar peduncles* are not certain. There is some evidence that an incoordination of fine limb movements and an ataxia of gait may result. In experimental lesions, circling may result.

References

Bucy, P. C., and Thieman, P. W.: Astrocytomas of the cerebellum. Arch. Neurol., *18*:14–19, 1968.

Dow, R. S., and Moruzzi, G.: *The Physiology and Pathology of the Cerebellum.* Minneapolis, University of Minnesota Press, 1958.

Eccles, J. C.: The Way in Which the Cerebellum Processes Sensory Information from Muscle, *In* Yahr, M.D., and Purpura, D. (eds.): *Neurophysiological Basis of Normal and Abnormal Motor Activities.* Hewlett, New York, Raven Press, 1967, pp. 379-414.

Eccles, J. C., Ito, M., and Szentagothai, J.: *The Cerebellum as a Neuronal Machine,* New York, Springer-Verlag, 1967.

Fox, C., and Snider, R. S. (eds.): *The Cerebellum.* Amsterdam, 1967.

Greenfield, J. G.: *The Spino-Cerebellar Degenerations.* Springfield, Ill., Charles C Thomas, 1954.

Holmes, G.: Clinical symptoms of cerebellar disease and their interpretation. Lancet, *1*:1177–1182, 1231–1237; *2*:59–65, 111–115, 1922.

Holmes, G.: The cerebellum of man. Brain, *62*:1–30, 1939.

Mettler, F. A., and Orioli, F.: Studies on abnormal movement: Cerebellar ataxia. Neurology, *8*:953–961, 1958.

Orioli, F. L., and Mettler, F. A.: Consequences of section of the Simian restiform body. J. Comp. Neurol., *109*:195–204, 1958.

Oscarsson, O.: Functional significance of information channels from the spinal cord to the cerebellum. *In* Yahr, M. D., and Purpura, D. (eds.): *Neurophysiological Basis of Normal and Abnormal Motor Activities.* Hewlet, New York, Raven Press, 1967, pp. 93–117.

Oscarsson, O.: Functional organization of spinocerebellar paths *In* Iggo, A. (ed.): *Handbook of Sensory Physiology,* Vol II: *Somatosensory System.* Berlin, Springer Verlag, 1970, pp. 121–127.

Victor, M., Adams, R. D., and Mancall, E. L.: A restricted form of cerebellar cortical degeneration occurring in alcoholic patients. Arch. Neurol., *1*:579, 1959.

26

The Electroencephalogram: Seizures, Sleep, Coma, and Consciousness

ELLIOTT M. MARCUS

THE NORMAL ELECTROENCEPHALOGRAM

The continuous oscillating electrical activity of the cerebral cortex was first observed in the laboratory in 1875, by the English physician Caton. Although considerable investigation on the electrical activity of the non-human brain had been undertaken, it was not until 1929 that Berger first published his studies of the electroencephalogram recorded through the scalp of man. Berger also noted that changes in the human electroencephalogram occurred with age, with sensory stimulation, and with seizure discharges. The clinical role of the electroencephalogram in the diagnosis and differentiation of the various seizure disorders in man was first defined by the studies of Gibbs, Davis, and Lennox in 1935 and elaborated by the studies of Jasper and Kershman in 1941. The value of the electroencephalogram in the localization of focal lesions, such as tumors, of the cerebral hemisphere, was first clearly indicated by the studies of Walter in 1936.

RECORDING METHODS

The electroencephalogram (EEG), as indicated in Chapter 20, records the variable

potential differences between two electrodes placed on the scalp. In bipolar recording, both electrodes are on the scalp over electrically active tissue. In monopolar or unipolar recording, one electrode (the active) is on the scalp, the other (the reference) is over a presumably electrically inactive tissue (e.g., ear lobe, vertebral spinous process). Each pair of electrodes is plugged into the input stage of an amplifying system. The potential difference is then displayed on a moving paper by means of an ink-writing oscillograph. Usually a series of electrode pairs is displayed simultaneously (in general eight at a time) by combining into a single machine, sets of amplifiers and ink-writing oscillographs. (Machines capable of displaying 16 pairs at a time are available.) Each set of amplifiers and oscillograph is referred to as a channel.

There are various schemes or systems of display in grouping the electrodes to be recorded at any single time. Thus, one may record alternate hemispheres in alternate channels as has been done in many of the illustrations which follow, e.g.,

Channel (1) LT frontal-central
Channel (2) RT frontal-central
Channel (3) LT central–occipital
Channel (4) RT central–occipital

710

Channel (5) LT frontal–temporal
Channel (6) RT frontal–temporal
Channel (7) LT temporal–occipital
Channel (8) RT temporal–occipital

On the other hand, in many laboratories it is standard procedure to record all of the leads from one hemisphere in the first four channels and then all of the leads from the contralateral hemisphere in the last four channels.

The placement of electrodes is also variable. At the present time, the most widely accepted electrode placement system is the International Federation System illustrated in Figure 26-1. This system uses certain landmarks—the nasion, the inion, and the tragus of the ear—to standardize electrode placement.

NORMAL ADULT RECORD

The usual electroencephalogram is recorded with the patient awake, but resting recumbent on a bed with his eyes closed. Under these conditions, in the normal adult, there is recorded a dominant activity (Fig. 26-2) in the parietal occipital areas (posterior hemisphere recording sites) of 8–13 cps sinusoidal waves of 50–100 microvolts (uV) amplitude, referred to as *alpha rhythm*. In the frontal areas (anterior recording areas) dominant activity is of lower amplitude and a faster frequency (14–30 cps), referred to as *beta rhythm*, is often present in addition to the alpha rhythm. It is important to note that there is a relative symmetry of amplitude and frequency between the left and right hemispheres. (In the language of the clinical electroencephalographer, any wave-forms at a slower frequency than alpha are referred to as slow waves: 4–7 cps=theta rhythm; 1–3 cps=delta rhythm).

NONPATHOLOGICAL ALTERATIONS

Suppression of Alpha Rhythm. Several conditions may produce a *blocking* or suppression of the alpha rhythm with the appearance of low-voltage fast-activity. This is essentially an arousal or "desynchronization" effect discussed in a previous chapter (p. 475). It may be produced by eye opening (Fig. 26-3), intense sensory stimulation, alert attention, or mental activity, e.g., mental or arithmetic problems.

Sleep. Sleep normally produces a series of changes in the electroencephalogram (Fig. 26-4). Initially, with drowsiness there is a decrease in amplitude of the alpha rhythm and the appearance of low amplitude 4–5 cps activity. (Note the change in Fig. 26-4B compared to Fig. 26-4A.) Activity in the 4–7 cps range is referred to as *theta rhythm*. As drowsiness and light sleep continue, periods of 15 cps low amplitude activity alternate with 4 cps activity (Fig. 26-4C). As sleep deepens, high voltage diphasic or triphasic waves appear in the central (vertex) areas (Fig. 26-4D). These waves are termed *K complexes* or biparietal sleep humps or vertex sharp waves.

As an additional increase in the depth of sleep occurs (Fig. 26-4E), bilateral 2–3 cps slow waves begin to appear. (Activity in the 1–3 cps frequency range is termed *delta rhythm*.) Only the beginnings of this stage are shown in the sequence, as arousal occurred shortly after section F began. In general, sleep electroencephalograms as performed in the clinical laboratory are usually not carried beyond this point.

In actuality, the *slow wave stages of sleep* (theta and delta activity) are usually found in the early part of a full night's sleep. Although the patient is asleep, considerable tone is still present in neck and other muscles. After a variable period (usually 90 minutes in man) a different plane of sleep is attained. In this stage, the patient shows the behavioral components of deep sleep with marked relaxation of muscles. However, the electroencephalogram is composed of low-amplitude fast-activity (not unlike that shown in Fig. 26-3). Taken alone, the electroencephalogram would be mistaken for an alert state.

Because of this marked discrepancy between the behavioral state and the electroencephalogram, the term *paradoxical sleep* has been applied. Since rapid eye movement can also be recorded during this stage of sleep, as opposed to slow wave sleep, the term *REM* (rapid eye movement) sleep has also been employed. In addition, since much of dreaming apparently occurs during this stage of sleep, the term *D-state* has also been applied.

Anesthetic Agents. Anesthetic agents and various drugs will produce a series of changes in the electroencephalogram. The successive stages obtained with cyclopropane anesthesia are demonstrated in Figure 26-5. Similar changes would also be noted with

(Text continued on page 716)

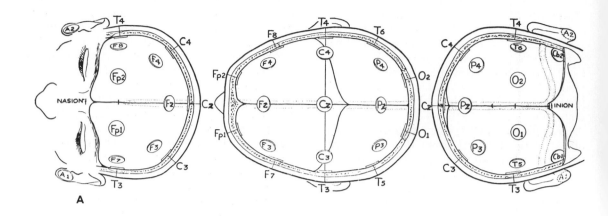

A

B

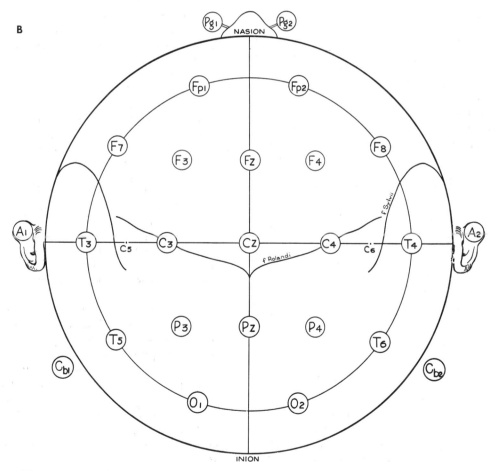

Figure 26–1 The International Federation ten-twenty electrode placement system. *A*, Frontal superior and posterior views; *B*, a single plane projection of the head demonstrating the standard positions and the Rolandic and Sylvian fissures. The term ten-twenty is based on the placement of electrodes at particular percentages of the distance between nasion and inion. (From Jasper, H. H.: Electroenceph. clin. Neurophysiol., *10*:374, 1958.)

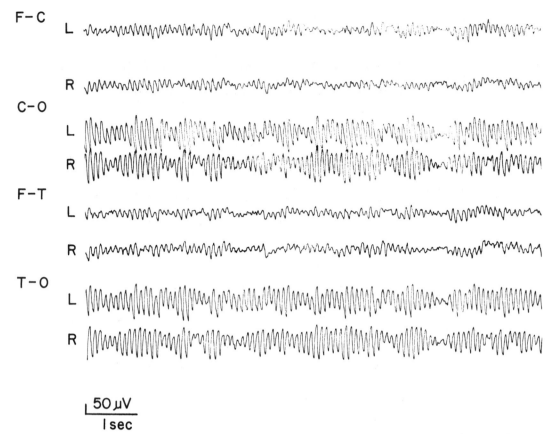

Figure 26–2 The normal adult electroencephalogram. The patient is awake but in a resting state, recumbent with eyes closed. F = frontal, T = temporal, C = central, and O = occipital. (Bipolar recordings.)

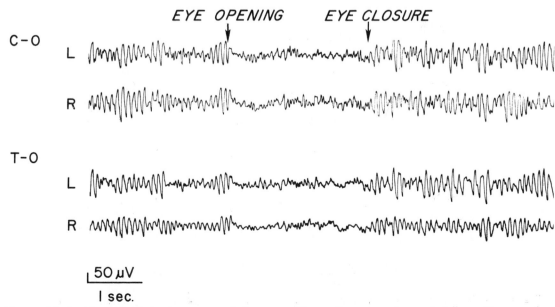

Figure 26–3 Normal adult electroencephalogram: effects of eye opening and closure. Eye opening is associated with a blocking or suppression of the *alpha rhythm* of 10 cps and with the appearance of a low-voltage fast-activity of 20 cps (*beta rhythm*). With eye closure, there is a return of the alpha rhythm. C-O = central occipital; T-O = temporal occipital. (Bipolar recordings.)

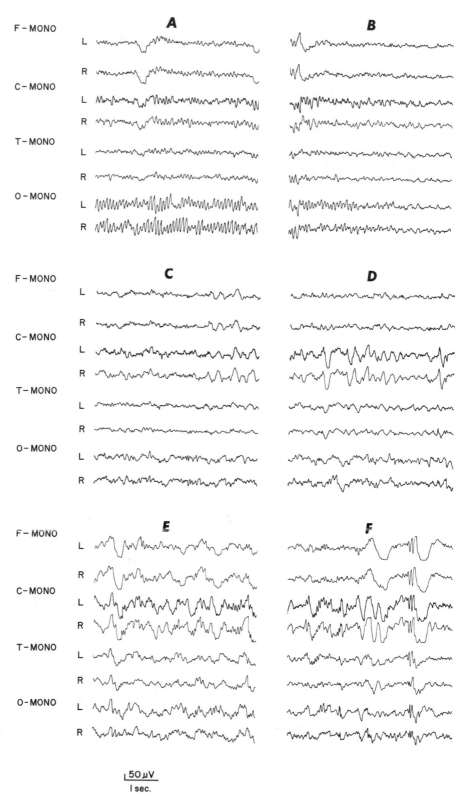

Figure 26–4 Successive stages of sleep in a young adult. Successive stages from awake but resting record (*A*), to drowsiness (*B*), to deeper stages of sleep (*E*) are shown. (See text for more detailed description.)

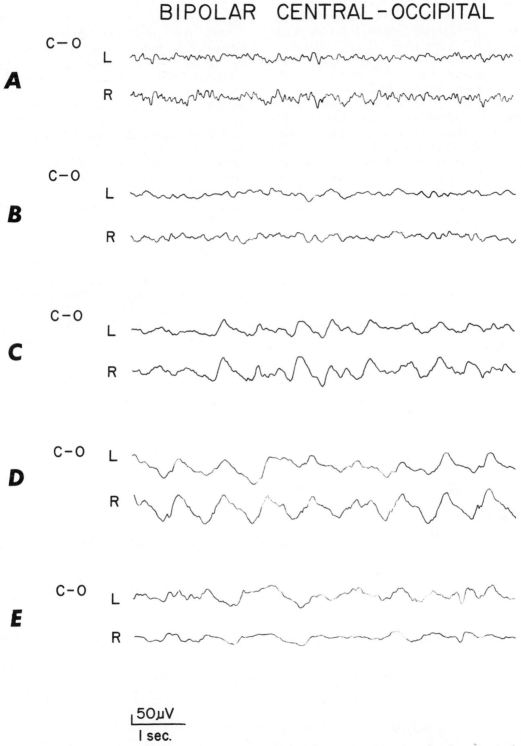

Figure 26–5 Changes in the human electroencephalogram with increasing depths of anesthesia. Beginning with a very light stage (*A*), progressively deeper stages are demonstrated (*B–E*). The anesthetic agent was cyclopropane.

agents such as ether and the intravenous barbiturates (e.g., thiopental or pentobarbital). As the depth of anesthesia is increased, there is, to a relative degree, a correlated change in the electroencephalogram from an initial stage of 8–13 cps alpha rhythm and low-voltage fast-activity to a stage of light anesthesia characterized by 4–7 cps activity (B) to a stage of high amplitude 2–3 cps slow wave activity (C). In this latter stage (C), a moderate depth of anesthesia is present with moderate relaxation of abdominal muscles and a mild depression of respiration. As depth of anesthesia is deepened, irregular 1–2 cps low waves are prominent (D). At deeper levels, periods when electrical activity is absent (isoelectric period) (E) alternate with periods of slow wave activity ("suppression burst phenomenon").* At these

*A more typical example of suppression burst phenomenon is presented in Figure 26–25, p. 743.

deeper stages (D and E) there is, from a clinical standpoint, a marked depression of respiration and good relaxation of abdominal muscles.

Age. Age produces variations in the otherwise normal electroencephalogram. At any given age, some activity in the alpha, theta, or delta range may be found. However, a particular frequency range usually predominates within a particular age range. Thus, in the 13-month-old infant demonstrated in Figure 26–6, the dominant awake activity is 4–5 cps. In the 5-year-old child, demonstrated in Figure 26–7, the dominant awake activity is 6–7 cps. In the 12-year-old, demonstrated in Figure 26–8, the dominant awake activity is 8–9 cps alpha rhythm.

EEG ABNORMALITIES

Two general statements may be made concerning the normal electroencephalogram:

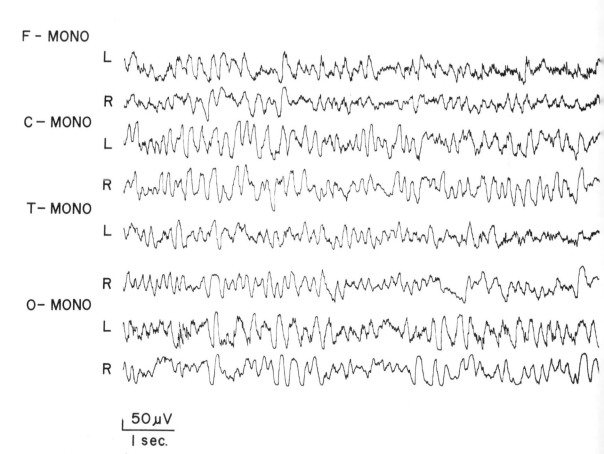

Figure 26–6 Effects of age on the electroencephalogram: A normal, awake, 13-month-old infant. The dominant activity is 4–5 cps. Monopolar recordings with ear as reference. F = frontal, T = temporal, C = central, and O = occipital.

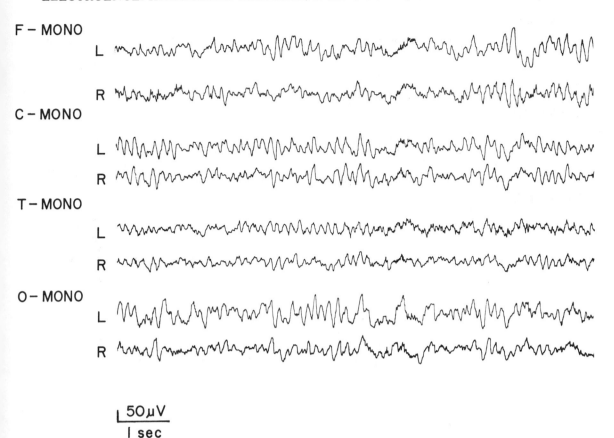

F – MONO

L

R

C – MONO

L

R

T – MONO

L

R

O – MONO

L

R

50 μV

1 sec

Figure 26–7 Effects of age on the electroencephalogram: a normal, awake, 5-year-old child. The dominant activity is 7 cps. Monopolar recordings with ear as reference. F = frontal, T = temporal, C = central, and O = occipital.

1. Homologous areas of the two hemispheres have a similar pattern. Thus, there is a relative symmetry of frequency and voltage amplitude.

2. At a given age, the state of alertness and consciousness (the dominant activity) falls within a particular frequency range and has a particular form (alpha rhythm in the awake adult).

In a sense, all abnormalities of the electroencephalogram represent a deviation from these two general rules.

In considering the correlation of electrical phenomena with clinical states, it is important to point out repeatedly that we will be speaking of relative correlations. There is no one-to-one correlation.

TYPE I ABNORMALITIES

In this type of abnormality the activity of the two hemispheres differs, i.e., asymmetry is present.

FOCAL SLOW WAVES

Focal slow waves imply focal cortical dysfunction having the quality of damage (Fig. 26–9). A number of additional examples have been provided in the chapters on cortical localization and diseases of the cerebral hemispheres, demonstrating focal slow wave activity in relation to infarction (Figs. 22–11, 22–17), abscess (Figs. 21–18, 22–35), glioblastoma (Fig. 21–25B), metastatic tumor (Fig. 21–14) and meningioma (Figs. 22–48, 22–51). The presence of focal slow wave activity when taken in isolation may allow for localization of the pathology but does not indicate the cause of the focal damage. The underlying nature of the pathology can only be predicted when clinical information and serial records are available.

FOCAL SPIKES

Focal spikes (Fig. 26–10) imply a focal cortical dysfunction having the quality of

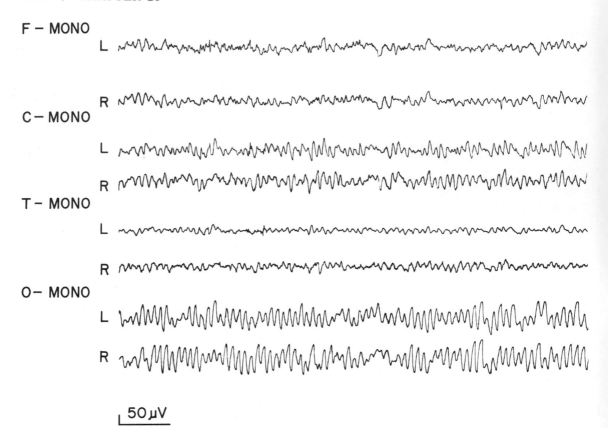

F — MONO

L

R

C — MONO

L

R

T — MONO

L

R

O — MONO

L

R

50 µV

1 sec

Figure 26–8 Effects of age on the electroencephalogram. A normal, awake, 12-year-old. The dominant activity is 8 cps. Monopolar recording with ear as reference. F = frontal, T = temporal, C = central, and O = occipital. Dominant alpha rhythm is usually attained by age 6–7 years.

sudden excessive neuronal discharge. The focal spike is the electrical correlate of the seizure of focal origin (also termed the partial or symptomatic seizure). Additional examples of focal spike discharges have already been presented (Figs. 21–25*A*; 22–24). In general, however, single focal spikes may occur in interictal (interseizure) periods without the occurrence of the actual focal seizure. In general, the focal seizure is likely to occur when frequent repetitive focal spikes occur or when the focal spike is followed by an after discharge. The usual duration of a spike discharge is 15–80 millisec. *Sharp waves* (blunt spikes, that is, spikes of longer duration—greater than 80 millisec) have the same general significance as spikes.

The pathological causes of focal seizures are variable, dependent in part on the age of the patient. A variety of patients presenting focal seizure disorders have been discussed in the chapters on cortical localization and diseases affecting the cerebral hemispheres.

We may specify the major causes of *focal* seizures beginning at particular ages as follows:

Within the first 48 hours of life—acute birth trauma (poor prognosis)

Within the first 2 years—birth trauma and congenital malformations (e.g., porencephalic cyst)

From 2 to 10 years—birth injury and head trauma

From 10 to 20 years—head trauma

From 20 to 35 years—head trauma and neoplasms

Over 50 years—tumor and vascular infarcts

The incidence of seizures (usually focal) following specific pathological processes has been variously estimated as follows:

*Cerebral cortical infarction—25%

---

*The overall incidence in all infarcts involving the cerebral hemispheres is much lower—perhaps in the area of 3 per cent.

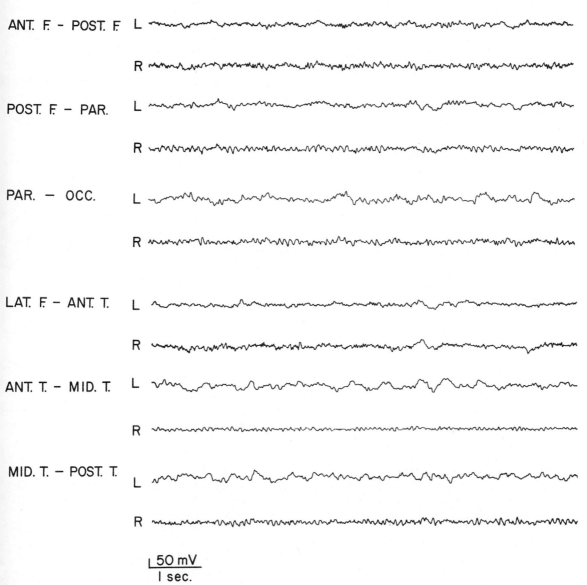

ANT. F. – POST. F. L

R

POST. F. – PAR. L

R

PAR. – OCC. L

R

LAT. F. – ANT. T. L

R

ANT. T. – MID. T. L

R

MID. T. – POST. T. L

R

50 mV

I sec.

Figure 26–9 Focal 2–5 cps slow wave activity in left temporal-parietal area. This 42-year-old patient had a glioma arising in the left middle-posterior temporal and posterior parietal area. His detailed case history has been presented in Chapter 21 (p. 529). This record was obtained approximately 3 months following partial resection of the tumor.

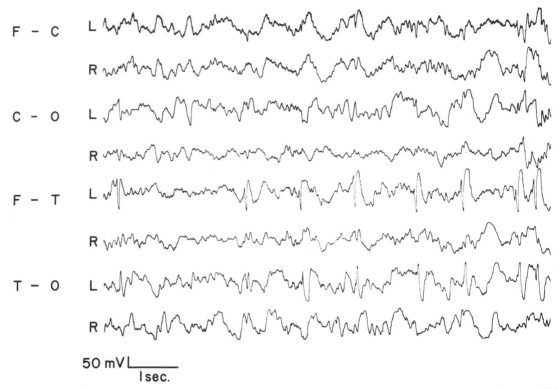

F − C   L

R

C − O   L

R

F − T   L

R

T − O   L

R

50 mV

1 sec.

Figure 26–10   Focal spike discharge left temporal area (with phase reversal in temporal area). This 4-year-old male had focal seizures manifested by psychomotor automatisms in addition to repetitive twitching of the right side of face and hand. Etiology could not be established.

*Penetrating head injuries—40–50%
Brain abscess—50%
Supratentorial tumors
         †Extracerebral (meningiomas)—62%
         Intracerebral (gliomas)—51%
Porencephalic cyst—44%

The common feature of all of these pathological processes is the fact that they primarily involve the cerebral cortex. In contrast, in the studies of Penfield and Jasper (1954), the incidence of seizures in infratentorial tumors was 0 per cent.

A given pathological process is more likely to cause seizure discharge if it involves an area of low threshold (motor cortex) rather than an area of high relative threshold (prefrontal area). A given pathological process is more likely to produce seizures if it produces partial damage rather than total destruction. That is, an excessive discharge represents the discharge of disordered neurons and synapses. Totally dead neurons cannot discharge. Epileptogenic foci, then, tend to be generated at the periphery of areas of tissue necrosis and not at the center of total necrosis.

There is often but not always a time factor in the development of epileptogenic foci. Occasionally focal seizures may occur in acute relationship to penetrating head injuries or to the cortical ischemia which follows a cerebral embolus. (In the laboratory, of course, acute epileptogenic foci may follow within minutes after the direct application of a convulsant agent to the pial surface of the cortex.) In clinical neurology, however, it is more often the case that a period of time —weeks, months, years (usually less than 2 years in posttraumatic cases)—has passed following the actual insult to the cerebral cortex.

The more specific pathological nature of the focus is often not clear in terms of what specific tissue alteration results in an epileptogenic focus. Damage to capillaries, fibroblastic and capillary ingrowth from menin-

_____

*The overall incidence in all blunt (nonpenetrating) head injuries is closer to 5 per cent.
†The actual incidence in meningiomas has been variously estimated—from 10 to 70 per cent.
  The actual incidence will depend on the location of the tumor, with a high incidence when occurring close to the motor cortex.

geal adhesions, gliosis, mechanical deformation of neuronal processes, and the effects of partial neuronal deafferentiation have all been suggested. There is usually not only the factor of evolving pathological changes at the focus but also the factor that these changes may be occurring in a nervous system that is evolving from a maturational standpoint. Thus, the effects of birth trauma or of cerebral edema in infancy, with regard to the temporal lobes, may not be evident until psychomotor seizures develop in late childhood, adolescence, or early adult life. The pathological findings in many of these cases of neuronal loss and gliosis (sclerosis) in medial temporal areas do not really indicate to us the nature by which the pathophysiological process evolved.

Experimental studies of the focal seizure and the epileptogenic focus have been concerned with two aspects: (1) the electrical behavior of neurons and synapses within the focus, and (2) the spread of discharge from the focus. As regards the electrical activity at focus, we have already indicated that much of what is recorded in the electroencephalogram represents the summated postsynaptic potentials of the apical dendrites. Since the duration of the spikes seen in the epileptic discharge is far longer than the potentials produced by axon or cell body discharge, it has been suggested (Brazier, 1955) that the epileptic spikes may be dependent on the postsynaptic discharge of the apical dendrites of pyramidal cells. The spike then represents summated excitatory postsynaptic potentials. Spike discharges at the cortical surface, then, are recorded as predominantly surface negative waves. More recent studies of cellular behavior at the epileptogenic focus have been summarized by Schmidt and Wilder (1968). The focus is defined as a group of abnormal cells ("epileptic neurons") with certain unique properties. These include the generation of autonomous paroxysmal discharges (which can be triggered by afferent stimulation), increased electrical excitability of the cell, and initiation of volleys of very high frequency impulses by sudden depolarization of the resting membrane potential. Detailed consideration of this topic is beyond the scope of this book. The reader is referred to the papers by Ward (1969) and Ajmone-Marsan (1969).

As regards the propagation of discharge from the focus, such spread occurs via several pathways: (1) short intracortical pathways—involving synapses and neurons within the adjacent neuropil, (2) long fiber systems to other cortical areas within the same cerebral hemisphere, (3) callosal and other commissural pathways to the contralateral cerebral hemisphere, and (4) descending pathways to basal ganglia, thalamus, reticular formation of the brain stem, and spinal cord. Obviously, the specific pattern of spread will depend on the location of the focus and on the anatomical connections or projections from the particular cortical area (see Chapters 20 and 21). Preferential patterns of spread are reviewed by Walker (1970) and by Wilder and Schmidt (1965).

It is important to realize that any focal spike discharge may become secondarily generalized (Fig. 26–11). From a clinical standpoint, any focal seizure may become a generalized seizure.

Figure 26–11 Generalization from a focal spike discharge. The discharge in this cat began at an experimental spike focus in left suprasylvian area (ss). After-discharge of repetitive spikes then occurred at the focus with subsequent spread to other recording areas of the same and contralateral cerebral hemispheres. P.S. = posterior sigmoid gyrus (sensory cortex); V. = visual projection area of marginal gyrus. (Calibrations: 1 second and 100 u volts.) (From Marcus, E. M., Watson, C. W., and Goldman, P. L.: Arch. Neurol., *15*:525, 1966.)

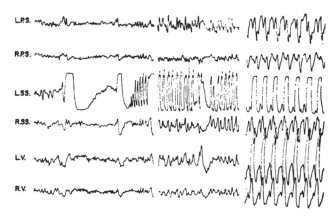

L.P.S.

R.P.S.

L.SS.

R.SS.

L.V.

R.V.

10 SEC. INTERVAL   50 SEC. INTERVAL

FOCAL DEPRESSION OF VOLTAGE AMPLITUDE

This implies electrically inactive tissue or material between the recording electrode and the active source of electrical activity. Thus, the electrically active tissue (cortex) is at a greater distance than usual from the recording electrode, and the amplitude of voltage detected is reduced. Blood or fluid in the subcutaneous tissue of the scalp, in the epidural space, in the subdural space, or in the subarachnoid space would produce this effect. A focal reduction in amplitude may also occur when both recording electrodes are located over a large intracerebral hematoma, over a large intracerebral fluid collection (e.g., a porencephalic cyst), or over a large area of necrotic dead tissue (as in a large cortical infarction as demonstrated in Figure 22–11).

MULTIFOCAL ABNORMALITIES

This represents a subcategory of type I abnormalities. Many of the disease processes affecting the cerebral hemisphere do not produce limited focal damage. Thus, a blow to the occipital area of the skull may not only produce injury to the occipital cortex at the site of the blow, but may also produce contusions of the cortex at a distance from the site of injury—anterior temporal poles and frontal poles and orbital frontal surfaces. The end result may be multifocal slow waves, implying multifocal damage or multifocal spikes, which in turn implies the evolution of multifocal areas of excessive neuronal discharge (Fig. 26–12).

TYPE II ABNORMALITIES

In type II abnormalities either the frequency of the dominant awake activity does not fall within the normal frequency range for the age, or the form of the dominant activity differs from the normal wave form and rhythm. All of the abnormalities to be discussed are essentially generalized abnormalities and imply a disease process affecting

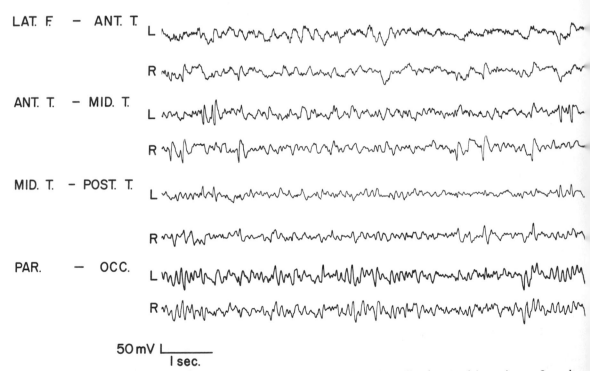

Figure 26–12 Multifocal spikes. At age 9, this patient had a generalized convulsive seizure. In subsequent years he experienced seizures which were multifocal in origin; most often psychomotor in type with automatisms and distortions of perception. At other times, discrete focal motor or sensory seizures involved, selectively, the right side of face, tongue, arm, throat, or chest. No definite etiology for the seizures was ever established. Neurological examination has remained normal and school performance has continued at a high level (now age 17). The electroencephalogram over the years has demonstrated multiple independent blunt spike foci of discharge, at times most prominent in the left or right temporal areas; at other times most prominent in the frontal central or occipital areas.

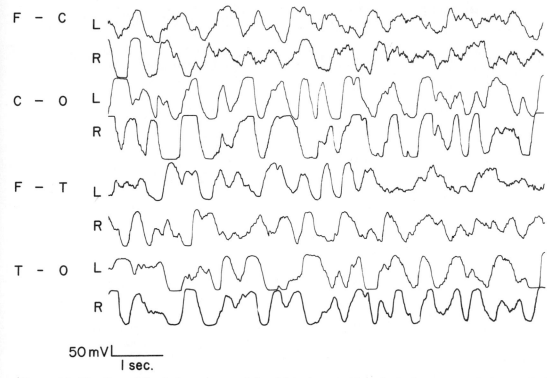

Figure 26–13 Generalized slow wave activity. This 4-year-old male had an acute viral encephalitis. The electroencephalogram demonstrated a dominant awake activity of 1–2 cps slow waves, despite attempts at arousal.

the cerebral cortex in a generalized or diffuse manner. We have included within this category bilateral symmetrical and relatively synchronous abnormalities which may be generalized or predominant in particular recording areas (e.g., bilateral frontal).

GENERALIZED SLOW WAVE ACTIVITY

This implies a generalized cortical dysfunction having the quality of damage. The dysfunction may reflect an actual generalized structural damage (Fig. 26–13) or may simply be indicative of a toxic or metabolic state (Fig. 26–14). An actual generalized structural damage may occur in anoxia, in encephalitis, or in a diffuse degenerative disease. A transient dysfunction may occur in hepatic or renal failure. Generalized slow wave activity may also occur transiently during the postictal state which follows a generalized convulsive seizure.

GENERALIZED PAROXYSMAL DISCHARGES

We refer in this category to generalized bursts of: (1) spike and slow wave complexes (correlated with the petit mal seizure); (2) polyspike and slow wave complexes (correlated with myoclonic seizures); (3) repetitive fast spikes (8–12 cps) (correlated with generalized seizures), and (4) rhythmic slow waves.

All of these electrical abnormalities suggest a generalized dysfunction having the quality of excessive neuronal discharge. These abnormalities are in general correlated with seizure disorders which are nonfocal in origin and which in the past have been variously termed idiopathic, essential, non-symptomatic, or cryptogenic. In the recent international classification of the epilepsies (Gastaut, 1965), this category is referred to as seizures which are generalized from their onset. This refers to the fact that no focal origin is evident for the electrical discharge and to the fact that the clinical seizure is characterized from its onset by the loss of consciousness.

The type of electrical abnormality and the correlated clinical seizure disorder should be contrasted to the focal spike and the focal (or symptomatic or partial) seizure disorder where a focal origin is clearly evident and

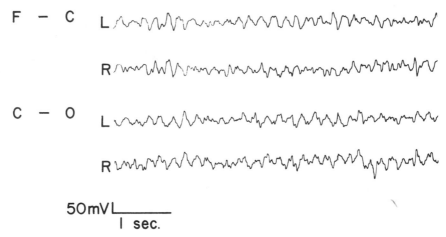

Figure 26–14 Generalized slow wave activity in a metabolic encephalopathy. This 67-year-old house-wife had a long history of impaired hepatic function secondary to cirrhosis with recurrent episodes of coma. During episodes of hepatic coma, the degree of electroencephalographic abnormality correlated in general with the severity of coma. When the patient was semicomatose in a stuporous state, the dominant awake activity was slow at 5 cps as illustrated. When the patient was more deeply comatose, the awake activity was even slower at 4 cps. When the patient was alert during intervening periods of recovery, the dominant activity was in alpha range.

where loss of consciousness is not the initial sign of the seizure.

We will describe in somewhat greater detail the various subcategories within this group and will discuss current theories concerning the anatomical and pathophysiological basis of the seizure type.

THE SPIKE SLOW WAVE COMPLEX AND THE PETIT MAL SEIZURE

Clinical Features. Generalized bursts of 3 cps (2½–4 cps) spike slow wave complexes correlate with the petit mal seizure (Fig. 26–15). The petit mal seizure consists of a short (5–30 seconds) interruption of consciousness in which general postural tone is relatively well preserved. During this brief period, the patient is observed to stare, oblivious to stimuli introduced into his environment. He interrupts his ongoing activities. For example, if in the midst of eating, the patient may stop with his spoon in midair. The interruption is relatively abrupt in onset and relatively abrupt in cessation. The patient's awareness and motor activities return promptly at the end of the episode. Memory is defective only for the period of the seizure. It is as though the patient, although physically present, has been absent as regards his higher cortical functions for the brief interval of the seizure.

The term *absence seizure* is sometimes used then to refer to the episode. In actuality, the impairment of awareness, the impairment of response capacity, and the impairment of motor activity is a relative phenomenon, occurring in variable degree. Thus, some patients may be unaware of phrases or numbers which are provided as auditory or visual stimuli during the episode. Other patients are aware of these same stimuli and are able to repeat them during the episode or during questioning at the end. Some patients are able to continue a familiar recitation during the petit mal seizure. Whether a response to a stimulus occurs during these brief seizures may, in part, depend on the intensity of the stimulus and the motivation and past experience of the patient. As we will see demonstrated repeatedly, there is no strict one-to-one correlation as regards the electroencephalogram and behavior; there are only relative degrees of correlation.

Short bursts of spike slow wave complexes (1–2 seconds) in general do not have any definite clinical accompaniment. Bursts of 6–30 seconds duration are in general accompanied by some interruption of consciousness (Mirsky and Pragay, 1967; Geller and Geller, 1970). It is the degree of interruption that is variable.

There may be little external evidence that the patient is in the midst of a seizure. Parents and associates may fail to note the 50 seizures a day that may occur in the untreated patient until the patient's schoolteacher brings short episodes of unattentiveness to light. There are minor motor phenomena which may often accompany the seizure: eye opening, eyelid myoclonus, and, at times, other extraocular movements. Myoclonus of the face and repetitive chewing may also occur. Some minor loss of postural tone in the neck muscles may occur, causing the head to drop onto the chest. Automatisms involving the hands may occur; at times these are to some extent appropriate to the environmental situation.

From the standpoint of differential diagnosis, the petit mal seizure must be distinguished from the focal seizure originating in the temporal lobe. In general, the duration of the temporal lobe seizure is longer; consciousness does not return abruptly, but rather the seizure is followed by a variable period of postictal confusion. The petit mal seizure must also be differentiated from focal seizures beginning in the prefrontal and premotor areas of the frontal lobes.

Several general statistics concerning petit mal seizures should also be considered. Onset of this type of seizure occurs in childhood or early adolescence (age 4–16). These seizures tend to diminish in frequency as adulthood is reached. However, at least 50 per cent of the patients will also exhibit generalized convulsive seizures at some time in life. The predisposition to petit mal seizures in many families, as judged by electroencephalographic studies of relatives, is apparently inherited as an autosomal dominant trait with variable penetrance (Metrakos and Metrakos, 1961). In some cases (a minority) there is little evidence of a genetic background and the seizures apparently reflect perinatal or other multifocal and diffuse pathological processes beginning in child-

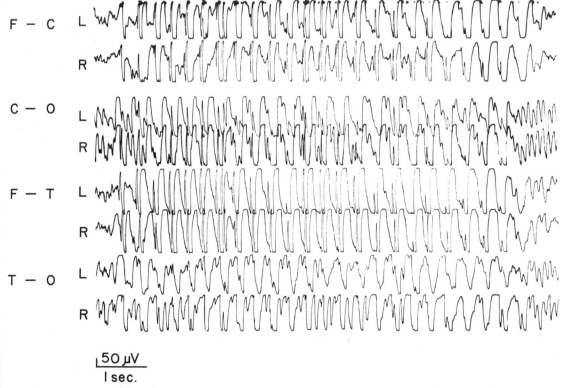

50 μV
I sec.

Figure 26–15 Generalized bursts of 3 cps spike-slow wave complexes in petit mal epilepsy: This 19-year-old male had frequent absence seizures, characterized by a blank stare, flickering of the eyelids (myoclonus) and a failure to respond to instructions. The record during a relatively short absence is demonstrated (total duration, 8 seconds). Many seizures were of longer duration (20–40 seconds). Note the abrupt onset and the abrupt cessation of the bilaterally synchronous and relatively symmetrical discharge. Spike components are usually most prominent in frontal and central recording areas.

hood. In such cases, mental retardation and positive findings may be present on neurological examination. The majority of patients with petit mal seizures are of normal intelligence and do not have significant abnormalities on neurological examination.

Pathophysiology of Petit Mal Seizures. As regards the anatomical substrate for the electrical and behavioral phenomenon of the petit mal seizure, several explanations have been advanced. These explanations based on experimental models differ as regards the emphasis given to the role of intralaminar nuclei of the thalamus and the mesencephalic reticular formation (the *centrencephalic hypothesis*) as opposed to the cerebral cortex.

A stimulus-related 3 cps spike-and-wave pattern may at times be produced in the cat on stimulation of the midline nuclei or of the intralaminar system of the thalamus as originally demonstrated by the studies of Jasper and Droogleever-Fortuyn (1946) (Fig. 26–16). The studies of Pollen (1963, 1964) have indicated that the spike of the thalamic-induced spike and wave corresponds to the recruiting response, discussed previously (p. 473). The long duration surface negative slow wave of the complex is the surface reflection of inhibitory postsynaptic potentials generated at axosomatic synapses in the deeper cell layers. Arrest of movement may also occur from stimulation within the intralaminar system of the thalamus but this is nonspecific, for a similar response may also occur on stimulation at a number of cortical, subcortical, and brain stem sites.

A series of recent experiments has reexamined the question of the pathophysiology of petit mal epilepsy from the standpoint of two central questions: (1) What is the essential locus of pathological lesion responsible for the bilateral spike slow wave discharges and the associated behavioral absence of petit mal epilepsy? (2) Irrespective of where the responsible lesions may be located, are the brain stem and diencephalic structures essential for the development of the bilateral discharges; that is, to what extent is the presence of these structures necessary for the evolution of the bilateral spike wave discharge?

As regards the first question, concerning the locus of pathological lesion, these studies have demonstrated that it is not necessary to implicate the thalamus or brain stem. Thus it has been possible to reproduce both the electrical and behavioral characteristics of petit mal epilepsy by directly increasing the excitability of particular areas of the cerebral cortex in a bilateral manner without the necessity of thalamic or brain stem pathology. Thus, in the studies of Marcus and Watson (1968) bilateral symmetrical foci of discharge in the anterior premotor areas of the monkey (areas 8 – anterior 6) resulted in well-developed bilateral bursts of 3 cps spike slow wave complexes (Fig. 26–17). In behavioral correlation experiments, these discharges were often correlated with an interruption of ongoing motor activities and an alteration in response capacity for visual and tactile stimuli. As in the human case, eyelid opening and extraocular myoclonus were prominent in the experimental case. This would be predictable since the bilateral epileptogenic foci were produced in the

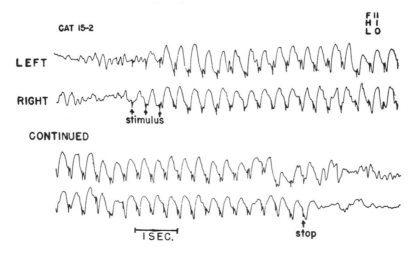

Figure 26–16 Experimental 3 cps spike wave discharges following midline thalamic stimulation. A stimulus-related bilaterally synchronous spike and wave discharge is produced in cat cerebral cortex by repetitive 3 cps stimulation of the massa intermedia. (From Jasper, H., and Droogleever-Fortuyn, J.: Res. Publ. Ass. nerv. ment. Dis., 26:272–298, 1947.)

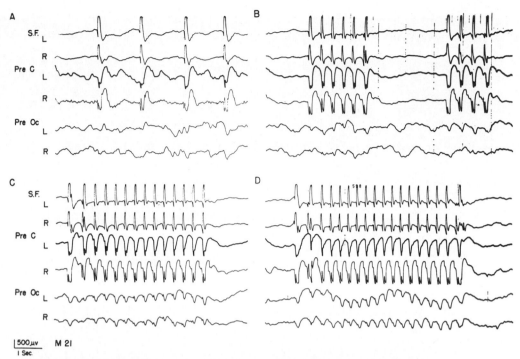

Figure 26–17   Experimental 3 cps spike wave discharge following production of bilateral epilepto-genic foci in anterior premotor cortex of monkey. Repetitive bursts of synchronous and symmetrical 2½–3 cps spike-wave complexes occurred frequently in this animal following a 3-minute period of minor hyperventilation. Similar bursts occurred during periods of normal ventilation but were less frequent. A similar effect of hyperventilation is noted in the human patients with petit mal epilepsy. S.F. = superior frontal-gyrus in prefrontal area, Pre C = precentral gyrus, and Pe O = preoccipital area, *A,* Just prior to hyperventilation; *B, C, D,* Two to three minutes after beginning of hyperventilation. (From Marcus, E. M., and Watson, C. W.: Arch. Neurol., *19*:103, 1968.)

frontal eye fields. The polysensory projection to this area of frontal cortex about the arcuate sulcus in the monkey has already been noted (p. 506). It is important also to indicate the significant projection from this area about the arcuate sulcus to the reticular formation of the brain stem. (Area 8 had been implicated as a suppressor area for motor activities, as discussed previously, p. 494.)

The behavioral components of the petit mal seizure such as arrest of movement and myoclonus are obviously represented and rerepresented at various levels of the neural axis. However, as regards the electrical discharge of bilateral spike slow wave complexes, from the standpoint of the experimental model with bilateral cortical foci, it is possible to demonstrate that the electrical phenomenon is essentially arising at a cortical level without the mediation of thalamic or brain stem structures. Thus, in considering the role, if any, of brain stem structures the following observations are relevant (question 2). A unilateral spike and slow wave discharge may be generated in an isolated island of cerebral cortex to which a convulsant agent has been applied. A bilateral discharge of 3 cps spike slow wave complexes may be generated following the production of bilateral foci in a preparation in which large islands of cerebral cortex in each hemisphere have been isolated from subcortical structures but remain connected to each other via the corpus callosum (Fig. 26–18). Moreover, in the intact animal with bilateral foci, synchrony of bilateral discharge is markedly disrupted by section of the corpus callosum. These observations do not rule out the demonstrated role of brain stem structures in synchronizing other types of cortical electrical activity.

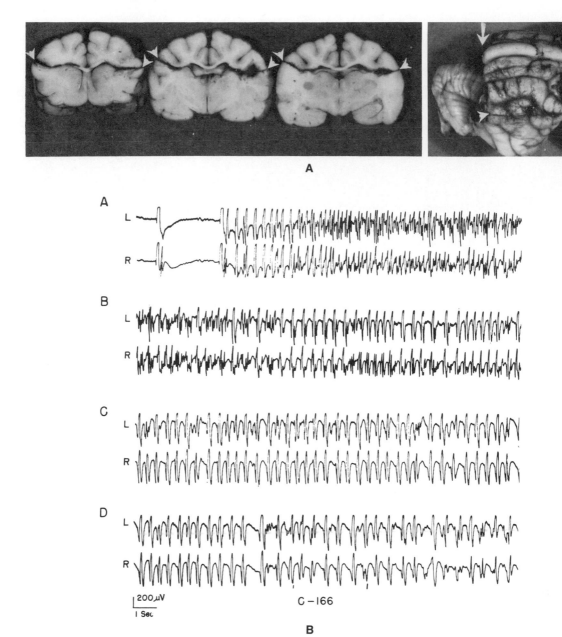

Figure 26–18A Bilateral isolation of cerebral cortex and corpus callosum: the cortical callosal preparation (cat). The coronal section demonstrates bilateral isolation of cerebral cortex. This was produced by dissection to the floor of each lateral ventricle at anterior and posterior poles. A curved spatula was then introduced into each lateral ventricle and the cortex was undercut to the pial surface. Pial blood supply remained intact. Cortex, anterior and posterior to the isolation, was then removed. In some animals rostrum of corpus callosum, septum, and dorsal hippocampus were also ablated. In the view of lateral surface, the total area of cortex included within the isolation is demonstrated. A similar procedure may also be performed in the monkey. (From Marcus, E. M., and Watson, C. W.: Arch. Neurol., *14*:602, 1966.)

Figure 26–18 B Bilateral synchronous spike-slow wave discharges following the production of bilateral epileptogenic foci in the cortical callosal preparation. Frequent prolonged bursts of 2-2½ cps spike slow wave complexes occurred in the preparation. (From Marcus, E. M., Watson, C. W., and Simon, S. A.: Epilepsia, *9*:243, 1968.)

GENERALIZED DISCHARGE POLYSPIKE SLOW WAVE COMPLEX AND MYOCLONUS

Generalized bursts of polyspike slow wave complexes correlate, in a general sense, with myoclonus and myoclonic seizures (Fig. 26–19). Bursts of this paroxysmal discharge may be accompanied by a sudden bilateral myoclonic jerk of the extremities or by myoclonus of the eyelids and facial muscles. At times when the discharge is prolonged an absence seizure may occur in addition to the myoclonus. At times the discharge may occur without any accompanying behavioral phenomenon but the patient will have a clinical history of generalized convulsive seizures or of morning myoclonic jerks.

Myoclonus: Definition and Anatomical Substrate. Myoclonus may be defined as a sudden rapid jerk or twitch resulting from the sudden contraction of one or more muscle groups. The jerks may be bilateral and symmetrical or multifocal. Facial muscles, extraocular muscles, and head or limbs may be involved. The intensity of the contraction may be strong enough to throw the patient to the floor or isolated and weak enough to result in the twitch of a finger.*

The anatomical substrate for myoclonus is variable. In the monkey myoclonus may occur as a result of bilateral epileptogenic foci in the motor cortex or the adjacent premotor cortex. Myoclonus may also occur in various extrapyramidal diseases involving the basal ganglia or ventrolateral nuclei of the thalamus. Myoclonic jerks may occur in decorticate or midbrain animal preparations. In a spinal cord preparation, myoclonic jerks may also be noted following the administration of a convulsant agent.

In the noncortical varieties of myoclonus, it is possible to have the behavioral phenom-

---

*Obviously the definition of myoclonus is somewhat imprecise. We usually do not employ the term to describe the focal clonic movements of a focal motor seizure. Nor do we usually employ the term to describe the local jerking of a limb which may occur in relationship to compression of a peripheral nerve or nerve roots.

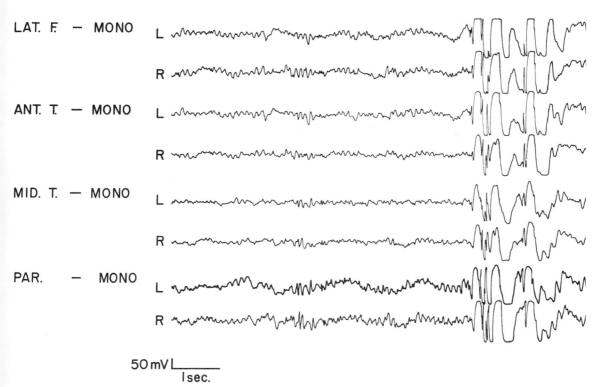

Figure 26–19 Generalized bursts of polyspikes and slow waves. This patient had the onset at age 13 of sudden single generalized myoclonic jerks, which initially were sufficiently violent to throw the patient to the floor. These jerks were *not* accompanied by any definite impairment of consciousness. Neurological examination has remained normal and the patient has never (now age 22 years) experienced generalized convulsive seizures or petit mal absences.

enon without the occurrence of accompanying spike or polyspike discharges in the electroencephalogram. In the cortical variety of myoclonus, conduction of discharges to the brain stem and spinal cord occurs along both pyramidal and nonpyramidal pathways. Stimulus sensitive myoclonus refers to the precipitation of myoclonic jerks by sound, light flash, proprioceptive or tactile stimuli. Usually the underlying disease is a diffusely distributed process. In some cases it is primarily cortical; in others it is primarily noncortical. The disease process usually involves neurons primarily rather than white matter.

From an etiological and prognostic standpoint, myoclonus may be seen under a variety of circumstances.

Benign Nonprogressive Myoclonus. Sudden *myoclonic jerks on falling asleep* or awakening occur in a large part of the normal population. Many have had the experience of sitting in a lecture at about 2:00 or 3:00 P.M. and beginning to drowse as the lecturer drones on, only to awaken with a sudden jerk

of the legs. Myoclonus may also occur in a family setting as *essential myoclonus.*

Nonprogressive Myoclonus and Idiopathic Epilepsy. Many patients with generalized convulsive seizures of the idiopathic variety will present a history of single or repetitive myoclonic jerks occurring frequently in relation to the drowsy state of approaching sleep or in relation to arousal. At times when repetitive jerks occur, the patient will proceed into a generalized convulsive seizure.

As noted, nonprogressive myoclonus also may occur as a component of the other seizure type of idiopathic epilepsy: the petit mal seizure.

In idiopathic epilepsy, a significant proportion of the patients will have the electrical discharges and accompanying myoclonus induced by the use of repetitive photic stimulation with a high intensity short duration flash of light (stroboscopic) at a frequency of 10 to 20 flashes per second (Fig. 26–20). The precipitation of similar electrical dis-

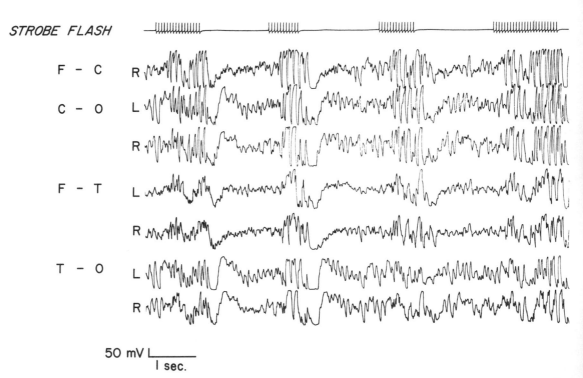

STROBE FLASH

F – C

C – O

F – T

T – O

50 mV

1 sec.

Figure 26–20 Generalized bursts of polyspikes and slow waves triggered by photic stimulation. This young woman at age 13 had the onset of generalized convulsive seizures and of frequent myoclonic seizures involving eyelids and arms. The myoclonic seizures were clearly triggered by bright flickering light. The bursts of polyspikes and slow waves illustrated in the record were often accompanied by myoclonus of eyelids, facial muscles, and limbs.

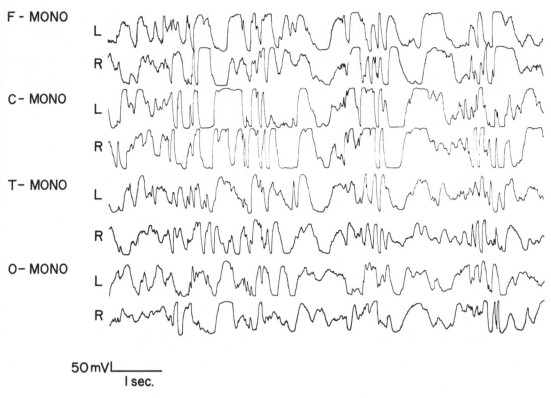

F - MONO

C - MONO

T - MONO

O - MONO

50 mV

1 sec.

Figure 26–21   Hypsarrhythmia in an infant with myoclonic spasms.

charges in the electroencephalogram by photic stimulation is also found to occur in a high percentage of the relatives of affected individuals and, as such, may serve as a possible index of the predisposition to idiopathic seizures. The transmission of this trait occurs as an autosomal dominant with a variable penetrance, dependent in part upon age and sex determined factors (Watson and Marcus, 1962). A similar response to photic stimulation of electrical discharge and myoclonus occurs in high frequency among a variety of baboons: papio papio. In the animal model, the discharge appears to originate at a cortical level in premotor areas.

Myoclonus in Diffuse Metabolic or Toxic Disturbances of the Nervous System. Myoclonic jerks may occur in relation to a variety of metabolic disturbances, e.g., the uremic state following renal failure, carbon dioxide narcosis in respiratory insufficiency, hypocalcemia, the pyridoxine deficiency state of infancy, and the postanoxic or posthypoglycemic state. Following recovery from anoxia, myoclonus may also remain as a chronic manifestation.

Myoclonus and Mental Retardation in Infancy. We refer in this context to infantile myoclonic spasms also called "massive spasms." This condition is usually first noted at 6 to 9 months of age and usually persists until 2 to 3 years of age. In addition to the frequent myoclonic jerks which may be generalized and massive or multifocal, retardation of psychomotor development also becomes apparent in most cases. The etiology is variable, reflecting a diffuse or multifocal pathology: perinatal brain damage, tuberous sclerosis, phenylketonuria, pyridoxine deficiency.

The electroencephalogram demonstrates a characteristic pattern referred to as hypsarrhythmia (Fig. 26–21), consisting of continuous high amplitude generalized but often asynchronous spikes and slow waves. At other times, particularly during drowsiness and sleep, the record may be characterized by generalized periodic bursts of polyspikes and slow waves, with intervening periods of relative electrical silence. (Similar to the pattern demonstrated in Fig. 26–25.)

In many cases both the myoclonus and the

electroencephalographic abnormality will be decreased by the use of ACTH (adrenocorticotrophic hormone) or of adrenal cortical steroids (such as prednisone). The mental retardation, however, persists. Even without treatment, the myoclonic seizures and the electroencephalographic abnormality tend to disappear with increasing age. Although myoclonic seizures tend to disappear, other seizure types may emerge: generalized convulsive seizures, akinetic seizures, or multifocal seizures. As the patient becomes older, the electroencephalogram may reveal other types of abnormality: generalized bursts of 1–2 cps spike slow wave complexes or multifocal slow waves and spikes.

Myoclonus and Progressive Diffuse Disease of the Central Nervous System. At each age period in life, there may develop neurological disorders, characterized by myoclonus, generalized convulsive seizures, progressive dementia, plus or minus progressive corticospinal dysfunction, plus or minus progressive extrapyramidal dysfunction.

In this group are considered the disorders grouped together as the *lipidoses,* in which neurons are swollen with collections of lipid. The lipid is not neutral fat, but rather a more complex glycolipid substance such as the ganglioside found in the *infantile form, Tay-Sachs disease.* In this latter form often labeled "cerebromacular degeneration," there is usually a characteristic "cherry red spot" in the macular area. This is the most frequent and best studied variety. The usual age of onset is 3 to 10 months of age. The disease occurs as an autosomal recessive — primarily in Jewish families from Eastern Europe. Less common forms are the late infantile type of Bielschowsky, the juvenile form of Spielmeyer-Vogt and the adult form of Kufs-Hallervorden. In general, the later the age of onset, the slower the rate of progression.

Other causes of progressive myoclonus in late childhood and adolescence are the myoclonus epilepsy of Unverricht and Lundborg, in which large amyloid inclusions (Lafora bodies) composed of polymers of glucose are found within neurons. Some cases of myoclonic epilepsy overlap the progressive spinocerebellar degenerations.

Other acute and subacute causes of progressive myoclonus should also be considered. Thus, myoclonus is a prominent symptom in acute herpes simplex encephalitis and also may be noted in other forms of acute encephalitis. Myoclonus is also prominent in the syndrome of subacute inclusion body encephalitis (SSPE), an uncommon disease which affects children and adolescents and in which the measles virus has been recently implicated (see p. 592). The question of subacute slow viral infection has also been raised with regard to Jakob-Creutzfeldt disease, a progressive disorder which affects middle-aged and older adults and which includes, among other symptoms, myoclonus and generalized seizures (see p. 592).

REPETITIVE FAST SPIKE DISCHARGES AND GENERALIZED CONVULSIVE SEIZURES

Clinical Aspects of Grand Mal Seizure. The stereotype of the generalized convulsion, the grand mal seizure, consists of two phases: the tonic and clonic. Unless the tonic-clonic convulsion represents a secondarily generalized seizure, the onset is abrupt, with loss of consciousness the initial sign. The patient stiffens and, if standing erect, is thrown to the floor. Respiration is arrested and the pupils dilate. After a short but variable period of 10 to 30 seconds the tonic stage then passes into the clonic stage. The symmetrical jerks of clonus than slow in frequency and cease. The total duration of the actual seizure is usually a matter of 2 to 5 minutes. This stage is followed by a variable period of coma, followed by stupor, confusion, and drowsiness. The total duration of confusion and drowsiness is usually 30 to 60 minutes. The patient will be amnesic about the onset of the attack, about subsequent events of the seizure, and about the postictal period of confusion. If the bladder has been full, incontinence of urine will have occurred during the seizure. The plantar responses are usually extensor during the attack and will remain extensor during the early part of the postictal period.

EEG Correlation. From the electroencephalographic standpoint, the electrical correlate of the tonic phase of the seizure is the fast spike discharge at 8–20 cps (Fig. 26-22A). The clonic phase correlates with a repetitive spike wave or polyspike wave discharge of gradually decreasing frequency (Fig. 26–22B, C, D). The initial postictal period is usually correlated with a short period of relative electrical silence in the electroencephalogram (Fig. 26–22E). Slow

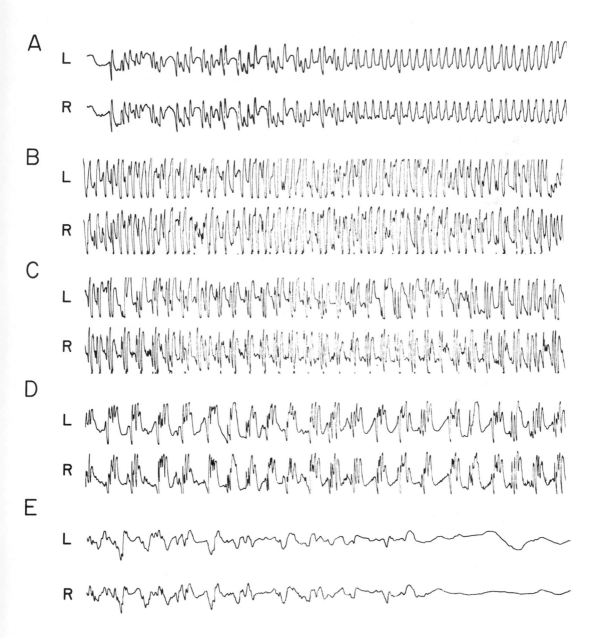

1 sec.

Figure 26–22 Experimental generalized convulsive seizure (without focal onset) in a monkey. The animal was tonic during segment *A* (corresponding to the fast spike discharge of 6–8 cps). During segments *C* and *D*, the animal had repetitive clonic jerks, gradually decreasing in frequency. The period of relative electrical silence shown at the end of segment *E* and the subsequent periods of 1–2 cps slow wave activity corresponded to the postictal depression of consciousness. The generalized seizure followed the production of bilateral epileptogenic foci in the premotor area. This monkey also had frequent petit mal seizures.

wave activity of 1–3 cps is then apparent and is correlated with the period of depression of consciousness. With clearing of confusion, the electroencephalogram gradually returns to a normal frequency range.

During interictal periods, the electroencephalogram in patients who are subject to generalized convulsive seizures may present a variable appearance. The record often may be normal. Generalized bursts of polyspikes and slow waves may occur. In some cases, focal or multifocal abnormalities may be present even though a clinical focus of seizure onset was not apparent.

Etiology of Grand Mal Seizures. The causes of generalized convulsive seizures are many. The tonic-clonic seizure represents the response of the brain to a number of events which alter excitability. Thus, any individual could experience a generalized convulsive seizure in relation to electroshock therapy (although the threshold voltage required might vary from one individual to the next). Febrile convulsions are frequent in the age group under 5 years and occur predominantly between 6 months and 3 years of age. It has been estimated that 4 to 7 per cent of all children under the age of 5 years will have at least one generalized convulsive seizure (the majority febrile). Children with febrile seizures have a high familial incidence of seizure disorder suggesting a factor of genetic predisposition. A significant proportion of these children will be found later to also have nonfebrile convulsions.

Various metabolic disorders may also be associated with generalized convulsive seizures, the more specific causes varying with the age of the patient, e.g., hypoglycemia, hypocalcemia, alkalosis, aminoaciduria (such as phenylketonuria), pyridoxine deficiency, water intoxication, uremia, and anoxia. Lead encephalopathy frequently includes among its manifestations generalized convulsive seizures. In the infant and child, meningitis and encephalitis usually include among their clinical effects generalized convulsive seizures. Recurrent generalized and focal and psychomotor seizures, of course, may remain as a residual effect of both types of central nervous system infections.

In the adult, withdrawal from the chronic usage of large amounts of alcohol (in its various tastier forms) is a frequent cause of isolated generalized convulsive seizures. Such seizures are most likely to occur 7 to 48 hours after abrupt withdrawal (Victor and Brausch,

1967). The postictal state may then merge into a more prolonged agitated and confusional state of delirium tremens. This same clinical state may also follow withdrawal from barbiturates, meprobamate, diazepam (Valium), and chlordiazepoxide (Librium) (see Essig, 1967; and Wikler and Essig, 1970).

Having eliminated these various transient toxic or metabolic alterations as causes of generalized seizures, there still remain the majority of patients who experience recurrent generalized convulsive seizures. In some of these patients, the seizure although generalized represents the residual effects of focal or multifocal damage incurred in relation to development or perinatal pathology, head trauma in childhood or adult years, brain tumors involving the cerebral hemispheres, or vascular disease involving the cerebral cortex. Such focal or multifocal pathological processes are usually considered in association with focal seizures, but at times (see case history 14, p. 606) focal onset may not be apparent. In addition to these various focal and multifocal pathological processes, various diffuse progressive diseases already considered may be associated with generalized convulsive seizures. Senile and presenile dementia should also be considered among these diffuse processes. Such diffuse diseases are in general, with the exception of the presenile and senile dementia, not commonly encountered.

Having considered and eliminated all of the forementioned causes, there will still remain the majority of patients with recurrent generalized convulsive seizures in whom an underlying pathological process cannot be clearly defined. These cases have been variously referred to as essential, cryptogenic, idiopathic, or primarily generalized or unlocalized generalized convulsive seizure. Such cases usually begin during childhood or adolescence. Intelligence is usually normal and the neurological examination unremarkable. There is often a family history of a seizure disorder, and genetic predisposition must be presumed. In some cases, as previously discussed, a history of petit mal seizures may be present in the patient or in other family members.

However, even when those seizures which begin in adult life are considered, the most frequent diagnostic category is that of "cryptogenic" (cause as yet hidden). This is true even if grand mal seizures beginning after the age of 35 years are considered (Berlin,

1953). This is also the most frequent diagnostic category if all patients with any type of seizure disorder beginning in the adult years of life are considered. Although the possibility of a brain tumor such as a meningioma or glioma always looms large in the diagnostic considerations of such a patient, this suspicion is usually not borne out by the actual statistics. Thus, in the studies of Raynor, et al. (1959) only 14 per cent of patients with onset of seizures after age 20 years were found to have a tumor. In the studies of Woodcock and Cosgrove (1964), only 36 per cent of patients with onset of seizures after age 50 years were found to have tumors. In both studies, the probability of brain tumor was markedly increased by the presence of (a) focal components to the seizure, (b) focal abnormalities on neurological examination, or (c) focal abnormalities in the electroencephalogram. These considerations will then determine whether the diagnostic evaluation in the adult patient includes such specialized studies as brain scan, arteriography, and pneumoencephalography.

Pathophysiology of Grand Mal Seizures.
The anatomical substrate of the generalized convulsive seizure may be briefly considered. As in the petit mal seizure, two aspects of the question must be considered: the behavioral phenomena and the cortical electrical discharge. As regards the behavioral components, the earlier work of Muskens (1928) clearly indicated the capacity of the midbrain preparation and the decerebrate preparation to develop both myoclonus and generalized convulsive seizures. More recently, Rodin, et al. (1971) have demonstrated that the onset of the myoclonic jerks and the tonic phase of a generalized convulsive seizure induced in the cat by the convulsant agents, Megimide, or pentylenetetrazol, coincided with bursts of high voltage, high frequency discharge in the brain stem reticular formation (at mesencephalic and pontine levels). (Such considerations, however, do not necessarily mean that in the intact animal the basic pathological lesion is located at the brain stem level; thus, the basic pathological lesion may be a cortical focus with the generalized convulsive seizure occurring as a secondary phenomenon.)

As regards the bilateral electrical discharge associated with the generalized convulsive seizure, experimental studies would suggest that this is primarily a cortical phenomenon.

If the generalized discharge which follows the intravenous administration of pentylenetetrazol is considered, it is possible to demonstrate (Fig. 26–23) that cerebral cortex isolated from all subcortical structures (or bilaterally isolated in the cortical callosal preparation) has the capacity for the generation of a discharge at threshold dosage which is identical to that obtained in the intact animal (Starzl, et al., 1953; Marcus, et. al., 1969). The explanation for the cessation of the seizures is not clear but presumably includes various inhibitory processes involving the cortex, subcortical nuclei, thalamus, and brain stem. In this regard we should note that the activity of isolated cerebral cortex is characterized by bursts of activity with intervening periods of relative electrical silence (Fig. 26–25).

CONDITIONS DISTINGUISHED FROM GENERALIZED CONVULSIVE SEIZURES

Several conditions in which a loss of consciousness and postural tone occur must be differentiated from grand mal epilepsy.

Syncope. Most frequently encountered is the condition of syncope (fainting), which may be defined as a transient loss of consciousness due to a general decrease in cerebral blood flow. The loss of consciousness almost always occurs when the patient is in an upright position; consciousness usually returns promptly when the patient assumes a recumbent position. The actual loss of consciousness is preceded by prodromal symptoms which last from seconds to minutes and which the patient usually remembers: light-headedness, weakness, dizziness, sweating, and blurring and dimming of vision. The patient often has time to reach a chair or bed. He is observed to slump limply to the ground (as opposed to the epileptic who usually stiffens and then falls violently to the ground). Tonic or clonic movements are rare but may occur. The period of unconsciousness is brief, a matter of seconds or a minute. During this time, the patient is noted to be pale and sweaty. The pulse is usually weak and the blood pressure often reduced. The return to consciousness is rapid, without a significant period of mental confusion.

The causes of syncope are several. In *vasovagal syncope,* a sudden loss of resistance in the peripheral circulation results in a pooling of blood in the periphery with a

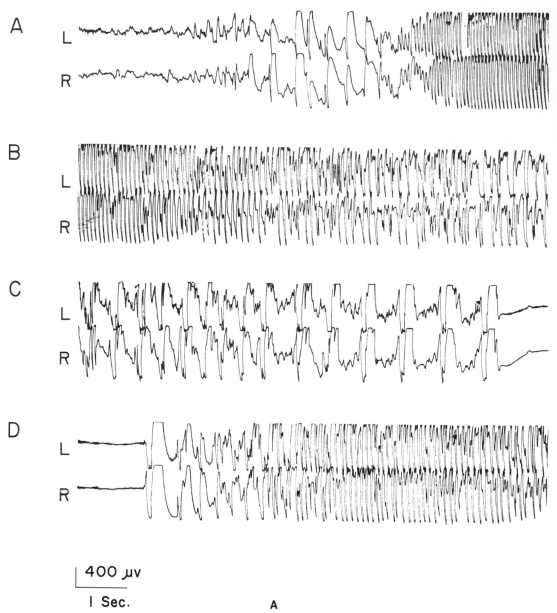

A

L

R

B

L

R

C

L

R

D

L

R

| 400 μv

I Sec.   A

Figure 26–23 The anatomical basis of the bilateral synchronous discharges of the generalized convulsive seizure. *A*, Intact adult cat. *B*, Cat with bilateral isolation of cerebral cortex and corpus callosum (see Fig. 26–18*A*). *C*, Cat with section of all major commissures. In each animal, the generalized discharge had been produced by the intravenous administration of the convulsant agent pentylenetetrazol (Metrazol) at a dosage of 20 mg/Kg (slightly above threshold for the cat). In each case the animal was paralyzed and artificially ventilated; if the animal were not paralyzed, a generalized convulsive seizure would be observed with this agent. Note the capacity for bilaterally synchronous fast spike discharge present in the isolated cortical callosal preparation. The animal with section of major commissures has the capacity for discharges in each hemisphere, but such discharges are independent in the two hemispheres. Note that the general form of the discharge in the isolated cortex corresponds to the intact animal. (From Marcus, E. M.: Unpublished experiments, 1969.)

Illustration continued on opposite page.

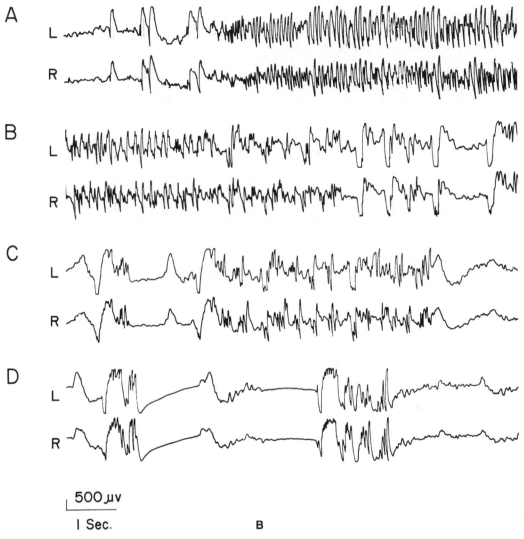

Figure 26–23 *Continued B.*

Illustration continued on following page.

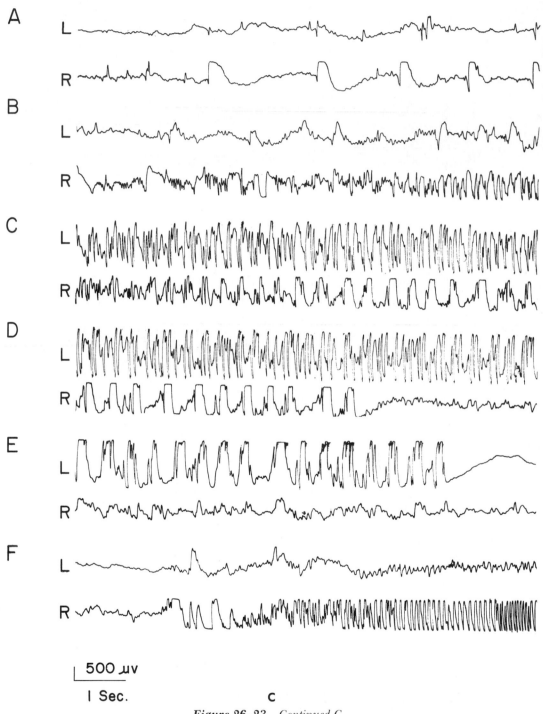

Figure 26–23 *Continued C.*

reduction in return of blood to the heart. The episode is usually precipitated by emotional or physical stress. In *orthostatic hypotension,* the reflex mechanisms for maintaining blood pressure on sudden standing are defective. In *cardiac syncope,* there is a reduction in cardiac output which may be chronic (as in aortic stenosis) or intermittent and paroxysmal as in various cardiac arrhythmias. In *carotid sinus syncope,* pressure on the carotid sinus produces an overactivation of the normal carotid sinus reflex with a slowing of the heart rate and a fall in blood pressure. *Hyperventilation syncope* is common and occurs in relation to anxiety. Hyperventilation produces both a relative respiratory alkalosis and a decrease in cerebral blood flow.

Akinetic Seizures and Drop Attacks. The other conditions which must be distinguished from generalized seizures are akinetic seizures in children or the drop attacks of basilar vertebral insufficiency in the adult.

Akinetic seizures are minor seizures in which the patient falls suddenly to the floor but then stands up again almost immediately. The loss of consciousness is brief. In some cases, there may be no definite evidence of an actual loss of consciousness. In some cases the fall represents a sudden loss of postural tone; in other cases, the fall represents a massive myoclonic jerk which throws the patient violently to the floor. In some cases, petit mal seizures are also present; in some cases, generalized convulsive seizures. There may be a previous history of infantile spasms, and mental retardation is often present.

Drop attacks in the adult may occur in relation to ischemia in the paramedian branches of the basilar artery with transient dysfunction in descending motor pathways and of the motor centers of the pontine or medullary reticular formation. In such cases, consciousness is usually preserved. Such patients often have other symptoms suggesting basilar vertebral insufficiency (see Chapter 15).

TREATMENT OF SEIZURE DISORDERS

The epileptic was formerly considered an incurable, in a sense marked by the gods or possessed by demons. Occasionally in history or in certain cultures, such a sacred stigma might convey some benefits. In general, however, the epileptic has been considered a social outcast subjected to various legal restrictions as regards employment, marriage, procreation, and immigration. These restrictions were usually imposed irrespective of the cause of the seizure disorder. With the introduction of successful methods of therapy, many of these restrictive regulations have now been removed. Many seizure patients, however, remain subjected to a form of discrimination in employment which is usually not imposed on workers with other types of disability or handicaps.

Specific methods of treatment may be briefly considered. Obviously, patients in whom seizures are secondary to a discrete metabolic disturbance require correction of the underlying biochemical or endocrine abnormality. Patients in whom seizures are secondary to a progressive space-occupying lesion will require additional evaluation and surgical therapy when indicated, in addition to anticonvulsant therapy.

Focal Seizures and Generalized Convulsive Seizures. The treatment of choice for focal seizures and generalized convulsive seizures is diphenylhydantoin (Dilantin) in a daily dosage of 4–7 mg./Kg. (300–400 mg. a day in an adult), or phenobarbital in a daily dosage of 1–3 mg./Kg. (90–180 mg. a day in an adult). The combination of diphenylhydantoin and phenobarbital may be employed. An alternate drug to be used when seizures persist is primidone (Mysoline) in a dosage of 10–25 mg./Kg. (750–1000 mg. a day in an adult).

Petit Mal Seizures. For petit mal (absence) seizures, the treatment of choice is ethosuximide (Zarontin) in a daily dosage of 20–30 mg./Kg. (750–1000 mg. a day). An alternate drug, but one with potentially fatal hematological complication (aplastic anemia), is trimethadione (Tridione) in a daily dosage of 10–25 mg./Kg.

Myoclonic Seizures. Myoclonic seizures are in general difficult to control. For *infantile myoclonic spasms* with the electroencephalographic pattern of hypsarrhythmia, the initial treatment of choice is adrenocorticotrophic hormone (ACTH) or corticosteroids such as prednisone. Other myoclonic seizure disorders in association with diffuse disease may respond to diazepam (Valium). Where myoclonic jerks occur as a benign manifestation of a cryptogenic generalized seizure disorder (idiopathic grand mal), the indicated treatment with Dilantin or phenobarbital may also eliminate the myoclonic jerks. Nitrazepam (Mogadon), not available on the American market, is apparently very effective in many types of refractory myoclonic seizure disorders.

Status Epilepticus. This is a serious condition requiring acute treatment. One may encounter continuing focal, temporal lobe, or petit mal seizures. The latter two types may be manifested as prolonged confusional states. The condition, however, is usually defined, with regard to generalized convulsive seizures, as a state in which seizures continue beyond the usual duration of a single seizure or in which seizures recur so frequently that consciousness is not regained between seizures. If allowed to continue, grand mal status is a threat to life with cerebral anoxia, cerebral edema, aspiration pneumonitis, hyperthermia, hypotension, and cardiac arrest as possible complications. Prolonged grand mal status may be followed by prolonged confusion and a residual impairment of recent memory, due to damage to hippocampal areas (see Chapter 27). Temporal lobe seizures may be sequelae of such a prolonged state.

The causes of status epilepticus are several: (a) acute withdrawal of medication in a known seizure patient, (b) diffuse cerebral infections such as encephalitis, (c) massive cerebral infarcts, (d) metabolic disturbances in infancy, (e) hypertensive encephalopathy or uremia. Treatment consists in the acute administration of intravenous medication: barbiturates or diazepam in sufficient dosage to end the seizure. Sodium phenobarbital in a dosage of 200–400 mg. or sodium amytal in a dosage of 400–500 mg. may be employed. Diazepam (Valium) may also be employed—the single dose of 5–10 mg. is titrated so as to end the seizure. In each instance, effects on respiration must be carefully monitored; an airway must be maintained and various general measures employed as in the care of other comatose patients.

EXPECTED RESULTS OF TREATMENT

When all cases of recurrent seizures are considered, complete control can be obtained in 50 to 60 per cent. An additional 25 per cent will have a reduction in seizure frequency. Approximately 15 per cent will remain as a refractory group in whom seizure control will not be obtained with standard medications.

When cases are controlled on medication, treatment should be continued for at least a seizure-free period of 3 years before any consideration is given to a gradual discontinuation or reduction of medication.

In the refractory patient, if a persistent focal origin of the seizure is evident from a clinical or electroencephalographic standpoint, consideration may be given to the surgical removal of the focal cortical area of pathology (atrophic scar, cyst, glioma, vascular malformation).

Other cases, refractory to treatment, include the myoclonic and akinetic seizure types.

There are, however, various cases which represent apparent failures of treatment in a situation where control should be obtained or where seizure control, once established, has been lost. The following reasons then should be considered in their approximate order of frequency:

1. The patient is not taking his medication and fails to attain adequate blood level. A withdrawal effect can occur if the omission has been abrupt.

2. The patient is taking his medication but is not receiving a sufficient amount to establish an adequate anticonvulsant blood level.

3. The patient is receiving the wrong medication for the particular type of seizure. Diphenylhydantoin (Dilantin) has no effect on petit mal seizures. Ethosuximide (Zarontin) has no effect on focal or temporal lobe seizures.

4. Sleep deprivation has been present. Sleep deprivation significantly increases clinical and electrical discharges in seizure patients.

5. The patient has been ingesting alcohol with a subsequent alcohol withdrawal effect.

6. Significant emotional stress is present or has been added.

7. An underlying metabolic disorder is present.

8. An underlying progressive neurological disorder is present.

EEG IN RELATION TO CONSCIOUSNESS: ANATOMICAL BASIS

In this section we will discuss several interrelated questions dealing with the electroencephalogram and behavior: What is the anatomical basis for continuous electrical activity in the electroencephalogram? Why do we remain awake? To what extent does the electroencephalogram correlate with sleep and level of consciousness? What is the anatomical basis for the changes which occur in the electroencephalogram in relation to sleep? How does cortical electrical activity in the larger sense relate to the brain stem?

The student will have arrived already at some tentative answers to these questions. We have in Chapter 20 already considered some of the discrete effects of brain stem and thalamic stimulation as regards evoked responses in the cerebral cortex. We have already dealt earlier in the present chapter with the paroxysmal disturbances in consciousness and the correlated electrical discharges which occur in relation to seizure disorders. As we survey this area, it will be evident that there was an initial expectation that the electroencephalogram would provide a one-to-one correlation of behavior and personality with a physiological variable (in a sense a resolution of the mind-body problem which had long concerned philosophy and psychology). It will already be evident to the student from our discussion that this hope has not been realized, the electroencephalogram does not provide a simple one-to-one correlation with behavior, although certain general correlations are possible.

DEFINITIONS

Before beginning a consideration of the relevant experimental data, it is necessary to provide some definitions of what is meant from a clinical standpoint by terms such as consciousness, unconsciousness, coma, and sleep. These are not easy terms to define. Various authors have provided different definitions depending on their background and orientation. Some, for example, would include in a definition of consciousness the total capacity of the brain to provide awareness, insight, thought, and communication. From this standpoint, obviously, the highest integrative functions of the cerebral cortex are required.

A more specific operational approach defines *consciousness* in terms of *alert wakefulness* meaning that the patient or animal "responds immediately, fully, and appropriately to visual, auditory, and tactile stimuli" (Plum and Posner, 1966).

Coma then defines a state at the other end of a continuum in which psychological and motor responses to stimulation are impaired.* Various gradations of coma exist. In *deep coma* these responses are completely lost. In *moderately deep coma*, rudimentary responses of a reflex nature only are present (e.g., corneal reflex, withdrawal of a limb to a painful stimulus), but psychologically understandable responses to external stimuli and inner need are absent.

Various terms have been employed to describe lesser degrees of impairment of consciousness. Thus, the term *semicoma* has been employed to describe a state in which response (e.g., change in facial expression, attempts to brush away offending objects) are present, but this response is elicited only by painful or other disagreeable stimuli such as pinching the skin or vigorous shaking (Denny-Brown, 1957). *Stupor* has a similar meaning.

Less marked impairment of consciousness has been described in terms of *obtundation* or *lethargy* (Plum and Posner, 1966). *Obtundation* is defined as a state of dull indifference in which wakefulness is barely maintained. *Lethargy* refers to a state of drowsiness or indifference in which responses to stimulation may be delayed or incomplete and in which increased stimulation is required to evoke the response. Others have designated varying degrees of confusion—severe, moderate, or mild—to describe these same states of impairment.

Confusion may be defined as an impaired capacity to think clearly and with customary speed and to perceive, respond to, and remember current stimuli. *Delirium* is a related state in which agitation (of motor activity) is present in addition to confusion. Confusion includes disorientation and memory impairment and will be considered again in Chapter 27 with regard to memory and dementia.

Additional terms, such as *akinetic mutism*, *coma vigil*, and *pseudoakinetic mutism*, which are sometimes used in connection with the comatose patient, will be defined and considered later in this chapter.

Sleep refers to a natural state in which consciousness (in the wakefulness-alertness

---

*Most definitions of consciousness and coma are imperfect. Thus, the patient paralyzed by curare and artificially ventilated may be alert and aware but unable to respond to stimuli. On regaining motor control the patient is able to relate that he was fully aware of stimuli but unable to respond.

sense) has been temporarily interrupted. In contrast to coma, however, the level of consciousness may be fully restored by an appropriate stimulus.

ACTIVITY OF CEREBRAL CORTEX IN ISOLATION

Before considering the effect of the brain stem on the electroencephalogram and consciousness, it will prove useful to return again to a consideration of the cerebral cortex in the sense of indicating certain capacities of the cerebral cortex.

We have already indicated that much of what we record in the electroencephalogram may be related to the summated postsynaptic potentials of the apical dendrites of cortical neurons. Now let us approach the problem from a somewhat different angle. Let us rephrase the question in the following terms: "What electrical activity is present if the cerebral cortex is considered completely isolated from subcortical structures?"

Early studies of isolated cerebral cortex tended to use only small islands and did not emphasize the "spontaneous" electrical activity. When a large block of cortex, however, is isolated from subcortical structures and adjacent cerebral cortex, but retains its blood supply, a considerable residual electrical activity is present.

In the studies of Kellaway, et. al. (1966), waves of variable frequency were present, e.g., 0.5–4 cps and 15–60 cps. Occasionally (Fig. 26–24) activity was continuous for one hour after isolation. More often (and eventually in preparations where initially continuous) electrical activity was discontinuous with silent periods alternating with bursts of electrical activity. The bursts of activity were in part related to unit discharges in the depths of cortex (1.0–1.5 mm.) at the level of pyramidal cell bodies. In contrast, the activity of isolated thalamus (a nonlaminar structure) was characterized by regular sinusoidal waves, 8 cps.

This approach may be extended to examine a preparation in which large blocks of cerebral cortex have been isolated from

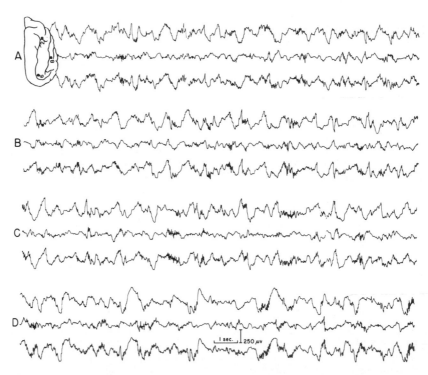

Figure 26–24 Electrical activity of the isolated cerebral cortex. *A, B, C,* and *D* are continuous strips illustrating the continuous slow and fast activity which may be recorded for approximately 1 hour in a preparation in which all cerebral cortex of one hemisphere has been isolated, when physiological conditions remain ideal. More often the activity obtained from such preparation resembled that shown in Figure 26–25. (From Kellaway, P., Gol, A., and Proler, M.: Exp. Neurol., *14*:292, 1966.)

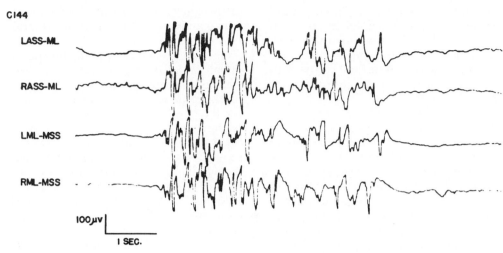

Figure 26–25 Activity of cerebral cortex in the isolated cortical callosal preparation. The spontaneous activity of this preparation (refer to Fig. 26–18*A*) was characterized by synchronous bursts of spikes, sharp waves, slow waves, and fast waves. These bursts alternated with periods of relative electrical silence. Had a large unilateral isolation been performed, similar activity would have been obtained from the unilaterally isolated island. All channels shown have been derived from the isolated blocks of cerebral cortex. (ASS=anterior suprasylvian gyrus, MSS=middle segment of suprasylvian gyrus, and ML= middle portion of lateral or marginal gyrus.) The activity recorded from nonisolated cortex (below the line of isolation) in this preparation was continuous. (From Marcus, E. M., and Watson, C. W.: Arch. Neurol., *14*:604, 1966.)

subcortical and adjacent cortex in each hemisphere but remain connected to each via the corpus callosum. The "spontaneous" activity of this preparation is characterized by bilateral relatively synchronous bursts of electrical activity with intervening periods of electrical silence (Fig. 26–25). The basic activity within the bursts (Marcus and Watson, 1966) is similar to that previously described above. Occasionally more continuous activity may be noted.

Similar burst-type activity is obtained when a preparation is examined in which all thalamic, hypothalamic, and nostral mesencephalic structures have been ablated.

In contrast when the ablation is limited to medial thalamic and medial mesencephalic structures, activity is relatively continuous. We should, however, note that a limited lesion of the basal diencephalon (hypothalamus) may produce the intermittent burst-type activity — perhaps by interrupting at this point an alternate pathway to the cortex from reticular formation.

From a clinical standpoint, the periodic burst activity, with intervening periods of electrical silence, is seen in several circumstances: (a) very deep anesthesia (Fig. 26–5), and (b) diffuse and progressive encepha-

lopathies in which the pathological process may serve to damage white matter, thus isolating cerebral cortex.

SUBCORTICAL AND BRAIN STEM STRUCTURES AND EEG AND CONSCIOUSNESS: EXPERIMENTAL STUDIES

Two differential theoretical concepts emerged early from the experimental studies of sleep:

1. Sleep and coma reflected a deafferentation of the cerebral cortex, that is, a lack of sensory input to the cerebral cortex. Sleep then was the lack of wakefulness and resulted passively from the withdrawal of influences which maintained a waking nervous system.

2. Sleep reflected the action of a system of related structures which produced cerebral inhibition. Sleep then would be an active process of inhibition rather than a passive state.

Studies of Bremer. The first concept, that of cerebral deafferentation, received considerable support from the studies of Bremer (1935) which demonstrated that transection of the neural axis in the cat at the spinal medullary junction resulted in an electroencephalogram resembling that obtained in the awake state. On the other hand, transection of the brain stem at the intercollicular level of the midbrain resulted in the electroencephalographic pattern of slow waves resembling sleep.

Stimulation Studies of Moruzzi and Magoun. The generalized arousal response to stimulation initially had been related to specific afferent stimulation over specific pathways. The subsequent studies of Moruzzi and Magoun (1949) refined these observations by indicating that the ascending reticular formation of brain stem and diencephalon (the extra lemniscal system), rather than the classical sensory pathways, were responsible for arousal of the electroencephalogram and behavior (see Fig. 20–28). Thus, electrical stimulation in the brain stem reticular formation at 200–300 cps or in the intralaminar nuclei of the thalamus at 200–300 cps will produce the same generalized desynchronization of the electroencephalogram as is produced by external stimuli such as sciatic stimulation.

It is important to note that this generalized response occurs with a latency of 40–60 ms. This generalized arousal response should, as discussed previously, be contrasted to the more specific and more localized cortical response to sciatic nerve or specific afferent system stimulation: the primary evoked response. The primary evoked response occurs with a latency of 10 to 15 milliseconds and is limited to a specific sector of the projection of the somatic sensory cortex. The primary evoked response for a particular cortical area is stimulus modality specific. In contrast the same generalized arousal response may occur from a variety of stimuli as early demonstrated in the studies of Rheinberger and Jasper (1937).

Ablation Studies of Lindsley et al. In related acute ablation-type studies, Lindsley, Bowden, and Magoun (1949) were able to demonstrate that a desynchronized (alert) electroencephalogram could still occur in the cat after transection of the brain stem at a medullary or pontine level but not after transection at the pontomesencephalic junction or higher levels in the midbrain. More selective lesions were then produced at the low mesencephalic level (Fig. 26–26). Lesions limited to the periaqueductal gray matter had little effect on behavior and on the alert electroencephalogram. Bilateral lesions

of the lateral tegmentum, involving the specific lemniscal pathways, also had little effect. However, lesions which destroyed the medial tegmental areas but spared the specific lemniscal pathways produced an alteration in electroencephalogram and behavior. Electroencephalographic activation no longer occurred. The slow wave pattern of sleep was present. From a behavioral standpoint, the cat was in a state of coma and could not be roused. Large lesions limited to the basal diencephalon (hypothalamus) produced similar effects. The findings of these studies led to a number of hypotheses which attempted to explain wakefulness, sleep, coma, and the anesthetic state in terms of a unitary concept of a reticular activating system.

MODIFICATION OF ORIGINAL CONCEPTS

In subsequent years, this useful concept has been modified by a large number of studies (many of which have originated from the laboratories of Moruzzi, Lindsley, and Magoun). These studies cannot be discussed here in detail; the reader is referred to the papers of Sprague (1967), Clemente (1967), Jouvet (1967), Magoun (1963), and Pompeiano (1967). The major modifications may be grouped and summarized as follows:

Acute vs Chronic. There are significant differences between acute and chronic preparations particularly when the cat or dog is considered. Thus, in chronic animals with transection of the mesencephalon, periods of arousal (desynchronization) occur in the electroencephalogram — often without clear temporal relationship to olfactory and visual stimuli, suggesting an autonomous periodicity of cortical electrical activity or neurohumoral influences. As we have already indicated in our discussion of the motor system, a chronic cat preparation with section at an intercollicular (decerebrate preparation) level or supracollicular (midbrain preparation) level is capable of and manifests periods of apparent behavioral wakefulness alternating with periods of sleep. In other studies, the effects of cumulative multiple stage procedures have been found to be less marked than the effects of a large single stage lesion. (Refer to Sprague, 1967.)

Interspecies Differences. There are significant interspecies differences. Thus, the chronic effects of lesions of the mesencephalic tegmentum (involving brain stem reticular formation) are more severe in the

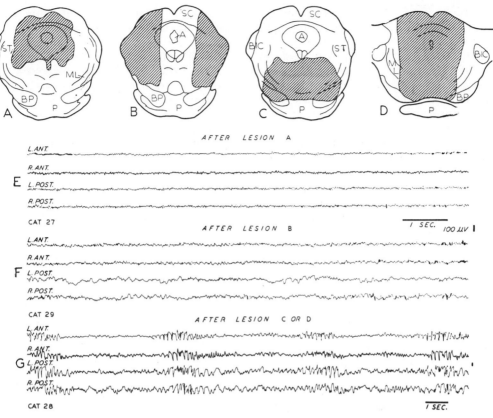

Figure 26–26 Effects of acute brain stem lesions on the cortical electrical activity of the cat. Transverse section through midbrain showing lesions of periaqueductal grey (*A*), lateral sensory (lemniscal) pathways (*B*), and tegmentum (*C* and *D*).

E shows persistence of activation following lesion A.

F shows persistence of activation 6 hours after lesion B and 3 hours after section of optic nerves and olfactory bulbs.

G shows occurrence of the spindle burst pattern of sleep with failure of activation shortly after ventral tegmental lesion C. Subsequently, spindle bursts become less frequent. Lesion D, which included dorsal as well as ventral tegmentum, was followed by more persistent spindle bursts. (From Lindsley, D. B., Bowden, D. W., and Magoun, H. W.: Electroenceph. clin. Neurophysiol., *1*:477, 1949.)

primate (the monkey) than in the cat, both as regards cortical electrical activity and behavior. (Refer to Magoun, 1963, and Sprague, 1967). The situation in man will be considered later.

Other Systems. There are other non-passive systems besides the ascending reticular formation involved in the slow wave stage of sleep. That is, there are observations which cannot be explained simply by postulating a decrease in the activating influences from the reticular formation on the cerebral cortex. Thus, as discussed by Clemente (1967), Pavlov in studying the development of negative or inhibitory conditioned reflexes (the dog learned not to respond) observed the sudden onset of sleep on presentation of the conditioned stimulus. In such an instance, sleep might be considered a process of active inhibition.

More relevant to our neuroanatomical considerations are the studies of Hess. In the cat, low frequency stimulation of the supraoptic and preoptic areas of the lateral-anterior hypothalamus produced a decrease in spontaneous activity and of muscle tone. Similar effects, with the actual induction of sleep, followed stimulation in medial thalamic areas. Stimulation of the caudal hypothalamus had the opposite effect—behavioral activation.

These results are consistent in general with the effects reported in many ablation experiments in cats and monkeys. Thus, lesions which destroy the posterior (and lateral) hypothalamus result in a somnolent state with a predominant slow wave pattern in the electroencephalogram. In contrast, lesions of the rostral hypothalamus (the suprachiasmatic, preoptic) result in a syndrome of hyperactivity, with constant wakefulness. The electroencephalogram remains in a desynchronized-aroused state.

More recently Clemente (1967) has demonstrated a system which includes the orbital frontal cortex and the rostral extension of the anterior hypothalamus (the preoptic and basal forebrain areas). Stimulation of this area results in the suppression of ongoing behavior, the induction of sleep, and the appearance of the slow wave stage of sleep in the electroenccphalogram. The anatomical projections from this area have been considered in Chapter 18 on the limbic system. The pathway involves hippocampus, septum, hypothalamus, anterior thalamic nuclei, mesencephalic tegmentum, and pontine reticular formation. The inhibitory effect on motor activity is mediated by the medullary reticular formation (the medullary inhibitory area already considered with regard to the motor system, Chapter 23). The effects on the electroencephalogram are mediated via corticocortical association fiber systems from orbital frontal cortex (as discussed in Chapter 20).

Paradoxical Sleep. The discovery of the paradoxical or rapid eye movement stage of sleep characterized by a "desynchronized" electroencephalogram indicated that the relationship between the electroencephalogram and state of consciousness was complex rather than a simple correlation. These studies have indicated that from a behavioral standpoint alone sleep is not a simple unitary stage. Thus, during this desynchronized stage of sleep, at a time when rapid eye movements are present, muscle tone is decreased and dreaming occurs.

Subsequent experimental studies have indicated a significant role of pontine and medullary structures in the genesis of sleep. Thus, midpontine section leads to a significant increase in the period of electroencephalographic wakefulness in the cat. As discussed by Jouvet (1967), more selective destruction of the midline raphe nuclei of the pons and medulla produces a marked increase in the total duration of wakefulness both from a behavioral and an electrical standpoint (total amounts of sleep are decreased by 80 to 90 per cent). The neurons of these nuclei contain large amounts of serotonin. Increase in brain serotonin has the opposite effect—slow wave sleep is increased. It has, therefore, been suggested that the raphe system may be involved in the onset of the slow wave stage of sleep by opposing the action of the reticular activating system.

These studies have also implicated another pontine area: the locus ceruleus, a collection of pigmented neurons below the floor of the fourth ventricle adjacent to the lateral pontine reticular formation. These neurons have a high concentration of noradrenalin. This area has been implicated in the triggering of the paradoxical stage of sleep, more particularly, the loss of muscle tone during this stage of sleep since destruction of these nuclei results in a loss of paradoxical sleep. These effects of the locus ceruleus may be mediated by the action of this nucleus on the inhibitory area of the medullary reticular formation.

A detailed discussion of neurotransmission within the central nervous system is beyond the scope of this chapter. It is sufficient to indicate that cholinergic mechanisms appear to be involved in the effects of the ascending reticular activating system on the cerebral cortex. Thus, electrical stimulation of the brain stem reticular formation produces an increased rate of liberation of acetylcholine from the surface of the cerebral cortex. Administration of the anticholinergic agent, atropine, prevents the effects of stimulation of brain stem reticular formation on cortical electrical activity. Desynchronization of the electroencephalogram fails to occur, although behavioral activation does occur (Shute and Lewis, 1967; Jasper, 1969).

COMA IN MAN

In discussing depression of consciousness in man, it is best to consider separately two aspects: (1) the patient who presents at the emergency room or on the general wards of the hospital with acute or subacute onset of coma; (2) the patient with prolonged depression of consciousness.

EMERGENCY ONSET OF COMA

In the emergency room evaluation of the patient in a coma of relatively acute onset, the specific etiologic factors will fall into three general categories:

1. Metabolic disorders, toxic disorders, diffuse infections, and other diffuse disorders of the central nervous system.

2. Supratentorial mass lesions.

3. Infratentorial lesions.

Diffuse Disorders of the Central Nervous System. The first group, diffuse disorders, is the most frequently encountered, particularly when unselected series derived from the emergency room of a large municipal hospital are considered. Included in this group are the following common *toxic and metabolic conditions:*

*a. Acute alcoholic intoxication

*b. Drug ingestions (barbiturates, opiates, salicylates, tranquilizers). In adults and adolescents these ingestions usually relate to suicide attempts or suicide gestures. In children, the ingestion may be accidental.

*c. Diabetic ketoacidosis

*d. Hypoglycemia including effects of exogenous insulin in diabetes

*e. Anoxia of various causes including chronic pulmonary disease

*f. Carbon dioxide narcosis (hypercapnia) in a setting of chronic pulmonary disease.

  g. Carbon monoxide poisoning

  h. Hepatic failure with encephalopathy

  i. Hyponatremia and hypernatremia

  j. Hypothyroidism (myxedema coma)

*k. Circulatory collapse (shock and severe congestive cardiac failure.

  l. Nutritional deficiency: Wernicke's encephalopathy

Diffuse infections include entities such as acute bacterial meningitis and encephalitis which directly and primarily involve the central nervous system. In addition, *severe systemic infections* such as pneumococcal pneumonia, typhoid fever, malaria, and other severe febrile illnesses are often associated with coma, stupor, or delirium.

Other diffuse conditions which may present as coma include such diverse problems as: (a) continuing epileptic status (status epilepticus); (b) postictal state following a generalized convulsive seizure; (c) concussion following head trauma; (d) acute toxic encephalopathy of childhood (acute cerebral edema of unknown etiology); (e) diffuse degenerative diseases of cerebral cortex or white matter. Case history illustrations of many of these conditions will be found in the monograph of Plum and Posner (1966).

---

*Most frequently encountered in the toxic-metabolic group.

Supratentorial Mass Lesions. These include a number of conditions already familiar to the student and are illustrated in the section on cortical localization (Chapter 21) and diseases of the cerebral hemispheres (Chapter 22). Specific examples include: massive cerebral infarcts, intracerebral hemorrhage, subarachnoid hemorrhage complicated by rupture into the substance of the brain or into the ventricles, brain abscess, epidural hematoma, subdural hematoma, meningiomas, gliomas, and other cerebral tumors. In some of these problems, the onset of coma is relatively acute (intracerebral hematoma). In others, the onset may be subacute (chronic subdural hematoma and infiltrating glioma).

Supratentorial lesions produce coma in several ways:

Uncal and Hippocampal Herniation. Expanding masses in the temporal lobe or lateral middle fossa produce uncal and hippocampal herniation through the tentorial opening compressing the ipsilateral third cranial nerve and the ipsilateral posterior cerebral artery and compressing and displacing the midbrain. The midbrain is then additionally compressed by the hard edge of tentorium on the contralateral side producing damage to the contralateral cerebral peduncle. Narrowing of the aqueduct of Sylvius occurs with an additional increase in intracranial pressure. Hemorrhages (Duret) occur in the substance of the brain stem (refer to Brain Stem, Chapter 15, Figs. 15–4, 15–5).

Central or Transtentorial Herniation. Other supratentorial masses, in a more parasagittal, or frontal or occipital location, produce a downward displacement and compression of the diencephalon and subsequently of the brain stem (central or transtentorial herniation). Narrowing of the aqueduct and secondary hemorrhages of the brain stem subsequently occur as complications in this state. The evolving symptoms will reflect the compromise of diencephalic and then of midbrain functions (both producing alterations in consciousness).

Cortical Dysfunction. Ipsilateral supratentorial lesions may at times produce involvement of the contralateral cerebral cortex. An infiltrating glioma may extend across the corpus callosum particularly in frontal areas to produce a widespread cortical dysfunction. An expanding swollen hemisphere may extend across the midline, compressing the contralateral hemisphere. The shift of the cingulate gyrus across the midline under the falx may compress the anterior cerebral arteries and associated veins over the surface of the corpus callosum producing additional ischemia and edema.

Diencephalic Involvement. Mass lesions in relation to the third ventricle and basal diencephalon may directly involve diencephalic structures (such as posterior hypothalamus) involved in consciousness. Such infiltrating lesions moreover usually involve the adjacent midbrain tegmentum and periaqueductal areas as well.

Infratentorial Lesions. The student should already be familiar with these lesions from his study of the brain stem in Chapter 15. The most common diagnostic entity in this group is the *infarct secondary to basilar vertebral arterial disease.** Also included in this group are: (a) infiltrating tumors of the brain stem; (b) tumor and abscess involving the cerebellum and producing a compromise of brain stem functions in their late stages; and (c) brain stem and cerebellar hemorrhage.

PROLONGED DISTURBANCES OF CONSCIOUSNESS

When cases of prolonged disturbance of consciousness are considered, a different frequency distribution is apparent as regards the anatomical location of the lesion and the specific pathological process. Thus, many of the metabolic and toxic diseases which constitute the most frequently encountered acute emergency room situation are self-limiting diseases or rapidly reversed by treatment.

When we consider supratentorial mass lesions in which tentorial herniation has occurred a relatively rapid progressive involvement of brain stem function may be expected. Thus, impairment of diencephalic functions is followed by an impairment of midbrain functions. With additional compression, edema, and hemorrhages, pontine and then medullary functions are impaired, resulting in death.

Thus, in considering the cases of prolonged impairment of consciousness, the intrinsic diencephalic and mesencephalic

problems constitute a disproportionately large percentage of cases. In the recent reported series of Barrett, Merritt, and Wolf (1967) seven of nine cases presented damage primarily to the mesencephalic pontine tegmentum with some damage to the adjacent posterior hypothalamus. Two of the nine cases had primary diffuse damage to the cerebral cortex and no brain stem lesions.

Thus, a relationship between the pathological lesions in the upper mesencephalon and drowsiness in Wernicke's encephalopathy was postulated shortly after the initial description of the disease.[†] Severe involvement of the posterior hypothalamus and the adjacent mesencephalon was noted in those cases of Von Economo's encephalitis lethargica manifesting prolonged hypersomnia. Periodic hypersomnia has long been noted in relation to tumors of the third ventricle and more prolonged somnolent states with tumors infiltrating the posterior hypothalamic and adjacent tegmental and periaqueductal areas of the mesencephalon.

However, prolonged depression of consciousness may also occur as a result of processes which produce a diffuse loss of neurons in the cerebral cortex, such as anoxia, or the diffuse degenerative diseases: presenile dementia, Jakob-Creutzfeldt disease, Huntington's chorea, and subacute inclusion body encephalitis. In these degenerative diseases, the depression of consciousness occurs as a late manifestation. A diffuse damage to white matter of the cerebral hemispheres may produce a similar picture. We should also note that apathetic-drowsy states may occur in relation to bilateral infarction of the frontal lobe territory within the distribution of the anterior cerebral arteries (as in occlusive disease or anterior communicating-anterior cerebral aneurysms).

It is evident then that from an anatomical standpoint, the conscious state reflects a complex interaction between brain stem structures, diencephalic structures, the basal forebrain areas on the one hand, and the cerebral cortex on the other.

Akinetic Mutism. The dual nature of this anatomical substrate is evident when one studies cases of akinetic mutism: a specialized type of impairment of consciousness. Thus, it is possible to distinguish a state of *apathetic or somnolent akinetic mutism* in which

---

*In such cases, there may often be a problem as to deciding whether coma or pseudocoma is present. Such a lesion may destroy all motor pathways. The patient could then be alert but unable to respond appropriately.

---

†We should, of course, note that the adjacent hypothalamus and thalamus are also involved.

the patient remains in a lethargic state most of the time. The patient may open his eyes in response to strong stimulation but soon closes them and returns to a lethargic state. Paralysis of vertical gaze and of other extraocular movements is usually found. Segarra (1970) has related this syndrome to occlusion of a penetrating branch arising from the proximal (mesencephalic artery) segment of the posterior cerebral artery at the basilar artery bifurcation. The territory of this relatively midline branch is bilateral and includes the diencephalic-mesencephalic junction: rostral midbrain tegmentum, the adjacent pretectal area, subthalamus, periventricular gray matter at the posterior end of the third ventricle; midline thalamic nuclei; reticular nucleus of the thalamus and intralaminar nuclei of the thalamus (centrum medianum).

This state should be contrasted to *hyperpathic akinetic mutism* to which the term *vigilant coma* has been applied. Although the patient lies immobile in bed, he provides some appearance of alertness in the sense that he is ready to be roused. He will often follow with his gaze whatever objects appear in his visual fields. He has no evidence of extraocular weakness. At times the akinesia will be interrupted by periods of restless motor agitation. If stimulated sufficiently, single words may penetrate the mute state. The anatomical substrate for this state relates to the medial, orbital, and anterior surfaces of the frontal lobes. The adjacent cingulate gyri or the septal area may also be involved.

Differential Diagnosis of Akinetic Mutism. In considering these akinetic mute states, the student should distinguish several other conditions. A patient with an acute massive infarct of the dominant hemisphere may appear mute because of destruction of Broca's area and seemingly akinetic because of a hemiparesis. Yet the patient may be quite alert. A patient late in the course of Parkinson's disease will demonstrate marked rigidity, akinesia, and mutism and yet also may be alert. A similar state may follow bilateral destruction of the putamen or globus pallidus as discussed in Chapter 24, p. 684.

Finally the student should realize that we measure apparent level of alertness (level of consciousness) by the response of the patient. If the descending motor pathways to the spinal cord and brain stem are interrupted and the cranial nerve motor nuclei destroyed, as in a massive pontine infarct following basilar artery thrombosis, we may be unable to communicate with the patient. In some instances, extraocular movements remain and a system of communication may be evolved employing eye blinking. Such a patient is alert and should be distinguished as being in a state of pseudoakinetic mutism (*pseudocoma*) (Kemper and Romanul, 1967). In such a patient, if eye movements were not preserved, a clinical dilemma would be present. We might not be able to really answer the question as to whether the patient was conscious and alert. Such patients without response capacity have at times been mislabeled as unconscious.

The electroencephalogram in patients with such large pontine lesions is often normal with a dominant alpha activity. The electroencephalogram in patients with infarcts of the rostral mesencephalon is usually abnormal with slow wave activity present. The actual degree of abnormality may appear minor in comparison to the clinical state. The difficulty in arriving at clear-cut correlations of such mesencephalic lesions will be evident when one recalls that the vessels involved are branches of the posterior cerebral artery. The posterior cerebral arteries also supply diencephalon, medial temporal, posterior temporal, and occipital areas of the cerebral cortex. Thus, the occurrence of slow wave activity in the electroencephalogram in such cases may have several explanations.

CARE OF THE COMATOSE PATIENT

Several general rules must be followed if life is to be preserved in the comatose patient until such time as recovery has occurred. The patient must be placed on his side and turned every 2 hours to avoid aspiration and passive congestion of the lungs. This will also serve to avoid decubitus ulcers. Joints must be manipulated passively through their full range of motion several times per day to avoid contractures. The legs should be protected from the weight of bed clothes by a cradle. Physiological ankle extension should be maintained by sand bags. Pressure areas should be protected by foam rubber to avoid decubitus ulcers. Suctioning is required at periodic intervals to avoid aspiration of nasal and oral secretions. An air way is often required when mouth and nasal passages are obstructed. Artificial respiration may be required depending on the level of pathology. Careful nasogastric feeding will be required to maintain nutritional status. While fluids and glucose may be administered temporarily by the intravenous route, this will not allow administration of adequate amounts of protein, lipids, and carbohydrates. Nutritional intake and urinary output must be recorded. A condom catheter or indwelling catheter will be required with periodic replacement. Urinary tract and respiratory infections must be treated with antibiotics but prophylactic antibiotics should not be administered. Constipation and fecal impaction should be avoided by the periodic use of mild cathartics. Enemas may be required.

OTHER DISORDERS OF SLEEP

Insomnia may be defined as inability to enter a state of sleep. *Hyposomnia* is defined as a reduction in sleeping time. Although both conditions may occur rarely on a neurological basis (following lesions of the rostral hypothalamus and preoptic area as previously discussed), most patients with these complaints do not have neurological disease. Instead the sleep disorder is psychologically determined.

Narcolepsy. Narcolepsy is a disorder characterized by paroxysmal attacks of sleep and of a desire to sleep. Following a period of sleep which varies from minutes to hours, the patient awakens refreshed. As in normal sleep, the patient can often be aroused from sleep by strong stimulation. Most cases have no known structural pathology and the neurological examination is normal. At times a family history of a similar disorder is present. Rarely onset of attacks has been related to the epidemic encephalitis of Von Economo or to head trauma.

Many of the patients with narcolepsy do manifest other periodic disorders which occur frequently enough to be grouped within the narcolepsy syndrome: cataplexy, sleep paralysis, and hypnagogic hallucinations. *Cataplexy* refers to a sudden loss of muscle tone and of postural reflexes, usually occurring in relation to laughter or sudden emotional stimulation. *Sleep paralysis* refers to episodes of inability to move and occurs in relation to the process of falling asleep or of awakening. *Hypnagogic hallucinations* are vivid sensory, dream-like experiences which occur upon awakening.

The paroxysmal nature of the narcolepsy might suggest at first view a relationship to epilepsy, but no such relationship exists. There is no evidence of sudden excessive neuronal discharge in the electroencephalogram. Seizure disorders do not occur in abnormal degree in the families of patients with narcolepsy.

Many aspects of the narcolepsy syndrome have been related to the desynchronized (rapid eye movement) stage of sleep. Thus, electroencephalographic studies have shown the early occurrence of periods of desynchronized sleep and rapid eye movements in these patients shortly after onset of sleep (as contrasted to normal where such episodes do not occur for 90 minutes). The desynchronized rapid eye movement stage of sleep is characterized by a depression of spinal reflexes (monosynaptic and polysynaptic) with a decrease in muscle tone as previously discussed. This could explain the cataplexy and the sleep paralysis. The hypnagogic hallucinations have been postulated to correspond to the dreaming which occurs during the rapid eye movement stage of sleep. The explanation for this facile triggering in the narcoleptic area of the brain stem centers involved in desynchronized sleep remains uncertain (Pompeiano, 1969; Rechtschaffer and Dement, 1967).

References

The Electroencephalogram in General and Seizures

Ajmone-Marsan, C.: Acute Effects of Topical Epileptogenic Agents *In* Jasper, H. H., Ward, A. A., and Pope, A. (eds.): *Basic Mechanisms of the Epilepsies.* Boston, Little, Brown & Company, 1969, pp. 299–319.

Ajmone-Marsan, C.: Pathophysiology of the EEG Pattern Characteristic of Petit Mal Epilepsy; A Critical Review of Some of the Experimental Data *In* Gastaut, H. et. al. (eds.): *The Physiopathogenesis of the Epilepsies.* Springfield, Illinois, Charles C Thomas, 1969, pp. 237–248.

Berger, H.: On the electroencephalogram of man. Electroenceph. clin. Neurophysiol., *28*:(Supplement H) 1969.

Berlin, L.: Significance of grand mal seizures developing in patients over 35 years of age. JAMA, *152*:794–797, 1953.

Brazier, M. A. B.: Neuronal structure, brain potentials and epileptic discharge. Epilepsia, Series III, *4*:9–18, 1955.

Essig, C. F.: Clinical and experimental aspects of barbiturate withdrawal convulsions. Epilepsia, *8*:21–30, 1967.

Gastaut, H., and Fischer-Williams, M.: The Physiopathology of Epileptic Seizures. *In* Field, J. (ed.): *Handbook of Physiology,* Section I, Vol. I, Neurophysiology. Washington, D.C., American Physiological Society, 1959, pp. 329–363.

Gastaut, H., et. al.: A proposed international classification of epileptic seizures. Epilepsia (Amst.), *5*:297–306, 1964.

Geller, M., and Geller, A.: Brief amnestic effects of spike-wave discharges. Neurology, *20*:1089–1095, 1970.

Gibbs, F. A., Davis, H., and Lennox, W. G.: The electroencephalogram in epilepsy and in conditions of impaired consciousness. Arch. Neurol. Psychiat., *34*: 1133–1148, 1935.

Gibbs, F. A., and Gibbs, E. L.: *Atlas of Electroencephalography*, Vol. II: *Epilepsy*. Cambridge, Massachusetts; Addison Wesley Press, 1952.

Halliday, A. M.: The electrophysiological study of myoclonus in man. Brain, *90*:241–284, 1967.

Holowach, J., Thurston, D. L., and O'Leary, J. L.: Petit mal epilepsy. Pediatrics, *30*:893–901, 1962.

Ingvar, D. H.: Electrical activity of isolated cortex in unanesthetized cat with intact brain stem. Acta. Physiol. (Scand.), *33*:151–168, 1955.

Jasper, H. H., and Droogleever-Fortuyn, J.: Experimental studies on the functional anatomy of petit mal epilepsy. Ass. Res. nerv. Dis. Proc., *26*:272–298, 1956.

Jasper, H. H., and Kershman, J.: Electroencephalographic classification of the epilepsies. Arch. Neurol. Psychiat., *45*:903, 1941.

Kooi, K. A : *Fundamentals of Electroencephalography.* New York, Harper & Row, 1971, 260 pp.

Lesse, S., Hoefer, P. F. A., and Austin, J. H.: The electroencephalogram in diffuse encephalopathies. Arch. Neurol. Psychiat., *79*:359–375, 1958.

Marcus, E. M., and Watson, C. W.: Bilateral synchronous spike wave electrographic patterns in the cat: Interaction of bilateral cortical foci in the intact, bilateral cortical-callosal and adiencephalic preparation. *Arch. Neurol.*, *14*:601–610, 1966.

Marcus, E. M., and Watson, C. W.: Bilateral symmetrical epileptogenic foci in monkey cerebral cortex: Mechanisms of interaction and regional variations in capacity for synchronous spike slow wave discharges. Arch. Neurol., *19*:99–116, 1968.

Marcus, E. M., Watson, C. W., and Jacobson, S.: Role of the corpus callosum in bilateral synchronous discharges induced by intravenous pentylenetetrazol. Neurology, *19*:309, 1969.

Marcus, E. M., Watson, C. W., and Simon, S. A.: An experimental model of varieties of petit mal epilepsy. Epilepsia, *9*:233–248, 1968.

Metrakos, K., and Metrakos, J. D.: Genetics of convulsive disorders: Part 2 (Genetic and EEG studies in centrencephalic epilepsy). Neurology, *11*:474–483, 1961.

Mirsky, A. F., and Pragay, E. B.: The relation of EEG and performance in altered states of consciousness. Res. Publ. Assoc. nerv. ment. Dis., *45*:514–534, 1967.

Morrell, F., Naquet, R., and Menini, C.: Microphysiology of cortical single neurons in papio papio. Electroenceph. clin. Neurophysiol., *27*:708–709, 1969.

Muskens, L. J. J.: *Epilepsy: Comparative Pathogenesis, Symptoms, Treatment.* New York, William Wood & Co., 1928.

Naquet, R.: Photogenic Seizures in the Baboon. *In* Jasper, H. H., Ward, A. A., and Pope, A. (eds.): *Basic Mechanisms of the Epilepsies.* Boston, Little, Brown & Company, 1969, pp. 565–571.

Penfield, W., and Jasper, H.: *Epilepsy and the Functional Anatomy of the Human Brain.* Boston, Little, Brown & Company, 1954.

Pollen, D. A.: Intracellular studies of cortical neurons during thalamic induced wave and spike. Electroenceph. clin. Neurophysiol., *17*:398–404, 1964.

Pollen, D. A.: Experimental spike and wave responses and petit mal epilepsy. Epilepsia, *9*:221–232, 1968.

Pollen, D. A., Perot, P., and Reid, K. M.: Experimental bilateral wave and spike from thalamic stimulation in relation to level of arousal. Electroenceph. clin. Neurophysiol., *15*:1017–1028, 1963.

Pollen, D. A., Reid, K., and Perot, P.: Micro-electrode studies of experimental 3/sec wave and spike in the cat. Electroenceph. clin. Neurophysiol., *17*:57–67, 1964.

Raynor, R. B., Paine, R. S., and Carmichael, E. A.: Epilepsy of late onset. Neurology, *9*:111–117, 1959.

Rodin, E., Onuma, T., Wasson, S., Prozak, J., and Rodin, M.: Neurophysiological mechanisms involved in nonfocal grand mal seizures induced by Metrazol and Megimide. Electroenceph. clin. Neurophysiol., *30*: 62–72, 1971.

Schmidt, R. P., and Wilder, B. J.: *Epilepsy.* Philadelphia, F. A. Davis, 1968.

Starzl, T. E. et al.: Cortical and subcortical electrical activity in experimental seizures induced by Metrazol. J. Neuropath. exp. Neurol., *12*:262–276, 1953.

Swanson, P. D., Luttrel, C. N., and Magladery, J. W.: Myoclonus: A report of 67 cases and review of the literature. Medicine, *41*:339–356, 1962.

Victor, M.: The role of alcohol in the production of seizures. Mod. Probl. Pharmacopsychiat., *4*:185–199, 1970. (Also in Niedermeyer, E.: *Epilepsy: Recent Views of Theory, Diagnosis and Therapy.* Basel, Switzerland, S. Karger.)

Victor, M., and Brausch, C.: The role of abstinence in the genesis of alcoholic epilepsy. Epilepsia, *8*:1–20, 1967.

Walker, A. F.: The propagation of epileptic discharge. Mod. Probl. Pharmacopsychiat., *4*:13–28, 1970. (Niedermeyer, E.: *Epilepsy: Recent Views on Theory, Diagnosis and Therapy of Epilepsy.* Basel, Switzerland, S. Karger.)

Walter, W. G.: The location of cerebral tumors by electroencephalography. Lancet., *2*:306, 1936.

Ward, A. A., Jr.: The Epileptic Neuron: Chronic Foci in Animals and Man *In* Jasper, H. G., Ward, A. A., and Pope, A. (eds.): *Basic Mechanisms of the Epilepsies*, Boston, Little, Brown & Company, 1969, pp. 263–288.

Watson, C. W., and Denny-Brown, D.: Myoclonus epilepsy as a symptom of diffuse neuronal disease. Arch. Neurol. Psychiat., *70*:151–168, 1953.

Watson, C. W., and Marcus, E. M.: The genetics and clinical significance of photogenic cerebral electrical abnormalities, myoclonus and seizures. Trans. Amer. neurol. Ass., *87*:251–253, 1962.

Weir, B.: Spike-wave from stimulation of reticular core. Arch. Neurol., *11*:209–218, 1964.

Wikler, A., and Essig, C. F.: Withdrawal seizures following chronic intoxication with barbiturates and other sedative drugs. Mod. Probl. Pharmacopsychiat., *4*:170–184, 1970. (Also in Niedermeyer, E.: *Epilepsy: Recent Views on Theory, Diagnosis and Therapy of Epilepsy.* Basel, Switzerland, S. Karger.)

Wilder, B. J., and Schmidt, R. P.: Propagation of epileptic discharge from chronic neocortical foci in monkey. Epilepsia, *6*:297–309, 1965.

Woodcock, S., and Cosgrove, J. B. R.: Epilepsy after the age of 50: a five-year follow up study. Neurology, *14*:34–40, 1964.

Sleep and Consciousness

Barrett, R., Merritt, H. H., and Wolf, A.: Depression of consciousness as a result of cerebral lesions. Res. Publ. Assoc. nerv. ment. Dis., *45*:241–272, 1967.

Bremer, F.: Cerveau "isole" et physiologie du sommeil. C. R. Soc. Biol. (Par.), *118*:1235–1241, 1935.

Clemente, C. D.: Forebrain mechanisms related to internal inhibition and sleep. Conditional Reflex, 3:145–174, 1968.

Clemente, C. D., and Sterman, M. B.: Basal forebrain mechanisms for internal inhibition and sleep. Res. Publ. Ass. nerv. ment. Dis., 45:127–147, 1967.

Dement, W. C.: Sleep and dreams In Freedman, A. M., and Kaplan, H. I.: Comprehensive Textbook of Psychiatry. Baltimore, Williams and Wilkins, 1967, pp. 77–88.

Denny-Brown, D.: Handbook of Neurological Examination and Case Recordings. Cambridge, Harvard Univ. Press, 1957.

Jasper, H. H.: Mechanisms of propagation: Extracellular studies In Jasper, H. H., Ward, A. A., and Pope, A.: Basic Mechanisms of the Epilepsies. Boston, Little, Brown and Company, 1969, pp. 421–438.

Jouvet, M.: Mechanisms of the states of sleep: a neuropharmacological approach. Res. Publ. Ass. nerv. ment. Dis., 45:86–126, 1967.

Kellaway, P., Gol, A., and Proler, M.: Electrical activity of the isolated cerebral hemisphere and isolated thalamus. Exper. Neurol., 14:281–304, 1966.

Kemper, T. L., and Romanul, F. C. A.: State resembling akinetic mutism in basilar artery thrombosis. Neurology. 17:74–80, 1967.

Lindsley, D. B., Bowden, J., and Magoun, H. W.: Effect upon the EEG of acute injury to the brain stem activating system. Electroenceph. clin. Neurophysiol., 1:475–486, 1949.

Magoun, H. W.: The Waking Brain. Springfield, Illinois, Charles C Thomas, 1963.

Moruzzi, G., and Magoun, H. W.: Brain stem reticular formation and activation of the EEG. Electroenceph. clin. Neurophysiol., 1:455–473, 1949.

Plum, F., and Posner, J. B.: The Diagnosis of Stupor and Coma. Philadelphia, F. A. Davis, 1966.

Pompeiano, O.: The neurophysiological mechanisms of the postural and motor events during desynchronized sleep. Res. Publ. Ass. nerv. ment. Dis., 45:351–423, 1967.

Pompeiano, O.: Sleep Mechanisms In Jasper, H. H., Ward, A. A., and Pope, A. (eds.): Basic Mechanisms of the Epilepsies. Boston, Little, Brown & Company, 1969, pp. 453–473.

Rechtschaffer, A., and Dement, W.: Studies on the relation of narcolepsy, cataplexy and sleep with low voltage random EEG activity. Res. Publ. Ass. nerv. ment. Dis., 45:488–505, 1967.

Rheinberger, M., and Jasper, H.: The electrical activity of the cerebral cortex in the unanesthetized cat. Amer. J. Physiol., 119:186–196, 1937.

Segarra, J. M.: Cerebral vascular disease and behavior. Arch. Neurol., 22:408–418, 1970.

Shute, C. C. D., and Lewis, P. R.: The ascending cholinergic reticular system: neocortical olfactory and subcortical projections. Brain, 90:497–821, 1967.

Sprague, J. M.: The effects of chronic brain stem lesions on wakefulness, sleep and behavior. Res. Publ. Ass. nerv. ment. Dis., 45:148–194, 1967.

27

Learning, Memory, and Instinctive Behavior

ELLIOTT M. MARCUS

LEARNING AND MEMORY

Learning may be defined as a relatively permanent change in behavior that results from practice. This definition implies a plasticity in central nervous system function and it also implies a plasticity in the formation of stimulus response connections. The definition excludes changes resulting from maturation, sensory adaptation, and fatigue.

Some would differentiate between memory and remembering. *Memory,* at times, has been defined as the "read in phase" of learning. More often the term memory is used to indicate the processes or neural mechanisms involved in the storage or representation of an experience. The term *remembering* is defined as the "read out phase" of learning. The term is often used to define the neural mechanisms involved in the retrieval of stored information.

Two types of learning have been distinguished in experimental studies: (1) classical conditioning (Pavlovian) and (2) instrumental conditioning.

CLASSICAL CONDITIONING

The terms employed in classical conditioning are as follows: the *conditioned stimulus* (CS) is a stimulus which prior to the procedure does not evoke the specific response under study. For example, the sound of a bell prior to conditioning fails to evoke salivation or withdrawal of a foot from an electrified grid.

The *unconditioned stimulus* (UCS) is that stimulus which normally evokes the particular reflex or response under study. For example, the sight or odor of food normally evokes salivation in a dog. (One might indicate parenthetically that initially, of course, the sight of food did not evoke the salivation but following a learning process the sight of food did come to evoke that response.) A shock to the foot is the normal unconditioned stimulus for withdrawal of the foot.

The *unconditioned response* (UCR) is the usual reflex or response to the unconditioned stimulus. Thus, the odor of food usually produces salivation. A shock to the foot usually produces withdrawal of the foot. The *conditioned response* (CR) is the response which results after the formation of the new conditioned stimulus-response connection. Thus, a conditioned response would involve the production of salivation to the sound of a bell and withdrawal of the foot on the sound of a bell.

We may conceptualize the process of conditioning as follows:

1. Prior to conditioning
   UCS $\longrightarrow$ UCR
   CS does not $\longrightarrow$ UCR

2. During conditioning
   CS prior to or + UCS——> UCR
3. After conditioning
   CS——> CR

Prior to conditioning, the unconditioned stimulus produces the unconditioned response. The neutral conditioned stimulus does not produce the unconditioned response. The process of conditioning involves the presentation of the conditioned stimulus just prior to the unconditioned stimulus on a series of occasions. The unconditioned stimulus on each occasion elicits the unconditioned response. When this has been done on a sufficient number of occasions, it is found that a process has occurred in which the conditioned stimulus now produces a conditioned response.

Several additional terms are used in conditioning. *Extinction* implies that, once established, if the conditioned stimulus is presented alone, repeatedly, without presentation of the unconditioned stimulus, it is found that the conditioned stimulus eventually fails to elicit the conditioned response. This implies that the unconditioned stimulus has a certain reinforcement value.

The term *generalization* implies that stimuli which are relatively similar will elicit the response once conditioning has occurred. Thus, once a circle has been established as a conditioned stimulus to elicit a response of salivation one may find that an oval whose axes are relatively similar, that is, an oval which is almost a circle will also elicit the conditioned response.

Discrimination implies that a process of differentiation among various categories of stimuli has occurred so that only particular classes of stimuli elicit the conditioned response. Thus, once a circle has become the conditioned stimulus, one finds that a long oval fails to elicit a conditioned response. The process of teaching a discrimination involves the manipulation of the unconditioned stimulus. Thus, if one wishes to establish discrimination concerning stimuli, one employs the unconditioned stimulus to reinforce those stimuli which one wishes conditioned. One fails to supply the unconditioned stimulus when a lack of response is desired to a particular stimulus.

INSTRUMENTAL CONDITIONING

In instrumental conditioning the animal must make some active response such as pressing a lever when a specific stimulus occurs. This instrumental response then determines whether the behavior will be reinforced. For example, pressing a lever in response to an appropriate stimulus results in the presentation of a reward in the form of a pellet of food.

Various types of instrumental conditioning may be considered. Pressing the lever in response to the appropriate stimulus with delivery of a food pellet may be considered *primary reward conditioning.*

In *secondary reward conditioning*, the animal receives an object which in the past has been associated with a biologically significant reward. For example, chimpanzees will learn to press a lever to obtain poker chips which they may later use to obtain fruit. The poker chips soon come to take on secondary reward value.

Escape conditioning occurs in a situation in which the response of the animal allows him to escape from what would otherwise be a painful situation. For example, an animal responds to a light which precedes an electrical shock to his foot. Response to a light opens a door which allows the animal to escape from the box in which he has been restrained.

Avoidance conditioning is a somewhat similar type of instrumental conditioning. In this situation the response of the animal in pressing a lever when the light flashes prevents the occurrence of the electric shock which the animal has learned follows the occurrence of the light.

We have mentioned the concept of *reinforcement* several times. This may be defined as any event contingent on the response of the organism that alters the future likelihood of that response. In simpler terms we may define reinforcement as reward or punishment. Thus, if one wished a particular response to be learned to a specific stimulus, rewarding the animal each time the correct response is made to the appropriate stimulus will increase the rate of learning for that stimulus-response combination. On the other hand, punishing an animal for incorrect responses will result in a decreased likelihood of occurrence of the incorrect responses to the specific stimulus.

NEURAL STRUCTURES INVOLVED IN CONDITIONING

Classical conditioning may occur in decorticate animals but the response is relatively gross. Classical conditioning may also occur during bilateral stimulation of the hippocampus in the cat. As will be evident later, such bilateral stimulation of the hippocampus does interfere with more complex types of learning. Moreover, in man and other primates, cortical lesions do interfere with certain types of more complex learning. We should note, however, that nonmammalian forms with relatively limited development of telencephalon (for example, the pigeon and the octopus) are capable of refined discrimination learning.

As regards the locus of stimulation, it has been demonstrated that direct stimulation of the sensory projection area of cerebral cortex may serve as the conditioned stimulus for classical stimulation. It may also be noted that it is possible to use direct stimulation of cerebral cortex as the unconditioned stimulus.

The studies of Olds, and of Delgado and Miller demonstrated that it was possible to use hypothalamic stimulation as the reward or punishment in instrumental conditioning. This implies that stimulation of specific areas of the hypothalamus has a certain reinforcement value as regards stimulus-response connections. (Refer to page 435.)

MEMORY IN MAN AND RELEVANT ANATOMICAL SUBSTRATE

Essentially three stages have been distinguished in human memory: (a) immediate memory, (b) second stage, or recent memory stage, or labile stage, and (c) long-term or remote memory. The distinctions are to some extent arbitrary; where one stage ends and another begins is often not clear.

Immediate Memory. This is a matter of seconds. At times this has been estimated as 10 seconds or less. It is best exemplified in simple digit repetition as in digit span testing. The patient is given a series of numbers which he immediately repeats. The neural substrate undoubtedly involves the reception in the appropriate primary sensory projection area with relay to the adjacent sensory association cortex; for example, areas 18, 22, 5, and 7 where, in combination with various nuclei of the thalamus, the appropriate response is selected. The pathways must then involve relay-to-motor association cortex and then to motor cortex if the information is to be recited to the examiner. In the monkey, bilateral ablation of the superior and middle temporal gyri eliminates the immediate stage of auditory memory.

Second Stage or Recent Memory. This stage may be considered a transcription and transduction stage. The duration of this intermediate process has been variously estimated in infrahuman species as a matter of 20 to 180 minutes. The time required is probably shorter as one ascends the phylogenetic scale.

Theoretically, this stage involves the transcription from a relatively localized reverberating neuronal circuit, indicated in the immediate memory stage, into a more permanent macromolecular form of recording. It has been hypothesized that RNA and protein synthesis are involved in this stage.

It should be noted that RNA turnover does increase in tissues undergoing learning-like experiences. RNA turnover also increases in areas of neural tissue subjected to repetitive stimulation. It is clear that interference with RNA synthesis or with protein synthesis (by the use of the antibiotic puromycin) interferes with this stage of memory.

The neural structures involved are the parahippocampal gyri, the hippocampus, the anterior and dorsal medial nuclei of the thalamus, and the mammillary bodies. From a clinical standpoint, we evaluate this stage of memory with the delayed recall test (list of 5 objects to be remembered for 5 minutes) and by asking the patient to recite a paragraph (cowboy or gilded boy story) which he has just read or heard.

This ability to learn and to retain new experiences and new material is often referred to as *retentive memory*. Disturbance of this stage in memory will be considered later under the topic of the amnestic-confabulatory syndrome.

Long-term Memory or Remote Memory. This phase is not discretely localized. Rather, it represents a diffuse storage throughout the cerebral cortex and possibly other areas of the central nervous system. Long-term memory would appear to relate more to the actual volume of cortex remaining intact than to any specific localized process (consistent with the concept of Lashley). Although not discretely localized, it must be recalled that the read out mechanism for such remote memories may be triggered by stimulation of the lateral aspect of the temporal lobe in the particular abnormal situation of patients who are subject to temporal lobe seizures. In such patients, ablation of the area which on stimulation produces the remote memory does not abolish this remote memory. From a clinical standpoint, we evaluate this stage of memory asking the patient to indicate his date of birth, date of marriage, dates of World War I and II, and so forth.

FACTORS INFLUENCING LEARNING AND MEMORY

In the consideration of the learning process, it is important to realize the influence of several additional factors. The *motivational level* of the subject alters the rate of learning. Thus, in animal experiments, a rat who has been deprived of food and has a high degree of hunger will rapidly learn a particular task or response in a test situation where for each correct response the animal receives a reward of food. In contrast, an animal who has been previously satiated with food will show a much slower rate of learning under these circumstances.

The term *drive* is sometimes used interchangeably with motivation. It is possible to speak of primary (by implication, instinctive) motivational forces or drives, such as hunger and thirst, and of secondary (by implication, learned) motivational forces or drives, such as achievement, anxiety, and dependency. These are learned drives in the sense that motivations, such as desire for acquiring money and fame, or particular fears and guilts are not present in the infant and are not present in all members of a species. (Refer to discussion of Dollard and Miller.) In contrast, primary drives are present in all members of a species, irrespective of cultural influences and in general are present in the infant. During the process of development, previously neutral cues may become attached to primary drives and take on the capacity to motivate performance. These stimuli or cues then serve as learned motivational forces. It is important to realize that in a particular situation, a high level of motivation may actually interfere with learning. Thus anxiety may trigger responses which are not goal-directed, thereby interfering with learning.

Motivation not only influences the learning process but also affects the central process of interpretation of stimuli (*perception*). In a sense, what we see depends upon what we wish to see and upon our frame of reference. These factors are much more likely to be operative in a situation where the stimuli are relatively unstructured or ambiguous. Thus in the studies of McClelland, a clear relationship could be demonstrated between the level of hunger and food deprivation and the interpretation of ambiguous visual stimuli as definite food objects.

How we perceive a stimulus will obviously in many situations determine which previously learned responses will be called forth. Whether stimuli are perceived will also depend on the general state of *attention* or *alertness* of the individual. Thus, in a state of drowsiness or fatigue, we may fail to perceive and to respond to stimuli which under conditions of alertness would trigger an instantaneous response. The reticular activating system has been proposed as providing the neuroanatomical substrate of attention. Central and peripheral effects of these nonspecific sensory systems on the reception and transmission of sensory information have been demonstrated.

We should also indicate that the ability to attend to a specific stimulus and to delay response to that stimulus is altered by lesions involving the prefrontal areas. (Refer to Chapter 21.)

In considering the learning process, it is important to realize that the *active performance* of a behavioral act is usually more effective than the passive observation of the response. For example, most individuals learn a new route better by having to drive over the route than by being passively driven over the route.

DISORDERS OF RECENT MEMORY

THE AMNESTIC-CONFABULATORY SYNDROME: WERNICKE-KORSAKOFF ENCEPHALOPATHY

Wernicke, in 1881, described a syndrome which is of relatively acute onset, occurring in alcoholics or nutritionally deficient patients and consisting of a triad: mental disturbance (confusion and drowsiness), paralysis of eye movements, and an ataxia of gait. The basic cause of the syndrome is a dietary deficiency of thiamine. As a deficiency of thiamine and of the other B-complex vitamins also results in a peripheral neuropathy, symptoms relevant to this degeneration of peripheral nerves often will be present as an associated finding. The metabolic activities of thiamine are discussed in Chapter 22.

The pathological findings involve the gray matter surrounding the third ventricle (anterior and medial thalamus and the hypothalamus), the aqueduct (periaqueductal gray matter and the ocular motor nuclei), and the fourth ventricle (nuclei of cranial nerve VI, the dorsal motor nuclei, and the vestibular nuclei) (Fig. 27-1). To a degree, pathological changes also occur in the anterior superior portion of the midline cerebellum. The basic pathological process consists of a necrosis of neural parenchyma and a prominence of blood vessels due to a proliferation of adventitial and endothelial cells. Petechial hemorrhages also occur about these vessels. Lesions in general are usually most prominent in the mammillary bodies and the medial thalamic areas (Fig. 27-2).

The various clinical findings may be correlated with the pathological lesions. The ophthalmoplegia is predominantly a bilateral involvement of cranial nerve VI, that is, weakness of the lateral rectus muscles. This clears rapidly on parenteral administration of thiamine (Fig. 27-3). Often improvement occurs within a matter of hours. The pathological changes in the extraocular nuclei are often minimal. It has therefore been postulated that the extraocular palsies are a reflection of a biochemical disturbance that has not yet progressed to a permanent structural change. The drowsiness also clears on treatment. This may reflect damage to the periaqueductal gray matter and to the diencephalic areas surrounding the third ventricle. The ataxia which involves gait and trunk at times resolves to a significant degree, although at times this clinical finding remains as a persistent disability. This symptom undoubtedly reflects involvement of the anterior superior portion of the cerebellum. This clinical finding and the pathology in this location are noted to a more severe degree in the "alcoholic cerebellar degeneration" (p. 703).

From the standpoint of our considerations of memory, those findings, which may be noted as the patient's drowsiness begins to clear with treatment, are of considerable interest. It will often be noted that a severe deficit in recent memory is present. This will be the case particularly if the patient has delayed seeking medical diagnosis and treatment. The patient will be unable to learn new material. He will have little memory of events surrounding his illness but will have little difficulty recalling events in the distant past. The patient may supply imaginary answers for questions concerning the recent past and for questions involving new material he has been requested to learn by the examiner.

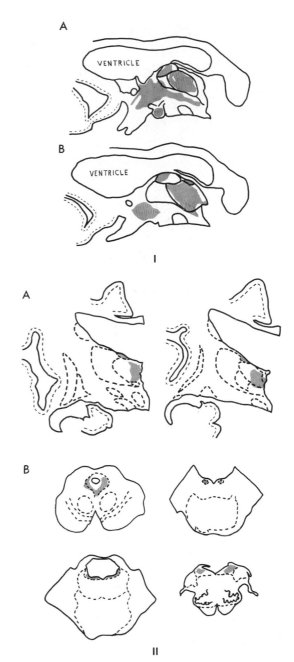

Figure 27-1 Wernicke-Korsakoff Syndrome: Anatomical Distribution of Lesions.

I Thalamic and hypothalamic involvement: *a.* Paramedian plane in sagittal section. *b.* 3 mm. more lateral.

II Thalamic and brain stem involvement: *a.* Lesions of dorsomedial and anterior thalamic nuclei shown in coronal sections. *b.* Brain stem lesions shown in horizontal sections. (From Victor, M.: The Effects of Nutritional Deficiency on the Nervous System, *In* Brain, Lord, and Norris, F. H. (eds.): *The Remote Effects of Cancer on the Nervous System.* New York, Grune and Stratton, 1965, p. 137, 138.)

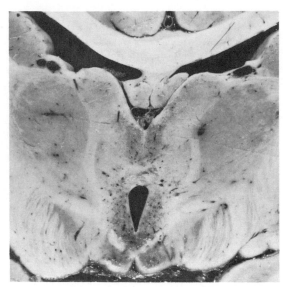

Figure 27-2 Wernicke's Encephalopathy. In the diencephalic areas surrounding the third ventricle, blood vessels are prominent and multiple small petechial hemorrhages are present. (From Foley, J.: In Robbins, S. L.: *Pathology*, 3rd Edition. Philadelphia, W. B. Saunders, 1967, p. 1424.)

These imaginary answers are termed *confabulations*. A significant disorientation for time is usually present. The memory disturbance involves both the retrograde amnesia (events prior to the illness) and anterograde amnesia (events since the onset of the illness). The

deficit in memory for recent events may be transient, clearing with continued treatment, or may be more persistent. The persistence of these disorders of recent memory and of the state of confusion as a chronic phenomenon is referred to as *Korsakoff's psychosis*. In the studies of Victor et al., pathological examination of the brain in these latter cases reveals persistent lesions in the dorsal medial and anterior nuclei of the thalamus. In contrast, cases coming eventually to autopsy after a history of Wernicke's encephalopathy but without the persistent memory deficits have not shown changes in these thalamic nuclei although lesions have been present in hypothalamic structures. The following case history illustrates the problem of Wernicke's encephalopathy.

Case History 1. NECH #157–865.
Date of admission: 7/26/63. (Patient of Dr. John Sullivan and Dr. John Hills.)

This 62-year-old, white, right-handed stonecutter (Mr. H. H.) had been a known heavy alcoholic spree drinker for many years. The patient would drink large quantities of wine for 6 to 8 weeks at a time. Two years previously, the patient had been admitted to the Boston City Hospital because of delirium tremens (tremor and visual hallucinations). In May 1963, shortly following the death of a brother-in-law, the patient began his most recent drinking spree. He unaccountably

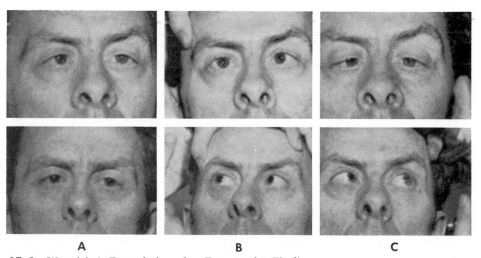

A **B** **C**

Figure 27-3 Wernicke's Encephalopathy: Extraocular Findings.
Top Row: Before therapy.
Bottom Row: After daily infections of 50 mg. of thiamine for 3 days in addition to a diet containing no other vitamins. *A*, primary position. *B*, gaze to right. *C*, gaze to left. A bilateral lateral rectus (nerve VIth) paralysis was present in addition to a lesser bilateral defect in adduction, which in this case was considered to reflect a defect in lateral conjugate gaze. With more severe involvement, there is actual paralysis of muscles supplied by third nerve. (From Victor, M.: Alcoholism. *In* Baker, A. B.: *Clinical Neurology*, 2nd Edition. Vol. II. New York, Hoeber-Harper, 1962, p. 1102.)

found himself in Florida, not knowing where he was and why he was there. Apparently, he had drifted aimlessly for 5 weeks with no definite food intake for a month. The patient was brought back by his family and hospitalized at his local community hospital on July 22, 1963 with diplopia, ataxia, and marked impairment of memory. The patient also complained of numbness of his finger tips and unsteadiness of gait. The patient was shortly thereafter transferred to the New England Center Hospital for additional neurological evaluation.

GENERAL PHYSICAL EXAMINATION:

No abnormalities were present except for an enlarged liver. The edge was palpated approximately 2½ fingerbreadths below the costal margin.

NEUROLOGICAL EXAMINATION:

1. *Mental status:*
   a. The patient was markedly disoriented for time and place. At times the patient thought that he was in New Jersey; at other times he stated correctly that he was in Boston. The patient with suggestion would recall his apparent travels that day to various other locations within and outside Boston. Confabulation was also evident when it was suggested that he had recently seen various fictitious persons.
   b. The patient was unable to state his age. At times the patient often indicated to visitors that his mother and father were still alive though both parents had been dead for over 20 years. He appeared to have little insight for his disorientation in time. He had no insight as to his condition or for the reason for his hospitalization.
   c. The patient's digit span was normal at 7 forward and 6 in reverse. The patient could name various objects correctly when these were presented to him and yet he was unable to retain any memory of which objects had been presented to him five minutes previously. He was unable to retain any information concerning a story which he had been requested to learn.
   d. The patient was able to provide his birth date correctly. He could not give his address or telephone number. When quizzed as to the president of the United States, he indicated

that Eisenhower was still president, (actually Kennedy).
   e. The patient was able to do 2 and 3 figure additions and multiplications without difficulty. He was able to do the initial subtractions in the serial 7 test but then lost track of the number to be subtracted.
   f. The patient was able to read and to write without difficulty. He showed no constructional apraxia and no left-right confusion.

2. *Cranial nerves:*
   a. There was horizontal diplopia on right lateral gaze. The minor degree of separation of images, however, did not allow precise identification of the muscle involved. A minor weakness of the right lateral rectus was suspected.* Horizontal nystagmus was present on lateral gaze bilaterally and vertical nystagmus on vertical gaze.

3. *Motor system:*
   a. Strength was intact except for a minor degree of weakness in the distal portions of the lower extremities evident on ankle dorsiflexion and toe dorsiflexion.
   b. The patient walked on a narrow base with eyes open and showed no evidence of an ataxia of gait. On a narrow base with eyes closed, the patient showed a positive Romberg test.
   c. No cerebellar findings were present.

4. *Reflexes:*
   a. Deep tendon reflexes in the upper extremities were normal, (triceps and biceps), and decreased at radial periosteal. Quadriceps and Achilles deep tendon reflexes were absent even with reinforcement.
   b. Plantar responses were flexor bilaterally.
   c. No grasp reflex was present.

5. *Sensory system:*
   a. Pain and touch were decreased in the lower extremities below the midcalf.
   b. Vibratory sensation was absent at the toes and decreased over the tibia to a marked degree and to a lesser de-

---

*The minor nature of the diplopia undoubtedly reflected the improved nutritional status which had occurred during the previous 5 days of hospitalization at his community hospital. We presume that if the patient had been examined prior to hospitalization, a more marked lateral rectus palsy probably would have been delineated.

gree over the knees. There was to a lesser extent, a decrease in the upper extremities at the fingertips and wrists.

c. Position sense was decreased at fingers and toes.

LABORATORY DATA:

1. Complete blood count was within normal limits.

2. Blood, urea, nitrogen, and liver function tests were within normal limits.

3. Lumbar puncture revealed spinal fluid with normal pressure of 120. Protein was 35 mgs./100 ml.

4. X-rays of the skull and chest were negative.

5. Electroencephalogram was normal.

HOSPITAL COURSE:

The patient was treated with thiamine, 50 mgs. daily. There was a significant improvement in extraocular muscle function. The patient had no diplopia after the day of admission. There was no significant change in his mental condition or peripheral neuropathy during the remainder of his hospital stay. The patient was then transferred to a Veterans Administration Hospital on August 1, 1963 for additional intermediate and chronic care. Evaluation 3 months later indicated persistent disorientation for time and place and severe selective deficits in recent memory. The patient was able to recite his serial number from World War II, but was unable to retain any new information.

COMMENT:

This patient presents a relatively typical history for the Wernicke-Korsakoff syndrome. He had been a heavy alcoholic spree drinker. We may assume that during his periods of heavy alcohol intake, his nutritional status was quite deficient. The major symptomatology that was apparent to the patient's family and to his physician related to his marked confusion and impairment of memory. The patient himself had no significant complaints and little insight into his disease. He appeared unaware of his marked disorientation for time and of his marked memory disturbances. Confabulation in this case was easily induced. In some cases the severe memory disturbances may be present without any definite evidence of confabulation. In this case the memory disturbance was quite severe. Not only was retentive memory for new material and recent material impaired, but it was quite evident that the patient's

distant memory also showed a significant but lesser degree of impairment. In such cases with severe impairment of memory, the prognosis for a complete recovery of mental status is very poor. The diplopia and nystagmus, as expected, resolved significantly with treatment with thiamine. The ataxia of gait which had been present early in the case had apparently resolved by the time of hospitalization. A significant peripheral neuropathy, mainly distal sensory, was present related to multiple B vitamin nutritional deficiency.

In many cases, the state of confusion in Wernicke's encephalopathy is preceded by or accompanied by a period of delirium tremens indicating alcohol withdrawal. The use of intravenous glucose feedings during such a withdrawal state may actually increase the requirements for thiamine, thus exacerbating the thiamine deficiency state. For this reason, all patients under treatment for alcohol withdrawal should be treated with high dosage vitamin therapy as well, on the presumption that they are candidates for nutritional deficiency.

In general, as we have indicated, the majority of patients with Wernicke's encephalopathy progress to a more persistent memory disturbance. Victor and Adams reported that 75 per cent of their 86 cases progressed to a permanent amnestic confabulatory syndrome.

The Korsakoff syndrome with its particular deficits in memory may also occur in other disease states involving the diencephalon. Thus, in the series of Williams and Pennybacker, tumors involving the posterior hypothalamus and third ventricle characteristically resulted in defects in recent memory. More anteriorly placed tumors in the hypothalamus apparently do not affect recent memory. The selective effect in this series of posterior hypothalamic tumors on recent memory was not a reflection of increased intracranial pressure, since in a control group of posterior fossa tumors with a significant degree of increased intracranial pressure, defects in recent memory were not an outstanding finding. These patients did have some general changes in mental status. Defects in recent memory have also been reported in tumors involving the posterior or anterior portion of the corpus callosum. In some of the anterior corpus callosum tumors, infiltration of both frontal areas has occurred.

BILATERAL LESIONS OF HIPPOCAMPUS (BILATERAL MEDIAL TEMPORAL LOBE LESIONS)

Bilateral destruction of the temporal lobe, particularly of the medial aspects of the temporal lobe, will produce a significant deficit in recent memory. Bilateral disease involving the temporal lobe may occur under a variety of circumstances.

Bilateral Ablation. Bilateral ablation of the anterior two-thirds of the hippocampus and the hippocampal gyrus with removal of the uncus and amygdala was performed by Scoville for treatment of temporal lobe epilepsy. Following surgery, a gross loss of the ability to retain current experiences and to learn new material was noted, in addition to a significant retrograde amnesia. Remote events were well recalled. It should be noted that a similar defect may follow unilateral ablation of the temporal lobe structures if disease is present in the contralateral temporal lobe. Such deficits in memory were reported by Penfield and Milner following unilateral surgical lesions.

Bilateral Infarction. Bilateral infarction of the hippocampal areas may occur with disease of the posterior cerebral artery. Often the basic disease process involves the basilar vertebral circulation. Thus stenosis of the basilar artery will produce decreased blood flow in both posterior cerebral arteries. The end result of insufficiency in the posterior cerebral artery circulation may be the bilateral infarction of the hippocampal areas as in the case reported by Victor et al. (1961) (Fig. 27–4).

In other cases, a transient ischemia of the medial temporal areas may occur as one aspect of more severe disease involving the distribution of the posterior cerebral artery to the calcarine cortex as illustrated in Case History 4, Chapter 22, page 554. In the illustrative case referred to, the patient had transient confusion and disorientation for time and place in relation to a bilateral blindness which receded into a unilateral homonymous hemianopsia with clearing of the confusional state. In still other instances, the ischemia apparently may be limited to the medial temporal area, that is, hippocampal areas, with little involvement of the occipital cortex. In these cases, transient episodes may occur and are identified as the *syndrome of transient global amnesia.*

This syndrome involves the sudden onset of a defect in memory. The deficit is similar to that which occurs in the amnestic confabulatory syndrome seen in Wernicke's encephalopathy. There is a significant retrograde amnesia for the events of the preceding days, weeks, and months. This retrograde amnesia slowly clears over a period of hours. The patient has a persistent amnesia for the period between the onset of the attack and the point of complete recovery.

During the period of the episode, the patient is unable to learn new material, that is, the patient is unable to register new memories. Apart from this defect, the patient usually shows no other abnormality of behavior during the episodes.

The actual vascular etiology of the syndrome has never been clearly proven but is strongly suspected. It is assumed that this ischemia involves in a bilateral manner the medial temporal areas.

We should note at this point that the posterior cerebral arteries via their penetrating branches also supply the medial diencephalic areas. Such ischemia in the posterior cerebral circulation, then, might well produce ischemia of the dorsal median nucleus, the anterior thalamic nuclei, and the mammillary bodies. Thus, in the case of persistent memory deficit following posterior cerebral artery lesions reported by Victor et al. (1961), the areas of infarction involved not only the hippocampal formation and fornix but also the mammillary bodies.

In the transient global amnesia syndrome, however, it is more likely that the actual disease process involves the hippocampal formation, rather than the diencephalic areas. As we will discuss later, the hippocampus is more likely to manifest a selective vulnerability to anoxia and would be expected to show functional impairment prior to the medial thalamic areas. The following case history illustrates this syndrome. A transient disease process involving the temporal areas is suggested but not proven.

Case History 2. NECH #75–50–10. Date of admission: 3/11/69.

This 55-year-old, right-handed, white male, college professor, (Mr. H. R.) awoke at 3 A.M. on the morning of admission in an uneasy and restless state. He asked his wife what day it was but then did not recall what she had told him. He did not know the month, kept repeating himself and asking the same ques-

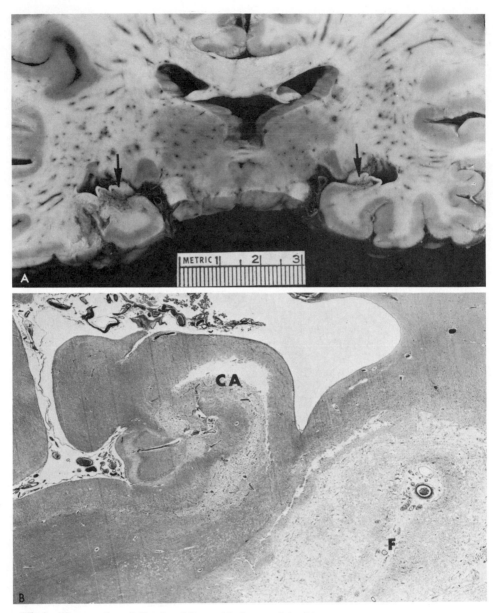

Figure 27–4   Memory loss following bilateral infarcts of the hippocampus.
A, Coronal section of brain at level of lateral geniculate bodies. Arrows point to discrete bilateral necrosis of hippocampus. Cortex facing collateral fissure on left shows a similar change (for normal gross appearance of hippocampus at this level see Fig. 17–29).
B, Left side. Chronic infarction of Ammon's horn (CA) and of parahippocampal and fusiform gyri along collateral fissure (F). (PTAH × 6.5). (From DeJong, R. N., et al.: Arch. Neurol., *20*:342, 343, 1969.)

tions. His wife arranged for him to be seen early in the morning by his family physician who lived a short distance away. The patient, who was familiar with the route, was unable to find his way there. When he arrived at the doctor's office, he was unable to explain why he had come. The patient apparently had forgotten about the incidents which had oc-

curred earlier that morning. He had no recollection that he had had a grandchild born to him 3 weeks before. He could remember no significant events from this 3-week period prior to the onset of his illness. The patient's more remote recall and other intellectual capacities remained intact. The patient drove into Boston later that day but became lost despite the usually familiar route.

PAST HISTORY:

The patient had a past history of gout with an elevated serum uric acid level.

NEUROLOGICAL EXAMINATION:

1. *Mental status:*

   a. When examined in the early afternoon, the patient was beginning to regain some of his ability to retain new information. The patient was generally oriented to person and place. However, he was disoriented for the day and month but was oriented for the year.

   b. The patient's store of information was quite intact suggesting a highly intelligent person.

   c. The patient had marked difficulty with delayed recall. He could recall none of the 4 objects after 5 minutes. He could not remember any of the three test phrases given to him when asked about these 5 minutes later. He did recall in a vague manner that a memory test had been given him. As regards recent memory, the patient was unable to remember his visit to his family physician earlier in the day.

   d. Digit retention, however, was relatively well preserved; 6 forward and 5 backward.

   e. The patient had no defects in calculation.

   f. There was no evidence of a constructional apraxia. Language function was entirely intact.

2. *Cranial nerves:* Nerves II through XII were intact.

3. *Motor system:* There was no weakness or disturbance of gait. Cerebellar tests were negative.

4. *Reflexes:*

   a. Deep tendon reflexes were symmetrical except for a minimal and questionable increase in the right quadriceps jerk compared to the left.

   b. Plantar responses were flexor.

   c. No grasp reflex was present.

5. *Sensory examination:* All modalities were intact.

LABORATORY DATA:

1. Complete blood count, blood urea nitrogen, total cholesterol, and uric acid were all within normal limits.

2. Skull x-rays and chest x-rays were normal.

3. Electroencephalogram was within normal limits.

4. Spinal fluid examination revealed normal pressure. No cells were present. There was a normal protein of 25 mg./100 ml.

5. The brain scan demonstrated a small area of increased uptake of radioisotope (Hg^{197}) in the left temporal region.

HOSPITAL COURSE:

Over the several hours following admission the patient gradually regained his ability to retain new information and to recall the events of the preceding 3 weeks, the more remote events being recalled first. The events of the day prior to admission were recalled last. The specific events that occurred on the morning of admission were never recalled. The following morning (March 12, 1969), delayed recall was 4-out-of-4 objects in 8 minutes. By the time of hospital discharge on March 13, 1969, the patient's mental status and neurological examination were otherwise within normal limits. The brain scan was repeated approximately 1 month later. This demonstrated an area of increased uptake of the isotope in the left anterior inferior temporal area and adjacent inferior frontal area (Fig. 27-5). The brain scan was repeated 2 months later in June 1969, and a significant degree of improvement had occurred. When repeated in August 1969 (Fig. 25-5*B*), the brain scan was entirely normal. It was the impression at that time, that the increased uptake noted previously was probably a small infarct undergoing resolution. Subsequent neurological evaluation has failed to reveal any significant neurological findings and the patient remains well now 1 year after the episode.

COMMENT:

This patient presented a selective deficit in memory which resulted in an inability to record and retain new memories (an anterograde amnesia) and an accompanying retrograde amnesia for a period of approximately 3 weeks preceding the onset of the disturbance. As was previously indicated, there was no sharp border between recent and remote memory. The process involved in the second stage or labile stage of memory has been estimated to be a matter of 20 to 180 minutes. And yet, these disturbances of "recent memory" are usually accompanied by significant retrograde amnesia that extends for a matter of days or weeks into the recent past. It may

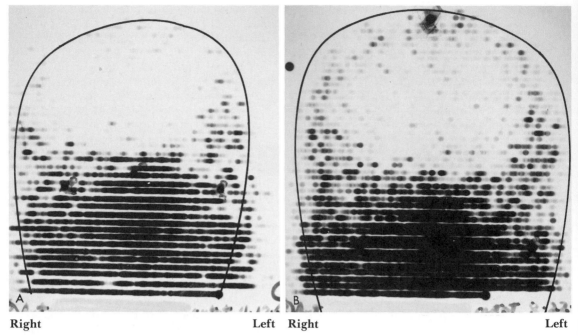

Right　　　　　　　　　　　　**Left**　**Right**　　　　　　　　　　　　**Left**

Figure 27–5　Transient global amnesia, from Case History 2.
A, In this anterior brain scan (Hg[197]), taken April 17, 1969, an increased uptake is noted in the left anterior temporal area. An increased uptake was apparent, as well, in the left lateral scan. *B*, In the brain scan taken on August 22, 1969 no significant difference in uptake was noted in the two hemispheres. (Courtesy of Dr. Bertram Selverstone.)

well be then that memories of the preceding day are somewhat labile but less labile than memories of 20 minutes previously. Memories of a week previously are also labile but certainly less labile than memories of the preceding day. The student should consider this primarily a defect in recent memory with a lesser impairment than of remote memory.

It should be noted that the patient was able otherwise to function intellectually in an intact manner. He was able to drive his automobile; he was able to answer many questions concerning general information on a level consistent with his intellectual ability and his profession as a teacher and educational administrator. The ability to do calculations and language functions was otherwise intact. This would suggest that lateral temporal areas were not involved. The electroencephalogram was normal and consistent with such a lack of involvement of the lateral aspects of the cerebral hemispheres.

The brain scan in this case did suggest a transient abnormality which would be consistent with an area of infarction which resolved over the succeeding months. Such an episode must be distinguished from epi-sodes of amnesia which may occur in relation to and following a temporal lobe seizure.

Stimulation.　Bilateral stimulation of the temporal lobe or unilateral stimulation with secondary spread to the contralateral hemisphere may occur during limited electrical stimulation of the medial temporal structures, during general stimulation of the brain (electrical shock therapy or a spontaneous generalized convulsive seizure), or during a temporal lobe seizure. Thus, it may be demonstrated that electrical stimulation of the depths of the temporal lobe in patients susceptible to temporal lobe seizures can produce a defect in memory for recent events without disturbing the patient's ability to recall remote memories.

In general, the longer the stimulation, the longer the duration of retrograde amnesia and the longer the recovery time before the new memories can be recorded. In the example cited by Doty (1967), *stimulation for 2 seconds* produced a retrograde amnesia for events just prior to stimulation and required a recovery time of 1 to 2 minutes before new memories could be recorded. *Stimulation for 5 seconds* produced a retrograde amnesia involving the events of the current day and required a period of 5 to 10 minutes before recent memories could be recorded. *Stimulation for 10 seconds* produced a retrograde amnesia that involved the events of the previous 3 weeks. A recovery time of 1 to 3 hours was required before new information could be recorded and retained.

In addition to these effects produced by limited electrical stimulation of the medial temporal areas, generalized electric shock producing a generalized convulsive seizure also produces a significant impairment of memory. The patient may be unable to recall events for a variable period of time prior to stimulation and may have difficulty recording new memories for a period of time after the electroshock therapy.

In a sense, a similar state is produced by an idiopathic generalized convulsive seizure or any focal seizure that is secondarily generalized as a tonic-clonic convulsion. The patient has amnesia for the events of the generalized seizure. The seizure is followed by a period of confusion during which the patient is unable to record new information and during which he is found to be confused and uncertain of memories prior to the seizure. In general, on recovery from this period of confusion the patient is amnestic for the entire period from the beginning of the seizure until the clearing of the postictal confusion. He usually, however, has no impairment of retrograde memories up to the point of the seizure.

The effects produced by electrical stimulation of the hippocampus may also occur as relatively selective ictal and postictal phenomena in a temporal lobe seizure as illustrated in the following case history in which focal temporal lobe seizure phenomena were followed by a period of impaired recent memory with an inability to record new memories.

Case History 3. NECH #185–160. Date of admission: 2/16/67.

This 68-year-old, white male (Mr. G. C.) in January 1966, fell, striking his occiput and transiently losing consciousness. Except for a persistent defect in his sense of smell, the patient had no apparent neurological defects following this injury.

Approximately 6 months later, the patient had the first of a series of recurrent episodes of amnesia. These episodes occurred most often on awakening. On some, but not all occasions, the episodes were preceded by a sensation of gastric upset, a strange odor, and a sensation of familiarity (deja vu). The episodes of total amnesia would last 30 to 60 minutes. There would then be an impairment of memory for approximately 1 to 2 days.

The patient was said during the episode of total amnesia and during the subsequent episode to behave in an otherwise normal and rational manner. For example, he would be able to converse with his wife and others. During the episodes, he was said to be unable to remember tasks which his wife had asked him to do during that day. A significant impairment of retentive memory would be apparent to his wife and to others. His memory for more distant and remote events was also impaired to a variable degree. The patient would then regain memory progressively over the course of the next 1 to 2 days. Apparently, memory was not regained in any orderly pattern from recent to remote or vice versa. The patient at no time had any abnormal movements suggestive of a generalized convulsion. No automatisms had been noted and to others the patient would appear fully conscious during the episodes.

GENERAL PHYSICAL EXAMINATION: No remarkable features were present.

NEUROLOGICAL EXAMINATION:

1. *Mental status:*
   a. The patient was oriented for time, place, and person.
   b. Delayed recall was intact. The patient could remember 4-out-of-5 objects in 5 minutes.
   c. Remote memory was intact.
   d. Digit span was slightly impaired at 6 numbers forward and 4 in reverse.
2. *Cranial nerves:* All areas were intact with the exception of cranial nerve I where olfaction was decreased for the odor of coffee grounds bilaterally.
3. *Motor system:* Strength, gait, and cerebellar tests were normal.
4. *Reflexes:*
   a. Deep tendon reflexes were symmetrical.
   b. Plantar responses were flexor.
5. *Sensory system:* All modalities were intact.

LABORATORY DATA:
1. Skull x-rays were normal.
2. Fasting blood sugar and glucose tolerance tests were normal.
3. Spinal fluid examination revealed no cells, normal pressure and a normal protein of 40 mg./100 ml.
4. The routine electroencephalogram was normal. However, the electroencephalogram

obtained after a period of sleep deprivation revealed occasional multifocal spikes during sleep in the right anterior temporal area and to a lesser degree the left frontal-anterior temporal area.

5. Brain scan (Hg^{197}) was normal.

6. Pneumoencephalogram was normal except for a minor degree of bilateral enlargement of the ventricles, and a slight widening of the sulci over the cortical surface.

SUBSEQUENT COURSE:

The patient was treated with anticonvulsant medication (phenobarbital). The episodes continued to occur once per month but the episode was now of shorter duration, lasting only 15 to 20 minutes. The impairment of memory was less marked and involved only the ability to learn new material without prolonged periods of retrograde amnesia. Follow-up evaluation in December 1968 and December 1969, indicated that the patient had had no definite episodes since September 1968. His neurological examination continued to be unremarkable except for the defect in olfaction. A follow-up electroencephalogram in December 1968 revealed no remarkable features.

COMMENT:

In this case, the episodes experienced by the patient could have posed a problem in identity were the occasional warning symptoms of olfactory aura, deja vu, and epigastric sensation not present. Most of the episodes experienced by the patient were not preceded by these clear symptoms of temporal lobe seizure discharge. Rather, these were episodes simply of amnesia with an inability to retain new information and inability to recall recent events and to some extent remote events. The patient's apparent behavior during these episodes was otherwise normal. Though the actual temporal lobe seizures apparently lasted only a matter of 30 to 60 minutes, some degree of impairment of memory was present for 1 to 2 days following the episode.

The etiology of the seizures in this case must relate to the patient's preceding head trauma. The loss of olfactory sensation following the trauma suggested that this trauma was of sufficient nature to tear the nerve filaments passing through the cribriform plate to the olfactory bulb on the orbital surface of the frontal lobe. We may also assume that this trauma may have been sufficient to produce some minor contusion of the anterior poles, inferior and medial

surfaces, of the temporal lobes against the bony walls of the middle fossa with a resultant scar and epileptogenic focus.

That these temporal lobe seizures beginning in this patient at age 68 were not indicative of more serious progressive pathology was shown by the lack of neurological findings on successive examinations and by the normal brain scan. The pneumoencephalogram suggested only a minor degree of cerebral atrophy but subsequent neurological examinations failed to reveal a progressive dementia. The electroencephalogram showed significant areas of discharge in the temporal lobe only under conditions of sleep deprivation. An overnight period of sleep deprivation acts to precipitate seizure discharges in individuals who have an underlying predisposition for seizure discharges.

Transient or Permanent Hippocampal Damage as a Result of Hypoxia or Hypo-Glycemia. The hippocampus demonstrates a relatively selective vulnerability to the effects of hypoxia and hypoglycemia with significant loss of pyramidal cells in sectors of the hippocampus (Fig. 27-6). Hypoxia may occur in relation to cardiac arrest, hypotension, defective aeration during anesthesia, and carbon monoxide poisoning, or in suicide attempts. Hypoglycemia may occur in relation to the use of insulin in the treatment of diabetes or in the use of insulin shock therapy. In such cases, the major deficits are in retentive memory with inability to form new associations and a variable impairment of memories formed in the recent past prior to the episode. While we have emphasized the effects of anoxia, hypoglycemia, and carbon monoxide poisoning on the hippocampus, we should not forget that these same insults may produce to a variable degree, involvement of neocortex (in the form of laminar necrosis) and of the globus pallidus (as in carbon monoxide poisoning).

Herpes Simplex Encephalitis. The virus herpes simplex, the common cold sore, may on rare occasions invade the central nervous system. When this occurs, several syndromes may occur. One syndrome is that of an overwhelming encephalitis with frequent generalized convulsive seizures and multiple myoclonic jerks progressing to death within a period of a week.

A second rare syndrome results from a more localized involvement of the medial temporal structures and is characterized by a subacute but progressive dementing process

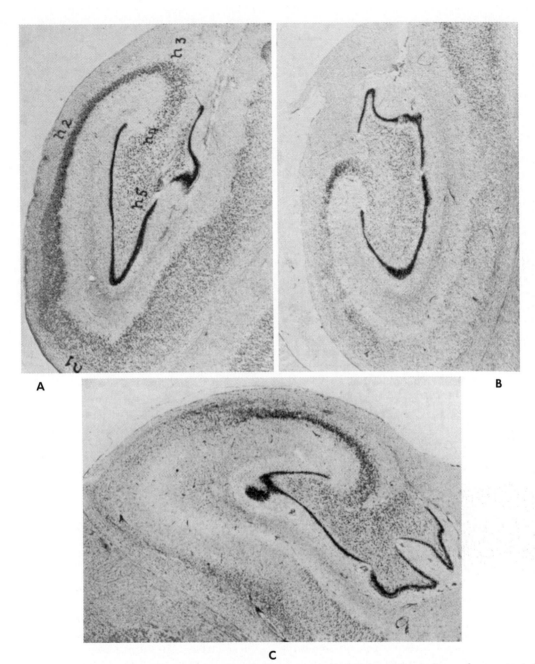

Figure 27–6 Necrosis of hippocampus in relation to anoxia and hypoglycemia, as demonstrated in Nissl stains. *A,* Normal Ammon's horn with fields h1-h5 of Rose inserted. *B,* Anesthetic death: recent necrosis in Sommer sector (h1) and partial loss of neurons in the end plate (h3, h4, h5). *C,* Hypoglycemic coma: there has been significant loss of pyramidal cells in sector h1. (From Meyer, A.: *In* Greenfield, J., et al., *Neuropathology,* 2nd Edition. Baltimore, Williams & Wilkins, 1963, p. 256.)

and temporal lobe seizures (Refer to Fig. 22–33). The disturbance of mental status is characterized by confusion and disorientation with a defect in memory for recent events and often for remote events as well. There is a marked inability to form new associations. The selectivity of the memory disturbance is less evident in these cases than in those cases of hippocampal disease previously discussed in detail.

TRAUMATIC AMNESIA

Perhaps the most common transient impairment of memory occurs in relation to head injury. When blunt trauma to the head occurs, consciousness is lost. As the individual recovers consciousness, there is a period of confusion before a return to normal behavior. The loss of consciousness and the subsequent period of confusion are often referred to as a concussion. Following this period of confusion, there is often a period during which behavior is otherwise normal but the ability to form new memories is defective.

Examination of the patient at that time will indicate that not only has he no memory of the actual period of unconsciousness and the following confusional state but also that he has defective memory for a period of time preceding the period of injury. The patient has then both an anterograde and retrograde amnesia. In general, the longer the period of retrograde amnesia, the more severe the head injury and in general the longer the period of time before memory will be regained. As recovery occurs, the period of retrograde amnesia is gradually reduced. The specific pathology and its location remain unknown in this condition.

PROGRESSIVE DEMENTING PROCESSES

Dementia refers to a progressive loss of mental faculties. In general, the loss involves initially the most severely recent memory and the ability to learn and retain new memories. To some extent, particularly as time passes, other areas of mental capability are also affected: remote memory, abstract reasoning, insight, arithmetic abilities, and language function.

In general, these processes involve the older adult population. However, certain rare disorders producing a progressive dementia affect infants, children, and adolescents. Some of these pediatric disorders reflect known or suspected inborn and genetic errors of metabolism: amino-aciduria, lipidosis, galactosemia, Hurler's disease (accumulation of mucopolysaccharides), and leukodystrophies. Other disorders are placed in the degenerative category because the etiology remains unknown; e.g., spongy degeneration. A detailed consideration of these various early onset problems is beyond the scope of this text.

The dementias must be distinguished from the *amentias*. The term *amentia* implies a nonprogressive congenital absence or relative deficiency of mental faculties. At times in the absence of an adequate history, the distinction may be difficult to make. The term *mental retardation* is somewhat less specific, referring to a retardation in the development of mental abilities or a retardation in the development of intelligence. The term mental retardation, as used, may reflect a congenital nonprogressive process, an acquired but nonprogressive process, or an early onset progressive dementing process.

The most common cause of a progressive impairment of mental faculties in the older adult population is the degenerative disease known as *presenile or senile dementia (Alzheimer's disease)*. Whether the process is called presenile or senile is arbitrary, based on the age of the patient. When the process begins before the age of 60 years (usually age 45 to 60), the designation presenile is used; when the process begins after the age of 60 years, the designation senile is employed. (Some authors place the dividing point at 65 years.)

The basic pathological process is, however, the same. Grossly, there is an atrophy of cerebral cortex, involving primarily in a diffuse manner the frontal and temporal areas, but sparing the motor cortex (Fig. 27-7). The process is most severe in the anterior frontal, anterior temporal, and medial temporal areas and at times appears to begin in these areas. In some cases, involvement of parietal areas is evident as well. In rare cases, the process appears to remain restricted to the frontal and temporal poles. These latter cases have been placed in a separate category as *Pick's disease*. They may be distinguished from Alzheimer's disease at autopsy, but there is no clinical distinction between the two.

From a microscopic standpoint, Alzheim-

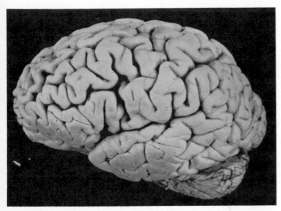

Figure 27–7 Cortical atrophy as found in presenile and senile dementia. There is widening of sulci and narrowing of the gyri, particularly in frontal areas.

er's disease is characterized by a loss of *neurons in all layers* of the cerebral cortex. Remaining neurons demonstrate degenerative changes, in particular, involving the neurofibrils with the formation of neurofibrillary tangles. In addition, amorphous silver staining clumps of material (senile plaques) of uncertain etiology are noted in the cortex between the nerve cells.

The clinical symptomatology in Alzheimer's disease relates to a progressive impairment of mental faculties, usually beginning with recent (retentive) memory. Initially, the social graces, remote memory, and rational reasoning capacities are well preserved. As the disease progresses, these aspects of mental function are also affected. In general, focal motor findings do not develop, deep tendon reflexes remain symmetrical and plantar responses are flexor. It is not unusual to have a significant degree of nominal aphasia present as the memory impairment becomes more severe. (The patient is unable to recall the names of objects.) Apraxias are also not unusual in these cases. The release of a grasp reflex is also often noted.

The following case history presents an example of presenile dementia.

Case History 4. Mrs. M. C. NECH #196–025.
Date of admission: 7/24/68. (Patient of Dr. John Sullivan.)
This 57-year-old, white housewife (Mrs. M. C.) was referred for evaluation of memory impairment of 1 year's duration.

In August 1967, the patient began to have difficulty remembering the price of items. This so interfered with her work as a clerk in a supermarket, that within a few weeks she was unable to continue her employment. The patient's husband indicated that this memory deficit had progressed slowly over a year. At the time of admission, she was beginning to have difficulty orienting herself in her own home and neighborhood. At home she would frequently put down objects and then be unable to recall their location.

There was no history suggesting episodes of cerebral ischemia. The patient had experienced no episodes of dizziness and no losses of consciousness. There was no past history of hypertension.

GENERAL PHYSICAL EXAMINATION: No remarkable features were present. Blood pressure was normal.

NEUROLOGICAL EXAMINATION:
1. *Mental status:*
   a. The patient was alert and cooperative.
   b. She was oriented for time, place, and person.
   c. As regards immediate memory, the patient was able to carry out one and two step commands but was unable to retain and carry out three stage commands.
   d. The patient was unable to recall 4 objects after a delay of 4 minutes. She was unable to recall what she had eaten for lunch.
   e. Remote memory was, in contrast, relatively intact. The patient was able to remember the high school that she had attended and the names of the teachers.
   f. The patient was able to read but comprehension was poor.
   g. Writing was intact. Calculations were poorly performed; the patient was unable to add or subtract anything more than the simplest figures.
   h. Occasional left-right confusion was present.
   i. Defects in constructional drawings were evident. When asked to draw a house, the patient forgot the walls and added a doorknob to one of the windows.
2. *Cranial nerves:* All areas were intact except for visual fields where there was an inconstant neglect of objects in the left field when simultaneous stimuli were presented.

3. *Motor system:*
   a. Strength and gait were intact.
   b. Cerebellar tests were normal.
4. *Reflexes:*
   a. Deep tendon reflexes were symmetrical and physiologic.
   b. Plantar responses were flexor.
   c. No abnormal grasp reflexes were obtained.
5. *Sensory system:* All modalities were intact except for occasional extinction of tactile stimuli on the left side when simultaneous stimuli were presented.

LABORATORY DATA:
1. Skull and chest x-rays were normal.
2. Electroencephalogram was normal.
3. Brain scan was normal.
4. Complete blood count, sedimentation rate, fasting blood sugar, blood urea nitrogen, calcium, electrolytes, and liver function tests were all normal.
5. The serum and cerebrospinal fluid serology (Hinton test for syphilis) was negative.
6. Free acid was present on gastric analysis suggesting that there was no defect in the ability to absorb vitamin B12.
7. Thyroid function was normal.
8. There were no detectable levels of barbiturates or bromides in the serum.
9. Cerebrospinal fluid was under normal pressure. No significant cells were present. The protein level was slightly elevated to 56 mg./100 ml. Cerebrospinal fluid sugar was normal.
10. Pneumoencephalogram revealed a mild dilatation of the ventricular system and evidence of probable cortical atrophy.

COMMENT:
In contrast to the very selective disturbance of recent and retentive memory presented in the previous illustrative case histories, this patient presents a somewhat more diffuse process. It is of course evident that the defect in recent memory and the inability to record new experiences were the initial features and remained the outstanding features of the patient's illness. In addition, however, severe impairment of the ability to perform calculations and of the ability to produce drawings was apparent. These findings, in addition to the inconstant ngelect of or inattention to visual and tactile stimuli on the left side, suggested that bilateral parietal lobe involvement was also present.
The progressive nature of the problem is evident from the history. The basic etiology remains uncertain and thus no specific treatment could be rendered in this case. The primary purpose of a complete evaluation in these cases is to rule out the treatable causes of dementia. In addition, several less frequent causes of dementia must be differentiated from Alzheimer's disease.

The treatable causes of dementia may be outlined as follows:

Chronic Infectious Processes. Tuberculous meningitis and cryptococcal meningitis can be ruled out by the lack of cells in the spinal fluid and the normal spinal fluid sugar. The tertiary complication of syphilis—generalized paresis—can be ruled out by the lack of cells in the spinal fluid and the normal blood and spinal fluid serology.

Nutritional Diseases

Wernicke's encephalopathy can be ruled out when there is no history of alcoholism or of nutritional deficiency.

Vitamin B12 deficiency is usually due to a defect in the production of intrinsic factor by the gastric mucosa. Since the same cells produce gastric acid, this problem may be ruled out by finding free acid on gastric analysis. Alternatively, measurements of serum vitamin B12 level or of the capacity to absorb orally administered radioactive vitamin B12 (the Schilling test) may be performed.

Chronic Intoxications. Such intoxications may produce a chronic confusional state with impairment of memory and judgement. An accompanying ataxia of gait may also be present. The responsible agents have varied with the popularity and availability of the various sedatives and tranquilizers. In the past, bromides were frequently implicated. Barbiturates remain high on the list of agents that are overused and misused. More recently, drugs such as meprobamate, chlordiazepoxide (Librium), and diazepam (Valium) have come into common usage. In some instances, intoxication with barbiturates and the other agents has reflected not an overdosage of the drug but rather an individual variation in the ability to metabolize the drug.

This treatable cause of dementia may be detected by determining the level of bromide or barbiturate present in blood or urine. The presence of ataxia and nystagmus in conjunction with the confusion and memory deficits should always raise suspicions as to a drug-related etiology. Finally, improvement of the confusion and dementia after a period of hospitalization should also lead to suspicions of such an etiology.

Metabolic and Endocrine Disorders. A number of systemic disorders such as hypoglycemia, hyponatremia, Addison's disease, hypercalcemia, renal failure, and hepatic failure may be associated with a transient disturbance of cerebral function. The neurologist is often called upon to evaluate the confusional state in such patients after the specific systemic diagnosis has been established. In the case of hypothyroidism (myxedema) the patient's complaints of a gradual slow down in mental capacities, memory defects, and a lack of energy may not have led to the establishment of a specific diagnosis and the patient is then referred for an evaluation of dementia. The diagnosis can be established by means of a determination of serum thyroxin (T4) of protein bound iodine (PBI) or of uptake by the thyroid of radioactive iodine (RAI).

Treatable Space-occupying Lesions. In this category must be considered mass lesions such as chronic subdural hematomas and meningiomas.

Chronic subdural hematomas, particularly when bilateral, may not be associated with clearly lateralizing or localizing findings but may present as a chronic progressive confusional state and dementia. (See Case History 11 (Mr. L. J.), Chapter 22, page 579). In general, the level of consciousness is also depressed or shows a fluctuating quality. Usually, the patient with Alzheimer's disease, although confused and disoriented, is alert.

The electroencephalogram, the brain scan, and arteriography in some cases will be helpful in differential diagnosis, but at times, these ancillary tests have little to offer or cannot be performed because of the patient's condition. The pneumoencephalogram may be helpful but offers a certain degree of risk, since the procedure must be performed in a patient with a supratentorial mass lesion where dangers of tentorial herniation exist. The best rule then in such cases in a situation where progressive confusion and dementia are associated with progressive alteration of consciousness is to suspect chronic subdural hematomas and perform the relatively simple procedure of trephine holes.

Meningiomas in several locations may produce slowly progressive syndrome of confusion and memory impairment: subfrontal and parasagittal. Thus, in the subfrontal olfactory groove meningioma illustrated in Case History 2 (Mrs. B. C.), Chapter 21, page 496, the patient for many years was incorrectly labeled as a presenile or senile dementia. Parasagittal frontal meningiomas may also show progressive alteration in memory in addition to the personality changes. (See Case History 15 (Mrs. E. N.), Chapter 22, page 614.)

In such cases, the brain scan will almost always show a dense uptake of radioisotope by the meningioma. Arteriography should then allow more specific delineation of the tumor mass.

Dementia Secondary to Late Onset Hydrocephalus. This is a rare syndrome of variable etiology and pathology resulting in a progressive dementia and gait ataxia (cerebellar and frontal lobe types). There may be some obtundation of consciousness as well. A block of the system at the aqueduct, an obliteration of subarachnoid cisterns, or a defect on passage from the cisterns to the superior sagittal sinus may be found. The diagnosis may be established by pneumoencephalography or by study of the rate of passage of radioactive iodinated serum albumin (RISA) from the cerebrospinal fluid. Treatment consists of shunting the cerebral spinal fluid in order to bypass the point of blockage in the system.

Other Essentially Nonremediable Entities to be Distinguished from Presenile or Senile Dementia. These entities may be outlined as follows:

The *lacunar state* (the syndrome of multiple little strokes). This syndrome is due to occlusion of small penetrating branches of the cerebral arteries and will be discussed in greater detail later.

Huntington's chorea occurs on a genetic basis with an autosomal dominant pattern of inheritance. This not uncommon entity involves progressive degeneration of neurons in the cerebral cortex (mainly frontal) and the basal ganglia (caudate nucleus and putamen). The resultant clinical syndrome of onset in the middle adult years of a progressive dementia, personality alteration, movement disorder, and gait disturbance has been illustrated in Chapter 24, Case History 2, page 688. The diagnosis is made on the basis of the clinical picture and family history.

Jakob-Creutzfeldt's disease is a rare subacute

disorder, possibly of viral etiology. (See Chapter 22, page 592.) In combination with rapidly progressive dementia of late adult onset, generalized seizures, myoclonic jerks, fasciculations, and rigidity are present. The diagnosis is made on the basis of the clinical picture of involvement of cerebral cortex, basal ganglia, and anterior horn cells in addition to a subacute history.

Glioblastomas (malignant astrocytomas), infiltrating the corpus callosum, prefrontal areas or diencephalic areas, may present a syndrome of progressive dementia. The diagnosis is made on the basis of brain scan and arteriography. Often the history suggests a relatively rapidly progressive process occurring in a middle-aged adult.

Metastatic carcinoma involving frontal lobe areas may also present a syndrome of relatively rapid progressive dementia and personality change. The diagnosis may be made on the basis of brain scan and arteriography. Metastatic carcinoma or sarcoma involving the meninges (*meningeal carcinomatosis*) may also present a progressive dementia. These are rare entities. Evidence of a meningeal process, with alterations in cellular count and morphology, will be evident on examination of cerebrospinal fluid. In addition, alterations in cerebrospinal fluid protein and sugar content will also be evident. (Refer to Chronic Meningitis, p. 585.)

Of these various nonremediable entities, perhaps the most common is the *lacunar state*, named from the multiple small old infarcts noted in the cerebral hemispheres at autopsy, primarily involving the internal capsule, basal ganglia, and subcortical white matter. As a cause of dementia this is second in frequency to the degenerative process of Alzheimer's disease. In such cases, there is often a previous history of hypertension. The basic pathological process involves the thickening and occlusion of small arteries, already considered in Chapter 22 in relation to diseases of the penetrating branches of the middle cerebral artery (page 545).

The clinical picture consists of multiple episodes of "relatively pure motor" hemiplegia with equal involvement of face, arm, and leg from which the patient appears to make an excellent recovery. Often additional episodes occur as apparent "dizzy" spells, or "faints" or "transient thickness of speech," each signifying a minor infarction. Many of the episodes may be so minor that the patient and his family attribute little significance to them until a significant degree of dementia is apparent. The dementia is usually accompanied by a significant apraxia of gait, a bilateral release of grasp reflex, an asymmetry of deep tendon reflexes, bilateral or unilateral Babinski signs and a moderate degree of extrapyramidal symptomatology (rigidity and akinesia). The latter is often labeled arteriosclerotic Parkinson's disease. A minor degree of tremor may be present but this is not usually a prominent symptom. Additional multifocal cortical signs may also be present; e.g., constructional apraxia.

The following case history illustrates this problem.

Case History 5. NECH #128–218. Date of admission: 7/9/59.

This 60-year-old, white housewife (Mrs. B. D. G.) was referred for evaluation of difficulty in walking. Four years prior to admission the patient was found to have a hypertension of 240/100 associated with anxiety, pounding headaches, and dizziness. Nineteen months prior to admission, the patient noted weakness of the left leg and was unable to walk for approximately 3 weeks. One year prior to admission her blood pressure was 190/80 and she was found to have bilaterally hyperactive deep tendon reflexes. Eight months prior to admission, the patient was again admitted to her local hospital because she had begun to experience intermittent falls with difficulty in walking. This was characterized by weakness of the legs and difficulty in getting up and out of a chair. Once walking was commenced, less difficulty was experienced. Depression and hypertension were again noted.

During hospitalization an anemia was found. Transfusions increased hematocrit from 30 per cent to normal but failed to modify either the patient's gait or her depression. At least 6 months prior to admission her husband noted that her memory was failing. Four months prior to admission, the patient was found to be losing her habits of cleanliness. In addition, the patient started to increase alcoholic intake in order to sleep at night. Nutrition also became poor. Two months prior to admission, increased unsteadiness of gait was noted. Three weeks prior to admission the patient had been noted to be quite tremulous, but had experienced no hallucinations or delusions. The present admission was precipitated by a fall in which the patient sustained a severe periorbital ecchymoses (a black eye). The patient attributed her falls to weakness of the right leg.

GENERAL PHYSICAL EXAMINATION:

1. The patient was obese, tremulous, anxious, and emotionally labile, with ecchymoses about the left eye and right elbow.

2. Fissures were present at the corners of the mouth; tongue was smooth and beefy.

3. Liver edge was one fingerbreadth below costal margin. Blood pressure was 190/90.

NEUROLOGICAL EXAMINATION:

1. *Mental status:*
   a. The patient was oriented for person and place but was only grossly oriented for time.
   b. There was poor attention with evidence of perseveration. The patient often neglected the questions of the examiners and instead picked at the bed clothes with her right hand. Constant chewing movements were present.
   c. The patient's store of information was poor.
   d. The patient was markedly impaired in her ability to learn new material. Delayed recall was 0-out-of-5 objects in 5 minutes.

2. *Cranial nerves:*
   a. Examination of the fundus demonstrated arteriovenous nicking.
   b. There were constant chewing movements of the jaw.
   c. The jaw jerk was hyperactive.
   d. A left central facial weakness was present.

3. *Motor system:*
   a. Strength was intact.
   b. A plastic cogwheel rigidity was present at the wrists, elbows, and knees.
   c. A tremor of the head and outstretched hands was present. This was rhythmical, increased by movement, and present at terminal sustained posture.
   d. The patient's gait was broad-based with shuffling movements of both feet. There was great difficulty in standing up from a chair and in beginning movement. Once underway, difficulty was less marked.
   e. The patient failed to swing the left arm in walking.
   f. Alternating movements were impaired bilaterally but were more marked on the left than right.
   g. In standing on a narrow base with eyes open, the patient swayed from side to side.

4. *Reflexes:*
   a. Deep tendon reflexes were hyperactive but symmetrical throughout.
   b. Plantar responses were flexor bilaterally.
   c. An excessive bilateral instinctive grasp was present. A suck reflex was also present bilaterally.

5. *Sensation:* Intact except for moderate decrease in vibration at toes.

LABORATORY DATA:

1. Complete blood count was normal.

2. Cerebrospinal fluid was under normal pressure with no cells present. Protein was 35 mg./100 ml. Serological test was negative.

3. No bromides were present in the serum.

4. Skull x-rays were negative.

5. The electroencephalogram demonstrated diffuse slow wave activity.

6. The bone marrow was normal and the Schilling test demonstrated normal absorption of vitamin B12.

7. The intravenous pyelogram demonstrated evidence of old pyelonephritis.

8. Blood urea nitrogen was elevated to 51 mg./100 ml.

SUBSEQUENT COURSE:

Nutritional status was improved, and renal infection was treated. The blood urea nitrogen returned to normal levels. Although the patient's anxiety and tremulousness disappeared, her memory impairment, ataxia of gait, and grasp reflexes remained unchanged. The patient was subsequently transferred to her local county hospital. Follow-up evaluation on October 7, 1959 indicated that she had adjusted well to life at the hospital. Ataxia was still present (frontal lobe in type), but the patient was somewhat more stable in walking and standing. A bilateral grasp reflex and tonic foot response were still present.

COMMENT:

The initial events in this case indicated multiple "small strokes" occurring on a background of severe hypertension. Each of the episodes involved motor function primarily. With repeated episodes, ataxia (of frontal lobe type), dementia, and depression became prominent. As these latter features emerged, the clinical picture was complicated in its later stages by poor nutrition and alcohol intake. These are not infrequent complicating features when depression and dementia in the elderly are considered. We should note that when depression begins in later life, the possibility of an underlying neurological disorder should always be considered.

INSTINCTIVE BEHAVIOR

As psychologists came to study learned behavior in animals, it soon became evident that not all behavioral patterns were learned. That is, not all behavioral patterns required a period of trial and error; not all behavior patterns required prior experience of the organism with his environment. Initially, all behavior that did not appear to be learned was described under the catch-all wastebasket phrase, instinctive behavior. As additional observations have been accumulated, it has become evident that several processes had been placed in this wastebasket. Some of these are clearly innate and do not require any prior experience. Other behavioral processes, although not clearly in the category of learning, do require at least one prior environmental experience.

Clearly innate instinctive behavioral response patterns* differ from learned stimulus response behavioral patterns as regards the following characteristics:

1. The behavior involved in a response occurs exactly the same way each time the stimulus is presented.

2. The complete response occurs at first presentation of the releasing stimulus before there has been a chance for learning to take place.

3. The response must occur in all members of a species.

4. Response must occur in individuals raised in isolation from species members.

Despite these rules for categorizing instinctive behavior, it is evident that variations in instinctive behavior do occur. Thus, Tinbergin (1951) has noted the relationship of the internal hormonal state in the release of

---

*Instinctive patterns of behavior can be clearly recognized in nonmammalian species, such as fish and birds, as regards activities such as mating, nesting, defense, and aggression. The role of innate instinctive factors in the behavior of primates such as man is less clearly defined.

instinctive behavioral patterns by environmental stimuli. He has also indicated that wherever there is a conflict of two instinctual behavioral patterns, an animal may exhibit a third behavioral pattern. It is also evident that as with learned behavior, with repeated performance of an instinctive behavioral pattern there is a weaning of the tendency to perform that behavioral pattern. In addition, as in learned behavior, the level of motivation will influence the frequency of performance of the behavioral response. Thus, with a strong motivation and an absence of the appropriate releasing stimulus for an instinctive behavioral pattern, one may have the performance of a behavioral act under inappropriate circumstances.

As regards the neuro-anatomical basis for innate instinctive behavioral patterns, it is of interest to note that complex instinctive behavioral reactions may be triggered by hypothalamic or midbrain stimulation in birds. In a sense these responses represent complex reflex activity.

IMPRINTING

Related to the concept of instinctive behavior patterns is the concept of imprinting. The initial concepts of imprinting evolved from the study of "following" behavior in newly hatched chicks. The response of following was released by the first object encountered after hatching. This object must fall within certain stimulus perimeters; that is, it must have certain distinctive stimulus characteristics. The specific stimulus object, however, which released the "following" could be variable. Thus, chicks will usually follow their natural mother since during the specific critical period after hatching they are usually exposed to the mother. However, if chicks do not encounter the mother but rather encounter a man, they will tend to follow the man. This pattern will persist even though they are later returned to the environment of the mother. Once the imprinting has occurred at this critical period, the specific stimulus-triggered behavioral pattern is difficult to alter. The essential purpose of imprinting in the natural environment should be evident. The following behavior which is evoked results in the immature chicks always being close to the protection of the mother. In addition, it has been found that that object which has become imprinted later in life releases sexual behavior.

Critical Periods. The concept of imprinting during the critical periods in the development of the organism has considerable relevance to various observations concerning human development.

It should be evident to the student from his study of embryology that there are critical periods in embryological development at which times organizers must induce a critical effect, i.e., the development and closure of the neural tube. It would not be unusual then to conceive of similar critical periods during the early postnatal period of development. Such a relationship is implied by Freud's theory of psychosexual development. That is, there are critical periods for the development of certain patterns of behavior and personality. Failure of exposure to appropriate stimuli during these stages of development will result in deviations from normal behavior and in conflicts at later stages of life as regards dependency, aggression, sexual behavior, and other aspects of social behavior.

EARLY EXPERIENCE AND POSTNATAL BRAIN DEVELOPMENT

Related to the subject of critical periods in development have been a number of studies which have demonstrated a significant effect of early environment of the infant animal or human on later brain development and function. In this category are the early studies of Spitz (1945) on hospitalism. Infants raised in a nonstimulating institutional environment (high walls about cribs, not fondled frequently) were compared to infants raised in a more stimulating institutional environment. Significant retardation and a higher mortality rate were noted in infants raised in the nonstimulating environment, even though the general health conditions and nuitrition of the nonstimulating environment were equal to those of the stimulating environment. These effects should be reversed if the infant was moved to a more stimulating environment early in life. However, the effects were irreversible after the age of 15 months, even if the infant at that time was moved to a more stimulating environment. Spitz related these effects to maternal deprivation. The results

of these experiments, however, have been reinterpreted in terms of stimulus deprivation during a critical period of development.

Experimental Studies. During the 1950's a number of studies dealt with the question of how early experience affected performance later in adult life. A number of studies, such as those of Hymovitch (1952) indicated that in developing rats, a wide environmental exposure as compared to a restricted environmental exposure resulted in a relatively permanent superior performance in various learning situations when these situations were tested in adult life. It was also demonstrated that monkeys or chimpanzees reared in darkness or in situations where no formed vision was possible (translucent bag was placed over the head) had difficulty perceiving forms and shapes. Even when the animals were exposed to light as adults, they were unable to acquire these capacities for discrimination and perception.

Anatomical, Physiological and Neurochemical Correlates. Later studies have demonstrated that such sensory deprivation or enrichment in the experimental animal produces significant changes of a structural and biochemical nature when specific sensory systems are considered. Thus, in the studies of Hubel and Wiesel (1963), deprivation of light by patching one eye in the kitten resulted in loss of cells in the lateral geniculate. In the occipital lobes there was an almost total absence of response in cells driven by the monocularly deprived eye. There is also some indication that cats reared in the dark developed fewer higher order branches in the dendrites of neurons and visual cortex than do visually experienced litter mates (refer to reviews of Riesen, 1966, and of Rosenzweig & Leiman, 1968). Significant increases in thickness of visual cortical areas have been found in rats raised in enriched environmental situations compared to normal or restricted environmental situations. Significant biochemical alterations also have been found in the cortex in an enriched environmental situation, particularly as regards cholinesterase. These and other biochemical studies are discussed in the review of Rosenzweig & Leiman and in the review of Russell (1966).

Significance for man. These various studies have obvious significance for man. It has been evident that children raised beyond a particular point in small, isolated, culturally deprived communities appear to have a long-term deficit in capacity for learning when tested at a later age. This apparently occurs even though they are switched at age 6 or 7 to a more enriched environment. There is an implication in these various studies that environmental and cultural deprivation may have long-lasting effects on the nervous system which cannot be reversed at a later point in time.* It is such considerations which have given rise to the use of "head-start" programs in preschool and primary grade students from culturally deprived backgrounds. (Refer to Hellmuth, 1968.)

References

Memory and Dementia

Adams, R. D., Fisher, C. M., Hakim, S., et al.: Symptomatic occult hydrocephalus with "normal" cerebrospinal fluid pressure. New Eng. J. Med., 273:117–126, 1965.

Bachrach, A. J.: Learning, In Freedman, A. W., and Kaplan, H. I. (eds.): Comprehensive Textbook of Psychiatry. Baltimore, Williams and Wilkins, 1967, pp. 166–171.

Barondes, S., and Cohen, H.: Puromycin: Effect on successive phases of memory. Science, 141:594–595, 1966.

De Jong, R. N., Itabashi, H. H., and Olson, J. R.: Memory loss due to hippocampal lesions. Arch. Neurol., 20:339–348, 1969.

Delgado, J. M. R., Roberts, W. W., and Miller, N. E.: Learning motivated by electrical stimulation of the brain. Amer. J. Physiol., 179:587–593, 1954.

Dollard, J., and Miller, N. E.: Personality and Psychotherapy. New York, McGraw-Hill, 1950.

Doty, R. W.: Limbic System, In Freedman, A. M., and Kaplan, H. I. (eds.): Comprehensive Textbook of Psychiatry. Baltimore, Williams and Wilkins, 1967, pp. 125–143.

Drachman, D. A., and Adams, R. D.: Acute herpes simplex and inclusion body encephalitis. Arch. Neurol., 7:45–63, 1962.

Fisher, C. M., and Adams, R. D.: Transient global amnesia. Acta Neurol. Scan., 40:(Suppl. 9) 7–83, 1964.

Flexner, L. B., Flexner, J. B., and Roberts, R. B.: Memory in mice analyzed with antibiotics. Science, 155:1377–1383, 1967.

Glickstein, M.: Neurophysiology of Learning and Memory, In Ruch, T., and Patton, H. (eds.): Physiology and Biophysics, 19th Edition. Philadelphia, W. B. Saunders, 1965, pp. 480–493.

James, A. E., De Land, F. H., Hodges, F. J., and Wagner, H. N.: Normal pressure hydrocephalus. J.A.M.A. 213:1615–1622, 1970.

John, E. R.: Neural Processes During Learning, In Russell, R. W. (ed.): Frontiers in Physiological Psychology. New York, Academic Press, 1966, pp. 149–184.

McClelland, D. C., and Atkinson, J. W.: The projective expression of needs. J. Psychol., 25:206, 1948.

McGaugh, J. L.: Time-dependent processes in memory storage. Science, 153:1351–1358, 1966.

Meyer, A.: Intoxications, In Greenfield, J., Blackwood, W., McMenemy, W. H., Meyer, A., and Norman, R. M. (eds.): Neuropathology. Baltimore, Williams and Wilkins, 1963, pp. 235–287.

Morrell, F.: Modification of RNA as a Result of Neural Activity. In Brazier, M. A. B. (ed.): RNA and Brain Function, Memory and Learning. (Brain Function Vol. II). Berkeley, University of California Press, 1964, 183–202, (Mirror Focus).

Nauta, J. H.: Some brain structure and functions related to memory. Neurosciences Research Symposium Summaries I: 73–107, 1966.

Olds, J.: Hypothalamic substrates of reward. Physiol Rev., 42:554–604, 1962.

Olds, J.: Self stimulation of the brain. Science, 127: 315–324, 1958.

Penfield, W., and Milner, B.: Memory deficit produced by bilateral lesions in the hippocampal zone. Arch. Neurol. Psychiat., 79:475–497, 1958.

Russell, R. W.: Biochemical Substrates of Behavior, In Russell, R. W. (ed.): Frontiers in Physiological Psychology. New York, Academic Press, 1966, pp. 185–246.

Scoville, W. B., and Milner, B.: Loss of recent memory after bilateral hippocampal lesions. J. Neurol., Neurosurg., Psychiat., 20:11–21, 1957.

Shuttleworth, E. C., and Morris, C. F.: The transient global amnesia syndrome. Arch. Neurol., 15:515–520, 1966.

Victor, M.: Alcoholism, In Baker, A. B. (ed.): Clinical Neurology, 2nd Edition., Vol. II. New York, Harper, 1966, pp. 1084–1129.

Victor, M.: The Effects of Nutritional Deficiency on the Nervous System, In Brain, Lord, and Norris, F. H. (eds.): The Remote Effects of Cancer on the Nervous System. Grune and Stratton, New York, 1965, pp. 134–161.

Victor, M.: Observations of the Amnestic Syndrome in Man and Its Anatomical Basis, In Brazier, M. A. B.: RNA and Brain Function, Memory and Learning (Brain Function, Vol. II). Berkeley, University of California Press, 1965, pp. 311–340.

Victor, M., Adams, R. D., and Collins, G. H.: The Wernicke Korsakoff Syndrome. Philadelphia, F. A. Davis, 1971, 206 pp.

Victor, M., Angevine, J. B., Mancall, E. L., and Fisher, C. M.: Memory loss with lesions of hippocampal formation. Arch. Neurol., 5:244–263, 1961.

Weiskrantz, L.: Impairment of Learning and Retention Following Experimental Temporal Lobe Lesions, In Brazier, M. A. B. (ed.): RNA and Brain Function, Memory and Learning (Brain Function, Vol. II). Berkeley, University of California Press, 1964, pp. 203–232.

Whitter, C. W. M., and Zangwill, O. L. Amnesia. London, Butterworths, 1966, 217 pp.

*There are of course factors of cultural background which may give rise to apparent differences in intelligence of an artifactual nature when performance on verbal tests alone is considered. Such tests have often had a bias in their design in favor of the upper- or middle-class Americans or Western Europeans. (Consider, for example, the general information subtest of the Wechsler-Bellevue Intelligence Test.) Such apparent differences can be corrected by learning. We are speaking here with regard to cultural deprivation in terms of deficits in *capacity for learning* which cannot be corrected by later experience.

Williams, M., and Pennybacker, J.: Memory disturbances in third ventricle tumors. J. Neurol. Neurosurg. Psychiat., *17*:115–123, 1954.

Instinctive Behavior and Related Topics

Hellmuth, J. (ed.): *Disadvantaged Child.* Vol. II: *Head Start and Early Intervention.* New York, Brunner-Mazel, Inc., 1968, pp. 613.

Hess, E.: Ethology *In* Freedman, H., and Kaplan, H. (eds.): *Comprehensive Textbook of Psychiatry.* Baltimore, Williams and Wilkins, 1967, pp. 180–189.

Hubel, D. H.: Effects of distortion of sensory input on visual system of kittens. Physiolog., *10*:17–45, 1967.

Hymovitch, B.: Effects of environmental variations on problem solving in the rat. J. Comp. Physiol. Psychol., *45*:313, 1952.

Riesen, A. H.: Sensory deprivation in progress *In* Stellar, E., and Sprague, J. M. (eds.): *Physiological Psychology.* New York, Academic Press, 1966, Vol. I, pp. 117–147.

Rosenzweig, M. B., and Leiman, A. L.: Brain Functions *In* Farnsworth, P. R. (ed.): Annual Review of Psychology, *19*:55–98, 1968.

Russell, R. W.: Biochemical substrates of behavior *In* Russell, R. W. (ed.): *Frontiers in Physiological Psychology.* New York, Academic Press, 1966.

Scott, J. P.: Critical periods in behavioral development. *Science, 138*:949–958, 1962.

Spitz, R.: Hospitalism. Psychoanal. Study of Child, *1*: 53, 1945.

Tinbergin, N.: *The Study of Instinct,* London, Oxford University Press, 1951, pp. 228.

Wechsler, D.: *The Measurement of Adult Intelligence.* Baltimore, Williams and Wilkins, 1944, pp. 258.

Wiesel, T. N., and Hubel, D. H.: Efforts of visual deprivation on morphology and physiology of cells in the cat's lateral geniculate lobes. J. Neurophysiol., *26*:978–993, 1963.

Wiesel, T. N., and Hubel, D. H.: Single cell responses in striate cortex of kittens deprived of vision in one eye. J. Neurophysiol., *26*:1003–1017, 1963.

Wiesel, T. N., and Hubel, D. H.: Extent of recovery from the effects of visual deprivation in kittens. J. Neurophysiol., *28*:1060–1072, 1965.

28

General Case History Problem Solving

ELLIOTT M. MARCUS

Case History 1. NECH #75–60–60.

This 63-year-old former bartender (Mr. J. F.) in 1967 had the onset of weakness and fatigue. The patient noted a change in his bowel movements. His stools became black and he was found to be anemic. He lost weight. When admitted to the hospital he was found to have a carcinoma arising from the rectosigmoid and infiltrating the bladder neck. A sigmoid colostomy was performed and the patient received high voltage x-irradiation directed to the tumor mass.

The patient did well for 8 months at which time multiple nodules were seen in the lung film, presumably metastatic disease.

In 1969, the patient experienced the first of a number of 30- to 60-second episodes of spontaneous twitching of the left corner of the mouth associated with a tingling sensation in the left thumb and index finger. These began to occur as often as twice daily and to last as long as 5 to 20 minutes. There was no aura and no loss of consciousness. There was no generalized convulsion. The patient was right handed.

NEUROLOGICAL EXAMINATION:

1. *Mental status* and language function were intact.

2. *Cranial nerves:* There was questionable flattening of the left nasolabial fold.

3. *Motor system:* Strength in the extremities appeared normal.

4. *Reflexes:* Deep tendon reflexes were slightly increased in the left upper extremity.

5. *Sensation:* Stereognosis and graphesthesia were impaired in the left hand.

SUBSEQUENT COURSE:

Appropriate medication was administered and the patient received x-irradiation. Three months later, the patient was reported as having a more pronounced left hemiplegia. The patient became more confused and gradually unresponsive, and his respirations ceased.

QUESTIONS:

1. Indicate the location of the pathology.
2. Indicate the nature of the pathology.
3. Characterize the nature of the episodes involving the left face and hand in 1969.

778

Case History 2. NECH #128–300.

Date of admission: 7/14/59.

This 59-year-old, white, married, plumbing contractor (Mr. J. R.), approximately 7 years prior to admission, had the onset of a tremor of the right hand occurring mainly at rest. One year prior to admission, the patient had noted progression so that tremor was now present at the wrist and shoulder in addition to the fingers. During this time, the patient had also noted a stiffness of the right leg when walking. During the 6 months prior to admission the patient had experienced short episodes of subjective vertigo resulting in a tendency to fall forward.

PAST HISTORY:

1. Poliomyelitis at age 2 with residual atrophy of gastrocnemius muscle of left leg.

2. Influenza in 1918.

3. Back injury one year prior to admission. Since then he had been unable to straighten up when walking and had to walk in a stooped over position.

NEUROLOGICAL EXAMINATION:

1. *Mental status:*
   a. Patient was depressed and anxious.
   b. There was mild impairment of digit span, of delayed recall, and of ability to retell stories. Some evidence of confabulation was present.

2. *Cranial nerves:*
   a. A fixed facies with minor facial asymmetry was present.

3. *Motor system:*
   a. *Strength* was intact except for plantar flexion at left ankle with associated atrophy of gastrocnemius and shortening of the left Achilles tendon.
   b. *Gait:* The patient walked stooped over with slow short steps. He turned *en bloc*. There was a lack of associated movements of the arms with greater impairment on the right side.
   c. There was a resting tremor of the right upper extremity at the shoulder, wrist, and fingers, rhythmical at 3-4 per second and pill-rolling in type.
   d. There was a plastic resistance to passive motion with intermittent cogwheel component of the right upper extremity at the shoulder, elbow, and wrist. To a lesser degree rigidity was present in the right lower extremity.

   e. Alternating movements were impaired bilaterally (right greater than left).

4. *Reflexes:*
   a. Deep tendon: biceps and triceps more active on left; quadriceps and Achilles more active on right.
   b. Plantars: extensor bilaterally.

5. *Sensation:* intact.

LABORATORY DATA:

1. PBI: normal

2. CSF: normal pressure, cells, protein, and Hinton.

3. EEG: negative.

4. Skull x-rays: negative.

QUESTIONS:

1. Indicate the diagnosis.

2. Where is the lesion? What significance do you attach to the bilateral Babinski signs?

3. Indicate the etiology.

4. Outline the diagnostic and therapeutic management.

5. Indicate the prognosis.

Case History 3. NECH #78–90–28.

Date of admission: 6/12/70.

This 53-year-old, right-handed, white housewife (Mrs. S. P.) had the onset of weakness in the lower extremities approximately 10 months prior to admission. At the same time the patient noted twitching of the muscles of the legs, that is, fasciculations. The weakness progressed so that the patient had difficulty in walking. Approximately 8 months prior to admission, the patient noted the onset of weakness and fasciculations in the upper extremities. This was noted most particularly with regard to the hands. The patient had had a progression of symptoms in the intervening months; approximately a 30-lb. weight loss had been experienced. Although the patient complained of fatigue and some lethargy, she had noted no definite change in mental status. She had not experienced any headaches or pains in the neck. She had had no diplopia or visual disturbances. No sensory symptoms had been noted; no urinary or bowel symptoms had been noted. Past history and family history were not remarkable.

NEUROLOGICAL EXAMINATION:

1. *Mental status:* intact.

2. *Cranial nerves:* All were intact except for 12. Ridges of atrophy were noted at the lateral borders of tongue; there were marked fasciculations of the tongue.

3. *Motor system:*
   a. There was marked atrophy of a diffuse nature involving the muscles of the hands and shoulders and present throughout the lower extremities.
   b. There was a diffuse weakness involving these muscles.
   c. Wide-spread fasciculations were present in all muscles of both upper and lower extremities.
   d. Gait and coordination were normal.
   e. No significant spasticity was present.
   f. No local muscle tenderness was present.
4. *Reflexes:*
   a. Deep tendon reflexes were hyperactive bilaterally.
   b. Plantar responses were equivocally extensor.
5. *Sensory system:* All modalities were intact.

LABORATORY DATA:
1. Complete blood count, blood sugar, blood chemistry and blood enzymes were within normal limits.
2. X-rays of skull, chest, cervical spine, upper gastrointestinal and barium enema were within normal limits.
3. Nerve conduction was normal.
4. Electromyography was consistent with the clinical diagnosis.

QUESTIONS:
1. What is the clinical diagnosis in this case?
2. What are the findings to be expected on electromyography?
3. What would a muscle biopsy reveal?
4. What is the prognosis in this specific case?

Case History 4. NECH #178–654.
Date of admission: 6/18/66.
This 45-year-old, right-handed male (Mr. S. S.) with a past history of elevated blood cholesterol (332 mg./100 ml.) awoke on June 14, 1966, to find "numbness" of the left side of the face and tongue. Diplopia was present particularly on looking to the left. When he arose from his bed, he noted objective vertigo (room spinning) and walked with a staggering gait with a tendency to fall to the left. Examination by the patient's physician indicated left lateral rectus weakness and intention tremor of the left hand. The patient was admitted to his local community hospital where improvement occurred. The numbness of face and tongue disappeared over several hours. The diplopia and ataxia improved over the next one to two days. The patient was subsequently transferred to NECH for additional evaluation.

PAST HISTORY:
Precordial pain in January 1966, with EKG changes of an acute myocardial infarction. Anticoagulation had been used since January 1966. In April 1966, the patient had a transient episode of left facial weakness and difficulty in remembering names.

NEUROLOGICAL EXAMINATION: 6/18/66, Blood pressure, 130/90; Pulse, regular.
1. *Mental status:* intact.
2. *Cranial nerves:*
   a. Extraocular movements: Some observers noted a moderate impairment of conjugate lateral gaze to the left side. When lateral gaze to the left occurred, there was a dissociated nystagmus with nystagmus greater in the abducting eye (the left eye). At times during red glass testing on left lateral gaze, a diplopia was reported. The pattern suggested possible weakness of right medial rectus although no actual weakness of right medial rectus was apparent.
   b. There was flattening of the left nasolabial fold with questionable deficit in forehead wrinkling on the left.
   c. Slight slurring of speech was noted.
3. *Motor system:*
   a. Strength was intact.
   b. Mild intention tremor of left hand with impairment of alternating movements. Mild heel to shin ataxia was present in the left lower extremity.
   c. Gait: Minimal ataxia on narrow base.
4. *Reflexes:*
   a. Deep tendon reflexes were symmetrical, except for questionable increase in left ankle jerk.
   b. Plantar responses flexor on right, equivocal on left.

HOSPITAL COURSE: Steady improvement over a 2-week period.

QUESTIONS:
1. Locate and diagram the lesion. Concern yourself with the history and findings of the present episode with regard to localization. Assume a single lesion.
2. Having decided on the location of the lesion, indicate the probable pathology. In

answering this question, you should be aware, of course, that the information concerning past history is relevant.

3. Discuss the localizing significance of the deficit in voluntary conjugate lateral gaze to the left (first in general terms and then in specific relationship to this problem).

4. Discuss the localizing significance of the dissociation of nystagmus on left lateral gaze (nystagmus greater in the abducting eye), both in general terms and in specific relationship to the present case.

5. Indicate the localizing significance of the tremor and incoordination involving the left arm and leg.

6. Indicate the localizing significance of the vertigo.

7. Why were the left side of the face and tongue numb?

Case History 5. NECH #132-348.
Date of admission: 2/15/60.

This 42-year-old woman (Miss R. C.) reported to the doctor with complaint of "trouble with my eyes." The history as it evolved was as follows: The patient stated she had had difficulty with her thyroid for 20 years. She believed that it was underactive, but she did not respond to thyroid medication. At around the age of 20, her menses ceased and she had not menstruated since. During the past few years, the patient had had some automobile accidents and noted that these accidents occurred with objects to her right. During the month before entry, the patient felt excessively tired and was sleeping more than usual but able to go to work. Her skin had become dry, she had gradually put on weight over the years, her hair was scant with loss of underarm hair, and scant pubic hair. Headaches—a bifrontal dull ache—had been present for one week. Examination during office consultation showed a normal, alert mental status. There was puffiness of hands and face and dryness of the skin. Blood pressure was 108/72; pulse, 82 and regular. Skin and mucous membranes were pale, and there was a bilateral pallor of the optic discs.

NEUROLOGICAL EXAMINATION:

1. *Mental status:* intact.

2. *Cranial nerves:* intact except the visual fields showed a bitemporal, upper quadrantic field defect, almost complete in the right eye, less marked on the left. There was also bilateral pallor of the optic discs. Pupils and ocular movements were normal.

3. *Motor system:* no abnormalities noted.

4. *Reflexes:* within normal limits.

5. *Sensory system:* normal.

SUBSEQUENT COURSE:

Patient returned the next day, having had an emotional upset at work with the onset of a severe pressure headache. She complained of sudden worsening of vision in the left eye and a film over the temporal fields. On examination, she was pale and sweating. Blood pressure was 100/70; pulse, 100. There was more marked cutting of visual fields, particularly on the left, with a true hemianopic defect (both eyes now demonstrated a full temporal hemianopsia). The patient was drowsy but could provide concise answers. Neurological examination was otherwise normal. The patient was immediately admitted to the hospital. Laboratory studies in the hospital confirmed the clinical impression of hypothyroidism with a protein bound iodine of 2.2; total iodine, 3.0. In addition, there was no FSH detected on an assay of 24-hour urine specimen. Plain skull films were positive and bilateral carotid arteriograms were performed. Patient was started on endocrine therapy and an operation was performed. Three days following surgery, it was noted that the patient was complaining of constant and excessive thirst and was consuming huge quantities of fluids.

QUESTIONS:

1. In this case, neurological evaluation many years previously would have established the diagnosis. Indicate the location of this lesion.

2. Indicate the most likely pathology. Speculate as to the other possible causes of this syndrome.

3. What is the localizing significance of the thyroid dysfunction?

4. What is the localizing significance of the ovarian dysfunction?

5. Why did the patient have excessive thirst and excessive consumption of fluids (polydypsia) after surgery?

6. Why was the patient sleeping more than usual with marked drowsiness at the time of admission? (Several explanations are possible in this case.)

Case History 6. NECH #76-75-71.
Date of admission: 8/18/69.

Three weeks prior to admission, this 69-year-old, right-handed white male (Mr. P. H.) had the onset of clumsiness of his right hand. Soon thereafter, he noticed weakness and numbness involving the right hand. He then noticed that his right leg was weak, and he fell to the floor. The weakness and numbness of the hand cleared in a matter of minutes. The patient, however, continued to have clumsiness of the right hand. On two subsequent occasions he had a recurrence of weakness of the right hand. The patient's history was also of significance in that over a 2-month period, he had had 3 episodes, each 3 minutes in duration, of a monocular blindness involving the left eye.

The patient had had diabetes mellitus for approximately 20 years. In February 1969, the patient had a sudden onset of weakness and coldness of the right lower extremity. This was due to sudden occlusion of the right femoral artery; a right femoral endarterectomy was performed with bypass. His symptoms in the right lower extremity improved. The patient had had episodes of chest pain (angina pectoris) for a number of years. The episodes never lasted longer than 5 to 10 minutes. Family history was significant in that the patient's mother, father, daughter, and son all had experienced severe diabetes mellitus.

GENERAL PHYSICAL EXAMINATION:

1. Blood pressure was 130/80 in both the right and left arms.

2. Light pressure on the left eyeball led to a blackout of vision; similar symptoms were not produced on the right side.

NEUROLOGICAL EXAMINATION:

1. *Mental status:* The patient was oriented for time, place, and person.

2. *Cranial nerves:* No significant findings were present.

3. *Motor system:*
   a. Strength was intact except for a minimal drift downward of the outstretched right arm when both arms were outstretched.
   b. Cerebellar tests and gait were intact.

4. *Reflexes:*
   a. Deep tendon reflexes were slightly increased in the right arm compared to the left. The Achilles' tendon reflexes were absent bilaterally, presumably related to the patient's diabetes.

5. *Sensory system:*
   a. Vibration was decreased bilaterally at the toes, presumably related to the patient's diabetes.
   b. Occasional errors were made in let-

ter and number recognition in the right hand (graphesthesia testing).

QUESTIONS:

1. What is the diagnosis? Be specific as to the vessel and area involved, if vascular in nature.

2. Outline your diagnostic approach to this problem.

3. Indicate possible therapeutic measures.

Case History 7. NECH #84–810.
Date of admission: 11/12/65.

This 80-year-old white male (Mr. G. C.) was referred for evaluation of increasing weakness about the lower extremities. This patient had had a prostatectomy in 1953 performed by Dr. Leadbetter for carcinoma of the prostate. Replacement of the femoral artery by graft was undertaken approximately 2 years later (10 years prior to admission). Several months prior to admission, the patient noted poor bladder control. Approximately three weeks prior to admission, the patient noted that he was becoming unsteady in gait, the left leg showing greater involvement than the right. The patient described this as being unable to know where to place the left leg. Shortly thereafter the patient awoke one morning and noted sudden weakness in both lower extremities.

The patient was admitted to the hospital on November 9 1965, at which time it was noted that he had insufficient strength to stand unassisted, but he could kick both legs about in bed and certainly could raise the legs from the bed. Vibration sensation was said to be absent in both legs as was pain sensation. There was loss of position sense in the left leg. According to the patient, since his admission to the hospital, he had experienced increased weakness in both lower extremities. Thus a steady progression of symptoms had occurred.

Past history is of additional significance. In the preceding 9 years the patient had been noted to have an essential or senile tremor. In June of 1963 he had an episode in which he awoke in a confused state and had difficulty in thinking. At that time he was noted to have increased reflexes on the right side with a right Babinski response. A diagnosis of cerebral ischemia was made and the patient was treated with heparin and then Coumadin. This has been discontinued. In May 1965 the patient had several bouts of aphasia. In August of 1965 several episodes of syncope were noted. The patient was admitted to Goddard Hospital on August 30, 1965 and stayed until September 5, 1965. A neurological examination at that time revealed a coarse tremor with reflexes more active on the right than on the left and an equivocal Babinski response.

NEUROLOGICAL EXAMINATION:

1. *Mental status:* This thin, well-developed white male was moderately disoriented for time, but oriented for place. The patient was able to provide a coherent history but the actual dates were somewhat vague. There was a mild nominal aphasia.

2. *Cranial nerves:* There was a suggestion of a right visual field deficit.

3. *Motor system:*

   a. Strength in the upper extremities was intact. There was a significant weakness in both lower extremities, more marked on the left than on the right. Dorsiflexion at the left ankle was less than 20 per cent of normal; at the right ankle less than 30 per cent of normal. The patient had less than 5 per cent normal dorsiflexion of the great toe on the left; approximately 30 per cent, on the right. On the left the patient was unable to raise the heel off the bed; on the right the patient was able to raise the heel off the bed to approximately 30°.

   b. There was a resistance to passive movement at flexion-extension of the elbows; this had some of the qualities of spasticity and possibly some of the characteristics of Gegenhalten.

   c. Coordination: there was the tremor of the outstretched hands present also on action and intention as noted previously.

4. *Reflexes:*

   a. Deep tendon reflexes: There was a reflex asymmetry in the upper extremities; right biceps was 3++, left, 3+. Triceps were both 1 to 2+. In the lower extremities quadriceps and deep tendon reflexes were 3+; ankle jerks were 2+.

   b. There were bilateral Babinski responses.

   c. There was a bilateral grasp present.

5. *Sensation:*

   a. There was a definite pain level on the anterior surface at the level of the xiphoid process; and on the posterior surface at the level of the T8 spinous process. There was no evidence of sacral sparing.

   b. Position sense was absent at left toe and ankle. Gross movement only was perceived at right ankle. Vibratory sensation could not be adequately tested.

6. On examination of the back there was local tenderness over the T7, T8 spinous processes.

7. There was evidence of some fecal and urinary incontinence as noted by soiled bed clothing.

8. Carotid pulses were present bilaterally; the right was greater than the left.

LABORATORY DATA:

1. Sedimentation rate: 40 mm. per hour.

2. Acid phosphatase: 1.5 units.

3. Alkaline phosphatase: 7.5 units.

4. X-rays of chest: negative except for possible destructive lesions at D8–D9.

QUESTIONS:

1. This patient has several neurological problems. Several of these problems are long-standing and do not present any immediate threat to neurological function. You should have no problem in dissecting off the findings relevant to these noncritical problems.

2. One problem requires immediate attention. What is the nature of this problem (location of and type of pathology)?

3. Which diagnostic procedures would you obtain and when?

4. Which therapeutic procedures should you undertake?

5. Indicate the etiology of the dementia in this case.

6. Why are the grasp and "Gegenhalten" present?

Case History 8. WAH #284–281.

Date of admission: 5/19/64.

This 23-year-old, white, right-handed, army recruit, (Private B. S.) on the day prior to admission was evaluated on sick call with an apparent upper respiratory infection. The patient was given a day of barracks rest. Early on the morning of admission, the patient apparently vomited. At reveille, the patient was found in his bed, unresponsive. He could not be roused; he was found to have been incontinent of urine and feces.

GENERAL PHYSICAL EXAMINATION:

1. The patient was febrile with a tempera-

ture of 102–103°. Blood pressure was 130/70; pulse 96.

2. There was a marked degree of nuchal rigidity.

3. Examination of the skin revealed a diffuse petechial rash with a number of ecchymotic areas on the extremities. Some of these areas had apparent necrotic centers.

NEUROLOGICAL EXAMINATION:

1. *Mental status:* The patient was in a coma; he did respond to painful stimuli by withdrawing his extremities.

2. *Cranial nerves:*
   a. The pupils were in midposition and responded poorly to light.
   b. Funduscopic examination was not remarkable.

3. *Motor system:*
   a. There was no definite lateralized weakness.
   b. Cerebellar system could not be tested.

4. *Reflexes:*
   a. Deep tendon reflexes were equal but hyperactive throughout.
   b. An extensor plantar response was present on the left side.

5. *Sensory system:* Could not be adequately tested.

LABORATORY DATA:

1. White blood count was markedly elevated to 42,000, with a differential count of 64 per cent neutrophils, 31 per cent bands, 5 per cent lymphocytes. Platelets were decreased to 95,000 per cubic mm.

2. Blood serology was negative.

3. Spinal fluid examination revealed a marked increase in pressure (500–600 mm. of water). The fluid was grossly cloudy. There were 7250 white blood cells per cubic mm.; 100 per cent of these were polymorphonuclear leukocytes. Spinal fluid sugar was 6 mg./100 ml.; spinal fluid protein was increased to 314 mg./100 ml.

4. Smears and cultures of spinal fluid were consistent with the clinical diagnosis.

SUBSEQUENT COURSE:

The patient was begun on specific therapy. As the patient's level of consciousness began to improve, it was apparent on the second hospital day that a left facial weakness was present. On the fourth hospital day, as the patient began to respond to questions by opening his eyes and moving his right hand, it became apparent that he had a left facial weakness, a weakness of the left arm and leg, and a left Babinski response. On the sixth hospital day, even though the patient was continuing to improve, he had the onset of focal seizures beginning on the left side of the body; some remained localized to the left side, some became generalized. Following readjustment of therapy, seizures disappeared. With physiotherapy, a significant improvement in function of the left arm and left leg occurred.

QUESTIONS:

1. Present a differential diagnosis and indicate the most likely specific diagnosis.

2. Indicate the specific findings of spinal fluid examination omitted from the protocol (as regards smears and cultures).

3. Outline the specific therapy which was probably used in the treatment of this problem.

4. Indicate the pathophysiology involved in the complications which developed during the patient's hospitalization.

Case History 9. #144–461.

Date of admission: 10/13/61.

This 62-year-old white divorcee (Mrs. M. McC.) was referred for evaluation of personality and memory change. The patient had a high school education and had been described in the past as a bright, alert, and intelligent lady. The patient was unable to provide a history. She showed little insight into her problem in the sense of being unaware as to any reason for her neurological evaluation. The patient's son indicated that the patient had begun to show some decline in intellectual capacity as long as 3 or 4 years prior to admission. During the preceding 12 months, a more marked change had occurred, particularly with regard to memory. In more recent months a lack of concern for her personal appearance and a lack of spontaneity had developed. She had lost interest in her home, friends, and activities.

PAST HISTORY: No significant cardiovascular disease or diabetes. No significant alcohol or drug ingestion.

GENERAL PHYSICAL EXAMINATION:

1. *Blood pressure:* 140/96; normal sinus rhythm.

NEUROLOGICAL EXAMINATION:

1. *Mental status:*
   a. The patient was pleasant and well mannered.
   b. She was disoriented for the day of the week, for the day of the month, for the month, and for the year.

c. She was unable to remember any of 4 test objects after a 5-minute period.

d. Moreover the patient was unable to remember the year she was born.

e. She was unable to recall any president but Kennedy.

f. She was able to follow very simple directions, but was unable to remember any instructions beyond these.

g. She was unable to comprehend subtraction of serial sevens and could not do even simple additions. She was unable to repeat numbers in reverse.

h. She was unable to draw a triangle but did recognize a circle.

i. There was a severe dysnomia for even common objects.

2. *Cranial nerves:*
   a. Pupillary reactions were normal.
   b. At times, the patient had extinction of simultaneously presented visual objects in the left field. At times on simultaneous presentation, objects in the right field were neglected.

3. *Motor system:*
   a. Strength and gait were intact.
   b. Minor tremulousness was present in the performance of hand and arm movements.
   c. Minor, variable resistance on passive motion existed and was described as "Gegenhalten."

4. *Reflexes:*
   a. Deep tendon: symmetrical and physiologic.
   b. Plantar: flexor bilaterally.
   c. Grasp: absent.

5. *Sensation:* negative.

QUESTIONS:

1. Does this patient have focal disease or a more generalized disease? If the latter, which areas are predominantly affected? What is the significance of the dysnomia in this case?

2. What is the most likely pathology in this case?

3. What treatable causes of this progressive syndrome must be considered? Discuss in terms of:
   a. infections
   b. nutritional diseases
   c. metabolic diseases
   d. intoxications
   e. other treatable etiologies

For each entity indicate the appropriate diagnostic tests.

4. How would you manage this patient as regards diagnosis and treatment?

5. What would you expect the electroencephalogram to demonstrate?

6. What would you expect the brain scan to demonstrate?

7. What x-ray procedures would you undertake?

8. What CSF findings are to be expected?

9. What is the prognosis?

10. What more restricted mental status changes would have been present early in the disease course?

Case History 10. NECH #80–11–51.
Date of admission: 12/7/70.

This 44-year-old, white, married, machine operator (Mr. G. D.) for several years had noted a general sensation of fatigue in his arms and legs at the end of a day. Approximately 6 to 7 weeks prior to admission, the patient began to have more significant difficulty with a marked increase in the degree of weakness of the arms and legs. At the same time, the patient noted significant slurring of words, difficulty in swallowing, and drooping of the lids. All of these symptoms were transient; they were not present in the morning; they were clearly precipitated by exercise. For example, although the patient would initially have strong chewing movements, as soon as he began to chew for a short period he would develop fatigue of jaw muscles. The degree of ptosis was sufficient enough to result in difficulty in driving.

PAST HISTORY: The patient had "spinal meningitis" at age 1 or 2 years. The patient apparently had a significant recovery, the only residual being minor weakness of the lateral rectus muscle and some decrease in vision of the right eye. The patient had a long-standing problem of marked obesity.

NEUROLOGICAL EXAMINATION:

1. *Mental status:* intact.
2. *Cranial nerves:*
   a. A significant bilateral ptosis of the eyelids was present. The degree of ptosis was markedly increased by exercise when complete closure of the left eyelid occurred.
   b. On repetitive upward gaze, a bilateral weakness of superior rectus developed.
   c. There was a bilateral facial weakness,

worse on exercise, more marked on the right than on the left.

    d. Jaw movements (opening, closing, and lateral movements) were weak. The degree of weakness was increased by exercise.

    e. Lateral tongue movements, particularly on sustained pressure, became weak.

3. *Motor system:*

    a. There was a significant weakness in shoulder abductors, elbow flexors and extensors, and hand grip. The degree of weakness was markedly increased by repetitive exercise.

4. *Reflexes:*

    a. Deep tendon reflexes were symmetrical.

    b. Plantar responses were flexor.

5. *Sensory system:* All modalities were intact.

LABORATORY DATA:

1. Chest x-ray and studies of thyroid function were normal.

2. A Tensilon test was performed (edrophonium). This demonstrated an almost immediate eye-opening effect with the disappearance of the bilateral ptosis. The ptosis, however, had reappeared 3 to 4 minutes after injection of 10 mg. of the agent.

QUESTIONS:

1. Indicate the most likely diagnosis and present a differential diagnosis of this problem.

2. Outline your diagnostic and therapeutic approach to this problem.

Case History 11. NECH #74–90–90.
Date of admission: 7/10/69.

This 51-year-old, white housewife, (Mrs. M. C. L.), one week prior to admission, developed episodic posterior headaches beginning in the neck and radiating to the vertex of the head. The headaches were usually related to and were definitely exacerbated by straining or coughing. At the same time the patient noted clumsiness of her left hand and a tendency to fall to the left side. The mechanical headaches, the clumsiness of the left hand, and the difficulty with gait progressed during the week prior to admission.

PAST HISTORY:

The patient had been admitted to the gynecology service in November 1968 with a 10-week history of postmenopausal vaginal bleeding. She was found to have an infiltrative anaplastic carcinoma of the uterine cervix. The patient was then treated with radiotherapy (4000-R to the pelvis), followed by vaginal insertion of radium. Re-evaluation in June 1969 revealed that this anaplastic epidermoid carcinoma of the cervix had spread to the anterior vaginal wall. In addition, metastatic nodules were now present in the lung.

NEUROLOGICAL EXAMINATION:

1. *Mental status:* The patient was an anxious white female who was cooperative, alert, and well-oriented.

2. *Cranial nerves:*

    a. There was coarse nystagmus on gaze to the left.

    b. There was a minor dysarthria for lingual and guttural sounds.

3. *Motor system:*

    a. Strength was intact.

    b. Gait was unsteady with tendency to fall to the left, especially when turning to the left. On a narrow base, the patient tended to fall backwards.

    c. Cerebellar tests revealed no definite truncal ataxia. There was a marked appendicular ataxia on the finger-to-nose test in the left upper extremity and the heel-to-shin test in the left lower extremity.

4. *Reflexes:*

    a. Deep tendon reflexes were active bilaterally. This, however, was felt to be consistent with the patient's degree of anxiety.

    b. Plantar responses were flexor.

5. *Sensory system:*

All modalities were intact except for a minimal decrease in vibratory sensation at the toes.

LABORATORY DATA:

The results of specialized studies were consistent with the clinical diagnosis.

QUESTIONS:

1. Where is the lesion? Be specific.

2. What pathological process is to be expected?

3. Outline your diagnostic and therapeutic approach for this case.

Case History 12.
Date of admission: February, 1965.

A 21-year-old, white, right-handed wife of an air force enlisted man had been married for 2 months and had just moved from her home in the South to an air force base in New Jersey. She had been complaining of increasingly severe right frontal temporal or bifrontal headaches for 3 to 4 weeks. During the 10 days prior to admission, she had been treated on several occasions at the base dispensary for these headaches which were relatively constant and were now accompanied by blurring of vision and frequent vomiting. Various medications had been prescribed for an upper respiratory infection or sinusitis. For the 48 hours prior to admission, the patient had been increasingly confused and ataxic.

PAST HISTORY: Negative as regards head injury or pulmonary, sinus, and ear infection.

GENERAL PHYSICAL EXAMINATION:

1. The patient was dehydrated and somewhat lethargic.

2. She was complaining of severe headache, particularly on head movement.

3. There was a moderate degree of hyperventilation.

4. No otitis media was present.

NEUROLOGICAL EXAMINATION:

1. *Mental status:* The patient was disoriented for time and place. She was unable to provide a history and was unable to cooperate for the examination, e.g., impersistent in fixing gaze or in maintaining eyes in open position.

2. *Cranial nerves:*
   a. Fundus: Bilateral papilledema was present with 2 to 3 diopters of disc elevation accompanied by fresh hemorrhages and venous engorgement.
   b. The right pupil was dilated and fixed in response to light. Extraocular movements were otherwise intact.
   c. A left central facial weakness was present to a marked degree.

3. *Motor system:*
   a. All limbs were moved spontaneously but there was a downward drift of the outstretched left arm.
   b. The patient was ataxic in a sitting position and in attempting to stand even on a broad base.
   c. There was a tremor of the outstretched hands, increasing to a minor degree on movement and intention.

4. *Reflexes:*
   a. Deep tendon reflexes were increased on the left in the upper and lower extremities.
   b. Plantar responses were extensor on the left, equivocal on the right.
   c. Grasp reflex was present bilaterally.

5. *Sensation:* Pain was intact.

6. *Neck:* Minor resistance to passive motion.

LABORATORY DATA:

1. Skull x-rays: negative

2. Chest x-rays: negative

3. EEG: Almost continuous focal 1–2 cps slow-wave activity was present.

QUESTIONS:

1. This patient was seen relatively late in her disease course. You should be able to localize the primary location of the pathology.

2. Indicate what secondary events have occurred.

3. The nature of the pathology may be somewhat uncertain to you. However, you should be able to present a differential diagnosis and then to indicate the most likely diagnosis. Keep in mind that the headaches had been present for only 3 to 4 weeks, the additional symptoms for only 2 to 10 days.

4. Was the papilledema long-standing?

5. What is the significance of the pupillary findings?

6. Assuming a cerebral hemisphere lesion, why was the patient ataxic in sitting and standing when examined late in her course?

7. What diagnostic studies would you perform in this case and when would you perform these?

8. Which diagnostic studies would you *not* perform? State reasons.

9. How would you manage this problem from a therapeutic standpoint? Indicate when you would institute this therapy.

Case History 13. NECH #79–48–38. Date of admission: November 1970.

This 38-year-old, right-handed, warehouse manager (Mr. W. R.) was in excellent health until 4 days prior to admission. On that day, the patient had a sudden loss of consciousness. He was found on the floor by his wife who witnessed a generalized convulsive seizure of approximately 10 minutes duration. When he regained consciousness, he had a severe generalized headache and some pain in the neck. Because of persistent headaches, the patient, on the following day, went to his local hospital for evaluation. A lumbar puncture demonstrated grossly bloody spinal fluid with an elevated pressure of 340 mm. of water. Following additional radiological studies, the patient was transferred to the New England Medical Center Hospital.

GENERAL PHYSICAL EXAMINATION:

1. The patient was restless and complaining of severe headache.

2. Marked nuchal rigidity was present.

3. Blood pressure was 150/90; pulse was 80 and regular; temperature was slightly elevated to 101° rectally.

NEUROLOGICAL EXAMINATION:

1. *Mental status:* The patient was lethargic but readily responded to his name and answered questions appropriately. No abnormality of memory was found.

2. *Cranial nerves:* all intact.

3. *Motor system:* There were no abnormalities except for a slight downward drift of the left upper extremity.

4. *Reflexes:*
   a. Deep tendon reflexes were symmetric and physiologic.
   b. Plantar responses were both flexor.

5. *Sensory system:* no abnormalities present.

SUBSEQUENT COURSE: The patient's condition remained unchanged until a surgical procedure was undertaken 2 days following admission.

QUESTIONS:

1. Present a differential diagnosis and then indicate the most likely diagnosis. There should be little question regarding the pathological nature of the diagnosis. Attempt to be specific as to the location of the lesion. If you cannot identify a specific location, present a listing of possible loci in terms of vessels involved, if you believe the process to be vascular.

2. Indicate your diagnostic and therapeutic approach to this problem.

Case History 14. NECH #116–061.
Date of admission: 12/57, Date of death: 12/30/66.

This right-handed, white housewife (Mrs. B. M.) had the onset of neurological symptoms in 1954 (at age 26) when, in relation to a febrile illness, she noted the onset of numbness of the left leg and a tendency to veer to the left when walking. These symptoms gradually subsided over a period of 7 months. In 1956, shortly following the birth of her first child, the patient developed urinary incontinence. This was occasional and occurred without the sensation of a full bladder. Bed wetting was frequent. Subsequently the patient developed weakness of the left leg and associated paresthesias of the left lower extremity. Over the subsequent months, the patient developed vertigo which was precipitated by a sudden change in position. She also experienced an un-

steadiness in gait which was more prominent at night or when in the dark. Difficulty in pronunciation of words had also been noted. The patient also reported diplopia occurring as a transient phenomenon when she was fatigued. In subsequent months, the patient noted a clumsiness of the left hand with difficulty in buttoning her clothes. Approximately 2 weeks before her admission to the hospital in November 1957, the patient developed the onset of a pins-and-needles sensation at the tips of the fingers of the left hand.

NEUROLOGICAL EXAMINATION:

1. *Mental status:* All areas were intact, except for a slowness in calculation and a moderate difficulty in delayed recall of 2-out-of-4 objects.

2. *Cranial nerves:*
   a. There was pallor of the temporal portion of the right disc.
   b. Diplopia was present on left and right lateral gaze.
   c. Nystagmus was present on gaze laterally to the right or left.
   d. There was dysarthria, with speech having a scanning quality.

3. *Motor system:*
   a. There was weakness in all muscle groups of the left arm and left leg.
   b. The patient had an ataxia of gait and walked on a wide base at times. The ataxia was exaggerated by turning. There was a marked ataxia on attempting to walk a tandem gait and on heel-to-toe test.
   c. There was an intention tremor on finger-to-nose testing of the left hand. There was also an impairment of rapid alternating movements of the left hand.

4. *Reflexes:*
   a. Deep tendon reflexes were symmetrical.
   b. There was an extensor plantar response on the left and an equivocal plantar response on the right.

5. *Sensory system:*
   a. Position and vibratory sensation were diminished in the left foot.
   b. Touch was poorly appreciated over the left arm and leg.
   c. Romberg test was positive.

LABORATORY DATA: Complete blood count, sedimentation rate, electroencephalogram, and spinal fluid examination were not remarkable.

SUBSEQUENT COURSE:

In January 1958, the patient had exacerbation of weakness in her left leg and increased thickness of speech. In February 1958, the patient developed diplopia and blurring of vision. In March 1958 the patient developed a tingling sensation in the right upper abdomen.

The patient was readmitted into the hospital in March 1958. Neurological examination now indicated bilateral enlargement of the blind spots with a large scotoma in the peripheral portion of the field of the right eye, confluent with the blind spot. Vertical nystagmus was now present on upward gaze. Dissociated nystagmus was present on right lateral gaze. On right lateral gaze there appeared to be a weakness of the right lateral rectus and left medial rectus. Speech was slurred to a greater degree. Weakness was now present in all four extremities, being of greatest degree in the left lower extremity. Deep tendon reflexes were now increased on the left although active bilaterally. Both plantar responses were now extensor. There was an absolute loss of pain and touch on the left below the level of D9; to a lesser degree a loss was also present on the right side below this level. Vibratory sensation was absent below the T6 spinous process. There was a marked ataxia on right heel-to-shin test and a marked bilateral intention tremor. Spinal fluid examination now demonstrated a protein of 55 mg./100 ml., 8 lymphocytes, and an elevation of the first zone colloidal gold curve. Following hospital admission, the patient developed an acute retention of urine which abated following treatment of a urinary tract infection. The patient was treated with ACTH with little improvement in her symptoms.

Re-evaluation in May 1959, indicated a complete paralysis of all voluntary movements of both lower extremities. There was a marked spasticity on passive motion of the lower extremities. Neurological symptoms were otherwise unchanged.

Re-evaluation in September 1962, indicated a bilateral internuclear ophthalmoplegia with the left eye failing to adduct on right lateral gaze and the right eye failing to adduct on left lateral gaze. In addition, a significant dissociated nystagmus was present with nystagmus on lateral gaze more marked in the abducting eye. On forward gaze the eyes were also dysconjugate, the right eye being deviated downward and outward and the left eye being deviated upwards. The patient was described as markedly euphoric. Although oriented for time, place, and person, her delayed recall was severely limited. The patient was unable to remember any of 5 objects in 3 minutes. There was now noted a significant defect in general information and calculations. Digit span was limited to 6 forward and 3 in reverse.

The patient continued in a bedridden state. In December 1966, she developed fever, abdominal distention, urinary tract infection, and septicemia.

QUESTIONS:

1. Indicate the diagnosis, specifying the pathological process and the location of lesion or lesions.

2. Review the expected prognosis in this disease state.

Case History 15. NECH #75-72-78.
Date of admission: 4/8/69.

This 49-year-old, white, right-handed, married male (Mr. E. W.) had the onset 7 to 8 months prior to admission of episodes characterized by a raising sensation beginning at the epigastrium, which lasted 45 to 60 seconds, and culminated in an inability to speak or even utter a sound. At this time he would also be unable to understand the speech of others. This impairment of language function would last for a minute or so and then clear. These episodes would occur at a frequency of 3 to 5 times a week. On some occasions, following an episode while driving, he would note a change in the appearance of the roadway. The road would appear desolate, empty, or strange and unfamiliar. This sensation of unfamiliarity would pass in a few minutes. The patient had never apparently sustained a generalized convulsive seizure. The patient did report some recent change in personality, which consisted of being depressed at times, cheerful at other times, and losing interest in his activity. He denied specifically any memory loss. The patient in the past had experienced rare episodes of diplopia, but the significance of this was never certain.

NEUROLOGICAL EXAMINATION:

1. *Mental status:* The patient was alert, oriented, and anxious, but all areas were intact. There was no evidence of any disturbance of language function.

2. *Cranial nerves:* All were intact except

for a minimal lag of the right side of the face on spontaneous smile.

3. *Motor system:* Strength, gait, and cerebellar tests were intact.

4. *Reflexes:*
   a. Deep tendon reflexes were slightly increased in the right upper extremity compared to the left.
   b. Plantar responses were flexor.

5. *Sensory system:* All modalities were intact.

6. *Hyperventilation:* A short episode was produced consisting of a smacking of the lips and tongue, a vacant stare, raising of the right arm with a clenched fist, and a failure to speak when asked to carry out a simple command. The patient remained standing during this episode which lasted for about a minute. Afterwards, he spoke in nonsense syllables for 30 to 45 seconds and then gradually regained full speech and the ability to carry out commands. The patient was amnesic for almost the entire episode. According to the patient's wife, this episode resembled the episodes which she had witnessed.

LABORATORY DATA: The electroencephalogram demonstrated a focal abnormality.

QUESTIONS:

1. Indicate the nature of the patient's episodes.

2. Indicate the location of the electroencephalographic abnormality.

3. Outline your diagnostic and therapeutic approach to this problem.

4. Present a differential diagnosis as regards the most likely pathological process.

Case History 16. NECH #80–08–73.
Date of admission: 11/14/70.

This 23-year-old, white, divorced, medical secretary (Miss. E. K.), 3 weeks prior to admission, noted the onset of paresthesias and pains on the dorsum of the hands accompanied by paresthesias of the distal portions of the lower extremities. The paresthesias spread into the hands and up the arms. The paresthesias also extended in a relatively symmetrical manner through the lower extremities to approximately the level of the knees. Approximately 2 weeks prior to admission, the patient noted a sensation of tightness in the shoulders and thighs. At the same time she began to note weakness in these areas. The weakness soon spread, involving the distal portion of the hands and feet. Initially, the patient had some sensations about the face, but these were poorly de-

scribed. She had had no actual urinary retention. Her symptoms progressed until the day prior to admission when a plateau was reached.

PAST HISTORY:

The patient had had "rheumatic fever" as a child, but she had had no significant rheumatic symptoms in the interim. The patient had had a minor upper respiratory infection approximately 3 to 4 weeks prior to admission. The patient had not received any medications except for a contraceptive pill which had been used for approximately one year (combination of estrogens and progestins).

NEUROLOGICAL EXAMINATION:

1. *Mental status:* The patient was a well-developed, anxious, white female who was oriented for time, place, and person.

2. *Cranial nerves:* Nerves 2-12 were intact except for rare fasciculations about the chin and corners of the mouth.

3. *Motor system:*
   a. A symmetrical weakness was present. In the upper extremities, this involved shoulder abductors and distal hand muscles to a relatively equal degree (approximately 40 per cent normal strength). In the lower extremities, proximal involvement was much greater than distal involvement. Hip flexors were approximately 20 to 30 per cent of normal.
   b. No spasticity was present.

4. *Reflexes:*
   a. Deep tendon reflexes were everywhere absent.
   b. Plantar responses were flexor.

5. *Sensory system:*
   a. Pain sensation was decreased in a glove-and-stocking manner to a moderate degree. Repetitive pain stimuli led to significant dysesthesias in the distal portions of the extremities.
   b. Vibratory sensation was slightly decreased in a distal manner at toes and fingers. Position sensation, however, was relatively well preserved.

6. Tenderness was present on palpation over the sciatic nerve and the brachial plexus.

LABORATORY DATA:

1. Complete blood count and sedimentation rate were normal.

2. Spinal fluid examination revealed normal pressure, no cells but a moderate elevation of spinal fluid protein.

HOSPITAL COURSE:

Within 48 hours of admission, the patient had had a significant improvement in strength and a recession of sensory symptoms. Within 3 weeks, strength had returned to normal.

QUESTIONS:

1. Present a differential diagnosis of this clinical problem and indicate the most likely diagnosis.

Case History 17. NECH #79–18–34.

Date of admission: 9/8/70.

This 63-year-old, white, female librarian (Miss. R. P.), 11 years prior to admission, experienced several generalized convulsive seizures. She experienced no additional difficulties until February 1970, when she had the first of recurrent focal seizures involving the left hand; uncontrollable jerking and twitching of the hand caused her to drop packages. In August 1970, the patient experienced a focal seizure in the left hand which spread up the arm and then involved the leg, resulting in a loss of consciousness. The patient was taken to the emergency room of her local hospital. There another seizure was observed. This began with focal movements of the left wrist and hand, then head turning to the left, and then clonic movements of the left leg.

NEUROLOGICAL EXAMINATION:

1. *Mental status:* intact.

2. *Cranial nerves:* All were intact including sense of smell.

3. *Motor system:*
   a. Strength was everywhere intact.
   b. Repetitive finger-thumb tapping was slightly slower on the left side than on the right. The patient, however, was right-handed.

4. *Reflexes:*
   a. Deep tendon reflexes were slightly asymmetrical in the upper extremities. Finger jerks were more active on the left than on the right. There was no asymmetry in lower extremities.
   b. Plantar responses were flexor.

5. *Sensory system:* No abnormalities were present.

LABORATORY DATA:

1. Skull x-rays were normal.

2. Electroencephalogram revealed minor borderline abnormalities.

3. Brain scan demonstrated significant local uptake of radioisotope.

4. Carotid arteriograms demonstrated significant focal abnormality.

QUESTIONS:

1. Where is the lesion located in this case?

2. Considering the history, the clinical findings, and the laboratory findings, present a differential diagnosis as to the pathology and indicate the most likely pathological process.

3. Outline your diagnostic and therapeutic management of this problem.

Case History 18. Nech #191–967.

Date of admission: 1/11/68.

This 55-year-old, white, widow (Mrs. B. P.), 6 to 8 years prior to admission, had the onset of a peculiar reeling gait. At the same time, she was noted to be "very nervous," having many peculiar restless movements. At other times she was described as constantly fidgeting. The patient's children felt that in recent years she had not been thinking as clearly as she once did. A personality change had also occurred.

FAMILY HISTORY:

The patient's mother died in her sixties with a disorder which had been labeled as parkinsonism. From the description of relatives, however, it was evident that the mother actually had restless movements which were similar to the patient's.

NEUROLOGICAL EXAMINATION:

1. *Mental status:*
   a. The patient was oriented and alert.
   b. General store of information was intact.
   c. Digit span was 6 forward and 3 in reverse.
   d. Object recall was 3-out-of-4 in ten minutes.

2. *Cranial nerves:* intact.

3. *Motor system:*
   a. Strength was intact.
   b. Gait showed a swooping quality of variable degree; there was also a decrease in associated arm movements.
   c. As the patient sat, she would move her head and neck and feet almost constantly.
   d. The patient was able to walk a tandem gait, and there were no abnormalities of cerebellar function.
   e. There was no significant spasticity or rigidity.

4. *Reflexes:*
   a. Deep tendon reflexes were symmetrical.
   b. Plantar responses were flexor.
   c. No grasp reflex was present.

5. *Sensory system:* intact.

LABORATORY DATA:

1. Routine laboratory studies were not remarkable.

2. Specialized neuroradiology studies were consistent with the clinical diagnosis.

QUESTIONS:

1. Present a differential diagnosis of this problem and indicate the most likely diagnosis.

2. Outline your diagnostic and therapeutic approach to this problem.

Case History 19. NECH #79–23–86.
Date of admission: 8/4/70.

This 39-year-old, white, married, airplane mechanic (Mr. S. C.) had the gradual onset of muscle weakness approximately 18 months prior to admission. This involved both arms and legs, with greater involvement of the proximal muscles than of the distal muscles. Gradual progression occurred so that by June 1969 significant difficulty in walking was experienced. Shortly thereafter, the patient experienced difficulty in swallowing, but this problem improved following his hospitalization in August 1969. Weakness of extremity musculature also improved following the use of cortisone. The patient at no time had difficulty in voiding. He had no sensory symptoms; he had had no actual pains or tenderness of muscles.

NEUROLOGICAL EXAMINATION:

1. *Mental status:* intact.

2. *Cranial nerves:* intact.

3. *Motor system:* The patient had severe weakness and atrophy of muscles (both proximal and distal) of all four extremities but with clearly more marked involvement of the proximal musculature. The patient was unable to lift his arms above the shoulder and unable to lift his legs off the bed. No fasciculations were present.

4. *Reflexes:*
   a. Deep tendon reflexes were everywhere absent except at the ankle where normal 2+ reflexes were found.
   b. Plantar responses were flexor.

5. *Sensory system:* No abnormalities were present.

LABORATORY DATA:

1. Sedimentation rate was elevated to 30–45 mm.

2. Electromyogram and muscle biopsy were consistent with the clinical diagnosis.

SUBSEQUENT COURSE:

Following treatment with prednisone in high dosage, the patient had a gradual improvement in strength.

QUESTIONS:

1. Present a differential diagnosis of this problem and indicate the most likely diagnosis.

2. Outline the expected findings on EMG and muscle biopsy.

Case History 20. NECH #183–943.
Date of admission: 6/27/67.

This 59-year-old, white, married male (Mr. E. J.) developed a disturbance in sensation of the right foot 12 days prior to admission. ("It felt funny.") Ten days prior to admission the patient developed a right hemiparesis and was admitted to St. Elizabeth's Hospital complaining of vertigo, nausea, and diplopia. At that time, examination revealed that the patient was oriented but confused and dysarthric. A possible left Horner's syndrome was present. Nystagmus was present on left lateral gaze and the patient was unable to look up or down. There was a dense right hemiparesis with a complete loss of pain and touch on the right side of the body. Lumbar puncture revealed xanthochromic CSF with 350 red blood cells in tube #1 and 850 in tube #3.

PAST HISTORY:

1. The patient had experienced three episodes of left leg weakness in December 1966.

2. Diabetes mellitus had been detected in December 1966.

GENERAL PHYSICAL EXAMINATION: The patient was well-nourished and slightly obese with a liver enlarged to 2 fingerbreadths but nontender.

NEUROLOGICAL EXAMINATION:

1. *Mental status:*
   a. Patient was disoriented for time and place.
   b. He was slightly lethargic but could be roused.
   c. Significant dyscalculia was present.
   d. Nominal aphasia was present with jargon, paraphasia, and the use of neologisms.
   e. Left-right confusion and finger agnosia were also noted.
   f. Although perseveration was noted, the patient was also at times impersistent.

g. Object retention was 0-out-of-4 in 5 minutes.

2. *Cranial nerves:*

a. He demonstrated extinction for objects in right visual field on double simultaneous stimulation.

b. Left pupil, 3 mm.; right, 4 mm. There was impairment of upward gaze and of convergence. Rotatory counterclockwise nystagmus was present on upward gaze to the right.

c. Right corneal reflex was absent and there was no deep or superficial sensation on the right side of the face.

d. A severe right central facial weakness was present.

e. Speech was described as dysarthric, thick, and slurred.

f. Right shoulder shrug was absent.

3. *Motor system:*

a. No voluntary movement of right arm and leg was present.

b. Right arm and leg were flaccid as regards resistance on passive motion.

4. *Reflexes:*

a. Deep tendon: slightly increased in right arm but decreased in right lower extremity compared to left.

b. Superficial plantar   abdominals
   right   extensor   0
   left   flexor   0

c. Grasp reflex: marked grasping of the left hand.

5. *Sensation:* complete absence of pain, touch, deep pain, position and vibration sense on the entire right side of the body.

LABORATORY DATA:

a. Sedimentation rate was 95 mm. in 1 hour. Hct 33, Hgb 10.2 gm.

b. Hinton: negative

c. CSF: xanthochromic; 25 RBC in tube #1; 22 RBC in tube #4. Protein 70 mg./100 ml.

d. Serum albumin low but liver functions normal.

e. Skull x-rays: 2 mm. shift of the pineal

f. EEG: focal slow wave activity

g. Brain scan on admission (6-30-67) positive. Later (7-18-67) brain scan negative.

h. Carotid angiogram: initial (7-3-67): mass lesion. Repeat (7-25-67): decrease in size of lesion.

HOSPITAL COURSE:

Over the course of hospitalization, upward gaze improved, and some improvement occurred in movement of the right arm and leg. Sensory deficits remained relatively unchanged. At the time of transfer to Rehabilitation Institute on July 27, 1967, a minimal aphasia and left right confusion were still present in addition to the aforementioned findings.

QUESTIONS:

1. Where is the lesion? (Assume a single large lesion.) Be specific. Is the lesion limited to the cerebral cortex or are deeper structures involved? Can a single lesion explain the symptoms?

2. What is the nature of the lesion?

3. Discuss the language disturbance, dyscalculia, left-right confusion, and finger agnosia in terms of localizing significance.

4. Why were upward gaze and convergence defective?

5. What is the localizing significance of the sensory disturbance?

6. What is the localizing significance of the extinction of right field on simultaneous stimulation?

7. What is the prognosis for eventual recovery of effective motor function in the arm and leg in the light of the relative lack of spasticity in the involved arm and leg approximately 10 days after onset of the hemiplegia?

Case History 21. NECH #179–255.
Date of admission: 5/17/66.

This 24-year-old, white, left-handed, male dental student (Mr. J. S.) was referred for evaluation of a right-sided weakness and numbness of a 48-hour duration. Since the age of 10, the patient had experienced throbbing left-sided headache (migraine type) preceded by scintillating scotomas (flashing lights and stars with deficit in area of vision) usually homonymous in the right field of vision. These symptoms were accompanied or followed by nausea and vomiting and at times (3 to 4 times per year) by numbness of the right face and arm or leg. The headaches would usually last for 24 hours; the sensory symptoms for 12 hours. Rarely, the patient had experienced a right-sided headache with numbness of the left side of the body.

Two days prior to admission, the patient experienced a vague faintness, and then noted numbness (tingling paresthesias) of the right upper extremity and right side of the face. Almost immediately the usual left-sided headache occurred accompanied by a disturbance in the right visual field. The patient took two tablets of cafergot (a vasoconstrictive agent) without relief of his symptoms and then went to bed. He woke in the morning to find that his right arm and, to a lesser extent, the right leg were weak. There was an associated sensory loss on the right side of the body. No difficulty in speech had been noted.

FAMILY HISTORY: One uncle had migraine headaches.

GENERAL PHYSICAL EXAMINATION: Not remarkable

NEUROLOGICAL EXAMINATION:
1. *Mental status:*
   a. Orientation and memory were intact.
   b. There was no evidence of a dysphasic disturbance, no left-right confusion, and no dyscalculia
   c. There was no constructional apraxia as regards drawing or copying.
2. *Cranial nerves:*
   a. A homonymous scotoma was present in the right visual field.
   b. An alteration without an actual loss of pain and touch was present on the right side of the face.
   c. A minor right supranuclear facial weakness was present.
3. *Motor system:*
   a. Strength: A marked weakness was present in the right upper extremity, particularly at the fingers and wrist where no voluntary movement was possible. In contrast only a minor degree of weakness was present in the right lower extremity.
   b. Marked spastic resistance was present at the right elbow. Ankle clonus was present on the right.
   c. Gait was hemiplegic in type.
4. *Reflexes:*
   a. Deep tendon reflexes were increased on right compared to left, particularly in the lower extremity.
   b. Plantar response was extensor on the right, flexor on the left.
5. *Sensory system:*
   a. Pain and touch were perceived but felt "different" on the right side.
   b. Position sense was markedly impaired at fingers and toes on the right with no perception of gross amplitude movements.
   c. Marked deficits were present in

tactile localization on the right over the face, arm, and leg.
   d. On simultaneous tactile stimulation of the right and left side, extinction of right-sided stimulus occurred over the right face, arm, and leg.
   e. Graphesthesia and stereognosis were defective in the right hand.

LABORATORY DATA:
1. Skull x-rays were normal.
2. Electroencephalogram revealed focal 4–7 cps slow wave activity consistent with focal damage.
3. Brain scan (Hg^{197}) revealed no abnormality.

SUBSEQUENT COURSE:
The patient had a moderate improvement in motor function. Re-evaluation 2 weeks after the initial examination indicated that voluntary movements in the fingers of the right hand were now 50 per cent of normal strength. On sensory examination, only gross amplitude movements could be perceived in the fingers and toes. Graphesthesia, tactile localization, and simultaneous stimulation were still defective in the right hand and fingers but were now intact over the face and leg. Pain, touch, and vibration were intact.

Re-examination 6 months after the episode indicated residual defects limited to the right hand but involving selectively position sense at the fingers, tactile localization, and graphesthesia.

QUESTIONS:
1. Localize the persistent deficits found at the time of follow-up examination. In considering this problem you should attend to:
   a. the selective involvement of certain modalities of sensation
   b. the much greater involvement of the hand than of the face or leg by the sensory and motor deficits.

2. This patient represents an example of classic migraine with a relatively uncommon complication. Discuss the pathophysiology of this lesion.

Case History 22. NECH #76–42–55. Date of admission: 6/29/69.

This 46-year-old, white, housewife (Mrs. G.A.) in May 1967 developed pain in the right posterior lateral neck radiating to the suboccipital area. Shortly thereafter she began to have symptoms of intermittent dizziness and ataxia. In addition, numbness and paresthesias of the left side of the face and hand were noted with clumsiness of the left hand. She was admitted to a hospital in October 1967 where her only neurological findings were a diminished pain sensation on the left side of the face, arm, and trunk.

Between October 1967 and January 1968, the patient noted increasing clumsiness of the left extremity and difficulty walking. In addition, the patient developed difficulty in swallowing (dysphagia), dysarthria, emotional lability, and acute urinary retention. The patient was admitted to another hospital in January 1968.

NEUROLOGICAL EXAMINATION:

1. *Mental status:* intact
2. *Cranial nerves:*
   a. Nystagmus was present on lateral gaze.
   b. A hyperactive jaw jerk was present.
   c. Dysarthria with slurring of all speech sounds was present.
   d. There was a bilateral paralysis of the vocal cords.
3. *Motor system:*
   a. A spastic left hemiparesis was present.
   b. A titubation of the head and a marked truncal ataxia were present.
   c. Finger-to-nose and heel-to-shin testing were stated to be impaired on the left. The significance of this, however, was uncertain in view of the left hemiparesis.
4. *Reflex system:*
   a. Deep tendon reflexes were increased on the left.
   b. Bilateral extensor plantar responses were present.
5. *Sensory system:* Sensory examination was apparently within normal limits.

SUBSEQUENT COURSE:

A temporary tracheostomy was required. The patient was treated with ACTH with some temporary improvement in neurological findings as regards walking, swallowing, and voiding. Within 1 month, however, the patient had had a progression of her symptoms. She had developed more persistent cervical occipital pain. Her neurological examination was now reported as revealing:

1. *Mental status:* There was a euphoric attitude.
2. *Cranial nerves:* There was now horizontal nystagmus on lateral gaze with a question of dissociated nystagmus. Pain sensation was diminished over the left face. Speech was slurred. Jaw jerk was hyperactive.
3. *Motor system:* A hemiparesis was present as previously. There was now a bilateral impairment of finger-to-nose testing with a bilateral intention tremor.
4. *Reflexes:* Deep tendon reflexes were hyperactive bilaterally, the left greater than the right. The left plantar response was extensor.
5. *Sensory system:* There was now diminished pain sensation over the left face, arm, and trunk.

In June 1969, the patient was readmitted for a tracheostomy and esophagostomy for feeding purposes. Because of continuing cervical occipital pain, a neurosurgical consultation was obtained. On neurological examination additional findings concerning the cranial nerves revealed:

1. hemiatrophy of the tongue
2. a bilateral decrease in palatal movements.

In addition, vibratory sensation was noted to be absent in the right lower extremity and decreased in the left lower extremity. Position sense was now decreased in the toes bilaterally.

QUESTIONS:

1. The diagnosis in this case may not be too apparent. You should, however, be able to localize the lesion and to provide a differential diagnosis as to the nature of this progressive neurological disorder. In addition, you should be able to rate the various possibilities as to which is the most likely explanation for the patient's complaints.

2. Indicate your diagnostic and therapeutic approach to this problem.

29

Descriptive Atlas of the Spinal Cord, Brain Stem, and Cerebrum

STANLEY JACOBSON

Text and illustrations appear on following pages.

SPINAL CORD SECTIONS

LEVEL: SACRAL II (FIG. 29-1)

Sacral levels can be identified by the large amount of gray matter in comparison to white matter.

Gray Matter. In this section there are two horns: one sensory (dorsal) and one motor (ventral). In the ventral horn the retrodorsal, dorsolateral, and ventrolateral nuclei innervate the inferior extremity.

White Matter. Most of the fibers from descending tracts have ended and the bulk of the white matter consists of ascending axons and intersegmental fibers. The dorsal columns at this level contain only fibers from regions innervated by the sacral cord; these form the fasciculus gracilis.

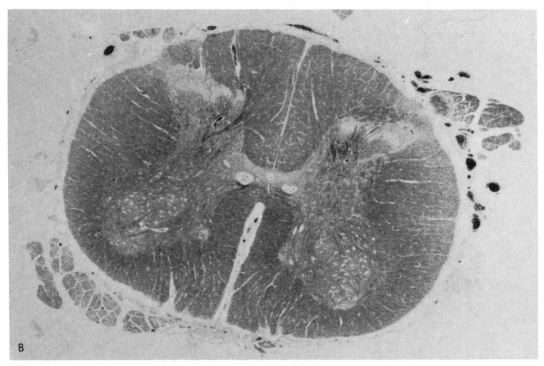

A

FASCICULUS GRACILIS
LATERAL CORTICOSPINAL TR.
CENTRAL CANAL
LATERAL RETICULOSPINAL TR.
LISSAUER'S TRACT
RUBROSPINAL TR.
SUBSTANTIA GELATINOSA
VENTRAL SPINO-CEREBELLAR TR.
DORSAL FUNICULAR GRAY
RETRODORSOLATERAL NUCLEUS
LATERAL SPINO-THALAMIC TR.
DORSOLATERAL NUCLEUS
VENTROLATERAL NUCLEUS
SPINO-OLIVARY TR.
LUMBROSACRAL NUCL.
VENTROMEDIAL NUCL.
VENTRAL RETICULO-SPINAL TR.
VENTRAL CORTICOSPINAL TR.
MEDIAL RETICULOSPINAL TR.
VENTRAL SPINOTHALAMIC TR.

B

Figure 29-1

LEVEL: LUMBAR I (FIG. 29-2)

Lumbar levels can be identified by the nearly equal amount of space taken up by the gray and white matter.

Gray Matter. In this level three horns are present: dorsal (sensory), ventral (motor), and intermediate (preganglionic sympathetic).

White Matter. The increase in the amount of white matter reflects the increasing number of ascending fibers in the dorsal column, the fasciculus gracilis, with some cuneate fibers, and the presence of the corticospinal fibers for the muscles in the thigh, leg, and foot.

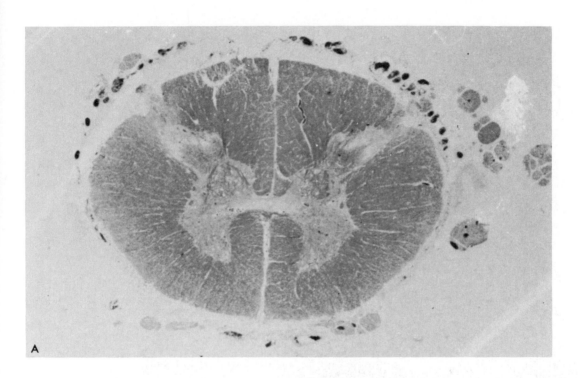

A

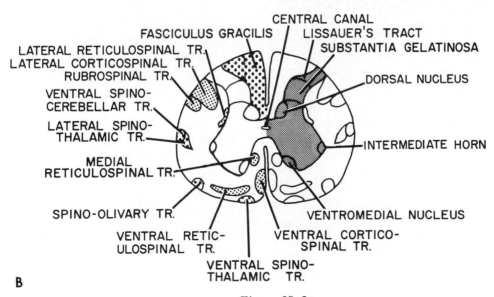

CENTRAL CANAL

FASCICULUS GRACILIS   LISSAUER'S TRACT

LATERAL RETICULOSPINAL TR.

LATERAL CORTICOSPINAL TR.   SUBSTANTIA GELATINOSA

RUBROSPINAL TR.

VENTRAL SPINO-CEREBELLAR TR.   DORSAL NUCLEUS

LATERAL SPINO-THALAMIC TR.

MEDIAL RETICULOSPINAL TR.   INTERMEDIATE HORN

SPINO-OLIVARY TR.

VENTRAL RETIC-ULOSPINAL TR.   VENTROMEDIAL NUCLEUS

VENTRAL CORTICO-SPINAL TR.

VENTRAL SPINO-THALAMIC TR.

B

Figure 29-2

LEVEL: THORACIC 7 (FIG. 29-3)

Thoracic levels are always identified by the small amount of gray matter and the vast bulk of white matter.

White Matter. The ascending and descending fibers for the lower limbs, abdomen, trunk, and pelvis provide the bulk of white matter for this section.

Gray Matter. There are three horns present in this level: dorsal (sensory), ventral (motor), and intermediate (preganglionic sympathetic).

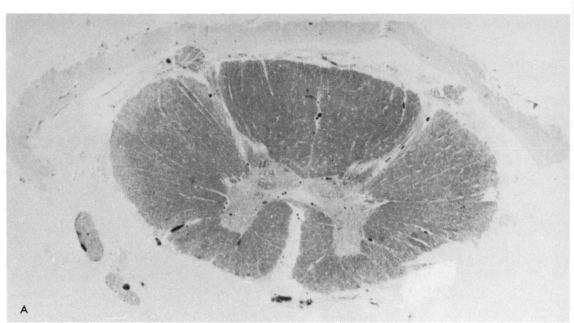

A

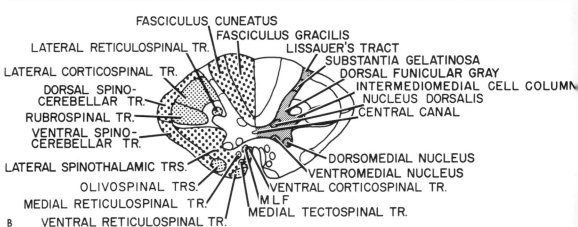

FASCICULUS CUNEATUS
FASCICULUS GRACILIS
LATERAL RETICULOSPINAL TR.
LISSAUER'S TRACT
LATERAL CORTICOSPINAL TR.
SUBSTANTIA GELATINOSA
DORSAL FUNICULAR GRAY
DORSAL SPINO-
CEREBELLAR TR.
INTERMEDIOMEDIAL CELL COLUMN
NUCLEUS DORSALIS
RUBROSPINAL TR.
CENTRAL CANAL
VENTRAL SPINO-
CEREBELLAR TR.
LATERAL SPINOTHALAMIC TRS.
DORSOMEDIAL NUCLEUS
OLIVOSPINAL TRS.
VENTROMEDIAL NUCLEUS
MEDIAL RETICULOSPINAL TR.
VENTRAL CORTICOSPINAL TR.
MLF
MEDIAL TECTOSPINAL TR.
B VENTRAL RETICULOSPINAL TR.

Figure 29–3

LEVEL: CERVICAL 7 (FIG. 29-4)

A cervical level can always be identified by the large amount of white and gray matter and the ovoid shape of the region.

White Matter. The bulk of this section consists of ascending and descending fibers to the extremities, thorax, abdomen, trunk, and pelvis. Note how the dorsal columns increase in bulk as one ascends. Re-examine:

(1) Figure 29-3 and note the decrease in bulk of the spinal cord white matter which results from innervating the cervical enlargements (provides innervations to superior extremity); and (2) Figure 29-2 and note the decrease in bulk which results from innervation to the throax, abdomen, and pelvis.

Gray Matter. In the ventral horn the retrodorsal, dorsolateral, and ventrolateral nuclei innervate the superior extremity.

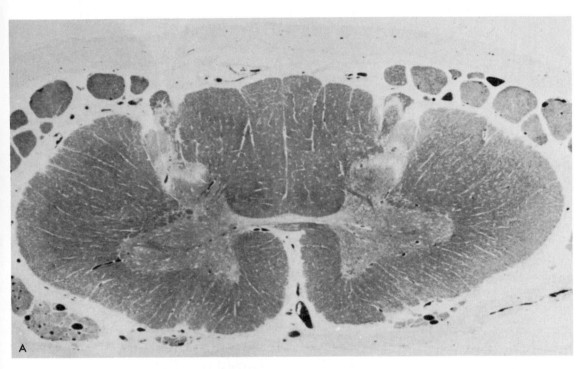

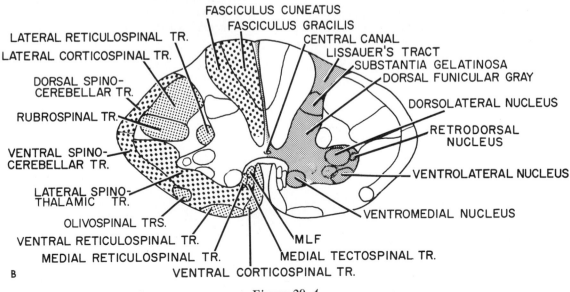

Figure 29-4

BRAIN STEM SECTIONS

LEVEL: MEDULLA – MOTOR DECUSSATION (FIGS. 29–5; 11–5)*

This section resembles a spinal cord section, but it is actually at the transition between the cervical spinal cord and the medulla. The most conspicuous feature is the crossing of the medullary pyramid from its anterior position in the medulla to a lateral position in the cord. A portion of the anterior corticospinal tract remains uncrossed and retains this position throughout the cord with the fibers slowly crossing. The fasciculus gracilis and the fasciculus cuneatus (fine touch, pressure, vibration, two-point discrim-

---

*The second figure number refers back to a more detailed analysis of the brain stem section in Chapter 11.

ination from the body) retain their same positions in the cord but now the nuclear masses of the secondary neurons in this system are appearing (nucleus gracilis and nucleus cuneatus). The descending nucleus and tract of cranial nerve V are also conspicuous lateral to the cuneate eminence. The dorsal and ventral spinocerebellar tracts will keep this same location through the lower medullary levels. The following tracts will retain the same position in the medulla and pons: (1) the medial longitudinal fasciculus at the midline in the tegmentum near the ventricular lumen, (2) the anterior spinothalamic tract (crude touch and pressure) and the lateral spinothalamic tract (pain and temperature) near the lateral margin of tegmentum, (3) the rubrospinal and rubrobulbar tracts near the lateral most extent of the tegmentum, (4) the tectospinal tract underneath the medial longitudinal fasciculus, and (5) the reticulothalamic tract in the reticular formation.

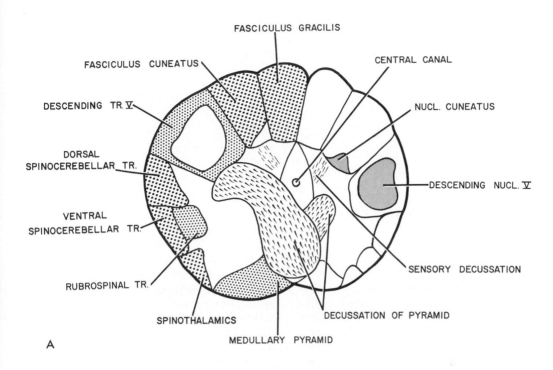

FASCICULUS GRACILIS

FASCICULUS CUNEATUS

CENTRAL CANAL

DESCENDING TR. Ⅴ

NUCL. CUNEATUS

DORSAL SPINOCEREBELLAR TR.

DESCENDING NUCL. Ⅴ

VENTRAL SPINOCEREBELLAR TR.

SENSORY DECUSSATION

RUBROSPINAL TR.

DECUSSATION OF PYRAMID

SPINOTHALAMICS

MEDULLARY PYRAMID

A

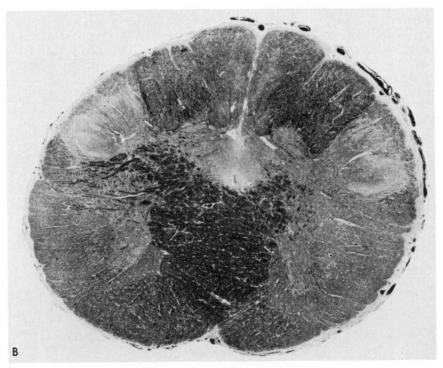

B

Figure 29–5

LEVEL: LOWER MEDULLA
(FIGS. 29-6; 11-6)

This section is representative of the medullary levels below the fourth ventricle with the ventricular system represented by a small canal. The most conspicuous feature is the massive medullary pyramids (corticospinal tracts). The axons in this heavily myelinated bundle synapse on motor neurons in the spinal cord; these motor neurons innervate the upper and lower limbs and trunk.

Cranial Nerves
Motor. The most inferior portion of nerves X (dorsal motor) and XII are found in relation to the spinal canal. The cell bodies of the ambiguous nucleus at this level represent the medullary portion of nerve XI innervating the trapezius and sternocleido-mastoid muscles.

Sensory. The descending nucleus and tract of nerve V are conspicuous throughout the medulla and upper pons.

Tracts. The nuclei gracilis and cuneatus are conspicuous, and secondary axons can be seen leaving their anterior surfaces, swinging around the ventricle, crossing the midline, and taking up a position posterior to the pyramids. These fibers, the sensory decussation, are forming the medial lemniscus, a specific discrete projection system to the thalamus. The central core of the brain stem consists of the reticular formation which is a nonspecific diffuse multisynaptic system important in maintaining our "posture" as regards the external and internal milieu.

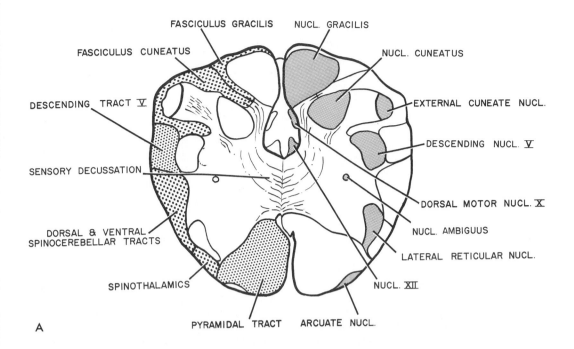

A

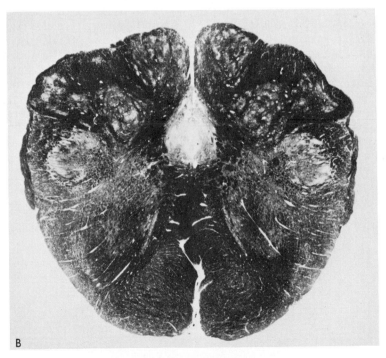

B

Figure 29–6

LEVEL: MEDULLA—OBEX
(FIG. 29-7)

This section is at the inferior margin of the fourth ventricle. The posterior surface of the medulla has opened and the medulla is beginning to expand laterally. The medullary olives which will become larger in the next sections are seen posterolateral to the medullary pyramids.

Cranial Nerves

Motor. The nucleus of nerves XII and X are conspicuous in the floor of the fourth ventricle. The hypoglossal (XII) nerve innervates the intrinsic muscles of the tongue, while the dorsal motor nucleus of nerve X innervates the thoracic and abdominal viscera up to the left colic flexure. The ambiguous nucleus is present in the lateral margin of the reticular formation and at this level the motor neurons are part of nerve X and innervate the pharynx and larynx.

Sensory. The axons subserving the gustatory and visceral sensations are carried via nerves X, IX, and VII and enter the tractus solitarius. The cell bodies in the solitarius form the secondary neurons in this pathway. The axons of these cells run bilaterally in the medial lemniscus up to the ventral posterior medial nucleus in the thalamus.

Tracts. The gracile nucleus is disappearing while the cuneate nucleus is still large. Numerous fibers are still seen entering the medial lemniscus which is prominent posterior to the pyramids, between the inferior olives. External to the cuneate tubercle and descending nucleus of nerve V, the spinocerebellar tracts and other fibers from nuclei in the brain stem are accumulating and starting to form the inferior cerebellar peduncle. The external cuneate nucleus is seen on the surface of the cuneate nucleus; it corresponds to Clark's nucleus in the spinal cord.

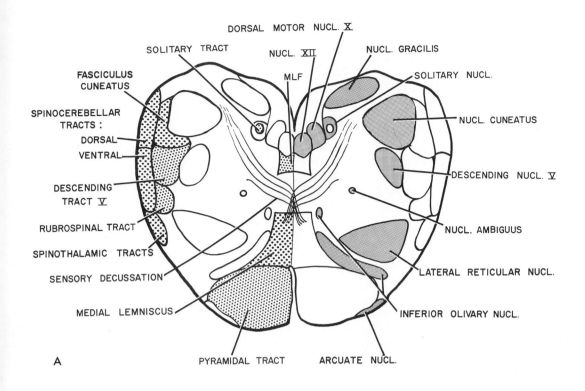

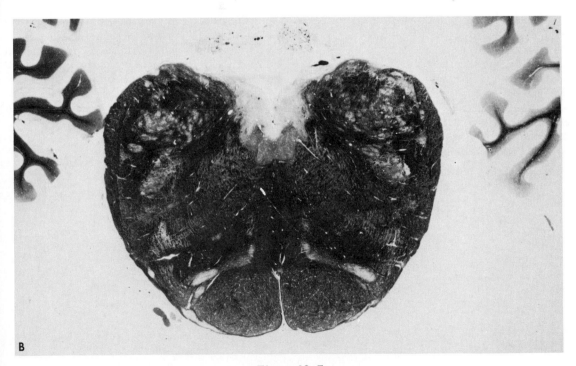

Figure 29–7

LEVEL: MEDULLA—LATERAL RECESS OF FOURTH VENTRICLE (FIGS. 29–8; 11–7)

The pyramids and olive are the most prominent structures at this level. The gracile and cuneate nuclei are no longer present, while the inferior cerebellar peduncle is prominent. At this level, the olivocerebellar fiber system is seen entering the inferior cerebellar peduncle. The prominent landmarks on the floor of the fourth ventricle are, medially, the medial eminence, and, laterally, the vestibular area (medial vestibular nucleus) and acoustic tubercle (dorsal cochlear nucleus).

Cranial Nerves

Motor. The dorsal motor nucleus of nerve X is no longer present and this section marks the superior extent of nerve XII. The ambiguous nucleus at this level still consists of nuclei of nerve X innervating the pharyngeal and laryngeal muscles.

Sensory. The nucleus and tractus solitarius are most conspicuous at this level. Nuclei associated with the vestibular and cochlear division of nerve VIII are present at this level. The medial and spinal divisions of the vestibular nuclei are seen near the floor of the fourth ventricle. Mixed in with the spinal vestibular nuclei are the descending rootlets of nerve VIII.

Tracts. The inferior cerebellar peduncle, the descending tract and nucleus of nerve VIII, and the solitary tract are conspicuous. On the floor of the fourth ventricle, the stria medullaris is seen; this tract connects the cerebellum with the brain stem. In the medial eminence of the fourth ventricle, many of the axons are descending fibers from the hypothalamus and limbic-midbrain nuclei, connecting to the cranial nerve nuclei and reticular formation.

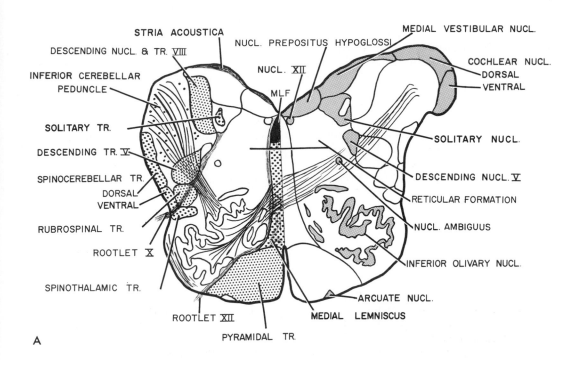

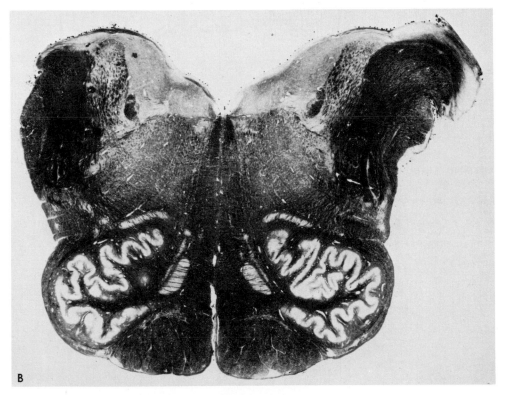

Figure 29–8

LEVEL: UPPER MEDULLA
(FIG. 29-9)

The most conspicuous structures in this section are the pyramids, the inferior olive, and the inferior and superior cerebellar peduncle. On the right side, the inferior cerebellar peduncle is seen connecting the cerebellum and brain stem. Medial to the restiform body, vestibular fibers (juxtarestiform body) are seen entering the cerebellum. Note the cerebellar cortex and the deep cerebellar nuclei (dentate and emboliform). The walls of the fourth ventricle here and through-out the pons are formed by the superior cerebellar peduncle (dentatorubrothalamic tract).

Cranial Nuclei

Motor. The only motor nerve present in this section is the nucleus ambiguus which, at this level, consists of cell bodies going to the stylopharyngeus muscle; note that for the first time, the position of the ambiguous nucleus is clearly seen.

Sensory. The vestibular, solitary, and ventral cochlear nuclei are present at this level. The spinal nucleus of nerve V has been displaced medially by the massive inferior cerebellar peduncle.

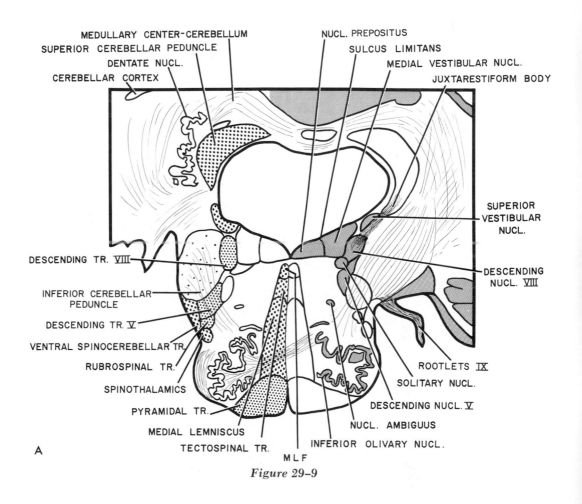

MEDULLARY CENTER-CEREBELLUM
SUPERIOR CEREBELLAR PEDUNCLE
DENTATE NUCL.
CEREBELLAR CORTEX

NUCL. PREPOSITUS
SULCUS LIMITANS
MEDIAL VESTIBULAR NUCL.
JUXTARESTIFORM BODY

SUPERIOR VESTIBULAR NUCL.

DESCENDING TR. VIII
INFERIOR CEREBELLAR PEDUNCLE
DESCENDING TR. V
VENTRAL SPINOCEREBELLAR TR.
RUBROSPINAL TR.
SPINOTHALAMICS
PYRAMIDAL TR.
MEDIAL LEMNISCUS
TECTOSPINAL TR.

DESCENDING NUCL. VIII

ROOTLETS IX
SOLITARY NUCL.
DESCENDING NUCL. V
NUCL. AMBIGUUS
INFERIOR OLIVARY NUCL.

A

M L F

Figure 29-9

(Illustration continued on opposite page)

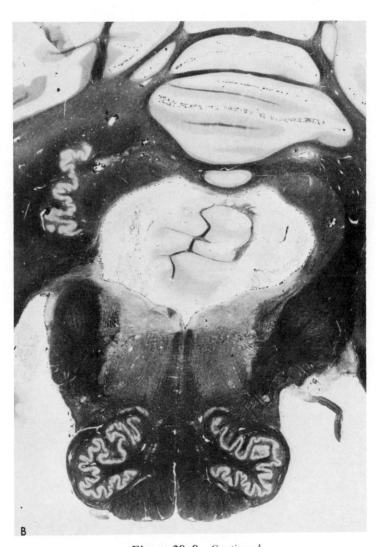

Figure 29–9 Continued.

See Filmstrip, Frame 17.

LEVEL: PONS—NUCLEI OF NERVES VI AND VII
(FIGS. 29–10; 11–8)

This section is at the most inferior portion of the pons and consists primarily of the middle cerebellar peduncle. The corticospinal tracts have just emerged from the pons and are forming the medullary pyramids. The walls of the fourth ventricle are formed superiorly by the superior cerebellar peduncle, and inferiorly by the superior vestibular nucleus.

Cranial Nerves

Motor. The motor nuclei of nerves VI and VII are present at this level. On the right, the rootlet fibers of nerve VII are seen leaving the medial surface of nerve VII, swinging around the nucleus of nerve VII, and passing laterally out into the tegmentum. On the left side is seen the genu and horizontal course of the nerve on the floor of the fourth ventricle and its position in the lateral margin of the tegmentum as it approaches the anterior surface of the brain stem.

Sensory. On the left side the rootlet of nerve V is seen on the pontine surface, while on the right side, the rootlets of nerve V are in the lateral margin of the tegmentum. The superior vestibulary nucleus is conspicuous on the wall of the fourth ventricle.

Tracts. At this most inferior level of the pons the tract position is still similar to that in the medulla. At this level, the ventral spinocerebellar tract is entering the cerebellum curving around the superior cerebellar peduncle. The tractus uncinatus connects the deep cerebellar nuclei with the reticular formation.

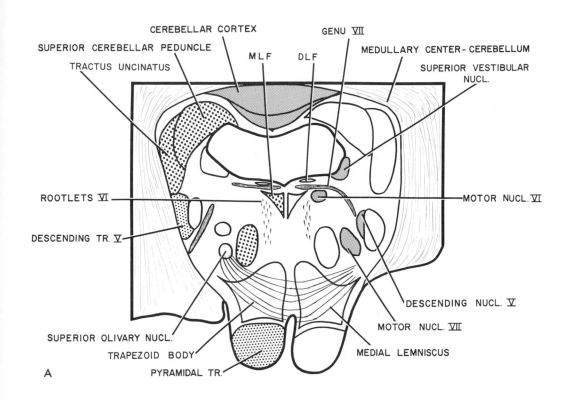

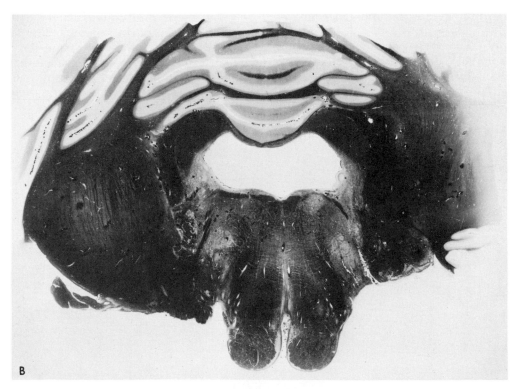

Figure 29–10

LEVEL: PONS—MOTOR NUCLEUS OF NERVE V (FIGS. 29-11; 11-9)

The most conspicuous structures in this level are the superior cerebellar peduncles forming the walls of the fourth ventricle and the massive middle cerebellar peduncle, forming the bulk of the pontine basis.

Cranial Nerves

Motor. The motor nucleus of nerve V is seen bilaterally medial to the rootlets of nerve V; it innervates the muscles of mastication.

Sensory. The mesencephalic nucleus and root of nerve V is visible at the lateral most margin of the fourth ventricle. It provides proprioceptive information on the muscles of mastication and all other muscles in the head. The chief sensory nucleus of nerve V is present lateral to the entrance of the root of nerve V; it carries fine touch for the face.

Tracts. The corticospinal tracts are covered by pontine white. In the inferior surface of the tegmentum, the secondary cochlear fibers are seen crossing the midline, then forming the trapezoid body, and entering the superior olivary nucleus where some axons synapse. The medial lemniscus is shifting laterally and now consists of trigeminothalamic fibers, secondary gustatory and visceral axons and spinothalamic fibers in addition to the dorsal columns. The medial longitudinal fasciculus (MLF) and the tectospinal, rubrospinal, and reticulothalamic fibers (central tegmental tract) still maintain the same position they have throughout the medulla.

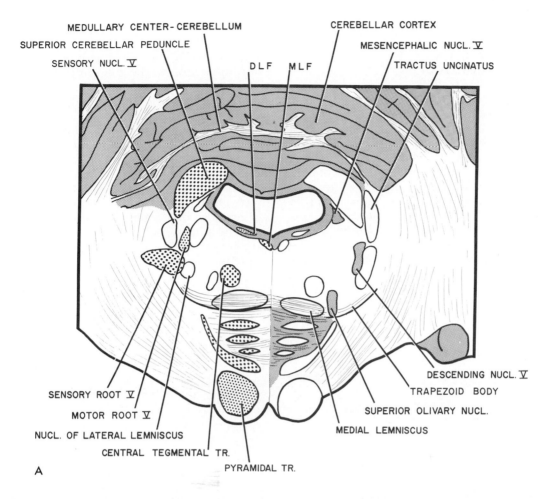

MEDULLARY CENTER-CEREBELLUM
CEREBELLAR CORTEX
SUPERIOR CEREBELLAR PEDUNCLE
MESENCEPHALIC NUCL. V
SENSORY NUCL. V
DLF MLF
TRACTUS UNCINATUS

DESCENDING NUCL. V
SENSORY ROOT V
TRAPEZOID BODY
MOTOR ROOT V
SUPERIOR OLIVARY NUCL.
NUCL. OF LATERAL LEMNISCUS
MEDIAL LEMNISCUS
CENTRAL TEGMENTAL TR.
PYRAMIDAL TR.

A

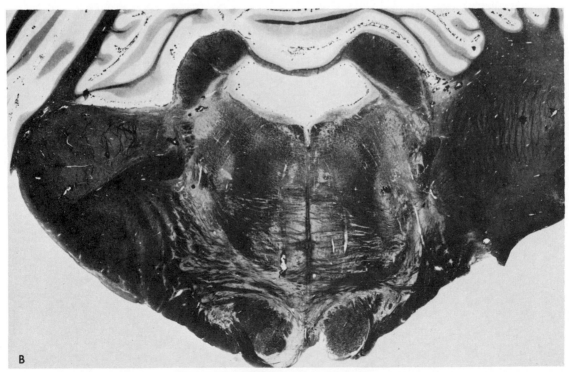

B

Figure 29–11

LEVEL: MIDBRAIN — INFERIOR COLLICULUS
(FIGS. 29-12; 11-10)

In this section the tectum and tegmentum are from the midbrain and the basilar part is from the pons. The tectum is the inferior collicular nucleus, an important relay station in the auditory pathway. Note the commissure of the inferior colliculus. The fiber bundle streaming up to the inferior border of the inferior colliculus is the lateral lemniscus which consists of secondary and tertiary auditory fibers.

Tegmentum. The dominant feature here is the superior cerebellar peduncle, which is starting to cross in the anterior portion of the tegmentum. The lateral margin of this region contains, anteriorly and laterally, the definitive medial lemniscus, which has migrated from its medial position in the pons. The medial longitudinal fasciculus (MLF) is conspicuous in the floor of the cerebral aqueduct.

Basis. The middle cerebellar peduncle covers the anterior surface of the midbrain.

Cranial Nerve. The rootlet fibers of nerve IV are seen on the floor of the aqueduct. The mesencephalic root and nucleus of nerve V are found at the lateral margin of the periaqueductal gray.

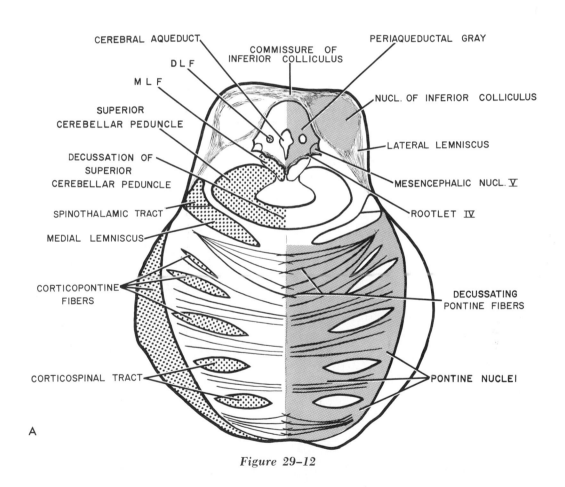

Figure 29–12

(Illustration continued on opposite page)

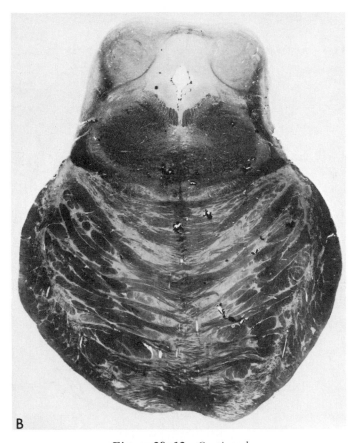

Figure 29–12 Continued.

LEVEL: MIDBRAIN—
SUPERIOR COLLICULUS
(FIGS. 29-13; 11-11)

In this section the tectum and tegmentum are of the midbrain and the basilar portion consists of pons and midbrain.

Tectum. The superior colliculus forms the tectum and consists of four layers; the tectospinal tract originates from the deepest layers. The superior colliculus is important in integrating eye movements to brain stem activity.

Tegmentum. The superior cerebellar peduncle is still crossing. The central tegmental tract (reticulothalamic) is conspicuous in the reticular formation. The medial longitudinal fasciculus (MLF) is seen with some fibers crossing the midline. On the right side, fibers of the auditory system, the brachium of the inferior colliculus, are seen entering

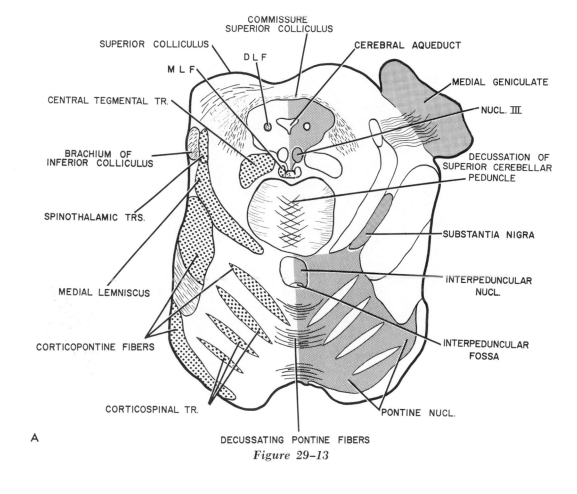

Figure 29-13

(Illustration continued on opposite page)

the medial geniculate nucleus of the thalamus. Most of these fibers originated in the inferior colliculus. The medial lemniscus is the conspicuous tract extending from the midline up to the lateral surface of the midbrain. A portion of the substantia nigra is seen on the left side between the medial lemniscus and cerebral peduncle. The lower half of the periaqueductal gray and other tegmental nuclei form the limbic-midbrain region important in our level of attentiveness.

Basis. Laterally the cerebral peduncles are present and fibers from the frontal cortex are seen entering the pons.

Cranial Nerves. Nerve III indents the medial longitudinal fasciculus (MLF) in the ventricular floor. A few cell bodies of the mesencephalic nucleus of nerve V are still seen in the lateral margin of the periaqueductal gray.

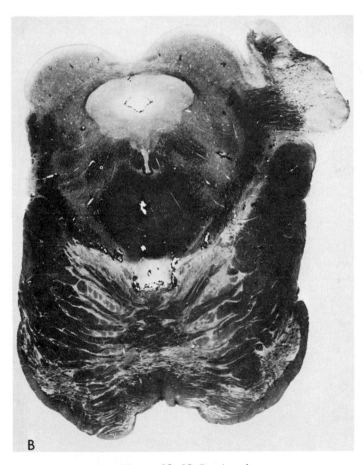

Figure 29–13 *Continued.*

LEVEL: MIDBRAIN—POSTERIOR COMMISSURE (FIG. 29-14)

This section contains the posterior horn of the lateral ventricles, the telencephalon (cerebral hemisphere), the diencephalon, and the mesencephalon.

Telencephalon. The splenium of the corpus callosum is seen above the brain stem. The temporal lobe is found lateral to the cerebral peduncles.

Diencephalon. The pulvinar and the medial and lateral geniculate nuclei are present on the right side. The medial geniculate is the last subcortical station for the auditory system, while the lateral geniculate is the final subcortical synaptic site for the visual system. The pineal gland of the epithalamus is seen at the midline above the posterior commissure.

Mesencephalon. This level of the midbrain is through the pretectal region, which mediates the light reflex and upward and downward gaze. The posterior commissure connects the pretectal region, the superior colliculus, and other nuclei in the midbrain. The cerebral peduncles are conspicuous on the anterior surface of the midbrain; internal to this tract is the substantia nigra. The red nuclei are seen in the tegmentum of the midbrain; some of the fibers of the superior cerebellar peduncle end here while others continue on to the thalamus (ventral anterior and ventral lateral nuclei). The medial lemniscus is seen lateral to the red nuclei.

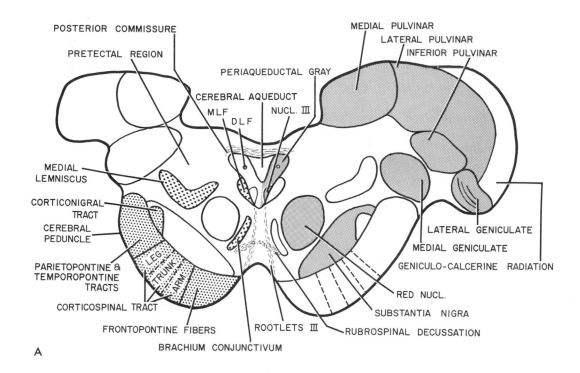

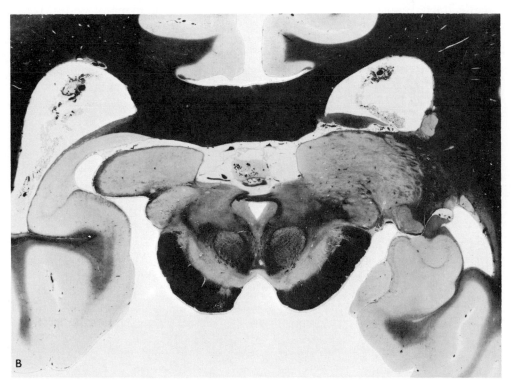

Figure 29–14

LEVEL: HABENULA (FIGS. 29–15; 11–12)

This section contains the lateral and third ventricles, the telencephalon, and the diencephalon.

Telencephalon. Same as in previous section.

Diencephalon. The lateral geniculate nucleus is conspicuous on the left side; the tertiary axons of the optic system synapse here. In the third ventricle, the habenular nuclei are seen protruding into the ventricle and the habenulopeduncular tract is seen connecting the habenula to the interpeduncular nucleus; note, this tract passes medial to the red nucleus. The conspicuous central medial nucleus near the ventricular surface is the thalamic site for the termination of fibers from the limbic-midbrain nuclei. The pulvinar and the most posterior portion of the ventral posterior medial nucleus are present. This nucleus receives the trigeminal and gustatory fibers.

Tracts. The cerebral peduncles are conspicuous on the inferior surface of the diencephalon; internal to the peduncles are the substantia nigra and red nucleus.

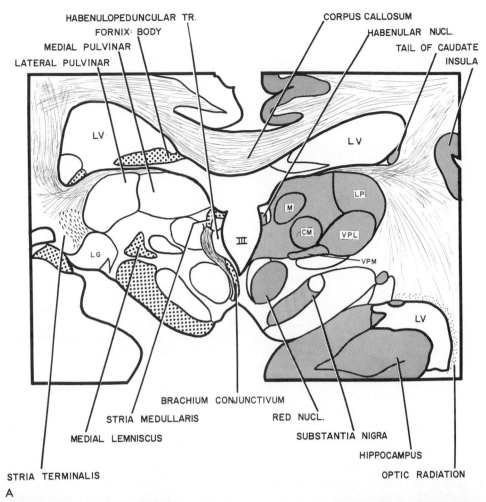

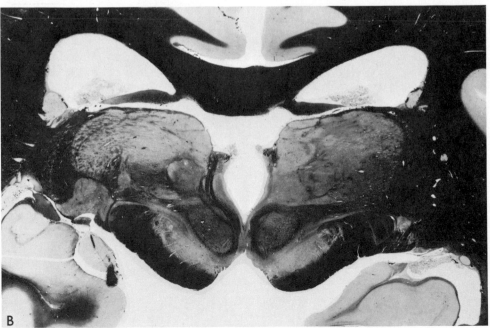

Figure 29–15

LEVEL: MIDTHALAMIC
(FIGS. 29–16; 11–13)

This section contains the telencephalon and diencephalon.

Telencephalon. The corpus callosum and tail of the caudate nucleus are present. The fornix is seen underneath the corpus callosum and in the mammillary nuclei of the hypothalamus. On the lateral margin of the thalamus, the posterior limb of the internal capsule separates the thalamus from the globus pallidus and putamen. The optic nerve is seen external to the cerebral peduncle.

Diencephalon. Two conspicuous nuclear groupings are seen: the medial and lateral complex. The medial nucleus projects to the frontal associational and orbital cortex. The superior half of the lateral complex consists of the lateral posterior nucleus while the lower half contains the ventral posterior lateral and the ventral posterior lateral nuclei. The ventral posterior lateral nucleus receives cutaneous proprioceptive and visceral sensations from the body, while the ventral posterior medial nucleus receives gustatory cutaneous and proprioceptive information from the head and neck. The subthalamus is conspicuous at this level.

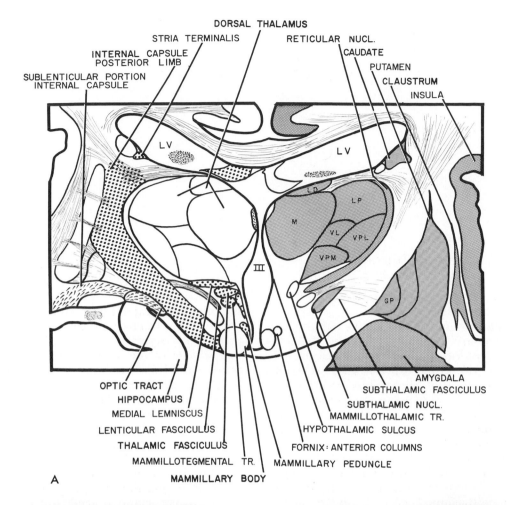

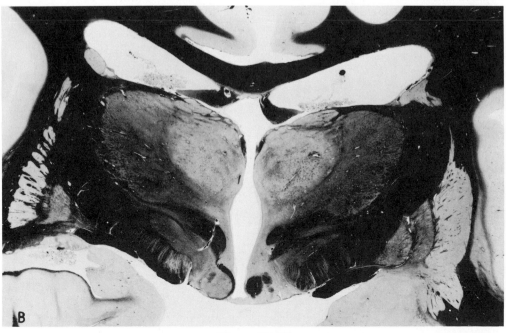

Figure 29–16

LEVEL: ANTERIOR TUBERCLE OF THALAMUS (FIGS. 29-17; 11-14)

This section contains the telencephalon and diencephalon.

Telencephalon. The globus pallidus and putamen are separated from the thalamus by the posterior limb of the internal capsule. The anterior commissure is seen on the inferior surface of the globus pallidus and putamen. A cellular bridge connects the caudate nucleus and putamen. The amygdaloid nucleus is seen on the medial surface of the temporal lobe.

Diencephalon. The inferior floor of the third ventricle is formed by the optic chiasm. The fornix is seen in the substance of the hypothalamus below the hypothalamic sulcus. The thalamus is divided into a medial and lateral nuclear complex by the internal medullary lamina of the thalamus which at this level contains many fibers of the mammillothalamic tract. The medial region consists of the anterior nuclei which forms a prominent elevation, the anterior tubercle, in the floor of the lateral ventricle. The anterior nuclei as they interconnect with the cingulate cortex are an important part of the visceral brain. The lateral region consists of the ventral anterior nuclei which receives fibers from the superior cerebellar peduncle and projects to the premotor cortices (areas 6 and 8). The ansa lenticularis sweeps around the anterior limb of the internal capsule interconnecting the globus pallidus and the ventral anterior and ventral lateral nuclei of the thalamus.

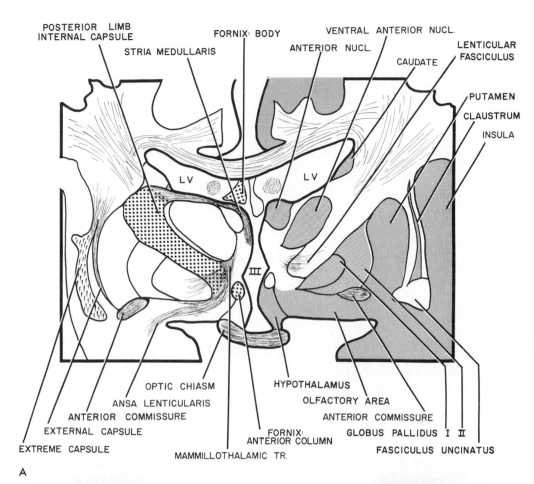

POSTERIOR LIMB
INTERNAL CAPSULE

STRIA MEDULLARIS

FORNIX: BODY

ANTERIOR NUCL.

VENTRAL ANTERIOR NUCL.

CAUDATE

LENTICULAR
FASCICULUS

PUTAMEN

CLAUSTRUM

INSULA

LV

LV

III

OPTIC CHIASM

ANSA LENTICULARIS

ANTERIOR COMMISSURE

EXTERNAL CAPSULE

EXTREME CAPSULE

MAMMILLOTHALAMIC TR.

FORNIX:
ANTERIOR COLUMN

HYPOTHALAMUS

OLFACTORY AREA

ANTERIOR COMMISSURE

GLOBUS PALLIDUS I II

FASCICULUS UNCINATUS

A

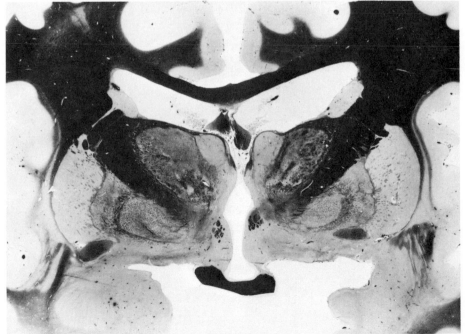

B

Figure 29–17

LEVEL: ANTERIOR LIMB OF INTERNAL CAPSULE (FIG. 29-18)

This section contains only the telencephalon. The anterior limb of the internal capsule separates the caudate nucleus from the putamen and globus pallidus. Note the cellular bridges between the caudate nucleus and the putamen. The septum which receives fibers from the hypothalamus and limbic cortex separates the anterior poles of the lateral ventricles.

The cerebral cortical regions are medially the gyrus rectus and, more laterally, the orbital gyri.

BRAIN SECTIONS

In the following figures only a few structures will be discussed. The student should identify the other structures and relate them to their function in the central nervous system.

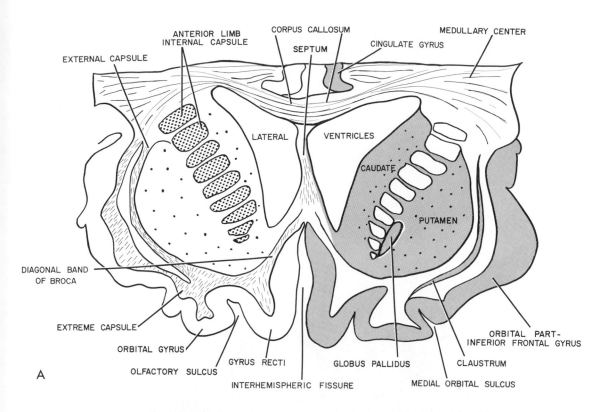

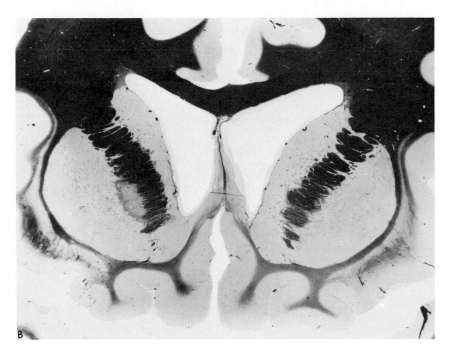

Figure 29–18

LEVEL: GENU OF CORPUS CALLOSUM – CORONAL SECTION (FIG. 29-19)

This section consists only of telencephalic regions with the genu of the corpus callosum prominent. The gray matter consists solely of frontal cortex.

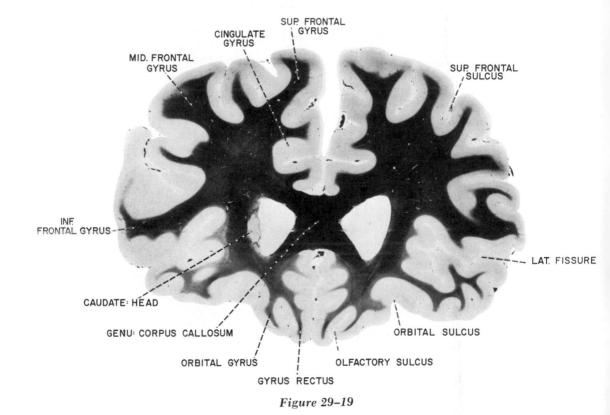

Figure 29–19

LEVEL: SEPTUM – CORONAL SECTION (FIG. 29-20)

This section consists of a portion of the basal nuclei and cerebral cortex which are subdivisions of the telencephalon. Note the thin membrane (septum pellucidum) which separates the anterior horn of the lateral ventricle. The temporal pole is visible inferior to the frontal lobe.

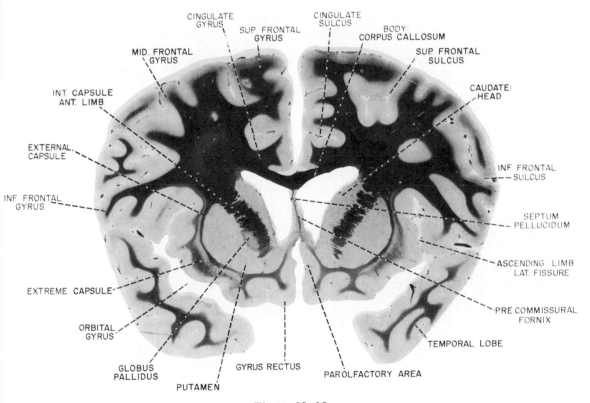

Figure 29–20

See Filmstrip, Frames 40 and 42.

LEVEL: ANTERIOR NUCLEI OF THALAMUS — CORONAL SECTION (FIG. 29-21)

This section consists of telencephalon (cerebral cortex, medullary center, and basal nuclei) and diencephalon (thalamus). The prominent anterior nucleus of the thalamus projects into the floor of the lateral ventricle. The anterior commissure is seen beneath the fornix adjacent to the midline. A labeled section of the thalamus at this level is found in Figure 29–17.

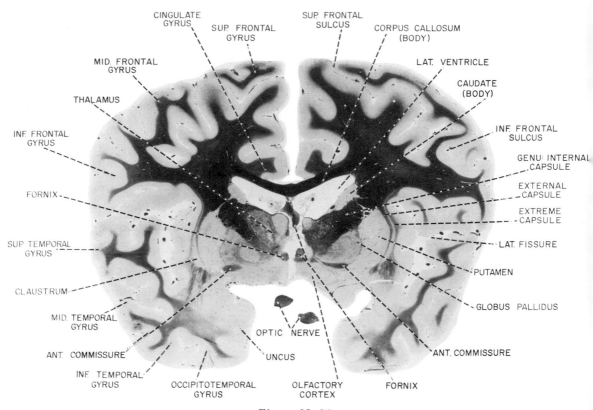

Figure 29–21

LEVEL: THALAMUS — CORONAL SECTION (FIG. 29-22)

This section consists of telencephalon (cerebral cortex, medullary center, and basal nuclei) and diencephalon (thalamus, hypothalamus, and subthalamus). All portions of the diencephalon are present in this section. A labeled section of the thalamus at this level is found in Figure 29–16.

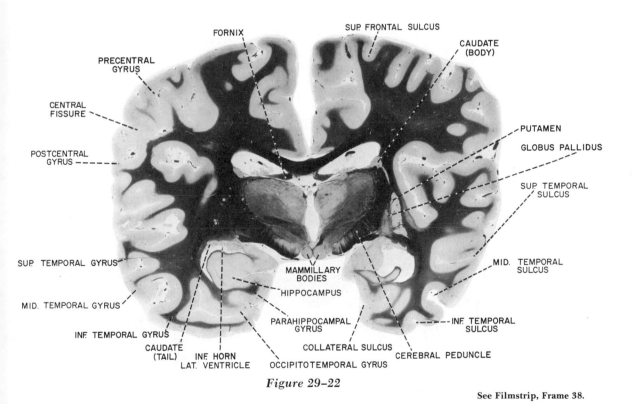

Figure 29–22

See Filmstrip, Frame 38.

LEVEL: HABENULAR NUCLEI — CORONAL SECTION (Fig. 29–23)

This section consists of telencephalon and diencephalon. All portions of the diencephalon (thalamus, subthalamus, hypothalamus, epithalamus, and metathalamus) are now present on this section. A labeled section which corresponds to this level can be seen in Figure 29–15.

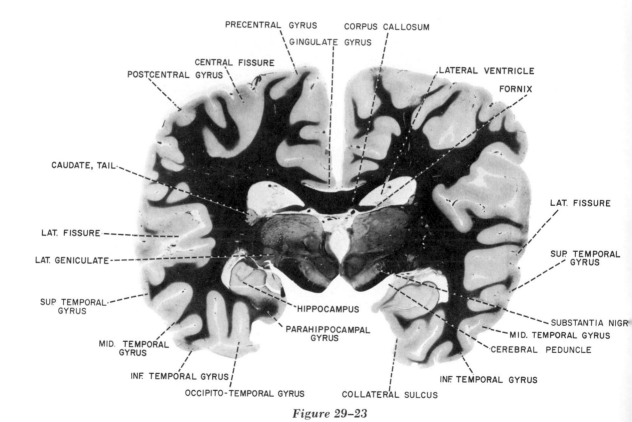

Figure 29–23

LEVEL: SPLENIUM OF CORPUS CALLOSUM – CORONAL SECTION
(Fig. 29-24)

This section consists of telencephalon and diencephalon, and midbrain (superior colliculus). Note the prominent cerebral peduncles and substantia nigra. In this section the inferior horn of the lateral ventricle is continuous with the body of the lateral ventricle. For detailed identification of the brain stem see Figure 29–14.

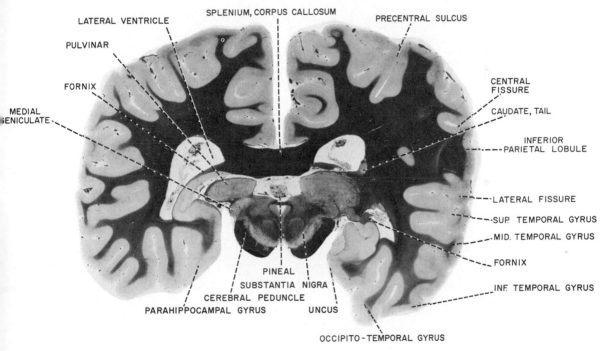

Figure 29–24

LEVEL: VISUAL CORTEX—CORONAL SECTION (Fig. 29-25)

This section consists of telencephalon (parietal and occipital lobe) and brain stem (pons) and cerebellum. Note the prominent myelinated stripe in the calcarine fissure; this represents the visual radiation.

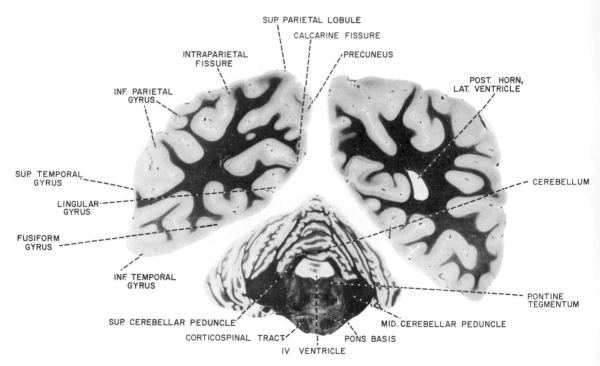

Figure 29–25

LEVEL: SPLENIUM – HORIZONTAL SECTION (Fig. 29-26)

This section consists of telencephalon (cerebral cortex, medullary center, and basal nuclei) and diencephalon (thalamus) separated by the limbs of the internal capsule. Note that in this section the head, genu, and posterior limb of the internal capsule are seen (review the relationships between the thalamus, internal capsule, and basal nuclei).

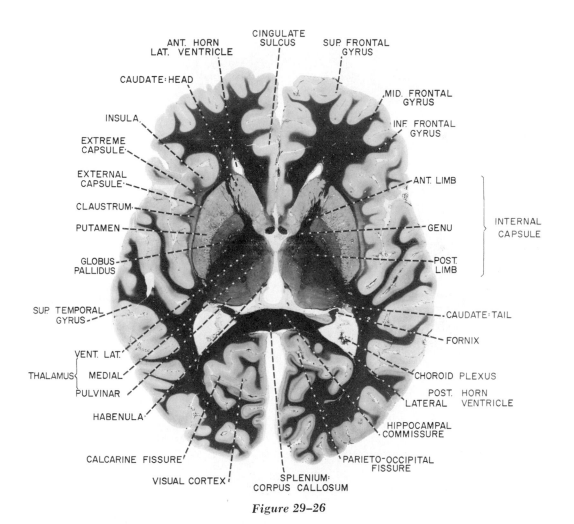

Figure 29–26

LEVEL: ANTERIOR COMMISSURE – HORIZONTAL SECTION (Fig. 29-27)

In this section two fiber commissures (anterior and habenular) and one gray commissure (massa intermedia) are present. Again review the relationships between the thalamus, internal capsule, and basal nuclei.

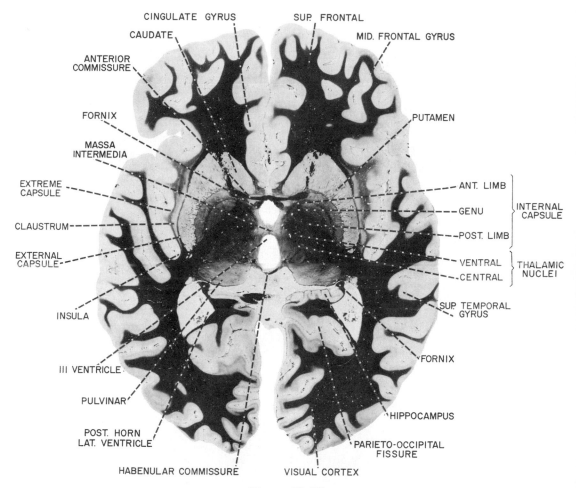

Figure 29–27

LEVEL: SUPERIOR COLLICULUS – HORIZONTAL SECTION (Fig. 29-28)

In this section locate the optic tract, mammillary bodies, and cerebral peduncles. Note the close proximity of the cerebral peduncles to the uncus.

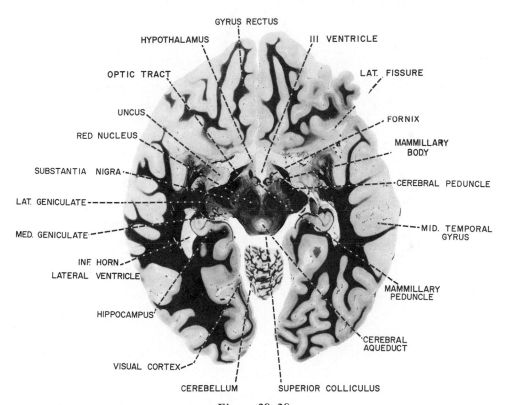

Figure 29–28

LEVEL: INFERIOR COLLICULUS— HORIZONTAL SECTION (Fig. 29-29)

In this section again identify the mammillary bodies, optic tract, and cerebral peduncles. Note that the cerebral peduncles are now disconnected from the cerebral hemispheres.

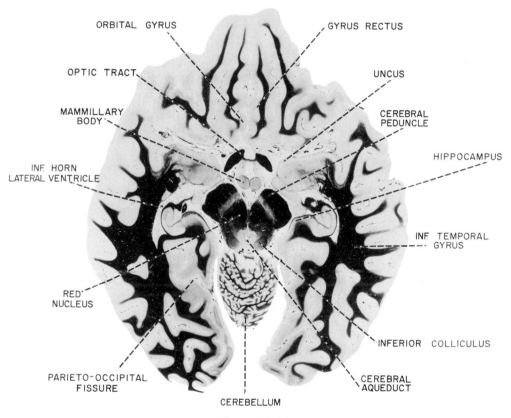

ORBITAL GYRUS

GYRUS RECTUS

OPTIC TRACT

UNCUS

MAMMILLARY BODY

CEREBRAL PEDUNCLE

HIPPOCAMPUS

INF. HORN LATERAL VENTRICLE

INF TEMPORAL GYRUS

RED NUCLEUS

INFERIOR COLLICULUS

PARIETO-OCCIPITAL FISSURE

CEREBRAL AQUEDUCT

CEREBELLUM

Figure 29–29

LEVEL: THALAMUS – SAGITTAL SECTION
(Fig. 29-30)

This section includes the telencephalon (cerebral cortex and corpus callosum), thalamus, hypothalamus, midbrain (superior and inferior colliculi), pons, medulla, and cerebellum. Identify the divisions of the corpus callosum and any functionally important tracts in the brain stem.

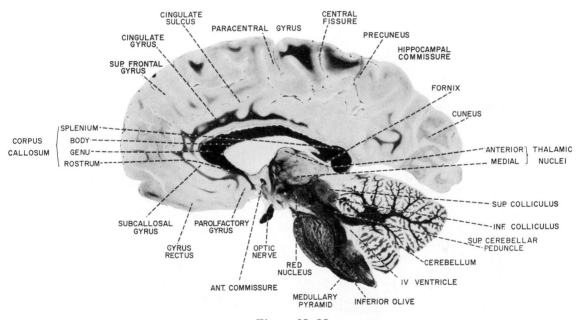

Figure 29–30

LEVEL: HIPPOCAMPUS – SAGITTAL SECTION (Fig. 29-31)

This section contains telencephalon and cerebellum. The bulk of this section contains the medullary center of the cerebral cortex. Note the relationship of the hippocampus to the inferior horn of the lateral ventricle.

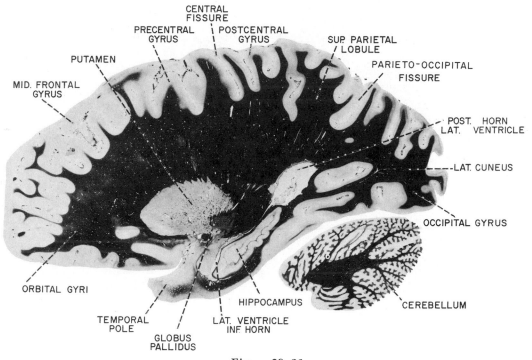

Figure 29–31

CRANIAL AND SPINAL NERVES
(Fig. 29-32)

The distribution of the cranial and spinal nerves in the head and neck.

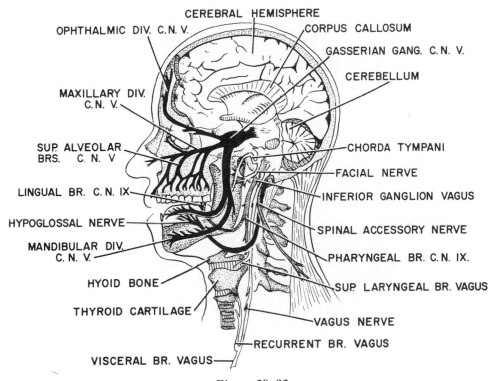

Figure 29–32

Index

Note: Page numbers in italics indicate illustrations. Those in **boldface** indicate case histories.

Outline of Supplementary Filmstrip

This color filmstrip of sixty-two frames whose individual descriptions follow is available from the publisher as is also an individual desk-top viewer.